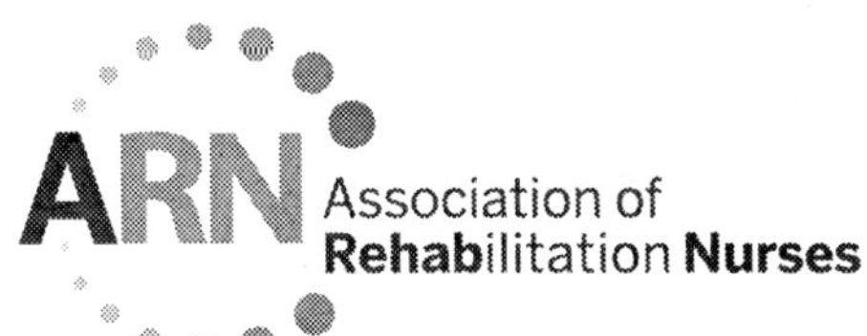

THE SPECIALTY PRACTICE OF REHABILITATION NURSING

A CORE CURRICULUM

SEVENTH EDITION

Cheryl Lehman, PhD RN CNS-BC RN-BC CRRN, Editor

THE SPECIALTY PRACTICE OF REHABILITATION NURSING

A CORE CURRICULUM

SEVENTH EDITION

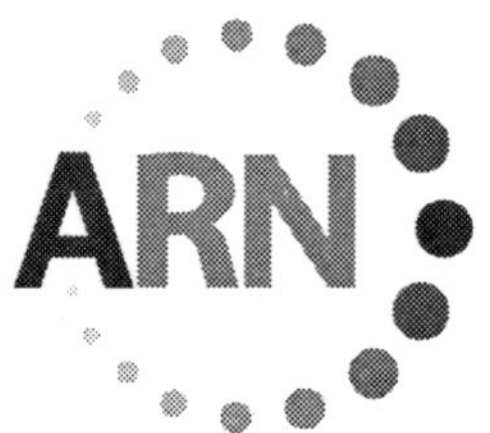

ISBN: 978-0-692-52035-2

CONTENTS

FOREWORD

I am honored to provide the foreword for the seventh edition of the Association of Rehabilitation Nurses' (ARN's) *The Specialty Practice of Rehabilitation Nursing: A Core Curriculum*. Each edition of the *Core Curriculum* reflects the evolving nature of rehabilitation nursing and the changing context of health care. This *Core Curriculum* is a reflection of all who have contributed to this and earlier editions that have been, published during the past 35 years. The 28 chapters have been divided into five sections and edited by Cheryl Lehman with contributions from 48 authors and 26 reviewers. It is a monumental task to manage this process, and my congratulations go to Dr. Lehman and her team of authors and reviewers. The *Core Curriculum* will serve as the guide to rehabilitation nurses in a time that is characterized by both challenge and change.

Rehabilitation nursing work brings us in close contact with many individuals (e.g., clients, families, and coworkers) from diverse backgrounds and experiences who may have very different values and behaviors. Many challenges arise when a nurse is confronted with such diversity. It is the hallmark of a professional rehabilitation nurse to work with clients from diverse backgrounds and help them achieve the highest level of wellness possible. To assist clients in achieving high-level wellness, rehabilitation nurses need openness, creativity, and a willingness to engage with the interdisciplinary team and the client to reach common goals.

ARN's mission is to promote and advance the professional rehabilitation nursing practice through education, advocacy, collaboration, and research to enhance the quality of life of those affected by disability or chronic illness. The *Core Curriculum* provides the roadmap for rehabilitation nurses to help clients navigate the journey toward recovery. Rehabilitation nurses must meet clients wherever they are along the way and help them move toward higher wellness. Knowledge, creativity, honesty, integrity, and caring are all attributes that are needed for success as a rehabilitation nurse. The *Core Curriculum* provides the basis for the working knowledge of rehabilitation diagnoses and practices that is necessary for the professional nurse.

This seventh edition provides essential knowledge and information for the specialty practice of rehabilitation nursing. This comprehensive guide is an important resource for rehabilitation nursing professionals to use their knowledge, skills, and leadership to adapt practice for their clients' changing health and wellness needs, and emerging changes in healthcare practice environments.

The contents of the *Core Curriculum* define rehabilitation nursing practice across settings. I hope it will be as well-used in your library as it is in mine. Leaders in the profession of rehabilitation will rely on the *Core Curriculum* and the other materials developed by ARN to demonstrate the unique practice focus and body of knowledge of rehabilitation nursing. I see the shared knowledge of many rehabilitation nurses when I look at *The Specialty Practice of Rehabilitation Nursing: A Core Curriculum*. As I review this text, I am proud to be a rehabilitation nurse and I hope it does the same for you.

Cynthia S. Jacelon, PhD RN-BC CRRN FAAN FGSA
September 2015

PREFACE

If you browse the Internet, you will find that most professions have developed a core curriculum. A core curriculum contains knowledge that is considered basic and essential for the profession. It serves as the basis for certification examinations, initial and ongoing training, evaluation, and competencies for a particular profession. A core curriculum is a statement of who the members of a particular profession are, what they should know, and even how they should behave.

This is the seventh edition of the Association of Rehabilitation Nurses (ARN) *The Specialty Practice of Rehabilitation Nursing: A Core Curriculum*. It defines the practice of rehabilitation nursing and serves as the framework for our specialty. If you begin with the first edition of the *Core Curriculum* and read through the six editions, which have spanned 4 decades, you will marvel at how rehabilitation nursing knowledge and practice has advanced. Research, technology, policy, and society have all shaped the development of our specialty. This newest edition of the *Core Curriculum* has been expanded to include newly developed competencies, discussion of *The Essential Role of the Rehabilitation Nurse in Facilitating Care Transitions* (an ARN white paper), and advances in knowledge and research.

The seventh edition of the *Core Curriculum* would not exist without a great number of people who contributed their time, effort, and talent to develop this up-to-date and valuable reference for rehabilitation nurses everywhere.

First, I would like to thank the authors and reviewers. Every chapter in this new edition was written or updated by volunteers and then reviewed and critiqued by even more volunteers. They graciously donated their time and expertise so that nurses everywhere could learn more about rehabilitation and rehabilitation nursing. The authors and reviewers are from all parts of the United States, are experts in their respective fields, and represent diverse settings such as academia, clinical practice, management, and business. I am proud to acknowledge that a clinically experienced, new Certified Rehabilitation Registered Nurse (CRRN®) who had not previously written for a publication was mentored through the process and became a chapter co-author! Way to go, Meghan Leah Leibas, BSN RN CRRN!

Next, I would like to acknowledge the ARN editorial staff. They developed the *Core Curriculum* work calendar and task list, helped find authors and reviewers, communicated with every volunteer and kept everyone on task, read and edited every chapter, obtained permissions for figures and tables, created a new cover design, and designed page layouts. This group of people went above and beyond in their work—the *Core Curriculum* would not exist without them. In particular, I would like to thank Katherine Wayne and Julie Enichen who led the ARN staff in this effort.

There were even more volunteers whose contributions were a bit more indirect, such as the ARN task force that developed the Competency Model for Rehabilitation Nursing and the ARN members who wrote the *The Essential Role of the Rehabilitation Nurse in Facilitating Care Transitions* white paper. Both of these works are incorporated into this new edition. I would also like to acknowledge the ARN Board of Directors who approved the expansion of the *Core Curriculum* and funding for its publication.

All of us have done our best to make sure that the seventh edition of the *Core Curriculum* is an up-to-date, evidence-based, and accurate professional resource. We offer it to you to support your learning, growth, and career as a rehabilitation nurse.

Cheryl Lehman, PhD RN CNS-BC RN-BC CRRN, Editor

AUTHORS

Chapter 1
Donna P. Jernigan, MS BSN RN CRRN

Chapter 2
Donna Williams, MSN RN CRRN

Chapter 3
Michele Cournan, DNP RN CRRN ANP-BC FNP
Denise Stiltner, MSN RNC-NIC
Donald D. Kautz, RN PhD CRRN CNE ACNS-BC

Chapter 4
Angela Stone Schmidt, PhD MNSc RNP RN

Chapter 5
Beverly S. Reigle, PhD RN
Andrea E. Berndt, PhD

Chapter 6
Stephanie Vaughn, PhD RN CRRN
Darpan I. Patel, PhD
Frank Puga, PhD

Chapter 7
Terrie Black, DNP MBA BSN RN CRRN FAHA
Anne Deutsch, PhD RN CRRN

Chapter 8
Stephanie Davis Burnett, DNP RN ACNS-BC CRRN
Elaine Tilka Miller, PhD RN CRRN FAHA FAAN

Chapter 9
Barbara J. Lutz, PhD RN CRRN FAHA FNAP FAAN
Michelle Camicia, MSN CRRN CCM
James Farrell, RN MBA

Chapter 10
Donna Williams, MSN RN CRRN
Kathryn Doeschot, MSN RN CRRN

Chapter 11
Paul Nathenson, RN HN-BC CTN CRRN

Chapter 12
Martha Acosta, PhD PT GCS MS
Bridget Piernik-Yoder, PhD OTR
Autumn Clegg, MSOT OTR
Cheryl Lehman, PhD RN CNS-BC RN-BC CRRN

Chapter 13
Anne Deutsch, PhD RN CRRN
James Farrell, MBA RN CRRN

Chapter 14
Mindi Miller, PhD MSN MA RN CRRN

Chapter 15
Deirdre F. Jackson, MSN RN APN CRRN CPN
Nicole C. Kelly, MSN RN CRRN CPN

Chapter 16
Kristen L. Mauk, PhD DNP RN CRRN GCNS-BC GNP-BC FAAN
Maria Radwanski, MSN RN CRRN

Chapter 17
Mary Sue Biggins, MBA BSN CRRN
Brenda R. French, MSN CRRN CBIS RN-BC
Paul Mittlesteadt, MSN LTC AN U.S. Army (Ret.)

Chapter 18
Kristen L. Mauk, PhD DNP RN CRRN GCNS-BC GNP-BC FAAN
Maria Radwanski, RN MSN CRRN

Chapter 19
Jill Rye, MA RN CRRN CNL
Mary Pat Murphy, MSN CRRN CBIST

Chapter 20
Margit B. Gerardi, PhD WHCNP PMHNP-BC

Chapter 21
Joan P. Alverzo, PhD CRRN
Kathryn Doeschot, MSN RN CRRN
Meghan Leah Leibas, BSN RN CRRN

Chapter 22
Linda L. Pierce, PhD RN CNS CRRN FAHA FAAN
Debbie Summers, MSN RN ACNS-BC CNRN SCRN FAHA

Chapter 23
Tiffany LeCroy, MSN RN CRRN FNP-C ACNS-BC
Joan McMahon, MSA BSN CRRN

Chapter 24
Paula Stangeland, PhD RN CRRN
Cheryl Lehman, PhD RN CNS-BC RN-BC CRRN

Chapter 25
Cheryl Lehman, PhD RN CNS-BC RN-BC CRRN

Chapter 26
Patricia A. Haldi, MS CRRN CDE
Susan Wirt, MSN RN CRRN CCM CLCP CRP CNLCP

Chapter 27
Pamela Masters-Farrell, MSN RN CRRN
Kathleen A. Stevens, PhD RN CRRN NE-BC

Chapter 28
Anne Leclaire, MSN RN CRRN
Gail L. Sims, MSN RN CRRN
Kathleen Stevens, PhD RN CRRN NE-BC

REVIEWERS

Chapter 1
Cynthia S. Jacelon, PhD RN-BC CRRN FAAN

Chapter 2
Maria Radwanski, MSN RN CRRN

Chapter 3
Teresa Thompson, PhD RN CRRN

Chapter 4
Aloma (Cookie) Gender, MSN RN CRRN

Chapter 5
Gail Powell-Cope, PhD ARNP FAAN

Chapter 6
Andrea Berndt, PhD

Chapter 7
Frank Puga, PhD

Chapter 8
Sherry Liske, MS RN CRRN

Chapter 9
Karen Preston, MS PHN CRRN FIALCP

Chapter 10
Karen Preston, MS PHN CRRN FIALCP

Chapter 11
Brenda McCall-Russell, MBA BSN RN CRRN

Chapter 12
Elizabeth Yetzer, MA MSN RN CRRN

Chapter 13
Carol A. Gleason, MM RN CRRN CCM LRC BCPC

Chapter 14
Cynthia S. Jacelon, PhD RN-BC CRRN FAAN

Chapter 15
Lyn Sapp, MN RN CRRN

Chapter 16
Brenda McCall-Russell, MBA BSN RN CRRN

Chapter 17
Leslie Neal-Boylan, PhD CRRN APRN-BC FNP FAAN

Chapter 18
Barbara Brillhart, PhD RN

Chapter 19
Pamela Masters-Farrell, MSN RN CRRN
Carolyn A. Sorensen, MSN RN CRRN CWOCN

Chapter 20
Pamala Larsen, PhD RN

Chapter 21
Carla J. Howard, MSN CRRN ACNP-BC FNP

Chapter 22
Patricia G. Martinez, BSN RN CRRN

Chapter 23
Catharine Farnan Kennedy, MS RN CRRN ONC CBIS

Chapter 24
Marcia Potter, MS RN CRRN RAC-CT

Chapter 25
Paula Stangeland, PhD RN CRRN

Chapter 26
Paddy Garvin Higgins, MN RN CRRN CNS

Chapter 27
Kristen L. Mauk, PhD DNP RN CRRN GCNS-BC GNP-BC FAAN

Chapter 28
Norma Clanin, MS RN CRRN

ARN COMPETENCY MODEL FOR PROFESSIONAL REHABILITATION NURSING

INTRODUCTION

We are excited to include and apply the Association of Rehabilitation Nurses (ARN) Competency Model for Professional Rehabilitation Nursing throughout the 7th edition of the *Specialty Practice of Rehabilitation: A Core Curriculum.* This section provides a brief overview of the Competency Model to support information that the reader will encounter throughout this book.

The specialty of rehabilitation nursing is practiced in multiple settings along the healthcare continuum; thus, a framework or model for professional rehabilitation nursing is needed to reflect all the competencies necessary for the rehabilitation nurse in the current healthcare environment. To meet this need, an ARN task force of experts representing clinical and academic settings developed an evidence-based framework to guide professional rehabilitation nursing practice. Four domains that highlight essential role competencies were created. The competencies were further separated into three levels of nurse proficiency: beginner (1–2 years), intermediate (3–5 years—CRRN), and advanced (5 years and more in varied roles, including educator, clinical nurse specialist [CNS], advanced practice registered nurse [APRN], and more). The Competency Model was finalized and published in 2014 (ARN, 2014).

ARN's *Core Curriculum* is an important educational and informational reference for the rehabilitation nurse who seeks to attain the identified rehabilitation nurse competencies. To help the rehabilitation nurse gain knowledge related to the competencies, new chapters on teamwork, equipment, medical complications, and transitions in care have been added to this edition. Existing chapters also have been updated to address the competencies.

At the beginning of most chapters, the editor and authors have identified domains and competencies from the Competency Model that align with each chapter's content. The reader is encouraged to refer back to this section for an explanation of the domains and competencies associated with each chapter.

Please note that this section does not include everything the reader should know about the competencies. The complete model with detailed explanations, including descriptors for the beginner, intermediate, and advanced proficiency levels of rehabilitation nursing, can be viewed on the ARN website at http://www.rehabnurse.org/profresources/content/ARN-Competency-Model-for-Professional-Rehabilitation-Nursing.html.

The following information has been excerpted and condensed from the ARN Competency Model for Professional Rehabilitation Nursing.

THE COMPETENCY MODEL

The ARN Competency Model for Professional Rehabilitation Nursing is depicted by a circle with the "Rehabilitation Nursing Professional Role" at the center, surrounded by the four domains and various competencies. The dotted lines illustrate the crossover of knowledge and skills that are represented in each domain, depicting a holistic practice that rehabilitation nurses espouse.

DOMAINS AND COMPETENCIES

Domain 1: Nurse-Led Evidence-Based Interventions to Promote Function and Health Management in Persons with Disability and/or Chronic Illness

1.1. Use supportive technology for improving quality of life for persons with disability.
1.2. Implement nursing and interprofessional interventions based on best evidence to manage the client's disability and/or chronic illness.
1.3. Provide client and caregiver education in relation to disability, chronic illness, and health management (DCIHM).
1.4. Deliver client- and family-centered care.

Domain 2: Promotion of Health and Successful Living in Persons with Disability or Chronic Illness Across the Life Span

2.1. Promote health and prevent disability across the life span.
2.2. Foster self-management.
2.3. Promote and facilitate safe and effective care transitions.

Domain 3: Leadership

3.1. Promote accountability for care.
3.2. Disseminate rehabilitation nursing knowledge.
3.3. Impact health policy for persons with disability and/or chronic illness.
3.4. Empower client self-advocacy.

Domain 4: Interprofessional Care

4.1. Develop interprofessional relationships.
4.2. Implement an interprofessional holistic plan of care.
4.3. Foster effective interprofessional collaboration.

ARN Competency Model for Professional Rehabilitation Nursing

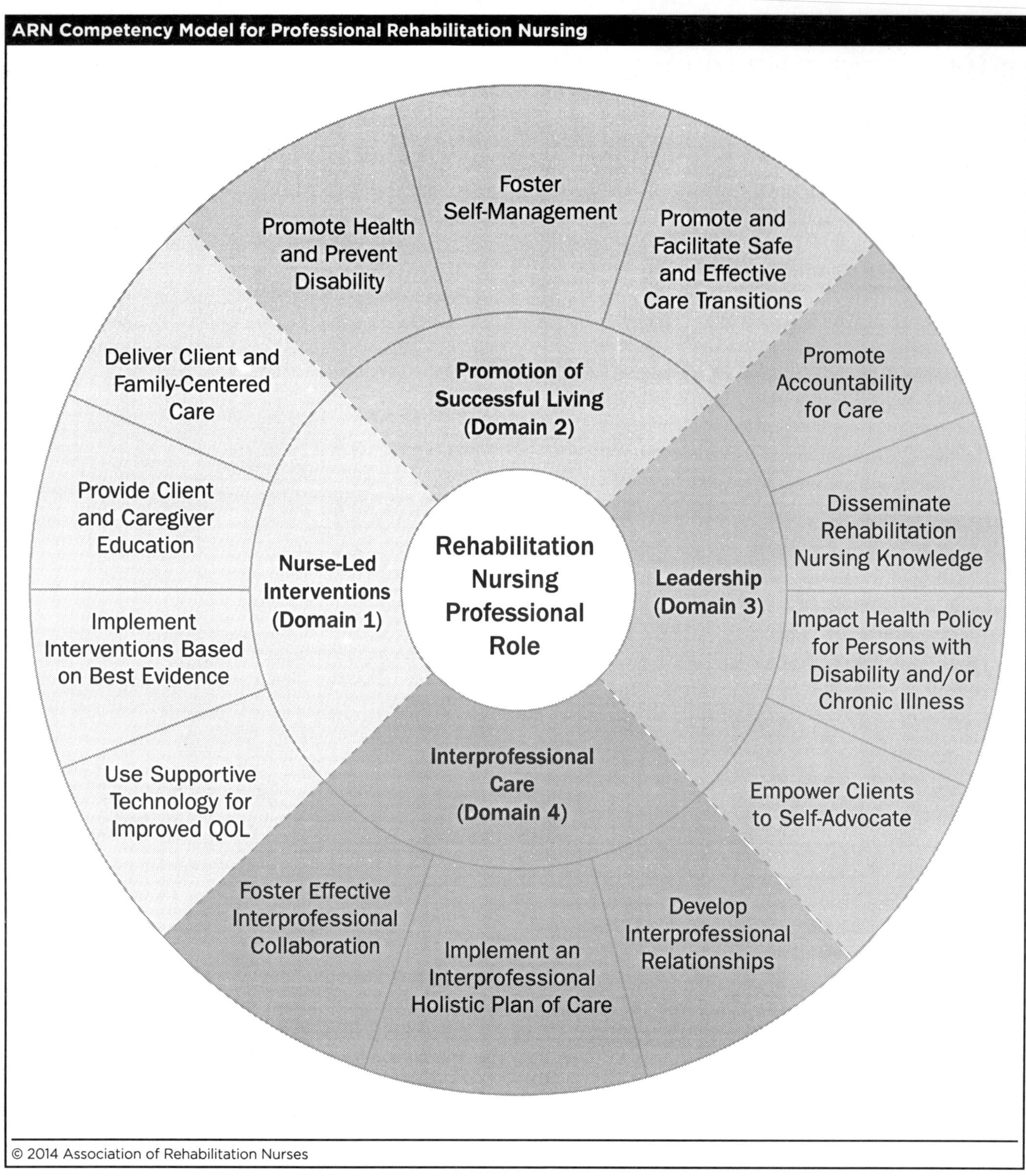

Domain 1: Nurse-Led Evidence-Based Interventions to Promote Function and Health Management in Persons with Disability and/or Chronic Illness

The practice of rehabilitation nursing is recognized as the specialty of managing the care of persons with disability and chronic health conditions across all ages. Rehabilitation nurses, whether novice or experienced, use current evidence and supportive technology to deliver the optimum patient- and family-centered care. Evidence-based best practices support these nurse-led interventions and all of the patient and caregiver education necessary for maximizing the quality of life for those we serve.

Rehabilitation nurses recognize that individuals are part of the family unit, and that families comprise the support structure in each community. They understand these relationships and work collaboratively with other professionals using nurse-led interventions to promote health for individuals, families, and communities.

Competency 1.1: Use supportive technology for improving quality of life for persons with disability.
Description/Scope: Uses appropriate technology (e.g., electronic monitoring, TENS, environment controls, telehealth) that improves self-management, functional improvement, and quality of life for individuals with disabilities and/or chronic illness.

Competency 1.2: Implement nursing and interprofessional interventions based on best evidence to manage the client's disability and/or chronic illness.
Description/Scope: Uses evidence-based interventions to manage common disabilities and chronic illness, such as traumatic brain injury (TBI), stroke, spinal cord injury (SCI), amputation, and neuromuscular disorders.

Competency 1.3: Provide client and caregiver education in relation to disability, chronic illness, and health management (DCIHM).
Description/Scope: Utilizes the nursing process to provide DCIHM education for individuals, families, interdisciplinary teams and communities. Areas of education include but are not limited to ADL management, mobility, communication, safety, and disease management.

Competency 1.4: Deliver client- and family-centered care.
Description/Scope: Demonstrates a collaborative approach to planning, delivering, and evaluating care that acknowledges and honors the client's and family's culture, values, beliefs, and care decision making.

Domain 2: Promotion of Health and Successful Living in Persons with Disability or Chronic Illness Across Life Span

The rehabilitation nurse provides education and plans for patients to manage disease and disability with maximal independence in the home-living environment. Rehabilitation nurses identify client and caregiver needs and integrate community care services that manage chronic disease and supports health over time.

This domain targets the role that the rehabilitation nurse plays in promoting overall successful living through risk reduction, harm prevention, and maintenance of optimal health.

Competency 2.1: Promote health and prevent disability across the life span.
Description/Scope: Uses risk reduction, harm prevention, and health management promotion strategies, such as helmet safety, transportation services, nutrition education, and lifestyle modifications, to promote and encourage wellness.

Competency 2.2: Foster self-management.
Description/Scope: Uses a collaborative approach that incorporates the client's self-efficacy, past experiences, and health literacy to problem solve and make decisions about his or her health care to achieve the highest quality of life while living with a chronic illness and/or disability.

Competency 2.3: Promote and facilitate safe and effective care transitions.
Description/Scope: Facilitates optimal collaboration and coordination among clients, families, and healthcare professionals to promote the safe and timely transition across care settings.

Domain 3: Leadership

Rehabilitation nurses at all levels are key in empowering clients and families to be self-advocates. They routinely collaborate with other professionals and organizations and influence health policy to promote optimum care across the continuum for individuals with disability or chronic illness.

The professional rehabilitation nurse is a qualified team leader and a competent key partner in a successful rehabilitation program. Client rehabilitation outcomes are maximized when the rehabilitation nurse takes a leadership role and collaborates with rehabilitation team members.

The Leadership domain highlights competencies which focus on accountability, advocacy, and the sharing of rehabilitation knowledge with clients and their families, and other members of the interprofessional team.

Competency 3.1: Promote accountability for care.
Description/Scope: Accountability for care is the continuous, multidimensional process that promotes ethical, cost-effective client- and family-centered quality outcomes in persons with disability and chronic illness.

Competency 3.2: Disseminate rehabilitation nursing knowledge.
Description/Scope: Disseminates rehabilitation nursing knowledge in diverse settings such as unit, agency, government, and academia. Dissemination activities include presentations, publications, government advocacy, student instruction, and professional organization engagement.

Competency 3.3: Impact health policy for persons with disability and/or chronic illness.
Description/Scope: Effectively champions the healthcare policy process in the legislative arena locally, regionally, or nationally. Presents ethical strategies for effective action.

Competency 3.4: Empower clients to self-advocate.
Description/Scope: Client advocacy is the safeguarding of a client's autonomy, acting on behalf of the client, and empowering the client through education, collaboration, and support for individuals living with chronic illness and/or disability (DCIHM).

Domain 4: Interprofessional Care

An integral part of the rehabilitation nurse's role is the ability to effectively communicate and collaborate within an interprofessional team. The rehabilitation nurse's role as a member of an effective interprofessional team is instrumental in the development and implementation of a rehabilitation plan of care that uses the best available evidence to promote desired quality outcomes in a diverse client population.

The Interprofessional Care domain explicates the rehabilitation nurse's role on the interprofessional team through relationship development, effective collaboration, and coordinated implementation of the plan of care.

Competency 4.1: Develop interprofessional relationships.
Description/Scope: The rehabilitation nurse builds and maintains interprofessional team relationships using effective communication and strategies such as client conferences and huddles.

Competency 4.2: Implement an interprofessional holistic plan of care.
Description/Scope: The rehabilitation nurse develops a plan of care for diverse clients, which prescribes strategies, alternatives, and interventions to attain desired outcomes.

Competency 4.3: Foster effective interprofessional collaboration.
Description/Scope: The rehabilitation nurse collaborates with the client, family, and other members of the interprofessional team in providing exemplary client care.

Reference

Association of Rehabilitation Nurses (ARN). (2014). ARN competency model for professional rehabilitation nursing. Retrieved from http://www.rehabnurse.org/uploads/files/education/ARN_Rehabilitation_Nursing_Competency _Model_FINAL_-_May_2014.pdf

Section I

The Specialty of
REHABILITATION NURSING

Chapter 1

Rehabilitation and Rehabilitation Nursing

Donna P. Jernigan, MS BSN RN CRRN

LEARNING OUTCOMES

- Define disability and rehabilitation.
- Describe the contents and relationships within the World Health Organization's (WHO's) International Classification of Functioning, Disability, and Heath (ICF) model of disability.
- Recognize the goals of the rehabilitation process.
- Identify the roles and responsibilities of the rehabilitation nurse.
- Discuss core competencies of the rehabilitation nurse, as defined within the Association of Rehabilitation Nurses (ARN) competency model.

KEY CHAPTER TOPICS

- Background and definitions
- Legislative initiatives
- Rehabilitation philosophy and goals across disciplines
- Educational preparation, licensure, and certification
- Role responsibilities for professional rehabilitation nursing
- Rehabilitation nursing competencies

Introduction

Rehabilitation is a philosophy of practice and a caring attitude toward people with disabilities and chronic health problems. Throughout the last few decades many trends have combined to increase the need for rehabilitation. Advances in health care have enabled people to survive serious injuries and illnesses and to live longer than in the past. Thus, the number of people with chronic illness and disability has been increasing. In addition, a large segment of the population is rapidly aging and living longer, so nurses and other healthcare professionals are seeing an increase in chronic health problems and disabilities related to old age.

The overall goals of rehabilitation are to improve quality of life and help people "who [have] a disability or chronic health problem in restoring, maintaining, and promoting his or her maximal health" (Association of Rehabilitation Nurses [ARN], 2014b, p. 7). Rehabilitation is not a place but a philosophy of care that is demonstrated by the rehabilitation team in the practice location. Rehabilitation is contingent on a team approach, and the discipline of nursing is integral to the team. Rehabilitation nursing is a specialty practice that confers a unique, holistic perspective to the care of clients with disabilities and chronic health problems. This unique perspective can be applied across the continuum of care.

The purpose of this chapter is to present an introduction to rehabilitation philosophy, goals, and processes and examine the role of nursing within the specialty. This chapter includes descriptions of the role responsibilities, educational preparation, competencies, certification, and resources for the specialty practice of rehabilitation nursing.

I. Background and Definitions

A. What Is "Disability"?

1. WHO (2014) defined *disability* as an umbrella term that includes impairments, limitations in activity, and participation restrictions.
   a. *Impairment* is defined as a problem in body function or structure.
   b. *Activity limitation* is defined as a difficulty in executing a task or action.
   c. *Participation restriction* is defined as a problem an individual

experiences with involvement in various life situations.

2. The WHO (2014) notes that disability is a complex interaction between the physical issues of the individual and the features of the society in which he or she lives.
3. The WHO (2001) has developed the International Classification of Functioning, Disability and Health (ICF).
   a. The ICF (**Figure 1-1**) is a model that acknowledges that disability is caused by features that are internal to an individual (e.g., disease, injury) and external to an individual (e.g., society).
   b. As shown in Figure 1-1, the health condition (disorder or disease), as well as contextual factors (environmental and personal), can affect not only body structure and function but also activity and participation.
      1) Environmental factors include societal attitudes, structural barriers, climate, terrain, and legal constraints, among other factors.
      2) Personal factors include gender, age, ethnicity and race, coping abilities, education, social background, profession, personal history and experiences, and other factors that influence how an individual interprets limitations caused by disability.
   c. The interaction of the health condition with contextual factors influences rehabilitation progress and healing.
   d. **Figure 1-2** outlines several definitions pertinent to impairment of function, activity, and participation.
   e. The WHO regards disability as dysfunction at the level of the body structure or part, at the level of the whole person, and at the level of the whole person in a social context.
      1) Dysfunction at the level of the body part is termed *impairment.*
      2) Dysfunction at the level of the individual is termed *activity limitation.*
      3) Dysfunction at the level of the person in society is termed *participation restriction.*
   f. The ICF model can be used as a basis for clinical care as well as research.

B. What Is Rehabilitation?

1. *Rehabilitation* is usually regarded as treatments or interventions that address injury, disease, or disability with the aim of restoring the individual to a fully functional status.
2. *Rehabilitation* has been formally defined as "a process of helping a person to reach the fullest physical, psychological, social, vocational, avocational, and educational potential consistent with his or her physiologic or anatomic impairment,

Figure 1-1. The ICF Model of Disability

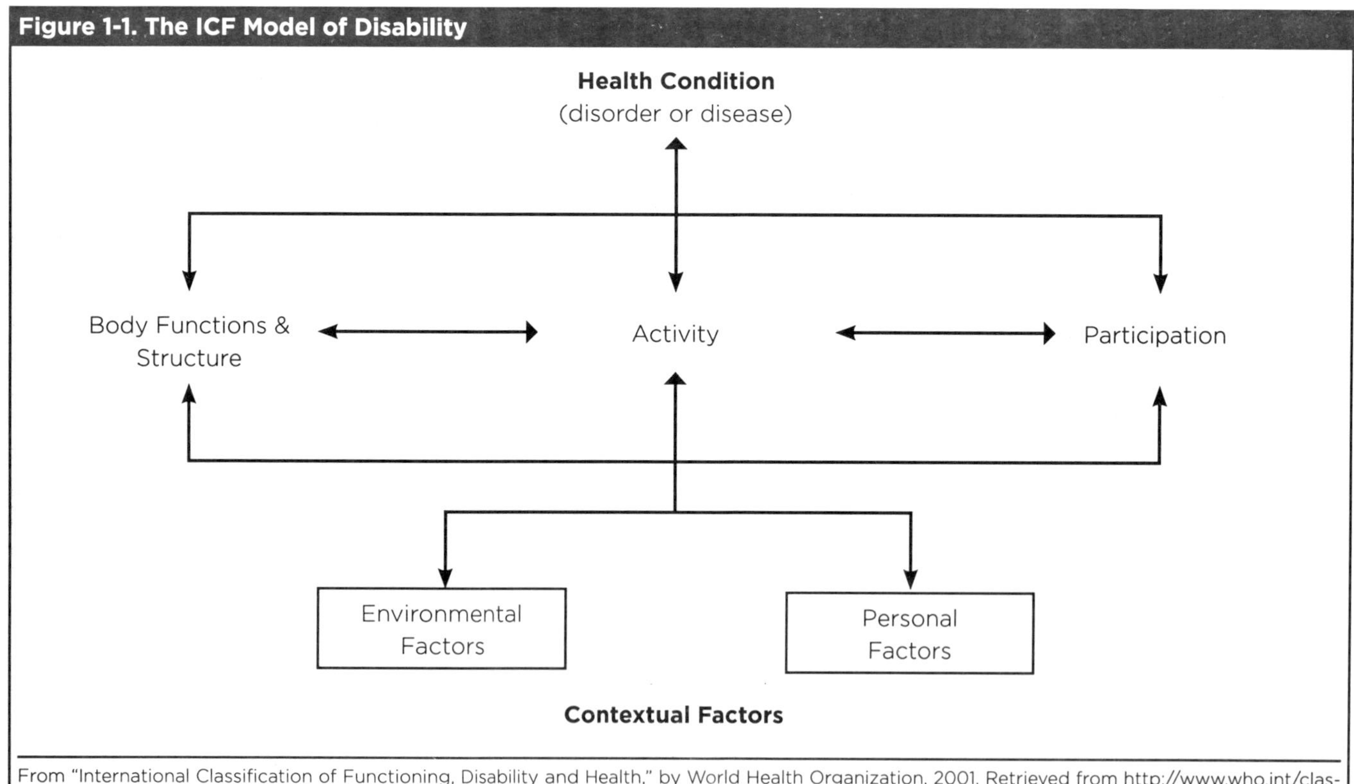

From "International Classification of Functioning, Disability and Health," by World Health Organization, 2001. Retrieved from http://www.who.int/classifications/icf/en/. Copyright 2001 by World Health Organization. Reprinted with permission.

Figure 1-2. WHO Definitions Within the ICF Model

Body Functions are physiological functions of body systems (including psychological functions).

Body Structures are anatomical parts of the body such as organs, limbs and their components.

Impairments are problems in body function or structure such as a significant deviation or loss.

Activity is the execution of a task or action by an individual.

Participation is involvement in a life situation.

Activity Limitations are difficulties an individual may have in executing activities.

Participation Restrictions are problems an individual may experience in involvement in life situations.

Environmental Factors make up the physical, social and attitudinal environment in which people live and conduct their lives.

From "International Classification of Functioning, Disability and Health," by World Health Organization, 2001. Retrieved from http://www.who.int/classifications/icf/en/.

environmental limitations, and desires and life plans" (DeLisa, Currie, & Martin, 1998, p. 3).

3. A related term is *habilitation,* often interpreted to mean training in skills and functions that have not been learned before.
   a. For example, habilitation could describe the process of training a congenitally disabled child to walk for the first time.

C. The Evolution of Rehabilitation

1. Advances in health care throughout the past century have enabled people to live longer and recover from injuries and illnesses that previously were fatal.
2. A consequence of saving lives is that clients are sometimes left with disabilities and chronic illnesses that profoundly change the way they live.
3. The field of rehabilitation emerged to help individuals and families integrate into their lives the adaptations needed for disability and/or and chronic health problems.
   a. Rehabilitation is a philosophy, an attitude, and an approach to caring for people with disabilities and chronic health problems that encourages self-management, improves the quality of life, and provides a meaningful context in which to live.
   b. The concept of rehabilitation as a philosophy and attitude is important.
   c. Attitudes toward people with disability, which arise from a philosophy, determine societal responsibilities and approaches.
      1) For example, in ancient Western civilization, disease and disability often were thought to be the result of evil spirits.
      2) Consequently, those so "possessed" were feared and shunned.
      3) Parents in ancient Rome could legally drown infants with congenital anomalies, and in Sparta such infants were left to die of exposure.
      4) This situation did not improve during the Middle Ages.
         a) Some people with disabilities were burned as witches, others were used as court jesters, and all who had disabilities were shunned from everyday societal functions.
      5) Even in more modern times, those living with disabilities or handicaps in Nazi Germany were considered "flawed" and were among the first people murdered during the Holocaust.
   d. Fortunately, philosophical approaches and attitudes toward disability have changed radically over time.
4. The interdisciplinary healthcare specialty of rehabilitation was a product of 20th-century wars.
   a. Many soldiers—young men for the most part—survived injury but faced serious disability after the two major wars of the 20th century.
   b. As a result, military hospitals established rehabilitation units that focused extensive efforts on returning these young men to society.
   c. Dr. Howard Rusk, head of the American Air Force Convalescent Training Program, was a strong leader in organizing rehabilitation programs (Rusk, 1972).
   d. Another influence on the development of rehabilitation was the polio epidemic.
   e. Civilians with disability were not a focus of attention until the latter half of the 20th century (Welch & Palamas, 1995).
   f. Rehabilitation units and hospitals began to spring up across the United States at this time, and the interdisciplinary specialty of rehabilitation gained importance.
   g. By 1974, ARN was formed, and nursing, which had always been involved in rehabilitation, became formally recognized as a rehabilitation specialty.

II. Legislative Initiatives

A. Legislation in the United States has been important in the development of the specialty of rehabilitation.

B. The result of these legislative acts has been to increase societal acceptance of people with disabilities and provide opportunities for them to maximize their potential.

C. Rehabilitation is a vital component of health care.

1. Although the root causes of disability may have changed over time, the need for rehabilitation is greater today than ever before.
2. Rehabilitation has moved from its era of research and development to one of scrutiny by the healthcare finance community.

D. Legislated Acts

Although this topic is covered in more depth in a later chapter, key legislation exists that deserves mention here.

1. After World Wars I and II and the Korean and Vietnam Wars, Congress enacted the Smith-Fess Vocational Rehabilitation Act (1920) and its amendments of 1943, 1954, and 1965 to address the rehabilitation needs of the wounded soldiers. The focus of this legislation was clinical care, and it benefited civilians as well (Welch & Palamas, 1995).
2. The Social Security Act (SSA), enacted in 1935, established an income maintenance system for those unable to work and included monies to provide medical and therapeutic services for handicapped children. The SSA also positively affected vocational rehabilitation programs (Colorado State University, 2014).
3. The Rehabilitation Act of 1973 (and its many amendments) was the first act to address equal access of people with disabilities (Colorado State University, 2014)
   a. Section 501: focused on affirmative action and nondiscrimination in employment in federal agencies
   b. Section 502: enforced the standards set under the Architectural Barriers Act of 1968
   c. Section 503: prohibited discrimination in employment on the basis of physical or mental handicap in federal contracts and subcontracts
   d. Section 504: prohibited discrimination on the basis of physical or mental handicap in programs that receive federal funding
   e. Section 508: required that electronic and information technology used by the federal government be accessible
4. The Education for All Handicapped Children Act ensured a free, appropriate public education for all students with handicapping conditions, and established the right of students to receive services such as speech therapy, audiology, physical and occupational therapy, psychological counseling, and medical counseling and care (Colorado State University, 2014).
5. The Americans with Disabilities Act (ADA) of 1990 (Colorado State University, 2014; U.S. Department of Justice, 2014) was a civil rights law that prevents discrimination based on disability.
   a. Title I
      1) Prohibits private employers, state and local governments, employment agencies, and labor unions from discriminating against qualified people with disabilities in job application procedures; hiring; firing; advancement; compensation; job training; and other terms, conditions, and privileges of employment
      2) Describes the traits of a person with a disability
         a) A physical or mental impairment that substantially limits one or more major life activities
         b) A record of such an impairment
         c) Regarded as having such an impairment
   b. Title II
      1) Provides comprehensive civil rights for qualified people with disabilities
      2) Addresses public entities and requires that all activities, services, and programs of public entities be covered by the ADA, including activities of state legislatures and courts, town meetings, police and fire departments, motor vehicle licensing, and employment
      3) Directly influences access, program integration, communication, construction, and alterations
   c. Title III
      1) Addresses the public sector
      2) Defines the private entities that must meet ADA requirements
   d. Title IV
      1) Telecommunication
   e. Title V
      1) Miscellaneous provisions to cover legal fees and to prohibit coercion and retaliation
   f. The impact of the ADA
      1) Allows people with disabilities to have equal opportunities, accessibility, and accommodations in employment, transportation, and public access

2) Has spawned litigation and clarification to further define its implementation and application (U.S. Department of Justice, 2014)
3) Has reinforced the advocate role of rehabilitation nurses based on their knowledge of the ADA as they inform clients, encourage ADA enforcement, and obtain resources

6. Healthcare funding (e.g., Medicare, Medicaid, and the Affordable Care Act) is discussed in a later chapter.

III. Rehabilitation Philosophy and Goals Across Disciplines

A. Rehabilitation is a philosophy that crosses the boundaries of practice disciplines.
1. It is an inherently collaborative endeavor, and it places the client and family in the center of the healthcare team.
2. Rehabilitation is contingent on a team approach.
   a. Indeed, most rehabilitation professionals would agree that the healthcare system would flourish if the ideals of rehabilitation permeated all aspects of health care.
3. These definitions provide a framework and a language—not only for rehabilitation but also for society.

B. Goal of Rehabilitation
1. The overall goal of rehabilitation is "restoring, maintaining, and promoting maximal health" (ARN, 2014b).

C. Who Provides Rehabilitation?
1. The rehabilitation team consists, first and foremost, of the individual and his or her family/significant others.
2. Other team members can vary depending on the needs of the person but typically include a physiatrist, rehabilitation nurse, social worker, physical therapist, occupational therapist, and speech-language pathologist.
   a. Others include a psychologist, pharmacist, chaplain, recreation therapist, music therapist, and dietitian as the need arises.
3. Insurers, vocational therapists, employers, case managers, audiologists, subacute and home-health providers, and medical consultants can be invited to contribute and share information at the appropriate times in the appropriate circumstances.

D. Nursing Focus and Core Values
1. Nursing brings a unique, holistic focus to rehabilitation. Whereas members of other disciplines treat particular aspects of a person, nurses focus on the person as a whole, providing continuity and integrity to the client's rehabilitation experience.
2. Fawcett (1984) defined the central foci (or metaparadigm) of nursing as person, health, environment, and nursing. The individual's philosophical view of these concepts is the foundation of how he or she approaches nursing care. The core values of rehabilitation as an interdisciplinary practice are congruent with those of nursing.
3. As a profession, nursing has stated its ethical foundation in the code of ethics for nurses (American Nurses Association [ANA], 2015).
4. Rehabilitation nursing arose as a specialty practice from the nursing discipline. Values and assumptions for the discipline are provided in nursing's social policy statement
   a. Humans manifest an essential unity of mind, body, and spirit.
   b. Human experience is contextually and culturally defined.
   c. Health and illness are human experiences. The presence of illness does not preclude health, nor does optimal health preclude illness.
   d. The relationship between nurse and patient involves both individuals in the process of care.
   e. The interaction between the nurse and the patient occurs within the context of the values and beliefs of the patient and the nurse. (ANA, 2010b, p. 3).
5. Rehabilitation nursing, as a specialty of the nursing discipline at large, embraces these values and further explicates its core values, which include the following:
   a. Individuals with functional limitations have intrinsic worth that transcends their disability and/or chronic illness.
   b. Individuals are complex yet unified, whole persons, who have the right and the responsibility to make informed decisions about their future.
   c. Individuals can benefit from rehabilitation nursing at any stage of the lifespan (ARN, 2014b, p. 5).

E. Definition of Rehabilitation Nursing
1. *Rehabilitation nursing* is defined as "the diagnosis and treatment of human responses of individuals and groups to actual or potential health problems relative to altered functional ability and lifestyle"(ARN, 2014b, p. 7).
2. Rehabilitation nursing interventions, in promoting maximal health, enhance the client's quality of life.
3. Essential in achieving this goal is collaboration with the client, his or her significant others, and other healthcare providers.

4. Rehabilitation nursing is client centered, goal oriented, and outcomes based.

F. The Specialty Practice of Rehabilitation Nursing

1. Both ARN and ANA view rehabilitation nursing as a specialty practice with a unique body of knowledge. Professional rehabilitation nursing practice is guided by philosophy, theory, and research and therefore can be practiced in any setting. When the client is at the center of care, and the goals are to optimize health (however it is defined) and improve the quality of life for those with disability or chronic disease, the boundaries of the healthcare system are less important. There are many resources that both justify and support the practice of rehabilitation nursing as a unique specialty. Three of the most important ones are
   a. *ARN Standards and Scope of Rehabilitation Nursing Practice* (ARN, 2014b)
   b. ARN's *The Specialty Practice of Rehabilitation Nursing: A Core Curriculum*
   c. *ARN Competency Model for Professional Rehabilitation Nursing* (ARN, 2014a)
2. Other evidence of a discrete body of knowledge for professional rehabilitation nursing practice includes
   a. ARN's peer-reviewed *Journal of Rehabilitation Nursing*
   b. Certified rehabilitation registered nurse (CRRN®) certification

G. What Is a Rehabilitation Nurse?

1. A rehabilitation nurse is a caregiver, teacher, collaborator, and patient advocate. He or she possesses specialized knowledge and skills in rehabilitation nursing, provides education and direction to ancillary staff, functions as a team member and team leader, and acts as a role model and resource for team members.
2. The following has been excerpted from ARN's (n.d.b) description of the role of the rehabilitation staff nurse:
   a. "The goal of rehabilitation nursing is to assist individuals with disability and/or chronic illness to attain and maintain maximum function. The rehabilitation staff nurse assists clients in adapting to an altered lifestyle, while providing a therapeutic environment for client's and their family's development. The rehabilitation staff nurse designs and implements treatment strategies that are based on scientific nursing theory related to self-care and that promote physical, psychosocial, and spiritual health. The rehabilitation staff nurse works in inpatient and outpatient settings that can be found in a range of acute to subacute rehabilitation facilities."
3. Rehabilitation nurses practice in many settings throughout the continuum of care. Practice settings for rehabilitation nursing can include settings of client employment, insurance companies, community centers, residential centers, daycare centers, clinics, skilled-care facilities, inpatient-rehabilitation centers, subacute or postacute units, and acute-care facilities.
4. Rehabilitation concepts are also applied by nurses in the emergency department, the intensive care unit, acute-care medical and surgical units, pediatrics, geriatrics, and the home setting.

IV. Educational Preparation, Licensure, and Certification

A. The public and other healthcare professionals consider rehabilitation nurses to be aides, licensed vocational (practical) nurses, and registered nurses.

1. Nursing aides
   a. Aides in the rehabilitation setting tend to be certified nursing aides (CNAs) or restorative aides (RAs).
   b. In most states CNAs take a course of several weeks' duration that consists of both didactic and clinical hours. They then take a certification examination.
   c. CNAs take vital signs, provide basic hygiene and bathing, assist with feeding, provide interventions to increase patient mobility out of bed, change linens, and document basic interventions and observations.
   d. CNAs report to the licensed nurse, who delegates activities to them based on the CNA's skills, knowledge, and experience and the patient's needs and acuity.
   e. RAs have further training in rehabilitation techniques, such as use of equipment, mobility interventions. They are also trained to support occupational therapy and physical therapy interventions. Requirements for RAs vary by state.
      1) A training manual and interactive online educational program for RAs, published by ARN, is available.
2. Licensed vocational/practical nurses
   a. Licensed vocational/practical nurses (LVNs/LPNs) generally are educated in programs requiring 9–14 months of study.
      1) The LVN/LPN practices under the supervision of a registered nurse, physician, or advanced practice nurse and assists clients in adapting to an altered lifestyle, while

providing a therapeutic environment for clients' and families' development.
   2) The LPN/LVN on the rehabilitation team contributes to and implements evidence-based treatment strategies that are related to self-care and promote physical, psychosocial, and spiritual health.
   3) The LPN/LVN on the rehabilitation team works in a variety of inpatient and outpatient settings that range from acute to subacute rehabilitation facilities (ARN, n.d.c).
   4) There are five areas in which the LPN/LVN can be a key member: teacher, caregiver, collaborator, client, and advocate.
   5) In some subacute settings such as a skilled nursing facility and nursing home, LVN/LPNs could have the additional responsibilities of patient assessment and rehabilitation nursing interventions.

3. Professional rehabilitation nursing
   a. Registered nurses (RNs) are prepared at the levels of associate's degree in nursing (ADN) and bachelor of science degree in nursing (BSN).
   b. Although both ADN- and BSN-prepared nurses are licensed as RNs, the BSN is recommended by many nursing organizations as the required credential for entry-level positions in professional practice.
   c. A BSN program includes nursing education in areas such as teamwork, public health, evidence-based practice, and research, thereby assisting the RN to manage and lead in increasingly sophisticated healthcare environments.
      1) RNs have many roles in the rehabilitation setting, as mentioned previously.
         a) These roles include bedside nurse, team leader, charge nurse, case/care manager, and nurse (unit) manager, among others.
4. Advanced practice nurse/advanced practice registered nurse
   a. Advanced practice nurses (APNs) and advanced practice registered nurses (APRN) commonly employed in rehabilitation settings have master's level education as clinical nurse specialists (CNSs) or nurse practitioners (NPs).
   b. In some states CNS and NP practices are the same, and in others they are completely different.
   c. CNSs typically undertake the roles of provider, educator, collaborator, researcher, consultant, and manager, whereas NPs most often undertake the roles of direct provider and consultant.
   d. NPs can assess, make medical diagnoses, and order interventions such as equipment and medications. In some states, CNSs may also perform those activities.
   e. A description of the role of the advanced practice nurse in the rehabilitation setting can be found in the members' area of the ARN website.
   f. The following has been extracted from ARN's description of the APN's role:
      1) "Advanced practice nurses in rehabilitation have a graduate degree in nursing. They conduct comprehensive assessments and demonstrate a high level of autonomy and expert skill in diagnosis and treatment. They manage complex responses of individuals, families, groups and communities to actual or potential health problems stemming from altered functional ability and altered lifestyle (resulting from physical disability or chronic illness). [APNs] in rehabilitation synthesize complex data to formulate decisions and plans that optimize health, promote wellness, manage illness, prevent complications or secondary disabilities, maximize function, and minimize handicap. Nurses in advanced practice integrate education, research, and consultation into their clinical practice role. They function in collaborative relationships with nursing peers, the Interdisciplinary team, and others who influence the healthcare environment" (ARN, n.d.a, PI).
5. Clinical nurse leader (CNL): The CNL is an advanced generalist clinician with education at the master's or post master's level in a formal CNL education program.
   a. In rehabilitation practice, the CNL oversees the coordination and integration of care for a distinct group of clients.
   b. The CNL puts evidence-based practice into action to ensure that clients benefit from the latest innovations in care delivery.
   c. The CNL evaluates client outcomes, assesses cohort risk, and has the decision-making authority to change care plans when necessary.
   d. The CNL is a leader and active member of the interdisciplinary healthcare team.
   e. The implementation of the CNL role varies across healthcare settings (American

Association of Colleges of Nursing [AACN], "What is CNL Certification?").

6. All nurses must be licensed by the state in which they practice.
   a. People who want to take the licensure exam for LPNs/LVNs or RNs may do so after they have successfully completed an accredited nursing program.
   b. Licensure for APNs varies from state to state.
      1) In general, persons who want to obtain licensure as an APN must be an RN; must have completed an approved educational program of advanced practice leading to a master's of science, doctor of nursing practice, or other approved degree; and they must meet the specific guidelines for licensure in the state in which they want to become licensed.
      2) Advanced practice licensure often relies on certification as an APN in the desired specialty area.
7. Certification is professional recognition of knowledge in a specialty practice.
   a. Certification programs are developed and maintained by professional nursing organizations such as the American Nurses Credentialing Center (ANCC) or ARN.
   b. Certification in rehabilitation nursing is a means of validating specialized knowledge and skills and communicates a sense of accountability to the public.
   c. Certification programs in many specialties are available for RNs and APNs.
   d. Fewer certification programs are available for LPNs.
8. Certified rehabilitation registered nurse (CRRN®): At the RN level of practice, ARN has developed and currently maintains a certification program in rehabilitation nursing.
   a. ARN's standards (2014b) do not mandate the type of professional nursing preparation (i.e., ADN or BSN) that is necessary for generalist practice or certification.
   b. The Rehabilitation Nursing Certification Board, a subsidiary of ARN, offered its first certification examination in 1984.
   c. Those who meet the criteria and pass the exam earn the CRRN credential. Currently, approximately 15,000 nurses hold the CRRN credential.
   d. Audrey Nelson, PhD RN, published research that found that a 1% increase in CRRNs on a unit was associated with a 6% decrease in length of stay. Other, more current, research about certified nurses in general has shown positive effects of certification including decreases in morbidity and mortality, and in length of stay and costs.
   e. Requirements for certification as CRRN include
      1) Current unrestricted RN license, plus:
      2) During the 5 years prior to the examination, 2 years of practice as an RN in rehabilitation nursing, OR
      3) During the 5 years prior to the examination, 1 year of practice as an RN in rehabilitation nursing and 1 year of advanced education at the post-BSN level
   f. The certification is good for 5 years and is renewable with either 60 points of credit or by retaking the examination.

V. Role Responsibilities for Professional Rehabilitation Nursing

American Association of Colleges of Nursing (American Association of Colleges of Nursing [AACN, 2008a]) described the role responsibilities for generalist nursing practice. They are discussed as follows in relation to rehabilitation nursing practice:

A. Provider of Care: "The nurse uses theory and research-based knowledge in the direct and indirect delivery of care . . . in the formation of partnerships with clients and the interdisciplinary healthcare team" (p. 16). Particular roles in rehabilitation with these responsibilities include caregiver, client advocate, client educator, counselor, nurse practitioner, expert witness, and researcher.

B. Designer, Manager, and Coordinator of Care: The nurse needs skills such as communication, collaboration, negotiation, delegation, coordination, and evaluation of interdisciplinary work. These are skills are particularly important for rehabilitation nurses who are team members or leaders. Rehabilitation roles that fulfill these responsibilities include care manager, case manager, consultant, administrator or manager, and CNS. Designing and coordinating care is assuming increasing importance in nursing, with today's healthcare systems' use of various skilled and semiskilled workers in direct care. Additionally, nurses are in a key position to provide leadership in the coordination of care across disciplines (AACN, 2008)

C. Member of a Profession: Professionals have a responsibility to value lifelong learning, identify with the profession's values, and incorporate professionalism into practice. Client advocacy is an important aspect of professional rehabilitation practice, and although this is an integral aspect of everyday practice, advocacy assumes a particularly important role in a larger societal sense. Rehabilitation nurses are responsible for helping to shape public policy in endeavors such as dismantling societal barriers for people with disabilities and educating the public to prevent disease and trauma. Although there are already many opportunities involving these roles, many more could be developed by creative and entrepreneurial nurses. In today's dynamic healthcare system, nurses have the opportunity to develop unique nursing roles that meet the goals of rehabilitation (AACN, 2008).

D. Rehabilitation Nurse as a Change Agent in Today's Healthcare Environment
   1. Change is a central concern for nursing, healthcare, and society.
      a. "Change in the rehabilitation setting can involve change in knowledge, attitude, behavior, or group organization or functioning" (Chin, Finocchiaro, & Rosebrough, 1998, p. 71).
      b. As a change agent, the rehabilitation nurse proactively helps the client or is involved in the change process in the organization.
      c. Change parallels the nursing process.
         1) Identify the problem to be addressed.
         2) Define the changes needed.
         3) Identify the purpose of the change.
         4) Gather and use the elements needed to accomplish the change.
         5) Implement actions to accomplish the change.
         6) Evaluate the change.
      d. Change is continuous, and the nursing process is not linear but is continually evolving, necessitating continuous reassessment.
   2. The demands of health care today have helped to make the healthcare field one of profound change.
   3. Rehabilitation nurses must have knowledge of barriers to change, identify internal and external barriers to openness to change, and make a commitment to change.
      a. Internal demands
         1) Reorganization
         2) Redesign
         3) Reengineering
         4) Continuous quality improvement
         5) Redeployment
      b. External demands
         1) New knowledge
         2) Competition
         3) Regulations
   4. Rehabilitation nurses must understand the external forces that drive change.
      a. Venue of care
      b. Expanded knowledge
      c. Upgrade of clinical knowledge and skills
      d. Fiscal accountability
   5. Rehabilitation nurses must recognize their own attitudes toward change or personality traits related to change. They must know the role that best describes their own viewpoints, and learn how to work with people who have different views.
   6. Rogers (1995) described six types of behavioral groups
      a. Innovators: Adventuresome
      b. Early adopters: Respected leaders in the organization
      c. Early majority: Deliberate
      d. Late majority: Skeptical
      e. Laggards: Hang on to traditional ways and ideas
      f. Rejecters
   7. Major hurdles to change-ready thinking (Kriegel & Brandt, 1996) include
      a. Fear
      b. Fatigue
      c. Comfort
   8. Reasons for taking a proactive approach to change and seeking out opportunities for change include
      a. Improving the quality of care
      b. Improving the cost-effectiveness of care delivery
      c. Making the adaptations needed to maintain change
   9. Resilience in facing change
      a. Attitudes and traits that are characteristic of change-resilient people (Conner, 1996; Giordono, 1997; Jacelon, 1997) include
         1) Positive thinking
         2) Sense of control
         3) Resourcefulness
         4) Focus
         5) Self-discipline
         6) Flexibility
         7) Organization
         8) Proactive behavior
      b. Resilience is needed to manage uncertainty (Porter-O'Grady & Malloch, 2003).
      c. Traits that limit resilience to change (Giordono, 1997) include
         1) Cynicism
         2) Distancing
         3) Avoidance

References

American Association of Colleges of Nursing. (2008). The essentials of baccalaureate education for professional nursing practice. Retrieved from http://www.aacn.nche.edu/education-resources/BaccEssentials08.pdf

American Nurses Association (2010a). *The code of ethics for nurses with interpretive statements.* Washington, DC: Author.

American Nurses Association (2010b). *Nursing's social policy statement.* Kansas City, MO: Author.

Association of Rehabilitation Nurses (2014a). ARN competency model for professional rehabilitation nursing. Chicago: Author. Retrieved from http://www.rehabnurse.org/profresources/content/ARN-Competency-Model-for-Professional-Rehabilitation-Nursing.html

Association of Rehabilitation Nurses (2014b). *Standards and scope of rehabilitation nursing practice* (6th ed.). Chicago: Author.

Association of Rehabilitation Nurses (n.d.a). The advanced practice rehabilitation nurse: Role description. Retrieved from http://www.rehabnurse.org/uploads/files/uploads/File/rdadvprac11.pdf

Association of Rehabilitation Nurses (n.d.b). The rehabilitation staff nurse: Role description. Retrieved from http://www.rehabnurse.org/uploads/files/uploads/File/rdstaffnurse11.pdf

Association of Rehabilitation Nurses (n.d.c). LPN/LVN on the rehabilitation team. Role description. Retrieved from http://www.rehabnurse.org/pubs/role/role-lpn_lvn.html

Chin, P. A., Finocchiaro, D. N., & Rosebrough, A. (1998). *Rehabilitation nursing practice.* New York: McGraw-Hill.

Colorado State University (2014). A Brief History of Legislation. Retrieved from http://www.rds.colostate.edu/history-of-legislation

Conner, D. R. (1996). How can you survive continuous change? *Medical Economics, 73*(8), 109–114.

DeLisa, J. A., Currie, D. M., & Martin, G. M. (1998). Rehabilitation medicine: Past, present, and future. In J. A. DeLisa & B. M. Gans (Eds.), *Physical rehabilitation medicine: Principles and practice* (pp. 3–32). Philadelphia: Lippincott-Raven.

Fawcett, J. (1984). The metaparadigm of nursing: Current status and future refinements. *Image: The Journal of Nursing Scholarship, 16,* 84–87.

Giordono, B. P. (1997). Resilience: A survival tool for the nineties. *AORN Journal, 65*(6), 1032–1034.

Jacelon, C. S. (1997). The trait and process of resilience. *Journal of Advanced Nursing, 25,* 123–139.

Kriegel, R., & Brandt, D. (1996). *Sacred cows make the best burgers: Developing change-ready people and organizations.* New York: Warner Books.

Porter-O'Grady, T., & Malloch, K. (2003). *Quantum leadership: A textbook of new leadership.* Boston: Jones & Bartlett.

Rogers, E. (1995). *Diffusion of innovation* (4th ed.). New York: Free Press.

Rusk, H. (1972). *A world to care for: The autobiography of Howard Rusk.* New York: Random House.

U.S. Department of Justice (2014). Information and technical assistance on the Americans with Disabilities Act. Retrieved from http://www.ada.gov/

Welch, P., & Palamas, C. (1995). A brief history of disability rights legislation in the United States. Retrieved from http://www.udeducation.org/resources/61.html

World Health Organization (2001). International classification of functioning, disability and health. Retrieved from http://www.who.int/classifications/icf/en/

World Health Organization (2014). Disabilities. Retrieved from http://www.who.int/topics/disabilities/en/

Suggested Internet Resources

Association of Rehabilitation Nurses: www.rehabnurse.org

Association of Rehabilitation Nurses history: http://www.rehabnurse.org/about/content/History.html

Association of Rehabilitation Nurses position statements and white papers: http://www.rehabnurse.org/advocacy/content/Position-Statements.html

About CRRN: http://www.rehabnurse.org/certification/content/About-CRRN.html

Chapter 2

Rehabilitation Nursing: Now and into the Future

Donna Williams, MSN RN CRRN

LEARNING OUTCOMES

- Appreciate societal influences on rehabilitation nursing practice.
- Review settings where rehabilitation care is delivered.
- Define community-based rehabilitation.
- Identify challenges to the delivery of rehabilitation nursing care.
- Consider the future of rehabilitation nursing.

KEY CHAPTER TOPICS

- The current face of rehabilitation
- Types of care
- Challenges to rehabilitation and rehabilitation nursing
- Association of Rehabilitation Nurses' (ARN's) assumptions about the future

---

I. Present: The 21st Century

A. The Practice of Rehabilitation Nursing in the 21st Century

1. Rehabilitation nursing continues to be an important specialty.
2. The value of rehabilitation nursing continues to increase as the healthcare system recognizes the positive impact of rehabilitation principles along the continuum of care.
3. ARN remains a strong voice for rehabilitation nurses in the healthcare community. ARN members—through grass roots efforts as well as contact with legislators are increasingly involved in efforts to raise public awareness of the value of rehabilitation nursing.
4. Rehabilitation nurses continue to use evidence-based practices to ensure they will be adequately prepared to provide for clients with greater levels of acuity and chronic conditions.
5. Client conditions continue to increase in complexity, and treatments are more technologically based.
6. Progressive modes of treatment and services are required, as advancing age affects the population and patients are moved more expediently through the healthcare system.
7. Rehabilitation nurses with advanced degrees, including doctorates, act in many capacities.
   a. As experts in research and evidence-based practice
   b. As advocates and managers for large populations needing restorative care
   c. As promoters of public policy for people with disabilities at the local and national levels
   d. As independent practitioners in offices, clinics, and other facilities
   e. As educators for the nursing workforce now and in the future

B. Populations Receiving Rehabilitation Services

1. Rehabilitation is appropriate for many and varied diagnoses. The basics of funding and eligibility for various settings is covered in a later chapter.
2. Many times, the availability of funding dictates whether a patient can receive rehabilitation at all, as well as the duration and setting of rehabilitation.

3. Availability of facilities also has an impact on the delivery of rehabilitation.
4. The Centers for Medicare & Medicaid Services (CMS) is deeply involved in rule setting for admission to rehabilitation facilities. For example:
   a. Persons with diagnoses in the following categories are eligible for inpatient rehabilitation facilities (IRF). The first 13 of the diagnoses, listed here with an asterisk, are under the CMS 60% rule, which mandates that 60% of those served fall into one of these 13 designated diagnostic categories for admission to rehabilitation. This rule does not apply to private insurers' plans and workers' compensation.
      1) Stroke
      2) Spinal cord injury
      3) Congenital deformities
      4) Amputation
      5) Major multiple trauma
      6) Hip fracture
      7) Brain injury
      8) Neurological conditions including multiple sclerosis, Parkinson's disease, and muscular dystrophy
      9) Burns
      10) Active polyarticular rheumatoid arthritis
      11) Systematic vasculidities with joint inflammation
      12) Severe or advanced osteoarthritis
      13) Bilateral knee or hip replacement with a body mass index of at least 50, or 85 years of age or older (see http://www.cms.gov/Outreach-and-Education/Medicare-Learning-Network-MLN/MLNProducts/downloads/InpatRehabPaymtfctsht09-508.pdf for more information)
      14) Cardiac disease
      15) Pulmonary disease
      16) Pain syndrome
      17) Orthopedic disorders
      18) Other disabling impairments
      19) Developmental disability
      20) Debility
      21) Medical complexity
5. The continuum of care starts in the emergency department and continues throughout the healthcare system and into the community. Rehabilitation nursing starts immediately so as to prevent complications.
6. Admission to rehabilitation services should occur as soon as possible after the event.
7. Rehabilitation care is best provided by nurses knowledgeable about the rehabilitation philosophy.

II. Models of Care

A. A "Model of Care" Is a Multifaceted Concept.
   1. It broadly defines the way in which health care is delivered and includes the values and principles, roles and structures, and care management and referral processes (NSW Government Health, 2015).

B. Rehabilitation Team Models
   1. The rehabilitation team consists, first and foremost, of the individual and his or her family. Other team members may vary, depending on the needs of the patient, but typically include a physiatrist, rehabilitation nurse, social worker, physical therapist, occupational therapist, speech-language pathologist, and case manager. Team members who contribute to a patient's rehabilitation vary with respect to specialty and are found across many disciplines.

C. Four Models for Team Functioning
   1. Medical, multidisciplinary, interdisciplinary, and transdisciplinary models have been described (Mauk, 2012). In all models, nursing is an integral part of the rehabilitation team.
      a. Medical model: The medical model is a physician-centered model of care in which all care is directed by the physician. This model is not consistent with rehabilitation philosophy or goals and is uncommon in rehabilitation practice.
      b. Multidisciplinary model: The multidisciplinary team model, which may be seen in rehabilitation, is one in which the professionals work in tandem; each discipline works toward particular client goals, with very little overlap between disciplines. Communication is more vertical than lateral, with the leader controlling team conferences. In a multidisciplinary model, the person working directly with the client does not always participate in team planning; rather, the department managers usually attend team conferences. This model is effective when the team membership is not stable (e.g., when there are different team members for different clients).
      c. Interdisciplinary model: The interdisciplinary model uses a more collaborative approach. The team works together in setting goals, providing treatment, making decisions, and conducting ongoing problem solving to ensure continuity of care and a holistic approach. From

the time of admission to discharge, the patient and team work together to establish, evaluate, and accomplish mutually agreed-upon goals (Behm & Gray, 2012). Mutual trust must be established between team members, and conflict resolution is an important skill that team members use. Team goal setting is an important feature of this model.

d. Transdisciplinary model: In the transdisciplinary model, the client has a primary provider from the team who is guided by the team in caring for the client. For example, the primary provider could be a nurse, who provides physical, speech, and occupational therapy based on the advice and counsel he or she receives from team members in those disciplines. This requires team members to be trained in disciplines in addition to their own. This model also raises many issues regarding licensure and accountability. It might be best suited for situations in which the client is stable and in need of long-term services.

D. Team Function

1. Regardless of the rehabilitation team model, all team members can increase their effectiveness by understanding their own roles and responsibilities as well as collaborative practice, group dynamics, conflict resolution, and team functioning.
2. Components necessary for effective team function include trust, knowledge, shared responsibility, mutual respect, communication, cooperation, coordination, and optimism.
3. Effective teams require a commitment from each member.

E. Models in Rehabilitation/Health Care

1. In the specialty of rehabilitation, no single model dominates and several models can coexist.
2. As health care continues to evolve, new models of providing services undoubtedly will emerge, and nurses are in an important position to lead the way.

F. Provision of Services

1. The rehabilitation philosophy can be infused into any healthcare setting.
   a. Collaboration within the team (through any of the team models) and between team members and the individual, family, and community is a vital aspect of rehabilitation.
   b. Mumma and Nelson (1996) offered a useful categorization of models for provision of services: client centered, setting centered, provider centered, and collaborative.
   c. Health care has been evolving away from a disease-centered model and toward the concept of patient- and family-centered care.
2. For the purposes of this chapter, a collaborative model (i.e., a team concept) is assumed in all rehabilitation models.
3. Models of care delivery
   a. Client-centered care
      1) Client-centered models are those that serve specialized populations.
      2) The focus can be on a specific developmental stage, such as childhood or older adulthood, or on a type of impairment, such as spinal cord injury or head injury.
      3) With a population-specific focus, providers can target their resources and gain extensive expertise through experience.
   b. Setting-centered care
      1) Acute, long-term, subacute, outpatient, home, and community care are the traditional models that focus on settings.
      2) Each describes where rehabilitation takes place.
      3) The trend away from inpatient care has accelerated in recent years as a result of changing funding practices.
   c. Provider-centered care
      1) Provider-centered models reflect how healthcare providers have decided to organize the provision of care.
      2) Many models have been used over the years with the goal of maximizing the use of human resources.
      3) The models within nursing have been the functional, team, and primary models.
         a) In functional nursing, the tasks are divided (e.g., one nurse delivers all the medications).
         b) In team nursing, a nurse oversees the care of a group of clients given by providers of various skill levels.
         c) Primary nursing (not to be confused with primary care) became popular in the 1980s as a means of providing client-centered care. One nurse provides direct total care to a group of clients and is responsible for planning and coordinating that care even when he or she is not on duty. This model generated several variations. Primary nursing has coordinated, client-centered care as its goal.

d. Patient-centered model
1) At the core of national and local efforts to improve the quality of healthcare, patients become active participants in their own care and receive services designed to focus on their individual needs and preferences, in addition to advice and counsel from health professionals, satisfying the full range of patient needs and preferences (Stanton, 2014).

e. Case management
1) Although not a new concept in nursing and health care, case management is an integral part of most models of care and is found in most settings.
2) Case managers coordinate a spectrum of care through patient transitions and across multiple practitioners and practice settings, although job descriptions can vary in different settings (Tomcavage & Garret 2010).

G. Focus on Outcomes
1. Outcomes, especially as they relate to function, are the most common measures across all levels of rehabilitation programs.
   a. The inpatient rehabilitation facility patient assessment instrument (IRF-PAI), used to document rehabilitation admission and reimbursement, is based on functional outcomes data.
   b. Skilled nursing facilities use the minimum data set (MDS) to assess the resident's physical and clinical conditions and abilities. The MDS can be used as a quality measure for consumers to review.
   c. Home health agencies use the outcome and assessment information set (OASIS) to measure patient outcomes.
2. Outcomes are used to communicate with consumers of rehabilitation services to describe the following:
   a. Comparisons between facilities and services
   b. Contracts between insurance companies and facilities
   c. Selection of a rehabilitation setting
   d. Marketing and competition for the rehabilitation client
      1) Consumers will consider quality and cost.

H. Recognition of a Transcultural Environment
1. Acknowledges rapidly changing demographics and increased awareness of cultural expectations
2. Promotes the delivery of nursing and rehabilitation care that is congruent with the patient's life practices and beliefs (Mauk, 2012).
3. Includes cultural self-awareness of values, beliefs, attitudes, and actions
4. Promotes conscious awareness of the individual, family, treatment team, and community
5. Confronts prejudices, biases, judgments, and generalizations.
6. Promotes culturally sensitive care, which allows for preservation and maintenance, accommodation and negotiation, education, and restructuring of care to meet clients' cultural and healthcare needs (Mauk, 2012).

I. Expectations of Health Care
1. The setting in which rehabilitation takes places is principally defined by the patient's changing needs over time and the availability of rehabilitation services.
2. Customer orientation
   a. There has been a shift from viewing the individual as the customer to viewing the population as the customer.
3. Wellness orientation
   a. With the movement toward focusing on client populations, the emphasis has become health promotion, which has redefined the health services that are provided and prioritized.
4. Cost versus revenue
   a. The emphasis is on managed care and capitation, and the responsibility for controlling costs lies with the provider.
   b. Evolution of reimbursement policies has continued to affect rehabilitation practice.
5. Approach to care
   a. There has been a shift from a departmental or an individual professional approach to an integrated, interdependent approach to care.
6. View of clients
   a. Clients are now viewed as consumers of cost and quality, which allows them to identify the types and cost of services needed to maintain wellness.
7. Continuity of information
   a. Information is now given to the client across time and discipline boundaries.
   b. Information is more readily available as electronic medical records are refined and their use increases.

J. Environments of Care
1. Acute care
   a. Clients in this setting require medical management.
   b. This setting might or might not provide care based on rehabilitation principles.
   c. Clients in an acute care setting might not be medically stable and able to tolerate intensive rehabilitation.

d. The role of the nurse includes teaching the client and the family and providing care focused on preventing complications to promote the client's ability to participate in and benefit from rehabilitation at a later time.

2. Acute care units for elders (ACE units)
   a. Understanding how older adults, the largest segment of the population receiving rehabilitation, are cared for (in preparation for rehabilitation) is important.
   b. The ACE model of care specifically addresses the needs of older adults in a safe, homelike physical environment.
   c. ACE is client and family centered, with discharge planning for the least restrictive environment.
   d. Staff has expertise in treating older adults and interdisciplinary teamwork (Amador, Reed, & Lehman, 2007).
   e. These units are located in acute care hospitals.
      1) These units are not rehabilitation units, but they provide age-appropriate care for older adults, with the possible result of transitioning to a rehabilitation setting.
      2) Functional outcomes are important in the ACE setting, and all patients are evaluated and treated by physical and occupational therapists.
      3) These units are not regulated like skilled nursing facilities and rehabilitation facilities; they are regulated and paid for like other acute-care hospital units (Amador et al., 2007).
      4) Research indicates that ACE units appear to be optimal for outcomes (Fox et al., 2013)
3. Inpatient rehabilitation facilities (IRFs)
   a. Overview
      1) Rehabilitation services can be provided by means of age-specific specialization (geriatric rehabilitation versus pediatric rehabilitation) or through diagnosis (e.g., stroke units, traumatic brain injury units, spinal cord injury units) (Lutz & Davis, 2008).
      2) Specialized units use standardized guidelines from the Commission on Accreditation of Rehabilitation Facilities (CARF) or model programs from the National Institute on Disability and Rehabilitation Research to treat clients and their families.
      3) Nationwide cost-containment measures have resulted in shorter client stays and lower reimbursement rates; this in turn has resulted in the shifting of care to less costly venues such as home health care and subacute or transition units.
      4) Nelson and colleagues' (2007) study on nurse staffing and client outcomes in IRFs revealed how staffing patterns affect client outcomes in IRFs.
         a) One pertinent finding of the study was that more certified rehabilitation registered nurses on staff correlated with better client outcomes as measured by Functional Independence Measure™ (FIM™) scores (Nelson et al., 2007).
      5) Acute rehabilitation can be provided in a specialized unit within a hospital setting or in a freestanding rehabilitation facility.
      6) Intensive inpatient rehabilitation with 24-hour nursing care is provided to address a range of issues including medication management, comorbidities, behavior, and the rehabilitative needs of the client and family.
      7) Clients are admitted to these facilities with a specific diagnosis.
      8) Much of the care provided in these settings focuses on the rehabilitation of older adults (Association of Rehabilitation Nurses [ARN], 2008).
      9) Medicare rules state that the necessity for intensive IRF services can be demonstrated by the client's need for at least 3 hours of skilled rehabilitative therapy for at least 5 days a week (Gage et al., 2009). The expectation is that these intensive services will yield significant improvement.
      10) Inpatient rehabilitation programs provide "coordinated and integrated medical and rehabilitation service that is provided 24 hours per day and endorses the active participation and choice of the persons served throughout the entire program" (Commission on Accreditation of Rehabilitation Facilities [CARF, 2006]).
      11) If only therapy is needed, this can be performed on an outpatient basis (Mauk, 2012).
      12) Documenting 24-hour rehabilitation nursing is critical, especially for IRFs that care for Medicare clients. Hentschke (2009) provided guidance on how facilities can better document this care.
4. Subacute care
   a. Subacute care emerged during the 1980s and 1990s as a lower-cost option for rehabilitative care (Lutz & Davis, 2008) for people who were

not ready for intensive, acute rehabilitation or who needed additional time to transition to the community (Quigley, 2007).

b. The definition of such care is inconsistent across the literature, and the CMS does not define subacute in its payment categories for rehabilitative services.

c. Subacute care units admit clients who cannot tolerate 3 hours of therapy per day and who need skilled medical and nursing care but not diagnostic or invasive procedures (Lutz & Davis, 2008).

d. For adults, subacute or postacute care units usually are inpatient settings and often are housed in an acute care, traditional rehabilitation unit, or a long-term care facility.

e. Data demonstrate that outcomes of subacute rehabilitation programs, at discharge and 6 months after discharge, are affected by the diagnosis, cognitive status, and level of independence at the time of admission to the facility (ARN, 2013).

5. Skilled nursing facilities (SNFs)

a. SNFs are also commonly called "nursing homes."

1) Skilled facilities provide daily skilled care given by, or under the direct supervision of, skilled nursing or rehabilitation staff.

2) Care is considered daily care even if these therapy services are offered only 5 or 6 days a week.

3) Medicare pays for these services with some restrictions involving requirements for previous hospital stays and length of stay at the facility.

b. Clients (called "residents" in long-term care) could need rehabilitation nursing and client and family education.

1) Typically these clients are medically stable and can participate in some rehabilitation as appropriate.

2) In a systematic review examining 41 randomized clinical trials (30 in the United States and 11 in Western Europe) and more than 3,000 clients in long-term care (e.g., nursing homes), physical rehabilitation was potentially effective when activity restriction was assessed as the primary outcome (Forster, Lambley, & Young, 2010).

c. Clients who no longer need skilled services can change to a custodial status and remain as long-term residents in some facilities or be discharged to home or assisted living.

d. The goal of care remains the same: optimal client wellness.

e. Clients at SNFs require less physician oversight than clients at IRFs, because typically they are less severely impaired.

f. SNFs vary in the acuity of clients they accept and generally provide a lower intensity of service (Gage et al., 2007).

1) However, some specialized SNFs provide intensive postacute treatment such as ventilator monitoring (Gage et al., 2009) and cardiopulmonary rehabilitation.

g. Orthopedic clients post fracture or joint replacement increasingly are admitted into the SNF setting.

6. Long-term care hospitals (LTCHs)

a. LTCHs are certified as acute-care hospitals but focus on clients who, on average, stay more than 25 days.

b. Extended medical and rehabilitative care is provided to people whose needs are clinically complex and who have multiple acute or chronic conditions (American Hospital Association, n.d.).

c. Clients are transferred to LTCHs from intensive- or critical-care units.

d. Services provided typically include comprehensive rehabilitation, respiratory therapy, head trauma treatment, and pain management (Centers for Medicare & Medicaid Services [CMS], 2009).

e. These facilities are commonly referred to as "long-term acute care."

7. Community settings

a. For cost-containment purposes, rehabilitative care increasingly is taking place in the community.

b. Home health care can provide a variety of rehabilitative services, including nursing, as well as physical, occupational, and speech therapy.

c. "Home healthcare nurses are the only group who can put 'feet on the ground' and who can understand and manage the complexities of providing care to some of the most vulnerable Americans" (Madigan, 2012).

d. Hospital at Home® programs discharge the patient from the hospital directly to home to receive medical care that traditionally would be have been delivered in the hospital. This can eliminate or decrease hospital stays.

e. Cost savings can be achieved only if the treatment is well defined and can be delivered in a feasible, safe, and efficient manner at home.

f. Care can be provided for chronically ill patients diagnosed with multiple illnesses who need acute episodic care, including patients who are elderly and disabled.
g. These patients often have difficulties with mobility and other activities of daily living and have trouble maintaining their households.
h. Many have caregivers who provide assistance (Paul, 2013).

8. *Patient-centered medical homes* are defined by the Agency for Healthcare Research and Quality as a model of the organization of primary care that delivers the core functions of primary health care:
   a. Comprehensive care that is patient centered, coordinated across the healthcare system, has accessible services, and is committed to quality and safety (Agency for Healthcare Research and Quality, 2014).
9. *Accountable Care Organizations* (ACOs) are groups of doctors, hospitals, and other healthcare providers who collaborate voluntarily to provide coordinated, high-quality care to their Medicare patients.
   a. The goal of coordinated care is to ensure that patients, especially those who are chronically ill, receive the right care at the right time, while avoiding unnecessary duplication of services and preventing medical errors (CMS, 2014).
10. Telemedicine is becoming more important to healthcare providers and patients around the world.
   a. The trend is already backed by many hospitals and major health insurers, and the U.S. government recently endorsed telemedicine through Medicare and Medicaid (Taylor, 2014). Telemedicine is widely used in the Veterans Administration (VA) hospital setting.
   b. Patients are able to see or communicate with doctors in their homes, offices, or a dedicated center, and doctors can remotely treat patients from hospitals, offices, homes, and other settings.

K. Roles of the Rehabilitation Nurse
1. ARN's (2014) *Standards and Scope of Rehabilitation Nursing Practice* provides the basis of practice for the rehabilitation nurse regardless of setting.
   a. Preventing medical and functional complications and readmission
   b. Engaging clients in care within medically indicated restrictions and precautions
   c. Promoting independence by increasing self-care actions
   d. Delegating and supervising aspects of rehabilitative and restorative care provided by licensed vocational nurses, technicians, and unlicensed assistive personnel
   e. Providing client and family education to support self-care and transitioning to home if feasible.
   f. Providing age- and developmentally appropriate care
   g. Educating older adults requires that the rehabilitation nurse be knowledgeable about geriatric principles to appropriately care for older clients and their families in IRFs, SNFs, the community, and other settings.

L. Community-Based Rehabilitation
1. Overview
   a. Community-based rehabilitation (CBR) focuses on enhancing the quality of life for people with disabilities and their families, meeting basic needs, and ensuring inclusion and participation.
      1) It is a multisectoral strategy that empowers persons with disabilities to access and benefit from education, employment, health, and social services.
         a) CBR is implemented through the combined efforts of people with disabilities, their families and communities, and relevant governmental and nongovernmental health, education, vocational, social, and other services (World Health Organization [WHO], 2014).
      2) CBR services typically are offered in a local community. Such services can include home healthcare, physical therapy, vocational rehabilitation, and others.
         a) The rehabilitation client's community is characterized in terms of the wider environment and geographic location and the availability of housing, transportation, healthcare providers, community buildings, and other resources (Boylan & Buchanan, 2008).
      3) CBR services in one community will appear different from those in another community, because the resources and services that are offered can vary.
      4) Community-based rehabilitation nursing combines the expertise of the rehabilitation nurse with the skills of a community health nurse.
         a) A nurse in this role can conduct home visits, act as a case manager, coordinate

care across settings, provide client and family education, and promote health.
    b) The ultimate goal of care is optimal health for the client and family (however it is defined).
    c) In community-based care, clients manage their care and daily activities independently, with assistance, or with supervision.
2. Types of community-based care
    a. Day care treatment programs and adult day services provide supervised care and therapeutic activities.
        1) This is a structured, comprehensive, nonresidential program that provides a variety of health, social, and related support services in a protective setting.
        2) The environmental design considers the impairments and limitations of the people served, promotes improvement and maintenance of their sense of control and self-determination, and provides them with a safe environment (CARF, 2006).
    b. Independent living centers and congregate living facilities offer independent living and opportunities to share activities of daily living with other residents.
        1) Congregate facilities include retirement and life-care communities.
        2) Shared activities in a congregate living setting can include meals, transportation, housekeeping, planned activities and outings, and religious services.
        3) Health monitoring might or might not be included in the setting.
    c. Community reentry programs and assisted-care living facilities provide coordinated, personalized, 24-hour assistance and support (both scheduled and unscheduled) in a congregate residential setting.
        1) The choices, privacy, independence, and rights of the people served are protected and promoted as an essential part of assisted living's core values and mission (CARF, 2006).
        2) The type of provider can vary.
3. Roles of the rehabilitation nurse in the community
    a. Direct care provider
        1) As the client's level of independence increases, the physical provision of care by the nurse decreases.
    b. Educator
        1) The nurse provides education to both the client and family.
    c. Care or case manager
        1) The nurse coordinates client care across settings, interacts with various care providers, and ensures that the client's treatment plan is carried out.
    d. Advocate
        1) The nurse advocates for the client and family.
    e. Consultant
        1) Rehabilitation nurses can act as a consultant for programs and individuals.
    f. Advanced practice nurse
        1) Nurse practitioners can work in a variety of community settings providing assessment, prescription, and supervision for clients who require management of chronic disease.
    g. Life-care planner
        1) Rehabilitation nurses have the knowledge and experience to consider the complex care/medical needs of patients throughout their life span.
4. A broader view of CBR
    a. CBR is an international concept originated by WHO's Disability and Rehabilitation Team, whose vision is that all people with disabilities live in dignity, with equal rights and opportunities.
    b. The focus of CBR, developed in the 1980s, is to enhance "the quality of life for people with disabilities and their families, meeting basic needs, and ensuring inclusion and participation." (WHO, 2010a).
    c. In 2004 a joint venture between the International Labour Organization (ILO), United Nations Educational, Scientific and Cultural Organization (UNESCO), and WHO repositioned CBR as a strategy for rehabilitation, equalization of opportunity, poverty reduction, and social inclusion of people with disabilities (WHO, 2010b). The goals of CBR are to ensure that the benefits of the United Nations' Convention on Rights of Persons with Disabilities reach the majority by
        1) Supporting people with disabilities to maximize their physical and mental abilities, access regular services and opportunities, and become active contributors to the community and society at large
        2) Activating communities to promote and protect the human rights of people with

disabilities; for example, by removing barriers to participation
3) Facilitating capacity building, empowerment, and community mobilization of people with disabilities and their families
4) CBR is a strategy with general community development. It is implemented through the combined efforts of people who themselves have disabilities, their families, organizations and communities, and the relevant governmental and nongovernmental health, educational, vocational, social, and other services (WHO, 2010b).

5. Community reentry and integration
   a. Focus: Transition to the community through a gradual acquisition of community skills, self-care, leisure and vocational activities, and psychosocial integration
   b. Community-based barriers
      1) Societal barriers such as reimbursement issues, ineligibility for services, cultural or attitudinal prejudices, and social stigma
      2) Internal barriers within the individual such as negative attitude, poor self-esteem, lack of motivation, poor self-image, feelings of dependence, insecurity, an inability to plan and meet goals, and unrealistic expectations
      3) Transportation problems that affect the client's environment and reintegration efforts
      4) Housing barriers such as lack of accessible housing
      5) Financial barriers
6. Conceptual model for nurses working in community reentry and independent living programs (Parker & Neal-Boylan, 2007, pp. 13–26)
   a. The client serves as manager of his or her life and care in a community-based or independent living setting. The nurse's role is that of an active participant who helps the client by providing education, coordinating resources, and understanding how the community's needs and resources affect the client's health.
   b. The client's lifestyle and needs are considered in terms of his or her environment. The nurse's role is to promote health and the ability to meet self-care needs and to facilitate communication and collaboration with other healthcare professionals.
   c. Client and family education is an ongoing process.
      1) Education is focused and goal directed.
      2) As the client reintegrates into the community, the focus of education changes to enhance the client's problem-solving skills.
      3) Preventive care is emphasized.
   d. The management of attendant care training and services facilitates independent living.
   e. Equipment and supplies should be evaluated before the client is discharged from the acute rehabilitation setting (the nurse coordinates the assessment and monitoring of equipment needed in the community).
   f. The client and family's financial resources must be assessed.
   g. The nurse, along with the client and family, identifies barriers and options in the community

III. The Future of Rehabilitation Nursing

A. Challenges in Rehabilitation Nursing
1. Leadership
   a. The Institute of Medicine's report *The Future of Nursing: Leading Change, Advancing Health* (2010) recognizes that leadership must unfold at every level of nursing practice and across every practice setting.
      1) The report clearly calls for nurses to assume primary responsibility for personal and professional growth through efforts that continue individual education and opportunities that develop and advance the exercise of leadership skills (Porter-O'Grady, 2011).
      2) ARN has responded to the need by offering leadership training at the ARN annual conference, and implementing competency-based leadership in elected and volunteer positions.
2. The effect of changing demographics on the demand for rehabilitation nurses and practice settings
   a. With more individuals and families buying their own coverage through the new health insurance marketplace exchanges, the voice of the consumer is becoming louder.
      1) Rehabilitation nurses need to understand their clients better, and recognize and understand how health care appears from the client's perspective (Harper, 2013).
   b. Many of the law's provisions also encourage greater collaboration between healthcare organizations and physicians and within the hospital environment itself, making cross-collaboration and transparency even more vital (Harper, 2013).

1) Consumers are starting to approach nurses with new expectations and demands as they take more direct responsibility for their coverage and care (Tyson, 2014).
2) As the population continues to age, the need for rehabilitation nurses who have the skills to treat chronic illnesses and their effects on function, quality of life, and access to care has grown significantly.
3) Rehabilitation nurses have seen a shift both in the distribution of illness from acute to chronic and in the kinds of injuries, especially in survivors of war and aging people.
4) The hospital is more acute, and the rehabilitation unit (acute and subacute) has changed as more clients arrive sooner after their event or are cared for in their homes, retirement centers, and other living arrangements in the community.

c. The nursing shortage and recruitment issues

1) A large number of nurses, both direct caregivers and educators, are reaching retirement age. In 2013, 55% of the registered nurse (RN) workforce was age 50 or older.
2) This decrease in the available workforce coincides with declining enrollment in nursing schools and declining interest in the nursing profession among young people.
3) The shortage of educators in colleges and universities has resulted in a waiting list for those interested in entering the profession.
4) Nursing schools turned away more than 79,000 qualified applicants from baccalaureate and graduate nursing programs in 2012 because of an insufficient number of faculty, clinical sites, classroom space, clinical preceptors, and budget constraints (American Association of Critical-Care Nurses, 2014).
5) Keeping nurses in the workforce into their retirement years at healthcare facilities and schools of nursing with flexible job descriptions, schedules, and benefits will be essential.

3. The healthcare crisis: access, equity, and reimbursement issues

a. There has been an increase in the number of insured Americans since the implementation of the Affordable Care Act (ACA), but many Americans remain uninsured or underinsured.

b. Health care continues to be in crisis mode, and the ongoing lack of, or inadequate, funding and other resources continues to affect the delivery system, admissions process, and length of stay.

c. Problems with environmental, financial, and geographical access to services and the availability of practitioners who understand the needs of clients who are older, chronically ill, and disabled are important issues to address.

d. Controversy continues regarding the role of the advanced practice registered nurse and other care providers that affects access to those most in need—the poor and those in rural areas and inner cities.

4. Ethical dilemmas

a. Nurses increasingly face the challenge of working with people who choose to end their own lives, and they have had to consider their positions on laws dealing with clients' rights and choices.

b. Nurses have had to assess their own feelings and attitudes related to ethical issues such as cloning, organ transplantation, and assisted suicide.

c. Nurses have to face the dilemma of providing lesser services than are needed because of financial constraints.

B. Nursing's Perspective on the Future of Health Care

1. Nurses have earned the trust of Americans and will use that trust, along with their health promotion expertise, to communicate with patients about the best prevention, timely care, and most efficient ways to obtain help as they navigate with patients through America's evolving system of care (Potempa, 2013).
2. The future of rehabilitation care must be considered within the context of the overarching health system and its evolution.
    a. The changing nature of the health system, along with the aging population, provides an ideal opportunity to develop a consistent model of care for rehabilitation services (NSW Government Health, 2015).
3. Technology, including computerized documentation systems, will make nurses' work more efficient, and preventive care will reduce the number of people experiencing catastrophic illness and injury.
4. Scientific advances in stem-cell therapy and genetics will be used to treat spinal cord injuries more effectively.
5. Harvesting body parts, cells, and limbs could make prosthetics obsolete.

6. Robotic, microscopic surgeries will prevent strokes and make repairs more effective.
7. Brain injuries will not be as common with the requirement that helmets be worn for sports participation.
8. The information availability in a high-technology world continues to expand rehabilitation nursing research beyond national borders and into an international collaborative research effort with colleagues across the globe.

C. Emphasis on Research and Evidence-Based Practice
1. ARN continues to focus on evidence-based practice with its 2014 publication *Evidence-Based Rehabilitation: Common Challenges and Interventions.*

D. Magnet Recognition Program for Nursing Excellence (American Nurses Association, 2010)
1. Magnet hospitals enjoy higher percentages of satisfied RNs, lower RN turnover and vacancies, improved clinical outcomes, and greater patient satisfaction.
   a. Approximately 7% of all registered hospitals in the United States have achieved ANCC Magnet Recognition (American Nurses Credentialing Center, 2014).
   b. The five components of the ANCC Magnet Recognition Model can be used as guides to strengthen rehabilitation nursing services and programs.
      1) Transformational leadership
      2) Structural empowerment
      3) Exemplary professional practice
      4) New knowledge, innovations, and improvements
      5) Empirical quality results
2. ANCC's Magnet program could be cost prohibitive for some rehabilitation hospitals and long-term care facilities.

E. Education Issues
1. With people aging and living longer with chronic disease, rehabilitation nursing should be a core requirement in every school of nursing (T. Black, personal communication, 2014).

F. Issues Related to Quality of Life and End-of-Life Decision Making
1. The foundation of rehabilitation nurse practice should be to value human life, promote health, and serve as a patient advocate (Bratcher, Farrell, Stevens, & Vanderground, 2012).
2. Rehabilitation nurses, along with the entire rehabilitation team, must attend to the wishes of the patients, and patients must receive treatment on a voluntary basis.
3. Pain management, alternative therapy, spirituality assessment, and bereavement counseling continue to be important parts of the plan of care for the aging population and for those who have experienced trauma or are dealing with loss and end-of-life issues related to medical diagnoses. Nursing research continues to be needed to develop and implement better therapy options.
4. Rehabilitation principles are of utmost importance to allow clients to live while dying and to help the family make this time productive and meaningful.

G. Changes in Practice and Care Settings
1. As the population ages and the home healthcare sector grows, the home health community must address deficiencies in care, and expand the use of evidence-based strategies to improve the quality and efficiency of care.
   a. Many promising innovations in service delivery exist, a wide variety of which have been tested and evaluated in postacute and long-term care settings (Parker, Zimmerman, Rodriguez, & Lee, 2014).
2. With advances in monitoring and telemedicine, care administered in the home, to properly selected patients, can approximate that delivered in the hospital.
   a. Appropriately selected qualified personnel deliver treatment at home, both individually and in teams, and patients understand the information communicated to them by providers.
   b. The benefits of treating chronically or terminally ill patients at home include significantly improved patient satisfaction and reduced costs.
   c. Numerous studies have shown that most patients prefer to spend their convalescence or their last days at home (Chandekar, Hungate, Purvis, Selby-Penczak, & Abbey, 2013).
3. Certified nurses demonstrate a more advanced level of rehabilitation nursing practice.
   a. It shows in the care and education they provide and in their level of confidence.
   b. Certified nurses also tend to do a better job with FIM scoring, which is critical for reimbursement (C. Gender, personal communication, August 14, 2014).
4. Rehabilitation nursing will be incorporated into all areas of health care, especially because rehabilitation is a process, not a place.
   a. Most nursing specialties are defined by a practice setting or body system.

b. Rehabilitation nursing's emphasis is on models of wellness, adaptation, and quality of life (D. Jernigan, personal communication, 2014).

H. ARN's Assumptions About the Future (ARN, 2013)

1. Global business and economic factors
   a. Uncertainty will continue regarding reimbursement for rehabilitation nursing services.
   b. Global outsourcing and influence on rehabilitation documentation and services will increase.
   c. Consumers will continue to expect high-quality care within all settings, despite decreases in reimbursement.
   d. It is unclear who will control healthcare spending (e.g., individuals, employers, insurance companies).
   e. The consumer will continue to be more active in healthcare decision making.
   f. More rehabilitation services will be home and community based.
   g. Consumers will continue to use discretionary funds to pay for healthcare services.
   h. Debate will continue over the creation of a single payer or universal healthcare coverage.
   i. The balance between the business model focused on productivity and the nursing model focused on quality and standards of care will continue to be an issue for nursing.
   j. Postacute bundling (i.e., who gets paid) will affect the number of future facilities.
   k. The continued uncertainty of funding could mean that disparity in care will persist.
   l. There will be an increase in custodial and palliative care.
   m. Practice will need to be evidence based to obtain funding.
   n. Continued global economic and political uncertainty will affect the future growth of the rehabilitation industry.
2. Social values and demographics
   a. As life expectancy continues to increase, the number of older persons living with chronic and disabling illnesses will increase.
   b. There will be a number of war veterans who will be aging with acquired disabilities and chronic illnesses.
   c. The population will be significantly more ethnically and culturally diverse.
   d. Obesity will continue to be a primary societal problem and will continue to increase in younger persons.
   e. Baby boomers will remain engaged, active, and desire self-care to remain independent into old age, and alternative approaches to keeping older people active and aging in place will be developed.
   f. Younger generations will
      1) Be more mobile
      2) Be more comfortable with changing technology
      3) Be more accustomed to diverse communities
      4) Expect more balance between work and personal life
      5) Change jobs and careers
      6) Be more likely to be self-employed (or employed in small companies and start-ups)
   g. Consumers will develop their own definitions of high-quality care that will be based on their increased access to information from a variety of sources (which may or may not be reliable).
   h. There will be an increase in the need for rehabilitation nursing along the continuum of care in both traditional and nontraditional settings such as spas and senior centers.
   i. The rehabilitation nursing workforce is aging, with an increase in rehabilitation nurses who are working beyond their expected retirement years.
   j. There will continue to be an increase in the number of nurses entering the profession as second-career professionals.
   k. Workplaces will need to develop adaptive strategies in response to the changing workforce (e.g., an aging workforce, experienced nurses becoming novice rehabilitation nurses).
   l. Time and convenience are considered to be highly important (i.e., valuable commodities), so consumers expect services to be available, convenient, and accessible.
   m. The debate about entry-level education for nursing is trending toward the bachelor of science in nursing.
   n. There is a shortage of qualified nursing faculty.
   o. There could be a continued lack of emphasis on rehabilitation even though the need is increasing.
   p. There will be an increase in the variety of rehabilitation practice settings.
   q. Patterns for referral and reimbursement for rehabilitation remain uncertain.
   r. Generational differences will necessitate strategies tailored to meet the needs of younger and older generations.
3. Technology and science
   a. Technology will continue to be dynamic.

b. Technology will become more complex and lead to a greater diversity of understanding.
c. The need to maintain an interface between technology and human behavior will continue.
d. There will be an increase in technology used in client care.
e. Scientific and technological advances affecting patient care will continue.
f. Patients and caregivers will continue to have greater access to medical and scientific information and will require more guidance in navigating and evaluating reputable sources.
g. Patients and caregivers will continue to be more knowledgeable as a result of greater access to information.
h. Scientific and technological advances will continue to have an impact on the cost of care.
i. The dependence on technology in clinical practice will continue to increase.
j. Technology is intended to create greater safeguards in care.
k. Technology is intended to create greater efficiencies.
l. The use of telemedicine will increase.
m. Technology will increasingly complement evidence-based practice, which, in turn, will drive the use of technology.
n. The dissemination or publishing of rehabilitation research results has the potential to increase.
o. The use of simulation technologies will increase.
p. Members will expect ARN to integrate technology into services and will desire seamless and simple experiences.
q. The use of electronic medical records will continue to increase. The outcome on impact of care is uncertain, although it will create a burden on staff while increasing the clinical information available.

4. Legislation and regulation
   a. Significant changes in reimbursement that affect rehabilitation health services will continue.
   b. There will be legislative activity that will promote nursing ratios.
   c. Research dollars will continue to be directed to selected and higher-profile institutions.
   d. The trend to cut research dollars will continue.
   e. The need for evidence-based research to drive public policy will continue.
   f. Other non-nursing professional organizations will have an impact on health policy.
   g. Healthcare coverage and policies will be influenced by political party changes, accountable care organizations' implementation of the ACA, legislation, and groups drafting legislation.
   h. The need for complete nursing documentation to illustrate the provision and need for rehabilitation nursing 24/7 to obtain Medicare funding for inpatient rehabilitation settings will continue.
   i. Increased lobbying efforts for funding rehabilitation services and nursing will be needed.
   j. Increased lobbying efforts for funding rehabilitation nursing research will be needed.
   k. The regulatory environment will result in fewer beds in IRFs and provide opportunities in all other parts of the postacute continuum.
   l. Quality indicators will increasingly influence rehabilitation reimbursement.
   m. The move toward accountable care means that freestanding facilities will increasingly align with larger gatekeepers of care.
5. Professional competition and structure
   a. CMS will introduce a screening tool to determine placements of patients in a level of care.
   b. There will be increased competition among specialties and professional nursing organizations for current rehabilitation nurses, drawing them to other specialties that acknowledge rehabilitation nursing philosophy.
   c. Nursing programs will need to integrate more educational content on rehabilitation.
   d. There could be an increase in the number of rehabilitation RN opportunities in alternative (i.e., nonhospital or nonfacility) settings.
   e. Rehabilitation RNs might need to seek alternative venues to provide services.
   f. There will be decreased dollars available for rehabilitation reimbursement.
   g. Demand for rehabilitation services continues to increase in response to an aging population.
   h. Magnet status will continue to drive an increase in the interest in specialty certification.
   i. The AACN Consensus Statement will expand opportunities for advanced practice nursing in rehabilitation.
   j. The Joint Commission's rehabilitation and advanced care accreditation will produce a greater need for educational resources and productivity.
   k. The Institute of Medicine's *The Future of Nursing: Leading Change, Advancing Health* (2010)

will encourage collaboration among nursing organizations.
l. The expectation that nurses will perform at the highest levels of practice is growing.
m. Accountable care organizations and bundled payment will foster development of formal business relationships across levels of care.

I. Thoughts from Nursing Colleagues Outside the Rehabilitation Setting
1. Technology will transform the nursing profession.
2. Technology will create a global professional community.
3. Many nursing functions will become automated (e.g., documentation and updating of client records, smart beds to monitor vital signs, bar codes, and automatic medicine carts).
4. As a result of nursing shortages, healthcare facilities will be forced to use their nurses judiciously.
5. Nurses will spend more time at the bedside as educators and care coordinators to refocus on the client (Peters, 2008).
6. Nurses will be the drivers, facilitators, and designers of delivery of care (Porter-O'Grady, 2014).
7. The increasing emphasis on quality and safety are trends that have benefited nursing.
   a. The National Database of Nursing Quality Indicators® tracks nursing impact on client care outcomes.
   b. The roles of clinical nurse specialist, clinical nurse leader, and doctor of nursing practice are quality focused.
8. Nursing workforce issues
   a. The demand for nurses will continue to grow, with only slow increases in supply affected by the availability of educators and those interested in the profession. Some new nurses are second-career nurses.
   b. The use of foreign nurses is increasing, and the nursing shortage is recognized worldwide.
   c. The physician shortage is increasing the demand for nurse practitioners.
   d. The push for staffing ratios and legislation on public reporting continues.
   e. Educational delivery and teaching methods continue to change with the use of distance learning, curriculum restructuring, and simulations.

J. Surviving in the New World
1. Be open to changing demographics and diversity.
2. Emphasize the need for continual learning; recognize that the consumer is increasingly well informed and wants to participate in life's decisions.
3. Know that alternative and complementary therapies can enhance health and healing and have entered the mainstream of healthcare delivery.
4. Move forward together! Nursing will continue to evolve, but the basics of human caring must remain. Nursing leadership must remain strong, and leaders must model change and mentor future nurse leaders.
5. Whatever the setting, rehabilitation is a partnership between the client, family, and care team.

ACKNOWLEDGMENTS

Thank you to Cynthia Jacelon, editor, and Pamela Larson, author, *Specialty Practice of Rehabilitation Nursing: A Core Curriculum* (5th ed.); and Terri Black; Cookie Gender; and Donna Jernigan, ARN past presidents, for sharing their insights on the future of rehabilitation nursing.

References

Agency for Healthcare Research and Quality (2014). Patient centered medical home resource center. Retrieved from http://pcmh.ahrq.gov/page/defining-pcmh

Amador, L.F., Reed, d., & Lehman, C. (2007). The acute care for elders unit: Taking the rehabilitation model into the hospital setting. *Rehabilitation Nursing, 32*(3), 126-132.

American Association of Critical-Care Nurses (2014). Nursing shortage resources. Retrieved from www.aacn.nche.edu/media-relations/nursing-shortage

American Hospital Association. (n.d.). Long term acute care hospitals. Retrieved from www.aha.org/aha_app/issues/Medicare/Long-Term-Care-Hospitals

American Nurses Association (2010). Magnet Recognition Program. Retrieved from www.nursecredentialing.org/Magnet.aspx

American Nurses Credentialing Center (2014). The Magnet Recognition Program: Growth of the program. Retrieved from http://www.nursecredentialing.org/Magnet/ProgramOverview/HistoryoftheMagnetProgram/GrowthoftheProgram

Association of Rehabilitation Nurses. (2008). *Standards and scope of rehabilitation nursing practice.* Chicago: Author.

Association of Rehabilitation Nurses (2013). Strategic Plan. Chicago: Author.

Association of Rehabilitation Nurses (2014). *Standards and scope of rehabilitation nursing practice.* Glenview, IL: Author.

Behm, J., & Gray, N. (2012). Interdisciplinary rehabilitation. In K. Mauk (Ed.). *Rehabilitation nursing: A contemporary approach to practice.* Valparaiso, IN: Jones & Bartlett.

Boylan, L. N., & Buchanan, L. C. (2008). Community-based rehabilitation. In S. Hoeman (Ed.), *Rehabilitation nursing: Prevention, intervention and outcomes* (4th ed., pp 178–191). St. Louis: Mosby Elservier.

Bratcher, R., Farrell, J. J., Stevens, K. A., & Vanderground, K. W. (2012). Ethical and legal issues. In Mauk, K. (Ed.). *Rehabilitation nursing; A contemporary approach to practice.* Valparaiso, IN: Jones & Bartlett.

Centers for Medicare & Medicaid Services. (2009). *What are long term care hospitals?* CMS Publication No. 11347. Retrieved from www.medicare.gov/publications/pubs/pdf/11347.pdf

Centers for Medicare & Medicaid Services (2014). Inpatient Rehabilitation Facility Prospective Payment System. Retrieved from http://www.cms.gov/Outreach-and-Education/Medicare-Learning-Network-MLN/MLNProducts/downloads/InpatRehabPaymtfctsht09-508.pdf

Chandekar, R., Hungate, B., Purvis, M., & Selby-Penczak, R., & Abbey, L. J. (2013). Improving outcomes and lowering costs by applying advanced models of in-home care. *Cleveland Clinic Journal of Medicine, 80*(e-Suppl. 1), eS7–eS14.

Commission on Accreditation of Rehabilitation Facilities. (2006). *2006 CARF accreditation sourcebook.* Retrieved from www.carf.org

Forster, A., Lambley, R., & Young, J. B. (2010). Is physical rehabilitation for older people in long-term care effective? Findings from a systematic review. *Age and Ageing, 39*, 169 175.

Fox, M. T., Sidani, S., Persaud, M., Tregunno, D., Maimets, I., Brooks, D., & O'Brien, K. J. (2013). Acute care for elders components of acute geriatric unit care: Systematic descriptive review. *Journal of American Geriatric Society, 61*(6), 939 –946. doi:10.1111/jgs.12282

Gage, B., Pilkauskasm, N., Dalton, K., Constantine, R., Leung, M., Hoover, S., et al. (2007). *Long term care hospital (LTCH) payment system monitoring and evaluation.* Phase II Report. Research Triangle Park, NC: RTI International.

Gage, B., Smith, L., Coots, L., Macek, J., Manning, J., & Reilly, K. (2009, September). *Analysis of the classification criteria for inpatient rehabilitation facilities (IRFs).* Research Triangle Park, NC: RTI International.

Harper, C. (2013). Central Valley Area Employee Orientation & Reorientation Playbook, Central Valley Area Public Affairs Department, Kaiser Permanente.

Hentschke, P. (2009). 24-hour rehabilitation nursing: The proof is in the documentation. *Rehabilitation Nursing, 34*(3), 128–132.

Institute of Medicine (2010). The Future of Nursing: Leading Change, Advancing Health. Retrieved from www.iom.edu/Reports/2010/The-Future-of-Nursing-Leading-Change-Advancing-Health.aspx

Lutz, B., & Davis, S. M. (2008). Theory and practice models for rehabilitation nursing. In S. Hoeman (Ed.), *Rehabilitation nursing: Prevention, intervention and outcomes* (4th ed., pp. 14–29). St. Louis: Mosby Elsevier.

Madigan, E. A. (2012). Views on the future of nursing and home healthcare: The future of nursing for home healthcare. *Home Healthcare Now, 30*(3), 149–151. Retrieved from http://www.nursingcenter.com/lnc/journalarticle?Article_ID=1314010#sthash.W47vuOGG.dpuf

Mauk, K. (Ed.). (2012). *Rehabilitation nursing; A contemporary approach to practice.* Valparaiso, IN: Jones & Bartlett

Mumma, C. M., & Nelson, A. (1996). Models for theory-based practice of rehabilitation nursing. In S. P. Hoeman (Ed.), Rehabilitation nursing. Process and application (2nd ed., pp. 21–31). St. Louis: Mosby.

Nelson, A., Powell-Cope, G., Palacios, P., Luther, S. L., Black, R., Hillman, T., et al. (2007). Nurse staffing and patient outcomes in inpatient rehabilitation setting. *Rehabilitation Nursing, 32*(5), 179–202.

NSW Government Health (2015). Rehabilitation Model of Care: NSW Rehabilitation Redesign Project. Final report—Model of care. Version 1.5, issued June 1, 2015. Retrieved from http://www.aci.health.nsw.gov.au/resources/rehabilitation/rehabilitation-model-of-care/NSW-Rehabilitation-moc-2014.pdf

Parker, B. J., & Neal-Boylan, L. (2007). Community and family-centered rehabilitation nursing. In K. L. Mauk (Ed.), *The specialty practice of rehabilitation nursing: A core curriculum* (5th ed., pp. 13–26). Glenview, IL: Association of Rehabilitation Nurses.

Parker, E., Zimmerman, S., Rodriguez, S., & Lee, T. (2014). Best practices in home health care: A review of available evidence on select innovations. *Home Health Care Management & Practice, 26*, 17–33.

Paul, D. (2013). An innovation in healthcare delivery: Hospital at home. *Journal of Management Policy and Practice, 14*(6), 73–91.

Peters, S. (2008). What is the Future of Nursing Careers? Retrieved from www.articlealley.com/article_645644_36.html

Porter-O'Grady, T. (2011). Future of nursing special: Leadership at all levels. *Nursing Management, 42*(5), 32–37. Retrieved from http://www.nursingcenter.com/lnc/journalarticle?Article_ID=1163290#sthash.BcwvfwJ0.dpufhttp://www.nursingcenter.com/lnc/journalarticle?Article_ID=1163290#sthash.BcwvfwJ0.dpuf

Porter-O'Grady, T. (2014, November). *Envisioning the future of rehabilitation nursing: Transforming practice in the age of reform.*

Paper presented at the meeting of Association of Rehabilitation Nurses, Anaheim, CA.

Potempa, K. (2013). Nurses will play a vital role in the enactment of the Affordable Care Act. Retrieved from http://thehealthcareblog.com/blog/2013/08/14/nurses-will-play-a-vital-role-in-the-enactment-of-the-affordable-care-act/

Quigley, P. A. (2007). Environment of care and service delivery. In K. L. Mauk (Ed.), *The specialty practice of rehabilitation nursing: A core curriculum* (5th ed., pp. 386–394). Glenview, IL: Association of Rehabilitation Nurses.

Stanton, M. (2014). Expanding patient-centered care to empower patients and assist providers. *Research in Action* (5). Retrieved from http://archive.ahrq.gov/research/findings/factsheets/patient-centered/ria-issue5/ria-issue5.html

Taylor, J. (2014). Why telemedicine is the future of healthcare. Retrieved from http://exclusive.multibriefs.com/content/why-telemedicine-is-the-future-of-healthcare/healthcare-administration

Tomcavage, J., and Garrett, M. (2010) Care coordination: Case managers "connect the dots" in new delivery models. Key finding from 2009 role and functions Survey. *CCMC issue Brief, 1*(2). Retrieved from ccmcertification.org

Tyson, B. (2014). Meeting the evolving needs of the health care consumer. Retreived from http://lookinside.kaiserpermanente.org

World Health Organization. (2010a). Community-based rehabilitation (CBR). Retrieved from www.who.int/disabilities/cbr/en/index.html

World Health Organization. (2010b). Community-based rehabilitation (CBR): What WHO is doing. Retrieved from www.who.int/disabilities/cbr/activities/en/

World Health Organization (2014). Community-based rehabilitation (CBR). Retrieved from www.who.int/disabilities/cbr/en/

Suggested Reading

Health2 Resources for the Commission for Case Manager Certification (2010). Care Coordination: Case managers "connect the dots" in new delivery models. *CCMC IssueBrief, 1*(2). Available at http://ccmcertification.org/sites/default/files/downloads/2011/4. Care coordination, case managers connect the dots - volume 1, issue 2.pdf

Chapter 3

Interprofessional Teamwork and Collaboration

Michele Cournan, DNP RN CRRN ANP-BC FNP
Denise Stiltner, MSN RNC-NIC
Donald D. Kautz, PhD RN CRRN CNE ACNS-BC

LEARNING OBJECTIVES

- Define interprofessional team.
- Discuss the roles of the various members of the interprofessional team.
- Identify potential roles of the registered nurse in the interprofessional team.
- Compare and contrast the various models of teamwork.
- Discuss Centers for Medicare & Medicaid Services and Commission on Accreditation of Rehabilitation Facilities regulations related to the team in the rehabilitation setting.
- Recognize the value of the nurse in the interprofessional team process.

KEY CHAPTER CONTENT

- Members of the interprofessional team and their roles
- Team models of function
- Characteristics of effective teams
- Regulations associated with teams in rehabilitation

PROFESSIONAL REHABILITATION NURSING DOMAINS AND COMPETENCIES

- Domain 4: Competencies 4.1, 4.2, 4.3 (Association of Rehabilitation Nurses [ARN], 2014)

Introduction

To be successful, rehabilitation requires teamwork. Rehabilitation, as a specialty, has one of the longest histories of utilizing teamwork to help meet patient goals, but teamwork is not always easy. The Institute of Medicine's (IOM's) 2001 report highlighted the challenge of continually advancing the effectiveness and efficiency of teams. "Team practice is common, but the training of health professionals is typically isolated by discipline. Making the necessary changes in roles to improve the work of teams is often slowed or stymied by institutional, labor, and financial structures, and by law and custom" (IOM, 2001, p. 12). The IOM has also issued a mandate for interdisciplinary education (Griener & Knebel, 2003) that focuses on the value of health professionals working together in an interdisciplinary manner in all settings. *Interdisciplinary* is the term most often used in rehabilitation; however, many prefer the term *interprofessional* to focus on the cooperation, coordination, and collaboration necessary to ensure patient-centered care among members of different healthcare professions. The goals of teamwork are enhanced patient safety, better communication during patient handoffs, and improved patient outcomes. A growing body of evidence links improved patient outcomes with more efficient use of resources by effective teams (Bosch et al., 2009; Zwarenstein, Goldman, & Reeves, 2009). As healthcare interventions and systems become increasingly more complex, the need for effective and efficient teams will continue to grow.

Dunn and Thompson (2013) pointed out that the IOM (2001) Quality and Safety Education for Nursing (Cronenwett et al., 2007), World Health Organization (2010), Interprofessional Education Collaborative Expert Panel (IPEC, 2011), and American Association of Colleges of Nursing (AACN, 2006, 2008, 2011) all call for more effective interprofessional healthcare teams.

This chapter provides an overview of teams and teamwork as they relate to rehabilitation and the rehabilitation nurse.

I. Members of the Interprofessional Team

A. A long list of potential team members is provided in section I.B. In reality, some team members will come and go, as patient need is identified and patient goals are attained. Some team members on the list will never be utilized, if the need for them does not arise. Note, however, that the patient and family or caregivers are listed first. When the patient and family or caregivers are informed and motivated and at the center of the team, everyone is more successful.

B. Constant* and Potential Team Members **(Table 3-1)**

1. Family or caregivers*
2. Physiatrist*
3. Physician*
4. Physician assistant
5. Advanced practice nurse: nurse practitioner, clinical nurse specialist
6. Registered nurse (RN), certified rehabilitation RN*
7. Licensed practical nurse (LPN), licensed vocational nurse*
8. Nursing assistant*
9. Physical therapist, physical therapy assistant, physical therapy aide*
10. Occupational therapist, certified occupational therapy assistant*
11. Speech-language pathologist
12. Recreation therapist
13. Vocational therapist
14. Neuropsychologist
15. Psychiatrist, psychologist
16. Social worker*
17. Audiologist
18. Discharge planner*
19. Care manager, case manager*
20. Dietitian*
21. Chaplain
22. Respiratory therapist
23. Minimum data set or prospective payment system coordinator*
24. Insurance companies*

II. Team Models of Function

A team model of function describes how the team structurally works: who leads, who follows, who communicates with whom, and so on. Team models vary from site to site and by type of rehabilitation. Team literature focuses on interdisciplinary teams as the ideal model, yet at some facilities, an interdisciplinary team may not be possible or even desirable, especially in outpatient settings, where there might be only one therapist and one nurse providing the care, or only one therapist and no nurses. However, in large facilities where the care is primarily inpatient, decades of multiprofessional, peer-reviewed literature supports the collaborative interface of an interdisciplinary/interprofessional team to achieve the best outcomes (Behm & Gray, 2012; Drinka & Clark, 2000; Momsen, Rasmussen, Nielson, Iversen, & Lund, 2012).

A. Interdisciplinary/Interprofessional Team Model
1. Members work together to determine goals and treatments.
2. Decision making and problem solving are shared.
3. There is a holistic approach to care.
4. Continuity of care is present.
5. The team is patient focused.

B. Transdisciplinary Team Model
1. One member is the primary provider of care.
2. Other team members guide the provider of care.
3. Team members are cross-trained in other disciplines.
4. There is blurring of roles.
5. Flexibility is present.
6. This model is common in restorative care programs.

C. Multidisciplinary Team Model
1. Members work independently toward discipline-specific goals.
2. An individual member might not have direct communication with other team members.
3. Communication is more vertical than lateral.
4. Team members do not participate in team conferences.
5. The team is task focused.

D. Medical (Primary Care) Team Model (Arcangelo, Fitzgerald, Carroll, & Plumb, 1996)
1. Physician driven
2. Vertical communication
3. Not patient focused

E. Unidisciplinary/Intradisciplinary Model
1. Focused solely on one's own profession

F. Collaborative Practice Team Model
1. Joint communication and decision making
2. No hierarchy
3. A common group of patients
4. Understanding of each role
5. Contribution of all care providers is essential.
6. Members function according to their expertise and education.

III. Characteristics of Effective Teams

A. The patient and family are the focus of care and work with the team to establish goals.
1. Clear goals are identified for everyone on the team to work toward.
2. Evidence of effective teams
   a. Clarity about each team member's role and contributions to each client
   b. Effective, clear, open, two-way communication

Table 3-1. Members of the Interdisciplinary Team	
Team Members	**Generalized Role**
Patient	Participates in care and decisions and plans for the next phase of rehabilitation. Understands and learns about his or her own disease process or injury and actively communicates with the interdisciplinary team.
Family members, care providers, and significant others	Explores available community resources. Becomes educated about the patient's disease process or injury. Openly communicates any problems or concerns to the interdisciplinary team. Adequately describes and explains the home environment where the patient will reside upon discharge.
Physiatrist	A physician who is specially trained in rehabilitation. Typically leads the rehabilitation team members. Identifies and explains any medical diagnoses. Communicates any set goals. Orders any necessary tests, procedures, and medical equipment and provides care after the patient is discharged. Establishes any restrictions on physical mobility and provides an impairment rating.
Physician (e.g., internal medicine, geriatrics, neurology)	Acts as "physiatrist" in some settings, managing the patient's rehabilitation process. Works in conjunction with the physiatrist in the rehabilitation setting as needed to manage the patient's medical issues or to follow up on surgical interventions.
Physician assistant	Provides a complete physical assessment. A decision about care is determined after all the data are collected from assessment findings, labs, X rays, and so on. Works in partnership with other members of the interdisciplinary rehabilitation team.
Psychiatrist or psychologist	Deals with emotional and mental disorders, including those resulting from the injury (e.g., posttraumatic stress disorder, intensive care unit syndrome) and premorbid conditions (e.g., bipolar disorder, schizophrenia). Helps individuals, including family members, to identify resources and personal coping mechanisms to deal with their illness or injury. All psychiatrists and in some states psychologists prescribe and monitor psychotropic medications. Through individual and group therapy, assists patients and families with the realization and acceptance of how the illness or injury has affected their lives.
Neuropsychologist	Understands and assesses for disorders involving the brain and nervous system. Offers appropriate strategies to deal with different behaviors and issues identified in neuropsychological assessment and in the clinical setting. Serves as an educator for the patient and care providers. Helps the interdisciplinary team understand and deal with patients who have behavioral problems. Assesses the mental well-being of the patient.
Nurse practitioner	Provides a complete physical assessment. Makes medical diagnoses and decisions about care after all the data are collected from assessment findings, and labs and X rays are complete. In conjunction with the physiatrist, orders any necessary tests, procedures, and medical equipment, and provides care after the patient is discharged. Works in partnership with other members of the interdisciplinary rehabilitation team.
Clinical nurse specialist	Provides direct or indirect patient care and consultation services to staff members to improve patient outcomes. Incorporates specific nursing skills, medical diagnoses, and specific treatment modalities for each patient to ensure quality care. Examines and addresses system and quality issues. Educates nursing staff. In some states, has same role as nurse practitioner.
Rehabilitation nurse (registered nurse; Certified Rehabilitation Registered Nurse® [CRRN®])	Manages and provides holistic rehabilitation-focused care for the patient on a daily basis. Meets the needs of the patient's mind, body, and soul based on the experiences and background of the individual nurse. Participates as a full member of the interprofessional team.
Licensed practical nurse	Works under the direction of the rehabilitation nurse, physician, physician assistant, or nurse practitioner. Provides direct patient care, offers appropriate education, emphasizes the care offered by other members of the interdisciplinary team, guides ancillary staff to provide quality care, establishes a bond with the family and the care providers, and organizes activities created by the interdisciplinary team to help the patient meet his or her outcomes goals.
Certified nursing assistant	Works under the direct supervision of the nurse. Assists the patient in meeting his or her goals. Follows the plan of care determined by the interdisciplinary team, encourages the patient to act independently, reports all responses to treatment modalities, assists with activities of daily living, observes the patient for any complications, assists with positioning and transferring the patient, provides range of motion exercises, and assists with bowel and bladder training.
Minimum data set (MDS) or prospective payment system coordinator	Ensures that the patient's assessment is completed and that guidelines established on the federal and state levels are followed when organizing each patient's care plan. Reviews patient's medical records to determine whether the MDS forms were filled out properly. Informs staff members of any issues that occurred with the documentation. Manages Medicare/Medicaid cases to help facilitate the reimbursement process. Works closely with insurance companies for reimbursement.

continued

Table 3-1. Members of the Interdisciplinary Team (Continued)	
Certified rehabilitation counselors	Helps patients live independently and accomplish goals. Understands the barriers that each individual faces. Explores individual needs and preferences. Conducts counseling sessions. Completes individual assessments to identify the abilities and interests of each patient. Helps individuals deal with their feelings and develop the strength to move forward with their lives.
Physical therapist (PT)	Supports the patient's ability to use and improve their gross motor skills and mobility. Assesses, diagnoses, and treats any disorders that can limit mobility. Serves as a patient educator. Helps the patient and care providers obtain needed assistive devices.
Physical therapy assistant	Works under the direct guidance of the PT. Assists in the treatment of patients and changes interventions based on the progress and comfort level of the patient.
Occupational therapist (OT)	Helps the patient improve his or her ability to perform activities of daily living (ADLs). Assesses, diagnoses, and treats any disorders that can limit the patient's ability to perform ADLs and instrumental ADLs. Serves as an educator. Establishes a plan to enhance the patient's ability to utilize his or her upper extremities.
Certified occupational therapy assistant	Works under the direct guidance of the OT. Carries out the interventions prescribed by the therapist.
Recreational therapist	Helps enable the patient to enjoy and participate in common leisure activities. Establishes leisure programs that benefit the patient. Offers resources to help facilitate the patient's transition back into the community.
Vocational therapist	Works with the patient to help determine a suitable occupation for him or her based on the patient's disability. Completes a thorough assessment to determine any specific work skills or abilities and training required.
Audiologist	Offers assessment, assistance, and treatment for patients who have alterations in their ability to hear. Can also assess and treat balance issues associated with the inner ear.
Speech-language pathologist	Assesses and provides treatment for problems with speech, swallowing, and cognition. Determines whether the patient can use alternative devices for communication. Serves as an educator.
Social worker	Acts as a support person and a liaison for the patient and care provider. Identifies any social issues that could potentially compromise recovery. Helps acquire needed resources. Can also counsel patient and family on issues related to family, role, finances, coping, and community reintegration.
Respiratory therapist	Assesses and treats disorders of the lungs, which includes the use of devices that promote ventilation.
Discharge planner	Coordinates the entire discharge process. Remains in close contact with all of the members of the interdisciplinary team to fully meet the needs of the patient.
Care manager	Helps with the process of transferring the patient to other facilities or discharging the patient home. Serves as a liaison. Helps the patient and care providers comprehend healthcare benefits. Fully explains what is expected during the rehabilitation process.
Case manager	Identifies the patient's desires, goals, and functional ability. Arranges a plan and needed resources. Establishes long- and short-term goals. Continually reevaluates the prognosis and outcome. Adjusts the plan according to the evaluation. Serves as a patient advocate to obtain the most cost-effective quality care available. Promotes the ability of the patient to become as self-sufficient as possible.
Dietitian	Manages the nutritional needs of each patient by performing an individualized assessment. Determines an appropriate nutritional treatment plan, which can include the following: specialized education, diets that meet the needs of the patient, and formulas for tube feedings.
Chaplain	Offers encouragement and religious and spiritual support for both the patient and care providers. Inspires others to identify and use spiritual resources to help them cope with their current situation. Works with individuals and families from a variety of faith traditions.

Note. This table was created from professional websites and general rehabilitation sources. Team member names and roles may vary within and between institutions. Rehabilitation nurses are encouraged to check professional websites and other sources for updates about each team members role.

c. Effective decision making
d. Trust among members
e. Development of positive working relations
f. Knowledge
g. Cooperative relationship between members
h. Coordination of care
i. Mutual respect
j. Commitment to the team concept
k. Shared responsibility and participative leadership
l. Willingness to compromise
m. Knowledge of the "where, what, who, and how" (Eggenberger, Sherman, & Keller, 2014; Kemp, Harris, & Comino, 2005; Lutz & Davis, 2008; Pellatt, 2005; Wagner, 2000; White et al., 2013)

B. Evidence of Core Competencies for Interprofessional Collaborative Practice (IPEC, 2011)
   1. Ethics and values of interprofessional practice
   2. Clear roles and responsibilities of team members
   3. Clear and effective interprofessional communication
   4. Commitment to team and teamwork

C. Outcomes Are Positive (Caldwell & Atwal, 2003; White et al., 2013)
   1. Effective delivery of effective services
   2. Focus on patient-care needs
   3. Efficient planning
   4. Minimal fragmentation
   5. Minimal duplication
   6. Employee satisfaction

IV. Ineffective Teams

A. Barriers to Team Effectiveness (Sargeant, Loney, & Murphy, 2008)
   1. Role conflicts
   2. Overload
   3. Heterogeneity
   4. Lack of knowledge
   5. Task or role confusion
   6. Poor leadership
   7. Inability to deal with conflict

B. Issues that Arise from Lack of Role Clarification (Drinka & Clark, 2000; Hilton, 1995)
   1. Role confusion: Members do not know what is expected of them and what they should expect from others.
   2. Conflict between members
   3. Ineffective communication
   4. Decisions are not carried out; individuals are not clear that they were to act.
   5. Crisis: results from members believing that other members are responsible, and consequently the work is not completed

C. Systematic Review (Buljac-Samardzic, Dekker-Van Doorn, van Wijngaarden, & van Wijk, 2010)
Forty-eight studies of interventions to increase healthcare team effectiveness found that the following four interventions showed moderate to high levels of evidence of effectiveness:
   1. Simulation training: Most research was aimed at team functioning in crisis situations and focused on information sharing, perception, and team task performance.
   2. Crew resource-management training: Focus on improving attitudes toward teamwork by improving communication, collaboration, team culture, and climate.
   3. Team-based training: Focus on team building, leadership, goal setting, and prevention of burnout.
   4. Continuous quality improvement: Focus on organizational interventions that indirectly affect team outcomes.

V. Essential Roles of the Rehabilitation Nurse and Nursing Staff in Effective Teams (Tables 3-2 and 3-3)

VI. Examples of Effective Interdisciplinary Teams in Providing Rehabilitation

A. Example 1: Improving the Nutritional Status of Stroke Patients with Swallowing Problems
   1. A concrete example of how nursing staff (RNs, LPNs, and CNAs) can contribute to a patient's team goals is summarized in Perry and colleagues' (2012) evidence-based guideline of nursing interventions for improving the nutritional status and outcomes of stroke patients with swallowing

Table 3-2. Specific Rehabilitation Nurses' Roles

Roles	Description
Rehabilitation admission liaison nurse	Has the responsibility of being a part of the screening process for patients admitted into rehabilitation. Visits patients in the setting of referral, performs assessment and reviews chart, and reports findings to physiatrist.
Patient care coordinator nurse	Has specific clinical experience in rehabilitation medicine and oversees the patient's care. Serves as a patient advocate and communicates any questions or concerns to the interdisciplinary team.
Rehabilitation nurse educator	Is experienced in rehabilitation medicine and provides the patient and care provider with the information necessary to help facilitate the transition to the rehabilitation facility and the discharge process.
Rehabilitation nurse case and care managers	Are typically certified in the field of rehabilitation. They oversee the entire rehabilitation process for each patient.
Clinical nurse specialist	Is an advanced practice nurse with a master's or doctoral degree in rehabilitation nursing. Provides direct or indirect patient care. Often serves as staff educator. Examines system and quality issues. Incorporates specific nursing skills, medical diagnoses, and specific treatment modalities for each patient to provide quality care.

Note. This table was created from professional websites and general rehabilitation sources. Roles may vary within and between institutions. Rehabilitaiton nurses are encouraged to check professional websites for updates about each team members role.

Table 3-3. Roles of Nursing Staff as Members of the Interdisciplinary Team

Roles	Description
Practitioner	Reviews medical records, coordinates the admission screening process, determines what care is appropriate, and completely documents all preadmission screen information.
Educator	Provides information about all aspects of the rehabilitation process.
Advocate	Provides support for the patient and family, serves as a liaison, and upholds ethical standards.
Consultant	Evaluates the patient's ability to participate in rehabilitation, evaluates the patient's progress in therapy, is involved in the discharge process, and determines the need for specialized equipment. Develops a plan of care for each patient and negotiates for reimbursement from external sources.
Marketer	Provides tours of the facility, fosters a relationship with the patient and care providers, establishes a rapport with referral sources, has a strong knowledge base of all aspects of the rehabilitation process, and is involved in preparing various reports.
Promoter	Endorses the rehabilitation facility and conducts himself or herself in a professional manner.
Collaborator	Serves as a contact person.
Negotiator	Negotiates for reimbursement with external sources, attempts to obtain approval for patients to remain in rehabilitation, formulates a patient expenditure plan that is financially viable and responsible, and generates outcomes data.

Note. This table was created from professional websites and general rehabilitation sources. Roles may vary within and between institutions. Rehabilitation nurses are encouraged to check professional websites for updates about each team members role.

problems. The speech-language pathologist, physical therapist, occupational therapist, and physiatrist do the diagnostic testing and provide the hand splinting and seating needs for the patient. Nursing staff assesses patient preferences; coordinates mealtime organization; provides mealtime supervision, assistance, and intake monitoring; and teaches family and caregivers about feeding skills. Thus, nursing staff members coordinate with each other to individualize care, manage meal delivery, and take responsibility for the dining environment, in addition to teaching staff, patients, and caregivers. Feedback on how the patient and family are doing at mealtimes is essential for the team to continue to assess progress and plan care.

B. Example 2: Bladder Management in Female Stroke Survivors
   1. Cournan's (2012) study showed that the implementation of evidence-based interventions with female stroke survivors on an inpatient rehabilitation unit significantly increased their functional independence measures scores for bladder function from the time of admission to discharge. This is a prime example of how the entire rehabilitation team needs to be involved with patients' basic activities of daily living.

C. Example 3: Nursing and Interdisciplinary Rehabilitation of the Stroke Patient
   1. The American Heart Association (Miller et al., 2010) published a scientific statement of the best available evidence and recommendations for interdisciplinary management of the needs of stroke survivors and their families during inpatient and outpatient rehabilitation and in chronic care and end-of-life settings.

VII. Regulations

A. Certain regulations apply to interdisciplinary team rounds (Centers for Medicare & Medicaid Services [CMS], 2009)
   1. CMS
      a. Acute inpatient rehabilitation (units and inpatient rehabilitation facilities)
         1) The CMS (2009) has published specific criteria for interdisciplinary teams.
         2) At a minimum, teams must consist of a rehabilitation physician with specialized training and experience in rehabilitation services, an RN with specialized training or experience in rehabilitation, a social worker or a case manager (or both), and a licensed or certified therapist from each therapy discipline involved in treating the patient.
         3) Members of the team must have up-to-date knowledge of the patient as documented in the medical record.
         4) Team conferences must be held once a week, at a minimum.
         5) The interdisciplinary team must be led by a rehabilitation physician. The rehabilitation physician is responsible for making the final treatment decisions. This physician must document concurrence with all decisions made by the team at each meeting.
         6) Team conferences must focus on assessing the patient's progress toward the rehabilitation goals, considering possible resolutions to any problems that could impede progress

toward the goals, reassessing the validity of the rehabilitation goals previously established, and monitoring and revising the treatment plan as needed.
   7) Review of each other's notes does not constitute a team conference.
   8) Treating professionals must be present at each conference. Absences should be infrequent and, if necessary, the absent treating professional should be represented by another professional from the same discipline who has current knowledge of the patient.
   9) The occurrence of the team conference and the decisions made during the conference, including discharge planning and a need for adjustment in goals or the treatment program, must be documented in the medical record.
   10) Documentation of the team conference must include the name and professional designations of the participants.
   11) Unfortunately, the patient is not a required member of the team, per CMS regulations.
 b. Subacute rehabilitation
   1) Interdisciplinary team conferences are held according to the individual facility's policy.
   2) Assessment and goal-setting conferences: The resident and family, significant other, or guardian should be invited.
   3) Assessment and goal setting should be documented in the medical record.
   4) An RN must sign off on completion of assessment and goal setting.
 c. Home rehabilitation
   1) Interdisciplinary team conferences can be logistically challenging in home care due to the geographic distance involved.
   2) There is an interdisciplinary team approach to coordinating services and setting goals.
   3) Teams do meet in person but might not discuss every patient receiving rehabilitation services. Patient cases to discuss are usually based on the complexity of the patient.
   4) Conferences are documented in the medical record.
   5) The designated team leader shares the outcomes of the conference with the patient.
2. The Commission on Accreditation of Rehabilitation Facilities (CARF) has specific criteria for certification related to the interdisciplinary team process.
 a. According to CARF (2013, pp. 99–100, 104), the team is determined by the assessment, individual planning process, predicted outcomes, and strategies used to achieve the predicted outcomes.
 b. The team must include
   1) The person served
   2) Members of the family or support system (as appropriate)
   3) Personnel with the competencies necessary to evaluate and facilitate the achievement of predicted outcomes in the following areas:
     a) Behavior
     b) Cognition
     c) Communication
     d) Functional
     e) Medical (e.g., physician, nursing, pharmacy, nutrition)
     f) Pain management
     g) Physical
     h) Psychological
     i) Recreation and leisure
     j) Social
     k) Spiritual
     l) Vocational
   4) The team provides services that address
     a) Impairments
     b) Activity limitations
     c) Participation restrictions
     d) Environmental needs
     e) The personal preferences of the person served.
   5) The responsibilities of the team include
     a) Reviewing relevant reports to facilitate assessment
     b) Identifying resources
     c) Integrating information on resources into program planning and implementation
     d) Conducting assessments
     e) Predicting outcomes
     f) Establishing the treatment plan
     g) Establishing the discharge or transition plan
     h) Providing services
     i) Modifying the treatment plan
     j) Ensuring that the disciplines change based on the needs of the patient
     k) Achieving the predicted outcomes
     l) Transferring the person served to the most appropriate level of care based on need
     m) Providing education and training
     n) Referring the person served to other services or programs as needed

o) Communicating with relevant stakeholders
p) Participating in performance-improvement activities
q) Considering the family and support systems: abilities, willingness, composition, communication, contingency plans, coping, expectations, educational needs, insight, interpersonal dynamics, learning style, problem solving, responsibilities, and health status
r) Considering cultural, financial, literacy, and social factors
s) Providing or arranging for service for family and support system as needed

6) All members of the team, regardless of shift, are aware of the importance of implementing and modifying the plan of care, and communicate decisions to all team members.
7) The team process is documented.
8) The team meets frequently enough to meet the needs of the person served, the program, and the external stakeholders (i.e., insurance companies).

VIII. Summary

Teams, and the rules governing teams, can be simple or complex, but the patient is always at the center of all interprofessional teamwork in rehabilitation. Professional members of the team do not work in isolation, but rather in a synergistic method that amplifies the contribution and value of each team member. Team function in rehabilitation seems like an equation of 1+1 = 3. Kautz (2013) presented a concrete example of all rehabilitation nursing staff working together to ensure that the patient and family's goals are met.

Nursing staff cares for inpatients 24 hours a day, 7 days a week, and often, many different staff members come in contact with a particular patient and family. Some certified nursing assistants (CNAs), LPNs, and RNs rarely see the therapists and physicians, and thus it is essential for all nursing staff to communicate the patient's progress and goals to every member of the nursing staff. Tables 3-2 and 3-3 outline the roles that all nursing staff can assume to help the patient achieve the team goals.

White papers published by ARN (Camicia et al., 2014) and the American Nurses Association (2012) outlined how rehabilitation nurses can best work with teams to facilitate care transitions. These publications contain excellent overviews of best practices for the team, patient, and family. Because nurses are present and accountable 24 hours a day, 7 days a week, and 365 days a year, they are responsible for the timely communication of essential information that enhances team function (Miller, Riley, & Davis, 2009). When this communication fails to happen effectively, the team's effectiveness is diminished.

It is essential that nursing staff actively participates in team meetings and patient team conferences. Experienced nurses must model the way for new nurses, so that nursing concerns are effectively addressed in team conferences, and all nurses are regarded as informed, professional, and effective team members. Use of a standardized form when participating in team conferences ensures that all essential aspects of the patient's care are reported and accurately convey the patient's progress toward team goals on the unit. All nursing staff, including RNs, LPNs, and CNAs, should be able to articulate their patient's functional status, progress toward discharge, and discharge plan.

References

American Association of Colleges of Nursing (2006). *The essentials of doctoral education for advanced practice nursing.* Washington, DC: Author.

American Association of Colleges of Nursing (2008). *The essentials of baccalaureate education for professional nursing practice.* Washington, DC: Author.

American Association of Colleges of Nursing (2011). *The essentials of master's education in nursing.* Washington, DC: Author.

American Nurses Association (ANA). (2012). *The value of nursing care coordination.* Silver Spring, MD: Author.

Arcangelo, V., Fitzgerald, M., Carroll, D., & Plumb, J. D. (1996). Collaborative care between nurse practitioners and primary care physicians. *Primary Care, 23*(1), 103–113.

Association of Rehabilitation Nurses (ARN). (2008). *Standards and scope of rehabilitation nursing practice.* Glenview, IL: Author.

Association of Rehabilitation Nurses (ARN). (2014). ARN competency model for professional rehabilitation nursing. Retrieved from http://www.rehabnurse.org/uploads/files/education/ARN_Rehabilitation_Nursing_Competency _Model_FINAL_-_May_2014.pdf

Behm, J., & Gray, N. (2012). Interdisciplinary rehabilitation teams. In K. L. Mauk (Ed.), *Rehabilitation nursing: A contemporary approach to practice.* (pp. 51–62). Sudbury, MA: Jones & Bartlett.

Bosch, M., Faber, M. J., Cruijsberg, J., Voerman, G. E., Leatherman, S., Grol, R. P. T. M.,...Wensing, M. (2009). Effectiveness of patient care teams and the role of clinical expertise and coordination: A literature review. *Medical Care Research and Review 66*(6), 5S–35S.

Buljac-Samardzic, M., Dekker-Van Doorn, C. M., van Wijngaarden, J. D. H., & van Wijk, K. P. (2010). Interventions to improve team effectiveness: A systematic review. *Health Policy, 94,* 183–195.

Caldwell, K., & Atwal, A. (2003). The problems of interprofessional healthcare practice in hospitals. *British Journal of Nursing, 12*(20), 1212–1218.

Camicia, M., Black, T., Ferrell, J., Waites, K., Wirt, S., Lutz, B., & Association of Rehabilitation Nurses Task Force (2014). The essential role of the rehabilitation nurse in facilitating care transitions: A white paper by the Association of Rehabilitation Nurses. *Rehabilitation Nursing, 39,* 3–15.

Centers for Medicare and Medicaid Services (2009). Medicare program; inpatient rehabilitation facility prospective payment system for federal fiscal year 2010. *Federal Register, 74*(151), 29762–39837.

Commission on Accreditation of Rehabilitation Facilities (2013). *Medical rehabilitation standards manual.* Tucson, AZ: Author.

Cournan, M. (2012). Bladder management in female stroke survivors: Translating research into practice. *Rehabilitation Nursing, 37*(6), 220–230.

Cronenwett, L., Sherwood, G., Barnsteiner, J., Disch, J., Johnson, J., Mitchell, P.,...Warren, J. (2007). Quality and safety education for nurses. *Nursing Outlook, 55*(3), 122–131.

Drinka, T. J. K., & Clark, P. G. (2000). *Health care teamwork: Interdisciplinary practice & teaching.* Westport, CT: Greenwood Publishing Group.

Dunn, D., & Thompson, T. C. (2013). Interdisciplinary collaboration and teams. In K. L. Mauk (Ed.), *Gerontological nursing: Competencies for care* (3rd ed.). (eChapter 31, pp. 1-22) Sudbury, MA: Jones & Bartlett.

Enggenberger, T., Sherman, R. O., & Keller, K. (2014). Creating high-performance interprofessional teams. *American Nurse, 9*(11), 12–14.

Greiner, A. C., & Knebel, E. (Eds.). (2003). The core competencies needed for healthcare professionals. In *Health professions education: A bridge to quality* (pp. 45–74). Washington, DC: National Academies Press. Retrieved from http://books.nap.edu/openbook.php?record_id=10681&page=R1

Hilton, R. W. (1995). Fragmentation within interprofessional work: A result of isolationism in health care professional education programmes and the preparation of student to function only in the confines of their own disciplines. *Journal of Interprofessional Care, 9*(1), 33–40.

Institute of Medicine (2001). *Crossing the quality chasm: A new health system for the 21st century.* Washington, DC: National Academy Press.

Interprofessional Education Collaborative Expert Panel (2011). *Core competencies for interprofessional collaborative practice: Report of an expert panel.* Washington, DC: Author.

Kautz, D. D. (2013). The power of touch. *Journal of the Australasian Rehabilitation Nurses Association (JARNA), 16*(1), 5–8.

Kemp, L. A., Harris, E., & Comino, E. J. (2005). Changes in community nursing in Australia: 1995-2000. *Journal of Advanced Nursing, 49*(3), 307–314.

Lutz, B. J., & Davis, S. M. (2008). Theory and practice models for rehabilitation nursing. In S. P. Hoeman (Ed.), *Rehabilitation nursing: Prevention, intervention, and outcomes* (pp. 14–29). St. Louis: Mosby Elsevier.

Miller, E. L., Murray, L., Richards, L., Zorowitz, R. D., Bakas, T., Clark, P., & Billinger, S. A. (2010). Comprehensive overview of nursing and interdisciplinary rehabilitation care of the stroke patient: A scientific statement from the American Heart Association. *Stroke, 41,* 2402–2448.

Miller, K., Riley, W., & Davis, S. (2009). Identifying key nursing and team behaviours to achieve high reliability. *Journal of Nursing Management, 17,* 247–255.

Momsen, A., Rasmussen, J., Nielson, C. V., Iversen, M. D., & Lund, H. (2012). Multidisciplinary team care in rehabilitation: An overview of reviews. *Journal of Rehabilitation Medicine, 44,* 901–912.

Pellatt, G. C. (2005). Perceptions of interprofessional roles within the spinal cord injury rehabilitation team. *International Journal of Therapy and Rehabilitation, 12*(4), 143–150.

Perry, L., Hamilton, S., Williams, J., & Jones, S. (2012). Nursing interventions for improving nutritional status and outcomes of stroke patients: Descriptive reviews of processes and outcomes. *World Views on Evidence-Based Nursing, 10,* 17–40.

Sargeant, J., Loney, E., & Murphy, G. (2008). Effective interprofessional teams: "Contact is not enough" to build a team. *Journal of Continuing Education in the Health Professions, 28*(4), 228–234.

Wagner, E. H. (2000). The role of patient care teams in chronic disease management. *British Medical Journal, 320*(7234), 569–572.

White, M. J., Gutierrez, A., McLaughlin, C., Eziakonwa, C., Newman, L. S., White, M., … Asselin, G. (2013). A pilot for understanding interdisciplinary teams in rehabilitation practice. *Rehabilitation Nursing, 38*, 142–152.

World Health Organization (WHO). (2010). *Framework for action on Interprofessional Education and Collaborative Practice.* (WHO/HRH/HPN/10.3).

Zwarenstein, M., Goldman, J., & Reeves, S. (2009). Interprofessional collaboration: Effects of practice-based interventions on professional practice and healthcare outcomes. *Cochrane Database of Systematic Reviews* (3):CD000072.

Chapter 4

Ethical, Moral, and Legal Considerations of Rehabilitation Nursing

Angela Stone Schmidt, PhD MNSc RNP RN

LEARNING OUTCOMES

- Describe ethical behavior.
- Review ethical models and theorists.
- Discuss models of ethical and moral decision making.
- Discuss barriers to ethical nursing care.
- Apply ethical principles to rehabilitation nursing.

KEY CHAPTER TOPICS

- Definitions
- Ethical models and theorists
- Ethical decision making
- Ethical conflict
- Ethical principles and rights
- Legal issues and considerations
- Professional codes of ethics

PROFESSIONAL REHABILITATION NURSING DOMAINS AND COMPETENCIES

- Domain 1: Competencies 1.2, 1.4
- Domain 2: Competencies 2.1, 2.2, 2.3
- Domain 3: Competencies 3.1, 3.3, 3.4
- Domain 4: Competencies 4.2, 4.3 (Association of Rehabilitation Nurses [ARN], 2014a)

Introduction

Specialty organizations provide recommendations and guidance for healthcare delivery, including ethical, moral, and legal considerations for nursing. According to the Association of Rehabilitation Nurses' (ARN) position statement (2014b) and the American Nurses Association (ANA; 2001), rehabilitation nurses have a moral obligation to provide ethical care. Determining what constitutes ethical care can be challenging, especially when conflicts arise between those who deliver care and those who seek care. Frameworks for ethical and moral decision making are needed to understand the reason and rationale for specific decisions that are made in ethical dilemmas. The ethical, legal, and social implications of care decisions demand further inquiry and discussion within healthcare delivery systems, communities, and the profession of nursing. Although laws, professional codes, and institutional policies help to guide practice, no guidelines exist that answer every ethical dilemma, even within legal constraints and scope of practice. Rehabilitation nurses are part of an interprofessional team that advocates for the care and services needed by those served, and nurses have a fiduciary relationship with the healthcare institution that obliges them to act as stewards of resources. The purpose of this chapter is to discuss the issues surrounding ethical dilemmas and to provide resources that assist with ethical resolution.

I. **Ethical and Moral Considerations**

Rehabilitation nurses' decisions and actions on behalf of clients must be made and performed in an ethical manner (ARN, 2008, 2014b). Frameworks for decision making in resolving ethical dilemmas are often found in ethical theories and principles. "Ethics involves the study of morals and moral evaluation, distinguishing right from wrong, beneficial from harmful, and virtuous from vicious" (Online Ethics Center for Engineering and Science, 2005). Ethics evolves from beliefs and values and has religious and cultural bases. Ethical behavior requires moral reasoning, problem solving, and decision making. In research studies, ethical behavior includes obtaining informed consent from participants and analyzing risks and benefits. Professional codes or standards, such as ANA's Code of Ethics for Nurses with Interpretive Statements (2010), guide expected ethical behavior for nurses. ARN (2003, 2014b) supports the ANA Code of Ethics and adds specific ethical expectations for rehabilitation nurses (Hoeman, 2008).

A. Definitions

1. *Ethics* is the study of "the nature and justification of general principles that can apply to special areas where there are moral problems" (McCourt, 1993, p. 230), such as human conduct, moral character, and motives inherent in deliberate human actions (Davis & Aroskar, 1991; Derstine & Hargrove, 2001). Ethics is a science of duty with a balance of values on either side of a moral dilemma that could result in conflict.
   a. *Normative ethics* is the study of what is right and wrong and examines ethical theories such as autonomy, beneficence, justice, and nonmaleficence and their application to rehabilitation health care or other disciplines (Butts & Rich, 2008; Morrison, 2008).
   b. *Metaethics* is the study of ethical concepts concerned with understanding the language of morality through an analysis of the meaning of ethically related concepts and theories (Butts & Rich, 2008; Morrison, 2008).
   c. *Descriptive ethics* is a scientific ethical inquiry that describes what people think about morality or how people actually behave (i.e., morals) (Butts & Rich, 2008).
2. Values or moral principles are relevant to an ethical issue in a clinical situation (Beauchamp & Childress, 2001; Hebert, 1996). Ethical issues are commonly viewed in health care as the conflict between two or more morally defensible alternative healthcare actions, including inaction. In the practice of rehabilitation, ethical issues exist that are specific to the nature of its treatments (Sliwa et al., 2002).
   a. *Morals* are specific beliefs, behaviors, and ways of being, providing boundaries for acceptable behaviors (Barrocas, Yarbrough, Bechnel, & Nelson, 2003; Butts & Rich, 2008).
   b. *Values* are beliefs that one considers meaningful and ideals that are good, worthwhile, and highly regarded. Values dictate how personal character is developed, and subsequently, how people behave (Butts & Rich, 2008; Grace, 2009).
      1) Values are usually derived from societal norms, family orientation, and religion (Guido, 2010).
      2) Values are subject to philosophical, moral, and individual interpretations (Butts & Rich, 2008).
3. "Morality is the tradition of belief about right and wrong moral conduct" (McCourt, 1993, p. 230). Common morality consists of normative beliefs and behaviors that members of society generally agree about and are familiar to most human beings (Butts & Rich, 2008).
4. Moral decision making involves using ethical principles to guide decision making through a rational course (Hoeman & Duchene, 2002).
   a. Ethical theories provide the foundation for understanding ethical dilemmas and are the basis for problem solving and decision making (Brillhart, 1995).
   b. Health care in the 21st century is affected by accelerating advances in technology and science, cost-containment efforts, and limited resources that compromise the provision of care for increasingly complex client healthcare needs. These factors combine to pose ethical dilemmas (Kalb & O'Conner-Von, 2007).
   c. *Philosophy* is the discipline of using reason and analysis to examine questions that are not answerable by empirical science (Grace, 2014).
5. Moral philosophy refers to the philosophical inquiry in ethics. As a theoretical endeavor, it concerns ethics with an understanding of human values that leads to the development of theories of value about the conditions of human beings living together within a society. In relation to a specific situation, different theories can give conflicting directions, depending on the theories' premises and assumptions, without providing concrete direction in healthcare settings (Grace, 2014).
6. Applied ethics uses the theoretical knowledge and assumptions gained as a result of ethical theorizing, as well as the skills and tools of moral philosophy or analysis to solve difficult problems (Grace, 2014). This application of moral philosophy to actual situations determines good or appropriate actions, in which a person or group is responsible for their actions.
7. *Bioethics* is the study of the relationships between biology, medicine, technology, and scientific advancements as related to ethical issues. Bioethical issues change with social changes (Ellis & Hartley, 2007). In rehabilitation, bioethical problems of conflicts of values are related to respect for autonomy, beneficence, nonmaleficence, and justice (Rudnick, 2010). Applied bioethical dilemmas in the practice of rehabilitation include
   a. Beneficence versus nonmaleficence, as exemplified by a leg prosthesis that could be beneficial in facilitating independent ambulation but could be harmful, resulting in complications or pain
   b. Autonomy versus justice, as exemplified by a poststroke elderly patient requesting to stay in

a rehabilitation inpatient unit longer than clinically necessary as a result of uncertainty and ineffective coping.

8. *Ethical practice* is the use of disciplinary knowledge, skills, experience, and personal characteristics to conceptualize what is needed for an individual or society (Grace, 2014). Ethical professional practice uses the goals and perspectives of the discipline, such as rehabilitation, to direct action.
9. Rehabilitation nursing ethics (**Figure 4-1**) are "judgments about decisions to act and subsequent actions based on the rules of conduct or precepts of rehabilitation nursing practice" (Graham-Eason, 1996, p. 35).

Figure 4-1. Savage Model for Facilitating Ethical Decision Making

1. Gather facts of the case and understandings of parties involved.
2. Identify the questions and goals.
3. Organize a meeting with key players—parents, physicians, nurses, social workers, therapists, and others who might assist in the decision making.
   a. Pose questions, clarify information, set goals.
   b. Explore options and their consequences and ethical ramifications.
   c. Make a plan for the future management of the case.
4. Provide information, referrals, education, and emotional support to the family.
5. Participate in implementation of the decision, if appropriate.
6. Review the process, evaluate your role, and revise the process as needed.

From "Ethical, legal, and moral issues in pediatric rehabilitation" (p. 67), by T. Savage and D. Michalak, 1999. In P. A. Edwards, D. L. Hertzberg, S. R. Hays, & N. M. Youngblood (Eds.), *Pediatric rehabilitation nursing*. Philadelphia: W. B. Saunders. Copyright 1999 by T. Savage and D. Michalak. Reprinted with permission.

   a. A fundamental principle that underlies all nursing practice, including rehabilitation nursing, is respect for the inherent worth, dignity, and human rights of every person. "The nurse, in all professional relationships, practices with compassion and respect for the inherent dignity, worth, and uniqueness of every individual, unrestricted by considerations of social or economic status, personal attributes, or the nature of health problems" (ANA, 2010, p. 7).

10. *Laws* are the established social rules for conduct; a violation of a law can result in criminal or civil liability. Laws can be generated by federal or state governments.
    a. Ethical decisions are guided by law, institutional policies and practices, policies of professional organizations, professional standards of care, fiduciary obligations, and management concerns.
    b. Risk management reduces the risk of liability through institutional policies and practices. Risk management is guided by legal parameters but has a broader institutional mission, including ethical applications (Brock & Mastroianni, 2008) (**Figure 4-2**).
11. Professional codes guide members of the profession in maintaining ethical practice. The ANA's *Code of Ethics for Nurses with Interpretive Statements* (2010) requires that professional and personal values be integrated (i.e., normative ethics).
12. Organizational codes of conduct are intended to serve as central guides and references to support daily decision making. Codes of conduct clarify an organization's mission, values, and principles, linking them with standards of professional conduct. A code is an open disclosure of the way an organization operates, and it provides guidelines for behavior. It "reflects the covenant that an organization has made to uphold its most important values, dealing with its commitment to employees, its standards for doing business and its relationship with the community" (Ethics Resource Center, 2009).
    a. The Commission on Accreditation for Rehabilitation Facilities (CARF) has written ethical codes of conduct in 13 identified areas, including these service delivery areas: exchange of gifts, money, and gratuities (1.A.6.a. (4) (b));

Figure 4-2. Two Models of Ethical Decision Making

Model 1 (Aiken & Catalano, 1994)	Model 2 (Blanchard & Peale, 1988)
1. Collect, analyze, and interpret data. 2. State the dilemma clearly. 3. Consider choices for action. 4. Consider and weigh choices 5. Analyze advantages and disadvantages of each choice. 6. Make decision from choices.	1. Ask "Is it legal?" If the answer is yes, then stop. If no, go on to Items 2 and 3. 2. Ask "Is it balanced?" This will help answer issues of fairness vs. giving advantages to one or more parties. 3. Ask "How will the decision make me feel?" This will help answer issues of personal standards of morality.

Model 1: Adapted with permission of F. A. Davis Company from Aiken, T., & Catalano, J. (1994). *Legal, ethical, and political issues in nursing* (pp. 31-35). Philadelphia: F. A. Davis. Copyright 1994 by F. A. Davis Company.

Model 2: Adapted with permission of William Morrow & Company, Inc., from Blanchard, K., & Peale, N. (1988). *The power of ethical management* (pp. 20-27). New York: William Morrow. Copyright 1988 by Blanchard Family Partnership and Norman Vincent Peale by William Morrow & Company, Inc.

personal fund raising (1.A.6.a. (4) (c)); personal property (1.A.6.a (4) (d)); and witnessing of documents (1.A.6.a (4) (f)) (CARF, 2013).

b. Corporate compliance programs were developed in response to the Sentencing Reform Act of 1984 (S 668), which created the United States Sentencing Commission in 1987 and led to the development of U.S. sentencing guidelines. The Sarbanes-Oxley Act of 2002 (HR 3763) required all publicly traded companies to submit an annual report of the effectiveness of their internal accounting controls to the Securities and Exchange Commission beginning in 2004 (O'Brien, 2006). Two provisions of the act also applied to nonprofit organizations:
   1) Standards relating to corporate compliance, ethics, and compliance with all legal and regulatory requirements were introduced in the CARF standards manuals in 2003.
   2) Organizations that receive direct or indirect federal funds must conform to corporate compliance standards, U.S. sentencing guidelines, and requirements of the Sarbanes-Oxley Act.

c. The Joint Commission (2009) adopted a code of conduct to provide standards to guide personnel in conducting themselves as a means of protecting and promoting organization-wide integrity. The principles and standards include legal compliance, business ethics, confidentiality, conflict and dualities of interest, core activity and relationships, and protection of assets.

B. Ethical Models and Associated Theorists (Ellis & Hartley, 2007): Ethical theories provide the foundation for understanding ethical dilemmas and the basis for problem solving and decision making (Brillhart, 1999; Derstine & Hargrove, 2001).

1. Deontology, also known as duty-based ethics (a proponent of which was the 18th-century philosopher Immanuel Kant). Decisions derive from moral rules and universal values that do not change; a categorical imperative exists. Consequences of decisions are less important than following the rules.
   a. "The science of right" specifies that there are definable principles of natural right associated with jurisprudence. In rehabilitation nursing, the nurse has a responsibility to provide competent care in accordance with the nurse practice act or scope of practice for the state. The duty consists of rational respect for fulfilling one's obligations to other human beings (Guido, 2010).
   b. Kant's moral law perspective that the issue of whether free will is possible is foundational in his metaphysical and epistemological ground of ethics in deontology (Morrison, 2008). The test of a good will is whether the person continues to act out of duty and reverence for the moral law even when doing so has no personal benefit.
      1) Virtue ethics: There is less emphasis on learning rules and regulations and more on the development of good character and habitual performance. Virtue ethicists' qualities include wisdom, courage, temperance, justice, generosity, self-respect, and sincerity (Guido, 2010). Virtue ethics can be applied in autonomy, beneficence, nonmaleficence, and justice principles (Morrison, 2008).
      2) Duty ethics: Obligations for human beings include duties to God, duties to oneself, and duties to others. Duties to self include avoiding wronging others, treating people as equals, and promoting the good of others (Frankena & Granrose, 1974). Ross (2002) considered qualities such as fidelity, reparation, gratitude, justice, beneficence, self-improvement, and nonmaleficence to be prima facie duties.
      3) Situation ethics: The decision maker acknowledges the unique characteristics of each individual, the caring relationship between the person and the caregiver, and the most humanistic course of action, given the circumstances.
   c. Deontology can be subdivided into act deontology and rule deontology (Guido, 2010).
      1) *Act deontology* is based on the moral values of the person making the ethical decision.
      2) *Rule deontology* is based on the belief that certain standards for ethical decisions transcend the individual's moral values.

2. Utilitarianism, consequentialism, and teleology
   a. Utilitarianism, also known as situational ethics (espoused by philosophers Jeremy Bentham, 1748–1832, and John Stuart Mill, 1806–1873), is based on the assumption that actions should lead to maximizing the overall good; the ends justify the means. Principles or actions can be proven to be good. The best principles or actions are those that result in good feelings, a premise known as "happiness theory," (Hinman, 2002; Hoeman, 2008) or teleological theory (Guido, 2010). What makes an action

right or wrong is its utility, with useful actions bringing about the greatest happiness, or the least harm and suffering, to an individual.

   1) *Rule utilitarianism* seeks the greatest happiness for all and appeals to public agreement as a basis for objective judgment about the nature of happiness.
   2) *Act utilitarianism* seeks to determine which action will bring about the greatest happiness or the least harm and suffering.

b. *Consequentialist* moral theories evaluate the morality of actions in terms of progress toward a goal or end and are a version of utilitarianism. Consequentialism is sometimes called teleology, with the goal being the greatest good for the greatest number (Morrison, 2008).
   1) *Classical utilitarianism* (or act consequentialism): Each act is considered based on its net benefit.
   2) *Rule consequentialism*: The decision maker develops the rules that will have the greatest net benefit.

3. *Objectivism* (espoused by St. Thomas Aquinas, 1225–1274): Actions are considered morally right when they are in accord with our nature, promote good, and avoid evil. Ethical egoism is the pursuit of one's own rational self-interest, and one's own happiness is the highest moral purpose of one's life (Morrison, 2008).
4. *Principalism* incorporates various existing ethical principles and attempts to resolve conflicts by applying one or more ethical principles rather than ethical theories (Guido, 2010; McCarthy, 2006).
5. *Relational ethics* moves decisions into the context of the environment in which decisions are made and create a more practical, action-oriented ethics (Bergum & Dossetor, 2005; Guido, 2010).
   a. The four components of relational ethics are engagement, mutual respect, embodiment, and environment.
   b. There is a shared relationship with obligations and responsibilities to other people, incorporating an understanding of culture and language. Relational ethics in nursing includes mutuality and caring (Gadow, 1999).
6. Normative ethical theories (Morrison, 2008) (**Figure 4-3**)

Figure 4-3. Normative Ethical Theories

Natural law theories	Egoistic theories	Authority-based theories	Teleological theories	Virtue ethics

   a. *Natural law theories:* The right thing to do is that which is in accord with the providentially ordered nature of the world.
   b. *Egoistic theories:* What is right is that which maximizes a person's self-interest.
   c. *Authority-based theories:* These can be faith based or purely ideological; the decision of the right thing to do is based in some authority.
   d. *Teleological theories* (consequentialism and utilitarianism): The decision depends on the consequences of the action and maximizes the good of a situation.
   e. *Deontological theories:* Act and rule (see I.B.1. Deontology)
   f. *Virtue ethics:* Habitual performance of wisdom, courage, temperance, justice, generosity, self-respect, and sincerity
7. Ethical relativism and objectivism (Butts & Rich, 2008)
   a. *Ethical relativism* is the belief that it is acceptable for ethics and morality to differ between people or societies. The two types are ethical subjectivism and cultural relativism.
      1) *Ethical subjectivism:* Individuals create their own morality, and there are no objective moral truths, only individual opinions.
      2) *Cultural relativism:* The moral evaluation is rooted in and cannot be separated from the beliefs and behaviors of a particular culture, and what is considered to be wrong in one culture may not be considered wrong in another.
   b. *Ethical objectivism* is the position that universal or objective moral principles exist. Examples include deontology, utilitarianism, and natural law theory.
8. Social equality and justice (espoused by philosopher John Rawls, 1921–2002): Supports justice and equal rights for all through development of positions that use a "veil of ignorance," so that decisions are not colored by the specific details of the people involved, thereby allowing disadvantaged persons to receive the same social and economic benefits as others.
9. Ideal observer (espoused by ethnologist Raymond W. Firth, 1901–2002): Decisions should be made by an impartial observer who is fully informed about the situation and the potential consequences of the decision.

C. Models of Ethical and Moral Decision Making

The process of moral decision making (Hoeman, 2008) (**Figure 4-4**) uses ethical principles to guide decision making through a rational course (MacDonald,

Figure 4-4. Process of Moral Decision Making

A. Recognizing the Moral Dimension The first step is recognizing the decision as one that has moral importance. Important clues include conflicts between two or more values or ideals.
B. Who Are the Interested Parties? What Are Their Relationships? Carefully identify who has a stake in the decision. In this regard, be imaginative and sympathetic. Often there are more parties whose interests should be taken into consideration than is immediately obvious. Look at the relationships between the parties. Look at their relationships with yourself and with each other and with relevant institutions.
C. What Values Are Involved? Think through the shared values that are at stake in making this decision. Is there a question of trust? Is personal autonomy a consideration? Is there a question of fairness? Is anyone to be harmed or helped?
D. Weigh the Benefits and the Burdens Benefits—broadly defined—might include such things as the production of goods (physical, emotional, financial, social, etc.) for various parties, the satisfaction of preferences, and acting in accordance with various relevant values (such as fairness). Burdens might include causing physical or emotional pain to various parties, imposing financial costs, and ignoring relevant values.
E. Look for Analogous Cases Can you think of other similar decisions? What course of action was taken? Was it a good decision? How is the present case like that one? How is it different?
F. Discuss with Relevant Others The merits of discussion should not be underestimated. Time permitting, discuss your decision with as many people as have a stake in it. Gather opinions and ask for the reasons behind those opinions. Remember that your ability to discuss topics with others may be limited by the other people's expectations of confidentiality.
G. Does this Decision Accord with Legal and Organizational Rules? Some decisions are appropriately made based on legal considerations. If one option is illegal, we should at least think very seriously before choosing that option. Decisions may also be affected by rules set by organizations of which we are members. For example, most professional organizations have codes of ethics that are intended to guide individual decision making. Institutions (hospitals, banks, corporations) may also have policies that limit the options available to us. Sometimes there are bad laws or bad rules, and sometimes those should be broken. But usually it is ethically important to pay attention to laws and rules.
H. Am I Comfortable with this Decision? Sometimes your "gut reaction" will tell you if you've missed something. Questions to be asked in this regard might include: 1. If I carry out this decision, would I be comfortable telling my family about it? My clergy? My mentors? 2. Would I want children to regard my behavior as an example? 3. Is this decision one that a wise, informed, virtuous person would make? 4. Can I live with this decision?
From *Guide to moral decision making,* by C. MacDonald, 2010. Retrieved from www.ethicsweb.ca/guide. Copyright 2010 by Chris MacDonald. Reprinted with permission.

2002). Ethical decision making includes important considerations in the daily practice of difficult situations that require the exercise of knowledge, experience, and skill, with a continued focus on the good of the client or family, without personal biases (Grace, 2009) (**Table 4-1**). The philosophical tools that can be applied to morally ambiguous situations are moral theories, moral perspectives, moral principles, and analytic techniques (Grace, 2014).

1. *Proxy decision making* is the act of deciding which healthcare actions might be permissible for a person who has lost decision-making capacity, either temporarily or permanently. Proxy decision making can also be done for a person who has never had decision-making capacity, such as someone with profound cognitive deficits or someone who lacks the maturity to make healthcare decisions, such as children (Grace, 2009) (**Table 4-2**)
2. Rest's processes (developed by James Rest of the University of Minnesota) for moral action with interfering factors includes interpretation of the situation and discerning the morally ideal action (determining what ought to be done, deciding what to do, and implementing and persevering) (Grace, 2014).
3. The Savage model (Savage & Michalak, 1999) for facilitating ethical decision making (Figure 4-1)
4. The clinical ethical decision-making model includes the medical considerations, patient preferences, quality of life, and contextual

Table 4-1. Ethical Decision Making in Difficult Situations: Important Considerations	
In the course of daily practice, what is needed for ethical action is the thoughtful exercise of knowledge, experience, and skill together with a constant focus on the good of the client or group in need of services and an understanding of one's own biases. In more complex situations, where what is good is not so clearly seen, a more in-depth analysis may be needed. This is not necessarily a linear process, nor will all of the following considerations always be pertinent. There are other decision-making models available, but all have similar considerations.	
Steps	**Questions**
Identify the major problem(s); relate them to professional goals.	What are the facts: clinical, social, environmental? What implicit assumptions are being made? What ethical principles or perspectives are pertinent? Examples: Autonomous decision making is in question, conflict of values between providers and client or significant others, economic versus client good. Are there power imbalances? What are these? Who has an interest in maintaining them?
Identify information gaps.	Do you need more information? From whom or where might you get this information?
Determine who is involved.	Who is the main focus? Is there more than one important party? Who has (or thinks they have) an interest in the outcome (relatives, staff, other)? Who will be affected by the outcome?
Identify the prevalent values. Determine whether an interpreter is necessary (for cultural or language issues). Who would be the most appropriate interpreter (knowledgeable and neutral)?	Values held by client, staff, institution. Are there value conflicts? Interpersonal, interprofessional, personal versus professional, client versus professional. Are there cultural perspectives? Who can help with these?
Identify possible courses of action and probable consequences.	Which course of action is likely to be the most beneficial and the least harmful to those involved, including you? Can safeguards be put in place in case of unforeseen consequences?
Implement the selected course of action. Conduct an ongoing evaluation.	Does the actual outcome correlate with the anticipated outcome? What was unexpected? Was this foreseeable given more data? Do similar problems keep reoccurring? If so, why (may require a look at underlying environmental or societal issues)? Does this point to the need for policy changes or development at the site, institution, or societal level? What further actions might be needed? Are there continuing provider education needs related to the issue?
Engage in self-reflection, reflection on practice (individually, in an interdisciplinary group debriefing session, or in a specialty group forum).	Could you have done things differently? What would you have liked to understand better? Would a consultation with colleagues or an ethics resource person have changed your understanding of the issue or the course of action taken? What valuable insights did you gain that should be shared with others and may be applicable to the approach used for future problems?

From *Nursing ethics and professional responsibility in advanced practice* (pp. 62–64), by P. J. Grace, 2009, Sudbury, MA: Jones & Bartlett. Copyright 2009 by Jones & Bartlett. Reprinted with permission.

features. The case-based approach to ethical decision making has been adapted, and the clinical ethical decision-making model has been applied (Jonsen, Siegler, & Winslade, 2010) (**Figure 4-5**)

5. Moral Ground Model: A virtue-based nursing model (Butts & Rich, 2008)
   a. The moral ground model was adapted from the Eightfold Path and the Four Immeasurable Virtues of Buddhism and was founded in Aristotle's approach to virtue ethics. The commonality is the alleviation of human suffering. As in teleological philosophies, the focus is on human morality moving toward a final purpose or goal (Butts & Rich, 2008; Keown, 2001). The model implies that nurses may start at an uneducated state of moral functioning and move toward moral ground along a path of intellectual and moral virtues.
   b. Intellectual virtues
      1) *Insight*: Awareness and knowledge of the moral nature of nurses' day-to-day work to transform moral suffering.
      2) *Practical wisdom*: Using deliberative reason to direct actions
   c. Moral virtues
      1) *Truthfulness*: Refraining from deception through false communication or self-deception

Table 4-2. Proxy Decision Making

Type	Explanation
A. Autonomy based: the person's previously expressed wishes	Written: Living will, advance directives Substituted judgment • Durable power of attorney for health care (person appointed to provide information about a client's previous wishes expressed while having decision-making capacity) • Informal (family member, friend, significant other)
B. Best interests	Surrogate determines the "highest net benefit among available options" (Beauchamp & Childress, 2001, p. 192). This is a quality-of-life (QOL) evaluation—it may or may not be based on a person's previously expressed desires. Previous values, beliefs, and wishes are considered to the extent that they give information about what would constitute QOL for the person. This may permit overriding a durable power of attorney's decision that does not seem to further client best interests and when there are no written instructions (from the incapacitated patient) to support the proposed course of action.
C. Reasonable person	A standard used when neither A nor B is applicable. It asks, "What would a reasonable person want?" The typical client was never competent (e.g., a baby or cognitively impaired person) and/or previous wishes cannot be determined. For example • Some permanently unconscious clients who might be said to have no interests and who cannot be "benefited" or "burdened." • Incapacitated, dying clients left on life support to preserve organs for transplantation (Medical College of Georgia, 2000).

From "Ethics in the clinical encounter" (pp. 295–332), by P. J. Grace, 2004. In S. K. Chase (Ed.), *Clinical judgment and communication in nurse practitioner practice*, Philadelphia: F. A. Davis. Copyright 2004 by F. A. Davis. Reprinted with permission.

2) *Gentleness*: Mildness in verbal and nonverbal communication
3) *Compassion*: The desire to separate others from suffering
4) *Loving kindness*: The desire to bring happiness and well-being to oneself and others
5) *Just generosity*: Giving and receiving based on need
6) *Courage*: Putting fear aside to act for a purpose that is more important than fear
7) *Sympathetic joy*: Rejoicing in others' happiness
8) *Equanimity*: An evenness and calmness of being

6. The PLUS (Policies, Legal, Universal, Self) Decision-Making Model is an alternative model that ensures that ethical issues inherent in practice can be effectively addressed by all persons in the healthcare team. This approach is a simplified process based on current theories and understandings of decision-making processes and ethics. The six steps are:
   a. Define the problem PLUS.
   b. Identify the alternatives.
   c. Evaluate the alternatives PLUS.
   d. Make the decision.
   e. Implement the decision.
   f. Evaluate the decision PLUS (Ethics Resource Center, 2009).
7. Three-step ACT (Anticipate, Clarify, Test) model (Graham-Eason, 1996)
   a. *A*: Anticipate obstacles to action.
   b. *C*: Clarify position related to planning action.
   c. *T*: Test choice.
8. There are four aspects of moral action and interfering factors. Affective (emotion) and cognitive (thought) components are included in moral action and can be applied to direct client care situations (Grace, 2009; Rest, 1982) (**Table 4-3**).
9. Reflective equilibrium as a decision-making model (Morrison, 2008) (**Figure 4-6**)
   a. Healthcare issue at hand is the middle of the model, containing the basic facts of the situation.
   b. Considered judgments or decision-making guides are used for making decisions about what to do.
      1) Intuitions or considered judgments about particular cases
      2) Regarding general moral rules
   c. Common morality influences the judgments and intuitions.
   d. Ethical theory examines people's motivations.
   e. Ethical principles include advancement of liberty, respect for autonomy, and acting out of beneficence to advance welfare. Also included is to ensure that, by following the principle of nonmaleficence and upholding principles of justice, we do nothing to harm others.
10. Josephson Institute of Ethics (Savage & Michalak, 1999) decision-making model
    a. All decisions must take into account and reflect a concern for the interest and well-being of stakeholders.

Figure 4-5. A Case-Based Approach to Ethical Decision Making

Medical Considerations ***The Principles of Beneficence and Nonmaleficence***	**Patient Preferences** ***The Principle of Respect for Autonomy***
What is the patient's medical problem? Is the problem acute? Chronic? Critical? Reversible? Emergent? Terminal? What are the goals of treatment? In what circumstances are medical treatments not indicated? What are the probabilities of success of various treatment options? In sum, how can this patient be benefited by medical and nursing care, and how can harm be avoided?	Has the patient been informed of benefits and risks, understood this information, and given consent? Is the patient mentally capable and legally competent, and is there evidence of incapacity? If mentally capable, what preferences about treatment is the patient stating? If incapacitated, has the patient expressed prior preferences? Who is the appropriate surrogate to make decisions for the incapacitated patient? Is the patient unwilling or unable to cooperate with medical treatment? If so, why?
Quality of Life ***The Principles of Beneficence and Nonmaleficence and Respect for Autonomy***	**Contextual Features** ***The Principles of Justice and Fairness***
What are the prospects, with or without treatment, for a return to normal life, and what physical, mental, and social deficits might the patient experience even if treatment succeeds? On what grounds can anyone judge that some quality of life would be undesirable for a patient who cannot make or express such a judgment? Are there biases that might prejudice the provider's evaluation of the patient's quality of life? What ethical issues arise concerning improving or enhancing a patient's quality of life? Do quality-of-life assessments raise any questions regarding changes in treatment plans, such as forgoing life-sustaining treatment? What are plans and rationale to forgo life-sustaining treatment? What is the legal and ethical status of suicide?	Are there professional, interprofessional, or business interests that might create conflicts of interest in the clinical treatment of patients? Are there parties other than clinicians and patients, such as family members, who have an interest in clinical decisions? What are the limits imposed on patient confidentiality by the legitimate interests of third parties? Are there financial factors that create conflicts of interest in clinical decisions? Are there problems of allocation of scarce health resources that might affect clinical decisions? Are there religious issues that might affect clinical decisions? What are the legal issues that might affect clinical decisions? Are there considerations of clinical research and education that might affect clinical decisions? Are there issues of public health and safety that affect clinical decisions? Are there conflicts of interest within institutions or organizations (e.g. hospitals) that may affect clinical decisions and patient welfare?

From *Clinical ethics* (7th ed.), by A. R. Jonsen, M. Siegler, and W. Winslade, 2010, New York: McGraw-Hill. Copyright 2010 by McGraw-Hill. Reprinted with permission.

b. Ethical values and principles always take precedence over nonethical ones.
c. It is proper to violate an ethical principle only when it is clearly necessary to advance another true ethical principle that, according to the decision-maker's conscience, will produce the greatest balance of good in the long run.

11. Critical thinking as a decision-making model: Paul and Elder, directors of the Foundation for Critical Thinking, defined critical thinking as "the art of analyzing and evaluating thinking with a view to improving it"; it is "self-directed, self-disciplined, self-monitored, and self-corrective thinking [that] requires rigorous standards of excellence and mindful command of their use" (Paul & Elder, 2006, p. 4). They proposed that critical thinkers do the following:
    a. Ask clear, pertinent questions and identify key problems.
    b. Analyze and interpret relevant information by using abstract thinking.
    c. Generate reasonable conclusions and solutions that are tested according to sensible criteria and standards.
    d. Remain open minded to consider alternative thought systems.
    e. Solve complex problems by communicating effectively with other people.
12. Nursing process as a decision-making model: Identify the problem, gather data, identify options, make a decision, act, and assess (Ellis &

Table 4-3. Four Aspects of Moral Action and Interfering Factors

Rest's Processes (1982)	Practical Implications	Interfering Factors
1. Interpretation of the situation	AP's understanding of the inherently ethical nature of any practice situation Assessment of this particular situation and what is needed	Personal troubles Energy level Time available Knowledge level No understanding of the inherently moral nature of practice Lack of connection with the client or inability to engage Perception or sensitivity affected by age and life experiences Lack of self-reflection
2. Discerning the morally ideal action (what should be done)	Using appropriate tools, methods, and resources for decision making Identifying the beneficiary, goal, and appropriate actions	Level of moral development Level of independence Level and types of education Personal values conflict with client's, significant other's, or other professionals' values Lack of reflection on practice
3. Deciding what to do	Deciding between competing courses of action What should be done may not always be possible or consensus may not be reachable	Situational ambiguity Theoretical ambiguity Uncertainty about outcome Lack of institutional or peer support
4. Implementation and perseverance	Envisioning steps and anticipating problems Addressing and overcoming problems and barriers Taking sociopolitical actions to get what is needed Keeping sight of the goal Reminding others of the goal	Too many obstacles Fear of personal consequences, peer or colleague disapproval Fatigue Frustration Lack of resources and supports

From *Nursing ethics and professional responsibility in advanced practice* (pp. 60–62), by P. J. Grace, 2009, Sudbury, MA: Jones & Bartlett.

Figure 4-6. Reflective Equilibrium at Work

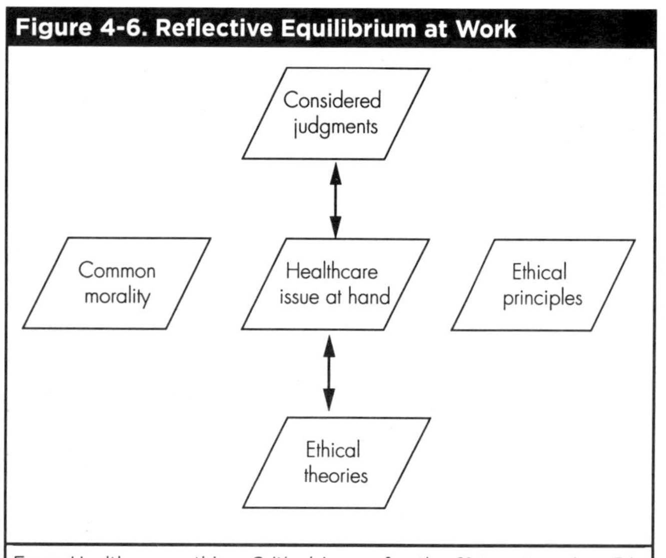

From Health care ethics: *Critical issues for the 21st century* (pp. 54–55; 2nd ed.), by E. E. Morrison, 2008, Sudbury, MA: Jones & Bartlett.

Hartley, 2007). The nursing process is a systematic, rational method of planning and providing individualized nursing care. The nursing process is based on a nursing theory developed by Ida Jean Orlando in the late 1950s as she observed nurses in action.

13. An *ethics committee* is an interdisciplinary group of healthcare professionals established specifically to address ethical dilemmas that occur in a particular setting. The group may include members of the community and people with formal ethics education and ethics consultation core competencies (Fletcher, Spencer, & Lombardo, 2005).
    a. Functions
        1) Provides a forum for ethical dialogue between people with ethical concerns

2) Ensures the presence of all stakeholders involved in the ethics issue, including client or surrogate
3) Provides education on ethical options; does not provide second medical opinion or render judgment about what actions should be taken
4) Is available to all areas of the institution, not just clinical areas
5) Reviews requests for ethics help for nonethics-related concerns and assists requester with appropriate referral to, for example, legal, compliance, and quality-improvement specialists
6) Is available for policy review for ethics content

b. Functions of a nursing ethics subcommittee (Marquis & Huston, 2009)
1) Addresses unique concerns of nursing
2) Helps nurses identify, explore, and resolve ethical issues in practice
3) Provides education and staff development
4) Develops and follows a defined model of critical thinking
5) Reviews departmental policies related to ethics

c. Ethics committees generally follow one or a combination of three distinct models or structures in ethical decision making.
1) The autonomy model facilitates decision making for the client who has capacity.
2) The client benefit model uses substituted judgment or best interest and facilitates decision making for a client who lacks maturity (e.g., a child) or one who lacks cognitive capacity.
3) The social justice model considers broad social issues and is accountable to the institution and society.

14. Other ethical decision-making models (see Figure 4-2)

D. Factors Influencing Actions in Decision Making
1. Individual beliefs, values, or philosophy
2. Sensitivity to cultural diversity and implementation of actions regarding respect for autonomy
3. Balancing medical and rehabilitative needs that present moral quandaries
4. Team contributions to decision making with regard to services for clients and clients' progress and outcomes
5. Definitions of quality-of-life issues
6. Resource allocation and cost effectiveness
a. Access to rehabilitative services regardless of the client's disability or funding level
b. Clinical decisions made by for-profit managed-care organizations
7. Laws and legal considerations for providing rehabilitation services
8. Standards and regulations imposed by various entities
a. Professional codes of behavior or codes of conduct
b. Institutional policies, including organizational codes of conduct and corporate compliance
9. Client decisions whether to adhere to recommended regimens as defined by the rehabilitation team
10. Clinical judgment in nursing as a nonlinear process of using knowledge, reasoning, experiential skills, and interpersonal skills to determine probable best actions (Butts & Rich, 2008; Grace, 2009) (**Table 4-4**).
11. Management and leadership that promotes ethical conduct by adherence to the following guidelines (Rice & Perry, 2013, pp. 38–44):
a. Establish ethical standards, expectations, and a written code of conduct, and reevaluate the code to ensure it is current with ethical demands.
b. Hire ethical people, presenting ethical dilemmas as part of the interview process.
c. Cultivate relationships to obtain honest feedback regarding professional conduct.
d. Serve as role models of ethical standards.
e. Complete an ethics self-assessment, and address areas that need improvement.
f. Establish an ethics committee to address both clinical and business ethics issues.
g. Require ethics training and education of all employees and staff.
h. Ensure compliance with ethical standards with reprimands and rewards.
i. Create an ethical environment with fair and equitable personnel practices.
j. Address impairment in the workplace with education, counseling, or other means.
k. Integrate patients' rights into operations, including patient advocacy and customer service programs.
l. Adopt a framework for ethical decision making consistent with the mission, vision, and values of the organization.

E. Ethical Conflict
1. Types of ethical conflicts (Fletcher et al., 2005)

Table 4-4. Clinical Judgment in Nursing

Definition: *Clinical judgment in nursing* is the nonlinear process of using knowledge, reasoning, tacit (experiential) skills, and interpersonal skills to determine—within the limits of available information—probable best actions given the inevitable existence of uncertainty about the possession of adequate knowledge and outcome of actions.

Components	Categories
Knowledge	The knowledge base of nursing • Nature of the discipline • Purposes and goals • Nature of people and environment • Characteristics of good practitioners • Scope and limits of practice Knowledge derived from other disciplines: philosophical (including ethical theory), physical, social, psychological, spiritual, biological Knowledge related to the situation • Primary subject (who is involved) • Subject's understanding of the situation, values, beliefs, and context • Goals
Experience	Previous experiences • Personal • Professional
Characteristics and skills	Perceptual • Grasp the nature and complexity of issues • Identification of needed and potential resources • Envision resolution • Reflection on practice and self-reflection • Creative, articulate Relational • Interpersonal • Collaborative • Mediation Motivation • Professional responsibility • Emotional engagement

From *Nursing ethics and professional responsibility in advanced practice* (p. 110), by P. J. Grace, 2009, Sudbury, MA: Jones & Bartlett. Copyright 2009 by Jones & Bartlett. Reprinted with permission.

   a. Conflicts of widely accepted moral duties or obligations
   b. Threats to important relationships
   c. Collisions of moral principles
   d. Collisions of values
   e. Conflicts of interest
2. *Ethical dilemma* is having to choose between two equally difficult actions because they are both right, both wrong, or both contain uncertainty (Butts & Rich, 2008).
3. Moral distress can occur in institutional ethics, professional practice, and clinical decision making.
   a. The state of being unable to follow the right course of action due to institutional barriers (Jameton, 1984)
   b. A moral decision has been made that cannot be acted on because of real or perceived limitations, such as moral constraint.
   c. The moral residue and crescendo effect describes the repeating of a moral distress being greater with a previously remembered moral distress (Epstein & Hamric, 2009).
4. *Moral residue* is that which remains when moral distress remains unresolved, resulting in increased job turnover and nurses leaving the workforce (Webster & Baylis, 2000).
5. Obstacles to ethical nursing care (Grace, 2014)
   a. Obstacles related to the individual patient
      1) Standardized patient care
      2) Bias toward or prejudgment of patient
      3) Interpersonal conflict, including conflicts involving provider-patient, patient-family, provider-provider
      4) Poor communication
      5) Power imbalances resulting in coercion or silencing
      6) Inadequate time or resources to evaluate and address needs
   b. Obstacles in the practice environment

1) Lack of primary focus on the good of the patient, including economic conflicts of interest
2) Autonomous practice constraints imposed by institutional mission, managed-care mandates, or other regulatory policies or agencies

c. Social injustices
1) Access and financing issues, including profit motive or fragmented services
2) Differing priorities
3) Socioeconomic disparities

F. Ethical Principles and Rights

1. Ethical principles: The relationship of ethical principles to situations encountered in the rehabilitation nursing practice or sphere of concern reflects issues common to rehabilitation settings (Hoeman, 2008) (**Table 4-5**).
a. *Autonomy*: Individual actions are independent of the actions and will of others.
b. *Nonmaleficence*: The concept of doing no harm
c. *Beneficence*: The concept of doing good for another
d. *Advocacy*: Championing the needs and interests of another
e. *Veracity*: Responsibility to speak the truth
f. *Fiduciary* (financial) responsibility: Ensuring there is sufficient benefit for the expense incurred
g. *Care*: Providing for and meeting the needs of others for compassion, empathy, and good
h. *Sanctity of life*: Value of life
i. *Quality of life*: Correlation between life and participation in activities and interests
j. *Consent*: Voluntary agreement
k. *Confidentiality*: Responsibility to keep information private
l. *Competence*: Ability or legal right to make appropriate decisions
m. *Values*: Positive qualities held by an object or outcome

2. *Rights* are the basis of professional, regulatory, and legal codes and judgments; they reflect the things society believes a person is entitled to. Rights can conflict with values (Ellis & Hartley, 2007; Masters-Farrell, 2006).
a. Self-determination rights: The Patient Self-Determination Act (1990), or the Danforth amendment, requires that clients be given an opportunity to decide on life support options on admission to any healthcare service. Organizations must supply documentation and education to support informed choice.
b. Patient rights: The American Hospital Association published "A Patient's Bill of Rights" in 1973, with a focus on confidentiality, privacy, and informed consent. Updated in 1992, it began to reflect the responsibilities of healthcare providers and reinforce the concept of collaborative care. In 2003, the document was rewritten and titled "The Patient Care Partnership," encouraging clients to be involved in their care and to ask questions (The American Hospital Association, 2003). The Joint Commission (2009) and the Commission on Accreditation of Rehabilitation Facilities (2013) require that clients receive information about their rights. The Joint Commission has expanded these rights to include the right to effective pain management. A federally mandated patient rights program is also under consideration. It includes the following rights:
1) The right to receive considerate and respectful care
2) The right to obtain relevant, current, and understandable information about diagnosis, treatment, and prognosis
3) The right to make decisions about the plan of care
4) The right to have advance directives about treatment
5) The right to privacy in all aspects of care
6) The right to expect that all communication and records will be treated confidentially
7) The right to review records pertaining to care
8) The right to expect reasonable responses to requests for appropriate and medically indicated care and services
9) The right to be informed about business relationships that could influence treatment and care
10) The right to consent to or decline participation in proposed research studies
11) The right to expect reasonable continuity of care
12) The right to be informed about hospital policies and practices that relate to client care, treatment, and responsibility

G. Professional Ethics Codes, Standards, and Statements

1. The ethical standard for the profession of nursing is established in the *Code of Ethics for Nurses: Provisions* (ANA, 2006). The ANA's *Code of Ethics for Nurses with Interpretive Statements* was developed as a guide for carrying out nursing responsibilities in a manner consistent with quality in nursing

Table 4-5. Relationship of Ethical Principles to Situations Encountered in Rehabilitation Nursing Practice or Sphere of Concern		
Ethical Principle	**Description**	**Examples**
Autonomy	An individual's actions are independent from the actions and the will of others. Individuals have the ability to form their own perspectives on right, wrong, and values.	Rehabilitation nurses must acknowledge that individuals for whom they care have freedom regarding their bodies and actions. Nurses may provide education on wellness and health promotion, but compliance with programs cannot be forced. Clients have autonomy in their healthcare programs.
Nonmaleficence	The concept of doing no harm	Rehabilitation nurses, like all healthcare practitioners, have a duty to do no harm to a client. To intentionally administer a lethal dose of medication to a client is an example of violation of the ethical principle of nonmaleficence. It is unthinkable for a nurse to intentionally harm a client.
Beneficence	The concept of doing good for another.	Nursing care is based on the concept of beneficence. Rehabilitation nurses intend to do good for others. The motivation that drives rehabilitation nurses to go the extra distance in care of their clients is an example of beneficence.
Advocacy	Loyalty: Championing the needs and interests of another	Rehabilitation nurses are in an ideal position to advocate for their clients. Nurses often see clients on a 24-hour basis and have an awareness for and appreciation of clients' abilities and energy levels that other disciplines may not. It is critical that such information be shared with team members in a way to advocate for the best plans for clients.
Veracity	Responsibility to speak the truth	Nurses have an obligation to speak truthfully in all aspects of their role.
Financial responsibility (cost-benefit analysis)	Stewardship: Ensuring there is sufficient benefit for the expense provided	There is an ethical responsibility to meet the client's needs as well as possible while using as few resources as possible. For example, extending lengths of stay in hospitals, home health care, and subacute programs when a cllient is capable of being discharged to a lesser level of care is not in line with the nurse's financial responsibility of care.
Care	Providing for and meeting the needs of others for compassion, empathy, and good	Care is a component of the rehabilitation nurse's role, regardless of setting.
Sanctity of life	Value of life, right to life	Rehabilitation nurses have an obligation to care for all clients, regardless of the extent of disability or potential for recovery, because all life is of value.
Quality of life	Condition of one's life, based on assessment of correlation between life and participation in valued activities and interests	Quality of life is a frequent question for individuals with devastating disabilities and chronic illnesses. Rehabilitation nurses can assist individuals and families in reframing situations to find quality of life in remaining abilities.
Consent	Voluntary agreement with a procedure, process, or treatment	The role of the rehabilitation nurse in informed consent is key. Because clients often confide in nurses, the rehabilitation nurse is in a position to validate understanding of a procedure, treatment, or course of therapy. As an advocate, the rehabilitation nurse supports the client's abilities to make decisions and participate in his or her plans of care.
Confidentiality	Responsibility to keep information private	Rehabilitation nurses are entrusted with substantial amounts of private information. Such information must be kept confidential, to be shared only as related to the nursing care and needs of the client.
Competence	The ability or legal right to make appropriate decisions	The need for rehabilitation sometimes follows a disability or illness that affects the clarity of the client's decision-making ability. This should not be confused with legal competence.
Values	Worthwhile or positive qualities held by an object or outcome; these should be chosen carefully but freely	The question of the value of life after a disability or chronic illness is sometimes placed in question. Rehabilitation nurses recognize the value of independence and of reframing prior values to achieve higher levels of life satisfaction.

From *Principles of normative ethics*, by D. Ursery, 2005, Austin, TX: St. Edwards University. Copyright 2005 by D. Ursery. Reprinted with permission.

care and the ethical obligations of the profession (ANA, 2010). The *Code of Ethics* provides a framework for nurses to use in ethical analysis and decision making. It establishes the ethical standard for the profession. It is not negotiable in any setting, nor is it subject to revision or amendment except by formal process of the ANA House of Delegates (ANA, 2010).

a. Provision 1: The nurse, in all professional relationships, practices with compassion and respect for the inherent dignity, worth, and uniqueness of every individual, unrestricted by considerations of social or economic status, personal attributes, or the nature of health problems.
b. Provision 2: The nurse's primary commitment is to the patient, which can be an individual, family, group, or community, and includes the significance of nurse-patient boundaries.
c. Provision 3: The nurse promotes, advocates for, and strives to protect the health, safety, and rights of the patient, including the nurse-patient relationship, to privacy and confidentiality.
d. Provision 4: The nurse is responsible and accountable for individual nursing practice and determines the appropriate delegation of tasks consistent with the nurse's obligation to provide optimum patient care.
e. Provision 5: The nurse owes the same duties to self as to others, including the responsibility to preserve integrity and safety, to maintain competence, and to continue personal and professional growth.
f. Provision 6: The nurse participates in establishing, maintaining, and improving healthcare environments and conditions of employment conducive to the provision of quality health care and consistent with the values of the profession through individual and collective action.
g. Provision 7: The nurse participates in the advancement of the profession through contributions to practice, education, administration, and knowledge development.
h. Provision 8: The nurse collaborates with other health professionals and the public in promoting community, national, and international efforts to meet health needs.
i. Provision 9: The profession of nursing, as represented by associations and their members, is responsible for articulating nursing values, maintaining the integrity of the profession and its practice, and shaping social policy.

2. The American Nurses Association's *Scope and Standards of Practice* (2004) acknowledges that the nurse's decisions and actions on behalf of clients are determined in an ethical manner. Standard V: Ethics measurement criteria are as follows:
   a. The nurse's practice is guided by *The Code for Nurses* and related ANA position statements, such as the *Position Statement on Nurses' Participation in Capital Punishment.*
   b. The nurse maintains client confidentiality.
   c. The nurse acts as a client advocate.
   d. The nurse delivers care in a nonjudgmental and nondiscriminatory manner that is sensitive to client diversity.
   e. The nurse delivers care in a manner that preserves and protects client autonomy, dignity, and rights.
   f. The nurse seeks available resources to help formulate ethical decisions.
3. ARN (2000, 2008) supported these standards and incorporated them into the *Standards and Scope of Rehabilitation Nursing Practice* (**Figure 4-7**). ARN contributes additional comments about standards of ethical rehabilitation nursing practice in its *Position Statement on Ethical Issues* (Pilkington & Strong, 2003). This statement presents concerns of rehabilitation nurses.
   a. ARN identified ethical issues applicable to those practicing rehabilitation nursing:
      1) Clients' rights, including the rights of minors. Minors may or may not be capable of understanding the decisions made in their name by their parents. If a minor was not involved in the decision-making process and does not agree with his or her parents' decision, the minor may have no recourse, a fact that can lead to an ethical and legal conflict
      2) The use of restraints
      3) Do-not-resuscitate orders
      4) Advance directives, which imply nursing intervention and responsibility regarding living wills and durable power of attorney
      5) Management of clients who are disposed to self destructive behaviors or suicidal gestures
      6) Issues related to healthcare reform and changes in how health care is allocated and delivered, including providing access to health care and rehabilitation, containing costs; ensuring quality of health care;

Figure 4-7. ARN Standards Regarding Ethics

Standard V. Ethics: The rehabilitation nurse's decisions and actions on behalf of clients are determined in an ethical manner.

- The rehabilitation nurse's practice is guided by *Code for Nurses with Interpretive Statements* (ANA, 2001) and by ARN's position statement on ethical issues (ARN, 2003)
- The rehabilitation nurse maintains a client's confidentiality within legal and regulatory parameters.
- The rehabilitation nurse advocates for patients and helps them develop skills so they can advocate for themselves.
- The rehabilitation nurse delivers care in a nonjudgmental and nondiscriminatory manner that is sensitive to patient diversity and supports patients' values.
- The rehabilitation nurse delivers care in a manner that preserves and protects patient autonomy, dignity, and rights.
- The rehabilitation nurse seeks available resources to formulate ethical decisions.
- The rehabilitation nurse maintains an awareness of his or her beliefs and value systems and the effect they may have on the care he or she provides to the patient and family.
- The rehabilitation nurse supports the patient's right to make decisions that may not be congruent with the values of the rehabilitation team, including those related to end-of-life care, and advocates for those rights with the team and the healthcare system..
- The rehabilitation nurse promotes the provision of information and discussion that allows the patient to participate fully in decision making.
- The rehabilitation nurse participates in decision making regarding allocation of resources.
- The rehabilitation nurse participates on interprofessional team.
- The rehabilitation nurse informs administrators of the risks, benefits, and outcomes of programs and decision that affect healthcare delivery.

From *Standards and scope of rehabilitation nursing practice* (6th ed.), by ARN, 2014. Chicago: ARN. Copyright 2014 by ARN.

determining length of stay, defining who meets the criteria for rehabilitation, dealing with clients' noncompliance with treatment and rehabilitation, teaching the client and family in preparation for discharge to home or another level of care, and discharging clients to a level of care in which appropriate skills are brought to bear for their needs

7) Confidentiality, security, and privacy related to client care
8) Substance abuse
9) Abused clients
10) The nurse-client relationship (e.g., when is intimacy between the nurse and the client appropriate or inappropriate?)

b. The Association of Rehabilitation Nurses' (2014b) *Position Statement: Ethical Issues* supports the ANA's *Code of Ethics for Nurses with Interpretive Statements* (ANA, 2001) and the American Hospital Association's *The Patient Care Partnership* (2003) as important guides for ethical decision making. ARN makes the following additional statements:

1) The rehabilitation nurse acts as a patient advocate.
2) The rehabilitation nurse recognizes the importance of the patient's participation in the decision-making process and realizes that some patients do not and will not value independence and wellness as much as the rehabilitation professional does.
3) The rehabilitation nurse is concerned about the rehabilitation patient's quality of life as defined by the patient, if advanced medical technology is compromising it. Advanced medical technology may prolong life but not improve its quality.
4) The rehabilitation nurse is responsible for providing information or assisting with the collection and interpretation of information that is necessary to resolve major ethical dilemmas and assist in the patient's decision-making process.
5) The rehabilitation nurse stays informed about ethical issues that might affect rehabilitation patients and is aware of his or her own values and attitudes.
6) The rehabilitation nurse practices with compassion and respect for the dignity and worth of every individual in a nonjudgmental and nondiscriminatory manner.
7) The rehabilitation nurse bases his or her decisions on the ethical principles of autonomy, beneficence, justice, and nonmaleficence.
8) The rehabilitation nurse participates in research and realizes that the benefits of research and human experimentation can be offset by certain threats to human rights. To protect these rights when a patient participates in research, the nurse considers the issues of informed consent, criteria for inclusion and retention of subjects, training of researchers, research dissemination, ethical supervision and accountability, and provision for subjects' privacy and the confidentiality of results and findings.
9) The rehabilitation nurse participates in decision making regarding allocation of resources used by or for the patient.

c. Regarding the rights of patients, ARN holds the following beliefs (ARN, 2014b).
   1) All people have the right to receive rehabilitation services regardless of their age, race, gender, ethnicity, religion, or economic status.
   2) All patients have the right to receive full resuscitation, request do-not-resuscitate orders, request the discontinuation of life-support measures, or refuse recommended treatment, as long as they fully understand what they are requesting.
   3) All patients' medications used to improve their ability to participate in rehabilitation will be accompanied by a defined plan of care with a targeted outcome.
   4) All patients have the right to expect modification to their environment to promote their safety. If environmental modifications prove unsuccessful, patients have the right to expect that the least restrictive restraint device be used to prevent risk of harm. Use of environmental modifications or restraints will be accompanied by a defined plan of care targeted at restraint reduction outcomes.
   5) All patients have the right to expect the patient education process to include health information and instruction that is applicable to the patient's care needs, as well as information needed to make decisions about discharge plans. These decisions can include resources for discharge to home or another level of care.

4. The International Council of Nurses' (ICN's) *The ICN Code of Ethics for Nurses* (2006) is a guide for action based on social values and needs. The code has served as the standard for nurses worldwide since it was adopted in 1953.
   a. According to *The ICN Code of Ethics,* nurses have four fundamental responsibilities:
      1) To promote health
      2) To prevent illness
      3) To restore health
      4) To alleviate suffering
   b. ICN (2006) stated the following:
      The need for nursing is universal. Inherent in nursing is respect for human rights, including cultural rights, the right to life and choice, to dignity, and to be treated with respect. Nursing care is respectful of and unrestricted by considerations of age, color, creed, culture, disability or illness, gender, sexual orientation, nationality, politics, race or social status. Nurses render health services to the individual, the family and the community and coordinate their services with those of related groups (p. 3). Elements of the ICN's *Code of Ethics* are
      1) Nurses and people
      2) Nurses and practice
      3) Nurses and the profession
      4) Nurses and coworkers

5. The Nuremberg Code specifies 10 basic requirements for medical experimentation (Hoeman, 2008) (**Figure 4-8**).

Figure 4-8. Nuremberg Code (Paraphrased)

1. Informed, voluntary consent of the subject is essential.
2. The study must be expected to have a result that will be of benefit to others.
3. The study must be based on an understanding of pathophysiology of the disease or problem or on prior animal studies.
4. Suffering of subjects will be prevented during the study.
5. Death or disability is not expected or predicted as a result of the study.
6. The degree of risk does not outweigh the potential good to be gained.
7. Subjects will be protected and safeguarded against problems that may occur during the study.
8. Researchers will have the appropriate credentials to complete the research.
9. Subjects may withdraw from studies if they cannot continue.
10. Researchers will stop the study if at any time they deem it in the best interests of the subjects to discontinue the study.

From *Rehabilitation nursing: Prevention, intervention, and outcomes* (p. 38), by S. Hoeman, 2007, St. Louis: Mosby Elsevier. Copyright 2007 by Mosby. Reprinted with permission.

   a. The Nuremberg Code was conceptualized and formulated to protect human rights. It codified crucial considerations, important safeguards, and guidelines related to research design, conduct, and human subject protections, including that research results should be likely to benefit humanity in some way; coercion of subjects to participate is forbidden; likely results should justify any risks; and risks should be minimized, including mental or physical suffering, which is not permissible (Grace, 2009).
   b. The National Institutes of Health specify the guidelines for clinical research involving human subjects, codified in Title 45, Code of Federal Regulations, Part 46 (National Institutes of Health, 2004).

II. Legal Issues and Considerations (Ellis & Hartley, 2007)

A. Laws: Laws govern the scope of nursing practice and delivery of care; protect licensure; define specifics of provision, access to services, and reimbursement; and finance education and research. Laws also provide the forum to test ethical issues related to healthcare dilemmas in rehabilitation (Hoeman, 2008).

1. The National Institute on Disability and Rehabilitation Research (2006) proposed a long-range plan for disability-related funding for 2005–2009 to support people with disabilities.
2. The No Child Left Behind Program and New Freedom Initiative
3. The Office of Special Education Programs offers support in special education, vocational rehabilitation, and research.
4. The Center for International Rehabilitation Research Information and Exchange facilitates the sharing of information between rehabilitation researchers in the U.S. and those in other countries.
5. The Americans with Disabilities (ADA) Act of 1990 (effective July 26, 1992) defined *disability* as a physical or mental impairment that substantially limits one or more major life activities. A record of a physical or mental impairment, or a patient who is regarded as having such an impairment, can also constitute a disability.
6. The Equal Employment Opportunity Commission issued guidelines for complying with the Americans with Disabilities law.

B. Summaries of Disability Laws (Hoeman, 2008) (**Figure 4-9**)

1. Employment
2. State and local government programs and services
3. Housing
4. Education
5. Travel and transportation
6. Technology and telecommunications

C. Other Legal Considerations

1. The Patient Self-Determination Act of 1990 requires that people receiving medical care be given written information about their right to make decisions about end-of-life issues.
2. Living wills and life-prolonging declarations allow people to make their wishes known before hospitalization regarding medical care, illness, or conditions resulting in incompetence.
3. A durable power of attorney enables a competent person to appoint a surrogate decision maker who is empowered to act legally for the client.
4. The Health Insurance Portability and Accountability Act of 1996 requires confidentiality.
5. Guardianship is a position of responsibility granted to a person by the court to make decisions about an incapacitated person's life.
6. Competency is determined by the court based on clinical opinions of a person's mental or cognitive fitness.
7. Informed consent is based on a full description of the risks and consequences of agreeing or refusing to have an operation or procedure.
8. Estate planning involves long-term planning for future care and expenses.
9. Legal death or brain death is based on the legal parameters defining the time at which life ceases.
10. Withholding or withdrawing treatment
11. Do-not-resuscitate orders allow people to indicate in advance that they do not want to be resuscitated in the event of cardiac or respiratory arrest.
12. Research on human subjects (Macrina, 2005)
    a. Basic rules and requirements for research studies can be found in various codes and regulations and focus on issues of informed consent.
    b. Participants should understand the purpose of the research and what is expected of them.
    c. Participants should be competent to decide to participate.
    d. Participants have the right to have their questions answered before they participate.
    e. Participants should be free to withdraw from the study at any time without fear of reprisal.

III. Ethical, Legal, and Moral Issues in Practice (Table 4-6)

A. Diagnosis and Prognosis: An Example

1. Cognition is altered.
2. The client lacks decision-making capacity and needs a surrogate decision maker.
3. Cognition may improve, eliminating the need for a surrogate.

B. Collaborative Decision Making and Effective Communication

1. Includes the client and family or social support, with the client's permission
2. Establishes a dialogue to determine cultural and socioeconomic attitudes related to learning, health, and wellness in defining an appropriate level of care
3. Identifies components of life support systems, policies of the healthcare setting, and support resources
4. Involves the entire rehabilitation team in communicating with the client and family and discussing their concerns about progress toward rehabilitation goals and treatment
5. Consults the ethics committee as needed for dilemmas in care delivery

Figure 4-9. Summaries of Disability Law

Employment

Americans with Disabilities Act, Title I: Prohibits discrimination in the workplace against people with disabilities

Section 501, Rehabilitation Act (1973): Requires affirmative action and nondiscrimination in employment by federal agencies of the executive branch

Section 503, Rehabilitation Act: Requires affirmative action and prohibits employment discrimination by federal government contractors and subcontractors with contracts of more than $10,000

Section 188, Workforce Investment Act: Prohibits discrimination against people with disabilities in employment service centers funded by the federal government

State and local government programs and services

Americans with Disabilities Act, Title II: Prohibits discrimination in the provision of public benefits and services (e.g., public education, employment, transportation, recreation, healthcare, social services, courts, voting, and town meetings)

Section 504, Rehabilitation Act: Requires that buildings and facilities that are designed, constructed, or altered with federal funds or leased by a federal agency comply with federal standards for physical accessibility

Housing

Fair Housing Act: Prohibits discrimination in any aspect of selling, renting, or denying housing on the basis of disability. Owners are further required to make reasonable accommodations in their housing policies to afford equal housing opportunities to those with disabilities

Americans with Disabilities Act, Title II: Prohibits discrimination by public housing authorities and other state and local government housing

American with Disabilities Act, Title III: Does not apply to regular privately owned residential dwelling units. However, it does apply to residences that are also public accommodations, such as nursing homes and school dorms. In addition, parts of residential facilities that serve a group of people or the public might be considered public accommodations, such as a swimming pool or a sales and leasing office.

Section 504, Rehabilitation Act: Prohibits discrimination by public housing authorities that receive federal funds, cities and towns that receive Community Development Block Grants or other federal funds, private for-profit or nonprofit housing developers that receive federal funds, and colleges and universities that receive federal funds (student housing)

Architectural Barriers Act: Applies accessibility standards to housing constructed with federal funding

Education

Individuals with Disabilities Education Act (IDEA): Requires public primary and secondary schools to make available to all eligible children with disabilities a free appropriate public education in the least restrictive environment appropriate to their individual needs

Section 504, Rehabilitation Act: Prohibits discrimination against students with disabilities in primary, secondary, or postsecondary schools receiving federal funds

Americans with Disabilities Act, Title II: Prohibits discrimination against students with disabilities in all educational institutions that receive funds from state or local government

Americans with Disabilities Act, Title III: Prohibits discrimination against students with disabilities in private schools

Travel and Transportation

Americans with Disabilities Act, Title II: Prohibits discrimination in transportation provided by state and local government entities such as bus, railway, subway, and other forms of ground transportation

Section 504, Rehabilitation Act: Prohibits discrimination in privately operated transportation services that receive federal funds

Americans with Disabilities Act, Title III: Prohibits discrimination in privately operated transportation such as limousines and hotel shuttle services

Air Carrier Access Act: Prohibits discrimination on the basis of disability in air travel. It applies only to air carriers that provide regularly scheduled services for hire to the public. Requirements address a wide range of issues, including boarding assistance and certain accessibility features in newly-built aircraft and new or altered airport facilities.

Technology and Telecommunications

Section 508, Rehabilitation Act: Requires federal agencies to make their electronic and information technology accessible to people with disabilities

Americans with Disabilities Act, Title IV: Requires telephone companies to establish telecommunication relay services for callers with hearing and speech disabilities. Title IV also requires closed captioning of federally funded public service announcements.

Section 255, Telecommunications Act: Requires manufacturers of telecommunication equipment and providers of telecommunication services to ensure that such equipment and services are accessible to and usable by people with disabilities and that people with disabilities have access to a broad range of products and services such as telephones, cell phones, pagers, call waiting, and operator services

From *Rehabilitation nursing: Prevention, intervention, and outcomes* (4th ed., p. 41), by S. Hoeman, 2007, St. Louis: Mosby Elsevier.

Table 4-6. Distinction Between Law and Ethics		
Concepts	**Law**	**Ethics**
Source	External to oneself; rules and regulations of society	Internal to oneself; values, beliefs, and individual interpretations
Concerns	Conduct and actions; what person did or failed to do	Motives, attitudes, and culture; why one acted as one did
Interests	Society as a whole as opposed to the individual within the society	Good of the individual within society as opposed to all of society
Enforcement	Courts, statutes, and boards of nursing	Ethics committees and professional organizations

C. Appropriate Level of Care Delivery
   1. Acute care, inpatient rehabilitation, long-term care, outpatient services, or home care services
   2. Involves making decisions based on the client's needs and available resources

D. Allocation of Resources
   1. *Microallocation*: Services are allocated for a specific client's care.
   2. *Macroallocation*: Distribution of available services across a client population
   3. Cost containment or cost effectiveness of care delivery
   4. Transparency of allocations
   5. Rationing of financial, clinical, or other resources
   6. Access based on need, ability to pay, and an identified discharge plan

E. Ethical Rehabilitation
   1. The client or surrogate by proxy participates in developing the plan of care.
   2. Independence and wellness are valued.
   3. Improvement in functional status and self-worth are key rehabilitation goals.
   4. Rehabilitation nurses are members of the interdisciplinary rehabilitation team and collaborate with other team members.
   5. The client is assessed for physical pain, and pain is treated.
   6. The client is assessed for emotional pain or depression, and treatment is provided.
   7. Rehabilitation services are delivered in the most appropriate setting in the shortest amount of time based on the needs of the client and available resources.

F. Team Issues
   1. The client is a member of the rehabilitation team and at the center of care.
   2. Measurable and objective goals are developed in collaboration with the client or surrogate.
   3. Team members demonstrate respect for each other and for the contribution each member makes.
   4. The team consults the ethics committee as needed for dilemmas in care delivery.

G. Ethical Issues Related to Alternative and Complementary Medicine and Therapies
   1. The client's right to choose and request alternative and complementary medicine and therapies
   2. Availability of alternative or complementary medicine and therapies
   3. Possible interactions between alternative or complementary medicine and traditional Western medicine

H. Ethics of Caring (Gergen, 2009; Gilligan, 1995)
   1. Care and services are delivered and received in the context of relationships.
   2. Relationships are reciprocal and occur in an environment of trust and transparency.
   3. Relationships exist between rehabilitation nurses and other team members, including the client or surrogate and the healthcare institution.

I. Ethical Foundations of Healthcare Reform (Butts & Rich, 2008; Cerise & Chokshi, 2009)
   1. Universal access: The client has access to health care regardless of the ability to pay.
   2. Comprehensive benefits: Care and services are provided across the healthcare continuum.
   3. Choice: Clients have choices about providers, plans, and treatments. They are informed about the risks and benefits of available treatments and are free to choose between them, or refuse treatment according to individual preferences and medical appropriateness.
   4. Equity of care: Care is based on need rather than individual or group characteristics.
   5. Fair distribution of costs: Costs and burdens of care are spread across the entire community, basing the individual contribution on ability to pay.
   6. Personal responsibility: Individuals assume responsibility for protecting and promoting health and contributing to the cost of care based on ability to pay.
   7. Age-based distribution: The unique needs of each stage of life are acknowledged, with the benefits and burdens shared fairly across generations.

8. Allocation of resources: The nation should balance prudently the amount it spends on health care against other important national priorities, including quality of life issues.
9. Effectiveness: The new system should deliver care and innovations that work and are desired by clients. It should encourage the discovery of improved and advanced treatments. It should enable the academic community and healthcare providers to exercise their responsibility to evaluate and improve health care by providing resources for the systematic study of healthcare outcomes.
10. Quality: The system should deliver high-quality care and provide people with the information necessary to make informed healthcare choices.
11. Effective management: By encouraging simplification and continuous improvement and making the system easier to use for clients and providers, the healthcare system focuses on care rather than administration.
12. Professional integrity and responsibility: The healthcare system should treat the clinical judgments of professionals with respect and protect the integrity of the provider-client relationship, while ensuring that health providers have the resources to fulfill their responsibilities for the effective delivery of high-quality care.
13. Fair procedures: To protect these values and principles, fair and open democratic procedures should underlie decisions about the operation of the healthcare system and the resolution of disputes that arise within it.
14. Local responsibility: The healthcare system should allow states and local communities to design effective, high-quality systems of care that serve all their citizens.

J. End-of-Life Issues
1. Cardiopulmonary resuscitation and do-not-resuscitate orders
2. Advance directives
3. Dying at home
4. Decisions to limit treatments
5. Withholding of nutrition and fluids
6. Palliative care
7. Euthanasia and assisted suicide

IV. Future Considerations and Directions

A. Genetic Research
1. Decoding genes that are responsible for specific diseases
2. Gene therapy
3. Genetic engineering
4. Use of genetic information
5. Cloning
6. Sharing of genetic information with all who are affected

B. Beginning-of-Life Issues
1. Abortion
2. Newborns with severe defects
3. Fetal tissue experimentation
4. Genetic counseling
5. Genetic manipulation
6. Surrogacy

C. End-of-Life Versus Quality-of-Life Issues
1. Technology advances, treatment options, and outcomes, including quality
2. Euthanasia and assisted suicide

D. Legislation Issues
1. Resource allocations for rehabilitation services across the continuum of care
2. Defining appropriate levels of cares and access to needed care.

References

Aiken, T., & Catalano, J. (1994). *Legal, ethical, and political issues in nursing*. Philadelphia: F.A. Davis Company.

American Hospital Association (AHA). (2003). *The patient care partnership* [Brochure]. Retrieved from http://www.aha.org/advocacy-issues/communicatingpts/pt-care-partnership.shtml

American Nurses Association (ANA). (1985). *Code for nurses with interpretive statements*. Washington, DC: Author.

American Nurses Association (ANA). (2001). *Code of ethics for nurses with interpretive statements*. Washington, DC: American Nurses Publishing.

American Nurses Association (ANA). (2004). *Nursing: Scope and standards of practice*. Silver Spring, MD: Author.

American Nurses Association (ANA). (2006). *Code of ethics for nurses: Provisions*. Washington, DC: Author.

American Nurses Association (ANA). (2010). *Code of ethics for nurses with interpretive statements*. Silver Spring, MD: Author. Retrieved from http://www.nursingworld.org/MainMenuCategoreis/EthicsStandards/CodeofEthicsforNurses/Code-of-Ethics.pdf

Association of Rehabilitation Nurses (ARN). (2000). *Standards and scope of rehabilitation nursing practice* (4th ed.). Glenview, IL: Author.

Association of Rehabilitation Nurses (ARN). (2003). *ARN position statement on ethical issues*. Glenview, IL: Author.

Association of Rehabilitation Nurses (ARN). (2008). *Standards and scope of rehabilitation nursing practice* (5th ed.). Glenview, IL: Author.

Association of Rehabilitation Nurses (ARN). (2014a). ARN competency model for professional rehabilitation nursing. Retrieved from http://www.rehabnurse.org/uploads/files/education/ARN_Rehabilitation_Nursing_Competency _Model_FINAL_-_May_2014.pdf

Association of Rehabilitation Nurses (ARN). (2014b). Position statement: Ethical issues. Retrieved from http://www.rehabnurse.org/advocacy/content/Position-Statement-Ethical-Issues.html

Barrocas, A., Yarbrough, G., Bechnel, P., & Nelson, J. E. (2003). Ethical and legal issues in nutrition support of the geriatric patient: The can, should, and must of nutrition support. *Nutrition in Clinical Practice, 18*(1), 37–47.

Beauchamp, R. L., & Childress, J. F. (2001). *Principles of biomedical ethics* (5th ed.). New York: Oxford University Press.

Bergum, V., & Dossetor, J. (2005). *Relational ethics: The full meaning of respect*. Hagerstown, MD: University Publishing Group.

Blanchard, K., & Peale, N. (1988). *The power of ethical management*. New York: William Morrow.

Brillhart, B. A. (1999). Ethics in rehabilitation nursing. *Rehabilitation Nursing, 20*(1), 44–47.

Brock, L., & Mastroianni, A. (2008). Law and medical ethics. University of Washington School of Medicine, Attorney General. Retrieved from http://depts.washington.edu/bioethx/topics/law.html

Butts, J., & Rich, K. (2008). *Nursing ethics: Across the curriculum and into practice* (2nd ed.). Boston: Jones & Bartlett.

Cerise, F., & Chokshi, D. (2009). Orienting health care reform around universal access. *Archives of Internal Medicine, 169,* 1830–1832.

Commission on Accreditation of Rehabilitation Facilities. (2013). Standards for written ethical codes of conduct. Retrieved from www.carf.org/about/becomeasurveyor/surveyorcommitment

Davis, A., & Aroskar, M. (1991). *Ethical dilemmas and nursing practice*. Englewood Cliffs, NJ: Prentice Hall.

Derstine, J. B., & Hargrove, S. D. (2001). *Comprehensive rehabilitation nursing*. New York: Saunders.

Ellis, J. R., & Hartley, C. L. (2007). *Nursing in today's world: Trends, issues & management* (9th ed.). Philadelphia: Lippincott, Williams & Wilkins.

Epstein, E. G., & Hamric, A. B. (2009). Moral distress, moral residue and the crescendo effect. *Journal of Clinical Ethics, 20*(4), 330–342. Retrieved from http://www.ncbi.nlm.nih.gov/pmc/articles/PMC3612701/

Ethics Resource Center. (2009). Why have a code of conduct. Retrieved from http://www.ethics.org/resource/why-have-code-conduct

Ethics Resource Center. (2009). The PLUS decision making model. Retrieved from http://www.ethics.org/resource/plus-decision-making-model

Fletcher, J., Spencer, E., & Lombardo, P. (Eds.). (2005). *Fletcher's introduction to clinical ethics* (3rd ed.). Hagerstown, MD: University Publishing Group.

Frankena, W. K., & Granrose, J. T. (Eds.). (1974). *Introductory readings in ethics*. Englewood Cliffs, NJ: Prentice Hall.

Gadow, S. (1999). Relational narratives: The post-modern turn in nursing ethics. *Scholarly Inquiry for Nursing Practice, 13*(1), 57–70.

Gergen, K. J. (2009). *Relational being: Beyond self and community*. New York: Oxford University Press.

Gilligan, C. (1995). Hearing the difference: Theorizing connection. *Hypatia, 10,* 120–127.

Grace, P. J. (2004). Ethics in the clinical encounter. In S. K. Chase (Ed.), *Clinical judgment and communication in nurse practitioner practice* (pp. 295–332). Philadelphia: F. A. Davis.

Grace, P. J. (2009). *Nursing ethics and professional responsibility in advanced practice*. Sudbury, MA: Jones & Bartlett.

Grace, P. J. (2014). *Nursing ethics and professional responsibility in advanced practice*. (2nd ed). Burlington, MA: Jones & Bartlett.

Graham-Eason, C. (1996). Ethical considerations for rehabilitation nursing. In S. Hoeman (Ed.), *Rehabilitation nursing: Process and application* (2nd ed., pp. 34–46). St. Louis: Mosby.

Guido, G. W. (2010). *Legal and ethical issues in nursing* (5th ed.). Upper Saddle River, NJ: Pearson.

Hebert, P. (1996). *Doing right: A practical guide to ethics for medical trainees and physicians*. Toronto, Canada: Oxford University Press.

Hinman, L. (2002). *Ethics: A pluralistic approach to moral theory* (3rd ed.). Belmont, CA: Thomson-Wadsworth.

Hoeman, S. (2008). *Rehabilitation nursing: Prevention, intervention, and outcomes* (4th ed.). St. Louis: Mosby Elsevier.

Hoeman, S. P., & Duchene, P. M. (2002). Ethical matters in rehabilitation. In S. Hoeman (Ed.), *Rehabilitation nursing: Process, application, and outcomes* (3rd ed., pp. 45–55). St. Louis: Mosby.

International Council of Nurses (ICN). (2006). *The ICN code of ethics for nurses*. Retrieved from www.icn.ch/images/stories/documents/about/icncode_english.pdf

Jameton, A. (1984). *Nursing practice: The ethical issues*. Englewood Cliffs, NJ: Prentice Hall.

The Joint Commission (2009). The Joint Commission code of conduct. Retrieved from htttp://www.jointcommission.org/assets/1/18/TJC_Code_of_Conduct_09.pdf

Jonsen, A. R., Siegler, M., & Winslade, W. (2010). *Clinical ethics* (7th ed.). New York: McGraw-Hill.

Kalb, K. A., & O'Conner-Von, S. (2007). Ethics education in advanced practice nursing: Respect for human dignity. *Nursing Education Perspectives, 28*(4), 196–202.

Keown, D. (2001). *Buddhism and bioethics*. New York: Palgrave.

MacDonald, C. (2010). Guide to moral decision making. Retrieved from www.ethicsweb.ca/guide/

Macrina, F. (2005). *Scientific integrity: Text and cases in responsible conduct of research* (3rd ed.). Washington, DC: ASM Press.

Marquis, B., & Huston, C. (2009). *Leadership roles and management functions in nursing: Theory and application*. Philadelphia: Wolters Kluwer Health/Lippincott Williams & Wilkins.

Masters-Farrell, P. A. (2006). Ethical/legal principles and issues. In K. L. Mauk (Ed.), *Gerontological nursing competencies for care* (pp. 589–618). Sudbury, MA: Jones & Bartlett.

McCarthy, J. (2006). A pluralist view of nursing ethics. *Nursing Philosophy, 7*, 157–164.

McCourt, A. E. (Ed.). (1993). *The specialty practice of rehabilitation nursing: A core curriculum* (3rd ed.). Skokie, IL: Rehabilitation Nursing Foundation of the Association of Rehabilitation Nurses.

Medical College of Georgia. (2000). Ethics syllabus glossary. Retrieved from www.mcg.edu/gpi/ethics/phlsyllabus/bioethic.htm

Morrison, E. E. (2008). *Health care ethics: Critical issues for the 21st century* (2nd ed.). Sudbury, MA: Jones & Bartlett.

National Institutes of Health, Office of Human Research Protection. (2004). Human Subjects Research. Title 45 Code of Federal Regulations, Part 46, 102 (d). Retrieved from www.hhs.gov/ohrp/humansubjects/guidance/

O'Brien, M. A. (2006). How corporate compliance helps your organization be accountable. *CARF Connection*. Retrieved from http://www.carf.org/WorkArea/DownloadAsset.aspx?id=22494

Online Ethics Center for Engineering and Science. (2005). Retrieved from www.onlineethics.org

Paul, R., & Elder, L. (2006). *The miniature guide to critical thinking concepts and tools* (4th ed.). Dillon Beach, CA: Foundation for Critical Thinking.

Pilkington, D., & Strong, S. (2003). *ARN position statement on ethical issues*. Glenview, IL: Association of Rehabilitation Nurses.

Rest, J. R. (1982). A psychologist looks at the teaching of ethics. *Hastings Center Report, 12*(1), 29–36.

Rice, J., & Perry, F. (2013). *Healthcare leadership excellence: Creating a career of impact*. Chicago: Health Administration Press.

Ross, W. D. (2002). *The right and the good*. Oxford, England: Oxford University Press.

Rudnick, A. (2010). Ethics in rehabilitation. In J. H. Stone & M. Blouin (Eds.), *International encyclopedia of rehabilitation*. Retrieved from http://cirrie.buffalo.edu/encyclopedia/en/article/16/

Savage, T., & Michalak, D. R. (1999). Ethical, legal and moral issues in pediatric rehabilitation. In P. A. Edwards, D. L. Hertzberg, S. R. Hays, & N. M. Youngblood (Eds.), *Pediatric rehabilitation nursing* (pp. 62–83). Philadelphia: W. B. Saunders.

Sliwa, J. A., McPeak, L., Gittler, M., Bodenheimer, C., King, J., Bowen, J., & American Academy of Pediatrics Medical Education Committee. (2002). AAP white paper: Clinical ethics in rehabilitation medicine: Core objectives and algorithm for resident education. *American Journal of Physical Medicine in Rehabilitation, 81*(9), 708–717.

Ursery, D. (2005). *Principles of normative ethics*. Austin, TX: St. Edwards University.

Webster, G., & Baylis, F. (2000). Moral residue. In S. Rubin & L. Zoloft (Eds.), *Margin of error: The ethics of mistakes in the practice of medicine* (pp. 217–230). Hagerstown, MD: University Publishing Group.

Suggested Resources

American Nurses Association. (2014). Ethics. Retrieved from http://nursingworld.org/MainMenuCategories/EthicsStandards.aspx

Andrews, M., Goldberg, K., & Kaplan, H. (2004). *Nurses' legal handbook* (5th ed.). Springhouse, PA: Springhouse.

Fry, S. T., & Johnstone, M. (2006). *Ethics in nursing practice* (3rd ed.). Englewood Cliffs, NJ: Prentice Hall.

The Hastings Center. (2014). About us. Retrieved from http://www.thehastingscenter.org/About/Default.aspx

Institute on Disability and Rehabilitation Ethics (2013). Retrieved from http://www.education.uiowa.edu/centers/idare/home

International Council of Nurses (2012). *Code of ethics for nurses*. Retrieved from http://www.icn.ch/about-icn/code-of-ethics-for-nurses/

Lachman, V. D. (2006). *Applied ethics in nursing*. New York, NY: Springer.

Lippincott's Nursing Center (2014). Focus on: Nursing ethics. Retrieved from http://www.nursingcenter.com/home/NursingCenterEthics1.asp

National Council of State Boards of Nursing (2014). Ethics of nursing practice [Online continuing education course]. Retrieved from http://learningext.com/nurses/p/ethics-of-nursing.aspx

NursingEthics.ca (2014). Nursing ethics resources. Retrieved from http://www.nursingethics.ca/

Perry, F. (2014). *Ethics and management dilemmas in healthcare* (2nd ed.) Chicago, IL: Health Administration Press.

Westrick, S., & McCormack-Dempski, K. (2009). *Essentials of nursing law and ethics*. Sudbury, MA: Jones & Bartlett.

Chapter 5

Building Rehabilitation Nursing Knowledge Through Research

Beverly S. Reigle, PhD RN
Andrea E. Berndt, PhD

LEARNING OBJECTIVES

- Describe the steps of the research process.
- Explain the importance of nursing research to the practice of rehabilitation nursing.
- Discuss the application of the research process to rehabilitation nursing practice.
- Foster the role of the nurse as a consumer of research.

KEY CHAPTER TOPICS

- The purpose and importance of nursing research and the steps of the process, which include
  - identifying the problem
  - stating the purpose
  - selecting a theoretical framework
  - conducting a review of literature
  - selecting the appropriate methodology
  - presenting the results
  - discussing the meaning of the findings, the limitations of the study, and recommendations for further research.

PROFESSIONAL REHABILITATION NURSING DOMAINS AND COMPETENCIES

- Domain 1: Competency 1.2 (Association of Rehabilitation Nurses [ARN], 2014a)

The Research Process

This chapter presents an overview of the research process and application of the information using rehabilitation nursing exemplars. The content is intended to foster the nurse's role as a consumer of research through activities such as reading research reports with greater understanding, participating in research studies as data collectors, or attending research conferences.

I. Introduction

A. What Is Rehabilitation Nursing Research?

1. Professional nursing is both an art and a science. The science component of nursing signifies a distinct body of knowledge that has been developed through scientific inquiry. Scientific inquiry is also considered research. According to Polit and Beck (2012), "Research is a systematic inquiry that uses orderly, disciplined methods to answer questions or solve problems" (p. 741) to "develop, refine and expand knowledge" (p. 3).
2. Nursing research uses the same scientific method of inquiry, but it is specific to questions important to nursing and the development of nursing knowledge. Research relevant to rehabilitation nursing implies use of the same scientific approach; however, the questions to be answered are specific to building the body of rehabilitation nursing knowledge (e.g., factors that have an impact on falls, interventions that prevent pressure sores).

B. Why Is Research Important to Rehabilitation Nurses?

1. As nurses, we have contracted with society to base our practice on the best evidence; specifically, research findings. According to the American Nurses Association (ANA) social policy statement (2010), "Nurses

apply research findings and implement the best evidence into their practice based on applicability to the individual, family, group, community, population, or system of care. These efforts generate knowledge and advance nursing science" (p. 15).

2. The contract also states that nursing actions are intended to produce beneficial outcomes and that research findings provide the scientific evidence for such nursing actions. Therefore, evidence-based practice (EBP) requires an understanding of research as noted in this *EBP* definition: "the process of finding, appraising and applying scientific evidence to the treatment and management of health care" and "the discovery of underlying trends and principles developed from the accumulation and refinement of a large body of studies" (Ledbetter & Stevens, 2000, p.102).
3. This definition stipulates that nurses who fully engage in EBP must be knowledgeable about the research process to evaluate a study's scientific rigor, and, based on adequate research findings (e.g., systematic review), nurses translate the findings into usable forms such as guidelines, protocols, and clinical pathways. They then integrate this usable form into practice. Additionally, such evidence is required when advocating for healthcare reform, both nationally and globally. Policymakers expect nurses to be experts in their field and provide sound evidence for the healthcare changes they propose.
4. The Association of Rehabilitation Nurses (ARN) promotes conduction of research that contributes to the body of rehabilitation nursing knowledge and has the potential to have an impact on rehabilitation nursing practice. This is evident in the third edition of the *ARN Rehabilitation Nursing Research Agenda* (ARN, 2014b).
5. Additionally, the first of four domains proposed in the *ARN Competency Model for Professional Rehabilitation Nursing* (ARN, 2014a) highlights the importance of research (Domain 1, Competency 1:2: Implement nursing and interprofessional interventions based on best evidence to manage the client's disability and/or chronic illness).

C. Major Approaches to Research

1. Researchers apply two major approaches or methods to answer research questions or address research problems. The approach depends on the question, and each approach is derived from a different philosophical background or paradigm (i.e., one's world view).
2. The first approach focuses on the objective and quantifiable and is called the *quantitative method* (Polit & Beck, 2012). In this approach, a reality exists and terms such as *cause* and *effect* are integral to understanding the types of designs used to answer quantitative research questions. This means that numbers are important, and this is most apparent in the use of statistical tests.
   a. Example: An example of the title of a quantitative study conducted by Hsieh and colleagues. (2008) is "The Effects of a Supervised Exercise Intervention on Recovery from Treatment Regimens in Breast Cancer Survivors."
3. The second approach focuses on multiple and subjective realities and is called the *qualitative method* (Polit & Beck, 2012). Methods such as phenomenology, ethnography, and grounded theory are employed to answer qualitative research questions. Statistical tests are not integral to this approach. Instead, themes are often derived from information obtained through personal interaction.
   a. An example of a qualitative study as conducted by Ligthelm and Wright (2014) is "Lived Experience of Persons with an Amputation of the Upper Limb."

D. The Research Process

1. The conduction of research is a process that involves several steps. The steps, presented in sequential order, are
   a. Problem identification
   b. Purpose statement including research question(s) or hypotheses
   c. Use of a theoretical framework (if appropriate)
   d. Review of the literature
   e. Methodology, which includes design, sample, setting, protection of human subjects, instruments (measurements), procedures, and data analysis
   f. Results or findings
   g. Discussion that includes interpretation, limitations, recommendations for further research, implications for practice and policy (if appropriate), and conclusions

II. Conceptualization of the Investigation

A. The Problem Statement

1. The *problem statement* is the researcher's articulation of the issue or enigma that he or she plans to investigate (Polit & Beck, 2012). The word *statement* can be misleading, because it is more than just a sentence; instead, it often consists of one or more paragraphs. It is the researcher's argument for conducting the research. Thus, the significance or importance of the research to nursing, and in this case, rehabilitation nursing, is included

in the argument. The problem could be derived from a practice situation, a social concern, the literature, an identified gap in the knowledge base, or an important interdisciplinary or nursing problem funded by an organization (e.g., the Rehabilitation Nursing Foundation [RNF]).

2. Six components typically are included in a problem statement (Polit & Beck, 2012):
   a. Identification of the problem
   b. Background or context of the problem
   c. Scope of the problem
   d. Consequences of the problem
   e. Knowledge gap in understaning the problem
   f. Proposed solution, or how the proposed study addresses or solves the problem
3. The researcher must define the problem clearly so that the purpose of the investigation is understood. In other words, the problem statement sets the stage for the investigation. The essence of the problem frequently is captured in the one or two sentences preceding the purpose statement. In fact, these one or two sentences pave the way for the purpose statement so that the researcher can state, "Therefore, the purpose of this study is...".
   a. Examples of sentences that capture the essence of the problem. "...Consequently, understanding relationships between cognitive factors of goal setting, motivation, and how they influence the exercise adherence of people with COPD warrant investigation. Goal setting and its influence on exercise motivation of people with COPD have not been studied" (Davis, 2007, p. 104). The phrase "have not been studied" constitutes the gap in the body of knowledge in this population.

B. The Purpose Statement

1. Unlike the problem statement, the purpose statement is written as one or perhaps two sentences. Polit and Beck (2012) state that it is a "broad declarative statement of the overall goals of the study" (p. 743). The purpose of a study is presented as a means of filling the gap in a body of knowledge.
2. The statement can begin with "the purpose is," "the aim is," or "the goal is." Sometimes the purpose statement can begin simply with "this study is designed to...". Importantly, the purpose statement should include the variables of interest (e.g., independent and dependent variables), the nature of the study, and the population involved.
   a. Example: The purpose statement, as articulated in the Davis (2007) study, serves as an example. Specific purposes of this study were to determine the relationship between motivation and goal orientation in participants with chronic obstructive pulmonary disease (COPD) and explore goal-setting behaviors of people with COPD, specifically their activity and exercise goals.
      1) The variables of interest in this purpose statement are motivation (independent variable) and goal orientation (dependent variable).
      2) The nature of the study is indicated by the term *relationship*, which suggests a nonexperimental, correlational design.
      3) The population of the study was participants with COPD (Davis, p. 105).
3. Definitions of terms used in this section
   a. *Independent variable:* First, the word variable indicates an item or concept that varies in numerical value. An independent variable is one that causes, contributes to, or influences the dependent variable (Polit & Beck, 2012). Using the above mentioned example, motivation is believed to influence goal setting. The independent variable precedes the dependent variable in time.
   b. *Dependent variable:* The dependent variable is the consequence or outcome of the impact of the dependent variable (Polit & Beck, 2012). Using the above mentioned example, goal setting would be the proposed outcome or consequence of motivation. From an epidemiological perspective, risk factors are viewed as independent variables that influence or increase the likelihood of a specific disease or health problem. For example, smoking (independent variable and risk factor) influences the development of lung cancer (dependent variable or consequence).
   c. *Population:* The population refers to the entire group of individuals or entities about which the researcher is interested. As noted in the example from the Davis (2007) article, the population was individuals with COPD. More detail about the population, eligibility criteria, and sampling is provided later in this chapter.

C. The Research Question

1. The *research question* is the question that the investigation is intended to answer.
2. The components of the question are similar to the purpose statement, but written in question form.
   a. Example: Using the example provided for the purpose statement, the research question could

be: Is there a relationship between motivation and goal setting in participants with COPD?

D. The Hypothesis

1. The *hypothesis* is the researcher's prediction about what he or she expects to be the outcome of the investigation. It is the expected answer to the research inquiry (Polit & Beck, 2012).
2. The two major types of hypotheses are research hypothesis and null hypothesis.
3. The *null hypothesis* is the statistical hypothesis and is written in the negative. In this case, the researcher hopes to reject the null hypothesis.
   a. Example: There is no difference in quality of life scores between men who have had a below-the-knee amputation and participate in a support group and those who do not participate.
4. The *research hypothesis* is written in a positive tone and indicates the outcome the researcher believes will occur.
   a. Example: There is a difference in quality-of-life scores between men who have had a below-the-knee amputation and participate in a support group and those who do not participate.
5. A research hypothesis consists of two types, directional and nondirectional.
   a. The *directional hypothesis* predicts the exact relationship between or among variables, or when discussing groups, it predicts which group will do better or worse on a particular dependent variable. If predicting a relationship, the directional hypothesis states whether the relationship is positive or negative. Although the Davis (2007) study did not specify a hypothesis, a directional hypothesis can be derived from the author's purpose statement.
      1) Example: There is a positive relationship between motivation and goal setting. *Positive*, in this case, means that as one of the variables increases, the other also increases. Thus, as motivation increases so will goal setting. If the two variables had a negative relationship, then one would expect that as motivation increases, goal setting would decrease. This is also called an inverse relationship.
      2) An example of a directional hypothesis that addresses differences in groups is as follows:
         a) Men who have had below-the-knee amputations and participate in support groups will have higher quality-of-life scores than those who do not participate. In this example, the researcher is predicting which of two groups will do better regarding the dependent variable, which is quality of life. (Note: The independent variable in this example is participation in a support group.)
   b. The *nondirectional hypothesis* states that a relationship exists but does not state the direction (i.e., positive or negative).
      1) Example: Using the Davis (2007) variables, the nondirectional hypothesis could be as follows: There is a relationship between motivation and goal setting in participants with COPD. In this hypothesis, the researcher is only predicting a relationship, not the type of relationship. The same approach fits when discussing differences between groups. The researcher would predict that a difference between the groups exists, but not which group does better or worse.
      2) Example: There is a difference in quality-of-life scores between men who have had a below-the-knee amputation and participate in a support group and those who do not participate.

E. The Theory or Theoretical Framework

1. Theories provide a conceptualization for a study. The goal of using theories in research "is to make findings meaningful, to integrate knowledge into coherent systems, to stimulate new research, and to explain phenomenon and relationships among them" (Polit & Beck, 2012, p. 148).
2. A *theory* is an "internally consistent group of relational statements that presents a systematic view about a phenomenon and that is useful for description, explanation, prediction, and prescription or control" (Walker & Avant, 2004, p. 28). The building blocks of a theory are called *concepts*, and statements of relationships between and among the concepts are called *propositions* (Polit & Beck, 2012).
3. Theories are often viewed as grand theories or middle-range theories.
   a. *Grand theories* are very broad in scope with concepts that might not be clearly defined and relationships that often are not clearly delineated.
   b. *Middle-range theories* are narrower in scope, have fewer concepts and propositions, have well-defined concepts, and clearly delineated propositions. Middle-range theories are testable and therefore are very appropriate for guiding research studies.

Figure 5-1. Hypothesis Model

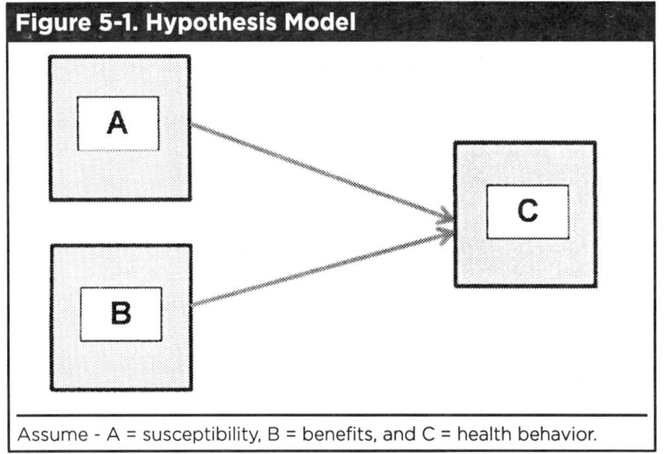

Assume - A = susceptibility, B = benefits, and C = health behavior.

4. Researchers test hypotheses, which often are derived from a theory.
   a. Example: In the visual depiction or schematic model (**Figure 5-1**), A, B, and C represent concepts and the arrows represent propositions or relationships. The point of the arrows indicate that A and B precede C; thus, A and B are considered independent variables when tested in a study, and C is the dependent variable (i.e., the outcome). Giving A, B, and C a label or name provides further explanation of the model.
   b. In this case, susceptibility and benefits have positive relationships with the health behavior. In using this theory to guide a study, the researcher might want to test it to determine the likelihood of women obtaining a mammogram. In this scenario, *susceptibility* would be defined as "a woman's risk for developing breast cancer"; *benefits* would be defined as "as a woman's beliefs about the value of obtaining a mammogram"; and the *health behavior* is "obtaining a mammogram."
   c. The researcher could then test two hypotheses:
      1) A woman's perceived susceptibility to breast cancer will be positively related to obtaining a mammogram.
      2) A woman's perceived benefits about obtaining a mammogram will be positively related to obtaining a mammogram. This means that the stronger a woman's belief that she is susceptible to breast cancer, the more likely she is to obtain a mammogram, and the stronger her belief that a mammogram is beneficial, the more likely she is to obtain a mammogram.
   d. If the results of the study indicate that the hypotheses are supported, then the theory is supported for that particular population.
      1) Example: Studies that are underpinned by a theory are often stated in the research report, as in the following example: "Using SCT as the framework, this study was designed to explore this gap in knowledge" (Davis, 2007, p. 104). The theory in this case is social cognitive theory (SCT).
5. Definitions of terms used in this section
   a. *Concept:* "an abstraction inferred from observation of behaviors, situations, or characteristics" (Polit & Beck, 2012, p. 722)
   b. *Proposition*: "a statement indicating relationships between or among concepts" (Polit & Beck, 2012)
   c. *Conceptual framework:* "interrelated concepts or abstractions assembled in a rational and often explanatory scheme to illuminate relationships among them" (Polit & Beck, 2012, p. 722). This framework has not been tested as extensively as a theoretical framework.
   d. *Model:* "a symbolic representation of concepts or variables, and interrelationships among them" (Polit & Beck, 2012, p. 734)

F. The Variables of Interest

1. A well-designed research study is one that clearly defines the variables of interest. Researchers usually begin by specifying a variable's conceptual definition, followed by its operational definition. The conceptual definition of a variable is often abstract and linked to a theoretical framework; it is also multifaceted and not easily measured. In contrast, an operational definition is very specific and provides information about exactly how a variable is measured or determined.
   a. A good example of an abstract variable is the concept of quality of life. Conceptual definitions for *quality of life* have included perceived satisfaction with present life circumstances; relative effectiveness of a patient's approach to solving problems associated with being seriously ill; and individuals' perceptions of their position in life within the context of the culture and value system in which they live and in relation to their goals, standards, and concerns (Jochan, Dassen, Widdershoven, & Halfens, 2006). An operational definition for quality of life might be a patient's perceptions regarding the ability to perform daily activities as measured by scores on the Klein-Bell Activities of Daily Living Scale (Bakas et al., 2012).
2. Definitions of terms used in this section

a. *Conceptual definitions:* "the abstract or theoretical meaning of the concept being studied" (Polit & Beck, 2012, p. 722)

b. *Operational definitions:* "the definition of a concept or variable in terms of the procedures by which it is to be measured" (Polit & Beck, 2012, p. 736)

G. The Literature Review

1. The researcher begins the process of accessing the literature to determine the current state of the science or knowledge relevant to the problem. The literature, in this case, refers to research reports and can be found by using online or library databases such as the Cumulative Index to Nursing and Allied Health Literature (CINAHL), Medical Literature On-Line (MEDLINE), and Cochrane Database of Systematic Reviews. Upon selecting seemingly relevant research reports, the researcher screens the reports by reviewing the abstracts, preferably of primary sources rather than secondary sources.
2. Abstracts provide a brief summary of a research study and help the reader to avoid reading an entire article that might have no relevance to the problem of interest.
3. Once the researcher selects the report, a review of the literature, or literature review, occurs. In a literature review, the researcher conducts "a critical summary of research on a topic of interest, often prepared to put a research problem in context" (Polit & Beck, 2012, p. 732). A critical appraisal requires knowledge of the research process and the importance of rigor. Researchers make decisions about the soundness of the study findings based on how rigorously the study was conducted (e.g., adequate sample size and representativeness, appropriate design for the research question, protection of human participants, psychometrics of the instruments, approach to data analysis, interpretation of results).
4. Ultimately, the literature review expands the problem statement and presents a critical summary of the research conducted in the problem area so that the gap in knowledge is clear. See an example of a literature review in Davis (2007, p. 106).
5. Definitions of terms used in this section

   a. *Abstract:* "a brief description of a completed or proposed study, usually located at the beginning of a report or proposal" (Polit & Beck, 2012, p. 719)

   b. *Critique:* "a critical appraisal—ideally one that analyzes both weaknesses and strengths—of a research report or proposal" (Polit & Beck, 2012, p. 724)

   c. *Primary sources:* "first-hand reports of facts or findings; in research, the original report prepared by the investigator who conducted the study" (Polit & Beck, 2012, p. 738)

   d. *Secondary sources:* "second-hand accounts of events or facts; in research, a description of a study prepared by someone other than the original researcher" (Polit & Beck, 2012, p. 742)

III. Methodology

Information about research methodology focuses on the research design, the sample and setting, the protection of human subjects, the instruments (measurements), the procedures, and the anticipated data analyses.

A. The Research Method and Design

1. The choice of methodology to use—either quantitative or qualitative (or a hybrid method)—depends on a variety of factors. The primary determinant should be linked to the research aims, purpose, questions, and/or hypotheses. For example, if the research aim is to test cause-and-effect relationships, the researcher should select a quantitative method and design. Other factors that can influence method or design choices include whether the researcher wants to be able to make comparisons between groups or wants to be able to measure changes in one or more outcomes over time. The degree to which a researcher can exert control over confounding variables is also likely to be an important factor in selecting one design over another.
2. Quantitative research designs

   a. *Quantitative studies* can be broadly classified as either experimental or non-experimental. Experimental studies are designed to test cause-effect relationships and are characterized by manipulation of an intervention or treatment. True experiments or randomized controlled trials (RCTs) are characterized by manipulation of an intervention or treatment, randomization, and the presence of control groups (Stanley, 2007). The combination of manipulation, randomization, and control groups provides the best evidence for cause-effect relationships. In some situations, researchers might be able to manipulate an intervention or treatment but lack randomization or a control group. Quantitative studies use quasi-experimental designs. In contrast to an RCT, quasi-experiments can have a comparison group rather than a control group, and they often lack randomization. Although a quasi-experiment can be used to test cause-effect relationships, the lack of a control group and randomization decreases the level of confidence in the findings due to the inability to rule out extraneous variables.

b. *Experimental designs* differ based on when data are collected (i.e., pretest and posttest, posttest only, pretest only, and multiple posttest measures), the introduction of one or more interventions, and group comparisons (Sun et al., 2014). An experimental design might compare an intervention group to a control group.

c. *Nonexperimental designs* explore relationships, investigate differences in subject characteristics, or describe the characteristics of a population without introducing an intervention. Examples of nonexperimental designs include descriptive research, correlational research, and comparative research. *Descriptive research* is used to determine the unknown characteristics of a population of interest. *Correlational research* is used to explore quantitative relationships among variables. *Comparative research* is used to compare groups to determine whether they differ on preexisting characteristics or study outcomes.

d. Definitions of terms used in this section
    1) *Experimental research:* "a study using a design in which the researcher controls (manipulates) an independent variable by randomly assigning subjects to different treatment conditions" (Polit & Beck, 2012, p. 727)
    2) *Nonexperimental research:* "studies in which the researcher collects data without introducing an intervention" (Polit & Beck, 2012, p. 735)

3. Qualitative research
    a. *Qualitative research* is used to elicit the experiences of participants to better understand the meaning of their situation by asking them open-ended questions. There are many types of qualitative research, but three of the most frequently used are ethnography, grounded theory, and phenomenology. *Ethnography* is derived from an anthropological framework and focuses on understanding cultural patterns and experiences. In ethnography, the researcher tries to understand participants by watching what they experience, listening to what they say, and collecting data about them. *Grounded theory* is derived from a sociological framework and focuses on processes that occur within a social setting. Based on the data collected, the researcher attempts to build a theory that explains the phenomenon observed. *Phenomenology* is derived from a philosophical framework and focuses on understanding the lived experience of a phenomenon based on the perceptions of those who live with the phenomenon.
    b. Definitions of terms used in this section
        1) *Ethnography:* "a branch of human inquiry, associated with sociology, that focuses on the way in which people make sense of their everyday activities and come to behave in socially acceptable ways" (Polit & Beck, 2012, p. 727)
        2) *Grounded theory:* "an approach to collecting and analyzing qualitative data that aims to develop theories grounded in real-world observations" (Polit & Beck, 2012, p. 729)
        3) *Phenomenology:* "a qualitative research tradition, with roots in philosophy and psychology, that focuses on the lived experience of humans" (Polit & Beck, 2012, p. 737)

B. The Research Sample and Setting

1. Determining the characteristics of a representative sample: Before the researcher can begin to recruit people to participate in a study, several questions need to be asked and answered. First, the researcher needs to determine the characteristics of the population to be studied. The researcher can determine these characteristics by answering the "who, what, when, where, and why" components of the research question or problem statement. These characteristics can be demographic and can include, for example, gender, age, ethnicity, race, geographic location, or education. Other characteristics could include health status; a diagnosis such as diabetes, hypertension, or stroke; or risk factors for alcohol or drug abuse.
2. The next question the researcher needs to ask and answer is: How can he or she draw a sample that will be representative of the population of interest? In other words, the sample should have the essential characteristics of the population. These essential characteristics will determine the researcher's inclusion criteria for the sample. The final question the researcher must ask and answer is: What population characteristics might interfere, confuse, or confound the study outcomes? These interfering characteristics will determine the researcher's exclusion criteria for the sample.

a. Example: Assume a researcher wanted to determine whether patients allowed to listen to music before having a procedure in a catheterization unit would report less anxiety than patients not allowed to listen to music. In this case, some probable inclusion criteria would be to choose patients who (1) are adults, (2) were admitted to the catheterization unit for a procedure, and (3) are not hearing impaired. Likely exclusion criteria would apply to patients who (1) are not adults, (2) were admitted to other nonsurgical units, and (3) are hearing impaired.

b. If the researcher is able to apply the inclusion and exclusion criteria and can randomly assign patients to the intervention group (i.e., listening to music) or control (i.e., no music) group, there is a strong likelihood that the patients who participate can be considered a representative sample of the population.

c. Definitions of terms used in this section
   1) *Exclusion criteria:* "sampling criteria specifying characteristics that a population does not have" (Polit & Beck, 2012, p. 727)
   2) *Inclusion criteria:* "criteria that specify population characteristics" (Polit & Beck, 2012, p. 274)
   3) *Representative sample:* "a sample whose key characteristics closely approximate those of the population of interest" (Polit & Beck, 2012, p. 275)

3. Sampling approaches for quantitative and qualitative research: After the researcher has identified the population of interest, decided how to acquire a representative sample, and chosen where the research will be conducted, a sampling plan is determined. The sampling plan specifies how individuals representative of the sample will be recruited and enrolled and how many individuals are needed to participate to answer the study question.

a. In quantitative research, two primary sampling methods are used. One of the methods, probability sampling, is chosen if the researcher wants to recruit and enroll a sample representative of the population using random procedures. Examples of probability sampling include simple random sampling, stratified sampling, and cluster sampling. Nonprobability sampling is chosen when the researcher is unable to use random procedures to recruit and enroll a sample. Examples of nonprobability sampling include convenience sampling and snowball sampling.

b. Example: Probability sampling would occur if a researcher wanted to collect a sample of nurses who are members of the Association of Rehabilitation Nurses. Every fifth name on the membership list could be contacted and asked to participate (systematic sampling). Nonprobability sampling would occur if, for example, a researcher attended a 2-day meeting for ARN and on the second day of the meeting asked attendees to participate in a study (convenience sampling).
   1) Definitions of terms used in this section
      a) *Nonprobability sampling*: "the selection of sampling...participants from a population using nonrandom procedures" (Polit & Beck, 2012, p. 735)
      b) *Probability sampling*: "the selection of sampling...participants from a population using random procedures" (Polit & Beck, 2012, p. 738)
      c) *Sampling plan*: "the formal plan specifying a sampling method, a sample size, and procedures for recruiting subjects" (Polit & Beck, 2012, p. 742)

c. In qualitative research, decisions about sampling are based on the enrollment of participants who can provide detailed information about the phenomena of interest. In contrast to quantitative researchers, qualitative researchers rarely use randomization procedures. Instead, qualitative researchers seek participants who are articulate and reflective and willing to be interviewed at length by researchers. Although many sampling techniques are used in qualitative research, two common techniques are purposive sampling and theoretical sampling.

d. *Purposive sampling* is used when the researcher wants to locate participants who possess characteristics that are representative of a group that could provide details about the phenomena of interest. Researchers also use purposive sampling when they want to make comparisons across participants on a specific dimension of interest. In such situations, participants are selected on the premise that each individual interviewed can provide maximal benefit to the study.

e. *Theoretical sampling* is used when the researcher wants to locate participants based on characteristics that form the basis for manifestation or representation of key theoretical constructs (Patton, 2002). These characteristics could be based on the ability of participants to provide unique details on aspects such as time periods, incidents or critical events, or slices of life.

1) Definitions of terms used in this section
   a) *Purposive sampling*: "a nonprobability sampling method in which the researcher selects participants based on personal judgment about which ones will be most informative" (Polit & Beck, 2012, p. 739)
   b) *Theoretical sampling*: "in qualitative studies, especially in grounded theory studies, the selection of sample members based on merging findings to ensure adequate representation of important theoretical categories" (Polit & Beck, 2012, p. 744)

4. Determining an appropriate sample size: The number of participants needed for a given study is based on practical and scientific considerations. Practical considerations could involve a researcher's access to participants or resources to provide incentives to participants. In contrast, the scientific consideration is focused on choosing a sample size large enough for the researcher to have confidence in the study findings.
   a. In quantitative research, researchers often use a formula (also called a "power analysis") to determine the total number of participants needed for their study (Hayat, 2013). A *power analysis* takes three components into consideration: (1) significance level, (2) power, and (3) effect size. Significance level has to do with the likelihood that the findings in a research study occurred by chance. In most nursing studies, the significance level is set to .05. This means that the likelihood that an identified difference or relationship in the findings is random or based on chance should occur only once in 20 occurrences. In contrast, power is the likelihood that the researcher will be able to identify a difference or relationship that actually exists. In nursing studies, power is usually set to .80 or .90. This means that if there is an actual difference between groups or an actual relationship between variables, the researcher can have 80%–90% certainty of identifying that difference or relationship.
   b. The final component considered for a power analysis is the effect size. The *effect size* is the expected magnitude for the effect of an intervention or condition. Effect sizes in nursing studies usually range from .20 to .40 (Polit & Beck, 2012). For example, a researcher might anticipate that a large increase in a drug dose (e.g., 50 mg) would result in a major improvement in patients' conditions. In contrast, a small increase in a drug dose (e.g., 5 mg) would result in only a minimal improvement.
   c. Example: A researcher wants to determine the number of participants needed for a study that will compare the recovery of patients who receive a new drug with those who will receive a placebo. The significance level is set to .05, so that the likelihood that the researcher will say the recovery of the groups is different when no difference actually exists is one time out of 20. The desired power for the study is set to .90, so that the likelihood that the researcher will be able to see true differences in recovery between the groups is nine times out of 10. Because the new drug has been shown repeatedly to result in substantial improvements, the researcher anticipates a large effect size (e.g., .40). If these values are plugged into the formula for a power analysis, the total sample size needed to compare patients' recovery in the drug group to those in the placebo group will be 172 (86 in each group).
      1) Definitions of terms used in this section
         a) *Effect size*: "a statistical expression of the magnitude of the relationship between two variables" (Polit & Beck, 2012, p. 726)
         b) *Power:* "the ability of a design or analysis strategy to detect true relationships that exist among variables" (Polit & Beck, 2012, p. 738)
         c) *Significance level:* "the probability that an observed relationship could be the result of chance" (Polit & Beck, 2012, p. 742)
   d. In qualitative research, the size of the sample is often not a fixed value. Instead, the size of the sample is based on the extent to which the researcher believes that new information can be obtained. Sample sizes are based on achieving data saturation, which is the point at which the information becomes redundant and no longer yields new information. Specifically, sample sizes in qualitative research are designed to increase the depth of the study findings. Achieving depth in study findings often means that researchers must interview participants more than once, or extend the length of interviews

so that more details about the phenomena of interest emerge.

5. Protection of human participants
   a. In any research endeavor that enrolls human participants, researchers are expected to meet two obligations. The first obligation is to generate knowledge that can contribute to society and provide a basis for subsequent knowledge building. The second obligation is to ensure that participants are protected with respect to their privacy, their decision making, and their safety. This is achieved by treating participants with dignity and respect and providing them with complete information to ensure their voluntary participation..
   b. Three ethical principles (i.e., beneficence, justice, and respect for persons) guide interactions in research with human participants. *Beneficence* focuses on the researcher's obligation to "do no harm" and ensures that benefit is to be had from the research. Although those participating in a study often do not benefit directly from the findings, hope exists that others can benefit from them over time. *Justice* is defined in the context of fairness relative to research participation. It is determined based on a consideration of who is participating in the research and who is carrying the burden of research relative to who will benefit from the research. Participants should be selected because they meet the study inclusion criteria, rather than because they are easy to access or can be persuaded to enroll. Finally, *respect for persons* is demonstrated when participants have the freedom and autonomy to make fully informed decisions about their initial and continued research participation. In situations in which participants have diminished authority (e.g., due to age, illness, incarceration), researchers are obligated to consider them a "vulnerable" population and follow the ethical guidelines for special populations.
   c. To ensure the protection of human participants, researchers at most institutions are required to submit complete information about their study and all related study documents to a formal committee, called an institutional review board, that reviews the proposed research plan. The duty of the committee members is to ensure that the proposed plan meets federal and institutional requirements for ethical research, and that all related study documents can be easily understood by the study participants.
   d. Definitions of terms used in this section
      1) *Beneficence:* "a fundamental ethical principle that seeks to maximize benefits for study participants and prevent harm" (Polit & Beck, 2012, p. 720)
      2) *Institutional review board:* "a term used primarily in the United States to refer to the institutional group that convenes to review proposed and ongoing studies with respect to ethical considerations" (Polit & Beck, 2012, p. 730)
      3) *Justice:* "participants' right to fair treatment and their right to privacy" (Polit & Beck, 2012, p. 155)
      4) *Respect for persons:* "participants' right to self-determination and the right to full disclosure" (Polit & Beck, 2012, p. 154)

C. Selecting and Using Instruments (Measurements)

1. To collect data on study outcomes, researchers take measurements. Measurement refers to the assessment, estimation, observation, evaluation, appraisal, or judgment of an event or series of events (Gavin, 1996). In many cases, a researcher can choose from a variety of available tools or instruments to measure outcome variables. Tools and instruments vary in terms of what they measure, how the data are collected, and the degree to which they are credible or appropriate.
2. In quantitative research, researchers often use instruments as tools for measurement. *Instrument* is the generic term that researchers use for a measurement device such as a survey, test, tool, or questionnaire. To help distinguish between the terms *instrument* and *instrumentation*, remember that an *instrument* is a device whereas *instrumentation* is a course of action (i.e., the process of developing, testing, and using the device).
   a. Physiological measures are those that collect data on a person's physical responses such as blood pressure, heart rate, or pulse. The tools used to collect this type of data are often specialized equipment that must be in good working order and calibrated on a regular basis. Individuals who use these tools could need training to use this equipment and to interpret the results correctly.
   b. Observational measures are those in which a researcher observes and records the behavior and comments of participants. Examples of behaviors that might be observed include hand washing, physical endurance, or workplace

communication. Key issues for observational measures include ensuring that clear definitions are provided regarding what is being observed and how behaviors should be observed and documented. Observers often need to be trained, and the consistency and correspondence of their scores need to be investigated.

c. Questionnaires or surveys are measures that gather data from individuals who provide responses to questions regarding their attitudes, knowledge, or characteristics. A multitude of questionnaires and surveys on a wide range of variables is available, including those involving patient satisfaction, quality of life, social support, anxiety, and depression. Some questionnaires have been used extensively and demonstrated excellent reliability and validity. Unfortunately, many questionnaires have been poorly developed and have very limited use and testing. The advantages of questionnaires or surveys are that they are often less expensive than other measures, and they can be administered to large groups of people. The disadvantages of questionnaires include poor response rates and high rates of missing data.

d. Clearly, all measures have inherent advantages and disadvantages. Therefore, the key is to select the best measure to answer the research question. Selecting a measure that does not capture data on the variable of interest is never useful, even if that measure is inexpensive or easy to administer. However, even when a measure is appropriate for a study outcome, it is incumbent on the researcher to ensure that the data collected are credible and appropriate.
   1) Definitions of terms used in this section
      a) *Physiological measures:* measures that collect data on individual body responses such as blood pressure, heart rate, or pulse
      b) *Observational measures:* measures in which a researcher observes and records the behavior and/or comments of participants
      c) *Questionnaires/surveys:* Measures "...to gather self-report data via self-administration of questions" (Polit & Beck, 2012, p. 740)

3. Concerns about quantitative instruments and measurements
   a. In quantitative research, the choice and strength of research instruments are key factors in assessing the quality of the study. A variety of factors can influence the scores obtained from quantitative instruments, which in turn can influence the interpretation of study analyses performed to address the research questions or hypotheses.
   b. *Reliability* refers to the extent to which a research instrument yields consistent and dependable results. For example, if an individual is weighed on a scale at 130 pounds and two minutes later is weighed at 130 pounds again, one would assume the scale is reliable. Knowing that the results of a study are reliable increases the researcher's confidence in the study findings. Reliability is evaluated in terms of the stability of the results over time (i.e., test-retest reliability), the equivalence of the results across observers or raters (i.e., interrater reliability), and extent to which items within an instrument measure a unidimensional concept (i.e., internal consistency reliability). In most situations, researchers assess reliability by computing and interpreting the magnitude of a reliability coefficient. The value for a reliability coefficient can range from .00 to 1.00. A value of .00 is interpreted as the complete absence of reliability, whereas a value of 1.00 is interpreted as perfect reliability. In general, values of .70 or greater are interpreted as evidence of adequate reliability.
   c. Any time a variable is measured, there is a possibility that the scores will be influenced by error. In fact, it is likely that most scores are at least somewhat influenced by measurement error. Some of the factors that can lead to measurement error are random, whereas other factors tend to be systematic and representative of bias.
      1) An example of random measurement error could be the degree to which an individual's cognitive, emotional, or physical state influences a given score. For example, if a participant had slept poorly the night before a knowledge test, his or her score might be substantially lower than it would be if he or she were well rested.
      2) In contrast to random measurement errors, systematic measurement errors can influence all participants' scores on an instrument, and as such are more serious problems. Examples of a systematic measurement error are when researchers interact with participants inconsistently or when instruments are administered to participants

inconsistently. The use of standardized procedures among researchers is often quite helpful in reducing systematic measurement error.

d. *Validity* refers to the extent to which a research instrument measures the concept it is intended to measure. For example, if an instrument is developed to measure anxiety, researchers need to be confident that scores on the instrument reflect anxiety rather something else, such as hypertension. The determination that an instrument is reliable is required for that instrument to be valid. An instrument that fails to yield consistent results can never be a valid indicator of a concept, because it is overly influenced by measurement error. However, there is no guarantee that an instrument will be valid just because it is reliable. For example, participants' weight can be consistently measured on a given scale. If researchers choose to use participants' weight as a proxy for their intelligence, their scores would not be valid indicators for intelligence.
   1) Unlike reliability, validity is not easily estimated through the application of formulas. Instead, validity is established by accumulating sufficient evidence for its inference. Four types of validity (i.e., face, content, construct, and criterion validity) can be assessed for quantitative instruments.
      a) *Face validity* refers to whether participants who are administered an instrument believe that the instrument measures the intended concept. For example, if participants are told an instrument was developed to measure their satisfaction with healthcare services, and they believe the items address satisfaction with healthcare services, the instrument possesses face validity. However, if the participants believe the items address use of healthcare services rather than satisfaction, the instrument lacks face validity.
      b) *Content validity* refers to the degree to which an instrument has adequate and sufficient coverage on the intended concept. As an example, a knowledge test is content valid if it covers the information students were told to study. Similarly, an instrument intended to measure anxiety is content valid if the items included are relevant, essential, and important for assessing anxiety.
      c) *Construct validity* refers to the degree to which results obtained from one instrument yield findings that are similar to findings obtained from other instruments that measure the same concept. For example, a participant's score on one intelligence test should be similar to his or her score on another intelligence test. By contrast, scores on that intelligence test should have little similarity to scores on a personality inventory.
      d) *Criterion validity* refers to the degree to which an instrument is predictive of an intended outcome. For example, if patients' scores on a fall risk scale correlate strongly with those of patients who subsequently fall in a rehabilitation unit, the instrument would evidence strong criterion validity.

e. Definitions of terms used in this section
   1) *Measurement error:* the degree to which scores on a measure vary as a function of random or systematic error
   2) *Reliability*: "the degree of consistency or dependability with which an instrument measures an attribute" (Polit & Beck, 2012, p. 741)
      a) *Internal consistency reliability:* "the degree to which subparts of a composite scale are all measuring the same attribute or dimension, as a measure of the scale's reliability" (Polit & Beck, 2012, p. 731)
      b) *Interrater reliability:* "the degree to which two raters or observers, operating independently, assign the same ratings or values for an attribute being measured or observed" (Polit & Beck, 2012, p. 731)
      c) *Test-retest reliability:* "assessment of the stability of an instrument by correlating the scores obtained on two administrations" (Polit & Beck, 2012, p. 744)
   3) *Validity:* "the degree to which inferences made in a study are accurate and well-founded" (Polit & Beck, 2012, p. 745)
      a) *Content validity:* "the degree to which items in an instrument adequately represent the universe of content for the concept being measured" (Polit & Beck, 2012, p. 723)

b) *Construct validity:* "the degree to which two methods of measuring a construct yield similar information" (Polit & Beck, 2012, p. 724)

c) *Criterion validity:* "the degree to which scores on an instrument are correlated with an external criterion" (Polit & Beck, 2012, p. 724)

d) *Face validity:* "the extent to which a measuring instrument looks as though it is measuring what it purports to measure" (Polit & Beck, 2012, p. 728)

4. Qualitative instruments and measurements
   a. In qualitative research, the primary sources of data collection are interviews (e.g., dyadic, focus group, and unstructured) and observations. Other sources of data collection can include participant diaries and/or journals, life or oral histories, and photographs or drawings. In contrast to quantitative studies, the expectation is that data collected across participants will not be consistent until data saturation is reached.
5. Concerns about qualitative instruments and measurements
   a. Evaluation criteria such as reliability and validity are not used to assess the strength of qualitative studies. Instead, qualitative researchers demonstrate trustworthiness to establish confidence in their study findings. Several components are evaluated to provide evidence of trustworthiness in a qualitative study. These components include but are not limited to: developing an audit trail, member checking, peer debriefing, establishing transferability, and using verbatim participant quotes.
   b. One way that trustworthiness can be established is through peer debriefing. In *peer debriefing*, a researcher other than the primary researcher analyzes the study data so the researchers can compare the themes each have identified. Next, the researchers continue to discuss and adjust these themes until they reach consensus.
   c. Another way to establish trustworthiness is to develop and follow an *audit trail.* An audit trail is created by the primary researcher and describes the data and themes and the methods used to develop those themes. The primary researcher provides the audit trail to another knowledgeable qualitative researcher to determine whether the process used to develop the themes was logical. The themes are further supported by using ample verbatim participant quotations.
   d. Researchers can ask participants whether the themes generated from interviews correspond with their experiences and meanings. Rechecking with participants is called *member checking.* Also, if participants indicate there are inconsistencies, the researcher can modify themes to improve correspondence to participants' experiences.
   e. A key criterion for determining trustworthiness is demonstrating evidence for transferability. *Transferability* is shown whenever the findings of a qualitative study can be applied to another situation or context.
      1) Definition of terms used in this section
         a) *Trustworthiness:* "the degree of confidence qualitative researchers have in their data, assessed using the criteria of credibility, transferability, dependability, confirmability, and authenticity" (Polit & Beck, 2012, p. 745)
         b) *Peer debriefing:* "sessions with peers to review and explore various aspects of a study, sometimes used to enhance trustworthiness in a qualitative study" (Polit & Beck, 2012, p. 737)
         c) *Audit trail:* "systematic documentation of material that allows an independent auditor to draw conclusions about the trustworthiness of a qualitative study" (Polit & Beck, 2012, p. 720)
         e) *Member checking:* "a method of validating the credibility of qualitative data through debriefings and discussions with informants" (Polit & Beck, 2012, p. 733)
         f) *Transferability:* "the extent to which qualitative findings can be transferred to other settings or groups" (Polit & Beck, 2012, p. 745)

IV. Discussion

Typically, the discussion portion of a research report includes the following information: the primary findings, interpretation of the findings, limitations that might threaten the validity of the findings, implications for nursing practice, and recommendations for future research.

A. Interpretation of the Study Findings

1. The discussion section is the opportunity for the researcher to interpret the results of the study. The results are summarized and then compared to previous studies discussed in the literature review.

They are evaluated as to whether the findings support or conflict with previous research findings. Findings that conflict with previous study findings require a tentative explanation (Polit & Beck, 2012). Additionally, if a theoretical framework was used to guide the study, the researcher discusses whether or not the results supported the theory.

   a. Example: An example of a statement in the discussion section that addresses the theory is found in Davis (2007): "Findings from this study support relationships predicted in SCT, demonstrating that motivation is linked with goals in people with COPD, suggesting that optimization of goal-setting behaviors may enhance motivation" (p. 108).

2. *Conclusions* refer to the researcher's attempt to demonstrate the knowledge that has been gained based on the study findings (Nieswiedomy, 2008). Conclusions are differentiated from findings in that findings are more concrete, and conclusions are more abstract. *Findings* specify the result. Conclusions suggest a broader, but cautionary, interpretation of the result.
   a. Example of a finding: There is a significant and negative relationship between age and frequency of exercise.
   b. Example of a conclusion based on the above-mentioned finding: Older individuals tend to exercise less frequently. The phrase "tend to" provides the tentative tone based on the finding, which refers to a correlational result.

B. Limitations of the Study Methodology

1. Methodological limitations can include but are not limited to the sample size, which could be too small; the sampling plan, which might not strongly support generalizability (e.g., nonprobability/nonrandom selection of the sample from the population); and the overrepresentation of one group and underrepresentation of another.
   a. Example of a limitation statement in a research report: "Because this is a small study with a convenience sample, generalizability to other people with COPD is limited" (Davis, 2007, p. 109).
2. Definitions of terms used in this section
   a. *Generalizability:* "the degree to which the research methods justify the inference that the findings are true for a broader group than the study participants; usually, the inference that the findings can be generalized from the sample to the population" (Polit & Beck, 2012, p. 729)
   b. *Randomization:* "the assignment of subjects to treatment conditions in a random manner (i.e., in a manner determined by chance alone)" (Polit & Beck, 2012, p. 740)

C. Implications for Nursing Practice

1. The researcher proposes ways in which the findings of the study could be appropriate for practice. However, most study findings, unless derived from a large randomized controlled trial, are not appropriate for translating into practice. Therefore, caution is necessary when a researcher suggests application of his or her findings to practice.
2. Typically, implications for practice should be futuristic so that, after further research is conducted, recommendations for practice can be proposed. Polit and Beck (2012) stated that implications "are speculative and so should be couched in tentative terms" (p. 687). For example, the researcher would use the phrase "the findings suggest" rather than "the findings prove."
   a. Example of an implication statement: "The findings of this study demonstrated that many of the participants were not setting exercise goals to achieve their activity goals. Nurses and other healthcare providers often are involved in the care of patients with COPD in a variety of settings. Nurses may also be directors of pulmonary rehabilitation programs, charged with developing education and exercise interventions and evaluating outcomes of rehabilitation. As clinicians, we have the opportunity to influence the cognition of our patients by providing education and direction" (Davis, 2007, p. 109).

D. Recommendations for Future Research

1. The researcher recommends that future studies be conducted that continue to build on the findings of the current study. Recommendations for the conduction of a study can include, but are not limited to, a different population, a larger sample size, or a different setting.
   a. Example of a recommendation: "Findings from this study may also inform future intervention studies with greater diversity in age, ethnicity, and randomization. Large and more diverse samples would have greater generalizability and provide more definitive recommendations for rehabilitation nursing practice" (Davis, 2007, pp. 109–110).

V. Summary

The content in this chapter addressed the purpose and importance of nursing research specific to rehabilitation nursing and the research process as it applies to an individual investigation or study. However, for application to practice, systematic reviews provide the strongest evidence (Stevens, 2001). "Systematic reviews provide the pivotal point for EBP because of their decided strength over single research studies. Systematic reviews are summaries that use a rigorous scientific approach to combine results from a body of original research studies into a clinically meaningful whole" (Stevens, 2001, p. 537).

References

American Nurses Association (ANA). (2010). *Nursing's social policy statement: The essence of the profession*. Silver Spring, MD: Author.

Association of Rehabilitation Nurses (ARN). (2014a). ARN competency model for professional rehabilitation nursing. Retrieved from http://www.rehabnurse.org/uploads/files/education/ARN_Rehabilitation_Nursing_Competency _Model_FINAL_-_May_2014.pdf

Association of Rehabilitation Nurses (ARN). (2014b). *ARN rehabilitation nursing research agenda* (3rd ed.). Chicago: Author.

Bakas, T., McLennon, S. M., Carpenter, J. S., Buelow, J. M., Otte, J. L., Hanna, K. M., . . . Welch, J. A. (2012). Systematic review of health-related quality of life models. *Health and Quality of Life Outcomes, 10,* 134. Retrieved from http://www.hqlo.com/content/10/1/134

Davis, A. H. T. (2007). Exercise adherence in patients with chronic obstructive disease: An exploration of motivation and goals. *Rehabilitation Nursing, 32,* 2014–2110.

Gavin, T. M. (1996). Research Forum–Methodology–Measurements, Part I: Principles and Theory. *Journal of Prosthetics and Orthotics, 8*(2), 45-49.

Hayat, M. J. (2013). Understanding sample size determination in nursing research. *Western Journal of Nursing Research, 35*(7), 943–956.

Hsieh, C. C., Sprod, L. K., Hydock, D. S., Carter, S. D., Hayward, R., & Schneider, C.M. (2008). The effects of a supervised exercise intervention on recovery from treatment regimens in breast cancer survivors. *Oncology Nursing Forum, 35,* 909–915.

Jochan, H. R., Dassen, T., Widdershoven, G., & Halfens, R. (2006). Quality of life in palliative care cancer patients: A literature review. *Journal of Clinical Nursing, 15*(9), 1188–1195.

Ledbetter, C. A., & Stevens, K. R. (2000). Basics of evidence based practice part 2: Unscrambling the terms and processes. *Seminars in Perioperative Nursing, 9,* 98–104.

Ligthelm, E. J., & Wright, S. C. D. (2014). Lived experience of persons with an amputation of the upper limb. *International Journal of Orthopaedic and Trauma Nursing, 18,* 99–106.

Nieswiadomy, R. M. (2008). *Foundations of nursing research* (5th ed.). Upper Saddle River, NJ: Pearson Education.

Patton, M. Q. (2002). Qualitative evaluation and research methods (3rd ed.). Thousand Oaks, CA: Sage Publications.

Polit, D. F., & Beck, C. T. (2012). *Nursing research: Generating and assessing evidence for nursing practice.* Philadelphia: Lippincott Williams & Wilkins.

Stanley, K. (2007). Design of randomized controlled trials. *Circulation, 115,* 1164–1169.

Stevens, K. R. (2001). Systematic reviews: The heart of evidence-based practice. *AACN Clinical Issues, 12,* 529–538.

Sun, X., Ioannidis, J. P. A., Agoritsas, T., Alba, A. C., & Guyatt, G. (2014). How to use a subgroup analysis: Users' guides to the medical literature. *Journal of the American Medical Association, 311*(4), 405–411.

Walker, L. O., & Avant, K. C. (2004). *Strategies for theory construction in nursing* (4th ed.). Upper Saddle, NJ: Prentice Hall.

Chapter 6

Evidence-Based Practice

Stephanie Vaughn, PhD RN CRRN
Darpan I. Patel, PhD
Frank Puga, PhD

LEARNING OUTCOMES

- Define key research/evidence-based practice (EBP) terms.
- Describe the role of the rehabilitation nurse in the EBP process.
- Discuss importance of EBP to the advancement of rehabilitation nursing as a specialty practice.

KEY CHAPTER TOPICS

- What is evidence-based practice?
- Research designs supporting EBP
- The EBP process: How to start improving practice
- Moving evidence to practice

PROFESSIONAL REHABILITATION NURSING DOMAINS AND COMPETENCIES

- Domain 1: Competency 1.2 (Association of Rehabilitation Nurses [ARN] 2014a)

The Need for Evidence-Based Practice in Rehabilitation Nursing Practice

The complex nature of health care poses a challenge for transformative change (Plesk & Greenhalgh, 2001). Such complexity stresses the need for strategies and solutions that are based on strong evidence and demonstrated outcomes. Therefore, rehabilitation nurses need to make evidence-based practice (EBP) decisions and implement evidence-based interventions and protocols to promote function and health management in persons with disability and chronic illness (ARN, 2014b). The process of searching for, critiquing, and synthesizing current knowledge and applying it to practice can be challenging. It can take decades for research findings to be translated into practice. With the influx of nursing research and knowledge having become more readily available, it is imperative that current evidence is quickly translated into rehabilitation clinical practice. Successful implementation of evidence-based interventions is facilitated by an understanding of the EBP process and confidence among rehabilitation nurses in using these strategies.

New knowledge gained from findings of rigorous research provides rehabilitation nurses and the interprofessional team with tools to translate evidence into practice (i.e., EBP), integrating it with the internal evidence (e.g., process improvement) to foster quality client outcomes in the clinical setting (Reigle et al., 2008). Without current salient evidence, clinical practice can quickly become outdated (Melnyk & Fineout-Overhult, 2011). Opportunities abound in the various clinical settings where rehabilitation nursing is practiced to facilitate EBP. Several models exist that describe how to use the best available evidence to address clinical questions or issues; for example, the ACE STAR Model (Stevens, 2004) the Stetler Model (Stetler, 1994), and Roger's Theory of Diffusion of Innovations (Rogers, 1995).

The revised Association of Rehabilitation Nurses Strategic Plan (ARN, 2013) highlights goals to promote the building of rehabilitation nursing research and its translation into evidence-based practice, which includes improving the knowledge and skills of the rehabilitation nurse and expanding the dissemination and translation of rehabilitation research knowledge into clinical practice. Research, which forms the foundation of EBP, is disseminated via a variety of methods. This research-generated information needs to be made available to rehabilitation nurses and other clinicians for application in practice settings and to other researchers for replication. Ideally, the results would be found in refereed journals such as *Rehabilitation Nursing, Western Journal of Nursing Research, Nursing Research*, or other recognized national and international journals.

The ARN/Rehabilitation Nursing Foundation research agenda reflects those strategic plan goals with priority research issues: (1) nursing and nursing-led interdisciplinary interventions to promote function in people of all ages with disability and/or chronic health problems, (2) experience of disability and/or chronic health problems for individuals and families across the life span, (3) rehabilitation in the changing healthcare system, (4) the rehabilitation nursing profession, (5) nursing and outcomes, (6) nursing and EBP evaluation, and (7) issues of quality and process improvement.

To foster and achieve the ARN research agenda and EBP goals, rehabilitation nurses must be knowledgeable about the basic research process and EBP, and its components, including evidence appraisal and implementation of EB interventions. This chapter defines key research/EBP terms; describes the EBP process, including identification of client issues; explains how to search for and appraise the evidence; and discusses how to move evidence into practice. It also highlights the importance of EBP to the advancement of rehabilitation nursing as a specialty.

I. What is EBP?

A. *Evidence* represents a collection of facts, external evidence generated through rigorous research that can be generalized to other settings, which is best disseminated via clinicians (i.e., rehabilitation nurses) (Melnyk & Fineout-Overholt, 2011). Internal evidence is usually developed by means of a performance improvement (PI) process within an organization, with the goal of improving a certain practice in the setting where it was generated. This section outlines key concepts that define EBP and describes a model that can be used to address a clinical question through the integration of evidence into the practice setting.

II. EBP: A Decision-Making Process Informing Clinical Practice That Integrates

A. Appraisal of High-Level External Evidence

1. Systematic reviews, randomized controlled trials (RCTs) about a specific clinical phenomenon/issue
2. Level of evidence and quality/strength of evidence (Melnyk & Fineout-Overholt, 2011; Polit & Beck, 2012) (**Figure 6-1**)
3. Internal evidence: performance or quality improvement results
4. ACE Star Model (Stevens, 2004)
   a. Discovery research: This is the knowledge-generating stage. In this stage, new knowledge is discovered through the traditional research methodologies and scientific inquiry. Research results are generated through conduction of a single study. This can be called a *primary research study*, and research designs range from descriptive to correlational to causal and from randomized control trials to qualitative trials. This stage builds the corpus of research about clinical actions.
   b. Evidence summary: Evidence summary is the first unique step in EBP—the task is to synthesize the corpus of research knowledge into a single, meaningful statement of the state of the science. The most advanced EBP methods to date are those used to develop evidence summaries (e.g., evidence synthesis, systematic reviews such as the systematic review methods outlined in the *Cochrane Handbook for Systematic Reviews of Interventions)* from randomized control trials. Some evidence summaries employ more rigorous methods than others, yielding more credible and reproducible results.
   c. Translation to guidelines: The aim of translation is to provide a useful and relevant package of summarized evidence to clinicians and clients in a form that suits the time, cost, and care standard. Recommendations are generically termed *clinical practice guidelines* (CPGs) and can be represented or embedded in care standards, clinical pathways, protocols, and algorithms.

Figure 6-1. Evidence Hierarchy: Levels of Evidence Regarding the Effectiveness of an Intervention

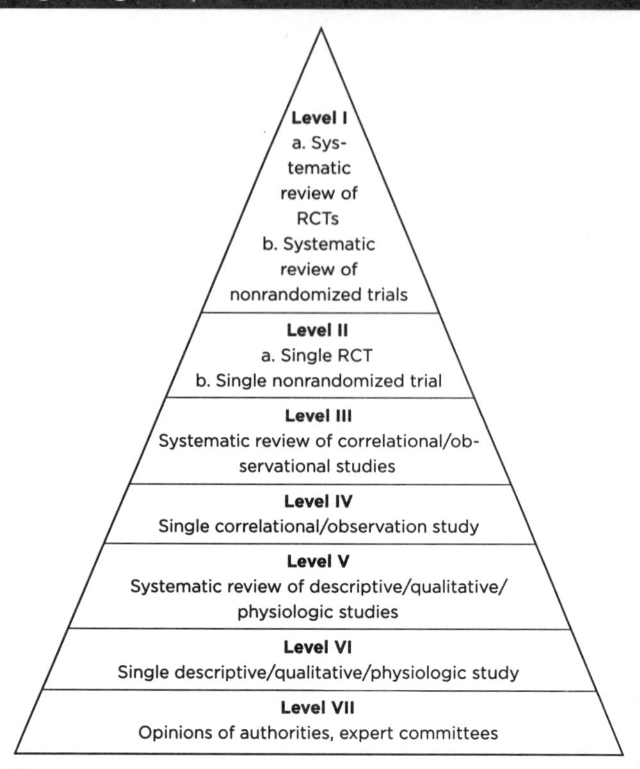

From *Nursing research: Generating and assessing evidence for nursing practice* (9th ed.), by D. F. Polit and C. T. Beck, 2011, Philadelphia: Lippincott Williams & Wilkins. Copyright 2011 by Lippincott Williams & Wilkins. Reprinted with permission.

d. Practice integration: Integration is perhaps the most familiar stage in health care because of society's long-standing expectation that health care be based on the most current knowledge; thus, it requires implementation of innovations. This step involves changing both individual and organizational practices through formal and informal channels. Major factors addressed in this stage are those that affect individuals' and organizations' rates of adoption of innovation and those that affect integration of the change into sustainable systems.

e. Process, outcomes evaluation: The final stage in knowledge transformation is evaluation. In EBP, a broad array of endpoints and outcomes are evaluated. These include evaluation of the impact of EBP on patient health outcomes, provider and patient satisfaction, efficacy, efficiency, economic analysis, and health-status impact. As new knowledge is transformed through the five stages listed here, the final outcome is evidence-based quality improvement of health care.

B. Rehabilitation Nurse Experience, Educational Level, and Evidence Appraisal Skills Influence EBP (Dalheim, Harthug, Nilsen, & Nortvedt, 2012)
   1. Nurse experience and knowledge, rather than evidence, influences practice.
   2. Nurse education levels and years in practice have an impact on research appraisal skills.

C. Consideration of Client/Family Preferences and Values
   1. Client/family culture/values/preferences need to be considered when making clinical decisions.
   2. Client concerns about clinical decisions and treatments need to be addressed.
   3. Client responses to interventions can vary.
   4. Client circumstance can be underdetermined.
   5. Client actions and preferences regarding care/treatment are dominant elements (Melnyk & Fineout-Overholt, 2011).

D. Evaluation of Available Resources and Organizational Barriers
   1. Organizational culture and support for EBP implementation
   2. Nurses' lack of time in locating research reports
   3. Nurses' lack of confidence in ability to appraise research/guidelines
   4. Limited time for implementing change (Dalheim et al., 2012)

E. Evaluation of Outcomes of Practice Change
   1. Impact on healthcare quality?
   2. Impact on client outcomes?
   3. Result in expected outcomes in clinical setting?
   4. Clinical expertise and client preferences integrated with evidence in implementation?

III. EBP Versus Research Utilization: Best Evidence versus Best Practice

A. Research involving clinical trials generally is equated with best evidence.

B. *Best practice* is that which results in the best possible client outcomes (Melnyk & Fineout-Overholt, 2011).
   1. Broader than research-based practice
   2. Integrates expertise of clinician/clients' needs and preferences (Burns & Grove, 2009; Melnyk & Fineout-Overholt, 2011)

IV. EBP Facilitators (Melnyk & Fineout-Overholt, 2011)

A. Organizational culture that supports EBP

B. EBP Mentors: nurse researcher, educator, or advanced practice nurse with EBP skills

C. EBP policies and procedures

D. Sufficient time to search for and evaluate research studies

E. Other Support Activities: journal clubs, EBP rounds, EBP staff education

V. EBP Terminology

A. Nursing Research: "To search again/examine carefully;" specific terminology needed to define nursing knowledge (Burns & Grove, 2011)

B. Clinical Phenomenon/Issue: Something that is observed (e.g., an increase in nocturnal falls in the stroke population) (Burns & Grove, 2011)

C. EBP: Integration of best research studies promoting quality/cost effective client outcomes

D. PICOT Questioning Format: Population, intervention/issue of interest/comparison intervention, outcome, time frame (Melnyk & Fineout-Overholt, 2011)

E. Qualitative Research: "The systematic, interactive subjective approach used to describe life-experiences and give them meaning" (Burns & Grove, 2011, p. 73)

F. Quantitative Research: "The formal, objective, systematic study process to describe and test relationships and to examine cause-and-effect interactions among variables" (Burns & Grove, 2011, p. 34)

G. Descriptive Research: "Research that has as its main objective the accurate portrayal of the characteristics of persons, situations, or groups, or the frequency with which certain phenomena occur" (Polit & Beck, 2012, p. 725)

H. Experimental Research: Objective, systematic, controlled study to test the effects of an intervention or treatment on selected outcomes (Burns & Grove, 2011; Melnyk & Fineout-Overholt, 2011). "This is the strongest design for testing cause-and-effect relationships" (Melnyk & Fineout-Overholt, 2011, p. 575)

I. RCT: A full experimental test of an intervention involving random assignment (an equal opportunity to be selected for either group); "Phase III of a full clinical trial" (Polit & Beck, 2012, p. 740).

J. Quasi-Experimental Research: "A type of experimental design that tests the effects of an intervention or treatment but lacks one or more characteristics of a true experiment (e.g., random assignment, a control or comparison group)" (Melnyk & Fineout-Overholt, 2011, p. 580)

K. Levels of Evidence: Ranking/hierarchy of research/evidence by research design/method (Melnyk & Fineout-Overholt, 2011)

1. Level I: systematic review or meta-analyses of RCT
2. Level II: RCTs
3. Level III: controlled trials without randomization (quasi-experimental)
4. Level IV: case control and cohort
5. Level V: systematic reviews of descriptive and qualitative studies
6. Level VI: single descriptive and qualitative studies
7. Level VII: expert opinion of authorities and/or committees (Melnyk & Fineout-Overholt, 2011, p. 12)

VI. Research Designs Supporting EBP

Quantitative and qualitative research and mixed methods are used to create scientific knowledge to enhance clinical practice and form the foundation of EBP. This section provides a brief overview of the differences between the two research paradigms and key elements to consider when examining the quality and relevance of the evidence generated and its generalizability or transferability to a specific practice situation. Even well-designed research targeted at different client populations might not be transferable to all practice settings. Rehabilitation nurses need to critically evaluate both the strengths and the limitations of a study to determine the feasibility of using the study in a particular setting with a designated client population. Critical appraisal and use of clinical expertise are pivotal aspects of EBP.

A. Quantitative Research Designs

This objective, structured, rigorous, systematic research process generating numeric or quantifiable data through description of phenomena, the

Table 6-1. Types of Quantitative Research Designs

Type of Design	Description	Strengths	Limitations	Examples
Experimental research	A type of research that predicts and controls phenomena , examining causality At least one variable is manipulated. Control exists over the experimental situation. Random assignment.	The most effective way to test hypotheses The most powerful and best-controlled research	Not all variables can be manipulated. Manipulation can create ethical problems. Artificiality is problematic. Generalizability can be limited.	Pretest-posttest design Solomon four-group design Factorial design Repeated-measures design
Quasi-experimental research	One independent variable is manipulated. Lacks at least one of the other two properties that characterize a true experiment.	Practical Feasible Generalizable	Control is lacking, so other hypotheses may exist.	Nonequivalent control group (no randomization) Time series One-group, pretest-posttest design
Nonexperimental research	Researcher collects data without introducing any treatment or changes.			Ex post facto Descriptive research Retrospective and prospective studies Survey research Evaluation research Need assessments Meta-analysis Delphi survey Methodological research Content analysis study

examination of the relationship between variables, or determination of the efficacy of interventions (Burns & Grove, 2011).

1. Quantitative Research Designs
    a. **Table 6-1** describes the most common quantitative research designs (Burns & Grove, 2011; Polit & Beck, 2012).
2. Appraising Quantitative Studies
    a. Quantitative research reports can be evaluated based on several criteria (Burns & Grove, 2011; Polit & Beck, 2012; Rempher & Silkman, 2007).
    b. Three overarching criteria
        1) Are results valid?
        2) What are the findings; are they reliable?
        3) Will the results improve care for my clients?
    c. Critical appraisal questions for quantitative studies (Melnyk & Fineout-Overholt, 2011)
        1) Why was the study done?
        2) What was the sample size?
        3) Was the sample size appropriate for the type of study that was conducted?
        4) Were measures valid and reliable?
        5) How were data analyzed?
        6) Did any issues/untoward events occur during conduction of the study?
        7) Are study results consistent with previous research?
        8) What are the implications for clinical practice?

B. Qualitative Research Designs

1. A systematic research approach is used to describe phenomena subjectively and give them meaning. Four qualitative research traditions are (1) phenomenology, (2) grounded theory, (3) ethnography, and (4) historical. Appraisal of qualitative studies focuses on the design integrity (Burns & Grove, 2011) (**Table 6-2**).
2. Appraising Qualitative Studies (Burns & Grove, 2011)
    a. What problem prompted the study?
    b. Were purpose and research questions consistent with identified research problem?
    c. Did the synthesis of literature identify what is known about the problem and the gaps in knowledge?
    d. What research tradition did the researcher use?
    e. What was the sampling method (e.g., purposive, snowball)?
    f. How were data collected (e.g., interview, focus groups)?
    g. How were human participants protected?
    h. How were data analyzed?
    i. What were the identified themes or concepts that emerged from the data?
    j. Was there evidence of rigor?
        1) Credibility: Do the participants recognize the experience as their own?
        2) Auditability: Can the reader follow the thinking of the researcher? Did the researcher document the research process?
        3) Fittingness: Can the findings be applied outside the study situation? Are the results meaningful to people not involved in the research?

VII. The EBP Process: How to Start Improving Practice

A. Employing EBP is a systematic process that involves developing an action plan, searching for evidence, and appraising the literature. There are many resources for searching for evidence on a topic. More information is becoming available online, and it is important to evaluate online evidence as thoroughly as evidence in print. This section provides an overview of the EBP process.

B. Steps of Evidence-Based Practice (Melnyk & Fineout-Overholt, 2011)

1. Develop a spirit of inquiry.
2. Ask the question in PICOT format.
3. Gather relevant evidence.
4. Appraise evidence (i.e., evaluate and synthesize, determining rigor and strength of studies).
5. Integrate evidence into clinical practice (using rehabilitation nurses' clinical expertise and client preferences).
6. Evaluate the outcomes or the effectiveness of the evidence-based interventions/practice change for a particular client or care situation.

Table 6-2. Types of Qualitative Research

Type	Description
Grounded theory	Develops theories and theoretical propositions that are based on real-world observations; focuses on process
Ethnography	Focuses on the culture of the people being studied
Phenomenology	Considers the lived experience of the people being studied
Historical research	Explores the past and applies findings to present and future
Case studies	In-depth studies on one particular case
Field studies	Examine people and how they function in real life

7. Communicate/disseminate outcomes of change/decision.

C. Searching the Literature/Gathering Evidence

1. Searching for the Evidence
   a. Traditional scholarly sources of evidence such as refereed/peer-reviewed journals, books, and non–peer-reviewed professional magazines.
   b. The World Wide Web is composed of interconnected documents that are available online (e.g., PubMed). Published articles; program descriptions; personal opinions; government documents; and information on businesses, organizations, and agencies are posted to websites.
   c. Essential steps of a search strategy
      1) Formulate a clear clinical question that contains no jargon or ambiguity.
      2) Determine the database, such as CINAHL or PubMED. Which is appropriate to use for the question?
      3) Decide which type of study design would best answer the question.
      4) Enter a subject heading or text word search guided by the PICOT components of the question.
      5) Start combining searches to find relevant evidence.
      6) Further restrict combined searches for study design, methods, indicators of clinical meaningfulness, or other appropriate, available limits. Consider limiting the search to English language and human subjects, depending on the question and the searcher.
      7) Apply a priori inclusion and exclusion criteria to studies gathered in the search to find the best available evidence (Melnyk & Fineout-Overholt, 2011).
      8) A librarian can be helpful in choosing search terms that aid in narrowing the topic (Pierce, 2009).
   d. Indexes and other sources
      1) The CINAHL index is "in nursing, the most relevant print database which contains citations of nursing literature published after 1955" (Burns & Grove, 2011, p. 94). The CINAHL database is available at www.ebscohost.com/CINAHL.
      2) The Cochrane Database of Systematic Reviews is prepared by the Cochrane Review Groups in the Cochrane Collaboration; each review is highly structured and systematic, with evidence included or excluded on the basis of explicit quality criteria to minimize bias (The Cochrane Library, 2010; Melnyk & Fineout-Overholt, 2011).
      3) Clinical practice guidelines are systematically developed statements based on the best available evidence to guide the management of persons or populations with specific conditions (Burns & Grove, 2011; Conway & Larson, 2012; Melnyck & Fineout-Overholt, 2011; Tricoci, Allen, Kranmer, Califf, & Smiyh, 2009)
      4) The National Guideline Clearinghouse (2010) includes summaries of evidence-based clinical practice guidelines and related documents. A condensed version of the guideline and a link to the full clinical practice guideline are available at www.guideline.gov.
      5) MEDLINE, from the National Library of Medicine, is the bibliographical database covering the fields of medicine, nursing, dentistry, veterinary medicine, the healthcare system, and the preclinical sciences (U.S. National Library of Medicine, 2010) and is available at www.ncbi.nlm.nih.gov/sites/entrez.
      6) PsycINFO: This database contains literature in behavioral and social sciences and mental health (American Psychological Association, 2010) and is available at www.apa.org/pubs/databases/psycinfo/index.aspx.
2. Outcomes of the Search: How Much Literature Is Enough?
   a. Use the most current literature in the search (i.e., from the last 5 years).
   b. Incorporate classic research literature related to a topic. If a researcher's name is in many or most of studies on a particular topic, refer to the seminal work.
   c. Once retrieved, research articles must be appraised and evaluated (Pierce, 2007).

D. Appraising the Literature for EBP

1. Literature Reviews (four types)
   a. *Narrative review*
      1) Summarizes different primary studies that support an author's point of view from which conclusions are drawn based on the reviewer's interpretation; presents a general background discussion for a particular issue or topic (Melnyk & Fineout-Overholt, 2011)
      2) Nonsystematic in approach to identifying articles and papers
   b. *Systematic review*: "A summary of evidence typically conducted by an expert or expert panel on a particular topic, that uses a rigorous process (to minimize bias) for identifying,

appraising, and synthesizing studies to answer a specific clinical question and draw conclusions about the data gathered" (Melnyk & Fineout-Overholt, 2011, p. 582).

c. *Meta-analysis*: "A statistical pooling of the results from several previous studies into a single quantitative analysis that provides one of the highest levels of evidence for an intervention's efficacy" (Burns & Grove, 2011, p. 541). A meta-analysis provides a single effect measure of all the summarized study results (Melnyk & Fineout-Overholt, 2011).

d. *Meta-synthesis*: "The interpretive translations produced from the integration or comparison of findings from qualitative studies" (Polit & Beck, 2012, p. 733). A meta-synthesis is neither a literature review nor a concept analysis (Polit & Beck).

2. Appraising the Quality of Systematic Reviews

a. Systematic reviews that themselves can identify and synthesize research based on a rigorous process that addresses a specific research question/topic are available to clinicians, policy decision makers, and clients (Burns & Grove, 2011; Melnyk & Fineout-Overholt, 2011).

b. Various instruments are available to evaluate the quality of the systematic review, such as the Appraisal of Guidelines for Research and Evaluation (AGREE) tool and the Conference on Guideline Standardization, among others (Melnyk & Fineout-Overholt, 2011).

c. AGREE tool (Melnyk & Fineout-Overholt, 2011)

a. Scope and purpose: Question and objectives were clearly described.

b. Stakeholder involvement: Professional groups, clients' views and preferences, and target users were identified.

c. Rigor of development: A strong link between recommendations and supporting evidence was found.

d. Clarity and presentation: Recommendations and specific options for management of condition were clearly presented.

e. Application: Organizational factors and cost implications of recommendations were noted.

f. Editorial independence: Any conflict of interest is noted.

3. Limitations of Systematic Reviews and Meta-Analyses

a. A disadvantage of systematic reviews is that the information cannot be generalized. A systematic review is so detailed that it can be applied only to the specific clinical question that is proposed.

b. A meta-analysis can be detrimental when the studies are too different to combine them in a statistically meaningful way (Melnyk & Fineout-Overholt, 2011).

VIII. Moving Evidence to Practice

To provide quality, cost-effective care in healthcare settings where rehabilitation nursing is practiced, interventions based on the best available evidence must be implemented. Strategies to implement evidence-based interventions into practice involve a systematic process that, as previously stated, begins with a PICOT question and the appraisal of the available evidence that addresses the question. Evaluation of the implemented evidence-based interventions is an essential component of this process. Models such as the reach efficacy-adoption implementation maintenance (RE-AIM) model (Glasgow, McKay, Piette, & Reynolds, 2001) can be used to systematically consider the strengths and weaknesses of the intervention(s).

IX. Using the Evidence: Creating an Environment for Translating Evidence into Practice (EBP)

A. EBP begins with a vision and organizational philosophy that reflect the goals of clinical excellence and EBP culture.

B. The impetus to create an EBP culture is grounded in regulatory and accreditation initiatives and mandated outcomes; for example, CMS's payment policy regarding hospitalized clients' "preventable complications," such as hospital-acquired infections and pressure ulcers.

C. The Magnet Recognition Program has also contributed to the creation of an EBP culture/environment to promote nursing excellence and quality innovations in practice (American Nurses Credentialing Center, 2014).

D. Although EBP advances the quality of care for clients and the practice of rehabilitation nursing, translation into clinical practice takes time.

1. Examples of strategies and issues regarding the uptake of EBP to promote practices that sustain quality care and improved health outcomes include the development and critical appraisal of clinical practice guidelines, adoption and spread of best practices, customization of best practices, institutional elements in adoption, defining best practice in the absence of evidence, consumers in EBP, and technology-based integration (Stevens & Ovretveit, 2013).

2. Approach: Although no uniform consensus exists on how to translate evidence into clinical practice,

the following steps capture the essence of a suggested approach:

a. Assess the need for change in practice.
b. Link the problem with interventions and outcomes.
c. Synthesize the best evidence.
d. Design a change in practice.
e. Implement and evaluate practice.
f. Integrate and maintain the practice change.

E. Integration of Evidence into Rehabilitation Nursing

1. EBP is critical to the present and future practice of rehabilitation nursing.
2. The commitment to EBP is reflected in the *ARN Professional Rehabilitation Nursing Domains and Competencies,* (ARN, 2014a) practice standards, and other publications.
3. According to the *ARN Competency Model for Professional Rehabilitation Nursing* (2014a), rehabilitation nurses, whether novice or experienced, use current evidence and supportive technology to deliver optimum patient- and family-centered care. Evidence-based best practices support these nurse-led interventions as well as all of the patient and caregiver education necessary for maximizing the quality of life for rehabilitation clients in a variety of clinical settings.
4. A key component of successful EBP outcomes is the recognition and initiation of interventions at the individual and organizational levels that consider the interaction between the individual, social, organizational, and economic factors that affect EBP.

F. Examples of EBP Implementation

1. CPGs are systematically developed statements that assist the practitioner and client in formulating decisions about appropriate health care. These can be based on expert opinion or consensus- or EBP as identified by research (Burns & Grove, 2011; Melnyk & Fineout-Overholt, 2011). Examples of clinical practice guidelines can be found at www.guideline.gov/ and strokeorganization.org. Another example is Miller and colleagues (2010) explicated guidelines for the management of stroke clients in the postacute setting.
2. Other real-life examples of evidence-based practices that have been implemented in clinical settings can be found at the Agency for Healthcare Research and Quality's Health Care Innovations Exchange (HCIE; 2012; http://www.innovations.ahrq.gov/). The Health Care Innovations Exchange (HCIE) is an expanding database of refereed, evidence-based innovations and quality tools used to improve practices across the country. The HCIE also accepts submission of new and novel innovations that are reviewed by an expert panel and submitted for publication into the HCIE.
3. Algorithms are "written guidelines to stepwise evaluation and management strategies that require observations to be made, decisions to be considered, and actions to be taken" (MacDermid 2008, p. 241). A good example of algorithms can be found in CMS's *Inpatient Rehabilitation Facility Patient Assessment Instrument Training Manual* (CMS, 2012) and scoring of the FIM™ instrument.
4. A clinical pathway is a framework or guide based on previous research, agency data, or clinical experience to define expected care actions and outcomes in a particular care situation (Burns & Grove, 2011). Interventions commonly included in a clinical pathway are consultations and referrals; assessments and observations; tests, treatments, measurements, and diagnostics; nutrition, medications, activity, and mobility; safety; client and family education or teaching; and discharge planning and follow-up, such as guidelines to manage specific stroke sequelae (e.g., poststroke urinary incontinence) (Vaughn, 2009).
5. Healthcare policies and laws are derived from evidence. Legislators cannot propose legislation without the necessary substantiation, based on various sources of evidence (Melnyk & Fineout-Overholt, 2011).

G. Using Interprofessional Teams to Facilitate Uptake of EBP

1. Improving care quality and practice is a complex process that requires partnerships between scientists and academicians.
2. Current frameworks suggest that transdisciplinary interaction promotes effective, sustainable intervention programs (Damschroder et al., 2009).
3. In team science, best practices exist to help foster collaborative efforts that promote effective transdisciplinary collaboration and readiness, establish shared mental models, and adopt effective project support and management (Puga, Patel, & Stevens, 2013; Stevens, Puga, & Patel, 2012).
4. Improvement and implementation science is a growing field, and new insights into adoption and uptake of EBP are gleaned from transdisciplinary research.
5. Roles for rehabilitation nurses in collaborative improvement/implementation research include
   a. Rehabilitation nurse researcher
      1) Serves as local site principal investigator
      2) Builds and coordinate research team
      3) Submits institutional review board protocol

4) Ensures scientific rigor

b. Rehabilitation nurse educator

1) Shares resources on improvement science

2) Educates nurses on study goals and implications

c. Rehabilitation nurse manager

1) Recruits participants

2) Coordinates data entry

3) Disseminates reports

d. Rehabilitation staff nurse

1) Provides the front-line voice

2) Collects data

3) Provides perspective on results context

6. Evaluation process (RE-AIM) (Glasgow et al., 2001)

a. Reach

b. Efficacy

c. Adoption

d. Implementation

e. Maintenance

X. Summary

A. New knowledge gained from findings of rigorous research provides rehabilitation nurses and the interprofessional team with tools to translate evidence into practice.

B. EBP is a systematic process that includes using current, relevant research findings to improve outcomes and sustain quality practice.

C. EBP is influenced by clinical expertise/opinions and client needs and preferences. The evidence is applied by nurses and other interprofessional team members to improve the delivery of cost-effective, collaborative rehabilitation care.

D. Rehabilitation nurses recognize that ultimately, individuals are part of the family unit, and families comprise the support structure in each community.

E. Rehabilitation nurses are responsible for providing client and family-centered care and contributing to the promotion of function and health management in persons with disability and/or chronic illness through the use of technology, client and caregiver education, and nurse-led, interprofessional interventions based on the best available evidence (ARN, 2014b).

References

Agency for Healthcare Research and Quality (2012). Health Care Innovations Exchange. Retrieved from http://www.innovations.ahrq.gov/index.aspx

American Nurses Credentialing Center (2014). Magnet Recognition Program. Retrieved from http://www.nursecredentialing.org/magnet.aspx

American Psychological Association (2010). *Publication manual of the American Psychological Association* (5th ed.). Washington, DC: Author.

Association of Rehabilitation Nurses (ARN). (2013). Strategic plan. Retrieved from http://www.rehabnurse.org/about/content/ARN-Strategic-Plan.html

Association of Rehabilitation Nurses (ARN). (2014a). ARN competency model for professional rehabilitation nursing. Retrieved from http://www.rehabnurse.org/uploads/files/education/ARN_Rehabilitation_Nursing_Competency _Model_FINAL_-_May_2014.pdf

Association of Rehabilitation Nurses (ARN). (2014b). *The rehabilitation nursing research agenda* (3rd ed.). Retrieved from http://www.rehabnurse.org/about/content/Research-Agenda.html

Burns, N., & Grove, S. (2011). *The practice of nursing research: Appraisal, synthesis, and generation of evidence* (5th ed.). St. Louis: Elsevier Saunders.

Centers for Medicare & Medicaid Services (2012). *Inpatient rehabilitation facility patient assessment instrument training manual.* Retrieved from http://www.cms.gov/Medicare/Medicare-Fee-for-Service-Payment/InpatientRehabFacPPS/Downloads/IRFPAI-manual-2012.pdf

The Cochrane Library (2010). About the Cochrane Collection. Retrieved from www.thecochranelibrary.com/view/0/AboutTheCochraneLibrary.html#CENTRAL

Conway, L., & Larson, E. (2012). Guidelines to prevent catheter associated urinary infections: 1980-2010. *Heart & Lung: The Journal of Acute and Critical Care, 41*(3), 271–283.

Dalheim, A., Harthug, S., Nilsen, R., & Nortvedt, M. (2012) Factors influencing the development of evidence-based practice among nurses: A self-report survey. *BMC Health Services Research, 12*, 367. Retrieved from http://www.biomedcentral.com/1472-6963/12/367

Damschroder, L. J., Aron, D. C., Keith, R. E., Kirsh, S. R., Alexander, J. A., & Lowery, J. C. (2009). Fostering implementation of health services research findings into practice: a consolidated framework for advancing implementation science. *Implementation Science, 4*(50). doi:10.1186/1748-5908-4-50

Glasgow, R., McKay, H., Piette, J., & Reynolds, K. (2001). The RE-AIM framework for evaluating interventions: What can it tell us about approaches to chronic illness management? *Patient Education Counselling, 44*(2), 119–127.

Melnyk, B. M., & Fineout-Overholt, E. (2011). *Evidence-based practice in nursing & healthcare: A guide to best practice* (2nd ed.). Philadelphia: Lippincott Williams & Wilkins.

MacDermid, J. (2008). Practice guidelines, algorithms, and clinical pathways. In M. Law, J. MacDermid (Eds), *Evidence-Based Rehabilitation. A Guide to Practice.* (2nd ed., 227–261). Hamilton, NJ: Slack, Incorporated.

Miller, E. L., Murray, L., Richards, L., Zorowitz, R. D., Bakas, T., Clark, P., & Billinger, S. A. (2010). Comprehensive overview of nursing and interdisciplinary rehabilitation care of the stroke patient. A scientific statement from the American Heart Association. *Stroke: A Journal of Cerebral Circulation.* doi:10.1161/STR.0b013e3181e7512b10A

National Guideline Clearinghouse (2010). About NGC. Retrieved from www.guideline.gov/about/index.aspx

Pierce, L. (2007). Evidence-based practice in rehabilitation nursing. *Rehabilitation Nursing, 32*(5), 203–209.

Pierce, L. (2009). Twelve steps for success in the nursing research journey. *Journal of Continuing Education in Nursing, 40*(4), 154–162.

Plesk, P. E., & Greenhalgh, T. (2001).Complexity science: The challenge of complexity in health care. *British Medical Journal, 323*, 625–628.

Polit, D. F., & Beck, C. T. (2011). *Nursing research: Generating and assessing evidence for nursing practice* (9th ed.). Philadelphia: Lippincott Williams & Wilkins.

Puga, F., Patel, D. I., & Stevens, K. R. (2013). Adoption of best practices in team science with a healthcare improvement research network. *Nursing Research and Practice*, 814360.

Reigle, B. S., Stevens, K. R., Belcher, J. V., Hugh, M. M., McGuire, E., & Mals, D. (2008). Evidence-based practice and the road to magnet status. *Journal of Nursing Administration, 38*(2), 97–102.

Rempher, K. J., & Silkman, C. (2007). How to appraise quantitative research articles. *American Nurse Today, 2*(1), 26–28.

Rogers, E. M. (1995). *Diffusion of innovations* (4th ed.). New York: Free Press.

Stetler, C. B. (1994). Refinement of the Stetler/Marram model of application of research findings to practice. *Nursing Outlook, 42*(1), 15–25.

Stevens, K. R. (2004). ACE Star Model: Knowledge Transformation. Academic Center for Evidence-Based Practice. The University of Texas Health Science Center at San Antonio. Retrieved from http://www.acestar.uthscsa.edu/acestar-model.asp

Stevens, K. R., & Ovretveit, J. (2013). Improvement research priorities: USA survey and expert consensus. *Nursing Research and Practice.* doi:10.1155/2013/695729

Stevens, K. R., Puga, F., & Patel, D. I. (2012). *Building successful research collaboratives for healthcare improvement.* San Antonio: Academic Center for Evidence-Based Practice.

Tricoci, P., Allen, J. M., Kramer, J. M., Califf, R. M., & Smith, S. C. (2009). Scientific evidence underlying the ACC/AHA Clinical Practice Guidelines. *Journal of the American Medical Association, 301*(8), 831–841.

U.S. National Library of Medicine (2010). MEDLINE Fact Sheet. Retrieved from www.nlm.nih.gov/pubsfactsheets/medline.html

Vaughn, S. (2009). The efficacy of evidence-based urinary guidelines in the management of post-stroke incontinence. *The International Journal of Urologic Nursing, 3*(1), 4–12.

Chapter 7

Quality and Safety: Performance Measurement and Accountability

Terrie Black, DNP MBA BSN RN CRRN FAHA
Anne Deutsch, PhD RN CRRN

LEARNING OUTCOMES

- Define key terms used in quality measurement and performance improvement.
- Identify four frameworks that are valuable to use when measuring quality and safety in health care.
- Describe the World Health Organization (WHO) International Classification of Functioning, Disability, and Health (ICF) framework for health and disability and its application to outcome measurement in the rehabilitation setting.
- Discuss federal quality measurement efforts throughout the rehabilitation continuum of care.
- Discuss models and tools used in process improvement.
- Identify key agencies that accredit rehabilitation programs.

KEY CHAPTER TOPICS

- Definitions
- Measuring quality and safety
- Medicare assessment tools
- Outcome measurement
- Process improvement
- Accrediting rehabilitation facilities

PROFESSIONAL REHABILITATION NURSING DOMAINS AND COMPETENCIES

- Domain 1: Competencies 1.1, 1.2, 1.3, 1.4
- Domain 2: Competencies 2.1, 2.2, 2.3
- Domain 3: Competency 3.1
- Domain 4: Competency 4.2 (Association of Rehabilitation Nurses [ARN], 2014)

Introduction

Performance measurement and accountability are essential for ensuring the delivery of high-quality health care and patient safety. Performance measurement focuses on measuring the quality and safety of care delivered by a clinician or team of clinicians. *Accountability* refers to sharing performance data through public reporting or performance-based payment. Reports from the Institute of Medicine (IOM) have documented quality gaps and the need to monitor quality using standardized quality measures. Rehabilitation programs have focused on measuring quality primarily through the outcomes of care, including improvement in patients' functional status. The Centers for Medicare & Medicaid Services (CMS) has begun several quality reporting programs and publicly reports quality data for nursing homes and home health agencies. Accreditation organizations, such as The Joint Commission and the Commission on Accreditation of Rehabilitation Facilities (CARF) International, also are responsible for ensuring the quality and safety of care provided by healthcare organizations. Rehabilitation nursing has responded to these initiatives by monitoring patient outcomes, including improvement in patients' functional status and the prevention of new and worsening pressure ulcers and hospital-acquired infections and injuries.

This chapter provides an overview of quality and safety in healthcare, frameworks for quality measurement, quality measurement in rehabilitation, and federal quality reporting efforts and profiles the agencies that accredit rehabilitation programs.

I. Quality and Performance Measurement in Health Care

A. Overview and Background

1. Key terms and definitions
   a. *Healthcare quality*: "Degree to which patient care services increase the probability of desired patient outcomes and reduce the probability of undesired health outcomes given the current state of knowledge" (Institute of Medicine [IOM], 2006, p. 468)
   b. *Patient safety*: Reporting, analysis, and prevention of medical errors that can lead to adverse healthcare events
   c. *Performance measurement*: Measuring the quality and safety of care delivered by a clinician or team of clinicians
   d. *Accountability*: Sharing performance data through public reporting or performance-based payment
   e. *Quality measure*: The "quantification of the degree to which a desired healthcare process or outcome is achieved or the extent that a desirable structure to support healthcare delivery is in place" (IOM, 2006, p. 42)
2. Key IOM reports
   a. *To Err Is Human: Building a Safer Health System* (IOM, 2000)
      1) Presented a roadmap to a safer healthcare system
      2) Reported that thousands of Americans die each year from preventable medical errors
      3) Proposed that improvement can be made with adequate leadership, attention, and resources
   b. *Crossing the Quality Chasm: A New Health System for the 21st* Century (IOM, 2001)
      1) This report concluded that there are quality gaps in the U.S. healthcare system and presented a comprehensive plan to reinvent the healthcare system to foster innovation and improve delivery of care.
      2) Presented 10 rules for healthcare system redesign
         a) Care is based on continuous healing relationships.
         b) Care is customized according to client needs and values.
         c) The client is the source of control.
         d) Knowledge is shared, and information flows freely.
         e) Decision making is evidence based.
         f) Safety is a system property.
         g) Transparency is necessary.
         h) Needs are anticipated.
         i) Waste is continuously decreased.
         j) Cooperation between clinicians is a priority.
   c. *Performance Measurement: Accelerating Improvement* (IOM, 2006): This report noted that the only way to know whether healthcare quality is improving is to document performance using standardized measures of quality.

B. Frameworks for Measuring Quality and Safety

1. Quality measures address several aspects of care, which have been classified by Donabedian (2005) as structure measures, process measures, and outcome measures.
   a. Structure measures track whether a particular mechanism or system is in place.
   b. Process measures track performance of a particular action.
   c. Outcome measures consider the end results of care, such as morbidity and mortality resulting from a disease.
2. The IOM identified six aims of healthcare delivery (IOM, 2001), sometimes referred to as STEEEP (Safe, Timely, Efficient, Effective, Equitable and Patient Centered):
   a. Safe care does not injure the clients; it is intended to help.
   b. Timely care is provided in a way that reduces wait times.
   c. Effective care involves services that are based on scientific knowledge and provided to all who could benefit but not to those not likely to benefit.
   d. Efficient care avoids waste, including waste of equipment, supplies, ideas, and energy.
   e. Equitable care does not vary in quality because of personal characteristics (e.g., gender, ethnicity, geographic location, or socioeconomic status).
   f. Patient-centered care is respectful of and responsive to individual client preferences, needs, and values.
3. National Quality Strategy (Agency for Healthcare Research and Quality; n.d.)
   a. The Affordable Care Act called for a National Quality Strategy to improve the delivery of healthcare services, patient health outcomes, and population health. After engaging both public and private stakeholders and collecting input, the National Quality Strategy was released in March 2011.

b. A central goal of the National Quality Strategy is to build a consensus on how to measure quality so that stakeholders can align their efforts for maximum results. The strategy is a framework for quality measurement, measure development, and analysis of where everyone can do more, including people in U.S. Department of Health and Human Services (HHS) agencies and programs and in the private sector.

c. The strategy presents three aims for the healthcare system

1) Better care: Improve the overall quality of care by making health care more patient centered, reliable, accessible, and safe.

2) Healthy people and communities: Improve the health of the U.S. population by supporting proven interventions to address behavioral, social, and environmental determinants of health in addition to delivering higher-quality care.

3) Affordable care: Reduce the cost of high-quality health care for individuals, families, employers, and government.

d. Six strategies

1) Making care safer by reducing harm caused in the delivery of care

2) Ensuring that patients and families are engaged as partners in their care

3) Promoting effective communication and coordination of care

4) Promoting the most effective prevention and treatment practices for the leading causes of mortality (e.g., cardiovascular disease)

5) Working with communities to promote wide use of best practices to enable healthy living

6) Making high-quality care more affordable for individuals, families, employers, and governments by developing and spreading new healthcare delivery models

C. Framework for Measuring Rehabilitation Outcomes

1. International Classification of Functioning, Disability, and Health (ICF) is a classification of health and health-related domains that describe body functions and structures, activities, and participation. It is the World Health Organization (WHO) framework for health and disability. It is a conceptual framework, not an assessment instrument. The domains are classified from body function, individual, and societal perspectives. Because a person's functioning and disability occur in a context, ICF also includes a list of environmental factors (WHO, 2001).

2. Body functions and structures: An abnormality of body structure, appearance, and organ or system function can result from any cause. Impairments occur at the organ level (e.g., dysphagia, hemiparesis).

3. Activities and participation: The consequences of impairment can be described in terms of a person's functional performance and activity or the nature and extent of function at the individual level. There may be activity disturbances at the level of the person bathing, dressing, communicating, walking, or grooming. The effects of impairments on work, family, and social roles determine the nature and extent of a person's involvement in life and various activities. Participation reflects interaction with and adaptation to one's surroundings.

4. Environmental factors: Examples of barriers and facilitators include climate and terrain, social attitudes, or physical elements such as curbs and steps.

5. **Figure 7-1** represents the model of disability that is the basis for ICF.

II. Quality Measurement in Rehabilitation and Postacute Care

A. Overview

1. Quality measures involve systematic collection, analysis, and use of data to evaluate and improve a particular program using items, instruments, and data sets.

2. When assessing the quality of rehabilitation care, an organization must collect data using items and instruments that have demonstrated reliability and validity so that accurate performance can be identified.

a. Reliability: Reproducibility of an item of instrument's scores

b. Validity: Ability of the item to measure what it was designed or intended to measure

3. Rehabilitation programs have traditionally measured quality in terms of outcomes achieved by clients. Measuring and monitoring outcomes are useful for the following reasons:

a. Track efficiency and effectiveness

b. Identify trends

c. Facilitate communication between the client, family, treatment team, payers, referral source, and other stakeholders

d. Assess follow-up measures to determine whether progress is continuing after discharge

e. Identify areas for improvement

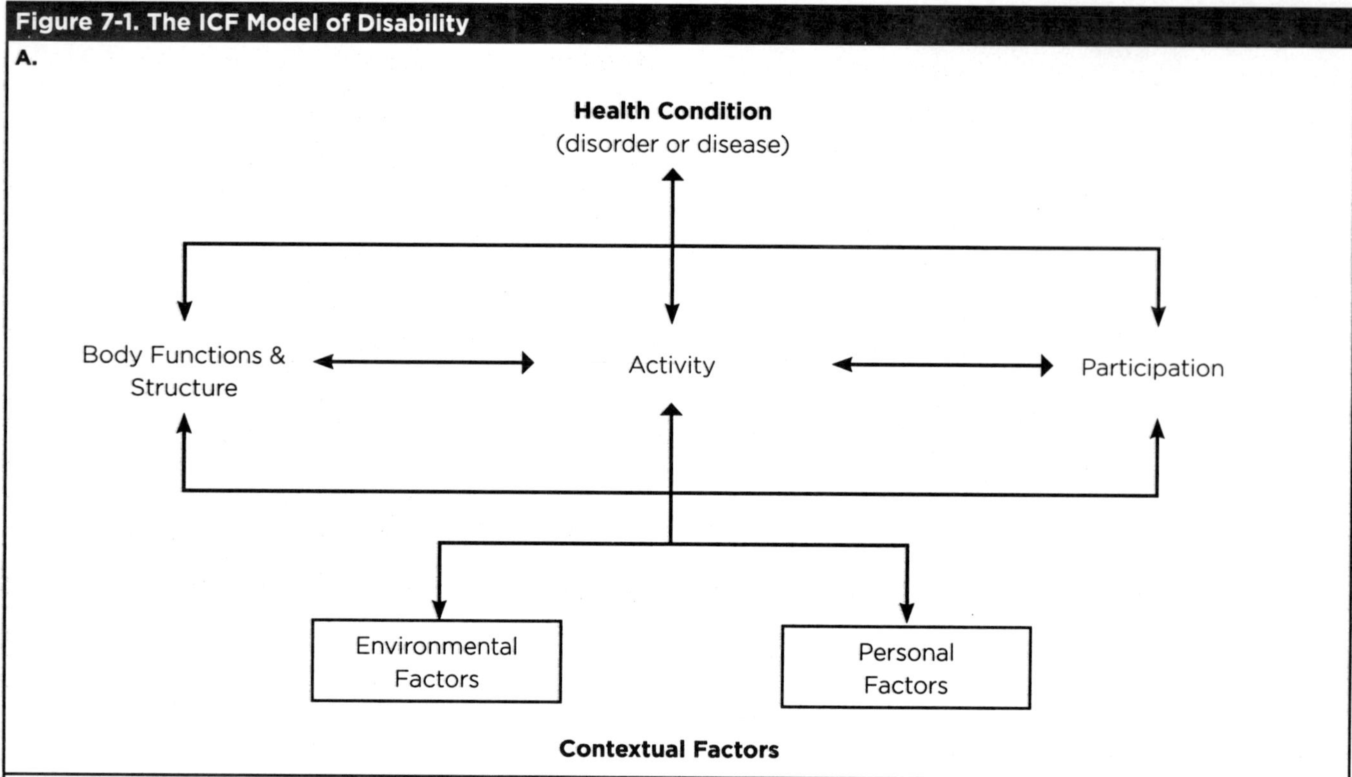

Figure 7-1. The ICF Model of Disability

B. Quick Reference of Terms Used in the ICF

Body functions are physiological functions of body systems (including psychological functions).

Body structures are anatomical parts of the body such as organs, limbs, and their components.

Impairments are problems in body function or structure such as a significant deviation or loss.

Activity is the execution of a task or action by an individual.

Participation is involvement in a life situation.

Activity limitations are difficulties an individual may have in executing activities.

Participation restrictions are problems an individual may experience in involvement in life situations.

Environmental factors make up the physical, social, and attitudinal environment in which people live and conduct their lives.

From "International Classification of Functioning, Disability and Health," by World Health Organization, 2001. Retrieved from http://www.who.int/entity/classifications/icf/en. Copyright 2001 by World Health Organization. Reprinted with permission.

4. Rehabilitation programs recognize that stakeholders are interested in quality and safety data. Therefore, there is a greater accountability to provide and share information about programs and outcomes with various stakeholders:
   a. Internal stakeholders include a rehabilitation program's case managers, administrator, board of directors, clinicians, and parties such as researchers and quality improvement practitioners who are interested in outcome data.
   b. External stakeholders who often evaluate programs and services using outcome data include case managers, payers, referral sources, and direct consumers of healthcare services.
5. Quality and safety data can be benchmarked according to past trends within an organization or corporation, national and regional standards or norms, and best practice standards. Benchmarking data can also be used to improve rehabilitation nursing care and serve as the basis for research. In addition, benchmarking data can provide insight into opportunities for performance improvement for a rehabilitation program.

B. Quality Improvement: Quality improvement for rehabilitation programs often focuses on the following key outcomes:
   1. Functional status at discharge: Improvement in motor and cognitive function
   2. Discharge destination: Discharge to the community or to the least restrictive environment
   3. Client experience: Satisfaction and perceptions of the client, family, and other stakeholders
   4. Follow-up functional status: Should improve or be maintained after discharge from the rehabilitation program

5. Readmissions: Clients readmitted to an acute care hospital soon after discharge from the rehabilitation program

C. Organizations Involved in Quality Measure Definitions and Endorsement

1. The National Database of Nursing Quality Indicators (NDNQI) contains data for the following indicators (www.nursingquality.org/):
   a. Nursing staff skill mix
   b. Nursing hours per client day
   c. Assault and injury rates
   d. Catheter-associated urinary tract infection rate
   e. Central line–associated bloodstream infection rate
   f. Fall and injury rates
   g. Hospital- or unit-acquired pressure ulcer rates
   h. Nurse turnover rate
   i. Pain assessment–intervention–reassessment cycles completed
   j. Peripheral intravenous line infiltration rate
   k. Physical restraint prevalence
   l. Registered nurse education and certification
   m. Registered nurse survey
   n. Practice environment scale
   o. Job satisfaction
   p. Ventilator-associated pneumonia rate
2. Exchanged Quality Data for Rehabilitation (EQUADR, n.d.)
   a. This rehabilitation-specific quality and safety organization database has a mission to improve overall quality and safety of healthcare services for rehabilitation patients in the United States before, during, and after their hospital stay.
   b. Hospital staff members can share information and conduct open discussions about quality and safety with other patient safety organization members without fear that the information will be shared externally or be subject to legal discovery.
   c. Quality indicators include rates of unassisted falls, restraint use, and pressure ulcers.
3. National Quality Forum (NQF, n.d.)
   a. The NQF is a voluntary consensus standard-setting organization. Its mission is to improve the quality of American healthcare by setting national priorities and goals for performance improvement, endorsing national consensus standards for measuring and publicly reporting on performance, and promoting the attainment of national goals through education and outreach programs.
   b. NQF-endorsed quality measures are used in 20 federal programs, including inpatient rehabilitation facilities, skilled nursing facilities, long-term care hospitals (LTCHs), and home health agencies.
   c. A list of endorsed quality measures can be searched at www.qualityforum.org/QPS.

D. Instruments That Measure Functional Status

1. Activity of Daily Living (ADL) Instruments
   a. FIM™ instrument (**Figure 7-2**)
      1) Measures severity of disability and the need for assistance (burden of care)
      2) Designed to promote a uniform language among the rehabilitation team and to describe the severity of disability
      3) Is included as part of the Inpatient Rehabilitation Facility Patient Assessment Instrument (IRF-PAI), which includes demographic, diagnostic, financial, and functional information about rehabilitation clients
      4) Includes 18 items (13 motor, 5 cognitive)
      5) Uses a 7-level scale in which 1 = *total assistance* (client performs less than 25% of an activity) and 7 = *total independence* (client performs an activity without an assistive device or a helper in a safe and timely manner); 0 (*activity does not occur*) is used for admission only for items not occurring during the 3-day admission assessment timeframe.
      6) Is used internationally
      7) Can be used by trained members of any discipline
      8) Provides the basis for predicting outcomes for various client populations
      9) Is the foundation for establishing case mix groups (CMGs), which are used as part of the IRF payment system
      10) Can be used to estimate the burden of care for ADLs (based on the FIM™ "Rule of Thumb Burden of Care" chart; Deutsch, Braun, & Granger, 1997; Uniform Data System for Medical Rehabilitation, 1996)
      11) Can be uploaded into a database to allow facilities to examine factors such as demographic data, diagnoses, and financial information. These databases also allow comparison of FIM™ data over time and with the data of others.
2. Instrumental Activities of Daily Living (IADLs) scale (Dittmar & Gresham, 1997)
   a. Encompasses activities that are more difficult than basic ADLs

Figure 7-2. Functional Independence Measure (FIM™) Instrument

FIM™ Instrument

LEVELS		
	7 Complete Independence (timely, safely) 6 Modified Independence (device)	**NO HELPER**
	Modified Dependence 5 Supervision (subject = 100%) 4 Minimal Assistance (subject = 75%+) 3 Moderate Assistance (subject = 50%+) **Complete Dependence** 2 Maximal Assistance (subject =25%+) 1 Total Assistance (subject = less than 25%)	**HELPER**

	ADMISSION	DISCHARGE	FOLLOW-UP
Self-Care			
A. Eating			
B. Grooming			
C. Bathing			
D. Dressing - Upper Body			
E. Dressing - Lower Body			
F. Toileting			
Sphincter Control			
G. Bladder Management			
H. Bowel Management			
Transfers			
I. Bed, Chair, Wheelchair			
J. Toilet			
K. Tub, Shower			
Locomotion			
L. Walk/Wheelchair	W Walk / C Wheelchair / B Both	W Walk / C Wheelchair / B Both	W Walk / C Wheelchair / B Both
M. Stairs			
Motor Subtotal Rating			
Communication			
N. Comprehension	A Auditory / V Visual / B Both	A Auditory / V Visual / B Both	A Auditory / V Visual / B Both
O. Expression	A Auditory / V Visual / B Both	A Auditory / V Visual / B Both	A Auditory / V Visual / B Both
Social Cognition			
P. Social Interaction			
Q. Problem Solving			
R. Memory			
Cognitive Subtotal Rating			
TOTAL FIM™ RATING			

NOTE: Leave no blanks. Enter 1 if patient is not testable due to risk.

b. IADLs include doing laundry, shopping, preparing meals, using a phone, and managing finances.

3. Participation scales

   a. Community Integration Questionnaire, a 15-item tool that assesses home integration, social integration, and productive activity (Willer, Ottenbacher, & Coad, 1994)

   b. Craig Handicap Assessment Reporting Technique (Hall, Dukers, Whiteneck, Brooks, & Krause, 1998)

      1) Designed to assess the reintegration of people with spinal cord injury
      2) Includes 32 items categorized into six dimensions (physical independence, cognitive independence, mobility, occupation, social integration, and economic self-sufficiency)
      3) Has a maximum score of 100 for each dimension

4. Pediatric tools

   a. WeeFIM™ instrument (**Figure 7-3**) (Braun, 1998)

      1) Designed for children age 6 months–7 years and older
      2) Derived from the FIM™ instrument
      3) Can be used by members of any discipline
      4) Measures actual performance across various settings
      5) The 0–3 Module (optional) of the WeeFIM™ instrument is designed to measure precursors to function in children ages 0–3 years who have a variety of disabilities.
      6) Intended to complement the FIM™ instrument by measuring early

Figure 7-3. WeeFIM™ Instrument

WeeFIM™ Instrument

LEVELS		
	7 Complete Independence (timely, safely) 6 Modified Independence (device)	NO HELPER
	Modified Dependence 5 Supervision (subject = 100%) 4 Minimal Assistance (subject = 75%+) 3 Moderate Assistance (subject = 50%+) **Complete Dependence** 2 Maximal Assistance (subject =25%+) 1 Total Assistance (subject = less than 25%)	HELPER

	ASSESSMENT	GOAL
Self-Care		
A. Eating		
B. Grooming		
C. Bathing		
D. Dressing - Upper Body		
E. Dressing - Lower Body		
F. Toileting		
G. Bladder		
H. Bowel		
Self-Care Total		
Mobility		
I. Chair, Wheelchair		
J. Toilet		
K. Tub, Shower		
L. Walk, Wheelchair	W Walk, C Wheelchair, L Crawl, B Combination	
M. Stairs		
Mobility Total		
MOTOR SUBTOTAL RATING		
Cognition		
N. Comprehension	A Auditory, V Visual, B Both	
O. Expression	V Vocal, N Nonvocal, B Both	
P. Social Interaction		
Q. Problem Solving		
R. Memory		
Cognition Total		
WEEFIM® TOTAL RATING		

NOTE: Leave no blanks. Enter 1 if patient is not testable due to risk.

functional performance and changes in performance over time

7) Used across many settings, including early intervention and preschool

b. Pediatric Evaluation of Disability Inventory (Haley, 1999)

1) Provides an assessment of key functional areas in children between the ages of 6 months and 7 years

2) Examines performance in three domains: self-care, mobility, and social function

III. Medicare Assessment Data Sets and Postacute Care Quality Reporting Programs

A. The HHS has implemented 20 performance measurement programs for clinician, hospital, postacute care, and long-term care.

1. These programs use quality measures in federal public reporting, performance-based payment programs, and other purposes.

2. The Measure Applications Partnership (MAP) is a public–private partnership convened by the National Quality Forum for the purpose of providing input to the HHS on the selection of quality measures for use in federal quality reporting programs.

3. The MAP includes varied stakeholders who are invested in the use of quality measures.

B. Inpatient Rehabilitation Facilities (IRFs)

1. The IRF standardized client assessment instrument is the IRF-PAI (**Figure 7-4**). Data include demographic, diagnostic, and FIM™ instrument (functional status) data. Data are collected on admission and discharge, and admission data are used to categorize each client into payment groups.

2. The CMS requires the IRF-PAI to be completed for all Medicare clients admitted to inpatient rehabilitation facilities.

3. IRF Quality Reporting Program

a. Medicare began an IRF Quality Reporting Program in 2012.

b. Failure to submit the required quality measure data as specified by CMS will result in a 2%-point reduction to the annual increase factor for payments made for discharges occurring during a future federal fiscal year.

c. In 2015, quality metrics focused on catheter-associated urinary tract infections, patients with new or worsened pressure ulcers, 30-day postdischarge readmissions, patient influenza vaccinations, influenza vaccinations of healthcare personnel, hospital-onset methicillin-resistant *Staphylococcus aureus* infections, and hospital-onset *Clostridium difficile* infections.

C. Home Care: Outcome and Assessment Information Set–C (OASIS-C)

1. The home health agency client assessment instrument is the Outcome and Assessment Information Set (OASIS-C). Data collected using the OASIS-C, such as clinical characteristics, functional status, and service use rates, are used to categorize each client into a payment group and to calculate facility-level quality indicators.

2. Data collection and submission of data are mandated by the CMS for use in home care as part of the home health prospective payment system (PPS).

3. Data used for calculating quality measures for home healthcare

a. Many quality measures are publicly reported on the Home Health Compare website (http://medicare.gov/homehealthcompare/).

b. These quality measures focus on timeliness of the start of home healthcare, teaching patients (or their family caregivers) about their drugs, taking their drugs correctly by mouth, fall risk assessment, depression screening, pain assessment, pain treatment, pain reduction when moving around, pressure ulcer risk assessment, prevention of pressure ulcers, improvement in walking or moving around, improvement in getting in and out of bed, improvement in bathing, frequency of urgent unplanned care in the hospital emergency room, readmissions, influenza vaccination, pneumococcal vaccination, treatment of heart failure symptoms for patients with heart failure, improvement in breathing for patients with breathing problems, wound improvement or healing after an operation, and foot care for patients with diabetes.

D. Skilled Nursing Facility (SNF): Minimum Data Set 3.0 (MDS 3.0)

1. The SNF client assessment instrument is the MDS 3.0. Data collected using the MDS 3.0, such as treatments provided and client characteristics, are used to categorize each client into a payment group and to calculate facility-level quality indicators.

2. Data collection and submission are mandated by CMS for use in long-term care settings; this serves as the data collection instrument for the skilled nursing facility prospective payment system.

Figure 7-4. IRF-PAI

Identification Information*

1. Facility Information
   A. Facility Name

____
____
____
____
____

   B. Facility Medicare Provider Number ______________________

2. Patient Medicare Number ______________________
3. Patient Medicaid Number ______________________
4. Patient First Name ______________________
5A. Patient Last Name ______________________
5B. Patient Identification Number ______________________
6. Birth Date ___/___/_____ MM / DD / YYYY
7. Social Security Number ______________________
8. Gender (*1 - Male; 2 - Female*) ______________________
9. Race/Ethnicity (*Check all that apply*)

American Indian or Alaska Native	A.	______
Asian	B.	______
Black or African American	C.	______
Hispanic or Latino	D.	______
Native Hawaiian or Other Pacific Islander	E.	______
White	F.	______

10. Marital Status ____________
    (1 - Never Married; 2 - Married; 3 - Widowed; 4 - Separated; 5 - Divorced)
11. Zip Code of Patient's Pre-Hospital Residence ____________
12. Admission Date ___/___/_____ MM / DD / YYYY
13. Assessment Reference Date ___/___/_____ MM / DD / YYYY
14. Admission Class
    (1 - Initial Rehab; 2 - Evaluation; 3 - Readmission; 4 - Unplanned Discharge; 5 - Continuing Rehabilitation)
15A. Admit From
    (01- Home (private home/apt., board/care, assisted living, group home, transitional living); 02- Short-term General Hospital; 03 - Skilled Nursing Facility (SNF); 04 - Intermediate care; 06 - Home under care of organized home health service organization; 50 - Hospice (home); 51 - Hospice (institutional facility); 61 - Swing bed; 62 - Another Inpatient Rehabilitation Facility; 63 - Long-Term Care Hospital (LTCH); 64 - Medicaid Nursing Facility; 65 - Inpatient Psychiatric Facility; 66 - Critical Access Hospital; 99 - Not Listed)
16A. Pre-hospital Living Setting ____________
    Use codes from 15A. Admit From
17. Pre-hospital Living With ____________
    (Code only if item 16A is 01- Home: Code using 01 - Alone; 02 - Family/Relatives; 03 - Friends; 04 - Attendant; 05 - Other)
18. DELETED
19. DELETED

Payer Information*

20. Payment Source
    (02 - Medicare Fee For Service; 51- Medicare-Medicare Advantage; 99 - Not Listed)
    A. Primary Source ________
    B. Secondary Source ________

Medical Information*

21. Impairment Group ________ ________
    Admission Discharge

    Condition requiring admission to rehabilitation; code according to Appendix A.
22. Etiologic Diagnosis
    (*Use ICD codes to indicate the etiologic problem that led to the condition for which the patient is receiving rehabilitation*)
    A. ______
    B. ______
    C. ______
23. Date of Onset of Impairment ___/___/_____ MM / DD / YYYY
24. Comorbid Conditions
    Use ICD codes to enter comorbid medical conditions

A.	________	J.	________	S.	________
B.	________	K.	________	T.	________
C.	________	L.	________	U.	________
D.	________	M.	________	V.	________
E.	________	N.	________	W.	________
F.	________	O.	________	X.	________
G.	________	P.	________	Y.	________
H.	________	Q.	________		
I.	________	R.	________		

24A. Are there any arthritis conditions recorded in items #21, #22, or #24 that meet all of the regulatory requirements for IRF classification (in 42 CFR 412.29(b)(2)(x), (xi), and (xii))? ________
    (0 - No; 1 - Yes)
25. DELETED
26. DELETED
    Height and Weight
    (While measuring if the number is X.1-X.4 round down, X.5 or greater round up)
25A. Height on admission (in inches) ______________________
26A. Weight on admission (in pounds) ______________________
    Measure weight consistently, according to standard facility practice (e.g., in a.m. after voiding, with shoes off, etc.)
27. Swallowing Status ________ ________
    Admission Discharge

    3- *Regular Food*: solids and liquids swallowed safely without supervision or modified food consistency
    2- *Modified Food Consistency/Supervision:* subject requires modified food consistency and/or needs supervision for safety
    1- *Tube/Parenteral Feeding:* tube/parenteral feeding used wholly or partially as a means of sustenance
28. DELETED

continued

Figure 7-4. IRF-PAI (continued)

Function Modifiers*

Complete the following specific functional items prior to scoring the FIM™ Instrument:

		Admission	Discharge
29.	Bladder Level of Assistance (Score using FIM Levels 1 - 7)	☐	☐
30.	Bladder Frequency of Accidents (Score as below)	☐	☐

7 - No accidents
6 - No accidents; uses device such as a catheter
5 - One accident in the past 7 days
4 - Two accidents in the past 7 days
3 - Three accidents in the past 7 days
2 - Four accidents in the past 7 days
1 - Five or more accidents in the past 7 days

Enter in Item 39G (Bladder) the lower *(more dependent) score from Items 29 and 30 above*

		Admission	Discharge
31.	Bowel Level of Assistance (Score using FIM Levels 1 - 7)	☐	☐
32.	Bowel Frequency of Accidents (Score as below)	☐	☐

7 - No accidents
6 - No accidents; uses device such as a ostomy
5 - One accident in the past 7 days
4 - Two accidents in the past 7 days
3 - Three accidents in the past 7 days
2 - Four accidents in the past 7 days
1 - Five or more accidents in the past 7 days

Enter in Item 39H (Bowel) the lower (more dependent) score of Items 31and 32 above.

		Admission	Discharge
33.	Tub Transfer	☐	☐
34.	Shower Transfer	☐	☐

(Score Items 33 and 34 using FIM Levels 1 - 7; use 0 if activity does not occur) *See training manual for scoring of Item 39K (Tub/Shower Transfer)*

		Admission	Discharge
35.	Distance Walked	☐	☐
36.	Distance Traveled in Wheelchair	☐	☐

(Code items 35 and 36 using: 3 - 150 feet; 2 - 50 to 149 feet; 1 - Less than 50 feet; 0 – activity does not occur)

		Admission	Discharge
37.	Walk	☐	☐
38.	Wheelchair	☐	☐

(Score Items 37 and 38 using FIM Levels 1 - 7; 0 if activity does not occur) See training manual for scoring of Item 39L (Walk/Wheelchair)

* The FIM data set, measurement scale and impairment codes incorporated or referenced herein are the property of U B Foundation Activities, Inc. ©1993, 2001 U B Foundation Activities, Inc. The FIM mark is owned by UBFA, Inc.

39. FIM™ Instrument*

	Admission	Discharge	Goal
SELF-CARE			
A. Eating	☐	☐	☐
B. Grooming	☐	☐	☐
C. Bathing	☐	☐	☐
D. Dressing - Upper	☐	☐	☐
E. Dressing - Lower	☐	☐	☐
F. Toileting	☐	☐	☐
SPHINCTER CONTROL			
G. Bladder	☐	☐	☐
H. Bowel	☐	☐	☐
TRANSFERS			
I. Bed, Chair, Wheelchair	☐	☐	☐
J. Toilet	☐	☐	☐
K. Tub, Shower	☐	☐	☐
LOCOMOTION (W - Walk; C - Wheelchair; B - Both)			
L. Walk/Wheelchair	☐☐	☐☐	☐
M. Stairs	☐	☐	☐
COMMUNICATION (A - Auditory; V - Visual; B - Both)			
N. Comprehension	☐☐	☐☐	☐
O. Expression (V - Vocal; N - Nonvocal; B - Both)	☐☐	☐☐	☐
SOCIAL COGNITION			
P. Social Interaction	☐	☐	☐
Q. Problem Solving	☐	☐	☐
R. Memory	☐	☐	☐

FIM LEVELS

No Helper

7 Complete Independence (Timely, Safely)
6 Modified Independence (Device)

Helper - Modified Dependence

5 Supervision (Subject = 100%)
4 Minimal Assistance (Subject = 75% or more)
3 Moderate Assistance (Subject = 50% or more)

Helper - Complete Dependence

2 Maximal Assistance (Subject = 25% or more)
1 Total Assistance (Subject less than 25%)

0 Activity does not occur; Use this code only at admission

Discharge Information*	Therapy Information

40. Discharge Date ___/___/_______ MM / DD / YYYY

41. Patient discharged against medical advice? __________ *(0 - No; 1 - Yes)*

42. Program Interruption(s) __________ *(0 - No; 1 - Yes)*

43. Program Interruption Dates
(Code only if item 42 is 1 - Yes)

A. 1st Interruption Date [ ] MM / DD / YYYY
B. 1st Return Date [ ] MM / DD / YYYY

C. 2nd Interruption Date [ ] MM / DD / YYYY
D. 2nd Return Date [ ] MM / DD / YYYY

E. 3rd Interruption Date [ ] MM / DD / YYYY
F. 3rd Return Date [ ] MM / DD / YYYY

44C. Was the patient discharged alive? __________ *(0 - No; 1 - Yes)*

44D. Patient's discharge destination/living setting, using codes below: (answer only if 44C = 1; if 44C = 0, skip to item 46) __________

(01- Home (private home/apt., board/care, assisted living, group home, transitional living); 02- Short-term General Hospital; 03 - Skilled Nursing Facility (SNF); 04 - Intermediate care; 06 - Home under care of organized home health service organization; 50 - Hospice (home); 51 - Hospice (institutional facility); 61 - Swing bed; 62 - Another Inpatient Rehabilitation Facility; 63 - Long-Term Care Hospital (LTCH); 64 - Medicaid Nursing Facility; 65 - Inpatient Psychiatric Facility; 66 - Critical Access Hospital; 99 - Not Listed)

45. Discharge to Living With __________
(Code only if item 44C is 1 - Yes and 44D is 01 - Home; Code using 1 - Alone; 2 - Family / Relatives; 3 - Friends; 4 - Attendant; 5 - Other)

46. Diagnosis for Interruption or Death __________
(Code using ICD code)

47. Complications during rehabilitation stay
(Use ICD codes to specify up to six conditions that began with this rehabilitation stay)

A. __________ B. __________
C. __________ D. __________
E. __________ F. __________

* The FIM data set, measurement scale and impairment codes incorporated or referenced herein are the property of U B Foundation Activities, Inc. © 1993, 2001 U B Foundation Activities, Inc. The FIM mark is owned by UBFA, Inc.

O0401. Week 1: Total Number of Minutes Provided

O0401A: Physical Therapy
a. Total minutes of individual therapy ______
b. Total minutes of concurrent therapy ______
c. Total minutes of group therapy ______
d. Total minutes of co-treatment therapy ______

O0401B: Occupational Therapy
a. Total minutes of individual therapy ______
b. Total minutes of concurrent therapy ______
c. Total minutes of group therapy ______
d. Total minutes of co-treatment therapy ______

O0401C: Speech-Language Pathology
a. Total minutes of individual therapy ______
b. Total minutes of concurrent therapy ______
c. Total minutes of group therapy ______
d. Total minutes of co-treatment therapy ______

O0402. Week 2: Total Number of Minutes Provided

O0402A: Physical Therapy
a. Total minutes of individual therapy ______
b. Total minutes of concurrent therapy ______
c. Total minutes of group therapy ______
d. Total minutes of co-treatment therapy ______

O0402B: Occupational Therapy
a. Total minutes of individual therapy ______
b. Total minutes of concurrent therapy ______
c. Total minutes of group therapy ______
d. Total minutes of co-treatment therapy ______

O0402C: Speech-Language Pathology
a. Total minutes of individual therapy ______
b. Total minutes of concurrent therapy ______
c. Total minutes of group therapy ______
d. Total minutes of co-treatment therapy ______

continued

Figure 7-4. IRF-PAI (continued)

	Quality Indicators- Admission Assessment		Quality Indicators- Discharge Assessment
Enter Code ☐	**Unhealed Pressure Ulcer(s)- Admission** **M0210.** Does this patient have one or more unhealed pressure ulcer(s) at Stage 1 or higher at Admission? **0. No →** skip to question **I0900 on Admission Assessment** **1. Yes →** continue to question **M0300A on Admission Assessment**	Enter Code ☐	**Unhealed Pressure Ulcer(s)- Discharge** **M0210.** Does this patient have one or more unhealed pressure ulcer(s) at Stage 1 or higher on Discharge? 0. **No→** skip to question **M0900A on Discharge Assessment** 1. **Yes →** continue to question **M0300A on Discharge Assessment**
	M0300. Current Number of Unhealed Pressure Ulcers at Each Stage- Admission		**M0300. Current Number of Unhealed Pressure Ulcers at Each Stage- Discharge**
Enter Number ☐	**M0300A. Stage 1:** Intact skin with non-blanchable redness of a localized area usually over a bony prominence. Darkly pigmented skin may not have a visible blanching; in dark skin tones it may appear with persistent blue or purple hues. **M0300A1. Number of Stage 1 pressure ulcers:** enter how many were noted at the time of admission	Enter Number ☐ Enter Number ☐ Enter Number ☐	**M0300A. Stage 1:** Intact skin with non-blanchable redness of a localized area usually over a bony prominence. Darkly pigmented skin may not have a visible blanching; in dark skin tones it may appear with persistent blue or purple hues. **M0300A1.** Enter **total** number of pressure ulcers currently at **Stage 1. If patient has no Stage 1 pressure ulcers at discharge, skip to Item M0300B1.** **M0300A2.** Of **these Stage 1** pressure ulcers present at discharge, enter number that were: (a) present on admission as a Stage 1 **and** (b) remained at Stage 1 at discharge. **M0300A3.** Of **these Stage 1** pressure ulcers, enter the number that were **not present on admission.** (i.e. – New stage 1 pressure ulcers that have developed during the IRF stay)
Enter Number ☐	**M0300B. Stage 2:** Partial thickness loss of dermis presenting as a shallow open ulcer with a red or pink wound bed, without slough. May also present as an intact or open/ruptured blister. **M0300B1. Number of Stage 2 pressure ulcers:** enter how many were noted at the time of admission	Enter Number ☐ Enter Number ☐ Enter Number ☐ Enter Number ☐	**M0300B. Stage 2:** Partial thickness loss of dermis presenting as a shallow open ulcer with a red or pink wound bed, without slough. May also present as an intact or open/ruptured blister. **M0300B1.** Enter **total** number of pressure ulcers currently at **Stage 2. (If patient has no Stage 2 pressure ulcers at discharge, skip to Item M0300C1.)** **M0300B2.** Of **these Stage 2** pressure ulcers present at discharge, enter the number that were: (a) present on admission, **and** (b) remained at Stage 2 at discharge. **M0300B3.** Of **these Stage 2** pressure ulcers present at discharge, enter the number that were: (a) present on admission as an **unstageable pressure ulcer** due to the presence of a **non-removable device and** (b) when it became stageable, the pressure ulcer was staged as a Stage 2, **and** (c) it remained at Stage 2 at the time of discharge. **M0300B4. Of these Stage 2** pressure ulcers present at discharge, enter the number that were: (a) not present on admission; **or** (b) were at a lesser stage at admission and worsened to a Stage 2 during the IRF stay

	Quality Indicators- Admission Assessment, Continued		Quality Indicators-Discharge Assessment, Continued
	M0300. Current Number of Unhealed Pressure Ulcers at Each Stage- Admission, Continued		**M0300. Current Number of Unhealed Pressure Ulcers at Each Stage-Discharge, Continued**
	M0300C. Stage 3: Full thickness tissue loss. Subcutaneous fat may be visible but bone, tendon or muscle is not exposed. Slough may be present but does not obscure the depth of tissue loss. May include undermining and tunneling.		**M0300C. Stage 3:** Full thickness tissue loss. Subcutaneous fat may be visible but bone, tendon or muscle is not exposed. Slough may be present but does not obscure the depth of tissue loss. May include undermining and tunneling.
Enter Number ☐	**M0300C1. Number of Stage 3 pressure ulcers:** enter how many were noted at the time of admission	Enter Number ☐	**M0300C1.** Enter **total** number of pressure ulcers currently at **Stage 3. (If patient has no Stage 3 pressure ulcers at discharge, skip to Item M0300D1.**
		Enter Number ☐	**M0300C2.** Of **these** **Stage 3** pressure ulcers present at discharge, enter the number that were: (a) present on admission, **and** (b) remained at Stage 3 at discharge.
		Enter Number ☐	**M0300C3.** Of **these** **Stage 3** pressure ulcers present at discharge, enter the number that were: (a) present on admission as an **unstageable pressure ulcer**, **and** (b) when it became stageable, it was staged as a **Stage 3**; **and** (c) it remained at **Stage 3** at the time of discharge.
		Enter Number ☐	**M0300C4.** Of **these** **Stage 3** pressure ulcers present at discharge, enter the number that were: (a) not present on admission; **or** (b) were at a lesser stage at admission and worsened to a Stage 3 during the IRF stay; **or** (c) were unstageable due to a non-removeable device at admission, initially became stageable at a lesser stage, , but then progressed to a Stage 3 by the time of discharge.
	M0300D. Stage 4: Full thickness tissue loss with exposed bone, tendon or muscle. Slough or eschar may be present on some parts of the wound bed. Often includes undermining and tunneling.		**M0300D. Stage 4:** Full thickness tissue loss with exposed bone, tendon or muscle. Slough or eschar may be present on some parts of the wound bed. Often includes undermining and tunneling.
Enter Number ☐	**M0300D1. Number of Stage 4 pressure ulcers:** enter how many were noted at the time of admission	Enter Number ☐	**M0300D1.** Enter **total** number of pressure ulcers currently at **Stage 4. (If patient has no Stage 4 pressure ulcers at discharge, skip to Item M0300E1.)**
		Enter Number ☐	**M0300D2. Of these** **Stage 4** pressure ulcers present at discharge, enter number that were: (a) present on admission at Stage 4 , **and** (b) remained at Stage 4 at discharge.
		Enter Number ☐	**M0300D3. Of these** **Stage 4** pressure ulcers present at discharge, enter the number that were: (a) present on admission as an **unstageable pressure ulcer**, **and** (b) when it became stageable, it was staged as a **Stage 4**, **and** (c) it remained at **Stage 4** at the time of discharge.
		Enter Number ☐	**M0300D4. Of these** **Stage 4** pressure ulcers present at discharge, enter the number that were: (a) not present on admission); **or** (b) were at a lesser stage at admission and worsened to a Stage 4 by discharge; **or** (c) were unstageable on admission, initially became stageable at a lesser stage, and then progressed to a Stage 4 by the time of discharge.

continued

Figure 7-4. IRF-PAI (continued)

	Quality Indicators-Admission Assessment, Continued		Quality Indicators-Discharge Assessment, Continued
Enter Number ☐	**M0300E. Unstageable Pressure Ulcers due to non-removable dressing/device:** Known but not stageable due to the presence of a non-removable dressing/device. **M0300E1. Number of unstageable pressure ulcers due to non-removable dressing/device**: enter how many were noted at the time of admission	Enter Number ☐ Enter Number ☐ Enter Number ☐	**M0300E. Unstageable Pressure Ulcers due to a non-removable dressing or device:** pressure ulcers that are known but not stageable due to the presence of a non-removable dressing or device. **M0300E1.** Enter **total** number of pressure ulcers currently **Unstageable** due to a **Non-removable dressing or device. (If patient has no pressure ulcers Unstageable due to Non-Removable Device at discharge, skip to Item M0300F1.)** **M0300E2.** Of **these Unstageable** pressure ulcers due to a **non-removable dressing or device** present at discharge, enter number that were:(a) present on admission as an unstageable pressure ulcer due to **non-removable dressing or device; and** (b) remained unstageable due to **non-removable dressing or device** until discharge. **M0300E3. Of these Unstageable** pressure ulcers due to **non-removable dressing or device** present at discharge, enter number that were (a) present on admission as a stageable pressure ulcer **and** became **unstageable due to non-removable dressing or device** during the IRF stay; and (b) remained unstageable due to a **non-removable dressing or device** until discharge.
Enter Number ☐	**M0300F. Unstageable Pressure Ulcers due to slough and/or eschar:** pressure ulcers that are known but not stageable due to coverage of wound bed by slough and/or eschar. **M0300F1. Number of unstageable pressure ulcers due to slough and/ or eschar**: enter how many were noted at the time of admission	Enter Number ☐ Enter Number ☐ Enter Number ☐	**M0300F. Unstageable Pressure Ulcers due to slough or eschar:** pressure ulcers that are known but not stageable due to coverage of wound bed by slough and/or eschar. **M0300F1.** Enter **total** number of pressure ulcers currently **Unstageable** due to a **Slough and/or Eschar. (If patient has no pressure ulcers Unstageable due to Slough and/or Eschar at discharge, skip to Item M0300G1.)** **M0300F2. Of these Unstageable** pressure ulcers due to **slough and/or eschar** present at discharge, enter number that were: (a) present on admission as an unstageable pressure ulcer due to **slough and/or eschar**; **and** (b) remained unstageable due to **slough and/or eschar** until discharge. **M0300F3. Of these Unstageable** pressure ulcers due to **slough or eschar** present at discharge, enter number that were: (a) present on admission as a stageable pressure ulcer **and** became unstageable due to **slough and/or eschar,** during the IRF stay; **and** (b) remained unstageable due to **slough and/or eschar** until discharge.
Enter Number ☐	**M0300G. Unstageable Pressure Ulcers with Suspected Deep Tissue Injury (DTI) in evolution:** suspected deep tissue injury in evolution. **M0300G1. Number of unstageable pressure ulcers with Suspected Deep Tissue Injury in evolution:** enter how many were noted at the time of admission	Enter Number ☐ Enter Number ☐	**M0300G. Unstageable Pressure Ulcers with Suspected Deep Tissue Injury (DTI) in evolution:** suspected deep tissue injury in evolution. **M0300G1.** Enter **total** number of **unstageable pressure ulcers with Suspected Deep Tissue Injury**. **(If patient has no Unstageable pressure ulcers with Suspected Deep Tissue Injury at discharge, skip to Item M0900A.)** **M0300G2. Of these unstageable pressure ulcers with Suspected DTI** present at discharge, enter number that were:(a) present on admission as an unstageable pressure ulcer due to a **suspected deep tissue injury; and** (b) remained unstageable due to a **suspected DTI** until discharge.

Quality Indicators- Admission Assessment, Continued

I0900. Pressure Ulcer Risk Conditions- Admission

Indicate below if the patient has any of the following pressure ulcer risk conditions:
(**NOTE:** You must also document the appropriate ICD codes for any pressure ulcer risk conditions documented below in Item 24 "Comorbid Conditions" above.)

Enter Number ☐ **I0900A**. Peripheral Vascular Disease (PVD)
0. No 1. Yes

Enter Number ☐ **I0900B.** Peripheral Arterial Disease(PAD)
0. No 1. Yes

Enter Number ☐ **I2900A.** Diabetes Mellitus (DM)
If I2900A = 0, skip I2900B-D
0. No 1. Yes

Enter Number ☐ **I2900B.** Diabetic Retinopathy
0. No 1. Yes

Enter Number ☐ **I2900C.** Diabetic Nephropathy
0. No 1. Yes

Enter Number ☐ **I2900D.** Diabetic Neuropathy
0. No 1. Yes

Quality Indicators-Discharge Assessment, Continued

M0900. Healed Pressure Ulcers- Discharge

Indicate the number of pressure ulcers that were: (a) present on **Admission**; **and** (b) have completely closed (resurfaced with epithelium) upon **Discharge.** If there are no healed pressure ulcers noted at a given stage, enter 0.

Enter Number ☐ **M0900A.** Stage 1

Enter Number ☐ **M0900B.** Stage 2

Enter Number ☐ **M0900C.** Stage 3

Enter Number ☐ **M0900D.** Stage 4

O0250. Influenza Vaccine – Discharge - Refer to current version of IRF-PAI Training Manual for current influenza vaccination season and reporting period.

Enter Code ☐ **O0250A.** Did the **patient receive the influenza vaccine *in this facility*** for this year's influenza *vaccination* season?

0. No → Skip to O0250C, If influenza vaccine not received, state reason
1. Yes → Continue to O0250B, Date influenza vaccine received

O0250B. Date influenza vaccine received → Complete date and skip to Z0400A, Signature of Persons Completing the Assessment

☐☐ ☐☐ ☐☐☐☐
MM DD YYYY

Enter Code ☐ **O0250C. If influenza vaccine not received, state reason:**

1. **Patient not in this facility** during this year's influenza vaccination season
2. **Received outside of this facility**
3. **Not eligible -** medical contraindication
4. **Offered and declined**
5. **Not offered**
6. **Inability to obtain influenza vaccine** due to a declared shortage.
9. **None of the above**

continued

Figure 7-4. IRF-PAI (continued)

Item Z0400A. Signature of Persons Completing the Assessment*

I certify that the accompanying information accurately reflects patient assessment information for this patient and that I collected or coordinated collection of this information on the dates specified. To the best of my knowledge, this information was collected in accordance with applicable Medicare and Medicaid requirements. I understand that this information is used as a basis for ensuring that patients receive appropriate and quality care, and as a basis for payment from federal funds. I further understand that payment of such federal funds and continued participation in the government-funded health care programs is conditioned on the accuracy and truthfulness of this information, and that I may be personally subject to or may subject my organization to substantial criminal, civil, and/or administrative penalties for submitting false information.

Signature	Title	Date Information is Provided	Time
A.			
B.			
C.			
D.			
E.			
F.			
G.			
H.			
I.			
J.			
K.			
L.			

3. Items assess the resident's physical and clinical conditions and abilities, preferences, and life care wishes.
4. Data are used to calculate quality measures.
   a. The Medicare program has been reporting quality measure data and other information about nursing homes, including short-stay skilled nursing facility residents, on their website (www.medicare.gov/NursingHomeCompare) for several years.
   b. In 2014, quality measures focused on residents who self-report moderate to severe pain, residents with pressure ulcers that are new or worsened, resident influenza vaccination, resident pneumococcal vaccination, and residents who are newly administered antipsychotic medications.
   c. Additional information about facilities provided on the site includes health inspection results and complaints, nursing home staffing data (number of registered nurses, licensed practical or vocational nurses, physical therapists and nursing assistants), and penalties levied against the nursing home.
   d. Five-Star Quality Ratings on the website provide a summary rating that considers health inspections, quality metrics, and hours of care provided per resident by staff performing nursing care tasks.

E. Long-Term Care Hospital (LTCH) CARE Data Set
1. The LTCH client assessment instrument is the LTCH CARE Data Set
2. Clinical data collection and submission are required by Medicare under the LTCH Quality Reporting Program.
   a. Medicare began an LTCH quality reporting program in 2012, which includes collection of standardized clinical assessment data on a patient assessment instrument called the LTCH CARE Data Set.

b. Failure to submit the required quality measure data as specified by CMS will result in a 2%-point reduction in the annual increase factor for payments made for discharges occurring during a future federal fiscal year.
c. The LTCH quality reporting program is expected to evolve to include additional quality measures and public reporting of quality metric data for each hospital.
d. In 2015, quality metrics focused on catheter-associated urinary tract infections, central line–associated bloodstream infection, patients with new or worsened pressure ulcers, 30-day postdischarge readmissions, patient influenza vaccination, influenza vaccination of healthcare personnel, hospital-onset methicillin-resistant *Staphylococcus aureus* infections, and hospital-onset *Clostridium difficile* infections. In 2016, data collection begins for two functional status quality measures and a fall with major injury measure.

F. Outpatient Therapy and Day Rehabilitation Programs
1. No standardized assessment required; several different assessments used voluntarily
2. Focus on Therapeutic Outcomes (Dobrzykowski & Nance, 1997)
   a. Created in 1992 as an outcome measurement system for outpatient orthopedic rehabilitation
   b. Monitors the efficiency and effectiveness of the outpatient orthopedic population
3. LIFEware℠ assessment tools (Granger, 1999)
   a. Designed for outpatient medical rehabilitation programs
   b. Examines physical function, pain, affective well-being, and cognitive functioning
   c. Customized for various client populations

IV. Performance Improvement

A. Tools for Performance Improvement (Brassard & Ritter, 1994)
1. Brainstorming allows team members to create as many creative ideas and solutions as possible; all suggestions are recorded to be evaluated at a later time.
2. A cause-and-effect diagram (fishbone diagram) allows team members to visually and graphically explore the relationship between the effects and possible causes of identified problems.
3. An affinity diagram gathers large amounts of data and helps organize the information into groups based on the relationships between the items.
4. A check sheet allows team members to record and collect data from various sources so patterns and trends may be identified.
5. A run chart is used to visually display data and to identify any changes that occur.
6. A histogram displays the distribution of data and reveals the amount of variation within a process.
7. A scatter diagram is used to study the possible cause-and-effect relationship between two variables.
8. A control chart is used to monitor, control, and improve variances in performance by identifying the source; it is similar to a run chart but with statistical upper and lower limits.
9. A flowchart is a pictorial representation of various steps of a process that allows team members to easily identify the flow of events.
10. A force field analysis identifies the forces in place that affect an issue or problem; ideally, it reinforces positives and eliminates negatives.
11. A Pareto chart is a display of bar graphs that can help focus on and determine which problems to solve and in which order so that efforts are directed to the problems that have the greatest improvement potential.

B. Models for Performance Improvement
1. Plan, Do, Check, Act approach
   a. Plan what you want to accomplish.
   b. Do what you planned to do.
   c. Check the results.
   d. Act on the information.
2. Failure Mode Effects Analysis: Systematic, proactive approach to evaluating a process
   a. Identify all steps of a process.
   b. Identify when and how the steps might fail.
   c. Assess the impact of each potential failure.
   d. Identify which steps are in most in need of change.
3. Six Sigma
   a. The focus is on reducing variation, then improving process capability.
   b. Certification is available through the Institute of Industrial Engineers and the American Society for Quality.
4. Lean approach
   a. A Toyota production system model designed to improve efficiency and effectiveness though process redesign
   b. Rules of lean
      1) Structure every activity.
      2) Clearly connect every customer or supplier.
      3) Specify every flow path.
      4) Improve through experimentation toward the ideal state.
   c. Lean requires that participants in the process come to high-level agreement.

d. Tools
   1) Waste elimination: Identify potential wastes (multiple handoffs, many people doing the same thing, paper versus automated processes).
   2) Five Ss: Separate, sweep, sort, sanitize, sustain
   3) Standardized work: Everyone does the process the same way.
   4) Process mapping (kaizen): A way of looking at a process by identifying every step of the process, then identifying wastes, and coming to high-level agreement on a new process
   5) Visual management: The use of signage to label spaces so that objects are put back in the same place every time
   6) Problem solving

V. Accreditation Overview

A. Primary Accreditation Agencies for Rehabilitation Providers
   1. CMS: Healthcare organizations that participate in and receive payment from Medicare or Medicaid must comply with Conditions of Participation set forth in federal regulations.
   2. The Joint Commission
      a. May serve as deeming authority on behalf of CMS
      b. Enforces standards that meet the federal Conditions of Participation
   3. The Commission on Accreditation of Rehabilitation Facilities (CARF): Uses a consultative accreditation process that centers on enhancing the lives of the people served
   4. State agencies: State health department

B. Benefits of Accreditation (The Joint Commission, 2014a)
   1. Helps organize and strengthen patient safety efforts
   2. Strengthens community confidence in the quality and safety of care, treatment, and services
   3. Provides a competitive edge in the marketplace
   4. Improves risk management and risk reduction
   5. May reduce liability insurance costs
   6. Provides education to improve business operations
   7. Enhances staff recruitment and development
   8. Provides deeming authority for Medicare certification
   9. Recognized by some insurers and other third parties
   10. Provides a framework for organizational structure and management
   11. May fulfill regulatory requirements in select states
   12. Provides practical tools to strengthen or maintain performance excellence

C. Benefits of Certification (The Joint Commission, 2014a)
   1. Improves the quality of patient care by reducing variation in clinical processes
   2. Provides a framework for program structure and management
   3. Provides an objective assessment of clinical excellence
   4. Creates a loyal, cohesive clinical team
   5. Promotes a culture of excellence across the organization
   6. Facilitates marketing, contracting, and reimbursement
   7. Strengthens community confidence in the quality and safety of care, treatment, and services
   8. Recognized by select insurers and other third parties
   9. Can fulfill regulatory requirements in select states

D. Impact on Patient Safety and Quality of Care
   1. Increases accountability
      a. Encourages and recommends proactive methods and models of quality and patient safety that will increase accountability, trust, and knowledge while reducing the impact of fear and blame
      b. Aligns existing standards from The Joint Commission with daily work in order to engage patients and staff throughout the healthcare system, at all times, in reducing harm
   2. Established metrics for benchmarking: Assists healthcare organizations with advancing knowledge, skills, and competence of staff and patients by recommending methods that will improve quality and safety processes

VI. Accrediting Agencies

A. The Joint Commission
   1. General
      a. Mission: To continuously improve healthcare for the public, in collaboration with other stakeholders, by evaluating healthcare organizations and inspiring them to excel in providing safe and effective care of the highest quality and value (The Joint Commission, 2014b)
      b. Vision: All people always experience the safest, highest-quality, best-value healthcare across all settings (The Joint Commission, 2014b)
      c. "Compliance": The Joint Commission's term for referring to meeting standards
      d. Organizational structure: Governed by a board of commissioners

e. The Joint Commission provides accreditation services for the following types of organizations:
   1) General, psychiatric, children's, and rehabilitation hospitals
   2) Critical access hospitals
   3) Home care organizations, including medical equipment services and hospice services
   4) Nursing and rehabilitation centers
   5) Behavioral healthcare organizations, addiction services
   6) Ambulatory care providers, including group practices and office-based surgery practices
   7) Independent or freestanding clinical laboratories

f. The Joint Commission also awards Disease-Specific Care certification to organizations that provide disease-specific care and chronic care services, and an advanced level of certification is offered for chronic kidney disease, chronic obstructive pulmonary disease, comprehensive stroke centers, heart failure, inpatient diabetes, palliative care, and primary stroke centers. The Joint Commission also has a Health Care Staffing Services certification program.

2. Historical perspective
   a. 1910: Dr. Ernest Codman proposed a system of hospital standardization in which hospitals track every client to determine whether treatment is effective.
   b. 1918: The American College of Surgeons began onsite inspections of hospitals.
   c. 1926: The first 18-page standard manual was published.
   d. 1951: The American College of Physicians, the American Hospital Association, the American Medical Association, and the Canadian Medical Association joined to create the Joint Commission on Accreditation of Hospitals (JCAH), whose primary purpose was to provide voluntary accreditation.
   e. 1953: JCAH published standards for hospital accreditation.
   f. 1966: Long-term care accreditation began.
   g. 1970: Registered nurses joined physicians in conducting surveys.
   h. 1982: The first public member began serving on the JCAH Board of Commissioners.
   i. 1987: The organization changed its name to the Joint Commission on Accreditation of Healthcare Organizations (JCAHO) to reflect its expanded scope of activities.
   j. 1988: Accreditation for home care organizations began.
   k. 1993
      1) The Accreditation Manual for Hospitals was reorganized around important patient care and organization functions from standards that measure an organization's capability to perform to those that look at actual performance.
      2) The number and nature of Type 1 recommendations against an organization became public information.
      3) JCAHO began making random, unannounced surveys of accredited organizations.
   l. 1996: The sentinel event policy was established.
   m. 1997: The JCAHO ORYX® initiative was launched to integrate outcomes and other performance measures into the accreditation process.
   n. 2002
      1) In June the 2002 National Patient Safety Goals were announced. The purpose of the National Patient Safety Goals is to improve safety. The goals focus on problems in healthcare safety and how to solve them.
      2) The JCAHO launched the Disease-Specific Care (DSC) certification program.
   o. 2007: The Joint Commission introduced its refreshed brand identity (name and logo) in support of its continuing efforts to improve the value of accreditation.
   p. 2009: The Joint Commission launched its Center for Transforming Healthcare in September, which develops solutions through the application of robust process improvement methods and tools.
   q. 2009: CMS approved the continuation of deeming authority for The Joint Commission's hospital accreditation program through July 2014.
   r. 2010: The Joint Commission launched its Leading Practices Library.
   s. 2012: The Joint Commission launched a Speak Up™ campaign to help people understand the importance of preventing strokes and seeking immediate treatment when they occur.
   t. 2012: The Joint Commission announced it would suspend reporting requirements for its ORYX noncore measures for accredited long-term acute care hospitals and inpatient rehabilitation facilities, effective January 1, 2013.

u. 2014: The Joint Commission and the American Heart Association/American Stroke Association announced, in September, the launch of the Disease-Specific Care Advanced Certification Program for Comprehensive Stroke Centers.

3. Accreditation process
   a. An organization submits an application to The Joint Commission.
   b. The organization prepares for the survey using the Survey Activity Guide.
   c. An initial conference with the organization's leaders is held on the first day of the survey to finalize the survey schedule.
   d. The survey includes a tour of the facility, reviews of medical records and documentation, observation of staff, and interviews with clients and staff.
   e. The major focus is on direct input from care providers, with the surveyors providing education while measuring compliance with standards.
   f. Elements of performance are the performance expectations for determining whether a standard is in compliance. Elements of performance are scored on a 3-point scale.
      1) 0 = Insufficient compliance
      2) 1 = Partial compliance
      3) 2 = Satisfactory compliance
4. Accreditation decisions or outcomes
   a. Preliminary accreditation: The organization demonstrates compliance with selected standards used in the surveys conducted under the Early Survey Policy.
   b. Accreditation: The organization is in compliance with all standards at the time of the on-site survey or has successfully addressed all requirements for improvement in an Evidence of Standards Compliance submission within 45 or 60 days after the posting of the Accreditation Survey Findings Report and does not meet any other rules for other accreditation decisions.
   c. Accreditation with follow-up survey: The healthcare organization is not in compliance with specific standards that require a follow-up survey within 30 days to 6 months.
   d. Contingent accreditation: The healthcare organization fails to successfully address all requirements of the accreditation with a follow-up survey decision.
   e. Preliminary denial of accreditation results when there is justification to deny accreditation to a healthcare organization for one or more of the following reasons: an immediate threat to health or safety for clients or the public, failure to resolve the requirements of an accreditation with follow-up survey status after two opportunities to do so, failure to resolve the requirements of a contingent accreditation status, or significant noncompliance with The Joint Commission standards.
   f. Denial of accreditation results when a healthcare organization has been denied accreditation.
5. The ORYX initiative
   a. Introduced in 1997
   b. Designed to help organizations strengthen their quality improvement efforts and to identify issues that warrant attention
   c. Uses data from organizations to monitor performance between on-site survey visits
   d. Supports The Joint Commission's mission and is a critical link between accreditation and client care outcomes
6. Benefits of The Joint Commission accreditation and certification
   a. Strengthens community confidence in the quality and safety of care, treatment, and services
   b. Provides a competitive edge in the marketplace
   c. Improves risk management and risk reduction
   d. Helps organize and strengthen client safety effort
   e. Provides education on good practices to improve business operations
   f. Provides professional advice and counsel, thereby enhancing staff education
   g. Provides deeming authority for Medicare certification
   h. Is recognized by insurers and other third parties
   i. May reduce liability insurance costs (The Joint Commission, 2014a)
7. Tracer method: The tracer method is an evaluation method in which surveyors select a resident or client and use that person's record as a roadmap to move through an organization to assess and evaluate the organization's compliance with selected standards and the organization's systems of providing care and services.
8. Unannounced surveys: The Joint Commission conducts unannounced surveys for accreditation. For Disease Specific Care (DSC) certification, organizations are provided a 30-day notice (initial certification) or a 7-day notice (recertification).

a. To help healthcare organizations focus on providing safe, high-quality care at all times, not just when preparing for a survey
b. To affirm the expectation of continuous standard compliance both by The Joint Commission of its accredited organizations and by these organizations of themselves
c. To increase the credibility of the accreditation process by ensuring that surveyors observe organization performance under normal circumstances
d. To reduce the unnecessary costs healthcare organizations incur to prepare for surveys
e. To address public concerns that The Joint Commission receives an accurate impression of the quality and safety of care

9. Sentinel events: In support of its mission to continuously improve the safety and quality of healthcare provided to the public, the Joint Commission reviews organizations' activities in response to sentinel events in its accreditation process. A sentinel event is an unexpected occurrence involving death or serious physical or psychological injury or the risk thereof. Such events are called "sentinel" because they signal the need for immediate investigation and response.

B. Commission on Accreditation of Rehabilitation Facilities (CARF)

1. General
   a. Mission: The mission of CARF is to promote the quality, value, and optimal outcomes of services through a consultative accreditation process that centers on enhancing the lives of the people served (CARF, 2014).
   b. *Conformance*: CARF's term referring to meeting standards
   c. Organizational structure
2. Accreditation programs (11 standard manuals)
   a. Aging Services: This includes Adult Day Services, Aging Services Network, Assisted Living, Person-Centered Long-Term Care Communities, Home and Community Services, Case Management, Independent Senior Living, Dementia Care Specialty Program, and Stroke Specialty Program.
   b. Behavioral Health: This includes Behavioral Health Field Categories (Alcohol and Other Drugs/Addictions, Mental Health, Psychosocial Rehabilitation, Family Services, Integrated Alcohol and Other Drugs (AOD)/Mental Health, Integrated Developlmental Disabilities (DD)/Mental Health, and Comprehensive Care), Behavioral Health Core Program Standards, Behavioral Health Specific Population Designation Standards, and Community and Employment Services (see www.carf.org for other specifics).
   c. Business and Services Management Network: This includes Network, Business Network, and Services Management Network.
   d. CARF–Continuing Care Accreditation Commission: This includes Adult Day Services, Aging Services Network, Assisted Living, Person-Centered Long Term Care Community, Home and Community Services, Case Management, Independent Senior Living, Continuing Care Retirement Communities, Dementia Care Specialty Program, and Stroke Specialty Program.
   e. Child and Youth Services: This includes Child and Youth Services Specific Program Standards and Child and Youth Services Specific Population Designation.
   f. DMEPOS: Durable Medical Equipment, Prothesis, Orthotics and Supplies
   g. Employment and Community Services: This includes Employment and Community Services, Specific Population Designations, and Psychosocial Rehabilitation Programs.
   h. Medical Rehabilitation: This includes Comprehensive Integrated Inpatient Rehabilitation Program, Outpatient Medical Rehabilitation Program, Home and Community Services, Residential Rehabilitation Program, Vocational Services, Pediatric Specialty Program, Amputation Specialty Program, Brain Injury Specialty Program, Cancer Rehabilitation Specialty Program, Spinal Cord System of Care, Stroke Specialty Program, Interdisciplinary Pain Rehabilitation Program, Occupational Rehabilitation Program, Independent Evaluation Services, and Case Management.
   i. One-Stop Career Center
   j. Opioid Treatment Program: This includes Court Treatment, Detoxification, Day Treatment, Health Home, Integrated Behavioral Health/Primary Care, Intensive Outpatient Treatment, Outpatient Treatment, Residential Treatment, and Criminal Justice.
   k. Vision Rehabilitation Services: This includes Comprehensive Blind Rehabilitation Services and Vision Rehabilitation Services.
3. Historical perspective
   a. 1966: Founded as a nonprofit organization
   b. 1993: Accredited its first program in Canada

c. 1995: Enacted new standards for occupational rehabilitation and comprehensive pain management programs in the medical rehabilitation division
d. 1996: Accredited its first program in Europe
e. 1999: Published standards for adult day services
f. 2000: Published standards for assisted living programs
g. 2001: Recognized by the Substance Abuse & Mental Health Services Administration as an approved accrediting organization for opioid treatment programs
h. 2003: Acquired the Continuing Care Accreditation Commission
i. 2005: Accredited first program in South America
j. 2008: CARF's ASPIRE to Excellence® framework is introduced.

4. Development and creation of standards
    a. National Advisory Committees (NACs): Each year, NACs are formed to review existing standards and create new standards. This is usually the starting point in the development of new standards. In years when there are no NACs, CARF solicits informal feedback from surveyors, consumers, other purchasers, and interested stakeholders.
    b. Field review: Proposed standards are sent to the rehabilitation field for review by national professional groups, third-party purchasers, consumers, surveyors, and advocacy groups. Feedback, suggestions, and requests are evaluated by CARF.
5. Accreditation process
    a. Contact a CARF office to verify which standard manual to use. Each standard manual year runs from July 1 to June 30.
    b. Perform a self-study. A facility may opt to complete a self-study and evaluation before and in preparation for the survey. CARF publishes numerous resources to help organizations in this process.
    c. Submit an application before the requested survey.
    d. Schedule the survey date. Surveyors are selected based on their expertise and knowledge of the programs being surveyed. Generally, there is an administrative surveyor and at least one program surveyor for medical rehabilitation programs.
    e. Have an orientation conference. This is done on the first day of the survey to allow surveyors to give an overview of the survey process and the organization to describe itself to the survey team.
    f. Have an exit conference. This provides immediate feedback to the organization about strengths, areas for improvement, suggestions, and any recommendations made by the survey team.
    g. The survey report with accreditation outcome is sent to the organization.
    h. The organization submits a quality improvement plan that addresses any recommendations in the survey report.
    i. Submit an annual conformance-to-quality report (CARF, 2006).
6. Key terminology related to CARF's survey process
    a. Standard conformance rating scale
        1) 0 = Nonconformance: The program does not even partially conform to a standard.
        2) 1 = Partial conformance: The program or service has achieved some components of a standard or made progress toward conformance yet does not meet expectations for full conformance.
        3) 2 = Conformance: The program or service fully meets the intent of a standard.
        4) 3 = Exemplary conformance: The program or service significantly exceeds the level of practice necessary to achieve conformance to a standard.
    b. Consultation: Suggestions from the survey team for improving services in the organization based on experience in the rehabilitation field. Suggestions are not linked to conformance to the standards in that an organization is not required to implement or act on them (CARF, 2006).
7. Accreditation decisions (2014)
    a. Three-year accreditation: The organization demonstrates substantial conformance to the standards.
    b. One-year accreditation: The organization is basically meeting the standards, but there are some significant areas of deficiency.
    c. Provisional accreditation: The organization received a 1-year accreditation on its immediately preceding survey, and although the organization is basically meeting the standards, there continue to be significant problem areas. Upon resurvey, an organization that has a provisional accreditation must achieve a 3-year accreditation or it will be nonaccredited.

d. Nonaccreditation: Major deficits exist in meeting standards, and concerns exist about whether the organization meets the needs of the people it serves.
e. Preliminary accreditation is awarded to allow new programs to establish demonstrated use and implementation of the standards (CARF, 2014).
f. Accreditation with stipulations: If an organization's accreditation status is displayed as having stipulations, CARF may require ongoing reporting or other action from the provider regarding its progress in maintaining conformance to the accreditation standards.

C. National Council on Quality Assurance
1. Oversees managed care companies
2. Uses the Health Employment Data Information Set (HEDIS) as its data set

D. Magnet Recognition Program
1. Recognizes healthcare organizations for quality patient care, nursing excellence, and innovations in professional nursing practice
2. Advances three goals within healthcare organizations
a. Promote quality in a setting that supports professional practice.
b. Identify excellence in the delivery of nursing services to patients/residents.
c. Disseminate best practices in nursing services.

VII. The Future of Quality Measurement

A. Increasing Importance of Outcome, Patient-Reported, and Cross-Cutting Quality Measures
1. Cross-cutting quality measures are aligned in order to be used across different settings or different populations.
2. Outcome quality measures, which focus on the benefits or end results of care, will increase. The durability of outcomes will become an even larger component of rehabilitation practice.
3. There is interest in using quality measures that incorporate the patient's voice. Patient-reported outcomes will gain higher priority in terms of what is important to patients.
4. Management of clients' needs across the continuum will be critical for successful chronic disease management. Measuring quality across the continuum will continue to have greater importance.
5. The emphasis of satisfaction will move from provider to payer to client or consumer (Jones & Evans, 1998).
6. Postacute care quality reporting programs will continue to evolve.

B. Greater Accountability to Stakeholders
1. Rehabilitation providers are experiencing an increase in accountability to demonstrate positive outcomes.
2. Rehabilitation providers are increasingly expected to share information about programs and outcomes.
3. Accountability depends on collaboration and shared goals by various stakeholders (Porter, 2010).
4. Shared accountability across providers (i.e., acute care and a postacute care setting) will increase.

References

Association of Rehabilitation Nurses (ARN). (2014). ARN competency model for professional rehabilitation nursing. Retrieved from http://www.rehabnurse.org/uploads/files/education/ARN_Rehabilitation_Nursing_Competency _Model_FINAL_-_May_2014.pdf

Agency for Healthcare Research and Quality. (n.d.) National Quality Strategy. Retrieved from www.ahrq.gov/workingforquality/

Brassard, M., & Ritter, D. (1994). The Memory Jogger II™: A pocket guide of tools for continuous improvement and effective planning. Methuen, MA: Goal/QPC.

Braun, S. (1998). The Functional Independence Measure for children (WeeFIM™ instrument): Gateway to the WeeFIM™ system. Journal of Rehabilitation Outcomes Measurement, 2(4), 63–68.

Carolinas Rehabilitation. (n.d.) EQUADR. Retrieved from www.carolinashealthcare.org/rehabilitation-healthcare-professionals-equadr

Commission on Accreditation of Rehabilitation Facilities (CARF). (2006). *Standards manual for medical rehabilitation*. Tucson, AZ: Author.

Commission on Accreditation of Rehabilitation Facilities (CARF). (2011). CARF's mission, vision, core values, and purposes. Retrieved from www.carf.org/about/mission/

Commission on Accreditation of Rehabilitation Facilities (CARF). (2014). Medical rehabilitation. Retrieved from http://www.carf.org/Programs/Medical/

Deutsch, A., Braun, S., & Granger, C. V. (1997). The Functional Independence Measure (FIM™) instrument. *Journal of Rehabilitation Outcomes, 1*(2), 67–71.

Dittmar, S., & Gresham, G. (1997). Appendix A: Description and display of selected functional assessment and outcome measures in physical rehabilitation. In *Functional assessment and outcome measurement for the rehabilitation healthcare professional* (pp. 90–138). Gaithersburg, MD: Aspen.

Dobrzykowski, E., & Nance, T. (1997). The Focus on Therapeutic Outcomes (FOTO) outpatient orthopedic rehabilitation database: Results of 1994–1996. *Journal of Rehabilitation Outcomes Measurement, 1*(1), 56–60.

Donabedian, A. (2005). Evaluating the quality of medical care. *The Milbank Quarterly, 83*(4), 691–729.

Exchanged Quality Data for Rehabilitation (EQUADR). (n.d.). EQUADR network. Retrieved from http://www.carolinashealthcare.org/rehabilitation-healthcare-professionals-equadr

Granger, C. (1999). The LIFEware system. *Journal of Rehabilitation Outcomes Measurement, 3*(2), 63–69.

Haley, S. (1999). The Pediatric Evaluation of Disability Inventory (PEDI). *Journal of Rehabilitation Outcomes, 1*(1), 61–69.

Hall, K., Dukers, M., Whiteneck, G., Brooks, C. A., & Krause, J. (1998). The Craig Handicap Assessment and Reporting Technique (CHART): Metric properties and scoring. *Journal of Rehabilitation Outcomes Measurement, 2*(5), 39–49.

Institute of Medicine. (2000). *To err is human: Building a safer health system*. Washington, DC: National Academy Press.

Institute of Medicine. (2001). *Crossing the quality chasm: A new health system for the 21st century*. Washington, DC: National Academy Press.

Institute of Medicine. (2006). *Performance measurement: Accelerating improvement*. Washington, DC: The National Academies Press.

Jones, M., & Evans, R. (1998). Outcomes in a managed care environment. *Topics in Spinal Cord Injury Rehabilitation, 3*(4), 61–73.

National Quality Forum. (n.d.) www.qualityforum.org. Accessed August 27, 2014.

Porter, M. (2010). What is value in healthcare? *New England Journal of Medicine* (pp. 1–5). Retrieved from www.nejm.org/doi/pdf/10.1056/NEJMc1101108

The Joint Commission (2014a). Benefits of Joint Commission accreditation. Retrieved from http://www.jointcommission.org/benefits_of_joint_commission_accreditation/

The Joint Commission. (2014b). Mission statement. Retrieved from www.jointcommission.org/assets/1/18/mission_statement_8_09.pdf

The Joint Commission on Accreditation of Healthcare Organizations. (2014). *2014 Accreditation manual for hospitals*. Oakbrook Terrace, IL: Author.

Uniform Data System for Medical Rehabilitation. (1996). *Guide for the Uniform Data Set for Medical Rehabilitation*. Buffalo: State University of New York.

Willer, B., Ottenbacher, K., & Coad, M. L. (1994). The Community Integration Questionnaire. *American Journal of Physical Medicine and Rehabilitation, 73*(2), 103–111.

World Health Organization. (2001). *International Classification of Functioning, Disability and Health (ICF)*. Geneva, Switzerland: Author.

Suggested Resources

Agency for Healthcare Research and Quality: www.ahrq.gov

American Nurses Association Nursing World: www.nursingworld.org

Institute for Healthcare Improvement: www.IHI.org

Medicare Payment Advisory Committee (MedPAC): www.medpac.gov

National Database of Nursing Quality Indicators: www.nursingquality.org

Section II

The Environment of Care in REHABILITATION

Chapter 8

Patient Education Across the Life Span

Stephanie Davis Burnett, DNP RN ACNS-BC CRRN
Elaine Tilka Miller, PhD RN CRRN FAHA FAAN

LEARNING OUTCOMES

- Identify key theories of learning.
- Recognize barriers to learning.
- Contrast teaching methods for the stages of development.
- Discuss teaching strategies for patients with disability/chronic illness.

KEY CHAPTER TOPICS

- Learning theories
- Assessing ability to learn
- Barriers to learning
- Developmental stages and learning
- Teaching strategies

PROFESSIONAL REHABILITATION NURSING DOMAINS AND COMPETENCIES

- Domain 1: Competency 1.3
- Domain 2: Competencies 2.1, 2.2 (Association of Rehabilitation Nurses [ARN], 2014)

Introduction

One of the central functions of the rehabilitation nurse is to care for and educate the patients and their families to promote maximum independence, prevent complications, and enhance patients' health statuses. *Pedagogy,* the art and science of teaching, is one of the central roles of the rehabilitation nurse. Patient teaching is vital to the healthcare process. Providing education to rehabilitation patients and their families or intended caregivers is an essential task of the rehabilitation nurse in all settings to effect a change in the learner's behavior. During an inpatient rehabilitation stay, the patient is prepared for the goal of returning to the community. When back in the community setting, the goal is to maintain or achieve maximum health and independence. This is especially important, because as hospital inpatient stays are shortened and reimbursement for care is reduced, more patients will need continued care provided by their family or identified caregivers. The goal of rehabilitation patients is to return to the community, so the more prepared they are to care for themselves, the more successful they can be in their community (Pryor et al., 2009).

Management of chronic conditions has shifted from a passive paternalistic model to one of more active patient/family involvement. In the passive model, the patient is an acquiescent recipient of care, participating marginally in his or her own direct care and decision making. In this model, the nurse essentially provides all of the direct care and assumes a dominant role, while the patient complies with whatever the nurse and other healthcare professionals deem appropriate. However, as we advance toward the more active model of rehabilitation nursing, the patient and family gradually assume more responsibility for day-to-day care management. Active participation in rehabilitation nursing care allows the patient the opportunity for performance, while offering encouragement, which is essential for self-efficacy in self-care (Bandura, 1986).

I. Domains of Professional Rehabilitation Competence

A. According to ARN (2014), two of the four domains for professional rehabilitation nursing competence relate directly to the importance of patient/family education.

1. Domain 1 (see the ARN Competency Model for Professional Rehabilitation Nursing chapter)—Nurse-Led, Evidence-Based Interventions to Promote Function and Health Management in Persons with Disability and/or Chronic Illness: Identifies the provision of patient/client and caregiver education related to disability, chronic illness, and health management (DCIHM)
   a. Family centered and dynamic
   b. Includes not only the needs of the patient/client, but the needs,

health, and welfare of the primary caregiver (Levin, 2011)

2. Domain 2 (see the ARN Competency Model for Professional Rehabilitation Nursing chapter)—Promotion of Health and Successful Living in Persons with Disability or Chronic Illness Across Life Span: Through education and preparation of the patient and family, health is promoted and disability is prevented across the life span. Self-management is fostered, and safe and effective care transitions are promoted and facilitated.
   a. Providing education in relation to DCIHM for population-appropriate care
      1) Population-specific competence of the rehabilitation nurse is necessary to meet the unique needs of the patient.
         a) Age appropriate
         b) Provided across the life span: From infancy to old age to death
         c) Growth and development considerations
         d) Ethnicity considerations
         e) Sensitivity to cultural differences and beliefs
         f) Sensitivity to health beliefs
         g) Sensitivity to dietary and religious practices
         h) Language translator (if possible)
         i) Promotion and facilitation of safe and efficient care transition

II. Overview of the Teaching and Learning Process and Learning Theories

A. The teaching and learning process encompasses dynamic, multifaceted, interactive, and ongoing communication between the patient, family, and healthcare provider that is focused on achieving a planned outcome.

B. *Learning* is defined as "a relatively permanent change in behavior or in behavioral potentiality that results from experience and cannot be attributed to temporary body states such as those induced by illness, fatigue, or drugs" (Olson & Hergenhahn, 2012, p. 6).
   1. Learning occurs as patients/families interact with their environment, incorporating new information into their knowledge base (M. M. Braungart, Braungart, & Gramer, 2014).
   2. Learning enables patients and families to acquire new knowledge (cognition), skills (psychomotor), and attitudes (affectivity) that can be measured (Bastable, 2014; McDonald, 2014).
   3. If learning is to be permanent, it must be treated as a process that occurs over time rather than an isolated event.
   4. Time and repeated contacts are required for an individual to acquire new knowledge, skills, and attitudes that are meaningful and significant (Bastable, 2014; McDonald, 2014).
   5. Learning is facilitated if information is provided in a manner that moves from simple to complex, from concrete to abstract, and from the known to what is not yet known.
   6. Learning is increased if the information is provided on a personal and individualized basis and is relevant to the learner's needs and problems.
   7. Learning is enhanced if the individual is attentive, and feedback is given soon after the educational event rather than later (Bastable, 2014; McDonald, 2014).

C. Teaching encompasses a deliberative, purposeful act of communicating information that focuses on a patient or family's educational need(s) and produces targeted measureable outcomes (Bastable, 2014; McDonald, 2014).
   1. Teaching requires that the educator be aware of the learning styles and needs of the patient and determines how capable the patient or family is of responding to the instruction provided.
   2. Learner expectations, attitudes, and motivation affect how productive the teaching can be and the subsequent outcomes.

D. The teaching and learning process can be learner centered or teacher centered.
   1. A learner-centered process specifies consistent communication between the patient/family and the healthcare provider (teacher) and the creation of an educational environment that is collaborative, cooperative, supportive, creative, and facilitative of learning (Blumberg, 2008).
   2. An educator-centered approach is one in which the educator speaks while the patient/family listens, and there is one-way communication in which the knowledge conveyed is not tailored to the patient and family's needs. The learning environment is nonparticipatory (Falvo, 2011).
   3. The educator's role is more facilitative than didactic (Blumberg, 2008).
   4. Students are actively involved in their own learning. They monitor their thinking, and with perceived control of their learning, they assume greater responsibility for their own learning and have better outcomes (Blumberg, 2008).

E. More than 40 evidence-based learning theories exist that offer various ways to assess the learning situation and key dynamics that affect learning, determine the educational objectives, design the educational interventions (teaching strategies), and determine the appropriate learning outcomes.

1. Major Learning Theories and How They View Learning
   a. Behavioral learning theories focus on what is directly observable in learners, with behavior outcomes regarded as a result of stimulus conditions.
      1) Ivan Pavlov (1849–1936) introduced his classical conditioning theory to differentiate it from the other types of stimulus-response associations. Thus, the conditioned stimulus is able to evoke the response (M. M. Braungart et al., 2014).
      2) B.F. Skinner (1904–1990) introduced the concept of operant conditioning, whereby a desirable behavior is more likely to be repeated or occurs more frequently because it is reinforced or strengthened by means of a reward.
   b. Cognitive learning theories focus on the operations of the mind and how thoughts influence the individual's actions in relationship to the environment (Candela, 2012).
      1) Kurt Lewin (1890–1947) believed that humans have a basic need to bring order to a situation, and their motivation to learn is stimulated by ambiguity of the situation. Motivation to learn is the key to this approach. Individuals can receive information but will not change their behavior if they are not motivated (McEwen & Wills, 2014).
      2) In information processing models, learning consists of strategies to transfer information from short- to long-term memory. Information in the short-term memory is lost within 5–20 seconds if action is not taken to reinforce it (Byrnes, 2008). It is important that the educator present information in an organized manner and to overlap that information with previously learned knowledge. Plus, in this framework, techniques such as visual imagery facilitate learning and recall of the information (Ormrod, 2012).
      3) Experimental learning entails interactions and postulates that individuals learn from their immediate experiences and that learning happens in all human settings (Kolb, 1984). Learning is how individuals adapt and cope with their environment, and each person's experience is unique in that individuals have preferred ways of learning. Jean Piaget (1896–1980), the best known developmental theorist, believed that cognitive development occurs in stages and affects what and how information can be learned. Piaget identified stages of learning from infancy to old age.
      4) Other developmental theorists include Abraham Maslow (1908–1970), who described the hierarchy of needs; Erik Erikson (1902–1994), who explored personality development; and Robert J. Havighurst (1900–1991), who described developmental tasks and life problems and how those lead to readiness to learn (McEwen & Wills, 2014).
      5) A more recent developmental theory growing in popularity is called constructionism and evolved from Piaget's research. *Constructionism* is the belief that knowledge has no existence outside an individual's mind and that learners always interpret what is presented to them using preexisting knowledge, history, and typical ways of perceiving and acting (Brynes, 2008).
      6) Albert Bandura's social learning theory (1986) focuses on the concept of reciprocal determinism and is concerned with the social influences that can affect learning (e.g., culture, ethnicity, groups). In this frequently applied theory, environment, cognitive factors, and behavior interact with one another. Individuals learn from each other through observation and role modeling.
      7) Malcolm Knowles (1913–1997) popularized the concept of *andragogy,* which is concerned with adult learning, as opposed to pedagogy, which focuses on youth learning. For Knowles, Holton, and Swanson (2005), the most important element in helping adults to learn is creating a climate of physical comfort, mutual trust, respect, openness, and acceptance of differences. By responding appropriately to the needs of the learner and providing the resources required for learning, educators facilitate learning. Knowles also asserted that adults need to know the reason for learning new information (Knowles et al., 2005).

III. Assessment of the Learner

A. The initial step in the nursing process for patient education is assessment.
   1. Use of an assessment tool can help focus the assessment (Levin, 2011).
   2. Identification of the caregiver is important.
      a. May need to be included in all teaching

3. Assessment of the learner should include
   a. Developmental stage
      1) Patients experience disability and chronic conditions throughout all stages of the life cycle. Each stage of the life span presents a different challenge based on the developmental stage; learning needs and skills; and the environmental, physical, emotional, and cognitive status of the patient/family.
   b. Learning needs and skills
      1) Patient's baseline knowledge about
         a) Disease or condition
            (i) Reason for admission
            (ii) Concurrent, chronic diseases or conditions
         b) Effects of disease or condition
         c) Potential complications
            (i) Recognition
            (ii) Prevention
         d) Medications
         e) Anticipated outcomes of stay
      2) Patient's baseline functional status
         a) Bladder, bowels, and skin in particular
   c. Health literacy
      1) *Health literacy* is the ability to obtain, process, and understand the basic health information and services needed to make appropriate health decisions (Lee, Arozullah, & Cho, 2004; U.S. Department of Health and Human Services, 2010).
      2) *Health literacy* is further defined as "the degree to which individuals have the capacity to obtain, process, and understand basic health information and services needed to make appropriate decisions" regarding their health, as adopted by Healthy People 2010 (Nielsen-Bohlman, Panzer & Kindig, 2004, p. 37).
         a) Low health literacy can be associated with poor patient-healthcare provider communications, poor decision making, poor patient outcomes, and the like.
         b) Instructions, such as medications or procedures, can be difficult to comprehend.
         c) Health literacy involves more than the ability to read and write.
         d) Marginal health literacy affects patients at every socioeconomic level and of all demographic groups (**Table 8-1**).
         e) Poor and minority groups are disproportionately affected.
         f) According to the National Assessment of Adult Literacy, there are four literacy levels (Kutner, Greenberg, Jin, & Paulsen, 2006):

Table 8-1. Testing for Health Literacy

Tool	Comments	Bedside Method	Comments
Newest Vital Signs	Quick tool, available in English and Spanish Consists of a nutritional label with related questions to test real-life understanding of label reading (Nigolian, 2011)	Universal Precautions Method	Due to differences in cultural, language, and ethnicity, assume all/most have health literacy problems, just as universal precautions are used for all patients to reduce infection risk. For example, all materials are presented at lowest reading level and use repetition.
Health Literacy Management Scale (HeLMS)	Assesses the individuals' broader social and environmental contest to determine their use of health information within the healthcare setting (Jordan et al., 2013)	Teach Back	Educational method for determining how well teaching concepts have been understood by the patient/family Involves asking learner in a nonshaming manner to repeat or demonstrate what they know or understand (Nigolian, 2011).
Test of Functional Health Literacy in Adults	Comprehensive test consisting of • a reading section that assesses the comprehension of health-related materials • a numeracy section, which tests understanding of numbers that would appear on prescriptions, appointments, etc. (Parker, Baker, Williams, & Nurss, 1995)		

(i) Below basic: able to comprehend no more than very simple, concrete, identifiable information
(ii) Basic: able to comprehend simple, everyday, uncomplicated information
(iii) Intermediate: moderately challenging, less common; able to summarize information
(iv) Proficient: complex and challenging; able to synthesize information

g) Health literacy should be assessed at baseline so that education can be adapted to best teach the patient/family. Key assessment points include
(i) Educational level
(ii) Reading level
(iii) Baseline knowledge
(iv) Past experiences with learning and health care
(v) Access to technology (e.g., computers)

d. Readiness to learn
1) Readiness to learn should be assessed and will depend on
a) Emotional state, relevance, and timing (Farrell & Raptosh, 2012)
b) Cognitive status
(i) Brain injury, stroke, depression, or confusion
c) Availability of resources
d) History of managing past health issues
e) Memory and recall
f) Energy level and health status
g) Application and pertinence of information

e. Ability to learn
1) Will depend upon
a) Patient acuity
b) Patient identification of need
c) Vision, hearing, mobility, and function
d) Timing
e) Medical status
(i) Brain injury
(ii) Confusion
(iii) Psychiatric issues
f) Conflicting stressors
(i) Therapy
(ii) Discharge planning
(iii) Worries about future

f. Learning style
1) Consider educational reading skills
a) Educational level
b) Computer skills and access
c) Consider available resources.
d) Auditory, visual, or kinesthetic learning preferences

B. Barriers to learning should be assessed before teaching so that they can be addressed or avoided.
1. Patient acuity
a. Patients who are ill will not learn well.
2. Reduced patient length of stay at facility
a. How much time will you have to teach complex topics?
b. What if time runs out?
3. Teaching skills of the educator
a. Pedagogical competence
b. Clinical experience
4. Available teaching resources
a. Patient resources
b. Organizational resources
5. Stress of situation for patient/caregiver
a. Learning will not take place if stress is great.
6. Cultural differences (Nigolian & Miller, 2011)
a. African Americans, Hispanics, and Asian Americans report that medical staff treat them unfairly and unfavorably and give them confusing instructions at the time of discharge.
b. Language differences: some patients believe that speaking a language other than English is viewed negatively
c. Nonverbal signals; for example, an Asian American patient may nod out of respect rather than to indicate understanding
7. Sensory deficits: visual or hearing limitations can affect communication; for example, understanding written information (e.g., the small print on medication labels), and have an impact on interactions with others
a. Ensure that eyeglasses and hearing aids are working and in place.
b. Ensure adequate lighting.
8. Cognitive status of the caregiver and patient
a. Brain injury or psychological issues

IV. Other Influences on Teaching and Learning Outcomes

A. Teacher communication style
B. Rapport and building relationship with the patient/family
C. Patient's prior knowledge or experience
D. Beliefs about health
1. Health belief model
2. Self-efficacy (confidence in abilities)
3. Locus of control
4. Dealing with change
E. Effectiveness of the communication between the educator and patient/family

F. Teaching is learner centered rather than educator centered.

G. Capability of the learner (e.g., cognitive, sensory, physical confidence, motivation) to understand and internalize the content and apply it

H. Develop a plan and attainable goals in conjunction with the patient and caregiver(s).

I. Communicate plan to team and discuss the feasibility of achieving the outcomes.

J. Technology
   1. Availability
   2. Lack of access and privacy
   3. Cost of maintenance
   4. Knowledge of effective operation
   5. Reliability
   6. Generational (i.e., version-related) differences that can affect use

V. Educational/Teaching Strategies for Achieving Planned Outcomes

A. What Do Rehabilitation Nurses Teach?
   1. Rehabilitation nurses teach patients, families, and caregivers about
      a. Diagnosis, plans, and outcomes
      b. Bowel and bladder management
      c. Skin care management
      d. Medication
      e. Self-care and mobility
      f. Health and wellness
      g. Nutrition
      h. Prevention of secondary complications
      i. Availability of resources (ARN, 2008)

VI. Other Topics, As Need Indicates

A. Fundamental Aspects Needed to Effectively Teach and Implement Appropriate Teaching Strategies (Bastable, 2014; Falvo, 2011; McDonald, 2014; Scruggs, Mastropieri, Berkeley, & Graetz, 2009).
   1. Educator's knowledge and skill with regard to the content and ability to effectively present content to achieve the planned outcome
   2. Educator's cultural competence and knowledge (best practices) pertaining to the multiple factors affecting a personalized educational approach (e.g., age; developmental stage; cognitive, sensory, motor, and emotional status)
   3. Required resources for effective teaching, follow-up, and evaluation of learning (e.g., equipment and technology, materials, space and time requirements)
   4. Coordination of educational activities that is consistent with discharge plan and other relevant patient/family information
   5. Recognize that teaching is not an exact science, and one approach does not work the same way with all learners.
   6. Effective teaching requires creativity and flexibility, and educators must continually monitor and adjust their teaching techniques.
   7. Timing and extent of the learning—and leveling of content from simple to complex—always need to be considered when planning.
   8. Engaging the student to participate, keeping him or her motivated to learn the content and/or skill, and making that knowledge or skill applicable as well as achievable with regard to short- and long-term outcomes (sustainable).
   9. Succinct and timely documentation of what was specifically taught and when, with measurable outcomes, so others can build on and reinforce prior teaching
   10. Evaluation of learning is essential, because it enables the educator to assess whether the outcomes were achieved.
      a. Formative evaluation occurs during the teaching process to allow a quick assessment if the learning appears to be occurring as intended.
      b. A summative evaluation occurs after all of the teaching is performed and if the specific outcomes are as planned.
      c. In most instances, the systematic evaluation of the learning process enables the educator and patient/family to reinforce elements, permitting the achievement of sustainable long-term learning outcomes.

B. Teaching Strategies to Consider When Educating Patients with Low Literacy or Other Cognitive or Learning Challenges (Bastable, 2014; Falvo, 2011; McDonald, 2014)
   1. Provide opportunity for a hands-on return demonstration and practice.
   2. Educational materials should not be beyond a 5th-grade level and should be culturally appropriate.
   3. Speak and write using short words with only one or two syllables whenever possible, and rely on common words that are easily recognized.
   4. Keep sentences short and limited to 15 words or fewer.
   5. Address the most important information first when teaching.
   6. Clearly state and define technical words (e.g., glucometer, fasting blood sugar) or replace with simpler words (e.g., use "high blood pressure" for hypertension).
   7. If the patient/family has low literacy skills, they could require more time to read and comprehend

the content. Asking them to repeat what they have just read or learned helps to assess their understanding.

8. Visual images, rather than a lot of reading material, can be very helpful.
9. The use of pictures closely associated with text and minimal distractions can be very effective for recall.
10. Avoid using abbreviations.
11. Use consistent words throughout the teaching process.
12. Present the information in "chunks" to facilitate learning and recall (e.g., signs/symptoms of hypoglycemia and what to do when it occurs).
13. Limit the number of items on a list to no more than seven.
14. Keep teaching sessions short—preferably 15 minutes or less.
15. Use teach-back method to ensure the patient/family understands. Never ask "Do you understand?" Instead, for example, ask the patient/family to state four signs or symptoms of hypoglycemia or four signs of a stroke.
16. Have a literacy expert review your written materials to determine the grading level.
17. Present information one step at a time to pace instruction, and permit the patient and family to understand and ask questions before proceeding to the next step of the teaching plan.
18. Remember that every interaction is an opportunity to teach.

C. Follow-up for Education
   1. Follow-up after teaching is important to ensure that necessary information was learned. Follow-up is done at intervals during the rehabilitation stay and after discharge.
      a. Follow-up phone call
      b. Patient portals
      c. Automated robocalls
      d. Doctor/nurse appointments
      e. Home health care

D. Use evidence-based teaching strategies that are applicable to most teaching and learning situations involving patients and families (Bastable, 2014; McDonald, 2014; Scruggs et al., 2009). It is highly recommended that, whenever possible, educators seek current research studies (preferably from the past 5 years) that pertain to their specific patient population, learning outcomes, and resultant level and quality of evidence.
   1. Patient/family establish with the educator the learning outcomes and feasible action plan to achieve them (highly effective).
   2. Explicit instruction, also referred to as *direct teaching* (the most effective approach of those studied), that is composed of three strategies: teaching in small steps, using guided practice, and fostering independent practice.
   3. Teaching strategies must take into consideration the developmental stage of the learner (highly effective) (**Table 8-2**)
   4. *Mnemonic strategies* are those that use patterns of letters, sounds, or associated ideas that all assist with remembering (highly effective).
   5. Classroom learning strategies refer to note taking, self-questioning, self-monitoring, and summarizing, permitting review of learning (highly effective).
   6. Hands on or activity-oriented learning that includes the patient returning to demonstrate what her or she has learned (highly effective)
   7. Peer or group interaction permits the patient/family to help teach each other and work together on learning and performing activities (effective).
   8. Computer-oriented instruction delivers a variety of applications, including drills and practice, strategy instruction, and simulation (moderately effective depending on the quality of the program and how well it is tailored to learning needs).
   9. Visual organizers help the learner understand and remember concepts, facts, and principles through the use of charts, diagrams, graphs, and other visual objects (effective).

Table 8-2. Appropriate Teaching Strategies for the Major Developmental Stages		
Learner Developmental Stage	**General Characteristics**	**Teaching Strategies**
Infant to toddler (birth to 2 years)	Dependent on others Explores self and environment	Focus teaching on caregiver. Use repetition and imitation. Stimulate all senses. Provide for safety and emotional security. Encourage play and manipulation.
Early childhood (3–5 years)	Egocentric Thinking concrete and literal Limited sense of time Can't generalize information Separation anxiety Active imagination, tends to be fearful Play is the child's work	Build trust. Provide a safe and calm environment. Have repetition of information. Reassure and do not blame. Encourage questions. Use play therapy. Stimulate senses.
Middle to late childhood (6–11 years)	Wants concrete information More realistic and objective Can compare objects and events Understands seriousness and consequences of actions Subject-centered focus	Encourage active participation and independence. Allay fears and be honest. Provide role models. Use analogies. Provide group activities. Be subject centered.
Adolescence (12–19 years)	Can build on past learning Abstract thinking Reasons by logic Motivated by social acceptance Peer group is important Strong personal preoccupation with appearance Feels invincible	Establish trust. Know their agenda. Include in plan of care. Focus on details and make information meaningful to them. Negotiate changes. Ensure confidentiality and privacy. Use peers for support and influence. Address fears and concerns pertaining to illness or condition.
Young Adulthood (20–40 years)	Self-directed, autonomous Intrinsic motivation Able to critically analyze Competency-based learner Uses personal experiences to enhance or interfere with learning	Center teaching on problems.. Encourage active participation. Focus on immediate application. Encourage to self-pace and be self-directed. Draw on meaningful experiences. Apply new knowledge and hands on practice.
Middle-Aged (41–64 years)	Sense of self is well developed Concerned with physical changes At peak of career Reflects on contributions to society and family Reexamines goals and values Has confidence in abilities Wants to modify unsatisfying aspects of life	Help maintain independence and reestablish normal life patterns. Assess positive and negative learning experiences. Determine motivational level for involvement and achievement of outcomes. Determine actual or potential sources of stress in life. Provide information that coincides with life concerns and problems.

continued

Table 8-2. Appropriate Teaching Strategies for the Major Developmental Stages (continued)

Older Adulthood (65 years and older)	Although there are common changes, healthcare providers need to assess each individual and not make assumptions. Reduced ability to think abstractly and process information. Increased reaction time Decreased short-term memory Sensory changes (e.g., reduction in vision and hearing, especially high-pitched tones and consonants) Fatigue and decreased energy Decreased risk taking Selective learning	Use concrete examples. Build on past life experiences. Make information relevant and meaningful. Use repetition and reinforcement. Use verbal exchange and coaching. Encourage active involvement. Keep explanations clear and brief. Avoid shouting. Use visual aids to supplement verbal instruction. Avoid glares and provide sufficient light. Use white backgrounds with black lettering (avoid pastel blues, greens, purples, and yellow). Increase safety precautions. Establish realistic short-term goals. Make learning positive, and demonstrate relevance to life. Integrate new behaviors with old ones.

Data from Bastable, 2014; Mauk, 2014; McDonald, 2014; Rankin, Stallings, & London, 2005; Scruggs, Mastropieri, Berkley, & Graetz, 2009.

Summary

In rehabilitation nursing practice, patients and their families frequently experience life-changing events that can have a profound effect on their physical, psychological, social, spiritual, and economic health. Education plays a pivotal role in helping patients and their families cope with their new reality. As illustrated in this chapter, patient and family education requires that the rehabilitation nurse have diverse knowledge and skills, a competency emphasized by ARN as essential for meeting the education needs of both the individual patient/client and the population group of rehabilitation patients. The evidence pertaining to the design, implementation, and evaluation of patient education is steadily expanding. Although it is clear that no perfect approach or formula exists for every educational encounter, a wealth of knowledge is available to help guide how to address the three domains of learning: cognitive, attitudinal, and psychomotor. Teaching and learning are complex processes that demand consideration of numerous elements such as culture, gender, learning styles, readiness to change, self-efficacy, developmental stage, literacy, resources, and ability to learn. In addition, rehabilitation nurses must be ever mindful of the importance of partnering with patients and families to establish short- and long-term educational goals. Evaluation of the teaching and learning processes is another critical task. It involves the systematic and continuous activity of collecting information to determine whether the educational objectives are being achieved. In conclusion, it is important to remember that every patient and family interaction can provide an opportunity for a teachable moment.

References

Association of Rehabilitation Nurses (ARN). (2008). *Standards and scope of rehabilitation nursing practice.* Glenview, IL: Author.

Association of Rehabilitation Nurses (ARN). (2014). ARN competency model for professional rehabilitation nursing. Retrieved from http://www.rehabnurse.org/uploads/files/education/ARN_Rehabilitation_Nursing_Competency _Model_FINAL_-_May_2014.pdf

Bandura, A. (1986). *Social foundations of thought and action: A social cognitive theory.* Prentice-Hall: Englewood Cliffs, NJ.

Bastable, B. B. (2014). *Nurse as educator: Principles of teaching and learning for nursing practice* (4th ed.). Burlington, MA: Jones & Bartlett Learning.

Blumberg, P. (2008). *Developing learner-centered teachers: A practical guide for faculty.* San Francisco: Jossey-Bass.

Braungart, M. M., Braungart, R. G., & Gramer, P. R. (2014). Applying learning theories to health care practice. In S. B. Bastable (Ed.), *Nurse as educator: Principles of teaching and learning for nursing practice* (4th ed., pp. 63–123). Boston: Jones & Bartlett Learning.

Brynes, J. P. (2008). *Cognitive development and learning in instructional contexts* (3rd ed.). Upper Saddle River, NJ: Prentice Hall Pearson.

Candela, I. (2012). From teaching to learning: Theoretical foundations. In D. M. Billings & J. A. Halstead (Eds.), *Teaching in nursing: A guide for faculty* (4th ed., pp. 202–242). St. Louis: Elsevier/Saunders.

Falvo, D. R. (2011). *Effective patient education: A guide to increased adherence* (2nd ed.). Burlington, MA; Jones & Bartlett Learning.

Farrell, P., & Raptosh, R. (2012). Educating clients and families. In K. Mauk (Ed.), *Rehabilitation nursing; A contemporary approach to practice* (pp. 176–199). Burlington, MA; Jones & Bartlett Learning.

Jordan, J. E., Buchbinder, R., Briggs, A. M., Elsworth, G. R., Busija, L., Batterham, R., & Osborne, R. H. (2013). The health literacy management scale (HeLMS): A measure of an individual's capacity to seek, understand and use health information within the healthcare setting. *Patient Education and Counseling, 91,* 228–235.

Knowles, M., Holton, E. F., & Swanson, R. A. (2005). *The adult learner: The definitive classic on adult education and human resource development* (6th ed.). Burlington, MA: Elsevier.

Kolb, D. A. (1984). *Experiential learning: Experience as the source of learning and development.* Englewood Cliffs, NJ: Prentice Hall.

Kutner, J., Greenberg, E., Jin, Y., & Paulsen, C. (2006). *The Health Literacy of America's Adults: Results from the 2003 National Assessment of Adult Literacy* (NCES 2006-483). US Department of Education. Washington, DC: National Center for Education Statistics.

Levin, C. (2011). The hospital nurse's assessment of family caregiver needs. *American Journal of Nursing, 111*(10), 47–51.

Lee, S. D., Arozullah, A. M., & Cho, Y. I. (2004). Health literacy, social support, and health: a research agenda. *Social Science & Medicine, 58*(7), 1309–1321.

Mauk, K. L. (Ed.). (2014). *Gerontology nursing: Competencies for care* (3rd ed.). Sudbury, MA: Jones & Bartlett Learning.

McDonald, M. E. (2014). *The nurse educator's guide to assessing learning outcomes* (3rd ed.). Burlington, MA: Jones & Bartlett Learning.

McEwen, M., & Wills, E. M. (2014). Theoretical basis for nursing (4th ed.). Philadelphia: Wolters Kluwer.

Nielsen-Bohlman, L., Panzer, A. M., & Kindig, D. A (Eds.). (2004). *Health Literacy: A Prescription to End Confusion.* National Academies Press: Washington, DC.

Nigolian, C. J., & Miller, K. L. (2011). Teaching essential skills to family caregivers. *American Journal of Nursing, 111*(11), 52–58.

Olson, M. W., & Hergenhahn, R. R. (2012). *An introduction to theories of learning* (9th ed.). Upper Saddle River, NJ: Pearson Prentice Hall.

Ormrod, J. (2012). *Human learning* (6th ed.). Boston: Prentice.

Parker, R. M., Baker, D. W., Williams, M. V., & Nurss, J. R. (1995). The test of functional health literacy in adults: A new instrumental for measuring patients' literacy skills. *Journal of General Internal Medicine, 10,* 537–541.

Pryor, J., Walker, A., O'Connell, B., & Worrall-Carter, L. (2009). Opting in and opting out: A ground theory of nursing's contribution to inpatient rehabilitation. *Clinical Rehabilitation, 23,* 1124–1135.

Rankin, S. H., Stallings, K. D., & London, F. (2005). *Patient education in health and illness* (5th ed.). Philadelphia: Lippincott, Williams, & Wilkins.

Scruggs, T. E., Mastropieri, M. A., Berkeley, S., & Graetz, J. E. (2009). Do special education interventions improve learning of secondary content? *Remedial and Special Education, 31*(6), 437–449.

U.S. Department of Health and Human Services, Office of Disease Prevention and Health Promotion. (2010). National Action Plan to Improve Health Literacy. Washington, DC: Author.

Web Resources

Adult learning

http://www.medscape.com/viewarticle/547417_4

http://www.aaace.org/adult-learning

http://nces.ed.gov/fastfacts/display.asp?id=89

Assessing learning styles

http://www.ncbi.nlm.nih.gov/pubmed/21791266

http://www.lib.miamioh.edu/multifacet/record/mu3ugb4210410

Barriers to learning

http://nursingworld.org/MainMenuCategories/ANAMarketplace/ANAPeriodicals/OJIN/TableofContents/Vol142009/No3Sept09/Cultural-and-Linguistic-Barriers-.aspx

Health literacy

http://www.health.gov/communication/literacy/quickguide/factsbasic.htm

http://www.cdc.gov/healthliteracy/

http://www.nih.gov/clearcommunication/healthliteracy.htm

Chapter 9

Care Transitions and the Role of the Rehabilitation Nurse

Barbara J. Lutz, PhD RN CRRN FAHA FNAP FAAN
Michelle Camicia, MSN CRRN CCM
James Farrell, MBA RN CRRN

LEARNING OUTCOMES

- Define and describe the importance of care transitions along the acute care to postacute care continuum for patients in need of rehabilitation.
- Review the role of the rehabilitation nurse in promoting and facilitating these care transitions.

KEY CHAPTER TOPICS

- Challenges in safe care transitions
- Legislative (federal) influence on care transitions in health care
- Definitions related to postacute care (PAC)
- Patient outcomes related to care transitions
- The role of the rehabilitation nurse in care transitions
- The role of the patient and family in care transitions

PROFESSIONAL REHABILITATION NURSING DOMAINS AND COMPETENCIES

- Domain 2: Competency 2.3 (Association of Rehabilitation Nurses [ARN], 2014a)

Content for this chapter was adapted from Camicia, M., Black, T., Farrell, J., Waites, K., Wirt, S., Lutz, B., and the Association of Rehabilitation Nurses. (2014). The essential role of the rehabilitation nurse in facilitating care transitions: A white paper by the Association of Rehabilitation Nurses. Rehabilitation Nursing, 39*(1), 1–13. Retrieved from http://onlinelibrary.wiley.com/doi/10.1002/rnj.135/pdf*

Introduction

Rehabilitation nurses are committed to promoting the health and welfare of clients with disabilities and ensuring that patients with disability as a result of injury or illness receive the right care at the right time by the right providers. Appropriate care transitions promote the greatest value and the most effective and efficient care for clients with disabilities. It is imperative that providers, health care policy makers, educators, payers, and other stakeholders in health care understand the value of the rehabilitation nurse's essential role in facilitating care transitions for patients with disabling conditions. A core competency of the rehabilitation nurse is to "promote and facilitate safe and effective care transitions" (Association of Rehabilitation Nurses [ARN], 2014b, p. 13).

It is important to note that patients who need rehabilitation services do not always move in a linear fashion from acute care through the postacute care continuum. Transitions can occur throughout the trajectory of an illness or disabling condition. For example, there are situations in which a person may transition from home or community to postacute care (PAC). However, the most common trajectory for those needing rehabilitation services is from acute care through the different levels of PAC. This continuum is under scrutiny as part of healthcare reform. Therefore, the focus of this chapter is on the transitions that occur from acute care to PAC to home or community. The term *postacute care* refers to care that does not occur in the acute care (i.e., hospital) setting and is defined more specifically later in this chapter.

I. Care Transitions

Care transitions are defined as the movement of patients with acute or chronic illnesses across the continuum of care between various healthcare providers and settings as care needs change (Coleman, n.d., para 1). The current process of care transitions for people with disabling conditions is often both ineffective and inefficient, especially as the patient moves from acute care to PAC. Decisions about care transitions to PAC settings for people with disabling conditions are complex. Clinicians are needed who have the necessary knowledge and skills to advocate and facilitate transitions that result in the greatest value to the patients, their families, and the healthcare delivery system. Rehabilitation nurses have the skills and expertise to fulfill this role.

A. Research reveals significant problems with PAC transitions.
   1. Care is fragmented, disorganized, and guided by factors unrelated to the quality of care or patient outcomes.
   2. Studies have demonstrated that the determination of PAC setting is influenced by multiple factors.
      a. Patient factors
         1) Gender
         2) Race
         3) Age
         4) Socioeconomic status
         5) Geographic proximity (Sandel et al., 2009)
      b. System factors
         1) Relationship between the acute care hospital, the PAC facility, and healthcare providers (Gage, 2009)
         2) Proximity of providers to PAC setting
         3) Payer source
         4) Variation in the interpretations of regulations regarding PAC

B. Decisions about care transitions to PAC involve many stakeholders, including the patient, family members, discharge planners, providers, insurance company representatives, social workers, and other healthcare providers.
   1. These stakeholders often have a poor understanding of the differences between the levels of PAC and lack adequate information to make the best decision during care transition planning.
   2. Decisions about the appropriate level of PAC affect long-term outcomes for patients and families and may result in the inappropriate use of resources.
   3. Care transitions are often disruptive for patients and their families, leaving them feeling overwhelmed, dissatisfied, and confused.
   4. Clinicians involved in PAC transitions for people with chronic diseases and disabling conditions must have the knowledge to provide patient-centered, goal-oriented, outcome-based care.

C. Historically, very little guidance has been provided to key decision makers in choosing the PAC setting that delivers effective and efficient care and results in optimal patient outcomes.
   1. In determining appropriate discharge placement, myriad factors should be considered.
   2. Nurses have a key role in guiding this decision making, as described in the American Nurses Association (ANA) white paper on "The Value of Nursing Care Coordination" (Camicia et al., 2013).
   3. Rehabilitation nurses have the skills to coordinate care and facilitate appropriate care transitions for patients who need rehabilitation services because of injury or illness causing disability.

D. Many factors must be considered when determining the appropriate PAC setting.
   1. System factors include the components of care and services, the intensity of services, and the structure and process of the program.
   2. Biological factors include a patient's medical needs, level of function before the injury or illness, and tolerance of rehabilitation.
   3. Social factors include psychological and community supports, both formal and informal.
   4. Financial resources include both the means and ability of the patient and family to pay for all costs incurred at the PAC setting and after discharge.

E. PAC is provided in various settings, including skilled nursing facilities (SNFs), inpatient rehabilitation facilities (IRFs), long-term acute care hospitals (LTACHs), home health (HH) agencies, and outpatient rehabilitation, which can be provided in a variety of settings.
   1. Rehabilitation is a key component of the care provided in each of these settings.
   2. Care in each of these settings is provided by a wide array of specialized clinicians, including physical therapists, occupational therapists, physicians, speech–language pathologists, neuropsychologists, social workers, discharge planners, and nurses with and without rehabilitation expertise.
   3. Clinicians must understand the differences between the levels of PAC, the roles of professionals in different PAC settings, and how these roles affect long-term patient outcomes.
   4. Determining the best setting for the patient requires a thorough understanding of rehabilitation services and evidence-based outcomes to evaluate appropriateness of care for the patient.

F. Rehabilitation nurses are defined by a unique skill set, enabling them to guide families in successful PAC transitions. These skills include the following:
   1. Knowledge and understanding of chronic illnesses and conditions that cause disability

2. A focus on helping patients recover as much function as possible
3. A comprehensive understanding of the resources available at each level of PAC
4. Advocating for the provision of appropriate services based on the patients and family's needs

G. Pilot studies have demonstrated that when a nurse with an understanding of care transitions is integrated into the decision process, hospital readmission rates decrease and outcomes are improved (Congressional Research Service [CRS], 2010).
1. Rehabilitation nurses have the training, knowledge, and experience to coordinate, support, and facilitate the discharge transition process and to promote high-quality outcomes and cost-effective care for people with disabling conditions (Camicia et al., 2014).
2. Rehabilitation nurses have the skills to educate and inform families about options and services available.

H. Studies are needed to evaluate the impact of rehabilitation nurses on the healthcare delivery system.
1. *Standards and Scope of Rehabilitation Practice* (ARN, 2014b) and the ARN white paper "The Essential Role of the Rehabilitation Nurse in Facilitating Care Transitions" (Camicia, et al., 2014) should be foundational documents for discharge planning education related to care transitions for people with disabling conditions.
2. ARN has developed a list of competencies at the novice, intermediate, and expert level to facilitate care transitions for patients with functional limitations (ARN, 2014a).

I. Because of their unique skill set, rehabilitation nurses must be involved in national policy decisions related to care coordination and transitions to improve cost efficiency and quality of patient care in the United States.

II. Background

The Patient Protection and Affordable Care Act (ACA) of 2010 seeks to improve quality and reduce costs of health care in the United States.

A. The U.S. Department of Health and Human Services (U.S. DHHS) developed the *National Strategy for Quality Improvement in Health Care*, which has three aims for improving the quality of health care in the United States (2012):
1. Better care: Improve the overall quality of care by making health care more patient centered, reliable, accessible, and safe.
2. Healthy people and communities: Improve the health of the U.S. population by supporting proven interventions to address behavioral, social, and environmental determinants of health in addition to delivering higher-quality care.
3. Affordable care: Reduce the cost of high-quality health care for individuals, families, employers, and government.
   a. To help achieve these aims, the report also established six priorities to help focus efforts by public and private partners:
      1) Making care safer by reducing harm caused in the delivery of care
      2) Ensuring that patients and families are engaged as partners in their care
      3) Promoting effective communication and coordination of care
      4) Promoting the most effective prevention and treatment practices for the leading causes of mortality, starting with cardiovascular disease
      5) Working with communities to promote wide use of best practices to enable healthy living
      6) Making high-quality care more affordable for individuals, families, employers, and governments by developing and spreading new healthcare delivery models
   b. *The National Strategy for Quality Improvement in Health Care* embraces a focus on quality as measured by clinical and patient-reported outcomes.
      1) The report recommends evaluation of care transitions and changes in functional status (U.S. DHHS, 2012), which are integral to PAC.
      2) To ensure high-quality health care, it is necessary to focus on PAC transitions to ensure effective care coordination as patients move from one site of care to another.

B. This increased focus on ensuring proper care coordination from acute care (hospital) to PAC is a result of reduced lengths of stay in acute inpatient care.
1. The average length of stay (ALOS) for hospital patients has steadily decreased since 1983 with the advent of the inpatient prospective payment system (IPPS) and the diagnosis-related group (DRG) system.
2. According to the American Hospital Association (AHA; 2013), from 1991 to 2011 the ALOS declined from 7.2 days to 5.4 days, a decrease of 25%.
3. Though patients are spending less time as hospital inpatients, the use of PAC services has increased.

C. PAC is a significant part of the overall care of many Medicare patients.
   1. About 30%–60% of the older patients develop new dependence in activities of daily living (ADLs) during an acute care hospital stay, which results in progressive disability after discharge (Huang, Chang, Liu, Lin, & Chen, 2013).
   2. Every year more than 10 million Medicare beneficiaries are transferred to a PAC setting (Grobowski, Huckfeldt, Sood, Escarce, & Newhouse, 2012).
   3. In a study of 200 PAC settings from 2008 to 2011, up to 35% of Medicare patients were discharged from acute care to a PAC setting (Gage, 2009).
   4. This increased use of PAC settings has made care transitions a critical component of favorable patient outcomes.
   5. Medicare's spending on these beneficiaries has increased significantly in the past decade, more than doubling from $26.6 billion in 2001 to $58 billion in 2010 (Medicare Payment Advisory Commission [MedPAC], 2011).
   6. According to a recent MedPAC report, Medicare paid for care in SNFs for 1.7 million beneficiaries.
   7. An estimated 3.4 million Medicare beneficiaries received home health care.
   8. IRFs treated 371,000 beneficiaries, and 123,000 Medicare beneficiaries received care in long-term care hospitals (LTCHs) (MedPAC, 2013).

D. Usage patterns alone are insufficient to determine whether a patient is receiving care in the setting most appropriate for his or her needs.
   1. Failure to determine the individual patient's appropriate site of care for PAC services has contributed to an unacceptable level of hospital readmissions.
   2. The CRS (2010) found that patients are readmitted to acute care providers from PAC settings often because the PAC setting lacks the ability to provide the appropriate level of care or lacks sufficient information to provide for the Medicare beneficiary's needs.
   3. A study of more than 11,000 stroke patients found that poorly coordinated care transitions led to disparities in care based on geographic proximities to providers and other factors unrelated to evidence-based practice (Sandel et al., 2009).
      a. Patients who experienced a stroke were more likely to go to an SNF if they were female and older.
      b. Patients who were Asian, black, from a higher socioeconomic class, or in close proximity to an IRF were more likely to receive PAC at an IRF.

E. According to the National Quality Forum (NQF), "care coordination is a vital aspect of health and health care services" (NQF, 2010, p. iv), and readmission measures can serve as an indicator of whether care coordination has been optimized (NQF, 2010).
   1. According to the MedPAC, unplanned readmissions to the hospital within 30 days of a patient's discharge cost the Medicare program approximately $15 billion annually (Tilson & Hoffman, 2012).
   2. The ACA requires that most acute care hospitals report their readmission rates. Hospitals with above-average readmission rates face a financial penalty.
   3. A similar readmission reduction program for PAC providers has been introduced.

F. The Centers for Medicare & Medicaid Services (CMS) Revised Appendix A "Interpretive Guidelines for Hospitals, Condition of Participation (CoP): Discharge Planning" (2013) notes that unplanned hospital readmissions can result from a variety of factors, including poor care transitions.
   1. Readmission is more likely if the patient is discharged from the hospital to an inappropriate setting or if the patient does not receive adequate information or resources to ensure continued progression of services.
   2. "System factors such as poorly coordinated care and incomplete communication and information exchanged between inpatient and community-based providers may also lead to unplanned readmissions" (U.S. DHHS, 2013, p. 4).
   3. Hospitals are now required to evaluate "the likelihood of a patient needing post-hospital services and the availability of services" and "the likelihood of a patient's capacity for self-care or the possibility of the patient being cared for in the environment from which he or she entered the hospital" (U.S. DHHS, 2013, p. 10).
   4. Hospitals are expected to be aware of the capabilities and limitations of PAC facilities to avoid readmissions.

G. Private insurance company contracts, often following the precedent of CMS Fiscal Intermediaries (FIs), create additional arbitrary guidelines for approval of admitting patients to various settings.

III. Care Transitions

A. The concept of care transitions and the use of PAC services is complex. The determination of postacute level of care is often driven by factors unrelated to producing the best possible outcomes of care.
   1. Discharge to PAC has been correlated with gender, race, age, socioeconomic background, and

geographic proximity to a PAC provider (Sandel et al, 2009).

2. Hospital relationship with a PAC provider also is related to discharge to a PAC setting. For example, if a hospital had a formal relationship with an IRF, SNF, or HH provider, patients were more likely to be discharged to one of those settings (Gage, 2009).

B. Throughout the decades since the advent of DRGs, acute care hospitals have implemented care coordination under the guidance of care management (CM).

1. In many settings CM has resulted in limited improvement in the quality of patient care.
2. Many of the early CM efforts were focused on utilization management, which focuses more on resource utilization rather than care or transition management.
3. When studying traditional models, the Agency for Healthcare Research and Quality (AHRQ) found that "CM had limited impact on patient-centered outcomes, quality of care, and resource utilization among patients with chronic medical illness" (2013, p. vii).
4. Care coordination and transitional care models have been proposed to reduce 30-day hospital readmissions, resulting in cost reductions and improved patient outcomes. In pilot studies conducted at an integrated healthcare network, coordinated care transitions resulted in significantly lower hospital readmission rates (CRS, 2010).

C. Failure to determine the appropriate site of care for PAC services has contributed to an unacceptable level of hospital readmissions. The CRS (2010) found that patients are readmitted to acute care providers from PAC settings often because they either lack the ability to provide the appropriate level of care or lack sufficient information to provide for the Medicare beneficiary's needs.

IV. Definition of Rehabilitation

Rehabilitation is a process, practice, and philosophy, not a care setting.

A. Rehabilitation is a philosophy of practice and an attitude toward caring for people with disabilities and chronic health problems (Larsen, 2011). The goal of rehabilitation is to restore mental or physical abilities lost to disease so that the patient can function in a normal or near-normal way (National Cancer Institute, 2013).

B. *Rehabilitation nursing* is defined as "the diagnosis and treatment of human responses of individuals and groups to actual or potential health problems related to altered functional ability and lifestyle" (ARN, 2008, p. 13).

C. Various levels and settings for rehabilitation services are available, including SNFs, IRFs, LTCHs, outpatient therapy (OPT), or HH.

1. Rehabilitation in each of these settings seeks to maximize the function of the person affected by the injury or disease.
2. The amount and type of care provided vary by setting.

V. Rehabilitation Levels of PAC

Each level of PAC has unique regulatory and admissions requirements, skill sets, abilities, and mission. It is important to be aware of the unique attributes of each when identifying the appropriate setting for the patient's needs. The differences between these settings are detailed in **Tables 9-1** and **9-2**.

A. Long-Term Care Hospitals (LTCHs)

1. LTCHs provide care for patients with complex medical problems, such as patients who are ventilator dependent or need intensive respiratory care, complex wound care, or multiple intravenous medications.
2. Care is provided in either a specialty hospital designated under LTCH licensure or a "hospital within a hospital," where a wing of a hospital has been contracted out to an LTCH provider.
3. For a facility to be considered an LTCH, the average length of stay for patients in long-term acute care must be 25 days, although patients may stay longer.

B. Inpatient Rehabilitation Facilities (IRFs)

1. IRFs are "designed to provide intensive rehabilitation therapies in an inpatient setting due to complexities of nursing, medical management, and rehabilitation needs" with an interdisciplinary approach to care (CMS, 2010, p. 23). This coordinated, interdisciplinary level of care is what distinguishes an IRF from other settings along the healthcare continuum.
2. IRFs are state licensed to provide an acute level of care and can provide general rehabilitation to patients with a variety of diagnoses or specialized care to a designated population, such as patients with spinal cord injury, traumatic brain injury, or stroke.
3. The scope of services may include patients of specified ages (e.g., geriatric, adult, or pediatric).
4. An IRF may be a freestanding facility or be contained and operated within an acute care hospital.
5. Care in IRFs is provided by an interprofessional team.
   a. A rehabilitation physician (typically a physiatrist) directs the rehabilitation team and provides services three or more times per week.

Table 9-1. Postacute Rehabilitation Levels of Care: Inpatient of Facility-Based Care				
	Long-Term Care Hospital (LTCH)	**Inpatient Rehabilitation Facility (IRF)**	**Skilled Nursing Facility (SNF)**	**Long-Term or Custodial Care**
Functional status	Medically complex needs that cannot be met at a lower level of care Have complex wounds *OR* Failure of 2 or more major organ systems *OR* Failed ventilator weaning after more than 3 weeks at a prior hospitalization	Patient has some degree of impairment in ADLs and mobility Cognitively able to participate in therapy Significant practical functional improvement is expected	Patient has some degree of impairment in ADLs and mobility or other skilled need Cognitively able to participate in therapy Some functional improvement is expected	Patient has some degree of mobility or ADL impairment and cannot be managed at a lower level of care Patient may or may not have cognitive deficits Patient has not reached independent level to be able to be managed at home setting Patient is no longer making progress where he or she can benefit from skilled intervention
Nursing and medical services needed	Needs ongoing acute medical management Needs 24-hour licensed nursing care	Needs ongoing acute medical management Needs 24-hour rehabilitation nursing care Needs coordinated, interdisciplinary care	Involvement of skilled nursing staff is needed to meet patient's medical needs, promote recovery, and ensure medical safety	Involvement of nursing staff does not require daily skilled nursing observation or intervention, but staff ensure that the patient's medical safety needs are met
Therapies needed	Therapy as an adjunct to medical treatment	Needs two or more therapies, one of which must be physical or occupational therapy	Needs one or more therapies *OR* Patient has daily skilled nursing need	May need therapy, but the total must be less than five times per week May benefit from Part B therapy if skilled therapy intervention is needed
Number of therapy hours needed and tolerated	No minimum hours required "Medically complex needs" is sufficient for admission	Tolerates at least 3 hours per day of therapy, 5 days per week	There is no minimum number of tolerated hours required for SNF admission; skilled need is sufficient	N/A
Discharge plan and social support	N/A	Probable discharge to community Adequate community support resources are available to meet needs based on functional prognosis	Completed psychosocial needs assessment Warm handoff completed between SNF and SNF coordinator or SNF physicians Possible discharge to community	SNF transfer must include long-term plan of care Completed psychosocial needs assessment and discussion with family regarding financial requirements Medi-Cal application completed if private funds are not available Warm handoff completed between SNF and SNF coordinator or SNF physicians

b. Nurses specializing in rehabilitation provide care 24 hours per day.
c. Physical therapists, occupational therapists, and speech–language pathologists provide treatment a minimum of 3 hours per day for 5 days per week, or a total of 15 hours per week.
d. Allied professionals: Social workers, case managers, neuropsychologists, psychologists, registered dietitians, therapeutic recreation therapists, respiratory therapists, seating and wheelchair specialists, prosthetists, orthotists, and other rehabilitation specialists provide treatment based on the patient's needs.
e. Support staff: Patient care technicians or aides, unit clerks, housekeepers, and dietary staff provide essential support to the care team. These staff members help facilitate the overall care provided to patients and families.

Table 9-2. Postacute Rehabilitation Levels of Care: Community-Based Care

	Integrated Outpatient Therapy/Day Treatment	**Home Health (HH) Care**	**Standard Outpatient Therapy**
Functional status	Patient is able to be cared for at home Needs skilled multidisciplinary intervention with potential to make significant functional improvement in ADLs, mobility, or cognition and language Able to participate in a home exercise or activity program	Patient has some degree of impairment in ADLs and mobility Completed cognitive evaluation	Patient has impairments and needs only supervision or minimal assistance with mobility or ADLs Cognitively able to participate in therapy
Nursing and medical services needed	Outpatient rehabilitation nurse, physical medicine and rehabilitation specialist, case manager, and medical social worker are part of the multidisciplinary team as needed	May need home health nursing	Referred to outpatient rehabilitation nurse, case manager, and medical social worker if needed
Therapies needed	Needs at least two therapies	Needs one or more therapies with a nurse or social worker	Needs one or more therapies
Number of therapy hours needed and tolerated	Tolerates at least 1 hour per day *OR* Patient has a skilled need and a functional goal with good rehabilitation prognosis	Tolerates at least 0.5 hour per day *OR* Patient has a skilled need and a functional goal with good rehabilitation prognosis	Tolerates at least 0.5 hour per day either in the clinic or doing at-home exercises *OR* Patient has a skilled need and a functional goal with good rehabilitation prognosis
Discharge plan and social support	Patient must have transportation to therapy location Has accessible environment at home and appropriate durable medical equipment to meet needs Has support to continue exercise or activity program at home	Patient must be able to get to and from therapy visits Has accessible environment at home and appropriate durable medical equipment Has social support to continue exercise or activity program at home	Confined to home Has accessible environment at home and appropriate durable medical equipment

Abbreviations. ADLs, activities of daily living; N/A, not applicable.

C. Skilled Nursing Facilities (SNFs)
1. SNFs often provide subacute level rehabilitation care (U.S. DHHS, 1994). Medical management in the SNF is provided by a physician with or without rehabilitation training.
2. Staffing in SNFs
    a. Physicians are required to see the patients within the first 30 days and every 30 days thereafter.
    b. Nursing specialization in rehabilitation is not required. A registered nurse is not required on site but must be available 24 hours per day, 7 days per week.
    c. Rehabilitative therapies (e.g., physical therapist, occupational therapist, and speech–language pathologist) are available, although they are provided less frequently and at a lower intensity than in the IRF.
    d. The providers in an SNF also include other disciplines, such as an activity or recreational therapist, registered dietitian, and pharmacist.
3. Long-term care is available for medical and nonmedical care for people with chronic illness or disability (CMS, 2012). This level of care helps clients meet health and personal care needs (e.g., ADLs) and can be provided at home, in community-based settings, or in SNFs for custodial residents.

D. Home Health (HH)–Based Rehabilitation Care
1. HH rehabilitation provides nursing and rehabilitation therapies in the home setting.

2. The patient may receive physical therapy (PT), occupational therapy (OT), or speech therapy (ST).
3. The intensity and frequency are lower at 0.5–1 hour per day, 1–3 days per week.
4. Nursing services are available but not necessarily specialized in rehabilitation.

E. Comprehensive Integrated Outpatient Programs
1. These integrated programs provide more intensive rehabilitative therapies in the community setting.
2. Therapy is provided at the intensity and frequency determined by the program. This ranges from 1 to 3 hours per day, 3–5 days per week.
3. To participate in this type of care, patients and their families must be able to manage care at home and travel to and from the program daily. More than one therapy is required.
4. Care management services are an integral part of comprehensive integrated outpatient programs.

F. Outpatient Therapy (OPT)
1. OPT is provided at various settings and may be a part of a specialty clinic or part of larger organizations including acute care hospitals.
2. Patients can receive PT, OT, or ST. The amount of therapy provided varies according to the care plan established between the therapist, patient, and physician.
3. The typical amount of therapy is 1 hour per day, up to 3 days per week for PAC after a joint replacement or up to 2 hours per day and up to 5 days per week for complex conditions.

VI. Postacute Settings and Patient Outcomes

A. Each level of PAC serves as a valuable component in the care continuum. However, external pressures from payers often result in selection of settings to minimize costs rather than optimize outcomes.

B. The appropriate level of care with the associated intensity of services and resources tailored to the client's needs is achieved through effective care coordination during transitions.

C. As previously noted, the amount of therapy a patient may receive varies by PAC setting.
1. Patients receive as little as 1 hour per day, 3 days per week in OPT or as much as 3 hours or more per day, 5 or more days per week in an IRF.
2. The amount of care provided is dictated by financial constraints and rules that govern the requirements for licensure and certification.

D. Outcomes vary by settings. For example, an evaluation of ventilator-dependent patients with the goal of weaning off the ventilator and returning to a community setting or lower level of care in an LTCH demonstrated that cost savings for transferring to an LTCH were more than $20,000 per patient. Also, patients transferred to an LTCH had a longer mean survival time than patients who did not receive transitional care in an LTCH (Seneff, Wagner, Thompson, Honeycutt, & Michael, 2000).

E. Another factor related to postacute transitions that may affect outcomes is the number of days it takes for a patient to begin care in a PAC setting. For example, patients who began rehabilitation at an IRF within 21 days had significantly better functional gains than patients whose PAC was delayed (Wang, Camicia, Terdiman, Hung, & Sandel, 2011) even in the most severely impaired patients.

VII. Rehabilitation Nursing

Rehabilitation nurses work in a variety of roles across the healthcare continuum to help patients achieve optimal outcomes through care management and coordination. Rehabilitation nurses use their expertise in effective communication to optimize collaboration and coordination between patients, family members, and the rehabilitation team to promote safe and timely transitions across the continuum of care (ARN, 2014b).

VIII. The Role of the Rehabilitation Nurse in Facilitating Care Transitions

According to the ARN Competency Model for professional rehabilitation nursing, the rehabilitation nurse has an essential role in promoting and facilitating safe and effective care transitions to promote health and successful living in people with disabilities or chronic illness across the lifespan (ARN, 2014a). The fulfillment of this role contributes significantly to optimal patient and family outcomes. This role transcends all other roles, practice settings, and populations served and requires optimal collaboration and coordination between clients, families, and healthcare professionals to promote the safe and timely transition across care settings.

A. Roles of the Rehabilitation Nurse
1. Staff nurse
2. Case manager
3. Clinical liaison
4. Advanced practice nurse
5. Nurse leader
6. Researcher

B. Practice Settings
1. Acute care
2. IRF
3. LTCH
4. SNF
5. HH
6. Community
7. Insurance company
8. Government agency

C. Populations
1. Pediatric

2. Adult
3. Geriatric

IX. Rehabilitation Nursing Proficiencies Related to Care Coordination and Care Transitions

According to the *ARN Staff Nurse Role Description* (ARN, 2006) and the *ARN Competency Model for Professional Rehabilitation Nursing* (ARN, 2014a), the rehabilitation nurse should possess the following competencies:

A. The rehabilitation staff nurse demonstrates, at a minimum, the beginner level proficiency for care coordination by
   1. Coordinating educational activities and use of appropriate resources to develop and implement an individualized teaching and discharge plan with clients and their families
   2. Coordinating nursing care activities in collaboration with other members of the interdisciplinary rehabilitation team to facilitate the achievement of overall goals
   3. Assessing the client and family regarding cultural values and health literacy as applicable to care transitions
   4. Participating in the development of an interprofessional plan for care transitions
   5. Contributing to the development and implementation of the goals for care transitions
   6. Participating in the care conference that evaluates the care transition plan.

B. In addition to the competencies of a beginning rehabilitation nurse, intermediate-level rehabilitation nurses must demonstrate proficiency for care coordination and facilitating care transitions by
   1. Identifying the barriers that could influence the care transitions
   2. Modifying the plan of care based on additional data collection
   3. Coordinating the resources needed for a seamless care transition
   4. Contributing to the interprofessional evaluation of the client and family care transition plan.

C. The advanced rehabilitation nurse competencies include additional proficiencies in care coordination and care transitions by
   1. Synthesizing client and family data and resources needed for a seamless care transition
   2. Coordinating the interprofessional plan for care transition
   3. Facilitating the interprofessional care transition plan
   4. Collecting program data to evaluate the client and family care transition experience for the purpose of program management and improvement.

X. Influence of the Certified Registered Rehabilitation Nurse® (CRRN®) on Resource Use

A. The CRRN is a rehabilitation or restorative nurse who has demonstrated a combination of experience and knowledge in this specialty practice area.

B. The value of the CRRN was illustrated in a multisite study by Dr. Audrey Nelson (2007), who found an inverse relationship between the number of CRRNs and length of stay in inpatient rehabilitation facilities.

XI. Other Members of the Rehabilitation Team

Rehabilitation nurses are key contributors to the care of people with chronic conditions and disability. However, rehabilitation care is provided by members of an interprofessional team who collaborate with each other and the patient and family to develop goals and objectives. This approach values all team members, with the patient and family in the center of the team. The composition of the rehabilitation team depends on the needs of the patient and the treatment setting. It is critical that patients with chronic and disabling conditions are served in a PAC setting that includes the services needed to optimize health outcomes and quality of life. Not every rehabilitation team will consist of representatives of each of these professions; rather, the makeup of the team is based on the needs of the patient and family. The members of the team include the following:

A. Patient: The patient is at the center of the rehabilitation team.

B. Family/Caregiver: The patient is joined by his or her family in the center of the rehabilitation team.

C. Physician: The rehabilitation physician (physiatrist) specializes and holds a board certification in physical medicine and rehabilitation (PM&R).

D. Physical Therapist: The physical therapist is a professional with skills in promoting optimal mobility and function.

E. Occupational Therapist: The occupational therapist works with patients who have disabling mental, physical, developmental, or emotional conditions to restore function for optimal participation in ADLs, including work, school, family, community, and leisure activities.

F. Speech–Language Pathologist: Speech–language pathology (SLP), otherwise known as a *speech therapy*, is the profession devoted to assessment, rehabilitation, counseling, and prevention services for people with some type of speech, voice, language, cognitive–communicative, or swallowing disorder.

G. Neuropsychologist: The role of neuropsychologist is to assist patients with adjusting to their new injury or disabling condition.

H. Social Worker: The role of the social worker is to provide psychosocial support to patients and their families or caregivers throughout the rehabilitation process.

I. Recreational/Activity Therapist: The role of the recreational or activity therapist is to work with the rehabilitation team to improve the patient's cognitive and physical functioning and promote social skills and constructive use of leisure time.

J. The roles of team members are further defined in Chapter 3.

XII. The Role of the Patient and Family: PAC Transitions

Transitions across care settings are a time of "heightened vulnerability" (Chugh, Williams, Grigsby, & Coleman, 2009, p. 11) for patients and confusion and uncertainty for family members. The key points of transition are between acute care and postacute levels of care and the transition to home. Transitions home can be particularly overwhelming and have been defined as a time of crisis for family caregivers, especially those who are new to the caregiver role (Lutz, Young, Cox, Martz, & Creasy, 2011).

A. Transitioning patients who qualify for rehabilitation services to the appropriate setting throughout the continuum of care is important to achieve the best possible patient outcomes (Chan et al., 2013).

1. Acute care hospitalizations are often a time of crisis for patients and their families, so cognitive decision making is often difficult.
2. The acute hospital average length of stay (ALOS) is often short (5 days), necessitating quick decisions about the next level of care.
3. Families often believe the patients' healthcare providers are the most appropriate people to make the decision about the next level of care, especially if the family is overwhelmed, is in crisis, or lacks the knowledge to make such decisions.
4. If the patient or family places a high value on the expertise of healthcare providers' knowledge about appropriate levels of care, they will rely heavily on that expertise. In many cases, when given a choice they will defer to the healthcare provider to make a recommendation. However, many healthcare providers do not have the necessary information to make decisions about the appropriate level of PAC.

B. Engagement of the patient and family in this decision making is essential, although the degree to which patients and families are involved varies.

1. Health literacy is an important consideration that is often overlooked. According to Dossa, Bokhour, and Hoenig (2012), discharge information must be legible, be in large type, and provide accurate information to patients about contact information for questions.
2. Discharge education and instruction must be thoroughly reviewed by both patients and their caregivers.
3. Patient and family engagement in decisions about care has been defined as "essential to improving quality" of care (Nursing Alliance for Quality of Care, 2013, p. 2) and is key to providing patient-centered care.
4. Rehabilitation professionals have identified the importance of including patients and their family members in the decision-making process regarding the most appropriate location for PAC.

C. Often the healthcare provider (e.g., physician, nurse, social worker, or case manager) makes the decision about the next level of care and the facility to which the patient transitions. This may depend on which facilities have space available, the healthcare provider's opinion on what the appropriate level of care is, or the provider's preference for a particular setting or institution.

D. Families and patients often indicate that they were not informed about their options or were not included in the decision-making process. When choices are provided, they often are not explained in sufficient detail for families and patients to make an informed choice (Lutz, Young, Cox, Martz, & Creasy. 2011).

XIII. The Role of the Patient and Family: Transitions from Institutionally Based Rehabilitation to Home

One of the principles of rehabilitation care is to include the patient and family members in the rehabilitation team and to integrate the patient's goals into care planning. However, in many inpatient rehabilitation programs, patients and families are not included in team conferences, where most team goal setting occurs. The common process is that a member of the rehabilitation staff talks with patients and family members to determine patients' goals, and then the staff addresses these goals during the team conferences (without patient or family present).

A. In the care of adults, patients' preferences are considered primary, and family members are often viewed as resources to help the rehabilitation team and the patient progress toward his or her goals (Lutz et al., 2011).

B. Patient preferences may outweigh family preferences. With adults there may be tension between a patient who wants autonomy and family members who want to be involved.

C. In the care of pediatric patients, the family is generally included because the child cannot provide consent, and the family is viewed as a social unit.

1. According to the American Academy of Pediatrics, "Families are the most central and enduring

influence in children's lives" (Schor & American Academy of Pediatrics Task Force on the Family, 2013, p. 1541).

2. Parents also play an integral part in pediatric care because the role of the parent is to make decisions about the child's care, so their inclusion is essential. Pediatric programs tend to be more family centered.
3. Training and education strategies for family members and patients focus on the skills family members need to provide physical care and continue the treatment plan (e.g., learning to do transfers, managing medications and therapies). The needs and preferences of the family members are seldom systematically assessed unless the family members advocate for themselves (Lutz et al., 2011).

D. "Nurses can assist older adults to achieve successful transitions of care by taking a systematic approach and individualizing care to meet patient and family health literacy, cognitive, and sensory needs" (Enderlin et al., 2013, p. 47).

E. Successful transitions are supported when a designated person is assigned to return patients' phone calls when they have questions related to their recovery (Dossa et al., 2012).

F. Home care providers need to communicate with primary care providers and other specialists regarding patient recovery and problems to improve continuity of care, and they need to ensure proper patient follow-up (Dossa et al., 2012).

G. Rehabilitation nursing is client centered. Rehabilitation nurses:

1. Understand the significance of patient and family engagement in decision making related to care transitions
2. Understand the needs of patients and their families and the resources that are available in the different levels of PAC to promote positive health outcomes
3. Possess skills to provide effective patient and family caregiver education
4. Are experts in collaborating with other professionals
5. Advocate for high-quality, cost-effective care that is of value to patients, their families, and the greater society.

XIV. Care Transition Models

Several evidence-based care transition models have been successfully implemented for patients transitioning from acute care to home. For example, Naylor and colleagues (1994, 2004) have conducted several randomized controlled trials testing an advanced practice nursing transitional care intervention for patients with congestive heart failure and chronic obstructive pulmonary disease and in general geriatric populations. These trials have demonstrated that the intervention improves patient outcomes and reduces costs (Naylor et al., 1994, 2004). Coleman and colleagues (2006) have tested a transitional care intervention that uses "coaches" who work with patients after an acute hospital stay. The coaches meet with the patients before discharge, make one home visit, and conduct one to three follow-up phone calls in the first 30 days after discharge (Coleman, 2003; Coleman, Parry, Chalmers, & Min, 2006). By facilitating care coordination and postdischarge care management, these interventions have shown promise in reducing costs and improving patient outcomes. However, there is almost no evidence related to transitional care interventions for patients in need of PAC. Studies are needed to test interventions to assist patients with functional limitations and their family members as they transition through the care continuum.

XV. Discussion

Care transitions to PAC settings for people with disabling conditions are often ineffective and inefficient. The patient and family are often overwhelmed and unable to process information. They do not have the necessary information and support to participate in decisions about care transitions to PAC. Furthermore, providers and other stakeholders involved in PAC decisions are often guided more by geographic proximity or formal relationships with the PAC settings, and they do not have a clear understanding of the different levels of PAC and associated patient outcomes. Clinicians involved in PAC transitions for people with chronic disease and disabling conditions must be client centered, goal oriented, and outcome based. They must understand the available levels of PAC and roles of other professionals and how each role determines long-term success in the patient's care.

Through specialty certification (CRRN) or experience in rehabilitation nursing, nurses can obtain this knowledge and skill. It is the role of the rehabilitation nurse to advocate on behalf of patients, understand the scientific basis for healthcare decisions, and partner with patients and families to integrate their preferences into healthcare decisions. Rehabilitation nurses have the skills and expertise to integrate the preferences of patients with complex medical and psychosocial conditions with relevant evidence to facilitate successful care coordination and care transitions (ARN, 2006).

XVI. Conclusion

The rehabilitation nurse has the training, knowledge, and experience to effectively coordinate, support, and oversee the transitions of care across the continuum to promote high-quality outcomes and cost-effective care for people with disabling conditions. The role of rehabilitation nurses in care transitions for people with disabling conditions can be summarized as follows:

A. Practice
   1. Rehabilitation nurses have the training, knowledge, and experience to effectively facilitate appropriate care transitions for people with disabling conditions.
   2. The rehabilitation nurse educates and informs families about options and services available, evaluating and summarizing scientific evidence and applying it in meaningful ways so families can make informed decisions about care transitions.

B. Policy
   1. Rehabilitation nurses should be actively involved in national policy decisions to ensure that cost-cutting measures do not compromise the quality of patient care in the United States.
   2. Greater use of rehabilitation nurses in policy making may facilitate balancing cost efficiency and healthcare quality.

C. Research
   1. Studies are needed to evaluate the impact of rehabilitation nurses on the healthcare delivery system.
   2. Studies are needed on the effectiveness of rehabilitation nursing interventions in planning and implementing care transitions with a focus on improving functional status, community reintegration, and health-related outcomes.

D. Education
   1. ARN's *Standards and Scope of Rehabilitation Nursing Practice* (2014) and the ARN white paper "The Essential Role of the Rehabilitation Nurse in Facilitating Care Transitions" (Camicia et al., 2014) should be foundational documents for discharge planning education related to care transitions for people with disabling conditions.

References

Agency for Healthcare Research and Quality (AHRQ). (2013). *Outpatient case management for adults with medical illness and complex care needs.* Washington, DC: Author. Retrieved from www.ahrq.gov

American Hospital Association (AHA). (2013). *Trendwatch chartbook. Trends affecting hospitals and health systems.* Washington, DC: Author. Retrieved from http://www.aha.org/research/reports/tw/chartbook/2013/13chartbook-full.pdf

Association of Rehabilitation Nurses (ARN). (2006). *Staff nurse role description.* Glenview, IL: Author. Retrieved from http://www.rehabnurse.org/uploads/files/uploads/File/rdstaffnurse11.pdf

Association of Rehabilitation Nurses (ARN). (2010). *Rehabilitation: The rehabilitation nurse case manager role description.* Glenview, IL: Author. Retrieved from http://www.rehabnurse.org/uploads/files/uploads/File/rdcasemgmt11.pdf

Association of Rehabilitation Nurses (ARN). (2014a). ARN competency model for professional rehabilitation nursing. Retrieved from http://www.rehabnurse.org/uploads/files/education/ARN_Rehabilitation_Nursing_Competency _Model_FINAL_-_May_2014.pdf

Association of Rehabilitation Nurses (ARN). (2014b). *Standards and scope of rehabilitation nursing practice.* Chicago: Author.

Camicia, M., Black, T., Farrell, J., Waites, K., Wirt, S., Lutz, B., and the Association of Rehabilitation Nurses. (2014). The essential role of the rehabilitation nurse in facilitating care transitions: A white paper by the Association of Rehabilitation Nurses. *Rehabilitation Nursing, 39*(1), 1–13. Retrieved from http://onlinelibrary.wiley.com/doi/10.1002/rnj.135/pdf

Camicia, M., Chamberlain, B., Finnie, R., Nalle, M., Lindeke, L., Lorenz, L., . . . Cisco, M. (2013). The value of nursing care coordination: A white paper of the American Nurses Association. *Nursing Outlook, 61*(6), 490–501.

Centers for Medicare & Medicaid Services (CMS). (2010). *Medicare benefit policy manual.* Washington, DC: Author. Retrieved from http://www.cms.gov/Regulations-and-guidance/Guidance/Manuals/downloads/bp102c01.pdf

Centers for Medicare & Medicaid Services (CMS). (2012). *What is long-term care?* Washington, DC: Author. Retrieved from http://www.medicare.gov/longtermcare/static/home.asp

Centers for Medicare & Medicaid Services (CMS). (2013). *Revisions to state operations manual (SOM), hospital appendix A: Interpretive guidelines for 42 CFR 482.43, discharge planning.* Washington, DC: Author. Retrieved from http://www.cms.gov/Medicare/Provider-Enrollment-and-Certification/SurveyCertificationGenInfo/Downloads/Survey-and-Cert-Letter-13-32.pdf

Chan, L., Sandel, E. M., Jette, A. M., Appelman, J., Brandt, D. E., Cheng, P., . . . Rasch, E. K. (2013). Does post acute care site matter? A longitudinal study assessing functional recovery after a stroke. *Archives of Physical Medicine and Rehabilitation, 94*(4), 622–629.

Chugh, A., Williams, M. V., Grigsby, J., & Coleman, E. A. (2009). Better transitions: Improving comprehension of discharge instructions. *Frontiers of Health Services Management, 25*(3), 11–32.

Coleman, E. (n.d.). *The Care Transitions Program® health care services for improving quality and safety during care hand-offs.* Denver, CO: The Care Transitions Program. Retrieved from http://www.caretransitions.org/definitions.asp

Coleman, E. A. (2003). Falling through the cracks: Challenges and opportunities for improving transitional care for persons with continuous complex care needs. *Journal of the American Geriatrics Society, 51*(4), 549–555.

Coleman, E. A., Parry, C., Chalmers, S., & Min, S. J. (2006). The Care Transitions Intervention: Results of a randomized controlled trial. *Archives of Internal Medicine, 166,* 1822–1828.

Congressional Research Service (CRS). (2010). *Medicare hospital readmissions: Issues, policy options and PPACA.* Washington, DC: Author. Retrieved from www.crs.gov

Dossa, A., Bokhour, B., & Hoenig, H. (2012). Care transitions from the hospital to home for patients with mobility impairments: Patient and family caregiver experiences. *Rehabilitation Nursing, 37*(6), 277–285. doi:10.1002/rnj.047

Enderlin, C. A., McLeskey, N., Rooker, J. L., Steinhauser, C., D'Avolio, D., Gusewelle, R., & Ennen, K. A. (2013). Review of current conceptual models and frameworks to guide transitions of care in older adults. *Geriatric Nursing, 34*(1), 47–52. doi:10.1016/j.gerinurse.2012.08.003

Gage, B. (2009). *Post-acute care: Moving beyond the silos* [PowerPoint slides]. Raleigh, NC: RTI. Retrieved from www.RTI.org

Grobowski, D. C., Huckfeldt, P. J., Sood, N., Escarce, J. J., & Newhouse, J. P. (2012). Medicare post-acute care payment reforms have potential to improve efficiency of care, but may need changes to cut costs. *Health Affairs, 31*(9), 1941–1950. doi:10.1377/hlthaff.2012.0351

Huang, H. T., Chang, C. M., Liu, L. F., Lin, H. S., & Chen, C. H. (2013). Trajectories and predictors of functional decline of hospitalized older patients. *Journal of Clinical Nursing, 22*(9–10), 1322–1331. doi:10.1111/jocn.12055

Larsen, P. (2011). The environment for rehabilitation nursing. In C. Jacelon (Ed.), *The specialty practice of rehabilitation nursing: A core curriculum* (6th ed., pp. 507–511). Glenview, IL: Association of Rehabilitation Nurses.

Lutz, B. J., Young, M. E., Cox, K. J., Martz, C., & Creasy, K. R. (2011). The crisis of stroke: Experiences of patients and their family caregivers. *Topics in Stroke Rehabilitation, 18*(6), 786–797. doi:10.1310/tsr1806-786

Medicare Payment Advisory Commission (MedPAC). (2011). *Report to the Congress.* Washington, DC: Author. Retrieved from http://medpac.gov

Medicare Payment Advisory Commission (MedPAC). (2013). *Report to the Congress.* Washington, DC: Author. Retrieved from http://medpac.gov

National Cancer Institute (NCI). (2013). *NCI dictionary of cancer terms.* Washington, DC: Author. Retrieved from www.cancer.gov/dictionary

National Quality Forum (NQF). (2010). *Preferred practices and performance measures for measuring and reporting care coordination: A consensus report.* Washington, DC: Author. Retrieved from http://www.qualityforum.org/Publications/2010/Preferred_Practices_and_Performance_Measures_for_Measuring_and_Reporting_Care_Coordination.aspx

Naylor, M. D., Brooten, D. A., Campbell, R. L., Maislin, G., McCauley, K. M., & Schwartz, J. S. (2004). Transitional care of older adults hospitalized with heart failure: A randomized, controlled trial. *Journal of the American Geriatric Society, 52,* 675–684.

Naylor, M. D., Brooten, D., Jones, R., Lavizzo-Mourey, R., Mezey, M., & Pauly, M. (1994). Comprehensive discharge planning for the hospitalized elderly. *Annals of Internal Medicine, 20*, 999–1006.

Nelson, A. (2007). Nurse staffing and patient outcomes in inpatient rehabilitative settings. *Rehabilitation Nursing, 32*(5), 179–202.

Nursing Alliance for Quality of Care (NAQC). (2013). *Fostering successful patient and family engagement.* Washington, DC: Author. Retrieved from www.naqc.org/Main/Resources/Publications/March2013-FosteringSuccessfulPatientFamilyEngagement.pdf

Sandel, E. M., Wang, H., Terdiman, J., Hoffman, J. M., Ciol, M. A., Sidney, S., . . . Chan, L. (2009). Disparities in stroke rehabilitation: Results of a study in an integrated health system in northern California. *PM&R, 1*(1), 29–40. doi:10.1016/j.pmrj.2008.10.012

Schor, E. L., & American Academy of Pediatrics Task Force on the Family. (2003). Family pediatrics: Report of the Task Force on the Family. *Pediatrics, 111*(6 Pt 2), 1541–1571.

Seneff, M. G., Wagner, D., Thompson, D., Honeycutt, C., & Michael, R. (2000). The impact of long-term acute-care facilities on the outcome and cost of care for patients undergoing prolonged mechanical ventilation. *Critical Care Medicine, 28*(2), 342–350.

Tilson, S., & Hoffman, G. J. (2012). *Addressing Medicare hospital readmissions. CRS Report for Congress Congressional Research Service (CRS).* Washington, DC: Congressional Research Service. Retrieved from http://op.bna.com/hl.nsf/id/bbrk-8url4c/$File/CRSMedicareReadmission.pdf

U.S. Department of Health and Human Services (U.S. DHHS). (1994). *Sub-acute care: Review of the literature.* Washington, DC: Author. Retrieved from http://aspe.hhs.gov/daltcp/reports/scltrves.htm#intro

U.S. Department of Health and Human Services (U.S. DHHS). (2012). *National strategy for quality improvement in health care.* Washington, DC: Author. Retrieved from www.ahrq.gov/workingforquality/nqs/nqs2012annlrpt.pdf

U.S. Department of Health and Human Services (U.S. DHHS) Centers for Medicare and Medicaid Services (CMS). (2013). *CMS manual system, revised Appendix A, interpretive guidelines for hospitals, condition of participation: Discharge planning.* Pub. 100-07. Washington, DC: Author. Retrieved from www.cms.gov/Regulations-and-Guidance/Guidance/Transmittals/Downloads/R87SOMA.pdf

Wang, H., Camicia, M., Terdiman, J., Hung, Y. Y., & Sandel, E. (2011). Time to inpatient rehabilitation hospital admission and functional outcomes of stroke patients. *PM&R, 3*(4), 296–304.

Chapter 10

Rehabilitation Nursing and Case Management

Donna Williams, MSN RN CRRN
Kathryn Doeschot, MSN RN CRRN

LEARNING OUTCOMES

- Define case management.
- Describe the role of the rehabilitation nurse case manager.
- Outline the scope of practice of the rehabilitation nurse case manager.

KEY CHAPTER TOPICS

- Historical perspectives on case management
- Standards of practice
- Goals of case management
- Models of case management
- Role functions and processes
- Certification
- Accreditation and regulation
- Life care planning
- Implications for practice

PROFESSIONAL REHABILITATION NURSING DOMAINS AND COMPETENCIES

- Domain 1: Competencies 1.3, 1.4
- Domain 2: Competencies 2.1, 2.2, 2.3
- Domain 3: Competency 3.4
- Domain 4: Competencies 4.1, 4.2, 4.3 (Association of Rehabilitation Nurses [ARN], 2014)

Introduction

Case management, an integral part of models of care delivery, has been shown to be a key strategy and innovative approach to managing healthcare services and improving client care. Case management is comprehensive, client centered, and promotes continuity of care across all settings. Our rapidly changing healthcare system demands financial and clinical outcomes within an appropriate time frame and with appropriate use of resources. Case management provides a framework for assessing, planning, implementing, and evaluating care, and is an effective process for working in the increasingly complex, fragmented, and constrained system of healthcare delivery. The practices of case managers and life care planners exemplify the four domains of the rehabilitation nursing professional role outlined in the *ARN Competency Model for Rehabilitation Nursing* (ARN, 2014).

The objectives of this chapter are to define case management, describe the role of the nurse case manager, and explore the scope of case management. Models, functions, and the processes that affect the quality and cost-effectiveness of healthcare services will be identified. The rehabilitation nurse is in a unique position to serve as a case manager because of his or her specialized knowledge, experience, and holistic approach.

I. Historical Perspectives on Case Management

A. Early 1900s: Social and Legislative Changes

1. 1920: The Smith-Fess Act, the first public rehabilitation program, provided funds for vocational guidance, training, occupational adjustment, prosthetics, and placement services.
2. 1943: The Vocational Rehabilitation Act updated the Smith-Fess Act and included physical restoration and services to people with mental and psychiatric disabilities. It required states to submit a written state care plan to the federal government.
3. 1945: Liberty Mutual hired nurses to coordinate care for insured patients.
4. 1965: The Vocational Rehabilitation Act amendments placed an emphasis on the workplace.
5. 1965: Medicare and Medicaid were established and required discharge planning.
6. 1970s: The Insurance Company of North America became the first private-sector rehabilitation company.
7. 1973: Public awareness of the needs of disabled people increased, and the

Vocational Rehabilitation Act was renamed the Rehabilitation Act, the foundation for the subsequent Americans with Disabilities Act. The Individual Written Rehabilitation Program amendment ensured the involvement of the consumer in developing a rehabilitation plan of action.

B. Insurance Industry
   1. 1970: Nurses and vocational rehabilitation counselors coordinated care and created long-term plans for people with disabilities.
   2. 1970s: Entrepreneurs began independent practice, mostly for workers' compensation.
   3. 1993: Boston Consulting Group coined the term *disease management,* an approach to managing specific diseases and client populations.

C. Facility-Based Case Management
   1. 1980s: Case management was developed in facilities to avoid duplication of services, evaluate care, and contain costs while improving the effectiveness of care (Cohen & Cesta, 2005).
   2. Roots in primary nursing

D. Government Case Management Programs
   1. 1973: The Health Maintenance Organization Act focused on prevention, wellness, and case management of costs.
   2. 1983: The Social Security Act, amended to include diagnosis-related groups (DRGs), propelled case management into acute settings as hospitals received reimbursement in the form of a fixed DRG-specific amount for each client treated.
   3. 1980s: The Department of Veterans Affairs and TRICARE, health insurance for military dependents and retirees, established the use of case management to optimize services and achieve high-quality care.
   4. 1990s: The Joint Commission, Commission on Accreditation of Rehabilitation Facilities (CARF), and the American Health Care Commission/Utilization Review Accreditation Commission all developed standards and processes regarding discharge planning and case management.

II. Definitions of Case Management

A. ARN's Definition: "the process of assessing, planning, organizing, coordinating, implementing, monitoring, and evaluating the services and resources needed to respond to a person's healthcare needs" (ARN, 2010).

B. Case Management Society of America's (CMSA's) Definition: "a collaborative process of assessment, planning, facilitation, care coordination, evaluation, and advocacy for options and services that meet an individual's and family's comprehensive health needs through communication and available resources to promote high-quality, cost-effective outcomes" (CMSA, 2010).

C. American Nurses Association's (ANA's) Definition: "a dynamic and systematic collaborative approach to provide and coordinate healthcare services to a defined population. It is a participative process to identify and facilitate options and services for meeting people's health needs while decreasing fragmentation and duplication of care and improving cost-effective clinical outcomes. The framework for nursing case management includes five essential functions: assessment, planning, implementation, evaluation, and interaction" (ANA, 2007).

III. Standards of Practice

A. ARN: Standards were developed in 1994 and updated in 2008 and 2014. Rehabilitation nursing is viewed as a specialty practice guided by philosophy, theory, and research.
   1. Scope of practice
   2. Standards of care
   3. Standards of professional performance
   4. Case manager role description

B. CMSA: Standards were developed in 1995 and updated in 2010. Standards provide a parameter for knowledge, skill, behavior, and practice.
   1. Voluntary practice guidelines
   2. Define practice settings, roles, and functions
   3. Identify standards and how they are demonstrated
   4. Encourage use of evidence-based practice

C. ANA: *Nursing: Scope And Standards of Practice,* updated in 2010, articulated the "who, what, when, where, and how" of practice. The *Code of Ethics for Nurses,* updated in 2010, established guidelines for carrying out nursing responsibilities in a manner consistent with quality in nursing care and the ethical obligations of the profession (visit www.nursingworld.org) (ANA, 2010).

D. International Academy of Life Care Planners (IALCP): Standards of practice for this subspecialty role were developed in 2002 and revised in 2006 and 2014.
   1. Standards of practice
   2. Philosophical overview and goals
   3. Roles and functions
   4. Standards of performance

IV. Goals of Case Management

A. The goal of case management is the provision of high-quality, cost-effective health and social services. The nurse case manager realizes this goal by organizing rehabilitation and other necessary healthcare services to promote outcomes that will encourage the highest possible level of independence and quality of life for the client (ARN, 2010).

1. Improve quality through appropriate and timely use of services and resources
   a. Meets expected outcomes and promotes optimal functioning and independence in the least restrictive environment
   b. Reduces risk of complications by facilitating communication between team members and ensuring that needed services are provided in a timely manner
   c. Improves coping with injury, illness, or disability
   d. Facilitates successful return to work, school, and community by identifying and including all appropriate team members
2. Facilitate outcomes of case management
   a. Coordinates care by ensuring access to healthcare services and monitoring all health care provided to the client
   b. Promotes collaborative practice through ongoing communication with the identified team in each practice setting along the continuum
   c. Educates or promotes the education of clients in relation to their health status and prevention of complications or further disability. Emphasis is placed on self-management and responsibility for healthcare needs.
   d. Advocates for the client's optimal functioning and independence in the community by providing the tools necessary to achieve that level of functioning

V. Models of Case Management

A. Models of case management can be determined by a number of factors. A facility or company can determine its own model or process for how case management is completed. Case management is determined in part by the setting, and factors that can include whether the case management is episodic or is needed for a specific illness, injury, disease, or event.

1. Setting: Case management services are provided in institutional, residential, outpatient, and community settings. These settings can include acute-care facilities, rehabilitation facilities, outpatient facilities, skilled nursing facilities or nursing homes, residential facilities, day-care agencies, private residences, or the workplace.
2. Employment: Case managers can be employees, contractors, or private practitioners. Many organizations develop their individual model, or process, of case management.
   a. *Facility- or agency-based case manager:* A case manager employed by a healthcare facility, government or private agency, or healthcare provider. This case manager is responsible for quality and cost-effectiveness of care delivery from admission to discharge. Research has shown that case management promotes organizational success by reducing length of stay and improving reimbursement.
   b. *Insurance-based case manager:* A case manager employed by a third-party payer (e.g., an insurance company)
      1) The case manager could be responsible for managing acute or chronic disease or incident-based injury or illness. In disease management, specific diseases are managed along the continuum, and aggressive prevention of complications and treatment of chronic conditions is promoted.
      2) In workers' compensation, the case manager is responsible for coordinating the medical care with a goal of return to work, and the file can close after return to work or at the time of settlement.
   c. *Employer-based case manager:* A case manager retained by an employer to provide case management services directly to employees
      1) The case manager could be involved in cases of industrial illness or injury.
      2) The case manager could be responsible for coordinating medical benefits provided by the employer and for promoting wellness.
   d. *Independent case manager:* A private case manager whose services are retained by a third-party payer, facility, attorney, agency, or individual or family. Responsibilities can include all those of other case manager types, depending on the referral source.

VI. Role Functions and Processes

A. Client Identification

1. Early identification of clients who would benefit from case management is essential to successful achievement of outcomes and should occur at the onset of injury or diagnosis of chronic illness. Clients of all ages are served by rehabilitation nurse case managers. In assigning a nurse case manager, consideration should be given to the client's age, diagnosis, and severity of the illness or injury, because specialized knowledge can be an important factor in achieving goals.
2. Facility-based case managers, inpatient and outpatient, typically serve all admitted clients and initiate services upon admission.
3. External case managers can receive referrals from insurance carriers; other third-party payers; attorneys; physicians; or concerned parties such as family members, agencies, or protective services.

Individual clients can also self-identify and self-refer. Case managers can help referral sources establish appropriate criteria for identifying those who would benefit from case management.

4. Insurance case managers can identify potential recipients of case management with diagnoses of chronic disease or catastrophic injury. Insurance companies often establish triggers for case management referral, such as high-dollar cases, excessive or inappropriate use of resources, or presence of comorbidities.

B. Data Collection and Assessment

1. Obtains all necessary authorizations to contact the client and family for an initial interview and assessment
2. Reviews and analyzes referral information in consultation with the client, health team members, employers, family, legal representatives, and claims and insurance personnel as indicated
3. Reviews and assesses the client's personal, social, economic, and environmental information and medical history; current status; diagnosis; prognosis; current treatment plan; and care provider's level of knowledge. For catastrophic injuries or illness, an onsite assessment of the client and anticipated or actual provider is highly recommended to determine whether the provider will be able to meet the client's needs.
4. Assesses the client's learning needs related to the medical diagnosis and prognosis, treatment providers, treatment options, financial resources (including specifics of insurance coverage), psychosocial adjustment and coping mechanisms, and vocational rehabilitation needs and potential
5. Assesses the family's knowledge, health status, expectations, and the potential for or actuality of a family member acting as the primary caregiver if necessary
6. Identifies the team members appropriate for each client

C. Data Analysis and Problem Identification

1. Identifies temporary or permanent alterations in function that have resulted from the injury or illness
2. Identifies potential challenges or complications of physiological or psychosocial function
3. Identifies potential challenges in community reintegration when appropriate
4. Identifies the learning needs of the client and significant others
5. Considers the vocational and historical prognosis for entering or reentering the workforce when appropriate

Figure 10-1. Case Management Variables in Achieving Optimal Outcomes

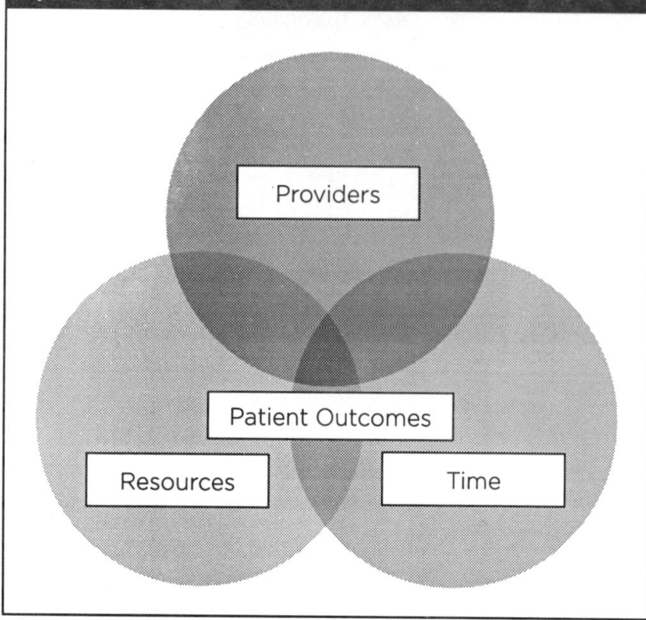

D. Establishment of Goals and Plan of Care

1. Establishes realistic goals to achieve optimal outcomes for the client within available resources; this is done in collaboration with the client and family and the interdisciplinary team
2. Helps the client, family, and team identify the variables that could influence the accomplishment of goals (**Figure 10-1**)
3. Develops a comprehensive plan that includes short- and long-term goals and preventive treatment measures for potential complications and health maintenance; identifies alternatives for the client's treatment when appropriate, including consideration of options of treatment site and potential use of resources, both private and public
4. Establishes target dates for achievement of goals
5. Includes evidence-based practice

E. Implementation and Coordination

1. Uses rehabilitation principles to plan an individualized program for maximizing function to promote identification of optimal outcomes for the client
2. Provides ongoing assessment of the progress of the client and the participation and educational needs of the client, family, and caregivers to evaluate the effectiveness of the treatment plan
3. Coordinates access to accelerated or alternative care options when appropriate
4. Coordinates access to appropriate government and community programs and resources
5. Coordinates and evaluates in a quality-conscious, cost-effective manner the client and family's use

of medical equipment, supplies, medications, and the full spectrum of services

6. Provides instruction to the client and family based on identified learning needs
7. Coordinates referrals for instruction or counseling for the client and family based on identified learning needs
8. Provides education, guidance, and recommendations to the payer about alternatives for care and services when appropriate
9. Intervenes promptly when necessary to promote optimal functioning and prevention or treatment of complications
10. Facilitates and collaborates with the healthcare team for timely discharge planning to an alternative level of care or return to the community when appropriate
11. Coordinates the discharge plan with the healthcare team and providers
12. Educates the client and family on care options and choices, allowing informed decisions even when the decisions are suboptimal or different from the case manager's recommendations

F. Monitoring

1. Ongoing assessment to promote awareness of potential or real complications and the need for plan revision
2. Adherence to the plan
3. Achievement of benchmarks

G. Evaluation

1. Goals and outcomes are monitored continuously.
2. Progress toward goals is evaluated and modified if necessary.

H. Quality Management

1. *Quality measurement* is a method for assessing how the case manager changes the structure and process of care, and identifying which clinical, administrative, physiological, and client outcomes are influenced by those changes. The goal is to ensure that case management activities are effective and efficient.

I. Outcomes

1. *Outcomes measurement* is a systematic method of assessing the extent to which a program has achieved its intended result and provides professionals with feedback that helps them ensure goal achievement. Measurements can vary depending on the information sought, but a standard tool that includes treatment trends, history, clinical decisions, and results of treatment allows review or alternative options for the treatment plan.
2. Categories of outcomes measurement include physiological, psychosocial, functional, behavioral, knowledge, home functioning, family strain, safety, symptom control, quality of life, goal attainment, client satisfaction, use of services, and nursing diagnosis resolution (Cohen & Cesta, 2005). Case management practitioners can apply these categories to clarify and specify the results of intervention for individuals and groups.

J. Cost Management

1. The case manager's role in cost management depends on the setting, expected function, and situation. Case managers can recommend and arrange for the purchase of services and supplies and negotiate and coordinate care and services, so that resources are used effectively. This provides an opportunity for creativity and development of nontraditional options to meet individual client needs.

VII. Certification

A. Certified Rehabilitation Registered Nurse (CRRN®): First offered in 1984 by ARN; requires 2 years of experience as a registered nurse in rehabilitation nursing

B. Certified Case Manager (CCM): First offered in 1993 by the Commission for Case Manager Certification; requires licensure in professional health care and 2 years of experience in case management

C. Nursing Case Management (registered nurse–board certified): First offered in 1998 by the American Nurses Credentialing Center (ANCC). Focused on facility-based practice, the application criteria include licensure as a registered nurse with a minimum of 2 years' full-time work and 2,000 hours of practice.

VII. Accreditation and Regulation

A. In 1996, The Joint Commission determined measures for meeting discharge planning criteria, including documentation of a formal plan of care with expected client outcomes. Case managers can be assigned the responsibility of discharge planning.

B. The Commission on Accreditation of Rehabilitation Facilities (CARF) developed standards for medical rehabilitation case management that were implemented July 1, 1999. CARF believes that case management is an integral part of rehabilitation care. Coordination, communication, and advocacy are primary themes in the CARF standards.

C. The American Health Care Commission/Utilization Review Accreditation Commission developed a process in 1998 to accredit case management programs in organizations including hospitals, health maintenance organizations, preferred provider organizations, and third-party administrators that promote innovation and best practice in the case management industry.

IX. Life Care Plans

A. Life care plans were introduced into rehabilitation and the legal literature in 1981 as part of a rehabilitation evaluation to project the impact of catastrophic injury on a person's future. A life care plan was distinguished from a discharge plan by its projection of costs of medical and associated care over a person's lifetime. The life care planner can be a nurse, case manager, counselor, physician, or other allied health professional. The case manager can also be involved in overseeing the implementation of the plan.

1. Definition of life care plan
   a. The IALCP defined *life care plan* as a dynamic document based on published standards of practice, comprehensive assessment, data analysis, and research. It provides an organized, concise plan for current and future needs with associated costs for people who have sustained catastrophic injury or have ongoing healthcare needs (IALCP, 2006).
   b. Uses of life care plans
      1) Identification of future care needs and costs for attorneys working on personal injury cases, child custody and family law cases, death benefits cases, and other cases requiring analysis of future care needs and costs
      2) Identification of potential costs ("reserves") for insurance or reinsurance companies to specify damages resulting from injury
      3) Guidance of case management activities for catastrophic injuries and illnesses
      4) Tool for clients of any age and their families to anticipate and self-monitor care
      5) Tool for tracking expenditures from group healthcare plans and special needs trusts in catastrophic injury or illness
   c. Principles of life care planning
      1) Must be consistent with the clinical needs of the client and should reflect strategies to minimize potential complications
      2) Must include healthcare needs (e.g., evaluations, treatment, medications, supplies, equipment, and attendant or nursing care) and quality-of-life needs (e.g., recreation, housing, transportation)
      3) Must consist of comprehensive plans prepared by assessment of all medical records and other data that might affect the plan (e.g., school and employment records); interview or observation of the client and care provider; and collaboration with treating professionals
   d. Training programs
      1) Available online or through onsite classes and generally consist of about 120 hours of content
   e. Certifications
      1) Certified life care planner (CLCP): Administered through the International Commission on Health Care Certification
      2) Certified nurse life care planner (CNLCP): Offered through the American Association of Nurse Life Care Planners
2. Medicare Set-Asides: Regulated by the Centers for Medicare & Medicaid Services (CMS)
   a. Until 1980, Medicare was the primary payer for all beneficiaries except those involving workers' compensation (WC) (including black lung benefits) or for care funded by another government entity. Medicare secondary payer provisions and subsequent amendments enabled Medicare to be the secondary payer to a primary payer or insurance plan; group health plan insurance in specific circumstances, including workers' compensation, medical malpractice/personal injury liability cases, automotive injury accident, or illness.
   b. The Workers' Compensation Medicare Set-Aside Arrangement (WCMSA) allocates a portion of the workers' compensation settlement for payment of all future work-injury–related medical expenses that are covered and otherwise reimbursable by Medicare.
   c. The goal of WCMSA is to accurately estimate the total cost of all medical expenses otherwise reimbursable by Medicare for work-related conditions for the claimant's lifetime, and to set aside sufficient funds from the settlement, judgment, or award to cover that cost.
   d. CMS will review the proposed WCMSA amount if the claimant is a Medicare beneficiary and the total settlement amount is greater than $25,000—OR—the claimant has reasonable expectation for Medicare enrollment within 30 months of the settlement date, and the anticipated total settlement amount for future medical expenses and disability/lost wages over a lifetime or the duration of settlement agreement is expected to be greater than $250,000.
   e. After the CMS-approved WCMSA amount has been exhausted and accurately accounted for and reported to CMS, Medicare will pay as the primary source for future Medicare-covered expenses related to the WC injury that exceed the approved set-aside amount (CMS, 2014).

f. Case managers and life care planners can be involved in the preparation of a WCMSA.
g. Certifications
   1) Medicare Set-Aside Consultant Certified (MSCC): Administered through the International Commission on Health Care Certification
   2) Certificate training programs are available online and onsite.

X. Advanced Practice

A. ANA has recognized advanced practice as a specialization that involves an expansion of practice and knowledge and a graduate-level course of study. However, an active dialogue is ongoing between ANA and advanced practice nurses about the definition of the term *advanced practice nurse*. At this time, ANA does not recognize case managers as advanced practice nurses. Nurses with master's degrees, certified and noncertified, who work in the field of case management can have expanded responsibilities in that arena as their education takes their practice to an advanced level. It is recognized that these nurses conduct comprehensive assessments, function autonomously, have advanced skill in leadership and education, and demonstrate expert skill in the diagnosis and treatment of complex responses to actual or potential health problems caused by an altered functional ability and altered lifestyle secondary to a physical disability or chronic illness.

B. Expanded Nurse Case Manager Functions
   1. Clinician: Uses advanced assessment skills to determine healthcare needs, establish the plan of care, and monitor the progress and outcomes
   2. Educator: Provides information about the plan of care to team members and information on the diagnosis and plan of care to the client
   3. Manager: Manages, assigns, and delegates tasks to team members in a cost-effective manner; organizes appropriate treatments
   4. Consultant: Addresses factors that affect outcomes, ensures quality of care, and acts as a resource
   5. Collaborates with physicians and other healthcare professionals using effective communication styles
   6. Develops and coordinates the plan of care throughout the continuum of care
   7. Researcher: Redesigns plans of care based on outcomes and evidence-based practice and monitors the quality of each plan
   8. Fiscal responsibility: Is familiar with the pertinent financial, regulatory, and accreditation issues in the setting in which practice occurs

XI. Issues

A. Multistate Licensure
   1. Nurse licensure rules and regulations initially were formed when nursing was practiced primarily within the boundaries of one state and usually within a facility or agency. As access to health care, the mobility of the population, and coverage by insurance companies change, nurses could find themselves providing services to clients who travel or live across multiple state lines. Many state nursing licenses are not recognized by other states. This is problematic for case managers who provide telephonic services across state lines or onsite services that can cross state lines for border areas. The following are issues for case managers in multistate practice:
   2. There can be additional costs for licensure.
   3. Nurses without malpractice insurance can be more vulnerable. This can affect the employer as well.
   4. As of June 2010, 24 state boards of nursing have joined to form a nurse compact, in which states mutually recognize nurse licenses from other states.
   5. A CMSA position paper revised in 2006 addressed the issue and can be found at www.CMSA.org.

B. Education and Certification
   1. The process of case management continues to develop as healthcare systems change, definitions are refined, job functions evolve, and the needs of the consumer and payer increase. Requirements for basic education and continued education will continue to change. Confusion about eligibility for the roles and certification must be addressed, because the trend is moving toward increasing legislation, rules, and regulations in case management practice (Huber, 2006).

XII. Implications for Practice

A. Leadership
   1. Case managers are in a prime leadership position. The case manager assumes responsibility for communication, collaboration, negotiation, and resolution of conflict between team members while identifying and coordinating the treatment plan. Conflict can arise from difficulty in fulfilling the plan because of economic, time, or other resource limitations or lack of client or family understanding. In complex cases, multiple providers can be treating a client and each could be unaware of the concurrent work of the other providers. The case manager can be instrumental in identifying all current providers, establishing communication

between them, and leading them through the process of coordinated care.

2. Review of leadership theory and processes can be useful to a nurse seeking a case management position.

B. Potential Ethical Conflicts in Case Management

1. Interdisciplinary teamwork involves collaboration, typically through team meetings. Members work together and share resources to arrive at a decision or position that balances ethical and cost concerns. Through this synergistic process, the team model provides support, expertise, and guidance that would not otherwise be available to individual professionals. Many managed care organizations are structured to allow this type of professional interaction.
2. Characteristics of case management that can present barriers to ethically appropriate care
   a. Accountability for cost of care: When a physician or medical center is held financially accountable for a client's costs of care, the client-physician relationship can be significantly affected by attempts to contain costs at the expense of the client's health and wellbeing. The case manager could feel pressure to prioritize financial goals above care outcome goals.
   b. Proactive care planning: Consideration must be given to future needs. Professionals could be conflicted between their loyalty and commitment to provide necessary care and the need to promote individual autonomy or respect of the client's right to self-determination.
   c. Outpatient services: Such services, whether provided in the clinic or home, help to avoid more costly hospitalizations. Comprehensive assessments must be completed to ensure that care plan recommendations are practical and within the ability of the client and family to perform. Conflict can arise if disagreement exists about the ability to participate in a home or clinic setting.
   d. Interventions for the general population: Most managed care plans exclude inefficient or costly approaches or those that research has not found to be sufficiently efficacious. Therefore, treatments that can benefit clients with particular conditions might not be covered. Many payers are experimenting with various guidelines for treatment as they consider approval for plans of care.
3. Factors that influence the effectiveness of an interdisciplinary team
   a. One of the most basic barriers to the effectiveness of interdisciplinary team planning is related to autonomy and the goals and desires of the client and her or his family. When these goals and desires are at odds with those presumed by the team, recommendations are likely to produce little improvement.
   b. Some cases can make it difficult to use a team care approach. The overall effectiveness of a team can be compromised by a lack of clear and concise goals.
   c. The means of measuring and demonstrating savings are inadequate when a team approach is used to plan for high-risk clients, particularly older adults. Although it has been very difficult to evaluate outcomes in older adults with debilitating conditions or comorbidities by using existing measures, multiple studies and evidence-based programs for seniors are finding some success in keeping seniors healthier and in their own homes. Challenges include financial viability and sustainability.
   d. Because the team process is time consuming and costly, team members often are pressured to demonstrate that the approach meets clients' needs in a cost-effective manner.
4. Principles to promote organizational ethics
   a. Build on an organization's existing resources.
   b. Understand that initially all ethics programs experience growing pains and could meet with resistance.
   c. Establish a high level of ethical behavior and accountability.
   d. Encourage and support professionals' efforts toward spiritual growth.
5. Ethical concepts
   a. Elements of ethical competence
      1) Commitment to client well-being: Case managers must ensure that client-centered care and services are provided.
      2) Responsibility and accountability: Through coordination activities, case managers monitor the effectiveness of the plan and can reinforce the accountability of others who are responsible for achieving specific goals or performing specific tasks within the plan.
      3) Ability to act as an effective advocate: With access to and knowledge of the healthcare system, the case manager acts as an advocate for clients within the system and coordinates community-based services.
      4) Ability to mediate ethical conflicts: Case managers are in a position to

identify ethical conflicts and seek resolution through ethics consultations and other means.

5) Ability to recognize ethical dimensions of practice: Skill in identifying potential ethical dilemmas is derived from an ability to analyze situations from multiple perspectives.
6) Ability to critique the potential to influence a person's well-being: With the availability of new healthcare technologies, case managers must analyze the potential of various interventions (both positive and negative).

b. Ethical approaches

1) Generally, the principle-based approach consists of traditional principles of autonomy, beneficence, nonmaleficence, and justice. Ethical dilemmas arise when the case manager cannot uphold one or more of these principles. Case managers can be seen as both a client advocate for care and the gatekeeper of services.
2) The care-based approach is based on the professional/client relationship and focuses on the totality of the client's life. It attends to the client's needs and interests while attempting to resolve ethical conflicts by improving relationships between the client, professional, and family.
3) The shared decision-making model recognizes the importance of considering the expertise and opinion of both the client and the professional when making a decision. Professionals give the client the information, skills, data, and other support necessary to make an informed decision. The client and the professional are active participants in the discussion leading to a decision. Each voices his or her thoughts and can consider the perspective of the other before making a decision.
4) Criteria for identifying the appropriate ethical approach
   a) The client's ability to comprehend information that is relevant to the decision to be made
   b) His or her ability to deliberate using a consistent set of values and goals
   c) His or her ability to communicate preferences

C. Legal Issues in Case Management Based on Changes in Healthcare Delivery

1. More knowledge and access to information through technology such as the Internet can result in some clients feeling they are being denied care they consider to be their right.
2. Clients' expectations of service providers can increase because of their greater knowledge and access to health information. Case manager recommendations that result in suboptimal outcomes can place the case manager at risk.
3. Case managers can be exposed to lawsuits as they assume more responsibility, and if the focus is on cost containment, clients could suspect that the case manager is preventing access to care to save money.
4. Increased caseloads of case management professionals as healthcare organizations downsize necessitate greater attention to the details of diagnosis, treatment plans, goals, placement, and time frames.
5. Increased autonomy of case managers and other healthcare professionals in their practices necessitates an adherence to standards of practice.

D. Risk Factors in Case Management

1. Case managers are responsible for integrating care and services, advocating for clients and their families, and acting as risk managers. Case managers can reduce the risk of litigation by performing their duties as defined by established standards and relevant scope of practice.
2. Case managers have a responsibility to communicate with the client, family, and treatment team in a timely manner. This is particularly true when the condition of the client changes significantly and warrants immediate attention. Case managers must ensure that the treatment plan remains accurate and relevant to the changing needs of the client.
3. Case managers have a responsibility to integrate services. In doing so, they develop relationships with clients, family, service providers, and others involved in the care and rehabilitation processes. Ethical and liability issues arise when the professional cannot integrate necessary care and services because of conflicting obligations (e.g., client advocacy versus contractual obligations to the employer).
4. Case management is a specialty practice within which providers are held to professional standards of practice. The elements of proof remain the same as in any professional malpractice case (e.g., duty, breach), but for a finding of malpractice, evidence must go beyond the reasonable person

standard and establish that the professional did not meet the necessary standards of care.

5. The role and functions of case management according to relevant nurse practice acts, certification standards, standards of professional organizations, and other sources are well documented. The jury compares those standards with the actions of the professional and uses them as guides in the decision-making process in a court setting.

E. Future of Case Management

1. Illness, injury, chronic diseases, aging, increases in population and use of resources, and increased healthcare costs all are part of the future. If the healthcare reform of 2010 remains in effect, the number of insured will increase. If not, uninsured clients will still need services. Regardless, hospitals, insurance companies, and other providers will be under pressure to provide health care efficiently. The demand for high-quality care and improved outcomes will continue.
2. Case managers will need to continue research for evidence that case management practice provides high-quality, effective, and cost-efficient care.
3. Case managers will need to advocate for themselves and negotiate for job descriptions and roles or models that will be most effective for the system they are working in.
4. Case managers will need to continue the fine art of collaboration with the identified team, and learn to delegate tasks that can be done by others.
5. Case managers should be assigned early and be on site to promote the most efficient use of healthcare resources.
6. The population is aging, and older adults will benefit from the care coordination that case management provides as they strive to remain, independently, in their own homes.
7. Changes in payer protocols, such as Medicare readmission policies and noncoverage of adverse events, increase the importance of case management in care planning and implementation.
8. Health policy changes, such as the Affordable Care Act, which expanded access to care and coverage for prevention and health maintenance services, increase the importance of case management in care planning and coordination.

References

American Nurses Association (ANA). (2007). *Nursing: Scope and standards of practice.* Washington, DC: American Nursing Publishing.

American Nurses Association (ANA). (2010). Code of ethics for nurses. Retrieved from http://www.nursingworld.org/codeofethics

Association of Rehabilitation Nurses (ARN). (2010). *The rehabilitation nurse case manager: Role description.* Glenview, IL: Author.

Association of Rehabilitation Nurses (ARN). (2014). ARN competency model for professional rehabilitation nursing. Retrieved from http://www.rehabnurse.org/uploads/files/education/ARN_Rehabilitation_Nursing_Competency _Model_FINAL_-_May_2014.pdf

Case Management Society of America. (2010). *Standards of practice for case management.* Little Rock, AR: Author.

Centers for Medicare & Medicaid Services. (2014). Workers' Compensation Medicare Set-Aside Arrangement (WCMSA) Reference Guide. Retrieved from https://www.cms.gov/Medicare/Coordination-of-Benefits-and-Recovery/Workers-Compensation-Medicare-Set-Aside-Arrangements/Downloads/May-29-2014-WCMSA-Reference-Guide-Version-22.pdf

Cohen, E., & Cesta, T. (2005). *Nursing case management from essentials to advanced practice applications* (4th ed.). St. Louis: Elsevier.

Huber, D. L. (2006). *Leadership and nursing care management* (3rd ed.). St. Louis: Elsevier.

International Association of Life Care Planners (2006). International Academy of Life Care Planners standards of practice. Retrieved from http://www.rehabpro.org/sections/ialcp/focus/standards/ialcpSOP_pdf

Suggested Resources

American Nurses Association NursingWorld: www.nursingworld.org.

Association of Rehabilitation Nurses: www.rehabnurse.org

Blackwell, T. L., Kraus, J. S., Winkler, T., & Steins, S. A. (2001). *Spinal cord injury desk reference: Guidelines for life care planning and case management.* New York: Demos.

Books for Case Managers: http://books4casemanagers.com/casemanagement.html

The Care Planner Network: www.careplanners.net.

Carter, J. (2009). Finding our place at the discussion table: Case management and healthcare reform. *Professional Case Management, 14*(4) 165–166.

Case Management Society of America: http://CMSA.org

Commission on Accreditation of Rehabilitation Facilities: www.CARF.org

Continuing Ed for Certified Health Professionals: http://www.aaaceus.com/

Gutbezahl, C., & Mullahy, C. (2010). Case management role is likely to expand under healthcare reform. *Hospital Case Management, 18*(6), 81–84.

The Joint Commission: http://jointcommission.org

Mullahy, C. M. (2013). *The case manager's handbook* (5th ed.). Sudbury, MA: Jones & Bartlett.

Riddick-Grisham, S. (2004). *Pediatric life care planning and case management.* New York: CRC Press.

Tahan, H., & Campgana, V. (2010). Case management roles and functions across various settings and professional disciplines. *Professional Case Management, 15*(5), 245–277.

Thomas, P. (2009). Case management delivery models: The impact of indirect caregivers on organizational outcomes. *Journal of Nursing Administration, 39*(1), 30–37.

Weed, R. O. (2010). *Life care planning and case management handbook* (3rd ed.). New York: CRC Press.

Chapter 11

Integral Nursing Theory: A Framework for Complementary and Alternative Practices in Rehabilitation Nursing

Paul Nathenson, RN HN-BC CTN CRRN

LEARNING OUTCOMES

- Define holistic nursing.
- Explore the framework and metaparadigms of integrated nursing theory.
- Discuss the concepts of complementary and alternative therapy (CAM).
- Identify nursing's role in CAM.
- Outline research applications related to integral nursing theory.

KEY CHAPTER TOPICS

- Integral nursing theory
- Integral nursing theory: The four domains
- The concept of self-care
- Theoretical framework description and analysis
- Complementary and alternative medicine
- Nursing-based CAM practices
- Wellness coaching
- Botanicals and supplements
- CAM practices for mental health
- Metaparadigms in integral nursing theory

PROFESSIONAL REHABILITATION NURSING DOMAINS AND COMPETENCIES

- Domain 1: Competencies 1.1, 1.2, 1.3, 1.4
- Domain 2: Competencies 2.1, 2.2
- Domain 4: Competencies 4.2, 4.3 (Association of Rehabilitation Nurses [ARN], 2014)

Introduction

Holistic nursing includes any form of nursing practice that takes the whole person into account, including mind, body, and spirit. In holistic nursing, this is known as the bio-psycho-social-spiritual framework, which includes contextual factors of environment and social interaction and has evolved into the theory of integral nursing.

Integral nursing theory is a perfect fit for rehabilitation, because in rehabilitation nursing practice the nurse takes into account all facets of the patient. Rehabilitation nurses understand the mind-body-spirit connection and recognize the contextual factors of vocation, finances, family or caregiver support, and personal preferences and life goals. The theory of integral nursing is broad and based on a worldview framework to guide holistic nursing practice and any nursing practice that views the person as an energetic whole consisting of mind, body, and spirit.

The theory of integral nursing is centered on healing (**Figure 11-1**). It embraces the concept of an individual as an energy field that is connected with the energy fields of all humanity and the world.

I. Integral Nursing Theory

A. Healing includes knowing, doing, and being. It is a lifelong journey and process of bringing the deeper-level aspects of oneself into harmony and moving through stages of inner knowing that lead to integration.

B. In the healing process, we are in a space in which we can face our fears; seek and express the self in all its fullness; and learn to trust life, creativity, passion, and love. Each aspect of healing has equal importance and value and leads to more complex levels of understanding and meaning.

C. We are born with healing capacities. It is a process inherent in all living things. No one can take healing away from life, even though we often get stuck in our healing, or forget that we possess it because of life's continuous challenges and perceived barriers to wholeness.

D. Healing can take place at all levels of human experience, but it might not occur simultaneously in all of them.

E. Healing is not predictable; it can occur with the curing of symptoms, but it is not synonymous with curing. Curing may not always happen, but the potential for healing to occur is always present, even at one's last breath (Dossey & Keegan, 2013).

II. Integral Nursing Theory: The Four Domains

Figure 11-1. Healing

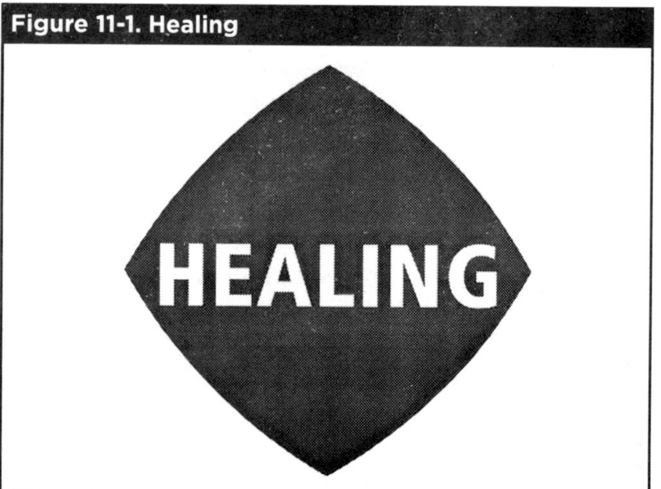

From Dossey, B. M., & Keegan, L. (2013). *Holistic Nursing: A Handbook for Practice* (6th ed.), Burlington, MA: Jones & Bartlett. Copyright 2013 by Barbara M. Dossey. Reprinted with permission.

A. The integral nursing theory provides a multifaceted approach to the metaparadigm of person described within four domains, or quadrants, that include the following: individual interior, individual exterior, collective interior, and collective exterior (**Figure 11-2**).

B. These four domains, developed by philosopher Ken Wilber, recognize the internal spiritual, emotional, and psychological self (our inner voice, so to speak).

C. The four domains also acknowledge the eternal environmental and social realms of our existence, as well as a collective oneness with spirituality and the realities of the world in which we live.

D. Integral dialogues consist of a transdisciplinary exchange of ideas to expand practice for the purpose of improving patient outcomes. The metaparadigms of nurse, patient, health, and environment are likewise fully integrated. Further, a change in any single domain of the self generates a change in all aspects of the self (Dossey, 2008).

E. The specifics of the four domains or quadrants are described as follows and are shown in Figure 11-2.

1. Upper-left (UL): In this "I" space (subjective; inside the individual) is found the world of the individual's interior experiences. These are the thoughts, emotions, memories, perceptions, immediate sensations, and states of mind (e.g., imagination, fears, feelings, beliefs, values, esteem, cognitive capacity, emotional maturity, moral development, and spiritual maturity). Integral nursing requires development of the "I."
2. Upper-right (UR): In this "It" (objective; outside the individual) space is found the world of the individual's exterior. This includes the material body (e.g., physiology [cells, molecules, neurotransmitters, limbic system] biochemistry, chemistry, physics); integral patient care plans; skill development (e.g., health, fitness, exercise, nutrition); behaviors; leadership skills; and integral life practices (see section II., A., 3 "Process"); and anything that we can touch or observe scientifically in time and space. Integral nursing among nursing colleagues and healthcare team members includes the "It" of new behaviors, integral assessment and care plans, leadership, and skills development.
3. Lower-left (LL): In this "We" (intersubjective; the inside of the collective) space is found the interior collective of how we can merge to share our cultural background, stories, values, meanings, vision, language, and relationships. It is also how we form partnerships to achieve a healing mission. This can decrease our fragmentation, and enhance collaborative practice and deep dialogue concerning matters of real significance. Integral nursing is built on "We."
4. Lower-right (LR): In this "Its" space (interobjective; the outside of the collective) is found the world of collective, exterior things. These include social systems/structures; networks; organizational structures; and systems (including financial and billing systems in health care); information technology; regulatory structures (e.g., environmental and governmental policies); and any aspect of the technological environment and the natural world. Integral nursing identifies the "Its" in the structure that can be enhanced to create more integral awareness and integral partnerships to achieve health and healing—both locally and globally.
5. On the outside of Figure 11-2, the left-hand quadrants (Upper-Left, Lower-Left) describe aspects of reality as interpretive and qualitative. In contrast, the right-hand quadrants (Upper-Right, Lower-Right) describe aspects of reality as measurable

Figure 11-2. The Metaparadigm of Person

UPPER LEFT	UPPER RIGHT
INDIVIDUAL INTERIOR (intentional/personal)	**INDIVIDUAL EXTERIOR (behavioral/biological)**
"I" space includes self and consciousness (self-care, fears, feelings, beliefs, values, esteem, cognitive capacity, emotional maturity, moral development, spiritual maturity, personal communication skills, etc.)	"It" space that includes brain and organisms (physiology, pathophysiology [cells, molecules, limbic system, neurotransmitters, physical sensations], biochemistry, chemistry, physics, behaviors [skill development in health, nutrition, exercise, etc.])
• Subjective • Interpretive • Qualitative — I / WE	IT / ITS — • Objective • Observable • Quantitative
COLLECTIVE INTERIOR (cultural/shared)	**COLLECTIVE EXTERIOR (systems/structures)**
"We" space includes the relationship to each other and the culture and worldview (shared understanding, shared vision, shared meaning, shared leadership and other values, integral dialogues and communication/morale, etc.)	"Its" space includes the relation to social systems and environment, organizational structures and systems (in healthcare—financial and billing systems), educational systems, information technology, mechanical structures and transportation, regulatory structures (environmental and governmental policies, etc.)
LOWER LEFT	LOWER RIGHT

From Dossey, B. M., & Keegan, L. (2013). *Holistic Nursing: A Handbook for Practice* (6th ed.), Burlington, MA: Jones & Bartlett. Adapted with permission from Wilber, K. (2000). *Integral Psychology: Consciousness, Sprit, Psychology, Therapy*. Boston: Shambhala. Copyright 2013 by Barbara M. Dossey. Reprinted with permission.

and quantitative. When we fail to consider these subjective, intersubjective, objective, and interobjective aspects of reality, our endeavors and initiatives are fragmented and narrow, and we often fail to reach identified outcomes and goals. The four quadrants are a result of the differences and similarities in Wilber's investigation of the many aspects of identified reality. The model describes the territory of our own awareness that is present within us and an awareness of all things outside of us. These quadrants help us to connect the dots of the process to understand more deeply who we are and how we are related to other people and to all things (Dossey & Keegan, 2013).

6. For example, the theory provides that a person's emotional state has an impact on his or her physical well-being, and because these concepts are multidirectional in relation to each other, it follows that spiritual well-being could have a healing effect on the emotional or physical health of the individual. In practice, the theory guides the nurse to assess the patient's spiritual belief system and incorporate it into individualized patient care planning.

III. Barbara M. Dossey: Holistic Nursing Visionary

A. Developed the theory of integral nursing to support the specialty practice of holistic nursing

B. Is the author and coauthor of several important works on holistic nursing and integral nursing theory. These include: *Holistic Nursing: A Handbook for Practice; AHNA Standards of Holistic Nursing Practice: Guidelines for Caring and Healing; Core Curriculum for Holistic Nursing (editor); AACN Handbook of Critical Care Nursing; Rituals of Healing; and Profiles of Nurse Healers*

C. Began contemplating her theory on holistic nursing in the 1970s while working as a cardiology nurse in critical care, when she and some of her colleagues began to search for something more to address the psychosocial needs of patients, such as the need for alleviation of anxiety and fear related to illness and hospitalization.

D. In her exploration of self-care modalities, Dossey began to learn about complementary and alternative therapies.

1. In a recent interview, Dossey defined self-care as attention to nutrition, stress management, and exercise (Medows, 2013). This notion of self-care became an important concept in holistic nursing.

IV. The Concept of Self-Care

A. Overlaps and integrates all of the domains of self

B. Self-care activities for physical well-being include whole foods nutrition and exercise. When exercise is performed with mindfulness and intention, the domain of mind becomes engaged.

1. For example, an activity such as yoga simultaneously engages the physical, psycho-emotional, and spiritual aspects of self and results in the multidimensional integration of self (Iyengar, 2007).

C. In the practice of integral nursing, the nurse engages in self-care practices such as personal reflection, evaluation, and a method to explore the principles of a higher self.

1. This results in self-awareness and the aspect of knowing.

D. There are six aspects, or patterns of knowing: empirical, personal, ethical, aesthetic, not knowing, and sociopolitical aspects. These patterns of knowing assist nurses in being present in the moment with self and others, to integrate aesthetics with science, and to develop the flow of ethical experience with thinking and acting (**Figure 11-3**) (Dossey & Keegan, 2013).

1. *Empirical knowing* is the assimilation of factual information. It is part of the science of nursing that focuses on formal expression, replication, and validation of scientific competence in both nursing education and practice. It is expressed in models and theories and can be integrated into evidence-based practice. Empirical indicators are accessed through the known senses and are subject to direct observation, measurement, and verification (Dossey & Keegan, 2013).
2. *Personal knowing* is self-knowledge and an emotional ability to have insights and relate to others. It can be developed through art, meditation, dance, music, stories, and other expressions of the authentic and genuine self in daily life and nursing practice (Dossey & Keegan, 2013).
3. *Ethical knowing* is related to moral values and an ethical framework for decision making. It includes valuing and clarifying situations to create formal moral and ethical behaviors that intersect with legally prescribed duties. It emphasizes respect for the person, the family, and the community, which in turn encourages connectedness and relationships that enhance attentiveness, responsiveness, communication, and moral action (Dossey & Keegan, 2013).
4. *Aesthetic knowing* is related to the holistic concept of presence. Aesthetic knowledge can be described as awareness of the current state or situation, or consciously being in the here and now (Paley, Cheyne, Dalgleish, Duncan, & Niven, 2007). It is the part of the art of nursing that focuses on how to explore experiences and meaning in life, alone or with another, that includes authentic presence, the nurse as a facilitator of healing, and the artfulness of a healing environment. The combination of knowledge, experience, instinct, and intuition connects the nurse with a patient or client to explore the meaning of a situation within the human experiences of life, health, illness, and death. It draws from the nurse the resources and inner strengths needed to help facilitate the healing process (Dossey & Keegan, 2013).
5. *Not knowing* is a concept that is more central and significant in integral nursing theory.
   a. The state of unknowing allows the nurse, when fully present, to use his or her intuition to discover new insights to solve problems and improve outcomes.
   b. Unknowing provides a cosmic link to the divine, which brings the aspect of spirituality into the holistic nursing process (Dossey, 2008b).
6. *Sociopolitical knowing* addresses the important contextual variables of social, economic, geographic, cultural, political, historical, and other key factors in theoretical, evidence-based practice and research. This pattern includes informed critique and social justice for the voices of the underserved in all areas of society, along with protocols to reduce health disparities (Dossey & Keegan, 2013).

V. Theoretical Framework Description and Analysis

A. A retroductive methodology was employed in the development of the bio-psycho-social-spiritual model, which is the underlying framework of integral nursing theory.

1. The framework is a hypothetical model used to describe a concept of reality that is not observable.
2. Consistent with a retroductive methodology, the concepts and metaparadigms are implicitly defined and well connected to the central framework (McNiel & Lopes, 2010).
3. The bio-psycho-social-spiritual framework is used to describe the holistic view of the person. These dimensions, which contain the subtle essence of the life force, are fully integrated and interconnected.

Figure 11-3. Healing and Patterns of Knowing in Nursing

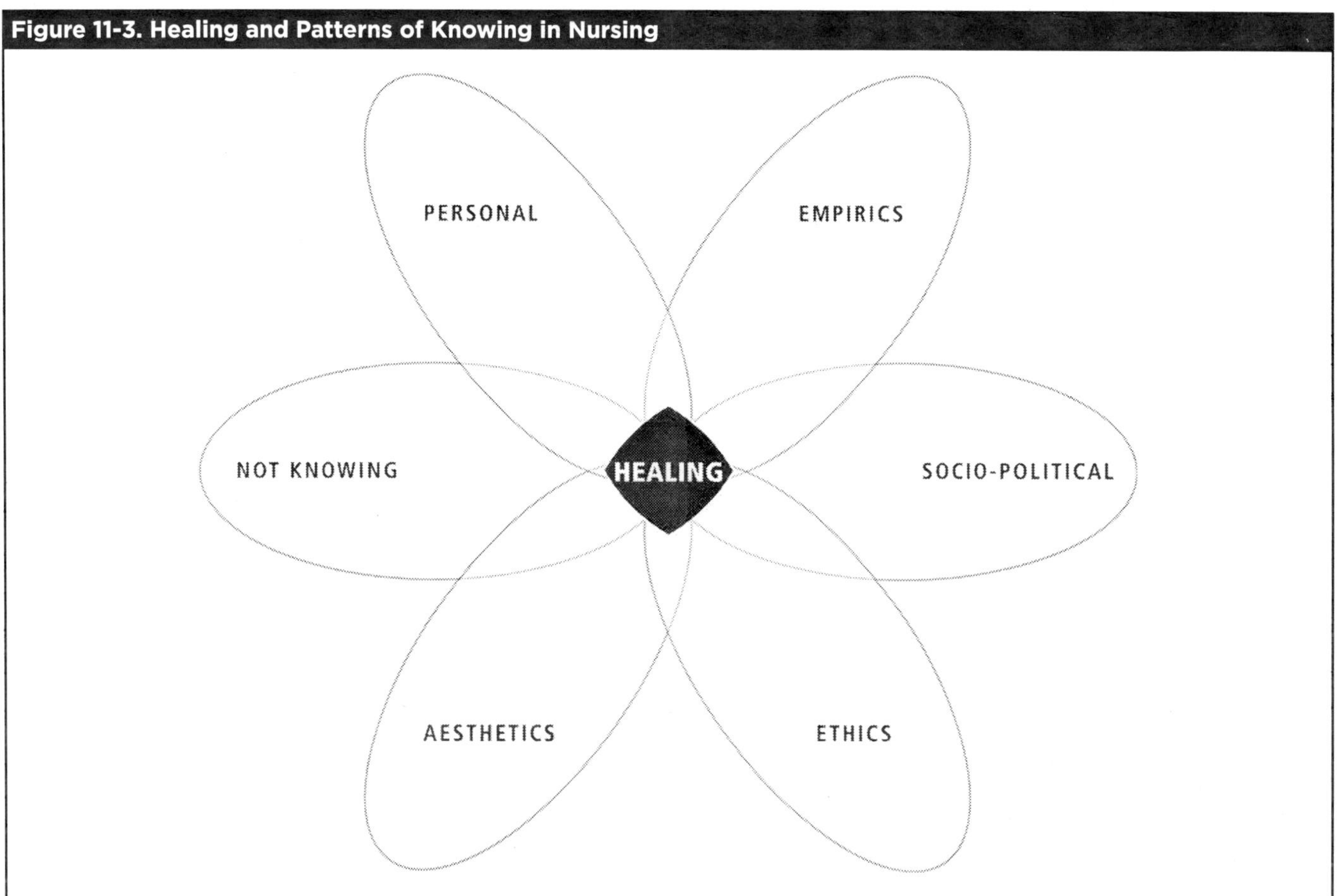

From Dossey, B. M., & Keegan, L. (2013) *Holistic Nursing: A Handbook for Practice* (6th ed.), Burlington, MA: Jones and Bartlett. Adapted from Healing and Patterns of Knowing in Nursing Source, by B. Carper, 1978. Copyright Barbara M. Dossey. Reprinted with permission.

a. One important concept in the model is that a change in any one dimension can have an impact on all dimensions (Dossey, 2008b).

4. The bio-psycho-social-spiritual model was first proposed by Dr. George Engel and Dr. John Romano at the University of Rochester in the 1970s.
   a. The model was developed to provide a more comprehensive systems approach to complement the traditional biomedical models of medicine, which focused on pathophysiology (Borrell-Carrió, Suchman, & Epstein, 2004).
   b. This model has application in wellness coaching and patient education in all areas of nursing.
      1) For example, a common teaching point in education for a patient who has had a stroke is the importance of stress management. In this example, the framework helps to illustrate how emotional stress can have an impact on physical health and well-being. This guides the nurse in explaining how stress management can help prevent future occurrence of stroke (Duncan et al., 2005).

VI. Metaparadigms in Integral Nursing Theory

A. A *metaparadigm* provides a global perspective on a profession.
   1. It is a way to define the profession as a whole, demonstrating how it is distinct and unique from other professions.

B. Four concepts in nursing are considered to be the metaparadigms of the profession.
   1. The four concepts include nurse, person, health, and environment (Butts, 2010) (**Figure 11-4**).
   2. The meaning of each metaparadigm is dynamic, and each concept has a specific meaning that is dependent on the specific nursing theory. In other words, the definition of each concept is context driven.
      a. The concept of *nurse*, as described by holistic nursing theory, considers the nurse a component of the therapeutic environment.
         1) This includes the concept of therapeutic use of self.
         2) This acknowledges that it is therapeutic to a patient for a nurse just to be with him or her. In holistic nursing, the nurse is mindful

Figure 11-4. Healing and Metaparadigm of Nursing Theory

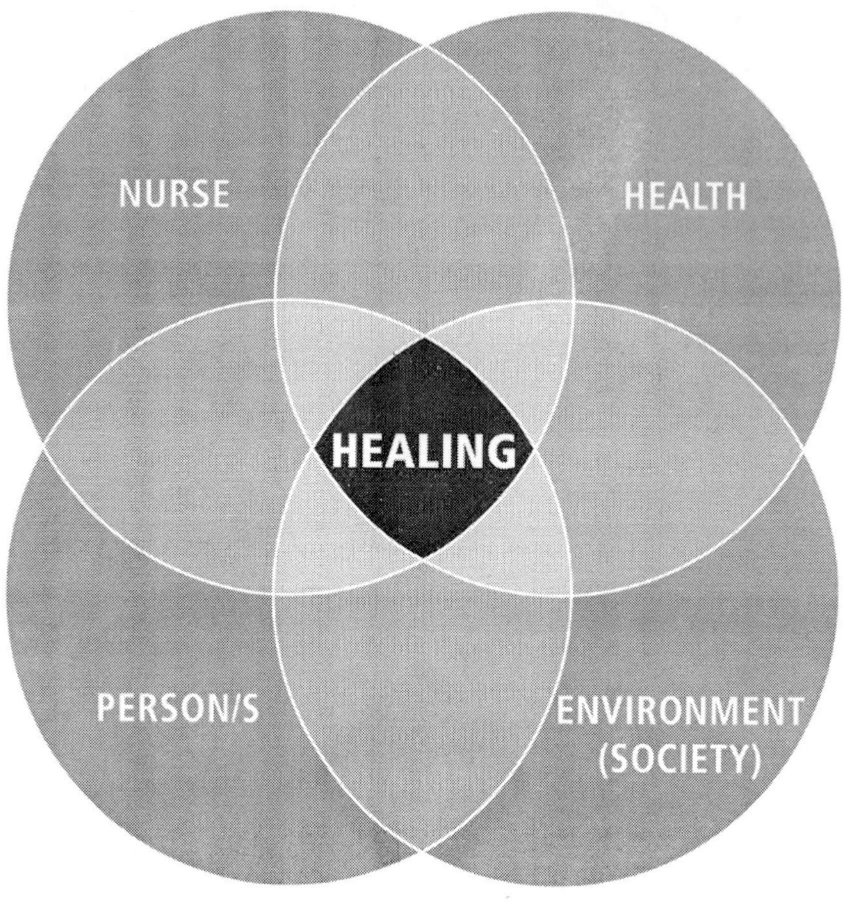

Adapted from *Holistic Nursing: A Handbook for practice* (6th ed.), by B. M. Dossey, and L. Keegan, Burlington, MA: Jones and Bartlett. Copyright 2007 by Barbara M. Dossey. Reprinted with permission.

of his or her presence and mentally extends that sense of presence to the patient.

3) The nurse enhances the therapeutic environment by practicing kindness and empathy (Sharoff, 2008).
4) This view of the metaparadigm of nurse builds on the concept definition found in nursing theorist Hildegard Peplau's (1909–1999) theory of interpersonal relations, wherein nursing is described as a therapeutic interpersonal process between the nurse and the patient.
5) There is a synergy between the nurse and the patient that facilitates growth in both parties (Schout, De Jong, & Zeelen, 2010).

b. The holistic concept of *patient* builds on Martha Rogers' (1914–1994) theory of unitary human beings, wherein the person (patient) is seen as being one with the universe and is an energetic being manifested as frequencies or energy waves.

1) The human energy field and the universal energy field are not dichotomous; rather, they are constantly interacting. In this context, illness is seen as an imbalance in the human energy field (Bramlett, Gueldner, & Boettcher, 2008).
2) Other important factors in regard to the concept of patient include the patient experience and the patient role.
   a) Patients can experience a loss of dignity in the patient role. This loss of dignity can result from a patient's perception of indifference and condescension on the part of the nurse.
   b) The nurse can facilitate the preservation of the patient's dignity by practicing self-awareness of verbal and nonverbal communication, as well as engaging the patient's participation in care through active listening and acknowledging the patient's input (Baillie & Gallagher, 2012).

c. The concept of *health* is described in terms of wellness, which is more than just the absence of illness, as is implicit in health used as a term.
   1) *Wellness* is defined as a self-directed quest for optimal well-being along a multidimensional continuum of mind, body, and spirit.
   2) Wellness in the mind, body, and spirit is influenced by contextual factors of social interaction and the environment.
      a) Social contextual factors include social support such as that provided by family and friends, as well as sociological determinants.
         (i) Studies have shown that low socioeconomic status is related to a greater incidence of adverse health outcomes. For example, women with a lower socioeconomic status had higher rates of low infant birth weight and a greater incidence of postpartum depression (O'Campo & Urquia, 2012).
         (ii) The nurse is thus guided by integral theory to assess contextual factors in the development of individualized patient interventions. Vigilant prevention and wellness interventions should help to prevent low infant birth weight. When an expectant mother is engaged in these strategies, the risk for postpartum depression is lower (Tomlinson, Cooper, Stein, Swartz, & Molteno, 2006).

d. The concept of environment in the theory is all-inclusive.
   1) The environment includes the physical surroundings of the patient. It also includes the things and people that are physically in that environment.
   2) Synergy exists between the people in the environment and the physical nature of the environment.
   3) A physical environment that has calming or healing colors, an absence of noxious sounds, and a presence of soft ambient sounds is conducive to healing for the patient and clinicians that interact within that environment.
      a) Call-light noises, overhead pages, and sounds from medical equipment are distracting and detract from the healing features desired in a therapeutic environment. Studies have noted that hourly rounding by nurses can reduce the occurrence of call lights, thus supporting a more therapeutic environment (France, Byers, Kearney, & Myatt, 2011).

VII. Complementary and Alternative Medicine

A. One of the centers of the National Institutes of Health is the National Center for Complementary and Alternative Medicine (NCCAM)
   1. NCCAM is the federal agency that funds research on complementary and alternative medicine (CAM).
      a. According to the 2007 National Health Interview Survey (NHIS), 38% of adults in the United States. reported using some type of complementary medicine modality (Barnes, Bloom, & Nahin, 2008).

B. *CAM* refers to methods, practices, and modalities that are outside of the realm of biomedicine.
   1. Some of the types of treatments and practices that are considered to be alternative include folk medicine, herbal medicine, homeopathy, faith healing, massage, energy healing, acupuncture, acupressure, supplements, naturopathy, and music therapy.
   2. Natural products are most commonly used (18%), followed by deep breathing (13%), meditation (10%), and chiropractic care (9%) (Basics, 2010).

C. There is much confusion about CAM and associated terms.
   1. It is generally accepted that alternative approaches are used instead of conventional biomedicine, whereas complementary approaches are used along with, but are not necessarily part of, biomedicine.
   2. *Integrative medicine* is the use of conventional biomedicine in conjunction with complementary approaches.
   3. The term *complementary health approaches* is used by NCCAM to describe complementary approaches (Basics, 2010).

VIII. Nursing-Based CAM Practices

A. Energetic healing through touch and the laying on of hands are complementary practices that have been developed by nurses in recent years.
   1. Different forms of energetic touch practices are used by nurses, including therapeutic touch, healing touch, and comfort touch.
   2. All of the techniques are based on the interaction of the human energy fields between the provider and client with the purpose of removing blockages in the energy field to promote healing.

3. Energetic touch therapies have been a nursing practice for more than 30 years. One of the earliest programs was developed in the 1970s by Dr. Dolores Krieger, PhD RN, and Dora Kunz.
4. Therapeutic Touch International Association provides for two levels of credentialing—qualified therapeutic touch practitioner (QTTP) and therapeutic touch teacher (QTTT) (Therapeutic Touch International Association, 2003).
5. Therapeutic Touch Practitioners typically work in the human energy field as it extends a few inches from the body.
   a. The practitioner uses gentle strokes to rebalance energy and restore energetic dynamics by removing energy blockages (Krieger, 1993).
6. Support for therapeutic touch becoming mainstream is evidenced by the inclusion, since 2004, of the nursing diagnosis Disturbed Energy Field (00050) in the North American Nursing Diagnosis Association's *Nursing Diagnosis: Definitions and Classification.*
   a. This diagnosis is defined as an imbalance in the human energy field (Herdman, 2011).

B. Janet Mentgen, BSN RN, developed a method called healing touch in 1989.
1. The program was supported by the American Holistic Nurses Association through a training program that began in 1993.
2. Training and certification responsibility was transferred to the new organization, Healing Touch International, after it was chartered in 1996.
   a. The organization offers two credentials: at the practitioner level, it offers the certified healing touch practitioner (CHTP) credential, and for teacher/trainers, it offers the certified healing touch instructor (CHTI) credential. Five levels of education and training are required for practitioner certification. This is followed by a written examination.
3. In healing touch, the practitioner works with the human energy field. The practitioner's hands are placed within the energy field of the client for certain techniques and in contact with the recipient's body for other techniques.
   a. The basic maneuvers are comprised of an eight-step process called the *healing touch sequence.*
      1) This sequence begins with asking for and receiving permission from the recipient to use healing touch to identify and treat health needs. The practitioner prepares with a self-centering technique and sets an intention to treat the recipient.
      2) The intention can be generalized to improve wellness, or it can be specific to work on a particular health issue as requested by the recipient. The practitioner then performs a body scan by passing his or her hands palm down, several inches above the recipient's body, with a focused awareness for body temperature, vibrational rate, magnetism or vibrational attraction, and density of energy flow.
      3) A magnetic pass can then be performed. The practitioner holds his or her hands palm down, a few inches from the recipient's body. With a sweeping motion of the hands, the practitioner begins to pass through the energy field, brushing away areas of density and smoothing out the energy flow from the recipient's head toward and slightly past the feet.
      4) After the assessment and magnetic pass, the practitioner holds his or her hands palms down over any area of concern or where the recipient has been experiencing pain.
      5) This position is held until the practitioner perceives a change in density or vibrational rate or a "letting go" on the part of the recipient.
      6) A reassessment scan is then completed, and the practitioner grounds the recipient by holding his or her feet and gently calling the recipient's name. The practitioner asks the recipient how the treatment went for him or her and remains available to discuss any feelings, sensations, or issues that surfaced for the recipient during the treatment.
   b. Additional techniques include magnetic clearing, chakra connection, trauma release, and different techniques to clear headaches (Hover-Kramer, Mentgen, & Scandrett-Hibdon, 1996).

C. In a systematic review of the literature, touch therapies were noted to achieve decreased pain response, as well as reductions in stress and anxiety. Improvements in well-being and quality of life were also reported.
1. Several studies indicated accelerated healing time and decreased use of medications.
2. Although overall results were inconclusive, the authors determined that there were sufficient positive results to warrant both continued use and further study of these energetic treatments and techniques (Wardell & Weymouth, 2004).

IX. Wellness Coaching

A. Nurse coaching and nurse wellness coaching are distinct competencies that are critical for the implementation of nursing's role in improving the landscape of health care.

1. *Nurse coaching* is an interactive experience between a nurse and a client, patient, family member, or colleague.
2. It is a purposeful and time-limited endeavor with the purpose of identifying and working through knowledge or experience gaps or to resolve issues that could impede the intended journey of the person with whom the nurse is working (Donner & Wheeler, 2009).
3. The purpose of nurse wellness coaching is to utilize coaching and mentoring competencies to improve patient care and the patient experience.
4. The nurse wellness coach sets the intention in a wellness session to engage and empower the patient through meaningful dialogue. This dialogue helps the patient to understand his or her health and wellness goals and to work collaboratively on a plan designed to achieve those goals in a step-by-step fashion.
5. When working with a patient to set goals, the goals must be measurable to establish parameters for success. It is often helpful to break down a long-term goal into smaller achievable steps to reinforce the patient's ability to take ownership of and progress toward health and wellness pursuits (Gulino-Schaub, Luck, & Dossey, 2012).
6. For more information, a workbook and study guide, *Coaching in Nursing: An Introduction*, is available online, free of charge. The workbook was developed by the International Council of Nurses (ICN), the International Center for Human Resources in Nursing (ICHRN), and the Sigma Theta Tau International Honor Society of Nursing.

X. Botanicals and Supplements

A. When evaluating any type of treatment regimen, patient safety is the primary concern; in other words, "first, do no harm."

1. When evaluating efficacy and safety of supplement use, it is worth noting that the Centers for Disease Control (CDC) report that prescription drug abuse is responsible for some 36,000 deaths annually, more deaths than those caused by heroin and cocaine combined (Centers for Disease Control and Prevention [CDC], 2011).
2. On the other hand, in the case of nutritional supplements, the American Association of Poison Control Centers' National Poison Data System reported that no deaths were caused by nutritional supplements in 2010 (Bronstein et al., 2010).

B. More than half of all adults in the United States have reported using some type of supplement. The most commonly used supplements include multivitamins, vitamin C, vitamin E, vitamin B-complex, or calcium (Radimer et al., 2004).

1. Supplement use in the United States is intended to promote health and prevent or treat chronic disease.
2. Although supplements are intended to increase health, evidence from the Iowa Women's Health Study indicated that in some cases, supplementation (e.g., iron supplements) can increase the risk of mortality.
3. Regardless whether the supplement is part of a conventional or complementary treatment, drug interactions, efficacy, and adverse effects must be carefully researched.
   a. For example, in the conventional treatment of osteoporosis, calcium supplementation is often prescribed. A meta-analysis of 15 clinical trials indicated that calcium supplementation of more than 1,500 mg daily increases the risk of cardiovascular disease. Further, the authors recommended a reevaluation of current treatment for osteoporosis (Bolland et al., 2010).
   b. An earlier, 2-year longitudinal study on the effects of magnesium on osteoporosis prevention and bone density demonstrated a significant increase in bone density and prevention of fractures (Sojka, 1995). Magnesium facilitates absorption of calcium by balancing parathyroid hormone—which leaches calcium out of the bones—with calcitonin, which increases calcium uptake in the bones. This results in a better balance of resorption and bone formation (Fuchs, 2002).

C. Pain is the primary reason that people seek medical attention.

1. Pain is linked to inflammation, and many people take nonsteroidal antiinflammatory drugs (NSAIDs) for their antiinflammatory action to relieve pain.
2. NSAID-related mortality rates are estimated to be as high as 16,500 deaths per year due to gastrointestinal bleeding (Cryer, 2005).
3. The anti-inflammatory effect of NSAIDs is achieved by the inhibition of prostaglandin, a cellular mediator that helps to initiate the inflammation response. Prostaglandin synthesis is interrupted by blocking the COX-2 enzyme; unfortunately, NSAIDs also inhibit the COX-1 enzyme,

which functions to create the protective lining of the stomach.

a. As NSAIDs degrade the integrity of the gastric mucosal lining, susceptibility to gastric ulcer rises exponentially (Hawkey, 2001).

4. A botanical alternative to NSAID therapy is the Indian spice turmeric (*Curcuma longa*).
   a. The use of turmeric has been a part of Ayurvedic medicine for centuries and is used mostly for its antiinflammatory activity. People may be familiar with turmeric as a spice and component of curry.
   b. The active ingredient is curcumin, which is a mild COX-2 inhibitor, but it does not possess COX-1 inhibition action. Because turmeric does not possess COX-1 inhibition action, there is no risk of the gastropathology that is a problem with the use of NSAIDs.
   c. Curcumin works not only by inhibiting inflammation by preventing the production of prostaglandins, but also by promoting activation of inflammation-regulating genes through its effects on cell signaling (Nieman, Cialdella-Kam, Knab, & Shanely, 2012).
5. Another botanical that is used for its antiinflammation effects is ginger (*Zingiber officinale*).
   a. *Zingiber officinale* possesses analgesic, antiinflammatory, antinausea, and sugar-moderating effects in the body.
   b. Like curcumin, ginger suppresses the synthesis of the proinflammatory molecules known as prostaglandins.
      1) Emerging research shows how ginger extract can actually inhibit or deactivate genes in the body that encode the molecules involved in chronic inflammation (Grzanna, Lindmark, & Frondoza, 2005).
6. Omega-3 fatty acids have received much attention for their positive effects on cholesterol modulation. The medical journal *Surgical Neurology* reported that omega-3 fatty acids have an anti-inflammatory action equal to or greater than that of NSAIDs for discogenic pain (Maroon & Bost, 2006).
7. Drugs such as gabapentin and pregabalin are often used in the treatment of neuropathic pain. These drugs were originally approved for the treatment of seizures.
   a. These drugs are very dangerous because of the severity of side effects.
      1) For example, the U.S. Food and Drug Administration (FDA) has reported that side effects of Neurontin® (gabapentin) include thoughts about suicide or dying, new or worsened depression, panic attacks, aggressive behavior, feelings of anger, or violent acting out of dangerous impulses (Irving, Tanenberg, Raskin, Risser, & Malcolm, 2014)
   b. A supplement alternative to drugs such as gabapentin and pregabalin is gamma-aminobutyric acid (GABA).
      1) GABA is the chief inhibitory neurotransmitter in the mammalian central nervous system. It plays a role in regulating neuronal excitability throughout the nervous system.
      2) GABA functions to turn down the nociceptive pain signal. Research data on the mode of action accumulated are providing evidence that GABA, as well as adenosine-related mechanisms, is involved in the pain amelioration in neuropathic pain conditions related to spinal cord injury (Meyerson & Linderoth, 2006).

XI. CAM Practices for Mental Health

A. Depression is highly prevalent in the United States. Estimates indicate that 10% of the adult U.S. population suffers from depression.

1. Depression is the leading cause of disability, excluding fatal illnesses.
   a. The cause of disability in depression is the severity of symptoms that impair one's ability to function at work. Functioning is impaired because of an inability to concentrate, to interact in a socially appropriate manner, to achieve restful sleep patterns, and to participate in everyday activities (Wang, Simon, & Kessler, 2008).
2. CAM recommendations for mental health include mindfulness practices, acupuncture, and supplements.
   a. Mindfulness practices include breathing techniques, meditation, yoga, and most important, living in the present moment.
      1) Mindfulness-based cognitive therapy uses a series of exercises to help dispel irrational and self-critical thinking by focusing on the present reality. By becoming more aware of one's thought patterns, negative self-thoughts can be transformed into positive affirmations (Coelho, Canter, & Ernst, 2013).
   b. Acupuncture is used as a stand-alone or concomitant treatment for depression. The role of acupuncture is to identify and treat the

underlying cause or imbalance that is contributing to the depression.

1) In a large-scale trial, the underlying organ system imbalance was found to be liver or liver qi (life energy in Chinese philosophy) stagnation, followed by spleen deficiency syndrome. Two thirds of the study participants were given lifestyle management counseling on nutrition and the use of herbs, as well as recommendations for relaxation (e.g., doing needlework) and stress-management techniques. (MacPherson, Elliot, Hopton, Lansdown, & Richmond, 2013).

c. Several supplements appear to be helpful in the treatment of depression.

1) A meta-analysis indicated that St. John's wort (*Hypericum perforatum*) had an efficacy equal to that of antidepressant medications.

a) St. John's wort is a perennial herb that was originally grown in Europe, Western Asia, and North Africa, but it is now widely cultivated in the United States. It can be recognized by its bright yellow flowers.

b) St. John's wort has been approved by the German Commission E (equivalent to the FDA), for the treatment of anxiety disorders and depression.

(i) In Germany, St. John's wort is prescribed more frequently than antidepressants.

2) S-adenosylmethionine (SAM-e) is a synthetic amino acid that was shown to reduce depression scores in 80% of randomized trials.

3) Omega-3 fatty acids, noted for their health effects on cholesterol, were shown to decrease depression scores in 16 clinical trials (Nahas & Sheikh, 2011).

XII. Research Applications

A. In holistic nursing, it is important to use research in clinical practice.

B. For nurses to be able to incorporate holistic nursing theory and research into practice, it is essential that research efforts on alternative and complementary interventions and treatments be expanded.

1. Such research efforts are necessary to validate the safety and efficacy of alternative and complementary approaches.

C. A series of questions are relevant to the consideration of research regarding complementary and alternative interventions aimed at wellness, prevention, and treatment.

1. The first question examines the physical sciences. For example, what is the biological and chemical basis of the intervention?
2. Second, what is the physiological basis for action and intended outcome?
3. Third, is the treatment or substance safe for humans?
4. If there are positive findings for these questions, the next step is an ethical determination for human trials for qualitative or quantitative testing.
5. Qualitative testing is relevant, because holistic health finds value in the perception or subjective elements of well-being in addition to the quantitative and empirical evidence (Smith, 2012).

a. For example, one of the techniques used by holistic nurses is therapeutic touch for pain control. To provide evidence-based care, the issue of the efficacy of this practice must be addressed.

1) A recent study indicated that therapeutic touch was effective in treating patients with fibromyalgia. Fibromyalgia is an autoimmune disorder known for its significant neuropathic pain. In the study, patients with fibromyalgia not only had significant improvement in pain levels after a series of therapeutic touch treatments, they also reported improved quality of life (Denison, 2004).

Conclusion

Approximately 40% of the adult U.S. population uses some form of CAM (Barnes et al., 2008). To provide patient-focused care, rehabilitation nurses have a responsibility to be well versed in CAM practices and have an understanding of research findings and limitations related to CAM use. In addition, different cultures have differing views on conventional medicine and hold beliefs vested in CAM practices. To be culturally competent, rehabilitation nurses should be open to listening, understanding, and integrating the culturally held health beliefs of their patients into the plan of care.

References

Association of Rehabilitation Nurses (ARN). (2008). *Standards and scope of rehabilitation nursing practice*. Glenview, IL: Author.

Association of Rehabilitation Nurses (ARN). (2014). ARN competency model for professional rehabilitation nursing. Retrieved from http://www.rehabnurse.org/uploads/files/education/ARN_Rehabilitation_Nursing_Competency _Model_FINAL_-_May_2014.pdf

Baillie, L., & Gallagher, A. (2012). Raising awareness of patient dignity. *Nursing Standard, 27*(5), 44–49. Retrieved from http://journals.rcni.com/doi/abs/10.7748/ns2012.10.27.5.44.c9333

Barnes, P. M., Bloom, B., & Nahin, R. L. (2008). Complementary and alternative medicine use among adults and children: United States, 2007. *National Health Statistics Reports, 10*(12), 1–23.

Basics, C. A. M. (Ed.) (2010). NCFCA Medicine. National Institutes of Health, U.S. Department of Health and Human Services, 1–7.

Bolland, M. J., Avenell, A., Baron, J. A., Grey, A., MacLennan, G. S., Gamble, G. D., & Reid, I. R. (2010). Effect of calcium supplements on risk of myocardial infarction and cardiovascular events: Meta-analysis. *British Medical Journal*, 341.

Borrell-Carrió, F., Suchman, A. L., & Epstein, R. M. (2004). The biopsychosocial model 25 years later: Principles, practice, and scientific inquiry. *The Annals of Family Medicine, 2*(6), 576–582.

Bramlett, M., Gueldner, S., & Boettcher, J. (2008). Reflections on the science of unitary human beings in terms of Kuhn's requirement for explanatory power. *Visions: The Journal of Rogerian Nursing Science, 15*(2), 7–22.

Bronstein, A. C., Spyker, D. A., Cantilena, J. R., Green, J. L., Rumack, B. H., & Giffin, S. L. (2010). 2009 annual report of the American Association of Poison Control Centers' national poison data system (NPDS): 27th annual report. *Clinical Toxicology, 48*(10), 979–1178.

Butts, J. (2010). Components and levels of abstraction in nursing knowledge. In J. B. Butts, & K. L. Rich, (Eds.), *Philosophies and theories for advanced nursing practice*, (pp. 89–112). Sudbury, MA: Jones & Bartlett.

Centers for Disease Control and Prevention (2011). Policy Impact: Prescription Painkiller Overdoses. Retrieved from http://www.cdc.gov/homeandrecreationalsafety/rxbrief/?iframe=true&width=80%&height=100%

Coelho, H. F., Canter, P. H., & Ernst, E. (2013). Mindfulness-based cognitive therapy. *Psychology of Consciousness: Theory, Research, and Practice, 1*, 97–107.

Cryer, B. (2005). NSAID-associated deaths: The rise and fall of NSAID-associated GI mortality. *American Journal of Gastroenterology, 100*(8), 1694–1695.

Denison, B. (2004). Touch the pain away: New research on therapeutic touch and persons with fibromyalgia syndrome. *Holistic Nursing Practice, 18*(3), 142–151.

Donner, G. J., & Wheeler, M. M. (2009). *Coaching in nursing: An introduction*. Indianapolis, IN: International Council of Nurses, Sigma Theta Tau International.

Dossey, B. M. (2008a). Nursing: Integral, integrative, and holistic: Local to global. In B. Dossey & L. Keegan (Eds.), *Holistic nursing: A handbook for practice* (5th ed., pp. 3–56). Sudbury, MA: Jones & Bartlett.

Dossey, B. M. (2008b). Theory of integral nursing. *Advances in Nursing Science, 31*(1), E52–E73. Retrieved from http://www.thhin.nursing.arizona.edu/PDF/DosseyTIN.pdf

Dossey, B. M., & Keegan, L. (2013). *Holistic nursing: A handbook for practice* (6th ed., pp. 1–58). Subury, MA: Jones & Bartlett.

Duncan, P. W., Zorowitz, R., Bates, B., Choi, J. Y., Glasberg, J. J., Graham, G. D.,...Reker, D. (2005). Management of adult stroke rehabilitation care: A clinical practice guideline. *Stroke, 36*(9), e100–e143. Retrieved from http://stroke.ahajournals.org/content/36/9/e100.short

France, N., Byers D., Kearney, B., & Myatt, S. (2011) Creating a healing environment: Nurse-to-nurse caring in the critical care unit. *International Journal for Human Caring, 15*(1). 44–48.

Fuchs, N. K. (2002). Magnesium: A Key to Calcium Absorption. Retrieved from http://www.spiritofhealthkc.com/wp/wpcontent/uploads/Health%20Library/Food%20and%20Herbs/Vitamins%20and%20Minerals/Magnesium/MAGNESIUM14%20%20A%20Key%20To%20Calcium%20Absorption.pdf

Grzanna, R., Lindmark, L., & Frondoza, C. G. (2005). Ginger—an herbal medicinal product with broad anti-inflammatory actions. *Journal of Medicinal Food, 8*(2), 125–132.

Gulino-Schaub, B., Luck, S., & Dossey, B. (2012). Integrative nurse coaching for health and wellness. *Alternative & Complementary Therapies, 18*(1), 14–20. doi:10.1089/act.2012.18110

Hawkey, C. J. (2001). COX-1 and COX-2 inhibitors. *Best Practice & Research Clinical Gastroenterology, 15*(5), 801–820.

Herdman, T. H. (Ed.). (2011). *Nursing diagnoses: Definitions and classification 2012-2014*. Hoboken, NJ: Wiley-Blackwell.

Hover-Kramer, D., Mentgen, J., & Scandrett-Hibdon, S. (1996). *Healing touch: A resource for health care professionals*. Albany, NY: Delmar Publishers.

Irving, G., Tanenberg, R. J., Raskin, J., Risser, R. C., & Malcolm, S. (2014). Comparative safety and tolerability of duloxetine vs. pregabalin vs. duloxetine plus gabapentin in patients with diabetic peripheral neuropathic pain. *International Journal of Clinical Practice, 68*(9), 1130-1140.

Iyengar, B. I. (2007). *B.K.S. Iyengar yoga: The path to holistic health*. New York: DK Publishing.

Krieger, D. (1993). Accepting your power to heal: The personal practice of therapeutic touch. Rochester, VT: Inner Traditions/Bear & Co.

MacPherson, H., Elliot, B., Hopton, A., Lansdown, H., & Richmond, S. (2013). Acupuncture for depression: Patterns of diagnosis and treatment within a randomized controlled trial. *Evidence-Based Complementary and Alternative Medicine, 10*(9). doi:e1001518

Maroon, J. C., & Bost, J. W. (2006). Omega 3 fatty acids (fish oil) as an anti-inflammatory: An alternative to nonsteroidal anti-inflammatory drugs for discogenic pain. *Surgical Neurology, 65*(4), 326–331.

McNiel, J., & Lopes, V. L. (2010, December). *Relational human ecology: Reconciling the boundaries of humans and nature* [Abstract]. Paper presented at the meeting of the American Geophysical Union. Retrieved from http://adsabs.harvard.edu/abs/2010AGUFMED43A0674M

Medows, C. (2013). Interview with Barbara Dossey. Retrieved from http://www.takingcharge.csh.umn.edu/interviews/interview-barbara-dossey

Meyerson, B. A., & Linderoth, B. (2006). Mode of action of spinal cord stimulation in neuropathic pain. *Journal of Pain And Symptom Management, 31*(4), S6–S12.

Nahas, R., & Sheikh, O. (2011). Complementary and alternative medicine for the treatment of major depressive disorder. *Canadian Family Physician, 57*(6), 659–663.

Nieman, D. C., Cialdella-Kam, L., Knab, A. M., & Shanely, R. A. (2012). Influence of red pepper spice and turmeric on inflammation and oxidative stress biomarkers in overweight females: A metabolomics approach. *Plant Foods for Human Nutrition, 67*(4), 415–421.

O'Campo, P., & Urquia, M. (2012). Aligning method with theory: A comparison of two approaches to modeling the social determinants of health. *Maternal & Child Health Journal, 16*(9), 1870–1878. doi:10.1007/s10995-011-0935-1

Paley, J., Cheyne, H., Dalgleish, L., Duncan, E. A., & Niven, C. A. (2007). Nursing's ways of knowing and dual process theories of cognition. *Journal of Advanced Nursing, 60*(6), 692–701.

Radimer, K., Bindewald, B., Hughes, J., Ervin, B., Swanson, C., & Picciano, M. F. (2004). Dietary supplement use by US adults: Data from the National Health and Nutrition Examination Survey, 1999–2000. *American Journal of Epidemiology, 160*(4), 339–349.

Schout, G., De Jong, G., & Zeelen, J. (2010). Establishing contact and gaining trust: An exploratory study of care avoidance. *Journal of advanced nursing, 66*(2), 324–333.

Smith, G. (2012). Editorial: Consensus on CAM methods for nursing research? *Journal of Clinical Nursing, 21*(5/6), 599–600. doi:10.1111/j.1365-2702.2011.03982.x

Sojka, J. E. (1995). Magnesium supplementation and osteoporosis. *Nutrition Reviews, 53*(3), 71–74.

Sharoff, L. (2008). Holistic nursing and medical-surgical nursing: A natural integration. *Medsurg Nursing, 17*(3), 206–208.

Teixeira, M. E. (2008). Self-transcendence: A concept analysis for nursing praxis. *Holistic Nursing Practice, 22*(1), 25–31.

Therapeutic Touch International Association (n. d.) Credentialing. Retrieved from http://therapeutic-touch.org/credentialing/

Tomlinson, M., Cooper, P., Stein, A., Swartz, L., & Molteno, C. (2006). Post-partum depression and infant growth in a South African peri-urban settlement. *Child: Care, Health & Development, 32*(1), 81–86. Retrieved from http://web.ebscohost.com.southuniversity.libproxy.edmc.edu/ehost/pdfviewer/pdfviewer?sid=e4eaaa52-edf5-4694-8f59-3d1b086e5f6d%40sessionmgr112&vid=4&hid=126

Wang, P. S., Simon, G. E., & Kessler, R. C. (2008). Making the business case for enhanced depression care: The National Institute of Mental Health-Harvard Work Outcomes Research and Cost-effectiveness Study. *Journal of Occupational and Environmental Medicine, 50*(4), 468–475.

Wardell, D. W., & Weymouth, K. F. (2004). Review of studies of healing touch. *Journal of Nursing Scholarship, 36*(2), 147–154.

Suggested Resource

Barbara Dossey's biography: http://www.dosseydossey.com/barbara/default.html.

Chapter 12

Technology and Adaptive Equipment in the Rehabilitation Setting

Martha Acosta, PhD PT GCS MS
Bridgett Piernik-Yoder, PhD OTR
Autumn Clegg, MSOT OTR
Cheryl Lehman, PhD RN CNS-BC RN-BC CRRN

LEARNING OUTCOMES

- Identify the indications for adaptive equipment and technology in the rehabilitation setting, including mobility, activities of daily living (ADL), communication, and community reintegration and socialization, among others.
- Discriminate between indications and contraindications for adaptive equipment and technology for the rehabilitation patient.
- Discuss safety issues that arise when using adaptive equipment and technology in the rehabilitation setting.

KEY CHAPTER TOPICS

- Physical therapy equipment and technology for mobility
- Occupational therapy equipment and technology for ADL and IADLs
- Equipment for communication
- Other adaptive aids and technology

PROFESSIONAL REHABILITATION NURSING DOMAINS AND COMPETENCIES

- Domain 1: Competencies 1.1, 1.2, 1.3, 1.4
- Domain 2: Competency 2
- Domain 4: Competency 4.2 (Association of Rehabilitation Nurses [ARN], 2014)

Introduction

Rehabilitation nurses encounter many types of adaptive equipment and forms of technology in the rehabilitation setting. Although the majority of this equipment is prescribed for the patient by the physical or occupational therapist or the speech language pathologist, it is the nurse's responsibility to help the patient use the equipment or technology in an appropriate, safe manner. The rehabilitation nurse must understand the purpose of the equipment and its proper application, techniques for use, safety monitoring, and removal, and any other methods of use prescribed by the therapist.

Nurses do learn about canes, walkers, and crutches in nursing school, but a vast array of other equipment is also employed in the rehabilitation setting. This equipment is changing rapidly as technology advances, and the rehabilitation nurse must stay up to date with any equipment that he or she may become responsible for in rehabilitation.

This chapter reviews equipment and technology prescribed by physical and occupational therapists. The goal is that this information will be useful in the clinical practice of the rehabilitation nurse.

I. Physical Therapy Equipment and Technology for Mobility

Prior to admission into healthcare settings (e.g., acute care inpatient hospitals, rehabilitation hospitals, skilled-nursing facilities), a majority of patients present with limited mobility, particularly older adults, who report limitations while still residing within the community (Merrill, Seeman, Kasl, & Berkman, 1997). Such limitations interfere with the safe navigation of the environment and can often lead to a need for additional support or compensatory strategies. Safe mobility is the overarching goal for the patient and all members of the healthcare team. As such, rehabilitation efforts are directed toward providing optimal security and safety with a minimal expenditure of energy. This section provides a broad overview of various forms of assistance that patients in a rehabilitation setting can use to attain safe mobility with a minimal expenditure of energy.

A. Preparation Concepts for Mobility

1. Patients may have physiological issues that can have an impact on their safety.
   a. Immobility and hypotension are two such issues.
      1) Transitioning to an upright position too quickly can trigger orthostatic hypotension, whereby the patient feels light-headed and must resume a recumbent position to avoid fainting.
      2) To address this problem, the physical therapist can use equipment such as a tilt table (**Figure 12-1**) to help accommodate the patient into an upright position if orthostatic hypotension persists or when the patient's physiological status is precarious.
         a) Nurses typically do not use a tilt table unless they are assisting physical therapy (PT).
         b) The tilt table gradually assists the patient's homeostatic mechanisms to adjust to an upright position without a drop in blood pressure or change in cardiac status.
2. Communication among rehabilitation team members also plays a key role in the rehabilitation setting.

Figure 12-1. Tilt and Standing Tables

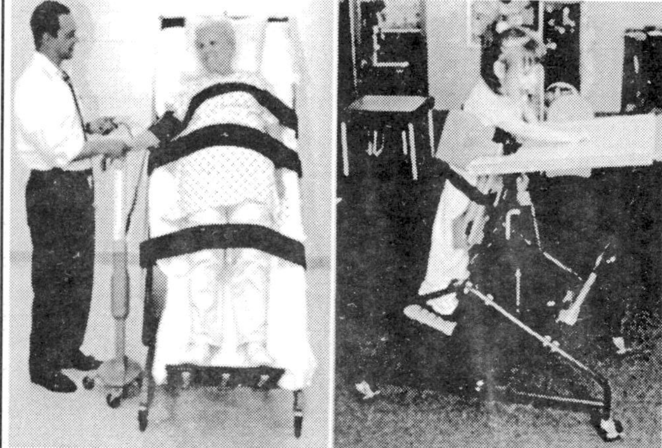

Dependent standing devices: tilt table (left), standing table (right).

From *Principles & Techniques of Patient Care* (5th Edition, Figure 9-2), by S. L. Fairchild, 2012, Stoneham, MA: Elsevier. Copyright 2012 by Elsevier. Reprinted with permission.

   a. The *medical record* is the permanent communication tool that reflects the past, current, and projected treatment plan and should be used accordingly by all who attend the patient.
   b. Interdisciplinary team meetings are critical opportunities to discuss patient mobility issues.
      1) However, the less formal, face-to-face interactions among team members are probably more vital in the daily functions of a rehabilitation setting.
   c. Adverse responses to treatment, atypical patient reactions, or even more subtle discrepancies that the therapist encounters should be documented and shared with the attending nurse for appropriate follow-up.
3. Rationale for use of assistive devices
   a. Healthcare professionals commonly identify an assistive device (**Figure 12-2**) as a means of promoting mobility independence.
   b. A person may need an assistive device to
      1) Improve functional mobility
      2) Compensate for decreased strength, impaired balance, uncoordinated movements, loss of a limb, or pain with weight bearing in one or both legs
      3) Balance an unstable gait pattern
      4) Enhance body functions
      5) Unload an extremity and assist with fracture healing (Fairchild, 2012).
   c. In the rehabilitation setting, such impairments can manifest as safety issues
      1) Patient falling while walking to the bathroom in the middle of the night
      2) Knees buckling when the patient tries to stand at bedside
4. When considering use of an assistive device in conjunction with ambulation activities, some basic preparation and organization are required.
   a. The caregiver must be aware of the patient's condition and personal ambulation goal, activity restrictions or limitations, and proper fit of the device.
   b. The patient with weight-bearing restrictions should be reminded to adhere to the specified weight-bearing status with upright positions and during gait to avoid compromising the healing process.
   c. For the patient with lines and tubes such as Foley catheters, care should be taken to secure the tubing by clipping it to the walker frame to prevent contact with the floor and keep the patient from tripping during ambulation.

Figure 12-2. Assistive Devices

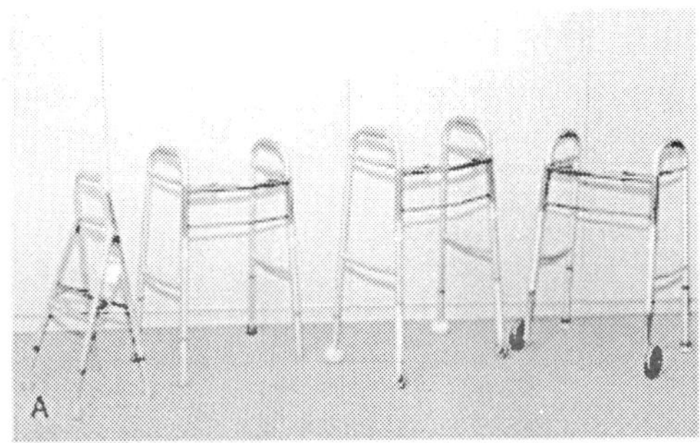

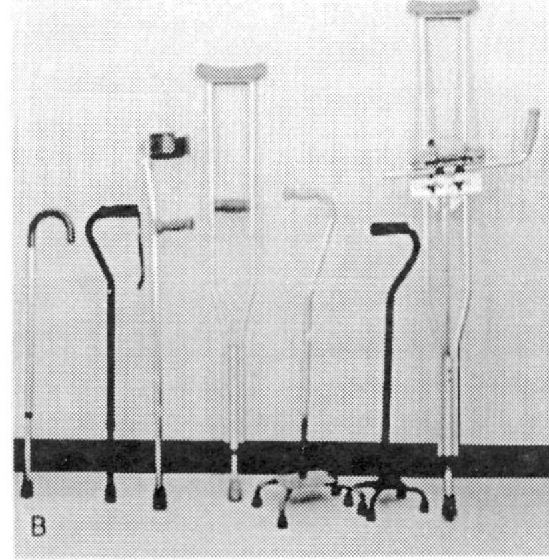

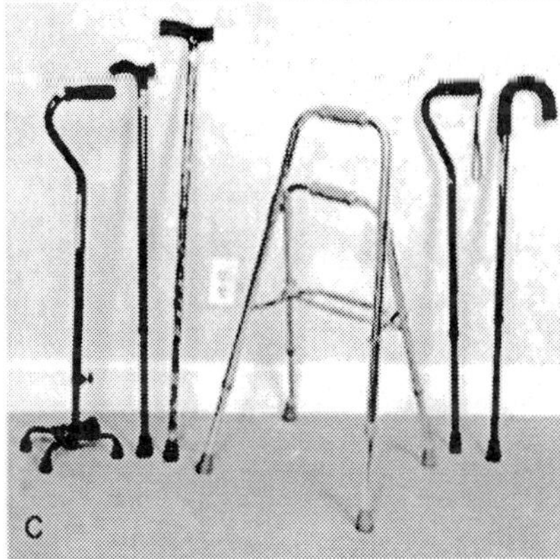

A. Types of walkers; B. An assortment of canes and crutches; C. An assortment of canes and a walker.

From *Principles & Techniques of Patient Care* (5th Edition, Figure 9-1), by S. L. Fairchild, 2012, Stoneham, MA: Elsevier. Copyright 2012 by Elsevier. Reprinted with permission.

d. A gait belt (**Figure 12-3**) fastened around the patient's waist facilitates proper guarding technique and helps protect the patient if he or she starts to fall or faint during movement.
   1) The gait belt should be securely fastened around the patient for optimal support.
   2) If the patient has a feeding tube (e.g., a percutaneous endoscopic gastrostomy [PEG]) or other drainage lines, placement of the belt could need to be adjusted either higher or lower on the trunk to avoid occluding or pulling the line.

Figure 12-3. Use of Gait Belt

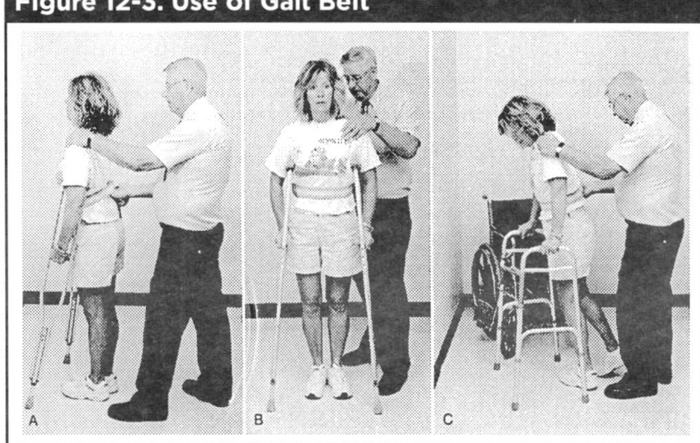

A. A caregiver holds the gait belt, which is securely fastened around the patient's waist. B., C. One of the caregiver's hands grasps the gait belt; the other hand controls the shoulder.

From *Principles & Techniques of Patient Care* (5th Edition, Figure 9-1), by S. L. Fairchild, 2012, Stoneham, MA: Elsevier. Copyright 2012 by Elsevier. Reprinted with permission.

   3) The surrounding area should be clear of any obstacles to maintain a clear, safe pathway for mobility.
   4) For healthcare worker safety, when assisting a patient who is unable to move independently, it is critical that proper body mechanics be maintained.
   5) Protecting the back (**Figure 12-4**) with good core stability, neutral spine alignment, and use of hip hinging is particularly important for a patient who has had bariatric surgery.
   6) Most rehabilitation hospitals provide back safety in-services as part of the orientation for all newly hired staff.
   7) A yearly review of safety strategies related to patient mobility is recommended for staff and patients.

5. Another aspect of preparation is the selection of equipment, including assistive devices.
   a. Selection is based on the physical therapist's findings, including examination, evaluation, and treatment goals as they relate to the functional outcomes.
   b. Factors that affect equipment decisions include a patient's cognition, vestibular function, judgment, physical endurance, and strength in both the lower and upper body.
   c. Also included in the decision are the patient's discharge destination, social environment, workplace, and home setting.
   d. Devices that provide assistance and safety vary and include single-point canes, four-point/quad canes, walkers with and without wheels (Figure 12-2), and even wheelchairs

Figure 12-4. Lifts

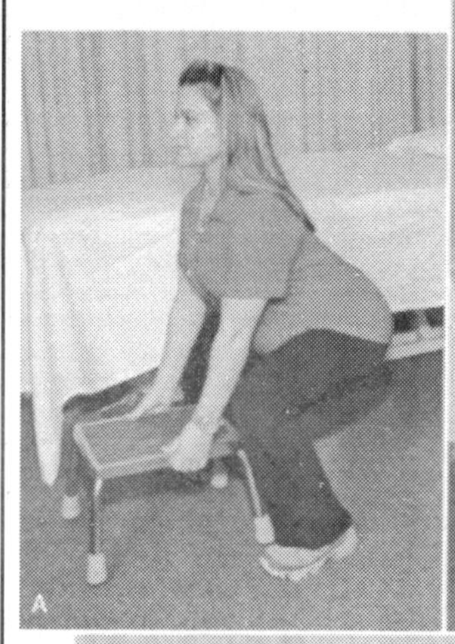

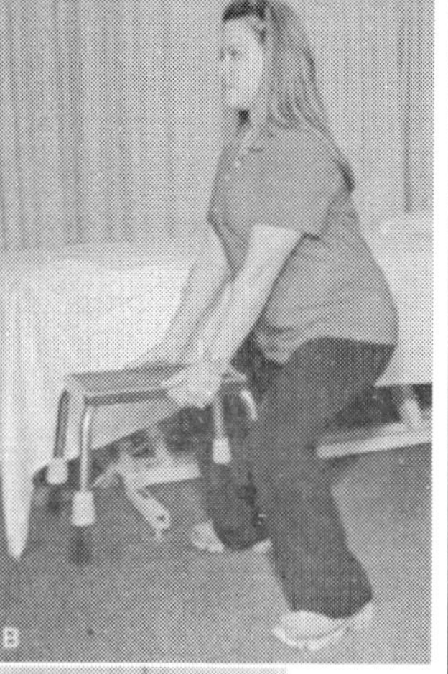

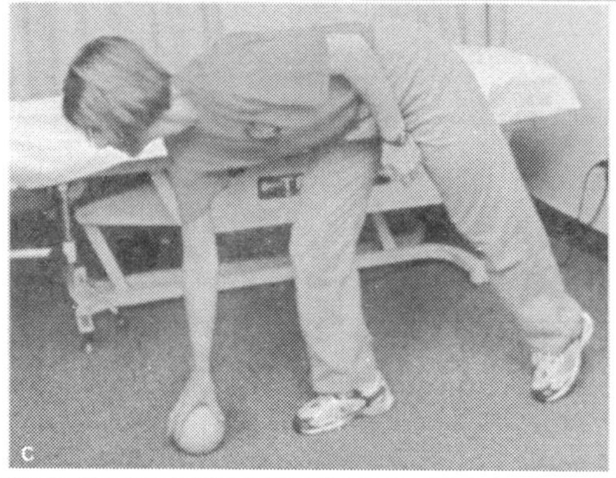

A. Start position; B. Continuation of lift; C. One-leg stance lift ("golfer's lift").

From *Principles & Techniques of Patient Care* (5th Edition, Figure 4-2), by S. L. Fairchild, 2012, Stoneham, MA: Elsevier. Copyright 2012 by Elsevier. Reprinted with permission.

Figure 12-5. Proper Stance During a Patient Transfer

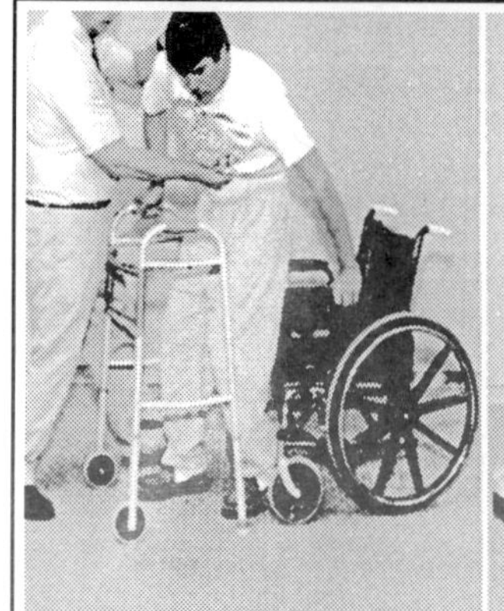

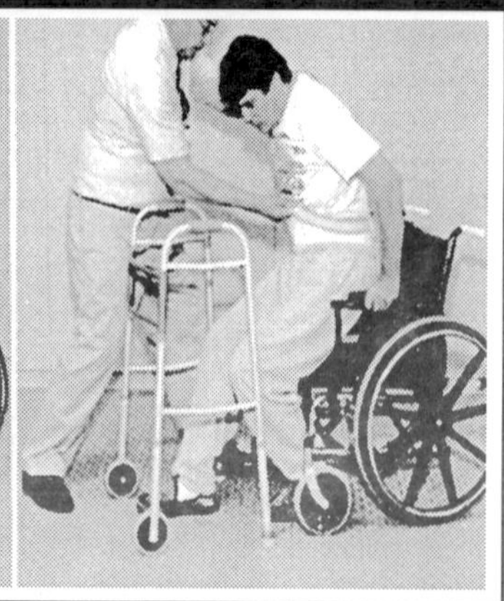

A caregiver with proper stance and use of a gait belt keeps the patient's body over the base of support during a transfer from walker to wheelchair.

From *Principles & Techniques of Patient Care* (5th Edition, Figure 9-20), by S. L. Fairchild, 2012, Stoneham, MA: Elsevier. Copyright 2012 by Elsevier. Reprinted with permission.

(**Figure 12-5**). All the factors listed thus far are preparatory issues that must be addressed to ensure effective patient intervention.

6. Safety during ambulation
   a. After deciding on the appropriate assistive device, several key points that protect the patient who will be ambulating should be considered (Fairchild, 2012).
   b. When ambulating, the patient should wear appropriate footwear with nonskid outsoles, as opposed to sandals, loose-fitting slippers, or shoes.
      1) This provides the patient with a sense of security and increases traction to prevent slippage on the floor.
   c. The caregiver should hold the patient's gait belt to control the patient's center of gravity in the event that a loss of balance occurs.
      1) Avoid holding the patient's arm, gown, belt, or clothing during gait activities.
   d. When guarding the patient (Figure 12-3), the caregiver should stand behind and slightly to the side of the patient with the hand gripping the gait belt.
      1) It is important to monitor the patient's physiological status during gait and check vital signs, general appearance, and level of alertness as he or she responds to the activity.
      2) The patient should not be left unattended while he or she is standing.
      3) If the patient has appliances (e.g., cast, drainage tubes, dressings), remember to protect the appliances.
   e. A good rule of thumb is always to expect the unexpected, such as the patient losing his or her balance, fainting while ambulating, or slipping during transfers from the bed to the wheelchair.
      1) If the nurse or therapist is holding onto the gait belt, the patient can safely be lowered to the floor in any of these scenarios if necessary.
   f. Specific instructions regarding safety during gait
      1) Always grip the gait belt.
      2) Guard the patient by standing behind and slightly to the side of the patient.
      3) Monitor the patient's physiological status: vital signs, general appearance, level of alertness, and response to activity
      4) Do not leave the patient unattended if he or she is standing.
      5) Protect appliances such as cast, drainage tubes, dressings, and the like.
7. Confirmation of fit of the assistive device

a. After the patient has been fitted for an assistive device by the physical therapist: Several key points that pertain to fit and usage should be kept in mind.
   1) When standing with any assistive device, the patient should be in a relaxed posture with the head and trunk erect, shoulders relaxed and level, and feet (foot) flat on the floor.

8. Specific instructions regarding safety during gait:
   a. Always grip the gait belt.
      1) The gait belt should be worn by the patient during all gait activities, particularly a patient with impairments in balance, strength, coordination or weight bearing (i.e., decreased ability to bear weight on one or both lower extremities).
      2) The belt is worn around the waist with adjustments as needed if the patient has a feeding tube (e.g., a PEG), as described previously.
      3) If the belt has a buckle, the buckle can be positioned to the side or back so it does not press against the skin.
      4) The gait belt should fit snugly and often needs to be retightened once the patient has assumed a standing position.
      5) By holding on to the gait belt, the healthcare provider can control the patient's center of gravity and therefore can facilitate maintenance of midline and a balanced position if the patient starts to fall during ambulation.
      6) Also, if indicated, the healthcare provider can safely lower the patient to the floor with better control of the descent.
      7) The caregiver might not be able to prevent a fall, but the risk of falling can be reduced by helping the person to a safe, secure position (e.g., midline in standing, floor, ground, chair, or stair step).
   b. When the patient is standing with a walker (e.g., rolling walker; four-point walker) and he or she grasps the hand pieces, the elbow should be flexed about 20 to 25 degrees.
   c. If the patient must lean forward, lock the elbows, or flex the elbows to more than 25 degrees when holding the walker, the walker might need to be adjusted or refitted.
   d. With a hemi-walker (used with patients who have use of only one upper extremity), the flexed elbow position is the same as with a walker (Figure 12-2).
   e. Fitting a patient with a cane or crutches requires additional features to be checked.
      1) The flexed elbow position is similar, and the 25-degree flexion applies to cane usage.
      2) A single-tip cane is held by the patient on the side opposite the affected lower extremity.
      3) With a quad cane (i.e., a cane with four tips), the position is the same.
      4) With axillary crutches, the fit can be confirmed (**Figure 12-6**) by having the patient stand while grasping the hand pieces and placing the crutch tips about 2 inches lateral and 4–6 inches in front of the tip of the shoe(s).
         a) From this position there should be approximately 2 inches between the axillary rest and the floor of the axilla; this means the healthcare provider should be able to place two fingers in the space between the top of the axilla rest of the crutches and the patient's axilla.
         b) When walking with crutches, the patient must be cued to not "hang" on them, as this can cause pressure on the nerves and vessels in the axillary area (Fairchild, 2012).

9. Transfer and gait safety concerns
   a. After a patient has obtained a properly fitted assistive device, he or she is ready for gait training.

Figure 12-6. Axillary Crutches: Measurement and Confirmation of Fit

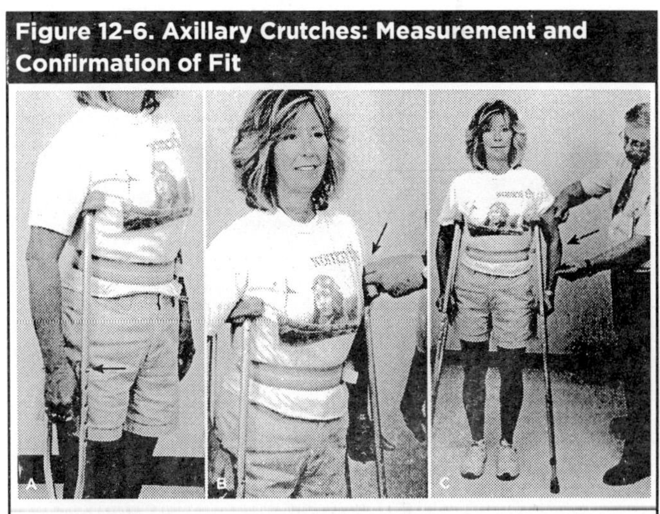

A. Axillary crutches: Correctly measured axillary crutches; B. Confirmation of fit using two-finger check; C. Confirmation of fit with elbow flexed approximately 25 degrees.

From *Principles & Techniques of Patient* Care (5th Edition, Figure 9-6), by S. L. Fairchild, 2012, Stoneham, MA: Elsevier. Copyright 2012 by Elsevier. Reprinted with permission.

b. Before the patient transfers to a standing position, he or she might need assistance shifting from a supine position to a sitting position.

c. Patients who have been recumbent or immobile should be allowed time to adjust to an upright position before transferring to standing.
   1) This can be accomplished by gradually raising the head of the bed.
   2) Raising the head of the bed allows time for the physiological responses to adjust to an upright position. Blood pressure can be monitored during this time to assess cardiovascular response.
   3) After the patient is safely sitting upright, the gait belt can be applied, and the assistive device can be placed in front of the patient ready for walking.

d. It is important to cue a patient to "stand tall," so that a stable, erect posture is maintained during movement.

e. If, while the patient is walking, you observe him or her leaning over the assistive device, use verbal cueing to correct the posture.

f. Always make note of the patient's physiological responses during the activity (e.g., pallor of skin, small perspiration beads over the eyebrows or upper lip, reports of light-headedness).
   1) Such signs and symptoms could require that the activity be stopped.

g. If the patient is transferring in or out of a wheelchair, it is imperative that the wheelchair brakes be locked at all times.
   1) Locking the brakes helps to maintain a safe, stable, nonmoving wheelchair position when the patient is not using it as a mobility device.

h. To come to standing from a seated position in the wheelchair, the patient needs to scoot to the edge of the seat before beginning to rise.
   1) This will keep the body over the base of support, and engage the powerful quadriceps and gluteal muscles for extending the trunk and legs to a standing posture. Feet should be placed on the floor about shoulder width apart to maintain a wide base of support for stability.

i. After the patient has ambulated and returned to the wheelchair, and he or she is close to the wheelchair seat, instruct him or her to turn around until the back of the legs are against the seat of the wheelchair.
   1) The patient then can reach for the arms of the wheelchair and safely lower into the seat.

j. Body mechanics and movement
   1) Activities related to transfers, stability in movement, safety with properly fitting equipment, and guarding the patient all are based on key foundational concepts.
   2) One of the most important of these concepts is good body mechanics for the healthcare provider as well as the patient.
   3) Both the healthcare provider and the patient should use good body mechanics at all times.
   4) By keeping the body over the base of support, the feet can distribute the weight evenly and produce more energy-efficient movements (Figure 12-5).
   5) For the rehabilitation worker, this involves planning before actually moving or assisting the patient, especially a patient who has had bariatric surgery.
   6) Assuming a standing posture with a wide base of support (feet about shoulder-width apart) and feet slightly staggered (one foot slightly in front of the other) provides a solid support for any unexpected changes.
   7) Maintaining a neutral spine and rotating the trunk as a unit, with the trunk/core muscles contracting, makes safer and stronger movements possible with less effort and decreased risk of injury.
   8) For an obese patient, mechanical lifts (**Figure 12-7**), operated manually, help a single worker to transfer the patient safely out of bed and to another location.
      a) The system uses a hydraulic fluid system to raise and lower the patient (Fairchild, 2012).
      b) Guidelines for use of this equipment should be available in the facility or should be obtained from the manufacturer.
      c) Similar types of lifts are electrically powered; however, they function in the same manner as mechanical lifts.

B. Orthotics and Prosthetics
   1. Another patient mobility consideration in a rehabilitation setting involves the variety of orthotics and prosthetics that patients wear.
      a. The types, designs, and technological complexity can vary considerably among these devices.

b. Each device is the result of an extensive assessment of the biomechanical, physiological, and kinematic (i.e., mechanical) principles of patients' presenting impairments.
c. The discussion that follows addresses the areas of orthotics and prosthetics separately, with clinical application focusing primarily on the rehabilitation setting.
d. Orthotics
   1) An external appliance that is worn to assist or restrict motion, or transfer the load from one area of the body to another, is an *orthotic* (formerly known as a *brace*) (O'Sullivan, Schmitz, & Fulk, 2014).
   2) A *splint* is an orthotic intended for short-term use.
   3) The healthcare professional who designs, fabricates, and fits orthoses for the limbs and trunk is the *orthotist*.
   4) The healthcare professional who designs, fabricates, and fits orthoses for the shoes and feet is the *pedorthist*.
   5) Orthesis nomenclature changes to indicate the joint involved and the type of motion. The older names were based on the name of the developer.
   6) As such, some of the names describe the use of the device and include
      a) Foot orthoses (FOs), appliances fitted to the foot and applied inside or outside the shoe (e.g., heel lifts or metatarsal pads [**Figure 12-8**])
      b) Ankle-foot orthosis (AFO) (Figure 12-8), fitted in the shoe and ending below the knee
      c) Knee-ankle-foot orthosis (KAFO) (**Figure 12-9**) extends from the shoe to the thigh

Figure 12-7. Mechanical Lift

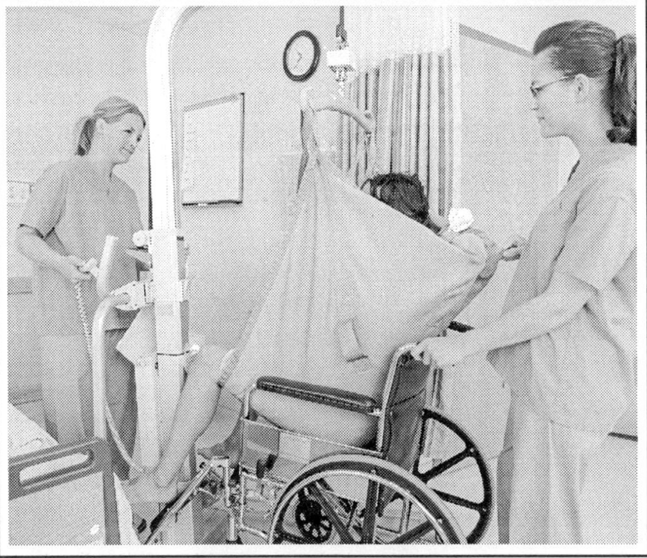

This is a type of electrical mechanical lift that can raise or lower the patient by pressing the control button on the unit. The lift includes a support/harness in which a totally dependent patient can be transferred with the assistance of only one person.

Figure 12-8. Foot Orthoses and Related Parts

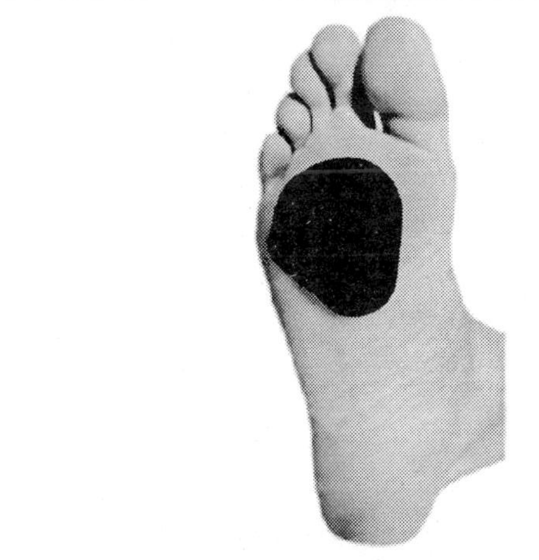

Copyright by Performance Foot. Reprinted with permission. Retrieved from http://www.performancefoot.com/ball-of-foot-pain-relief/81-gel-metatarsal-pad.html

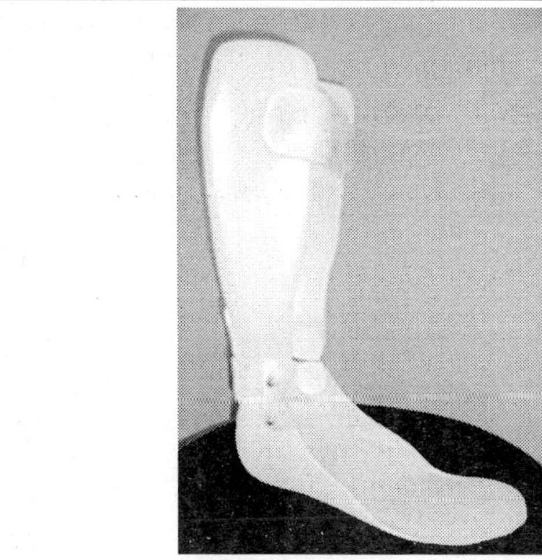

Copyright by Dagny Laur, C.O., American Limb & Orthopedic Company of Valparaiso. Reprinted with permission. Retrieved from http://www.americanlimbvalparaiso.com/orthoses.php

d) Hip-knee-ankle-foot orthosis (HKAFO) (**Figure 12-10**) is a KAFO with a pelvic band surrounding the lower torso

Figure 12-9. Conventional and Plastic Knee-Ankle-Foot Orthoses

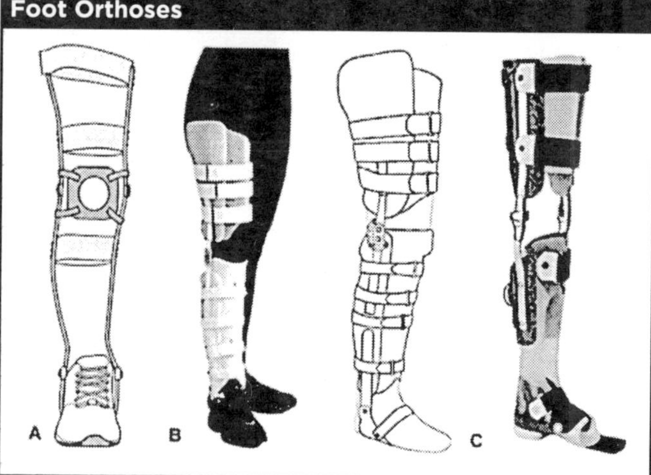

A. Conventional KAFO with knee cap; B. Plastic KAFO pictured on a subject together with schematic of same orthosis; C. This orthosis allows conversion between an AFO and KAFO based on patient requirements. The knee component that provides more proximal alignment and stability is detachable to create an AFO.

Figure 12-10. Hip-Knee-Ankle-Foot Orthosis

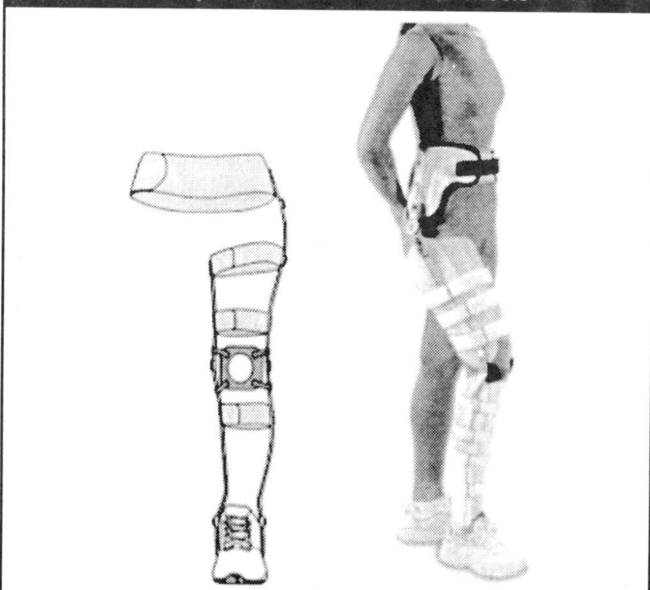

(Left) Conventional HKAFO with stirrup; uprights; hinged ankle, knee, and hip joints; drop ring locks at the knee and hip; and pelvic band. (Right) Plastic and metal HKAFO with hip and knee joints unlocked.

e) Trunk-hip-knee-ankle-foot orthosis (THKAFO) (**Figure 12-11**) covers the lower extremities and part of the trunk
f) Knee orthosis (KO) and hip orthosis.

7) A patient with a newly diagnosed condition, disease, or trauma may have his or her first exposure to an orthotic in a rehabilitation setting.
8) Depending on the intended function, orthoses can be constructed from any number of materials (e.g., metal, plastic, carbon fiber).
9) Some AFOs have spring-loaded ankle joints to assist walking for patient with hemiplegia and a drop-foot condition secondary to paralysis.
10) Other orthoses can be constructed from hard plastic and steel to provide static assistance where muscle power is lacking completely.
11) Computer-controlled KAFOs powered by lithium batteries (**Figure 12-12**) are available to support the knee joint during the rehabilitation process.
12) Other types of orthotics with more extensive components, such as silicon chips within the HKAFO, are available and typically used by patients with paraplegia.
13) Because orthotics such as the HKAFO and THKAO are more cumbersome to don/doff and add weight to the device, they are carefully analyzed before they are prescribed.
14) With any type of orthotic, skin integrity must be examined in the rehabilitation setting daily, particularly for patients who have a compromised sensory system.
15) If a patient reports problems with the fit of the orthotic, the information needs to be communicated to the physical therapist and the orthotist.
16) Trunk orthoses are used to support the trunk and control spinal motion.
    a) These arthoses can also be used in conjunction with lower-extremity orthoses.
    b) They can be worn to reduce the impact of disability caused by low back pain, scoliosis, neck pain, or other skeletal or musculoskeletal disorders (O'Sullivan et al., 2014).
    c) Trunk orthoses can be worn in rehabilitation settings by patients with spinal cord injury, in which vertebral motion is restricted, or the abdomen is

Figure 12-11. Trunk-Hip-Knee-Ankle-Foot Orthosis

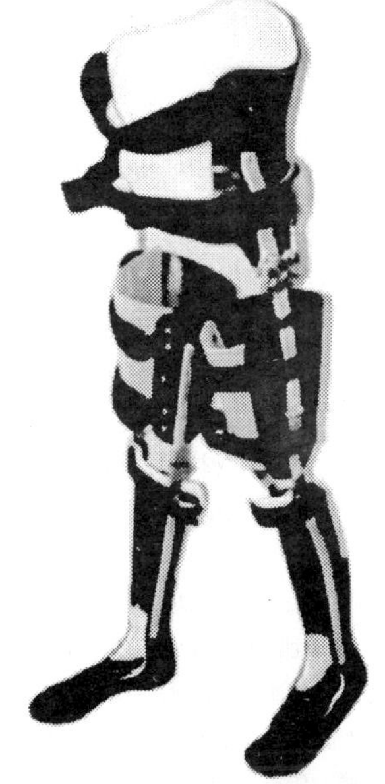

From *Most Common Types of Hip Knee Ankle Foot Orthotic* by M. Raney, 2015, Round Rock Orthotics and Prosthetics (RROP), Inc. Copyright 2015 by RROP, Inc. Reprinted with permission. Retrieved from https://rropinc.wordpress.com/2015/03/18/most-common-types-of-hip-knee-ankle-foot-orthotic/

compressed to improve respiration, or both.

17) Neck orthoses restrict neck motion until surgery or other approaches provide needed spinal stability.
18) Other types of orthoses in this trunk orthosis group include corsets (**Figure 12-13**) to increase intrabdominal pressure; lumbosacral or thoracolumbosacral orthoses (**Figure 12-14**) to restrict motion; cervical collar (soft or hard, such as a Philadelphia collar) (**Figure 12-15**); scoliosis orthoses such as a Milwaukee orthosis (**Figure 12-16**); and the halo cervical orthosis (**Figure 12-17**) for maximal stabilization of the head and neck, usually after cervical fractures.
19) Maintenance, routine inspection, and proper wear of the support device is critical to successful use of all these types of orthoses.
    a) Inspection of skin integrity upon removal of an orthotic allows monitoring of potential pressure areas and helps to avoid skin ulceration.

e. Amputation and prosthetics
   1) Along the healthcare continuum, rehabilitation hospitals typically are the setting for care of patients with a surgical, disease-related, congenital, or traumatic amputation.

Figure 12-12. Knee-Ankle-Foot Orthosis with Electronic Knee Control

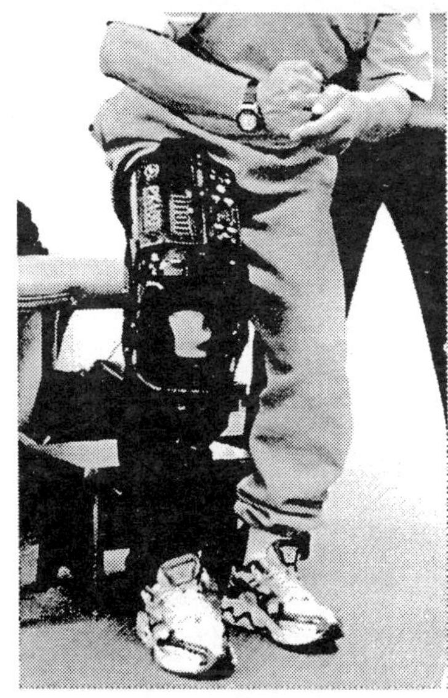

Patient moving from sit-to-stand wearing the Tibion Bionic Leg (Courtesy of Alter-G Corporation). This is a KAFO with electronic knee control designed to support the rehabilitation process. A computer allows the therapist to program the amount of support the orthosis is providing during various tasks.

From *Physical rehabilitation* (6th edition), by S. B. O'Sullivan, T. J. Schmitz, & G. D. Fulk, 2013, Philadelphia: F. A. Davis. Copyright 2013 by F. A. Davis. Courtesy of Alter-G Corporation. Reprinted with permission of F. A. Davis.

   2) After amputation, such patients are fitted for a prosthesis to replace the absent arm or leg.
   3) A *prosthetist* is the member of the healthcare team who designs, fabricates, and fits limb prostheses.
   4) The prosthetist and physical therapist work closely together, particularly during the initial phase of fitting, to ensure that the wear, comfort, and adaptability of a lower-extremity prosthesis is optimized for gait training.
   5) Key members of the full rehabilitation team for a patient with an amputation include the physician, nurse, physical therapist, occupational therapist, and prosthetist.
   6) Amputations in the lower extremity are more common than those in the upper extremity (O'Sullivan et al., 2014).
      a) The main lower-extremity prostheses include partial foot, transtibial, and transfemoral (**Figure 12-18**); Syme's (**Figure 12-19**); and hip and knee disarticulations.

b) Partial foot prostheses work to restore foot function or simulate the shape of the part of the foot that is missing (O'Sullivan et al., 2014).

c) A *Syme's amputation* is done by sectioning the lower extremity through the tibia and fibula at the distal end, and removing the foot while preserving the calcaneal fat pad.

  (i) Patients typically can bear a significant amount of weight through the distal end of the limb.

d) A *transtibial amputation*, formerly known as a below-knee amputation, is made by transecting the leg through the tibia and fibula.

  (i) The anatomical knee remains in place with its motor and sensory innervations intact.

  (ii) This type of procedure is typically performed on patients with vascular disease (Johannsson, Larsson, & Ramstrand, 2009).

7) With a *transfemoral amputation*, the leg is transected across the femur.

  a) If the amputation is at the distal end of the femur, the patient can wear a knee disarticulation prosthesis.

  b) If, however, the amputation is near the greater trochanter (i.e., near the hip joint), the patient will need a hip disarticulation prosthesis.

Figure 12-13. Corset

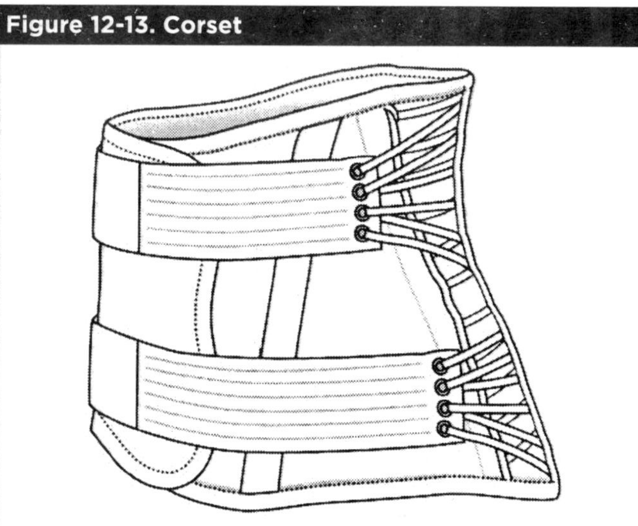

Lumbosacral corset (cotton/elastic polymer) with front hook-and-loop closure.

From *Physical rehabilitation* (6th edition), by S. B. O'Sullivan, T. J. Schmitz, & G. D. Fulk, 2013, Philadelphia: F. A. Davis. Copyright 2013 by F. A. Davis. Reprinted with permission.

Figure 12-14. Thoracolumbosacral Orthoses

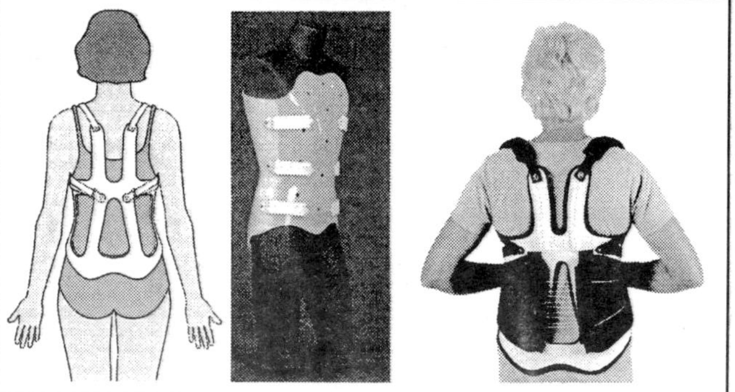

(Left) Conventional thoracolumbosacral flexion, extension, lateral (TLS FEL) control orthosis. (Middle) Custom-fabricated plastic TLS FEL. (Right) Prefabricated, adjustable TLS FEL.

Courtesy of Orthomerica Products, Inc. Copyright 2015 by Orthomerica Products, Inc. Reprinted with permission.

Figure 12-15. Philadelphia Collar

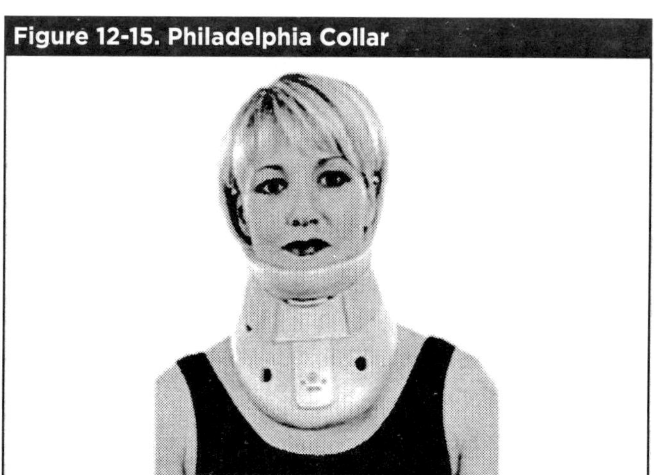

Copyright by Trulife. Reprinted with permission. Retrieved from http://trulife.com/all-products/orthotics/cervical/rigid-collar/philadelphia-trachea-collar

Figure 12-16. Milwaukee Orthosis

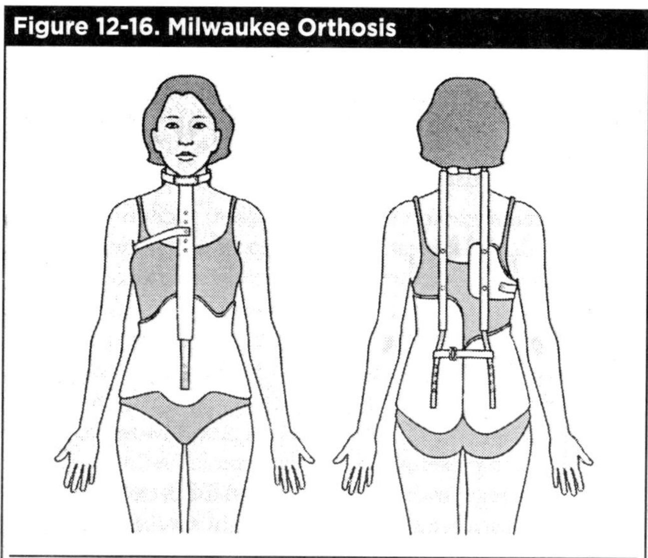

From *Physical rehabilitation* (6th edition), by S. B. O'Sullivan, T. J. Schmitz, & G. D. Fulk, 2013, Philadelphia: F. A. Davis. Copyright 2013 by F. A. Davis. Reprinted with permission.

Figure 12-17. Halo Cervical Orthoses

Halo cervical orthoses restrict movement in the upper cervical spine when more postoperative stabilization is required.

Copyright by Trulife. Reprinted with permission. Retrieved from http://trulife.com/all-products/orthotics/cervical/non-invasive-halo/lerman-non-invasive-halo

8) With any of these prostheses, optimal function depends on general health maintenance and proper care of the amputation limb, prosthesis, socks or sheaths, and the unaffected limb.
9) All rehabilitation team members interacting with a patient who sustained an amputation are likely to confront related psychological issues of one form or another.
    a) The support, encouragement, and education from all team members help empower patients to reach treatment goals.
    b) Communication among all rehabilitation team members is paramount with any of the abovementioned patient scenarios.
    c) Evidence supports the significance and role of clinical team management (Granville & Menetrez, 2010; Potter & Scoville, 2008).

2. In the rehabilitation setting, communication and collaboration are paramount for successful treatment outcomes. The coordinated exchange of information, done formally via the medical record and informally with face-to-face interactions, provides the groundwork for sound decision making in a patient-centered environment. Successful rehabilitation depends on the collaborative efforts of all team members to focus on the whole person.
3. **Table 12-1** summarizes the key points concerning equipment and technology used for mobility.

C. The Nurse's Role with Equipment Used to Aid Mobility
1. Communicate with PT department.
    a. How unfamiliar equipment works

Figure 12-18. Transfemoral and Transtibial Prostheses

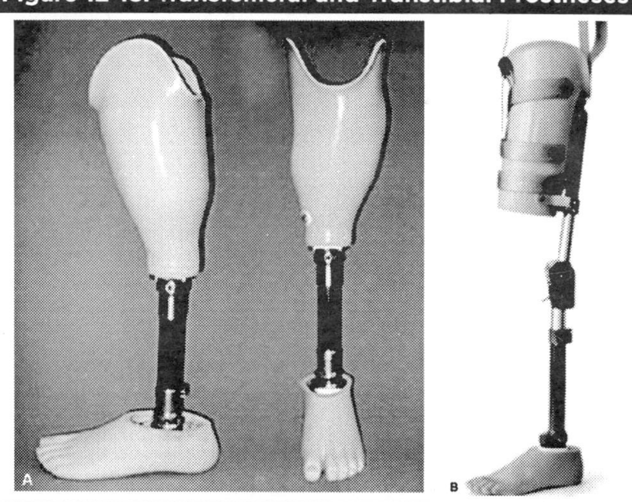

A. Transtibial Prosthesis; B. Tansfemeral Prosthesis.

A. Image courtesy of Center for Prosthetics Orthotics (CPO), Inc. Copyright by CPO, Inc. Reprinted with permission. Retreived from http://cpo.biz/transtibial-prosthesis/

B. Image courtesy of Ossur, Inc. Copyright by Ossur, Inc. Reprinted with permission. Retrieved from http://www.ossur.co.uk/prosthetic-solutions/products/post-operative-and-rehabilitation/femurett

Figure 12-19. Syme's Prostheses

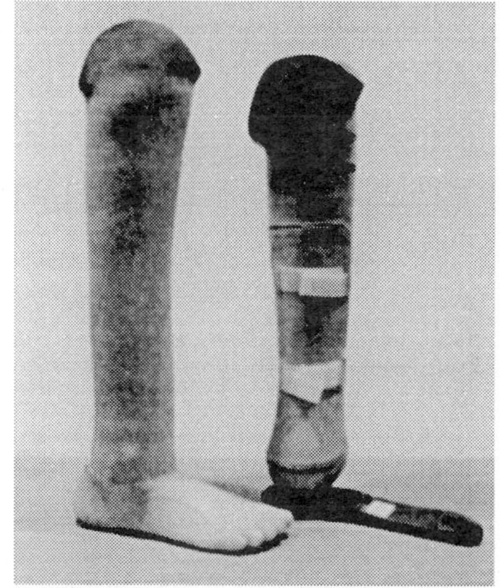

(Left) Socket with continuous walls. (Right) Socket with medial opening.

From *Physical rehabilitation* (6th edition), by S. B. O'Sullivan, T. J. Schmitz, & G. D. Fulk, 2014, Philadelphia: F. A. Davis. Copyright 2013 by F. A. Davis. Reprinted with permission.

    b. How to apply equipment
    c. When to use equipment
    d. How to clean equipment
    e. Safety monitoring points
    f. Potential complications to monitor
2. Share information with PT on the use of prescribed equipment.
    a. Patient's ability to don/doff
        1) Amount of assistance required

Table 12-1. Equipment and Technology Used for Mobility

	Description	Indications/ Benefits	Contraindications/ Disadvantages	Proper Techniques for Use	Safety/Monitoring
Gait Belt (see Figure 12-3)	A thick, strong strap/belt with a buckle fastener worn around the patient's waist during mobility activities	Patient wears gait belt during all mobility and transfer activities, so that the therapist or other assistant holding on to the belt can assist the patient back to a stable position in the event of a loss of balance or fall	For patients with a feeding tube (e.g., a PEG [percutaneous endoscopic gastrostomy]), the level of the gait belt must be adjusted to avoid disruption of the ostomy site at the PEG entrance.	Gait belt is securely fastened around the patient's waist; it could require adjustment once the patient has assumed an upright position.	Use of a gait belt is critical when ambulating a patient; although it does not prevent a fall, it does provide an optimal level of safety in the event of loss of balance or consciousness.
Cane: Single Tip (see Figures 12-2B and 12-2C)	Made of wood or aluminum; can be transported or stored more easily than crutches or a walker. Types can include "J," "T," pistol grip, or offset shaft	Used with patients who have impaired balance or need more stability; they are more functional on stairs and/or in small, confined spaces	Proper fit is essential for the safe use of this assistive device. The appropriate weight-bearing status must be maintained during mobility.	Physical therapist instructs patient on gait pattern and safety factors associated with this assistive device. Specific instructions on care and use of this assistive device is provided by the physical therapist.	Patient might need verbal cues for proper use of the device (as instructed by the physical therapist); the device should be used at all times to ensure stability and safety in mobility when navigating through the environment.
Cane: Quad (see Figures 12-2B and 12-2C)	Made of aluminum; can be transported or stored more easily than crutches or a walker; is four-legged or four-footed and often called a "quad cane"	Used with patients who have impaired balance or need more stability; they are more functional on stairs and/or in small, confined spaces	Proper fit is essential for the safe use of this assistive device. The appropriate weight-bearing status must be maintained during mobility.	Physical therapist instructs patient on gait pattern and safety factors associated with this assistive device. Specific instructions on care and use of this assistive device is provided by the physical therapist.	Patient might need verbal cues for proper use of the device (as instructed by the physical therapist); the device should be used at all times to ensure stability and safety in mobility when navigating through the environment.
Walker: With wheels (two or four wheels; standard and front-wheeled) (see Figure 12-2A)	Various styles available; most have four support legs ("feet"); most are adjustable for proper fit; most are light weight; some can be folded for storage; sizes range from child to bariatric	Used with patients who require maximal support and stability	Proper fit is essential for the safe use of this assistive device. The appropriate weight-bearing status must be maintained during mobility.	Physical therapist instructs patient on gait pattern and safety factors associated with this assistive device. Specific instructions on care and use of this assistive device is provided by the physical therapist.	Patient might need verbal cues for proper use of the device (as instructed by the physical therapist); the device should be used at all times to ensure stability and safety in mobility when navigating through the environment.

continued

Table 12-1. Equipment and Technology Used for Mobility (continued)

	Description	Indications/ Benefits	Contraindications/ Disadvantages	Proper Techniques for Use	Safety/Monitoring
Walker: without wheels (see Figure 12-2A)	Various styles available; all with four support legs ("feet"); most are adjustable for proprer fit and light weight; some can be folded for storage; sizes range from pediatric to bariatric	Used with patients requiring maximal support and stability.	Proper fit is essential for the safe use of this assistive device. The appropriate weight-bearing status must be maintained during mobility.	Physical therapist instructs patient on gait pattern and safety factors associated with this assistive device. Specific instructions on care and use of this assistive device is provided by the physical therapist.	Patient might need verbal cues for proper use of the device (as instructed by the physical therapist); the device should be used at all times to ensure stability and safety in mobility when navigating through the environment.
Walker: other (hemiplegic or one-handed walker) (see Figure 12-2C)	Redesigned for patients with use of only one upper extremity (postparalysis of one side); four legs of walker converge to a common base with single hand grip.	Used with patients requiring maximal support and stability.	Proper fit is essential for the safe use of this assistive device. The appropriate weight-bearing status must be maintained during mobility.	Physical therapist instructs patient on gait pattern and safety factors associated with this assistive device. Specific instructions on care and use of this assistive device is provided by the physical therapist.	Patient might need verbal cues for proper use of the device (as instructed by the physical therapist); the device should be used at all times to ensure stability and safety in mobility when navigating through the environment.
Crutches (axillary crutches) (see Figures 12-2B, 12-6)	Most are made of wood or aluminum and easily adjusted for proper fit; can be transported and stored; can use in narrow spaces or for stairs; can be slight differences among types.	Used with patients requiring less support or stability than a walker or parallel bars; patient has greater selection of gait speed and gait pattern; they provide support and stability.	Proper fit is essential for the safe use of this assistive device. The appropriate weight-bearing status must be maintained during mobility.	Physical therapist instructs patient on gait pattern and safety factors associated with this assistive device. Specific instructions on care and use of this assistive device is provided by the physical therapist.	Patient might need verbal cues for proper use of the device (as instructed by the physical therapist); the device should be used at all times to ensure stability and safety in mobility when navigating through the environment.
Crutches (forearm crutches; also called Lofstrand or Canadian crutches) (see Figure 12-2B)	Made of wood or aluminum; can be adjustable or non-adjustable; easy to transport and store; crutch remains on the forearm when reaching for object secondary to the forearm cuff.	Used when the stability and support of axillary crutches is not needed, but patient needs more support and stability than a cane can provide. They remove the potential for damage to axillary vessels and nerves; they are more functional on stairs and in small, confined spaces.	Proper fit is essential for the safe use of this assistive device. The appropriate weight-bearing status must be maintained during mobility.	Physical therapist instructs patient on gait pattern and safety factors associated with this assistive device. Specific instructions on care and use of this assistive device is provided by the physical therapist.	Patient might need verbal cues for proper use of the device (as instructed by the physical therapist); the device should be used at all times to ensure stability and safety in mobility when navigating through the environment.

continued

Table 12-1. Equipment and Technology Used for Mobility (continued)					
	Description	**Indications/ Benefits**	**Contraindications/ Disadvantages**	**Proper Techniques for Use**	**Safety/Monitoring**
Crutches (platform crutches) (see Figure 12-2B)	Platform is attached to an axillary or forearm crutch or to a walker; it is also known as a "trough" or "shelf."	Used with patients unable to bear weight through wrists and hands, who present with severe wrist or finger deformities that make it difficult to grasp the handpiece of a regular crutch, have a below-elbow amputation, or are unable to extend one or both elbows.	Proper fit is essential for the safe use of this assistive device. The appropriate weight-bearing status must be maintained during mobility.	Physical therapist instructs patient on gait pattern and safety factors associated with this assistive device. Specific instructions on care and use of this assistive device is provided by the physical therapist.	Patient might need verbal cues for proper use of the device (as instructed by the physical therapist); the device should be used at all times to ensure stability and safety in mobility when navigating through the environment.
Wheelchair (see Figure 12-5)	Many types and styles with varying features; can be manual or electric; most have armrests; wheels (large back and front casters); front rigging (leg rest, footrest); seating system (back rest and seat). Some recline; many fold for storage and transportation.	Is a means of transportation or mobility; also can provide support, stability, and safety for functional activities Proper fit paramount with patients who have decreased sensory awareness; limited ability to change position; loss of soft tissue (bony prominences at risk); impaired peripheral circulation in bilateral lower extremity; abnormal skin integrity; used when mobility device is needed for extended time as a mobility device.	Patient with open lesions over ischial tuberosities or posterior thighs, hips, and back.	Propulsion of wheelchair independently. The user grasps the hand rims at the top of the wheels (the 12 o'clock position) and pushes forward or pulls backward with equal force on each wheel. For a turn, patient holds one hand on one rim while pushing or pulling the other rim with the opposite hand. Every patient should be taught how to (a) operate the wheel locks and tighten them if needed; (b) remove and replace arm rests; (c) remove, replace, and swing away front rigging; and (d) elevate and lower the footplates prior to activity. More specific procedures required with specialized types; these require special training by physical therapist. Includes but not limited to navigating curbs, elevators, inclines, uneven surfaces.	Wheelchair brakes should be locked before transferring in or out of wheelchair; additional support or restraint could be necessary with poor trunk control or extraneous, uncontrollable movements; for proper usage, wheelchair parts must be cleaned and maintained on a regular basis.

continued

Table 12-1. Equipment and Technology Used for Mobility (continued)					
	Description	**Indications/ Benefits**	**Contraindications/ Disadvantages**	**Proper Techniques for Use**	**Safety/Monitoring**
Mechanical Lift (see Figure 12-7)	An electrical (battery powered) or manual (hydraulic), mechanical lift with a large, wide-based, C-shaped hoist to which is attached a large body sling that holds the patient.	Used for totally dependent patients or those who have had bariatric surgery; used for patients weighing up to 450 pounds, depending on the specification for the lift; user must follow weight limitations provided by the manufacturer.	If manufacturer's weight limits are exceeded, patient injury is possible. Recent surgical procedures (such as total joint replacements) can preclude the safe use of this lift.	Patient is positioned on the body sling while in bed; the wide, wheeled U-base of the lift is rolled into position at bedside. Sling supporting patient is attached to the lift; the lever of the lift is "pumped" as the body sling/ patient comes off the bed. Once cleared off the bed, the lift can be rolled to its destination.	Make sure all rings, or S-hooks, of the body sling are attached to lift arm before moving lift out of position. Caution patient not to reach for the spreader bar when being raised.
Orthotics (see Figures 12-8–12-17)	A group of orthoses or custom-made braces designed, fabricated, and fitted to patients with neuromuscular and musculoskeletal impairments. Can be made of leather, metal, wood, thermoplastic materials, foamed plastic, and visco-elastic polymers.	Used to assist patients with functional limitation and disability For persons with neuromuscular or musculoskeletal dysfunction, orthotics assist in support, gait, stability, and positioning to prevent contractures, minimizing the impact of abnormal movement. Many other benefits, depending on the orthotic design.	Improperly fitted orthotics can lead to skin breakdown and affect performance of functional skills; patient's tolerance for wear and/ or use of an orthotic affects overall performance in function. If patient is unable to don/ doff orthotic independently, another person will be required to do so.	Patient is instructed in proper use of the orthotic by the physical therapist (mobility or truncal/ spinal support devices) or the occupational therapist (ADL).	Patient's skin integrity should be monitored for potential pressure from the orthotic; patient is instructed by the therapist in the care and use of the orthotic. Patient reports of sensory changes (e.g., pressure, numbness, pain) at or near the area covered by the orthotic must be reported to the therapist or orthotist for follow-up.
Prosthetics (see Figures 12-18, 12-19)	A group of prostheses or custom-made artificial limbs designed, fabricated, and fitted to patients with partial or total loss of limbs. Can be made of leather, metal, wood, or thermoplastic materials, foamed plastic, and visco-elastic polymers.	Functions to replace the missing limb.	Improperly fitted prosthetics can lead to skin breakdown and affect performance of functional skills; patient's tolerance for wear or use of a prosthetic affects overall performance in function; if patient unable to don/doff prosthetic independently, another person will be required to do so.	Patient is instructed in proper usage of the prosthesis by the physical therapist (mobility or truncal devices) or by the occupational therapist (ADL).	Patient's skin integrity should be monitored for potential pressure from the orthotic; patient is instructed by the therapist in the care and use of the orthotic. Patient reports of sensory changes (e.g., pressure, numbness, pain) at or near the area covered by the orthotic must be reported to the therapist or orthotist for follow-up.

continued

Table 12-1. Equipment and Technology Used for Mobility (continued)					
	Description	**Indications/ Benefits**	**Contraindications/ Disadvantages**	**Proper Techniques for Use**	**Safety/Monitoring**
Standing Frame (see Figure 12-1)	Standing device with a metal framework that includes a standing platform with a forward tray and support straps for supported upright standing.	Patient is securely positioned in standing to perform functional activities with weight bearing in postural joints for proprioceptive input.	Patients who are intolerant of upright standing position for extended periods.	Used in physical therapy department.	Checking for pressure areas could be needed if sensation impairments are present; checking for vital signs to monitor patient's tolerance for upright position.
Tilt Table (see Figure 12-1)	Battery-powered table with a foot board that can be gradually and incrementally elevated from full horizontal position to full vertical position; straps positioned to prevent patient from falling forward as table is inclined.	Persons who need to gradually acclimate (physiologically) to an upright position secondary to conditions such as: prolonged recumbence, decreased proprioception; impaired balance, kinesthesia, or lower-extremity circulation; or generalized weakness. Table can be elevated gradually and maintained at any position.	If the person is non-weight bearing (NWB) on one lower extremity, a platform or wooden box can be placed under the weight-bearing extremity so the NWB extremity is not in contact with the footboard of the tilt table.	Used in physical therapy department.	Monitor vital signs and/or signs of distress when changing to an upright position.

Note. The devices listed here are most commonly used by patients in rehabilitation settings. This list is not all-inclusive; other devices available are tailored for specific conditions.

From *Orthotics and Prosthetics in Rehabilitation* (3rd Edition), 2012, by M. Lusard, M. Jorge, & C. Nielsen. St Louis: Elsevier. Copyright 2012 by Elsevier. Reprinted with permission.

b. Patient's ability to use safely
c. Patient's understanding of equipment purpose and function
d. If the nurse thinks the equipment is not functioning as planned
    1) Malfunctioning
    2) Poor fit
    3) Too complex for patient
    4) Complex wearing schedule that does not fit with patient routine
    5) Problems with maintaining cleanliness and hygiene

3. Collaborate with PT on communication method to share equipment information with all nursing staff.
    a. Day shift, evening shift, night shift
    b. Wearing schedules, safety issues
4. Sponsor a PT equipment fair at regular intervals.
    a. Competency training and testing of nursing staff
    b. Updates on the latest and best equipment

II. Occupational Therapy and Adaptive Equipment: Tools to Support Performance of Daily Occupations

Occupational therapists address a person's ability to perform daily occupations as successfully and independently as possible. In a rehabilitation setting, daily occupations of self-care are often a primary focus in intervention because a person's ability to participate in the self-care or activities of daily living (ADLs) is often a deciding factor in discharge destination and the amount of caregiver assistance that will be required.

A. *Adaptive equipment* refers to devices that facilitate a person's ability to complete daily tasks by compensating for impairments he or she has as a result of injury or illness (Thomas, Pinkelman, & Gardine, 2010).

B. Occupational therapists recommend specific pieces of adaptive equipment based on their assessment of a person's abilities and challenges, and the demands of the activity that will be performed in a specific context.

C. For many patients, adaptive equipment is important in assisting them to perform ADLs to the highest level of independence possible while in the rehabilitation setting.

1. Many patients will require assistance to set up the equipment for use, but then can perform an activity at their own pace.

D. Some patients use adaptive equipment until their skills or abilities improve, or until they no longer require the equipment for safety's sake. However, some patients will need to utilize adaptive equipment as a long-term, compensatory approach to help them perform their ADLs.

E. Key things to remember when assisting patients with adaptive equipment:
   1. Occupational therapists have selected specific adaptive devices for patients based on their patients' needs, requirements of their activities, and therapy goals.
   2. Never hesitate to contact a patient's occupational therapist to discuss why he or she has recommended a specific piece of adaptive equipment for the patient.
   3. Many types of adaptive equipment are individually fit and adjusted specifically for a patient; therefore, many pieces of equipment are not interchangeable among patients.
   4. Infection control practices are best observed by not using the same piece of equipment for more than one patient at a time.
   5. Patients and their families are often overwhelmed by the amount of information they receive in the rehabilitation setting.
   6. Most likely, an occupational therapist has trained a patient and family as appropriate on the use of a particular type of adaptive equipment. However, many patients need repetition in training, and this might not become evident until a patient attempts to use adaptive equipment away from a therapy session.
   7. If a patient appears to need additional education or training, do not hesitate to notify his or her occupational therapist.
   8. Research has indicated that patients can be resistant to developing new habits or routines, such as using adaptive equipment, because they fear it signifies that they will not progress or improve in their abilities (Wallenbert & Jonsson, 2005).
   9. If a patient seems resistant to using adaptive equipment, remind him or her that the equipment is intended to help him or her be more functional, and that it might not be needed in the future.

F. Equipment to Support Eating (**Table 12-2**)
   1. Eating is an activity of daily living that is very personal and important to most patients.
   2. Many patients are highly motivated to feed themselves as independently as possible rather than having a nurse or family member feed them.
   3. Adaptive equipment can help to enable a person to feed himself or herself, but most patients need to have the equipment set up.

G. Grooming and Hygiene
   1. Grooming and hygiene tasks are often initiated early in the rehabilitation process as they can be performed in brief sessions from a variety of positions.
      a. However, the requirement to manipulate small items can make these tasks a challenge for many patients.
   2. Occupational therapists can adapt grooming and hygiene tasks using readily available products (e.g., spray deodorant, electric razor, electric toothbrush) to reduce the demands of the activity.
   3. Adaptive equipment can also be used to assist in performing these tasks (**Table 12-3**).

H. Dressing
   1. Dressing as a self-care occupation, or ADL, is often a goal of most patients in rehabilitation.
   2. Adaptive equipment can assist in enabling a person to dress himself or herself, but most will require set up of the equipment or supervision for safety while using it during their dressing routine (**Table 12-4**).

I. Bathing (**Table 12-5**)
   1. Bathing is an advanced self-care activity addressed by occupational therapists because the requirements for safe bathing are comparatively stringent with regard to strength, balance, endurance, and safety awareness.
   2. Many commercially available products, such as handheld showers, pump dispensers for shampoo and soap, grab bars, and safety strips for the tub or shower floor, can aid a person in bathing.
   3. However, because these products are used in many households, they are not considered adaptive equipment.

J. Splints and Orthotics (**Table 12-6**)
   1. Splints and orthotics include a variety of devices that can be used to protect joints or an extremity, or provide support to enhance function.

K. The Nurse's Role with Tools to Support Performance of Daily Occupations
   1. Communicate with OT
      a. Equipment prescribed by OT
      b. How to use unfamiliar equipment
         1) Applying, removing
         2) Safety issues
         3) Potential complications

c. Wearing schedule
d. Needs identified by nursing
1) Aids for feeding, toileting, bathing, grooming, or other activities
2. Share information with OT on patient success with using adaptive equipment
a. Ability to don/doff
b. Assistance required
c. Complications seen
1) Pain
2) Skin breakdown
3) Restricted movement
3. Collaborate with OT in planning for the equipment needed and testing it with the patient.
a. Patient education
b. Fabrication of aids

III. Communication Technology

A. Speech language pathologists (SLPs) are the team members primarily responsible for assessment of communication and prescription of adaptive devices to facilitate communication.
B. Augmentative and alternative communication includes all forms of communication beyond speech.
C. Hundreds of methods and devices in use and on the market
1. Unaided communication
2. Body language, gestures, facial expressions
3. Aided communication
4. Pencil and paper
5. Books
6. Boards, letter boards
7. Electronics
8. Computers
9. Written (typed) text, speech generation
10. Speech-generating devices
11. Voice-output communication aids
a. Assist people unable to generate natural speech
b. Can generate word-to-speech common in modern computers or digitized human speech; prerecorded phrases that sound human rather than computerized
c. Growing number of voice-output communication aids becoming available in smartphone configuration applications
d. Depending on equipment, can access speech capabilities with hands/fingers, head pointing, eye pointing, or switch-access scanning
D. Baseline assessment by SLP vital to determine baseline and need
1. Vision
a. Must be able to visualize for many methods of communication
1) Computer screen
2) Picture boards
2. Hearing
a. To participate in oral/aural communication
b. To hear speech-generated voice
3. Cognition
a. Attention and focus
4. Language and literacy skills
5. Method of accessing and using equipment
a. Upper-extremity function
b. Lower-extremity function
c. Head and neck function
d. Oral, tongue function
e. Eye and facial-muscle function
6. Best equipment to use based on all of foregoing, plus
a. Cost
b. Equipment availability
c. Set up
d. Maintenance
e. Internet or telephone access if necessary
f. Accessibility
g. Environment
h. Social support
7. Occupational therapists often collaborate with SLPs to determine baseline function and equipment type.
8. Rehabilitation nursing responsibilities can include
a. Seeking education from SLP on specific devices and methods of communication aids
b. Device or equipment set up and monitoring
c. Basic troubleshooting
d. Referral to SLP as necessary
e. Recommending patients for SLP evaluation for augmentative communication aids
f. Patient and family teaching and ongoing support
9. Resources for learning more include
a. Augmentative and Alternative Communication at the University of Washington, Seattle: http://depts.washington.edu/augcomm/index.htm
b. Augmentative and Alternative Communication: Research Engineering Research Center: http://aac-rerc.psu.edu/index.php/site/index
c. American Speech, Hearing and Language Association: http://www.asha.org/

Table 12-2. Equipment to Support Eating

Adapted Utensils	Description
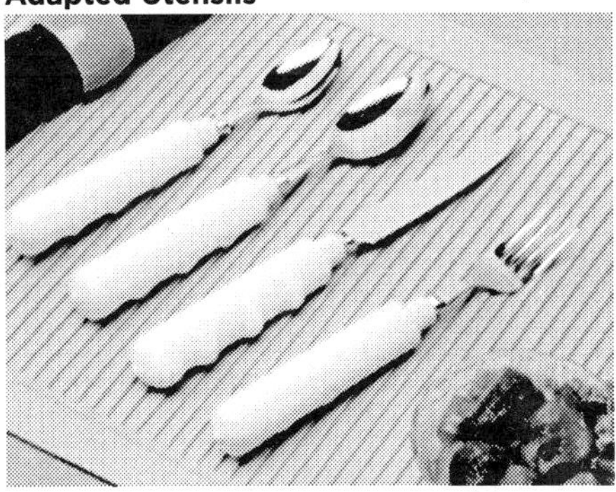 Copyright by RehabMart. Reprinted with permission. Retrieved from http://www.rehabmart.com/product/comfort-grip-utensils-6522.html	**Description** Adapted utensils include any type of utensil that has been modified for use during eating. The most common modification is an adapted handle. Adapted utensils can include those with large handles, angled handles, extended handles, or handles that are weighted. The utensils are commercially available, or the occupational therapist might fabricate an adaptation for the handle from various materials. **Indications/Benefit** Adapted utensils are selected by an occupational therapist to compensate for decreased strength or upper-extremity range of motion. They can be used for people with decreased grip strength, decreased hand or arm range of motion, or decreased coordination. They are beneficial in enabling patients to feed themselves a variety of food items. **Contraindications** Weighted utensils are appropriate only for patients with tremor or ataxia to help stabilize their hands as they feed themselves. Weighted utensils should not be used by patients with weakness, because they will tire quickly while feeding themselves. Do not use utensils if they have not been properly washed after prior use. **Proper Techniques for Use** Provide set-up assistance to ensure that utensils are available for patients at meal times. **Safety/Monitoring** Patients might need to be supervised while using feeding devices to ensure they are complying with prescribed dysphagia precautions. Patients could become fatigued during mealtimes, so monitoring could be required to ensure adequate nutritional intake.
Universal Cuff 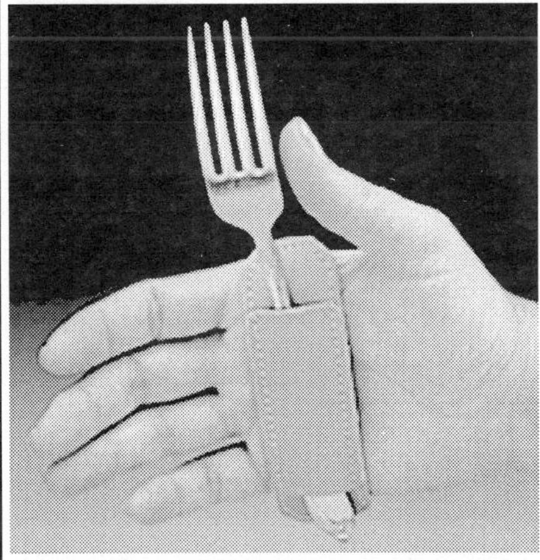 Copyright by The Wright Stuff, Inc. www.wright-stuff.biz. Reprinted with permission. Retrieved from http://www.wrightstuff.biz/unelcu.html	**Description** A universal cuff is a multipurpose piece of adaptive equipment that can be used in a variety of activities of daily living, including eating. The cuff contains a pocket that holds utensils to support self-feeding. **Indications/Benefit** Universal cuffs are used by patients who have decreased hand function and are not able to grasp the handles of objects such as utensils. **Contraindications** None **Proper Techniques for Use** The cuff is positioned so the pocket is placed in the palmar surface of the patient's hand with the opening toward the thumb. The cuff is secured in place by fastening the velcro strap over the dorsal surface of the hand. The utensil is slid into the pocket in preparation for eating. **Safety/Monitoring** The cuff might need to be adjusted or tightened during the meal to ensure best use.

continued

Table 12-2. Equipment to Support Eating (continued)	
Rocker Knife 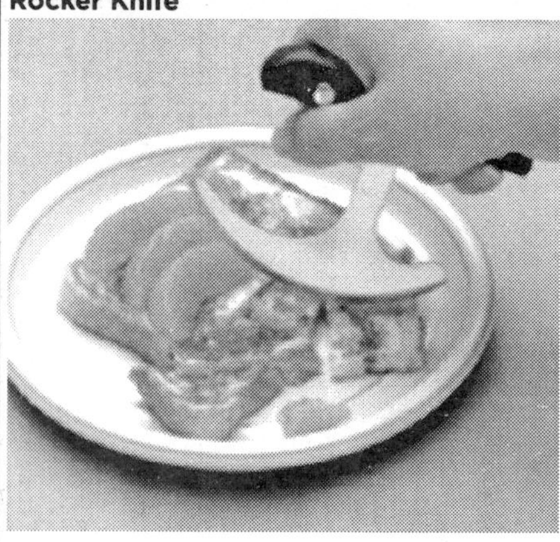 Copyright by RehabMart.com. Reprinted with permission. Retrieved from http://www.rehabmart.com/product/thandle-rocker-knife-135.html	**Description** A rocker knife has a curved blade with a handle. This type of adapted knife requires the use of only one hand, enabling a person to cut food items using a rocking motion. **Indications/Benefit** A rocker knife is utilized by patients who use a one-handed feeding technique. This can include those who have had a stroke or upper-extremity amputation. **Contraindications** Do not use adapted plates if they have not been properly washed after prior use. **Proper Techniques for Use** Food items must be set up on an adapted plate. This can be done in the kitchen or at the table. **Safety/Monitoring** Monitor patients for safe use of the knife because it has a sharp blade.
Adapted Plates 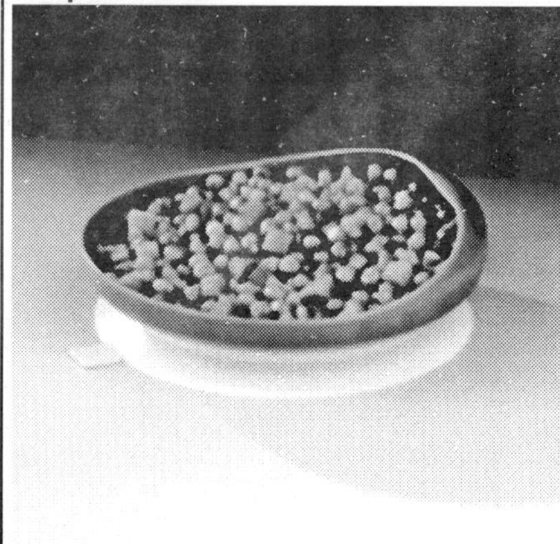 Copyright by The Wright Stuff, Inc. www.wrightstuff.biz. Reprinted with permission. Retrieved from http://www.wrightstuff.biz/blue-scooper-plate-suction-base.html	**Description** Adapted plates are modified to enable a person to more easily scoop food against the side of the plate onto a utensil. **Indications/Benefit** Adapted plates are used by patients who use a one-handed eating technique. They are beneficial in assisting them to place food onto a utensil, preventing food from being pushed off the edge of the plate. **Contraindications** Do not use adapted plates if they have not been properly washed after prior use. **Proper Techniques for Use** Food items must be set up on an adapted plate. This can be done in the kitchen or at the table. **Safety/Monitoring** Patients might need to be supervised while using feeding devices to ensure compliance with prescribed dysphagia precautions.
Plate Guard 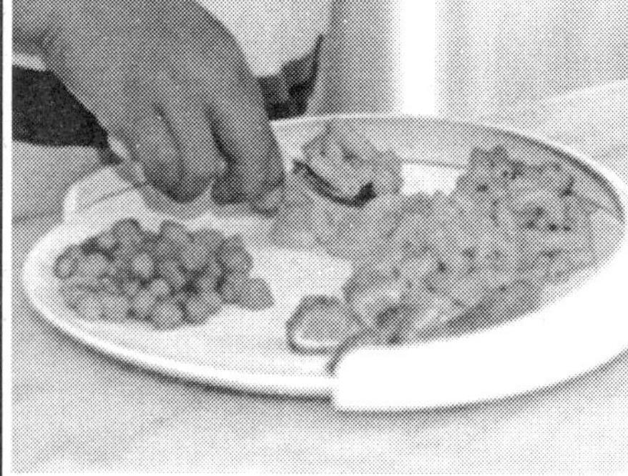 Copyright by The Wright Stuff, Inc. www.wrightstuff.biz. Reprinted with permission. Retrieved from http://www.wrightstuff.biz/myplatemate.html	**Description** Plate guards are metal or plastic devices that are attached to the rim of a plate to enable patients to more easily scoop food against the side of the plate onto a utensil. They are portable and can attach to a variety of plate sizes. **Indications/Benefit** Like adapted plates, plate guards are used by patients who use a one-handed eating technique. They are beneficial in assisting them to place food onto a utensil, and they prevent food from being pushed off the edge of the plate. **Contraindications** Do not use plate guard if it has not been properly washed after prior use. **Proper Techniques for Use** The plate guard needs to be affixed to the rim of the plate at the beginning of the meal. Be sure to remove the plate guard at the end of the meal, and wash it for the next use. **Safety/Monitoring** Patients might need to be supervised while using feeding devices to ensure compliance with prescribed dysphagia precautions.

continued

Table 12-2. Equipment to Support Eating (continued)	
Adapted Cup 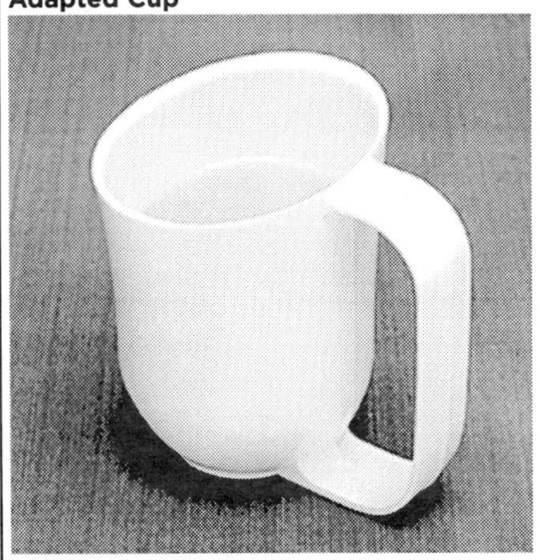 Copyright by The Wright Stuff, Inc. www.wright-stuff.biz. Reprinted with permission. Retrieved from http://www.wrightstuff.biz/dysphagiacup.html	**Description** Adapted cups include a variety of cups made of different materials or modified designs to support a patient's safe intake of liquids. **Indications/Benefit** Adapted cups are used by a variety of patients, including those with dysphagia or who have difficulty handling a traditional cup or glass. These cups might limit the amount of liquid that can be taken at one time, or allow a person to drink from them using a chin-tuck method. **Contraindications** Do not allow patients to use adapted cups if they have not been recommended by the occupational therapist or speech-language pathologist. Do not use cups if they have not been properly washed after prior use. **Proper Techniques for Use** Liquid is poured into cup. Liquid consistency may need to be modified to comply with dysphagia recommendations. **Safety/Monitoring** Patients might need to be supervised while drinking from adapted cups to ensure compliance with prescribed dysphagia precautions.
Nonskid Mats 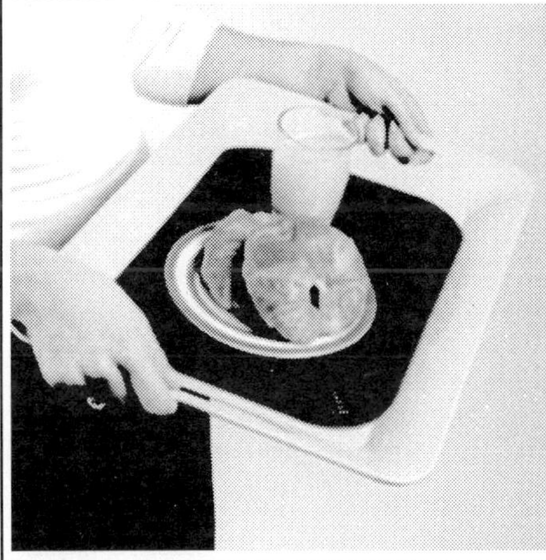 Copyright by The Wright Stuff, Inc. www.wright-stuff.biz. Reprinted with permission. Retrieved from http://www.wrightstuff.biz/dycem-non-slip-large-rectangle-mat.html	**Description** Nonskid mats are used to prevent dishes from sliding on the eating surface. Commercial products such as Dycem® can be used, as can a nonskid shelf liner. **Indications/Benefit** Nonskid mats are used during mealtimes for patients who have decreased coordination or difficulty modulating their movements. **Contraindications** Do not use if the nonskid mat has not been properly cleaned after prior use. **Proper Techniques for Use** The nonskid mat needs to be placed on the eating surface and dishes set on it at the beginning of the meal. **Safety/Monitoring** Patients might need to be supervised during the meal because it is difficult to reposition dishes on the nonskid mat if needed.

Table 12-3. Equipment to Support Grooming and Hygiene

Adapted Handles

Copyright by RehabMart. Reprinted with permission. Retrieved from http://www.rehabmart.com/product/easypull-hairbrush1-9821.html

Description

Adapted handles for grooming items may be fabricated by an occupational therapist using a variety of materials including foam, PVC, or plastic.

Indications/Benefit

Adapted handles can be applied to a variety of grooming items such as combs, brushes, or toothbrushes. A built-up or extended handle can assist a person with limited upper-extremity range of motion or strength to perform their grooming activities.

Contraindications

None

Proper Techniques for Use

The item with the adapted handle is used in a manner that is typical for that item.

Safety/Monitoring

Patients might need to have the item placed in their hand prior to use.

Table 12-4. Equipment to Support Dressing

Button Hooks

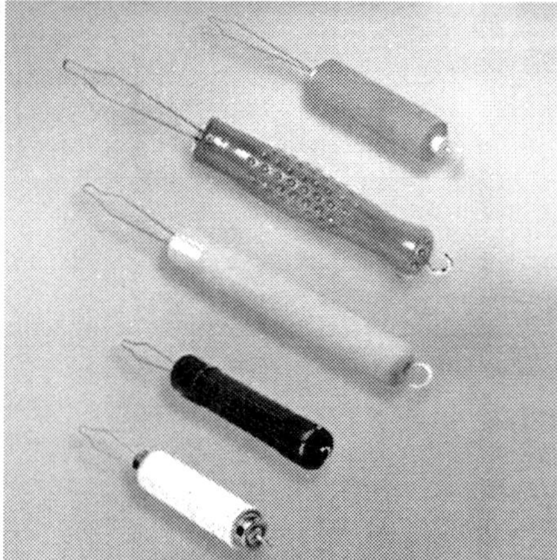

Copyright by Patterson Medical. Reprinted with permission. Retrieved from http://www.pattersonmedical.com/app.aspx?cmd=getProduct&key=IF_921029833

Copyright by Able2 UK Ltd. Reprinted with permission. Retrieved from http://www.able2.eu/product/pr55020/good-grips-button-hook

Description

A button hook is a tapered wire loop attached to a handle.

Indications/Benefit

A button hook will assist a person who has poor hand function to button.

Contraindications

None

Proper Techniques for Use

Direct the patient to slide the wire loop through the button hole. Hook the button in the wire loop. Pull the hooked button back through the button hole. If the patient with either upper extremity is able to stabilize the shirt, this will assist in pulling the button back through the button hole. When the button is pulled through the button hole, release the button from the hook.

Safety/Monitoring

Using a button hook takes practice, so some patients may become frustrated with the process.

continued

Table 12-4. Equipment to Support Dressing (continued)	
Reacher 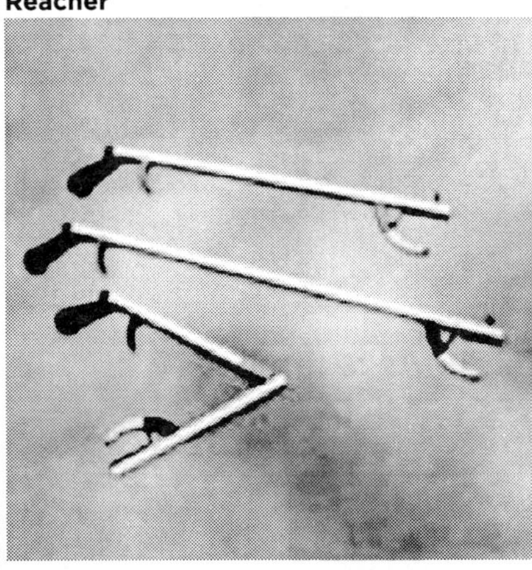 Copyright by Patterson Medical. Reprinted with permission. Retrieved from http://www.pattersonmedical.com/app.aspx?cmd=getProduct&key=IF_921002233	**Description** A reacher is a long-handled device with a grasp feature on one end that is operated by a trigger handle. Reachers come in various lengths and may fold for portability. **Indications/Benefit** Reachers extend the reach of a person, so they are useful when picking up items from low surfaces, retrieving items above shoulder level, and managing clothing for lower body dressing. **Contraindications** Patients with poor sitting balance may be at an increased risk for falls when reaching for items. **Proper Techniques for Use** When using a reacher to assist with dressing activities, have the patient grasp the waist of the pants with the reacher by positioning the material in the grasp end and closing the device using the trigger handle. While maintaining pressure on the handle to keep the grasp end closed, lower the pants toward the feet so the patient can insert one or both legs into the pants. It is usually recommended that the person dress the affected extremity first, particularly if there is weakness, limitations, or precautions in hip range of motion. While still maintaining pressure on the handle, the patient can pull the pants up until he or she is able to reach the waist of the pants. Set the reacher aside at this point so the patient can pull up the pants from either a seated or standing position. **Safety/Monitoring** Monitor the patient during dressing for fall risk and the need to maintain joint precautions.
Dressing Stick 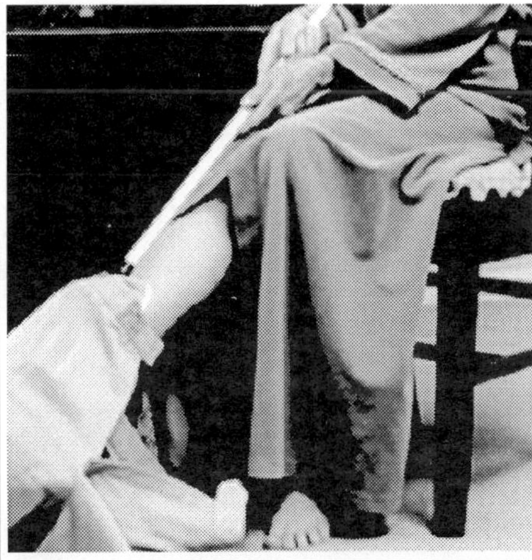 Copyright by NC Medical. Reprinted with permission. Retrieved from https://www.ncmedical.com/item_298.html	**Description** A dressing stick is a neoprene hook attached to a long, wooden stick. **Indications/Benefit** Dressing sticks extend the reach of a person to assist with pushing and pulling clothing off and on during lower extremity dressing. **Contraindications** Patients with poor sitting balance may be at an increased risk for falls when reaching for items. **Proper Techniques for Use** When using a dressing stick, have the patient hook the clothing with the hook end of the dressing stick. Lower the clothing toward the feet so the patient can insert one or both legs into the pants. It is usually recommended that the affected extremity be dressed first, particularly if the patient has weakness, limitations, or precautions in hip range of motion. Using the stick the patient can pull the pants up until he or she is able to reach the waist of the pants. Set the dressing stick aside at this point so the patient can pull up the pants from either a seated or standing position. Dressing sticks may be used for a variety of clothing items and may also be used to push clothing items down during undressing. **Safety/Monitoring** Monitor the patient during dressing for fall risk and the need to maintain joint precautions.

continued

Table 12-4. Equipment to Support Dressing (continued).

Sock Aid	Description
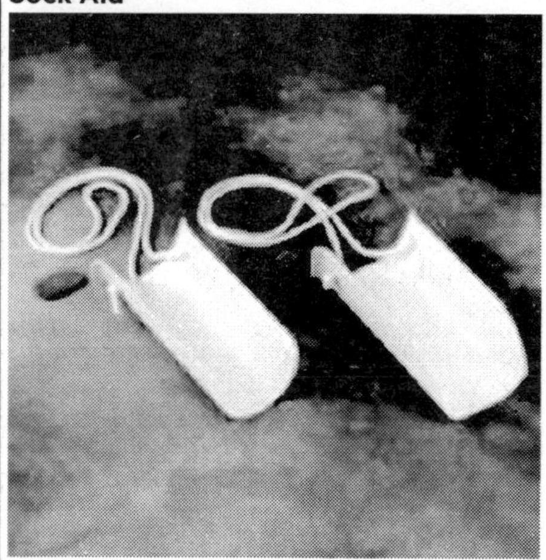 Copyright by Patterson Medical. Reprinted with permission. Retrieved from http://www.pattersonmedical.com/app.aspx?cmd=getProduct&key=IF_921028891 Copyright by Patterson Medical. Reprinted with permission. Retrieved from http://www.pattersonmedical.com/app.aspx?cmd=getProduct&key=IF_921000766	Sock aids may be made of rigid plastic or flexible plastic with long pull ropes attached. Sock aids are shaped so the sock may be placed over them and pulled onto the foot using the rope handles. **Indications/Benefit** Sock aids are used to assist patients with putting on their socks without requiring them to bend over, flex the hip, or cross the leg. **Contraindications** Patients with poor sitting balance may be at an increased risk for falls when using a sock aid during lower-body dressing. **Proper Techniques for Use** While holding the device between the legs, the patient will stretch the sock over the device with the heel of the sock on the solid underside of the device. Pull the sock onto the device until the sock meets the knots of the rope handles. Lower the sock aid to the ground while holding onto the rope handles. Place the foot into the mouth of the device and pull the rope handles while keeping the toes pointed into the sock. The device should slide over the heel while pulling the sock onto the foot. Applying powder to the inside of the sock aid may make it easier to slide it over the foot. **Safety/Monitoring** Monitor the patient during dressing for fall risk and the need to maintain joint precautions.
Long-Handled Shoe Horn 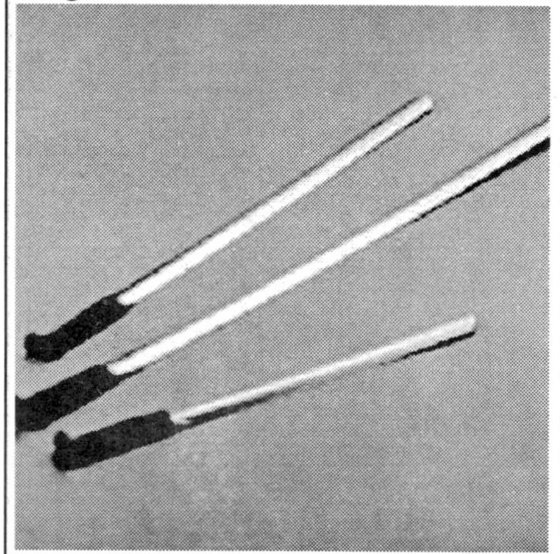 Copyright by Patterson Medical. Reprinted with permission. Retrieved from http://www.pattersonmedical.com/app.aspx?cmd=getProduct&key=IF_921000733	**Description** A long-handled shoe horn is a traditional shoe horn with an extension that enables it to be used from an upright, seated position. **Indications/Benefit** A long-handled shoe horn assists patients in putting on their shoes by enabling them to use the extended handle from an upright position in order to place the shoe horn at the heel of the shoe **Contraindications** Patients with poor sitting balance may be at increased risk for falls when using a shoe horn during lower-body dressing. **Proper Techniques for Use** The patient should grasp the long-handled shoe horn by the handle end and place the shoe horn end into the heel of the shoe. He or she can use the shoe horn to assist with sliding the foot into the shoe more easily. **Safety/Monitoring** Monitor the patient for fall risk and the need to maintain joint precautions.

Table 12-5. Equipment to Support Bathing

<table>
<tr><td>Transfer Tub Benches
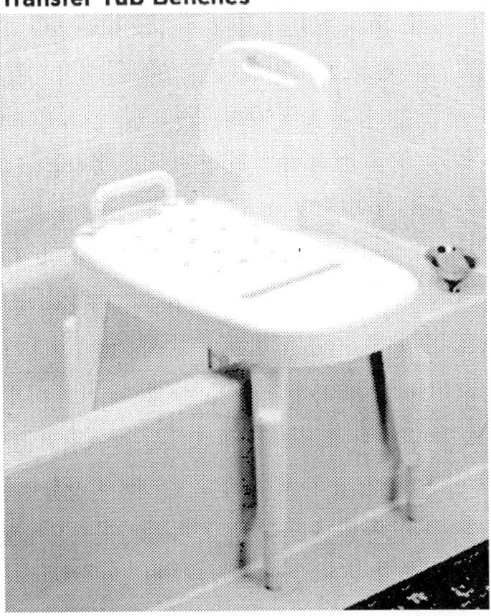
Copyright by The Wright Stuff, Inc. www.wrightstuff.biz. Reprinted with permission. http://www.wrightstuff.biz/miadtrbe.html</td><td>Description
Transfer tub benches provide a sturdy seat for patients in the bathtub and are best used in conjunction with a handheld shower. Unlike smaller shower chairs, tub transfer benches provide a bench surface that extends over the side of the tub, so that the person can sit on the bench first, and then safely move their legs (with assistance as needed) over the edge of the tub.
Indications/Benefit
Transfer tub benches are beneficial for patients with decreased standing tolerance, decreased standing balance, or decreased endurance, or for patients who are at an increased risk for falls in the shower.
Contraindications
Do not attempt bathing using a tub transfer bench if the patient's safety risk is not manageable by the person assisting with the bathing.
Proper Techniques for Use
A patient should be supervised or assisted as needed to move onto the transfer tub bench. The patient should be assisted to lift his or her legs over the tub as needed, and then scoot to the optimal position on the bench.
Safety/Monitoring
Provide supervision and physical assistance as needed during bathing for safety.</td></tr>
<tr><td>Long-Handled Sponges
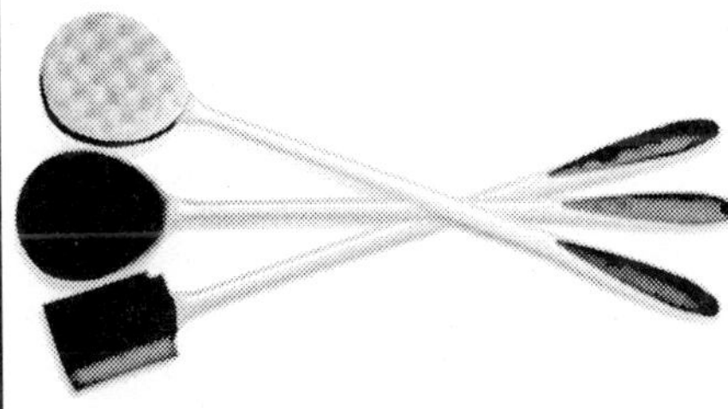
Copyright by RehabMart. Reprinted with permission. Retrieved from http://www.rehabmart.com/product/long-handle-bath-sponges-23685.html</td><td>Description
Long-handled sponges are foam sponges affixed to long plastic handles.
Indications/Benefit
Long-handled sponges extend a person's reach during bathing activities.
Contraindications
None
Proper Techniques for Use
The patient may require set-up of the sponge to apply soap.
Safety/Monitoring
Provide supervision and physical assistance as needed during bathing for safety.</td></tr>
<tr><td>Bath Mitt
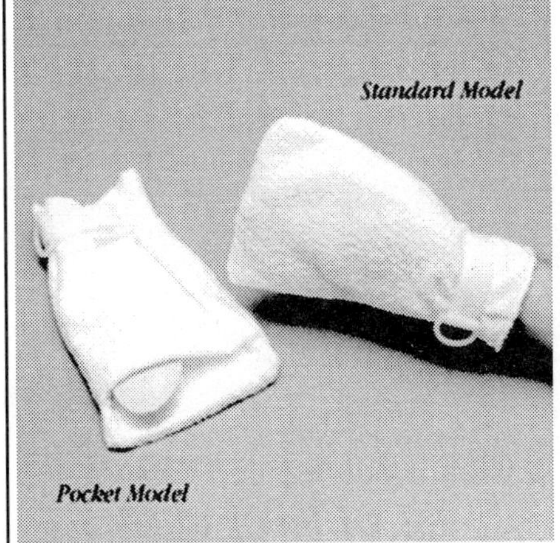

Copyright by RehabMart. Reprinted with permission. Retrieved from http://www.rehabmart.com/product/terry-cloth-wash-mitt-23.html</td><td>Description
Bath mitts are made from cotton or terry cloth. They are made to slide over and cover a person's hand. They contain a strap to secure the mitt to the wrist.
Indications/Benefit
Bath mitts are beneficial for people with limited hand function who would have difficulty grasping a cloth or sponge but who can still participate in bathing with gross motor movement of the upper extremity.
Contraindications
None
Proper Techniques for Use
The patient will require set-up of the bath mitt to secure the strap and to apply the soap.
Safety/Monitoring
Provide supervision and physical assistance as needed for safety during bathing.</td></tr>
</table>

Table 12-6. Splints and Orthotics

Splints 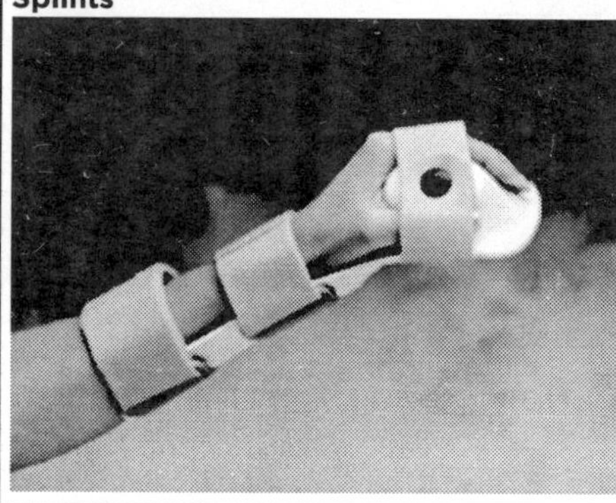 Copyright by RehabMart. Reprinted with permission. Retrieved from http://www.rehabmart.com/product/preformed-neutral-position-splint-4778.html 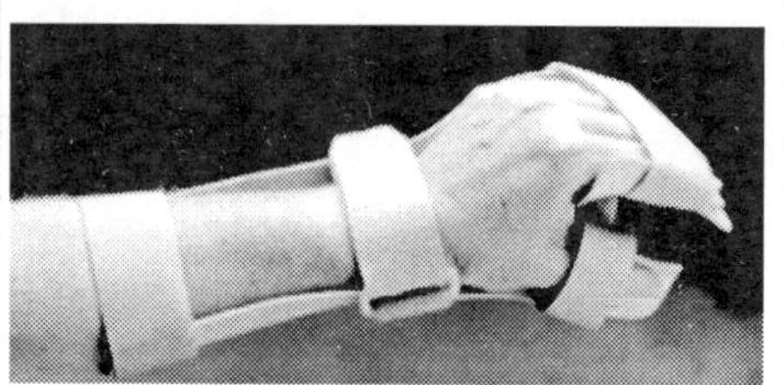 Copyright by RehabMart. Reprinted with permission. Retrieved from http://www.rehabmart.com/product/wanchik-neutral-position-resting-splint-3942.html	**Description** Splints can include a variety of orthoses used by occupational therapists. Some splints are commercially available, whereas others are fabricated specifically for the patient. Splints can be made from fabric, neoprene, or plastic. **Indications/Benefit** Splints can be used by a patient to immobilize a joint(s), maintain joint structures in the absence of motor function, reduce pain, reduce abnormal tone, or support function. **Contraindications** In general, contraindications specific to the individual patient are considered by the occupational therapist in the application of a splint. Therefore, it is important to be aware of the wearing requirements for each patient. **Proper Techniques for Use** The splint should be applied as directed by the occupational therapist. The occupational therapist also establishes a wearing schedule. The patient might require assistance from nursing to adhere to the established schedule. **Safety/Monitoring** Patients might need to be monitored for places of pressure or irritation caused by wearing the splint. These most commonly occur on edges or over bony prominences. If a patient complains of pain or pressure being caused by the splint, remove the splint to inspect the area. If the area appears red or irritated, contact the occupational therapist, as adjustment in the fit could be needed.
Functional Electrical Stimulation (FES) Orthosis 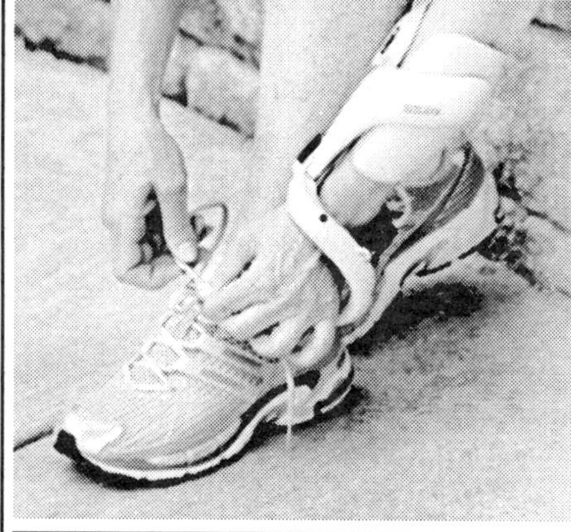 Copyright by Ectron. Reprinted with permission. Retrieved from http://www.ectron.co.uk/neuro-rehabilitation-functional-electrical-stimulation	**Description** FES orthoses provide low-dose electrical stimulation to a specific area to improve motor function. **Indications/Benefit** FES orthoses can be appropriate for patients who have sustained a central nervous system injury such as stroke, brain injury, or spinal cord injury. The FES helps to improve hand function by promoting motor learning or managing tone in the extremity. **Contraindications** FES orthosis should not be used where a cancerous lesion is present or suspected; if the patient has a pacemaker, implanted defibrillator, or other implanted metal or electronic device; or if the patient has another condition in the extremity, such as a fracture or dislocation that could be adversely affected by the electrical stimulation. Precautions should be taken when using with patients with a spinal cord injury at the T6 level or higher, epilepsy, or peripheral vascular conditions, or those who are pregnant. **Proper Techniques for Use** The therapist is the person primarily responsible for setting up the orthosis and can train others involved with the patient's care as appropriate. **Safety/Monitoring** Ensure the unit is turned off before removing the orthosis. After removing the orthosis, monitor the skin for redness, irritation, or indentation lasting longer than 1 hour. Do not allow the patient to bathe or shower with the orthosis on the extremity.

continued

Table 12-6. Splints and Orthotics (continued)	
Slings or Harnesses 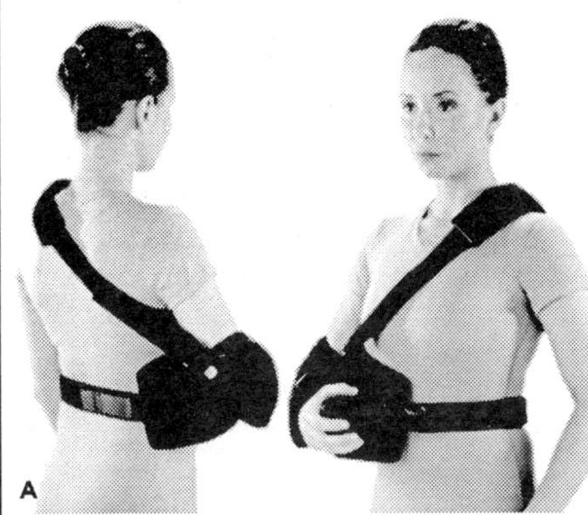 Copyright by RehabMart. Reprinted with permission. Retrieved from http://www.rehabmart.com/product/arm-sling-with-abduction-pillow-38662.html 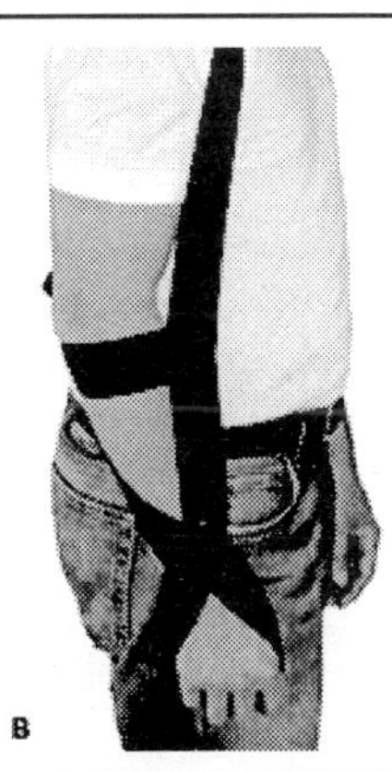 Copyright by GivMohr Corporation. Reprinted with permission. Retrieved from www.givmohr.com	**Description** Slings or harnesses are most often made of fabric and contain Velcro® straps to secure the device in place. **Indications/Benefit** Slings or harnesses can be used to immobilize an extremity for protection after injury or surgery (see Figure A which is used for patients with rotator cuff repair). In specific circumstances in which the patient has impaired motor function or hemiplegia, a sling or harness can be used to support the affected extremity (Figure B). However, the mere presence of hemiplegia is not sufficient reason to warrant the use of a sling or harness. **Contraindications** For patients who have had orthopedic surgery, slings and immobilizers must be worn as ordered. However, in general, slings are not recommended for full-time wear because the prolonged immobility of the extremity carries the risk of secondary issues. **Proper Techniques for Use** The sling or harness should be applied and worn as directed by the occupational therapist. The straps should be adjusted so the sling or harness fits properly and securely. **Safety/Monitoring** Ensure that the sling or harness is appropriately applied. If a patient complains of pain or pressure being caused by sling or harness, inspect the area. If the area appears red or irritated, contact the occupational therapist, as adjustment in the fit could be needed.

continued

Table 12-6. Splints and Orthotics (continued)

<table>
<tr><td>Mobile Arm Supports (MAS)
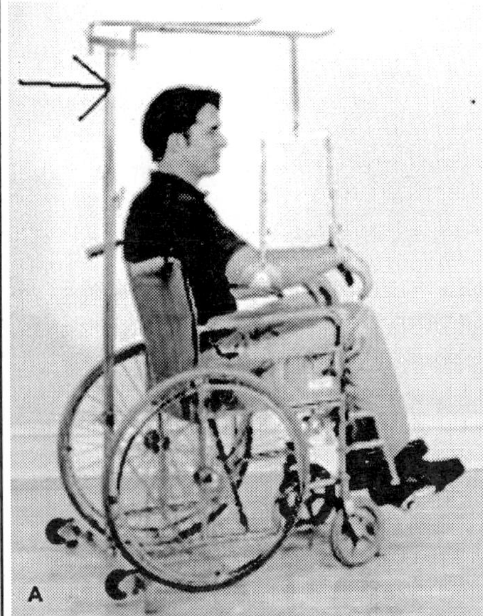
Copyright by RehabMart. Reprinted with permission. Retreived from http://www.rehabmart.com/product/folding-arm-suspension-frame-9886.html
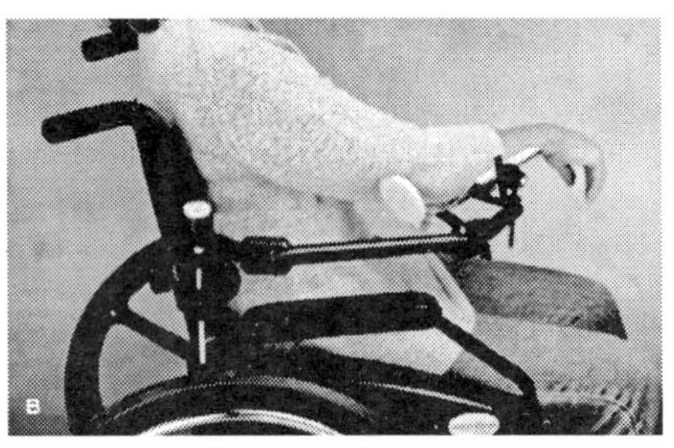
Copyright by RehabMart. Reprinted with permission. Retreived from http://www.rehabmart.com/product/jaeco-multilink-mobile-arm-supports-8009.html</td><td>Description
MAS consist of several types of devices that are used to support a person's upper extremities during functional activities. MAS are typically used by the patient while in a seated position. Some types of MAS are attached to a wheelchair and cradle the upper extremity to provide support (Figure B). Other MAS consist of slings suspended from a frame that is positioned behind the person (Figure A).
Indications/Benefit
MAS are beneficial for patients with limited shoulder function or strength, particularly in the deltoid and shoulder girdle musculature. They are most useful for patients with at least some ability to flex the elbow using bicep function. Therefore, MAS compensate for decreased shoulder function, but the person is able to flex his or her elbow to participate in eating, oral, hygiene, or other activities.
Contraindications
None
Proper Techniques for Use
MAS require effective set-up to be beneficial for the patient. The occupational therapist performs the initial set up and adjustment. After initial set-up and adjustment, the patient's upper extremity can be placed in the sling or on the support. Other adaptive equipment such as adaptive utensils or a universal cuff might need to be set up for the patient to use in conjunction with the MAS.
Safety/Monitoring
MAS might need to be adjusted during the activity to provide effective support.</td></tr>
</table>

IV. Other Assistive Services, Technologies, and Adaptations in Rehabilitation to Aid the Rehabilitation Process, Mobility, ADL, and Other Functions

A. Telerehabilitation

1. A method for extending rehabilitation care
   a. To underserved areas and populations
   b. For cost-effective ongoing therapy after inpatient rehabilitation
2. Can be facilitated in different settings
   a. Outpatient clinic
   b. Home
3. Utilizes information and communication technologies
   a. Telephone
   b. Internet-based videoconferencing
   c. Sensors and wearable devices
   d. Data transmitted to providers
4. Services offered are many and varied
   a. Consultation with specialists
   b. Assessment, diagnosis, goal setting, therapy, education, monitoring
   c. Counseling and support
   d. Case management
   e. Prevention activities
   f. Home assessments
   g. Still photography, video
5. Both real-time and asynchronous interaction used depending on goals of treatment
6. Stems from telehealth
7. Considered an alternative method of providing therapy
8. Challenges
   a. Infrastructure
   b. Both at-home and provider settings
   c. Cost

d. Availability of Internet providers and equipment
1) Skill of providers
2) Some things become more difficult
3) Muscle strength assessment
4) Security of data
5) Technical troubleshooting of equipment failure

9. Future research needed to explore
a. Who is most likely to benefit from this method of rehabilitation?
b. Cost-effectiveness
c. Most suitable types of therapies and interventions most suited
d. Outcomes from current programs (Laver et al., 2013)

10. The role of the rehabilitation nurse in telehealth
a. Deliver services to rural patients from distant sites.
b. Assessment
c. Case management
d. Patient education
e. Interventions
f. Assist at site where the patient is located.
g. Communicate with distant providers and facilitate interventions.
h. Perform assessments as guided by therapists and physicians.
1) Muscle strength
2) Range of motion
i. Set up and troubleshoot equipment.

B. Other
1. Virtual reality programs
2. Computer-based therapy programs

C. Electrical Stimulation
1. Mentioned briefly in section IV, electrical stimulation is a method used to increase muscle strength and function.
2. Provides low-voltage stimuli to the surface of the skin
3. Used with neurologic conditions or injuries, such as a spinal cord injury or stroke
4. Excites the peripheral nerve, creating a chemical reaction in the sodium-potassium pump, resulting in a muscle contraction
a. Peripheral nerve thus must be intact.
5. Combined with exercise therapy, it can contribute to neural plasticity and recovery of function.
6. Reorganization of central nervous system around a damaged area to find new pathways that can take over for damaged pathways
7. Even if function does not improve, electrical stimulation can be useful
a. Prevention of venous thrombosis
b. Maintaining muscle size (preventing disuse atrophy)
c. Improving tissue health
d. Reducing spasticity
e. Reducing progression of osteoporosis
f. Improving strength
8. Other uses for electrical stimulation
a. Cardiac/respiratory pacing
b. Trunk control
c. Pain management
1) Transcutaneous electrical nerve stimulation
d. Functional electrical stimulation
1) Utilizing electrical stimulation of muscles to restore functions, such as
a) Opening and closing hand and grip
b) Handwriting
c) Using kitchen utensils
d) Holding glass
e) Shaking hands
f) Limb movement
g) Standing
h) Walking
i) Aerobic exercise
j) Riding a bicycle.
2) Implantable functional electrical stimulation systems have been used for
a) Grasping and reaching
b) Standing/ambulation
c) Trunk stability
d) Cough
e) Bladder and bowel function
f) Diaphragmatic pacing
e. External components interface with internal components (Bryden, Ancan, Mazurkiewicz, McKnight, & Scholtens, 2012)

D. Assistive Technology for Access
1. Assists access to computers, environmental control units, mobility and communication devices
a. Mouse
b. Surface mounted, trackballs
c. Head-point mouse
d. Eye-gaze technology and eye-tracking mouse
e. Brain-computer interfaces
f. Keyboard access
g. Mouth stick
h. Head-pointing stick
i. Computerized word completion
j. Tablets/smartphones
k. Recording
l. Audio and visual
m. Uses for students and others
1) Lesson file downloading versus taking notes

2) Electronic textbooks
n. Personal schedules
o. Memory book
p. Speech recognition software
q. Eye-gaze technology
1) Uses cameras pointed at retinas of eyes
a) Camera translates eye movements into cursor movements.

E. Environmental Control Units
1. Use input from patient to electronically control television, telephone, light switches, computers, pagers, doors, curtains, alarms, etc.
2. Benefits
a. Increased independence and safety
b. Decreased caregiver time and effort
3. Disadvantages
a. Cost
b. Lack of availability
c. Troubleshooting
d. Provider lack of knowledge (Paul, Frank, Hanspal, & Groves, 2006)

F. Service Animals
1. Social supports with health benefits
a. Companions
b. Pets
c. Visitors
d. Animal-assisted therapy
e. Guide dogs
1) For the blind
f. Hearing dogs
1) For the hearing impaired
g. Service dogs
1) Trained to assist those with mobility and balance challenges, unstable medical issues, and psychiatric disabilities or autism
2) Help conserve energy and prevent injury
3) Activate devices, open doors
4) Retrieve items
5) Detect and respond to medical emergencies (e.g., seizures, hypoglycemia)
6) Retrieve phone
7) Carry medication
8) Activate emergency medical services
9) Benefits
a) Improved socialization and community participation
b) Decreased need for paid assistance
c) Increased independence and decreased reliance on others
d) Decreased burden on caregivers
e) Improved affect and sense of well-being
10) Disadvantages
a) Lengthy waiting list
b) Cost
c) Grooming
d) Veterinary bills
e) Challenges to public access and housing
f) Interference with working dog by public
g) Access to training facilities and animals (Winkle, Crowe, & Hendrix, 2012)

SUMMARY

The primary task of the rehabilitation nurse in the patient's use of adaptive equipment and technology is to provide support. The nurse applies and monitors adaptive equipment, troubleshoots malfunctioning equipment, reinforces patient education about the equipment (including proper use and safety precautions), and monitors for complications related to use. Through knowledge of the types of equipment and technology available for patients, the nurse is also responsible for recommending equipment that the therapists or medical providers might not have considered. Although the nurse's role is supportive with respect to adaptive equipment and technology, it is by no means minor. Rehabilitation nurses have a responsibility to stay up to date with and learn from therapists and others about the most current equipment and technology and their proper use.

References

Association of Rehabilitation Nurses (ARN). (2014). ARN competency model for professional rehabilitation nursing. Retrieved from http://www.rehabnurse.org/uploads/files/education/ARN_Rehabilitation_Nursing_Competency _Model_FINAL_-_May_2014.pdf

Bryden, A., Ancans, J., Mazurkiewicz, J., McKnight, A., & Scholtens, M. (2012). Technology for spinal cord injury and its application to youth. *Journal of Pediatric Rehabilitation Medicine, 5*(2012), 287–299.

Fairchild, S. L. (2012). *Principles & techniques of patient care* (5th ed.). Stoneham, MA: Elsevier.

Granville, R., & Menetrez, J. (2010). Rehabilitation of the lower-extremity war-injured at the Center for the Intrepid. *Foot and Ankle Clinics, 15*(1), 187–189.

Johannsson, A., Larsson, G., & Ramstrand, N. (2009). Incidence of lower limb amputation in the diabetic and nondiabetic general population: A 10-year population-based cohort study of initial unilateral and contralateral amputations and reamputations. *Diabetes Care, 32*(2), 275–280.

Laver, K. E, Schoene, D., Crotty, M. George, S., Lannin, N. A., & Sherrington, C. (2013). Telerehabilitation services for stroke (review). *CochraneiLibrary 2013(12),* 1–46.

Merrill, S. S., Seeman, T. E., Kasl, S. V., & Berkman, L. F. (1997). Gender differences in the comparison of self-reported disability and performance measures. *The Journals of Gerontology Biological Sciences & Medical Sciences, 52*(1), M19–M26.

O'Sullivan, S. B., Schmitz, T. J., & Fulk, G. D. (2014). Physical rehabilitation. In M. M. Biblis (Ed.). *Physical rehabilitation* (6th ed., pp. 1505). Philadelphia: F. A. Davis.

Paul, S. N., Frank, A. O., Hanspal, R. S., & Groves, R. (2006). Exploring environmental control unit use in the age group 10-20 years. *International Journal of Therapy and Rehabilitation, 13*(11), 511–516.

Potter, B., & Scoville, C. (2008). Amputation is not isolated: An overview of the US Army Amputee Patient Care Program and associated amputee injuries. *Journal of the American Academy of Orthopedic Surgeons, 14,* S188.

Thomas, W., Pinkelman, L., & Gardine, C. (2010). The reasons for noncompliance with adaptive equipment in patients returning home after a total hip replacement. *Physical and Occupational Therapy in Geriatrics, 28*(2), 170–180.

Wallenbert, I., & Jonsson, H. (2005). Waiting to get better: A dilemma regarding habits in daily occupations after stroke. *American Journal of Occupational Therapy, 59,* 218–224.

Winkle, M., Crowe, T. K., & Hendrix, I. (2012). Service dogs and people with physical disabilities partnerships: A systematic review. *Occupational Therapy International, 19*(2012), 54–66.

Bibliography

Pendleton, H., & Schultz-Krohn, W. (Eds.). (2013). *Pedretti's occupational therapy practice skills for physical dysfunction* (7th ed., pp. 157–232). St. Louis: Elsevier.

Web-Based Resource

Hip hinge: http://www.bsmpg.com/articles---resources-0/bid/63394/The-Hip-Hinge-The-Best-Exercise-You-re-Not-Teaching-In-Your-Rehabilitation-Program

Chapter 13

Healthcare Financing and Health Policy in Rehabilitation

Anne Deutsch, PhD RN CRRN
James Farrell, MBA RN CRRN

LEARNING OUTCOMES

- Discuss funding sources for healthcare and rehabilitation in the United States.
- Outline economic barriers to health care.
- Review funding for assistive technology.
- Describe how health policy is developed in the United States.
- Identify opportunities for rehabilitation nurses to become involved in health policy.

KEY CHAPTER TOPICS

- Medicare, Medicaid, worker's compensation, Children's Health Insurance Plan, Tricare, private insurance
- Reimbursement for healthcare services
- Funding for assistive technology
- Health policy and the future of healthcare delivery

PROFESSIONAL REHABILITATION NURSING DOMAINS AND COMPETENCIES

- Domain 3: Competency 3.3 (Association of Rehabilitation Nurses [ARN], 2014)

Introduction

This chapter provides an overview of healthcare financing and health policy making. The American healthcare system, including the delivery of rehabilitation services, is financed through a mix of federal and state programs and private health insurance. Because of rising healthcare costs, the reimbursement of healthcare services by insurance companies and government agencies have shifted from a fee-for-service model to managed-care and prospective-payment models with shared financial risks. Concerns that the U.S. healthcare delivery system is becoming increasingly fragmented have resulted in several initiatives to examine payment for episodes of care, also known as *bundled payment*. In addition to healthcare costs, healthcare quality is a key health policy issue that includes the development of standardized assessment data elements and quality measures for public reporting of quality information, quality improvement, and pay-for-performance activities.

The processes of developing and modifying health policy provide opportunities for rehabilitation nurses to share their expertise with local, state, and federal government agencies; legislators; and other key organizations. Rehabilitation nurses' unique knowledge and understanding of the needs of people with disabilities position them to advocate for health policy changes. A rehabilitation nurse's involvement can include a range of activities such as educating the public about health issues (e.g., at schools or senior centers, in local newspapers or magazines); commenting on draft policy statements, reports, legislation, and proposed rules; and participating in expert panels.

I. Economics: Financing the Delivery of Healthcare Services in the United States (Table 13-1)

A. Public Programs

1. Medicare: The federal health insurance program for people who are elderly or disabled under the authority of the U.S. Department of Health and Human Services (DHHS). It began with the enactment of Title XVIII of the Social Security Act of 1965. In 2012, Medicare provided health insurance coverage to 49 million people, of whom 40 million were age 65 years or older and 9 million had permanent disabilities and were younger than age 65 years. With total healthcare spending estimated at $2.28

Table 13-1. Funding Sources for Healthcare and Rehabilitation Programs

	Programs			
	Medicare (Federal)	**Medicaid (State)**	**Workers' Compensation**	**Private Health Insurance**
Eligibility Requirements	Must be older than 65 years, have end-stage renal disease, or have been disabled for 2 years	For people with low income	Workers injured in the course of employment	Policyholders
Benefits	Part A—Hospital Part B—Supplemental medical insurance Part C—Medicare Advantage plans Part D—Prescription drug coverage	Hospital costs and visits to a physician	Medical care for a work-related injury Income support during periods of disability	Hospital costs and outpatient treatment, as specified in policy Physician visits, as specified in policy May or may not cover rehabilitation care

From *The specialty practice of rehabilitation nursing: A core curriculum* (3rd ed., p. 227), by A. E. McCourt (Ed.), 1993, Skokie, IL: Association of Rehabilitation Nurses. Copyright 1993 Association of Rehabilitation Nurses.

trillion in 2011, the Medicare program accounted for 23% of national health expenditures (The Henry J. Kaiser Family Foundation, 2014b; Medicare Payment Advisory Commission, 2014).

a. Administration: Managed by the Centers for Medicare & Medicaid Services (CMS), which designates Medicare administrative contractors to process claims
b. Coverage
   1) Original Medicare plan
      a) Medicare Part A: A hospital insurance plan that covers inpatient services provided by hospitals, home healthcare agencies (skilled care only), hospice care, and short-term stays in skilled nursing facilities (SNFs); it does not cover custodian care. Most beneficiaries do not pay a monthly premium for Part A services but are responsible for the deductibles that are required for each benefit period; a benefit period ends after 60 consecutive days of no hospital or SNF care; there is no limit of benefit periods per year, so the cost to patients could be higher. Part A is financed through the CMS Hospital Insurance Trust Fund by taxes paid by employers and their employees (CMS, 2013).
      b) Medicare Part B: Supplemental medical insurance program that covers physician, outpatient, home health, and preventive services. It is financed through the CMS Supplementary Medical Insurance Trust Fund by federal taxes and monthly premiums from beneficiaries, typically $147 in 2014 (CMS, 2013).
      c) Medicare Part D: Outpatient prescription drug coverage offered through private companies. Coverage varies depending on the plan chosen. Enrollment requirements exist. If a beneficiary does not join a Medicare Prescription Drug Plan when first eligible, there could be a late enrollment penalty. It is financed through taxes, beneficiary premiums, and state payments for people with both Medicare and Medicaid coverage.
      d) Medicare beneficiaries in the original plan can buy private Medicare supplemental insurance (e.g., Medigap) to pay for the costs not covered (e.g., deductibles, coinsurance, vision, and dental services). In 2010, 14% of Medicare beneficiaries did not have supplemental insurance coverage through private insurance or Medicaid (The Henry J. Kaiser Family Foundation, 2014b).
   2) Medicare Part C: This Medicare Advantage program allows beneficiaries to enroll in private health plans. Plans include preferred provider organizations (PPOs), provider-sponsored organizations, private fee-for-service plans, high-deductible plans linked to medical savings accounts, and special needs programs for people who are dually eligible for Medicare and Medicaid. This program provides hospital and physician coverage. It often includes prescription drug coverage and is an alternative to Parts A, B, and D coverage. The plans receive payments from Medicare to provide Medicare-covered benefits. It is not separately financed from Parts A, B, and D. Medicare Advantage enrollees generally pay the monthly Part B premium and also often pay an additional premium directly to their plan (the

average was $65 per month in 2014) (CMS, 2013).

c. Eligibility

1) People age 65 years and older qualify for Medicare Part A if they or their spouses are eligible for Social Security payments, have made payroll tax contributions for 10 or more years (40 quarters), and are U.S. citizens or permanent residents. People age 65 years and older who are not entitled to Part A, such as those who did not pay enough Medicare taxes during their working years, can pay a monthly premium to receive Part A benefits. People entitled to Part A and those age 65 years and older can elect to enroll in Part B. People are eligible for Part C (Medicare Advantage) if they are entitled to Part A and enrolled in Part B. People are eligible for Part D (i.e., prescription drug coverage) if they are entitled to Part A or enrolled in Part B. Medicare is a secondary payer if the person also has private health insurance.

2) People younger than age 65 years with permanent disabilities are eligible for Medicare Part A after receiving Social Security Disability Income (SSDI) for 24 months. People with end-stage renal disease or Lou Gehrig's disease are eligible for Medicare Part A as soon as they begin receiving SSDI payments, with no waiting period. People entitled to Part A and those age 65 years and older can elect to enroll in Part B. People are eligible for Part C (Medicare Advantage) if they are entitled to Part A and enrolled in Part B. People are eligible for Part D (i.e., prescription drug coverage) if they are entitled to Part A or enrolled in Part B.

2. Medicaid: The health insurance program for certain individuals and families with low income and resources. It began with the enactment of Title XIX of the Social Security Act of 1965 and provides medical assistance to people and families receiving cash assistance (welfare). Medicaid has expanded to cover health and long-term care services for specific categories of low-income people and expanded farther in 2014 for states that opted into the Medicaid expansion to include the majority of people younger than age 65 years with an income up to 133% of the federal poverty level (The Henry J. Kaiser Family Foundation, 2014a). In 2010, Medicaid covered 66 million people, and in 2012, Medicaid spending was approximately $415 billion.

a. Administration: Managed by each state through a state agency with oversight from CMS; financed by a federal-state partnership in which the federal government matches state Medicaid spending

b. Coverage: Medicaid covers a wide range of healthcare and long-term care services but covered services vary by state. Medicaid managed care and nonmanaged care options are available. Some states require enrollment in a managed care plan. Covered services include long-term care, mental-health care, and services and supports for people with disabilities. Medicaid covers comprehensive services for children. It assists low-income Medicare beneficiaries, known as "dual eligibles." Medicaid is the largest funding source for coverage of long-term care, covering approximately 70% of all nursing home residents (The Henry J. Kaiser Family Foundation, 2014a). The federal government requires states to provide the following: inpatient and outpatient hospital, physician, laboratory, X-ray, prenatal, and preventive-care services; federally qualified health center and rural health clinic services; family planning services and supplies; pediatric and nurse practitioner services; nurse midwife services; nursing facility services for people older than 21 years; home health care for people eligible for nursing facility services; and medically necessary transportation. States can add services to this list and can place certain limitations on the federally mandated services. States can obtain federal waivers to operate their Medicaid programs outside federal guidelines.

c. Eligibility

1) Under the current law, people qualify for Medicaid if they meet the financial criteria and belong to one of the groups that are "categorically" eligible for the program. In addition, eligibility is limited to American citizens and certain lawfully residing immigrants. To be eligible for federal funds, states are required to provide Medicaid coverage for certain "mandatory" groups. The mandatory groups include the following:

a) Families with limited incomes with children who meet certain of the eligibility requirements in the state's Aid to Families with Dependent Children plan, which became effective on July 16, 1996

b) Most older adults and people with disabilities who receive Supplemental Security Income (SSI)
c) Children younger than age 6 years and pregnant women whose family income is at or below 133% of the federal poverty level
d) Children ages 6–18 years living below 100% of the federal poverty level

2) Under the Patient Protection and Affordable Care Act of 2010, most people younger than age 65 years with income below a national "floor" are eligible for Medicaid. Eligibility is limited to American citizens and certain lawfully residing immigrants.
3) States have the option to provide Medicaid coverage for other "categorically needy" groups. These optional groups share characteristics of the mandatory groups, but the eligibility criteria are somewhat more liberally defined. Examples of the optional groups that states can cover as categorically needy (and for which they will receive federal matching funds) under the Medicaid program include the following:
a) Pregnant women, children, and parents with incomes that exceed the mandatory thresholds
b) Older adults and people who are disabled and earn up to 100% of the federal poverty level
c) Working disabled people who earn up to 250% of the federal poverty level
d) People residing in nursing facilities with incomes below 300% of the SSI standard
e) People who would be eligible if institutionalized but who are receiving care under home- and community-based service waivers
f) Medically needy people who cannot meet the financial criteria but have high medical expenses relative to their incomes and who belong to one of the categorically eligible groups.

3. State Children's Health Insurance Plan (CHIP): Health insurance plan for children in families with incomes too high to qualify for Medicaid but too low for them to afford private health insurance. In 2014, the total enrollment was 9.6 million children (CMS, 2014).
   a. Administration
      1) Jointly financed by the state and federal government. States are given broad flexibility in tailoring programs to meet their own circumstances.
      2) States can create or expand their own separate insurance programs, expand Medicaid, or combine both approaches.
   b. Eligibility: States have the opportunity to set eligibility criteria for age, income, resources, and residency within broad federal guidelines.
4. Workers' compensation: Government-sponsored and employee-financed systems for compensating employees who incur an injury or illness in connection with their employment. Benefits provided include medical care, disability payments, rehabilitation services, survivor benefits, and funeral expenses.
   a. Administration: Each state, plus the District of Columbia, Puerto Rico, and the U.S. Virgin Islands, designates an agency to administer the program (e.g., state department of labor, independent workers' compensation agency, court administration).
   b. Eligibility: Workers who are disabled by injury or families of a worker whose death arose out of and during the course of employment
   c. Coverage: Provides both medical care related to the compensable injury and income benefits through the following sources:
      1) Private commercial insurance companies
      2) Self-insurance (corporations that are able to carry the risk)
      3) State funds
      4) State's second injury fund
   d. Medical care provisions
      1) Treatment and rehabilitative programs for work-related injury
      2) Reimbursement in full, or in certain states, according to a medical fee guide
      3) Life-care planning: The process of mapping out short- and long-term care needs, expenses, and resources for clients with a debilitating, chronic illness or injury. A life-care plan is created to ensure that the client receives consistent, comprehensive, cost-effective care from current and future caregivers (Barker, 1999).
   e. Vocational rehabilitation benefits: Most states provide job retraining, education, and job placement.

B. Private Health Insurance
1. Purchasing private health insurance plans
   a. Employers and other organizations can purchase private health insurance on behalf of a group of individuals. Purchasing groups often

negotiate coverage, so benefits often vary by group. Group members (e.g., employees) contribute to the insurance premium.

b. An individual can purchase private health insurance and pay the full premium.

c. Under the Affordable Care Act, health insurance coverage is required, except when a qualified exemption exists (e.g., for Indian tribes and short coverage gaps).

2. Types of health insurance and service plans

a. Indemnity plans: Provide comprehensive coverage for medical and hospital services

1) The employer or subscriber pays a premium, and the subscriber agrees to pay any required deductible, copayments, and amounts over the insurer's usual and customary rate for specific services.

2) The subscriber can receive services from physicians, hospitals, or other qualified providers of his or her choice for services that are medically necessary and meet accepted standards of medical practice.

3) Preapproval for coverage could be required.

4) Experimental and other noncovered services could be negotiable under certain circumstances.

b. Managed care plans (Kongstvedt, 2012)

1) Overview

a) Managed-care plans provide an identified set of medical or hospital care services for a fixed, predetermined premium.

b) The managed-care organization (MCO) can restrict the subscriber's choice of providers and control subscriber access.

c) Subscribers often choose or are assigned a primary care physician who is employed by or under contract with the MCO. In many cases, the primary care physician acts as a gatekeeper for all other medical and hospital services.

d) The different types of insurance plans were reasonably distinct until the late 1980s. Since that time, the differences between traditional forms of health insurance (e.g., indemnity plans) and managed care plans have decreased substantially.

e) MCOs vary greatly in terms of their focus on controlling costs and quality (**Figure 13-1**).

(i) Less controlled: Managed indemnity plans that can include precertification of elective admissions and case management of catastrophic cases

(ii) More controlled: Group and staff model health maintenance organizations (HMOs)

Figure 13-1. Continuum of Managed Care

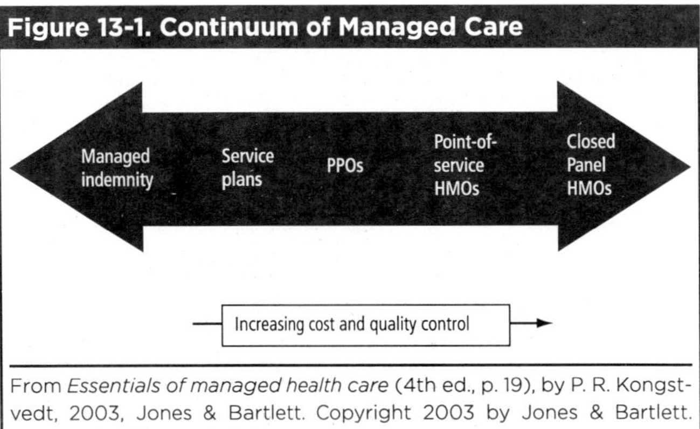

From *Essentials of managed health care* (4th ed., p. 19), by P. R. Kongstvedt, 2003, Jones & Bartlett. Copyright 2003 by Jones & Bartlett. Reprinted with permission.

2) Types of managed-care plans

a) HMOs: Organized healthcare systems that are responsible for both the financing and delivery of a broad range of healthcare services to an enrolled population. The original definition of HMO also included financing health care for a prepaid fixed fee. HMOs must ensure that their members have access to covered healthcare services and are responsible for the quality and appropriateness of these services.

b) PPOs: Employer health benefit plans and insurance carriers contract with PPOs to purchase healthcare services for covered beneficiaries from a selected group of participating providers who typically agree to follow utilization management and other processes implemented by the PPO, and agree to the reimbursement structure and payment models. PPOs offer incentives for enrollees to use participating providers. Enrollees are permitted to use non-PPO providers, but typically they must pay higher coinsurance or deductible amounts. Key attributes of a PPO include a selected provider panel, negotiated payment rates, rapid payment terms, utilization management, and consumer choice.

c) Point-of-service (POS) plans: POS plans offer enrollees some indemnity-type coverage but typically have high deductibles and coinsurance to encourage members to use the HMO-type services.
d) Consumer-driven healthcare programs: Many variations in these programs exist. Typically, employers provide employees with a personal care account of a fixed amount in the form of a voucher, refundable tax credit, higher wages, or some other transfer of funds. Employees choose their own services and providers and manage their own healthcare spending. Employees who use up all the funds in their account pay expenses up to a deductible, when catastrophic coverage begins. The employee can purchase health care through an intermediary.

c. Medicare supplemental benefits plan (Medigap): Purchased by Medicare beneficiaries to pay for expenses that are not covered by Medicare
d. Auto liability: Covers medical care needed as a result of a motor vehicle accident

C. Programs for Special Groups
1. Military personnel: TRICARE is the U.S. Department of Defense's health insurance program for military service members, retirees, and their families, formerly known as the Civilian Health and Medical Program of the Uniformed Services (CHAMPUS). TRICARE provides civilian health benefits for military personnel and military retirees and their dependents, including some members of the reserves. It is managed by TRICARE Management Activity under the authority of the U.S. assistant secretary of defense for health affairs. Veterans of any age, except those who have been dishonorably discharged, can apply for the medical benefits package at the Department of Veterans Affairs (VA). To receive benefits from the VA Medical Benefits Package, the person must be a veteran, be enrolled in the VA health system, and receive health care at VA facilities. People enrolled in the VA Medical Benefits Package may also have private health insurance or federally funded coverage through TRICARE or Medicare. The programs are independent and do not coordinate.
2. Indian Health Service (IHS): Administered by the U.S. DHHS to provide hospital care, dental and health benefits, substance abuse counseling, public health nursing, and other services. IHS services are administered through 12 area offices and 161 IHS and tribally managed service units. Eligibility is limited to members of the 564 federally recognized Indian tribes and their descendants; in 2010, the program included 1.9 million American Indians and Alaskan Natives living on or near reservations.
3. Railroad Retirement Act program
4. Black Lung Benefits Act of 1972
5. Longshoremen and Harbor Workers' Compensation Act

II. Reimbursement for Healthcare Services

A. Payment Terms
1. Prospective payment system (PPS): The rate of payment to the healthcare facility is predetermined based on the medical diagnosis, treatment, or other information, regardless of the cost for care for a specific client.
2. Per-discharge payment: The provider or hospital is paid one amount for all services delivered during one stay.
3. Per diem payments: The healthcare facility is paid one amount for all services delivered to a client during one day.

B. Medicare Payment Systems
1. Acute-care hospitals
a. Inpatient hospital acute care
b. Medicare implemented a per-discharge inpatient PPS in acute-care hospitals in 1983. PPS payments are expected to cover all operating and capital costs. PPS payments are determined based on client and facility factors.
1) The classification system for the inpatient PPS is Medicare Severity Diagnosis-Related Groups (MS DRGs). Data from the bill are used to assign each client into one of the MS DRGs (payment groups). There are 335 base DRGs, with many splitting into two or three MS DRGs based on the presence of a complication or comorbidity. Discharge destination and use of certain drugs are occasionally used with the principal diagnosis or procedure to assign the client into a base DRG.
2) Adjustments are made for a rural location, indirect medical education, the proportion of low-income population, geographic differences in labor costs, and outlier cases.
3) The base payment rate is updated each year.
2. Critical access hospitals (CAHs)

a. CAHs are small hospitals, limited to 25 beds, that operate primarily in rural areas. In addition to the 25 acute-care beds, CAHs can have distinct skilled nursing facilities, 10-bed psychiatric units, 10-bed rehabilitation units, and home-health agencies.
b. Each CAH receives 101% of costs for outpatient, inpatient, laboratory, therapy, and postacute care services in the hospital's swing beds.

3. Long-term care hospitals (LTCHs)
    a. LTCHs, also known as long-term acute-care hospitals, provide care to clients who are chronically critically ill, such as individuals who require invasive ventilator support and therefore need hospital care for extended periods. On average, LTCH clients must have a length of stay of 25 days. LTCHs are not distributed evenly across the United States.
    b. The 25% rule reduces payments for LTCHs that exceed the established percentage thresholds for clients admitted from certain referring hospitals during a cost-reporting period. Less stringent thresholds are applied to hospitals within hospitals and satellites in rural or urban areas, where they are the sole LTCH and there is a dominant acute-care hospital.
    c. Medicare implemented a per-discharge LTCH PPS in 2002. PPS payments are expected to cover all operating and capital costs, with certain high-cost ancillary services paid separately. PPS payments are determined based on client and facility factors.
        1) The client classification system for the LTCH PPS is the Medicare Severity Long-Term Care Diagnosis-Related Group (MS-LTC-DRG). The MS-LTC-DRGs are the same groupings used in the acute care inpatient PPS, but the relative weights for each group are different. Data from the hospital bill (e.g., diagnosis, procedures, client characteristics) are used to assign each client into one of the MS-LTC-DRGs (payment groups).
        2) Payments are adjusted for short-stay outliers and high-cost outliers.
        3) Adjustments are made for indirect medical education and geographic differences in labor costs.
        4) Transfer policies aim to discourage transfers between an LTCH and a co-located acute-care hospital and transfers to co-located SNFs, IRFs, and psychiatric facilities.
        5) The base payment rates are updated each year.
4. Inpatient rehabilitation facilities (IRFs)
    a. IRFs, which include freestanding rehabilitation hospitals and distinct rehabilitation units within general (acute care) hospitals, provide intensive rehabilitation services, such as physical, occupational, or speech therapy and hospital-level care to clients after an major illness, injury, or surgical care. Clients must be able to tolerate and benefit from 3 hours of therapy daily.
    b. The 60% rule (formerly known as the 75% rule) is a criterion used to define IRFs; it requires that 60% of clients admitted to an IRF have 1 of 13 qualifying medical conditions. The 13 conditions are stroke; spinal cord injury; congenital deformity; amputation; major multiple trauma; hip fracture; brain injury; neurological disorders (e.g., multiple sclerosis, Parkinson's disease); burns; three arthritis conditions for which aggressive and sustained outpatient therapy has not been effective; and joint replacement for both knees or both hips, when body mass index is 50 or higher or age is 85 years or older.
    c. The IRF standardized client assessment instrument is the Inpatient Rehabilitation Facility Patient Assessment Instrument (IRF-PAI). Data include demographic, diagnostic, and FIM™ instrument (functional status) data. Data are collected on admission and discharge, and admission data are used to categorize each client into payment groups.
    d. Medicare implemented a per-discharge IRF PPS in 2002 for Medicare fee-for-service clients. PPS payments are expected to cover all operating and capital costs, with certain high-cost ancillary services paid separately. PPS payments are determined based on client and facility factors.
        1) The client classification system for the IRF PPS is the case-mix group (CMG). In addition, payments are adjusted for the presence of a tiered comorbidity. Data from the IRF-PAI are used to assign each client into one of the CMG and comorbidity (payment) groups.
        2) A transfer rule aims to discourage IRFs from discharging clients to other institutional settings.
        3) Payments are adjusted for short-stay outliers and high-cost outliers.

4) Adjustments are made for rural or urban location, treatment of low-income clients, teaching status, and geographic differences in labor costs.
5) The base payment rate is updated each year.

5. Skilled nursing facilities (SNFs)
   a. SNFs provide short-term skilled care (nursing or rehabilitation services) on an inpatient basis. Medicare beneficiaries must have an inpatient hospital stay of at least 3 days to be eligible for SNF services coverage. The Medicare SNF benefit covers skilled nursing care, rehabilitation services, and other goods and services for up to 100 days, if the client meets established criteria.
   b. The SNF client assessment instrument is the Minimum Data Set 3.0 (MDS 3.0). Data collected using the MDS 3.0, such as treatments provided and client characteristics, are used to categorize each client into a payment group and to calculate facility-level quality indicators.
   c. Medicare implemented a per diem SNF PPS in 1998. PPS payments are expected to cover all operating and capital costs, with certain high-cost, low frequency ancillary services paid separately. PPS payments are determined based on client and facility factors.
      1) The client classification system for the SNF PPS is the resource utilization group (RUG IV). Data from the MDS 3.0 are used to assign each client to one of the 66 RUGs (payment groups).
      2) Adjustments are made for rural or urban location and geographic differences in labor costs.
      3) The base payment rates are updated each year.
6. Home-health agencies (HHAs)
   a. An HHA provides skilled care (from a nurse or physical or occupational therapist) on a part-time or intermittent basis in the person's home. To qualify for this benefit, Medicare beneficiaries generally are restricted to their homes. A face-to-face form signed by the attending physician attesting to the need for specific services must be obtained and submitted for billing.
   b. The HHA client assessment instrument is the Outcome and Assessment Information Set (OASIS-C). OASIS-C is a modification of the Outcome and Assessment Information Set. Data collected using the OASIS-C, such as clinical characteristics, functional status, and service-use rates, are used to categorize each client into a payment group and to calculate facility-level quality indicators.
   c. Medicare implemented a PPS for home health in 2000 that pays a predetermined rate to the agency for each 60-day episode. PPS payments are determined based on client and facility factors.
      1) The client classification system for the HHA PPS is the Home Health Resource Group (HHRG). Data from the OASIS-C are used to assign each client to one of the 153 HHRGs (payment groups).
      2) Payments are adjusted if fewer than five visits are delivered during the 60-day episode and for other special circumstances, such as high-cost outliers.
      3) Adjustments are made for geographic differences in labor costs.
      4) The base payment rate is updated each year.

III. Economic Barriers to Care

A. Lack of Health Insurance

1. Overview: The majority of Americans younger than age 65 years receive health insurance coverage through their employers or private or state programs. Almost all older adults receive coverage through Medicare, with many having secondary private insurance. Medicaid and the State CHIP provide insurance for millions of nonelderly low-income people, especially children. However, program limits and gaps in employer coverage have resulted in many people not having health insurance. The Affordable Care Act seeks to eliminate this increasing gap in health insurance coverage by making affordable coverage more accessible. It includes an expansion of the Medicaid program, and it requires people to obtain health insurance. In 2014, 49 million adults did not have health insurance (Levy, 2014).
2. Who does not have insurance?
   a. Low-income Americans (family incomes below 200% of the poverty level) are likely to be uninsured. More than one third of the poor and 30% of the near-poor do not have health insurance.
   b. Approximately 81% of the uninsured are in working families. Low-wage workers are likely to be uninsured, as are people employed in small businesses, the service industries, and blue-collar jobs.
   c. Medicaid covers low-income children; coverage for adults is more limited. Parent income eligibility levels are much lower than the levels

for children. There are also enrollment hurdles and lack of outreach.

d. The rate of uninsured among older adults is low (less than 2%) as a result of the Medicare program; however, underinsurance can be an economic barrier for older adults who must supplement their insurance coverage with out-of-pocket money. Black and Hispanic older adults are disproportionately uninsured (Okara, Young, Strine, Balluz, & Mokdad, 2005).

B. Underinsurance and Other Limitations of Access and Coverage

1. Health insurance does not guarantee access to care. An estimated 31.7 million adults between 19 and 64 years of age are underinsured (Schoen, Hayes, Collins, Lippa, & Radley, 2014). There are often limitations on coverage for special services, such as behavioral health care, preventive care, long-term care, catastrophic illnesses or accidents, and psychiatric care. Also, exclusions or waiting periods for illnesses or conditions can exist at the time the person enrolls in the health plan.
2. Most health insurance plans also include copayments or deductibles to discourage overuse of services and reduce premium costs. Copayments and high deductibles can discourage some clients from seeking preventive care (e.g., immunizations, mammograms) and managing chronic conditions effectively. This is particularly problematic for people with low incomes.
3. Substantial gaps in cost-sharing provisions and coverage exist in the traditional Medicare program. There are large deductibles and copayments for hospital care and restrictions on long-term care coverage.
4. Some low-income older adults could qualify for Medicaid in addition to Medicare. Although Medicaid is comprehensive, many physicians do not participate in the program because of its low level of payment. Therefore, barriers still exist for low-income older adults trying to access basic healthcare services.

C. Effects of a Lack of Adequate Health Insurance

1. Lack of adequate health insurance creates substantial barriers to obtaining timely and appropriate health care.
   a. More than 40% of nonelderly uninsured adults have no regular source of health care, and many delay seeking or go without needed care because of concerns about high medical bills.
   b. More than one third of the uninsured have a serious problem paying medical bills, and one quarter are contacted by collection agencies because of outstanding medical bills.
2. Delaying or not receiving treatment can lead to more serious illness and avoidable health conditions.
   a. People without insurance are less likely to receive preventive care and more likely to be admitted to a hospital for a preventable or avoidable condition than people with insurance.
   b. Researchers estimate that at least 18,000 Americans die prematurely each year because of lack of health insurance. A reduction in mortality of 5%–15% could be achieved if the uninsured had health insurance.
3. Uninsured and underinsured clients typically receive care from a select group of providers (e.g., community clinics and public hospitals) that are willing to provide care regardless of a person's ability to pay, such as hospital-based outpatient departments, emergency departments, and community-based clinics.
   a. Costs in these institutional settings often are high, increasing the total costs of delivering care.
   b. To cover the costs of caring for uninsured and underinsured people, providers must either shift fees to other payers or seek government or private subsidies.
   c. Current market forces, including managed care and fixed-fee schedules, make cost shifting difficult and result in decreased services provided to underinsured and uninsured people.
4. At a societal level, lack of adequate health insurance leads to more disability, lower productivity, and a greater burden on the healthcare system.

D. Responses to the Lack of Health Insurance

1. The Health Insurance Portability and Accountability Act of 1996 (HIPAA) prohibits group insurance plans from including eligibility criteria related to health status, medical history, genetic information, or disability and reduces exclusions for preexisting conditions when the person was previously covered by a group insurance plan.
2. The Consolidated Omnibus Budget Reconciliation Act of 1986 gives people in specific categories the right to continued health plan coverage for up to 18 months after voluntary or involuntary termination of employment or reduction in work hours. The person must pay the entire premium.
3. The Patient Protection and Affordable Care Act of 2010 seeks to eliminate this increasing gap in health insurance coverage by making affordable coverage more accessible, including an expansion

of the Medicaid program, and requiring individuals to obtain health insurance (see state-by-state links for coverage information at www.HHS.gov/HealthCare).

IV. Funding for Assistive Technology

A. *Assistive technology* refers to any item, piece of equipment, or product system—whether acquired commercially, off the shelf, modified, or customized—that is used to increase, maintain, or improve the functional capabilities of people with disabilities.

B. Why Funding for Assistive Technology Is a Significant Problem

1. Insurance and health programs do not pay for assistive devices if they are not considered medically necessary.
2. The Technology Related Assistance for Individuals with Disabilities Act of 1988 (PL 100-407) provided grants to states
   a. To increase the availability of assistive technology
   b. To conduct need assessments
   c. To develop innovative programs
   d. To manage public awareness
   e. To identify policies that promote the availability of assistive technology
3. In 1994 an amendment (PL 103-218) expanded and strengthened the 1988 act.

V. Health Policy: Overview

A. *Policy* refers to the decisions that are made about goals and priorities and the ways in which resources are allocated to reach these goals. The choice of policies reflects the values, beliefs, and attitudes of those designing the policy. Health policy includes the decisions made to promote the health of individual citizens.

B. Stakeholders: The healthcare industry has a variety of stakeholders who can have common or conflicting concerns about policies and policy changes.

1. Clients tend to favor comprehensive coverage, high-quality health care, and low out-of-pocket expenses, and oppose limited access to care and larger client payments.
2. Providers (individual and entities) tend to favor income maintenance, autonomy, and comprehensive coverage, and oppose limits on provider payments.
3. Taxpayers tend to favor limits on provider payments and oppose higher taxes.
4. Employers tend to favor cost containment, administrative simplification, and elimination of cost shifting, and oppose government regulation.
5. Regulators (i.e., government) tend to favor disclosure and reporting by providers, cost containment, access to care, and high-quality health care, and oppose provider autonomy.
6. Pharmaceutical manufacturers, biotechnology entities, assistive technology vendors, and suppliers tend to favor comprehensive coverage, and oppose limits on provider payments.
7. Private insurance companies tend to favor business autonomy.
8. Consumer organizations, such as the American Stroke Association and the Paralyzed Veterans of America, favor securing money for research and public education.

C. Key Healthcare Policy Issues

1. The delivery of healthcare services
   a. Access to care: Many people have limited ability to obtain necessary health services for two reasons:
      1) Individuals who have no health insurance or are underinsured might not seek care because of the high cost of healthcare services.
      2) Individuals might not have access because of limited healthcare personnel and lack of facilities near their homes; limited availability of transportation, including accessible transportation; limited healthcare personnel who can provide care that is culturally acceptable or use the language with which the client is most familiar.
   b. Costs of care
      1) In 1960, national health expenditures represented 5.1% of the gross domestic product (GDP); expenditures per capita were $141.
      2) In 2008, health care represented 16% of the GDP (i.e., 16 cents of every dollar was spent on health care).
      3) As a result, various cost-containment strategies (e.g., PPS, managed care) are now used.
   c. Quality of health care: *Healthcare quality* can be defined as the "degree to which patient care services increase the probability of desired patient outcomes and reduce the probability of undesired health outcomes given the current state of knowledge" (Institute of Medicine [IOM], 2006, p. 468). Although the United States offers advanced healthcare services, care is not always accessible, effective, safe, and efficient (IOM, 2006).
   d. Health disparities: Disparities in healthcare use and outcomes for people from racial and ethnic minority groups and people with low incomes result in significantly higher rates of chronic illness and disability among some

racial and ethnic groups and among low-income populations.

2. Nursing services and workforce
   a. Reimbursement for nursing services, including rehabilitation nurses
   b. Scope of practice (e.g., for advanced practice nurses), as defined by state licensure laws and regulatory bodies
   c. Emerging critical shortage of nurses and nursing faculty
   d. Funding for nursing education and research
3. Social issues related to populations that rehabilitation nurses serve
   a. The need for accessible communities that enable all individuals to participate in community activities
   b. Discrimination against people with disabilities in hiring practices or in the workplace
   c. Disincentives for people with disabilities to return to work
   d. Availability of vocational rehabilitation services
4. Privacy and confidentiality
   a. HIPAA privacy regulations on protected health information, effective April 2003
   b. Development and implementation of electronic medical records

VI. Process of Making Health Policy

A. Phases of Healthcare Policy Making (**Figure 13-2**)

1. Policy formulation (Longest, 2012)
   a. Agenda setting
      1) This first stage of policy development refers to identifying problems and possible solutions proposed by diverse political interests.
      2) Once issues become prominent in the political agenda, they can proceed to the next stage of policy formulation: the development of legislation. However, only a small percentage of issues reach that point.
   b. Development of legislation (**Figure 13-3**)
      1) The legislative process begins with proposals (i.e., bills), which can be drafted by senators or representatives and their staff members, members of the executive branch, political or special interest groups, or individual citizens.
         a) Only members of Congress can officially sponsor a bill.
         b) Occasionally, identical bills are simultaneously introduced in the Senate and the House of Representatives for consideration.
      2) Each bill is assigned to the appropriate committee(s) based on its content and the jurisdiction of the committees and subcommittees. Hearings are held and the bill is marked up. Once it is approved by the full committee, the House or Senate receives

Figure 13-2. A Model of the Public Policymaking Process in the United States

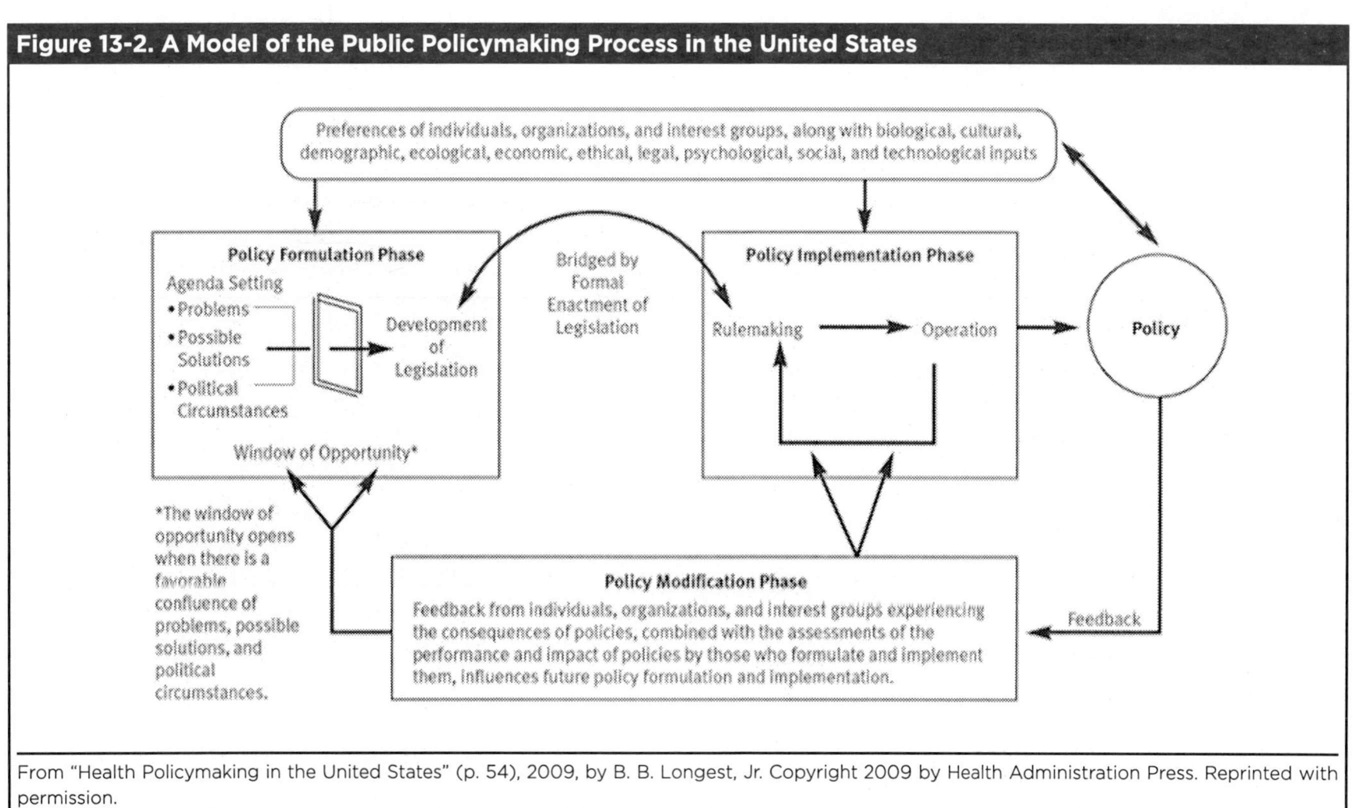

From "Health Policymaking in the United States" (p. 54), 2009, by B. B. Longest, Jr. Copyright 2009 by Health Administration Press. Reprinted with permission.

Figure 13-3. The Path of Legislation in the U.S. Congress

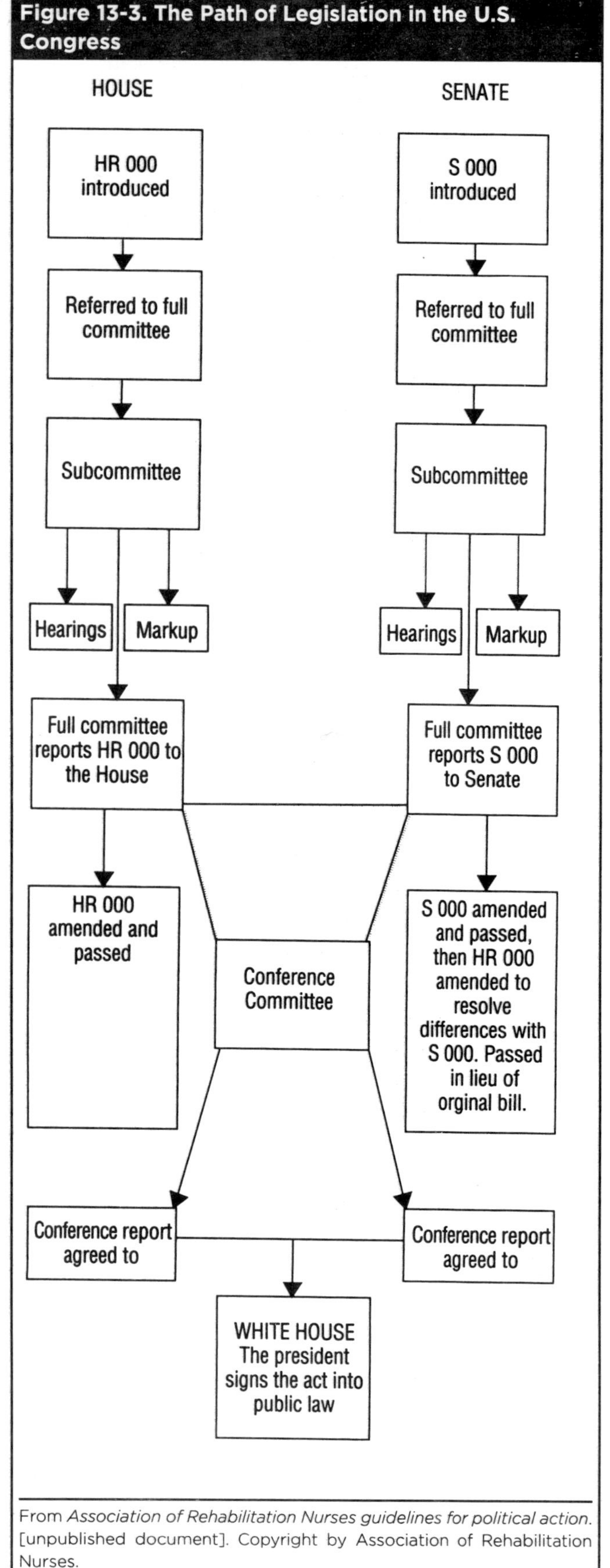

From *Association of Rehabilitation Nurses guidelines for political action.* [unpublished document]. Copyright by Association of Rehabilitation Nurses.

the bill and places it on the legislative calendar for floor action. The bill can be further amended during debate on the floor.

3) After the bill passes either the House or the Senate, it is sent to the other chamber of Congress, where the process is repeated. If the second chamber passes the bill, any differences between the House and Senate versions must be resolved before the bill is sent to the White House for presidential action.
4) The president has the option to sign the bill to make it a law or to veto the bill and return it to Congress with an explanation for the rejection. A presidential veto can be overridden by a two-thirds vote in both houses of Congress. If the president does not sign or veto the bill after 10 days, the bill automatically becomes law.

2. Health policy implementation (includes rule making and policy operation)
   a. Once a law is enacted, implementation rests primarily with the executive branch of the government. Cabinet departments such as the Department of Health and Human Services and agencies such as the CMS and the Centers for Disease Control and Prevention oversee the implementation.
   b. Other agencies such as the Government Accountability Office, the Congressional Budget Office, the Congressional Research Office, and the Office of Technology and Assessment have oversight responsibility.
   c. Laws often are vague on implementation details, so the organization responsible for implementing the law publishes a "Notice of Proposed Rule Making" and "Final Rule" in the Federal Register.
   d. Policy implementation involves the actual operation of programs that are described in the enacted legislation.
3. Policy modification: This stage allows all prior decisions to be modified once the outcomes, perceptions, and consequences of existing policies are discovered. Modifications to any legislation must begin with the agenda-setting stage.

B. Opportunities for Rehabilitation Nurses to Influence Health Policy Making

1. In policy formulation
   a. Agenda setting
      1) Define and document problems.
      2) Develop and evaluate solutions to problems.
      3) Shape political circumstances by lobbying and working through the legal system.

b. Legislation development
1) Participate in drafting legislation.
2) Testify at legislative hearings.
3) Participate in technical expert panels
2. In policy implementation or rule making
a. Provide formal comments on proposed rules published in the Federal Register.
b. Serve on and provide input to rule-making advisory bodies.
c. Work on policy operation by interacting with policy operators.
d. Provide comments and recommendations to draft reports from organizations such as the National Quality Forum.
3. In policy modification: Document cases for modification through operational experience and formal evaluations (i.e., research).

C. Reasons Why Nurses Should Become Involved in Developing Health Policy
1. Has a positive effect on clients and the healthcare delivery system as a whole
2. Enables participation in decisions related to the future of the profession and health care
3. Promotes the ability to provide input at policy-making and health-planning levels
4. Shows a commitment to maintaining healthcare standards
5. Ensures that the value and contribution of the rehabilitation nurse in all levels of care is understood and incorporated into healthcare policy.

D. Guidelines for Taking Political Action
1. Register and vote for the candidates of your choice.
2. Stay informed on issues.
3. Become involved in professional nursing associations and their health policy task forces.
4. Obtain lists of local, state, and national legislators (available from government offices, websites, or public libraries).
5. Join the Association of Rehabilitation Nurses (ARN) Health Policy Committee.
a. Be informed about ARN's position on legislation by contacting the ARN office or the ARN health policy committee chair, or by searching the ARN website (www.rehabnurse.org).
b. Communicate with the ARN health policy committee chair about local and state issues and personal activities.
c. Attend legislative conferences (e.g., Nurse in Washington Internship).
6. Do not act as a spokesperson for a national or local organization unless specifically authorized to do so.
7. Establish a relationship and communicate with federal, state, and local legislators to make them aware of positions on specific issues (see Chapter 9 of the Health Policy Tool Kit at www.rehabnurse.org/advocacy/content/Advocacy-Toolkit.html).
a. Call for information
b. Send e-mail.
c. Request in-person meeting in Washington, DC, or state office.

VII. Healthcare System's Response to Health Policy (Nosse, Friberg, & Kovacek, 1999; Relman, 1988; Roper, Winkenwerder, Hackbarth, & Krakauer, 1988)

A. Growth and Development of the Healthcare Delivery System (1965–1980)
1. The structure of the delivery system included small, independent physician group practices.
2. Larger multispecialty clinics were developing but were uncommon. Hospitals provided secondary and tertiary care.
3. The supply of and demand for healthcare services expanded in response to several factors
a. Introduction of Medicare and Medicaid programs
b. An increased need for the capacity, capabilities, and number and types of healthcare providers
c. A greater number of people accessing the delivery system
d. An increased amount of care provided
e. New and improved treatments and technology

B. Cost Containment in the Delivery of Health Care (1981–1991)
1. Cost containment was a concern for physicians, hospitals, and public and private insurers.
2. Acute care PPS began in 1983 and helped reduce the costs of inpatient hospital care by
a. Decreasing the average length of stay
b. Decreasing the use of routine diagnostic tests during inpatient hospitalizations
c. Shifting care to outpatient settings
d. Increasing the use of postacute care services (e.g., inpatient rehabilitation hospitals and units, SNFs and home care)
3. The decrease in inpatient hospital use resulted in excess acute-care bed capacity, decreased profits for hospitals and physicians, and imposed financial limits on purchasing new technologies and upgrading facilities.
4. These trends caused providers to compete for a larger share of the healthcare market and to react in many ways.

a. Reduced costs through reorganization and staff layoffs
b. Developed and modified alternative care options (e.g., rehabilitation services, home care, ambulatory care, long-term care)
c. Restructured the organization through vertical and horizontal integration with other providers so that hospital networks cover larger geographic areas and provide a full continuum of services
d. Focused new attention on marketing provider services

C. Value, Assessment, and Accountability (1990s to present)
1. Managed-care enrollment increased dramatically in the early 1990s.
2. National, publicly traded, for-profit healthcare corporations became more common.
3. Small independent providers joined together to form specialty service networks to capture and hold market shares.
4. Large physician groups joined with hospitals or contracted with managed-care organizations.
5. Interest in the quality of care and documenting the outcomes of health services, including publishing healthcare report cards, increased.
6. Consumerism increased.
7. Interest in evidence-based practice increased.
8. PPSs were developed for skilled nursing facilities, home-health agencies, inpatient rehabilitation hospitals, and long-term care hospitals.
9. Quality measures were developed for public reporting, quality-improvement activities, and pay-for-performance activities.
10. Accountable care organizations were formed to manage and provide coordinated care for Medicare patients.
11. Initiatives that examined paying for episodes of care (i.e., bundling) were implemented.

VIII. Key Forces Shaping the Future of Healthcare Delivery in the United States (Kovner & Knickman, 2011; Sultz & Young, 2013)

A. Changing Demographics
1. Aging of the population: Healthcare resource use and costs increase significantly with advancing age.
2. Increasing ethnic diversity: Racial and ethnic minority groups in the United States have poorer health than the White population. If the current disparities continue, the burden of illness will increase as the minority population increases.

B. Controlling of Spending for Medicare/CHIP and Medicaid Programs: Changes made to these programs will affect the entire healthcare marketplace, because these programs combined account for 39% of personal health expenditures, 44% of hospital expenditures, 32% of physician and professional expenditures, 56% of nursing home care, and 81% of home-health care (Medicare Payment Advisory Commission, 2014).

C. Public Belief That Our Own Behaviors Affect Our Health: There is increasing understanding that the determinants of health have less to do with the healthcare system than with the way we lead our lives and the environment in which we live.

D. Uninsured: The Affordable Care Act seeks to reduce the number of uninsured.

E. Adoption of Health Information Technology: Technology can facilitate accountability and increase productivity through the use of data collection, analysis, and utilization to guide patient care. It also raises concerns related to maintaining the privacy of health information.

F. *Genomics*: The linking of human diseases with variations in specific genes

G. Technological Growth and Innovation: New diagnostic and treatment modalities are expected to further shift care into outpatient settings and prolong life; telehealth could increase access to care.

H. Changing Professional Labor Supply: Shortages of key health professionals, redefinition of professional roles

I. Expanding Role of Nurses: Nurses' roles are expanding to address the need for care coordination and navigation of the healthcare delivery system. Nurses are therefore practicing in more than one state and need licenses in multiple states or multistate licensure. The National Council of State Boards of Nursing (www.NCSBN.org) has adopted a compact that grants one license that confers the ability to practice in participating states.

J. Globalization of the Economy: Increased scrutiny of healthcare costs

K. Greater federal government involvement in measuring and paying for positive outcomes, while penalizing providers with poor outcomes.

References

Association of Rehabilitation Nurses (ARN). (2014). ARN competency model for professional rehabilitation nursing. Retrieved from http://www.rehabnurse.org/uploads/files/education/ARN_Rehabilitation_Nursing_Competency _Model_FINAL_-_May_2014.pdf

Barker, E. (1999). Life care planning. *RN Journal,* 52(3), 58–61.

Centers for Medicare & Medicaid Services (2013). 2014 Medicare costs. Retrieved from www.medicare.gov/Pubs/pdf/11579.pdf

Centers for Medicare & Medicaid Services (2014). 2014 CMS Statistics. CMS Publication No. 03510. Retrieved from http://www.cms.gov/Research-Statistics-Data-and-Systems/Statistics-Trends-and-Reports/CMS-Statistics-Reference-Booklet/Downloads/CMS_Stats_2014_final.pdf

The Henry J. Kaiser Family Foundation (2014a). *Medicaid: A primer.* Menlo Park, CA: Author.

The Henry J. Kaiser Family Foundation (2014b). *Medicare: A primer.* Menlo Park, CA: Author.

Institute of Medicine (2006). *Performance measurement: Accelerating improvement.* Washington, DC: The National Academies Press.

Kongstvedt, P. R. (2003). *Essentials of managed health care* (4th ed.). Sudbury, MA: Jones & Bartlett.

Kongstvedt, P. R. (2012). *Essentials of managed health care* (6th ed.). Sudbury, MA: Jones & Bartlett.

Kovner, A. R., & Knickman, J. R. (2011). *Healthcare delivery in the United States* (10th ed.). New York: Springer.

Levy, J. (2014). In U.S., Uninsured rate lowest since 2008. Retrieved from http://www.gallup.com/poll/168248/uninsured-rate-lowest-2008.aspx

Longest, B. B. (2012). *Health policymaking in the United States* (4th ed.). Chicago: Health Administration Press.

Medicare Payment Advisory Commission (2014). *Data book: Healthcare spending and the Medicare program.* Washington, DC: Author.

Nosse, L. J., Friberg, D. G., & Kovacek, P. R. (1999). *Managerial and supervisory principles for physical therapists.* Baltimore, MD: Lippincott Williams & Wilkins.

Okara, C. A., Young, S. L., Strine, T. W., Balluz, L. S., & Mokdad, A. H. (2005). Uninsured adults aged 65 years and older. Is their health at risk? *Journal of Health Care for the Poor and Underserved, 16*(3), 453–463.

Relman, A. S. (1988). Assessment and accountability: The third revolution in medical care. *New England Journal of Medicine, 319*(18), 1220–1222.

Roper, W. L., Winkenwerder, W., Hackbarth, G. M., & Krakauer, H. (1988). Effectiveness in health care. An initiative to evaluate and improve medical practice. *New England Journal of Medicine, 319*(18), 1197–1202.

Schoen, C., Hayes, S. L., Collins, S. R. Lippa, J. A., & Radley, D. C. (2014). *America's underinsured: A state-by-state look at health insurance affordability prior to the new coverage expansions.* New York: The Commonwealth Fund.

Sultz, H. A., & Young, K. M. (2013). *Health care USA* (8th ed.). Sudbury, MA: Jones & Bartlett.

Suggested Resources

American Nurses Association Activist Toolkit: http://www.rnaction.org/site/PageServer?pagename=nstat_activist_toolkit

Bodenheimer, T. S., & Grumbach, K. (2012). *Understanding health policy: A clinical approach* (6th ed.). Norwalk, CT: Appleton & Lange.

Center for Medicare & Medicaid Services: www.cms.gov

Hoeman, S. P. (Ed.) (2002). *Rehabilitation nursing: Process, application & outcomes* (3rd ed., pp. 37–44). St. Louis: Mosby Elsevier.

Kominski, G. (Ed). (2014). *Changing the U.S. health care system: Key issues in health services policy and management.* San Francisco: Jossey-Bass.

Mason, D. J., Leavitt, J. K., & Chaffee M. W. (Eds.). (2014). *Policy & politics in nursing and health care.* St. Louis: Saunders.

Chapter 14

Theory and Practice Models for Rehabilitation Nursing

Mindi Miller, PhD MSN MA RN CRRN

LEARNING OUTCOMES

- Review theories pertinent to rehabilitation nursing.
- Compare and contrast the work of theorists within topical areas.
- Reflect on the application of theory to clinical practice in rehabilitation.

KEY CHAPTER TOPICS

- Developmental theories
- Behavioral theories
- Cognitive theories
- Moral theories
- Personality theories
- Family development and function theories
- Nursing theories and conceptualizations
- Application of theory to advanced practice

PROFESSIONAL REHABILITATION NURSING DOMAINS AND COMPETENCIES

- Domain 2: Competencies 2.1, 2.2, 2.3 (Association of Rehabilitation Nurses [ARN], 2014)

Introduction

Changes in viewpoints and priorities occur when theories are developed, tested, and refined. A rich history of theory building by various disciplines has been documented that addresses human growth across the life span. The motion of the life span involves more than chronological age. Numerous interdisciplinary models depict physical, cognitive, emotional, and social development under various conditions, whereas family concepts are tied to cultural beliefs and relationship values. In short, human growth and development involves a fluctuating milieu through which assorted tasks are accomplished. Choices and behavioral patterns lead to either successful or unsuccessful management of life and its circumstances. Issues of compliance and independence correlate with personality traits, learning preferences, and moral decision making.

Nurses select and create theories to improve the quality of life for their clients. Holistic care incorporates the client's developmental needs, social networks, and lifestyle preferences. Nurses plan interventions and perform research to measure outcomes related to various theories. As described within the Gestalt theory developed by Max Wertheimer in the 1920s, the whole is greater than the sum of its parts. Pieces and parts fit together to produce thoughts, actions, and structures, such as family units (Ellis, 1938; Goodman, 2009). Suppositions such as the Gestalt theory are invaluable to healthcare providers, as they advocate that the patient and the entire family are assisted back to wellness. A theory is more than a speculation; theories become methods for discovering the "whole."

Hypotheses that entail emotional elements are pertinent when coping methods and new skills are developed during rehabilitation. Theories such as cognitive dissonance (Festinger, 1957) are applicable when patients' belief systems clash with reality, thus influencing their coping abilities. The work of Gardner (1993, 2008) suggests that individuals have "multiple intelligences," and growth can occur beyond traditional expectations such as intelligence quotient (IQ) measurements. Efficacy theories (Bandura, 1997; Knight & Shea, 2014) are also relevant to life-span adjustments because independence correlates with opinions about self-care and situational control.

This chapter summarizes diverse viewpoints, theories, and models that are applicable to rehabilitation nursing. The frameworks and suppositions are interrelated, so categories are general and often follow branches of psychology. New to this edition is content from ARN's Domains and Competencies, specifically Domain 2: Promotion of Health and Successful Living in Persons with Disability or Chronic Illness Across the Life Span.

I. Developmental Theories

A. Overview

1. Theories provide systematic statements to explain human phenomena. Theories can be organized in a variety of ways, although traditional headings are psychoanalytic, learning, cognitive, behavioral, and interactive (Boyd & Bee, 2006). Several other categories of theories pertain to life span and rehabilitation, namely, interpersonal, dissonance, moral, family development, and personality theories.
2. Models provide structure for testing new hypotheses about human growth and development.
3. Models that relate to milestones of age, personality, multiple intelligence, social interaction, family function, and moral development add to the mix of traditional conceptual frameworks (Shenk, 2009; Townsend, 2014).
4. Nursing assessment, diagnosis, intervention, outcomes, and resultant reevaluation depend on a firm understanding of interdisciplinary theories (Doenges, Moorhouse, & Murr, 2013). (A summary of individual development and functional theories is provided in **Table 14-1**.)

B. Intrapsychic (Psychoanalytic) Theories

1. Sigmund Freud (1856–1939), the early and long-dominant theorist in the field of personality development, is responsible for the development of intrapsychic theory.
    a. People experience conflict between their natural instincts and society's restrictions on them.
    b. Conflict experienced in childhood influences one's adult personality (Freud, 1959; Gay, 2006).
    c. Four phases occur within set time frames during childhood.
    d. Fixation (e.g., oral, anal, phallic) can result if phases are not achieved successfully.
        1) Oral phase: first year of life
            a) Involves exploring the world orally, and the mouth, lips, and tongue are the center of existence for the infant.
            b) Begins development of the infant's personality, which depends on the mother's (or mothering person or caretaker's) sense of personal security in self and satisfaction in the mother role
            c) The infant experiences the mother's emotions, leading to vulnerability (e.g., if the mother has pervasive anxiety, the infant begins life with a deficit in adaptive abilities).
            d) Weaning from breastfeeding can be challenging.
        2) Anal phase: 18 months–3 years of age
            a) This phase centers on buildup and release of tension in the orifices; involves experiencing pleasure in expelling urine and feces.
            b) It is a challenge to parents' coping ability to allow their child to move away from them and seek freedom or a greater sense of self.
            c) This phase involves ambivalence related to complying with parental and societal values of elimination.
                (i) Complying through proper elimination on the part of the infant
                (ii) Complying through retention or inappropriate discharge of feces or urine by the infant, which brings retribution and further anxiety
                (iii) Toilet training by the parents and the infant's corresponding response, which can govern adult personality
        3) Phallic phase: 3–6 years of age
            a) Becomes aware of gender roles and how males and females differ
                (i) Has romantic attraction to the parent of the opposite sex (i.e., Oedipus complex, boys; Electra complex, girls)
                (ii) Experiences rivalry with the same-sex parent or resolves guilt and fear by identifying with the same-sex parent
            b) Develops a conscience
                (i) Represses sexual urges
                (ii) Imitates sex-related behaviors and beliefs of the parent of the same sex
                (iii) Learns standards of society from parents
        4) Latent and genital phase: 6–12 years of age (latent) and puberty (genital)
            a) Learns to hide sexuality or sublimate urges with hobbies and sports; also, during this time, children learn social rules while experiencing sexual gratification related to feelings toward others
            b) Involves responses from the preceding stages; can cause serious adjustment problems if the stages are not accomplished and instead are carried into

adulthood (e.g., the person is unable to turn away from the self to a more productive activity) and can produce sexual problems
        c) Brings out defensive measures used during earlier phases (e.g., denial and regression) (Freud, 1959)
  e. Other concepts developed by Freud include theories of personality and coping.
    1) Levels of awareness influence personality.
        a) The conscious mind is aware of the current moment.
        b) The preconscious mind pays attention to details that are brought to conscious awareness.
        c) The subconscious mind drives behavior.
    2) Transference: projecting onto another person
        a) Paternal transference (i.e., father figure) to promote feelings of security or authority
        b) Maternal transference (symbolizing unconditional love), or connection to a "fairy godmother" or "wicked witch" figure
        c) Sibling transference (i.e., brother or sister role development) to substitute for absent parental influences
        d) Nonfamiliar transference: treating others as stereotyped or envisioned entities rather than as actual persons
    3) Components of personality interrelate feelings, thoughts, and behaviors.
        a) The id is pleasure seeking, with primitive (animal-like) drives that do not perceive reality.
        b) The ego (agent of adaptation) is aware of reality and identifies consequences of behaviors.
        c) The superego (self-evaluation) houses values and recognizes social morals of right and wrong.
    4) Tension may cause various forms of anxiety.
        a) Reality anxiety is diminished by taking oneself out of an anxiety-producing situation.
        b) Fear of punishment is largely unconscious (from the id) and may result in neurotic anxiety.
        c) Moral anxiety caused by violation of values or moral codes may result in feelings of guilt and shame.
    5) Defense mechanisms and reality distortions result from conflicts between the id, ego, and superego.
        a) Denial: believing that something false is true
        b) Displacement: placing emotions elsewhere, onto a substitute
        c) Intellectualization: objectively analyzing an issue or situation
        d) Projection: blaming feelings on others
        e) Regression: displaying behavior that is younger than one's age or previous developmental phase
        f) Repression: unpleasant thoughts pushed into the subconscious
        g) Sublimation: redirecting bad or wrong urges into socially acceptable forms
  f. Freud's theory of phases has been criticized for lacking research data to support its suppositions, although his models of behavior have relevance as metaphors that depict his observations (Gay, 2006). Freud's models have served as a springboard for later theories and philosophies (Tauber, 2010).
  g. O'Driscoll (2014) suggested that Freud's underlying theory remains helpful when, for example, nurses caring for individuals with learning disabilities use psychoanalytical theory to promote therapeutic communication.
    1) Unconscious thoughts and motives are best assessed by both patients and staff with the use of open-ended discussions. This technique is similar to Freud's psychotherapy methods.
    2) Unplanned sessions encourage clients to speak their thoughts, allowing themes to surface; therefore, repression is exchanged for exploration to promote better insight.
2. Alfred Adler (1870–1937) researched the significance of birth order.
  a. Adler expanded theories of personality to include aspects of superiority, inferiority, and self-actualization.
  b. He identified a connection between illnesses/disabilities and the person's self-image and personality.
3. Carl Jung (1875–1961) developed analytical (or Jungian) psychology.
  a. Jung proposed the collective unconscious, which devised psychic or mental patterns.
  b. Dreams, religion, and other symbols influence a person's view of the world (Jung & Wolfgang, 1955).

Table 14-1. Summary of Individual Development and Function Theories						
				Periods		
Theory and Theorist*	**Description**	**Infancy (0–12 months)**	**Birth–2 years old**	**Toddler (12–36 months)**	**2–7 years old**	
Intrapsychic (Freud, 1959)	Conflict between individuals' natural instincts and society's restrictions on them experienced in childhood influence individuals' adult personality; children are thought to progress through four stages of psychosexual development (Glod, 1998; Whiting, 1997).	Oral	N/A	Anal	N/A	
Interpersonal (Sullivan, 1956, 1971)	Repeated experiences between parents or caretakers and children lead to development of a good self and a bad self, which is the basis for healthy development; six stages represent processes by which an individual's identity develops in the context of relationships (Glod, 1998; Whiting, 1997).	Infancy	N/A	Childhood	N/A	
Social Learning (Erikson, 1963)	Interaction between parents or caretakers and the child is essential to healthy psychological growth; each phase of normal development requires the individual to accomplish age-appropriate developmental tasks through eight phases of development from infancy to older adulthood (Glod, 1998).	Trust vs. mistrust	N/A	Autonomy vs. shame and doubt	N/A	
Behavioral (Pavlov, 1927; Skinner, 1953)	Individuals' development is influenced by stimulus-response interaction; individuals' behavior is shaped through the consistency of responding; two attributes of the human brain—flexibility and plasticity—allow for a developmentally significant variety of adaptive sequences (Glod, 1998).	N/A	N/A	N/A	N/A	
Interactional (Schaie, 1981)	Development of individuals in a progressive direction occurs when goodness of fit (consonance) exists; poorness of fit (dissonance) involves discrepancies between individuals and their environment, which results in distorted development and maladaptive functioning; starting with dependency in infancy, interference with development of independence in adolescence is likely to inhibit the establishment of interdependence in adulthood (Schaie, 1981; Whiting, 1997).	Dependency	N/A	N/A	N/A	
Cognitive (Piaget, 1952)	Motor activity involving concrete objects results in the development of mental functioning; children move through four general periods of cognitive development in the same sequence although not according to the same timetable (Glod, 1998).	N/A	Sensorimotor	N/A	Preoperational	

Major Points

- Human development is a complex, interactive, and multifaceted process that involves a variety of forces.
- Some older theories of development (Freud, 1959; Piaget, 1952) emphasize completion of development early in childhood.
- Other theories (Pavlov, 1927; Skinner, 1953) are not age-specific but allow for a developmentally significant diversity of adaptive sequences.

*Many theories (Erikson, 1963; Schaie, 1981; Sullivan, 1956, 1971) view individual development as a continuous process that unfolds throughout the lifespan rather than as a process that is limited to a few early years in relationships with limited numbers of people (Glod, 1998; Whiting, 1997).

	Periods								
	Preschooler (3–5 years old)	**School age (5–12 years old)**	**7–11 years old**	**11–15 years old**	**Childhood (1–12 years old)**	**Adolescence (12–18 years old)**	**Early adulthood (18–25 years old)**	**Adulthood (26–65 years old)**	**Older adulthood (older than 65 years old)**
	Phallic, oedipal	Latent and genital	N/A	N/A	N/A	N/A	N/A	N/A	N/A
	Childhood, juvenile	Juvenile, preadolescence	N/A	N/A	N/A	Early to late adolescence	Adulthood	Adulthood (continues)	Adulthood (continues)
	Initiative versus guilt	Industry versus inferiority	N/A	N/A	N/A	Identity versus role confusion	Intimacy versus isolation	Generativity versus stagnation	Integrity versus despair
	N/A	N/A	N/A	N/A	N/A	N/A	N/A	N/A	N/A
	N/A	N/A	N/A	N/A	Decreasing dependency	Dependency to independence	Interdependency (adulthood)	Interdependency (adulthood continues)	Interdependency (adulthood continues)
	N/A	N/A	Concrete operational	Formal operational	N/A	N/A	N/A	N/A	N/A

C. Interpersonal Theories
   1. Harry Stack Sullivan (1892–1949) developed the interpersonal theory associated with potential personality factor.
      a. Sullivan (1956; 1971) departed from Freudian concepts; he believed the personality is developed from interaction with social groups (Barton, 1996).
      b. The term *integrating tendencies* describes behavior in which one person gravitates toward another person.
      c. Healthy development is based on repeated experiences between parents or caretakers and children that lead to the development of a good self and a bad self.
      d. Seven stages of development represent processes by which the person's identity develops in the context of relationships.
         1) Infancy: Developing senses of sequential time and self-representations of good and bad
         2) Childhood: Beginning to develop interpersonal relationships with peers, language skills, and gender identity
         3) Preadolescence juvenile: Expanding interactions to social, group, and societal relationships
         4) Preadolescence: Same-sex relationship with ability to form meaningful, nondependent peer relationships
         5) Early adolescence: Developing sexuality and gender identity
         6) Late adolescence: Beginning to assume responsibility
         7) Adulthood: Containing these interpersonal themes that continue to emerge in new relationships
   2. Personality is shaped by relationships.
      a. Difficulties in development are viewed as manifestations of disordered interpersonal relationships (Sullivan, 1956).
      b. Psychotherapy aims to understand interactions to improve participation and facilitate connections (Barton, 1996; Goodman, 2009).
   3. Frieda Fromm-Reichmann (1889–1957) and Clara Mabel Thompson (1893–1958) wrote extensively on the topic of interpersonal development.
   4. Both worked with Harry Sullivan to establish the William Alanson White Institute, which trains psychotherapists.
   5. Both addressed cultural influences and humanistic aspects of psychoanalysis, concentrating on interpersonal relationships (Bradberry, 2007; Carducci, 2009).

D. Social Learning Theories
   1. Erik Erikson (1902–1994) suggested that interactions between parent or caretaker and child are essential to healthy psychological growth (i.e., parents raise the child, and the child influences the parents).
      a. Through satisfactory completion of the developmental task of each psychosocial stage, people become ready to move through the stages of development from infancy to adulthood (Erikson, 1963).
      b. There are eight sequential psychosocial stages.
         1) Trust versus mistrust (infancy)
            a) Viewing the universe as reliable
            b) Seeing relationships as stable and available
         2) Autonomy versus shame and doubt (toddlerhood)
            a) Understanding control over one's body and thoughts
            b) Understanding disappointment in self and others
         3) Initiative versus guilt (preschool years): Dealing with predominantly genital issues
         4) Industry versus inferiority (school age): Dealing with latency, school, and relationships outside the family
         5) Identity versus role confusion (adolescence)
            a) Clarifying personal identity
            b) Depersonifying internal representations
         6) Intimacy versus isolation (young adulthood)
            a) Rediscovering attachment
            b) Developing mature bonding
         7) Generativity versus stagnation (middle adulthood)
            a) Being creative and productive
            b) Carrying out parental responsibilities
         8) Integrity versus despair (older adulthood): Feeling a sense of completeness based on an integrated philosophy of one's unique life (Erikson, 1963)
   2. Joan Erikson (1920–1997) continued her husband's work on the eighth and the new, ninth stage (Erikson, Erikson, & Kivnick, 1986).
      a. Using notes and her own ideas, she articulated the gerotranscendence stage.

b. In the ninth stage, people experience a change of focus, shifting from valuing materialistic things to attaining life satisfaction goals.
c. This theory is relevant to the aging populating with longer life spans (Jarvis, 2012).

3. Albert Bandura (1925–present) theorized that behavior is learned by observing and modeling others.
   a. Social learning results from attention, retention, reproduction, and motivation.
   b. An additional theory was developed related to self-efficacy, a belief in one's own ability to manage situations and challenges (Bandura, 1997).
   c. Theories of belief, choice, and behavior may have dual classifications between developmental and behavioral frameworks (B. M. Newman & Newman, 2009).

E. Significance for Rehabilitation
1. Milestones of age and developmental tasks are taken into consideration within the treatment milieu.
2. Psychoanalytic theories assist with identifying appropriate age-specific coping mechanisms when dealing with life-changing events.
3. Domains are pertinent to developmental tasks.
   a. 2.1: Health promotion is lifelong as age-specific milestones are addressed.
   b. 2.2: Self-management is fostered within the context of age-appropriate development.
   c. 2.3: Transitions of care are juxtaposed with life-span transitions to optimize independence.

II. Behavioral Theories

A. Overview
1. Ivan Pavlov (1849–1936) and B. F. Skinner (1904–1990) studied how behavior is affected by its consequences. Behavior is reportedly developed through a stimulus-response interaction.
2. Human behavior is derived largely from childhood experiences (Sigelman & Rider, 2011; Skinner, 1953).
3. Dissonance (poorness of fit) involves discrepancies between the individual and the environment that result in distorted development or maladaptive functioning (Festinger, 1957).

B. Classical Conditioning Theory
1. Conditioning occurs when a once-neutral stimulus becomes analogous with a response after the stimulus and the response have been associated with each other (Pavlov, 1927).
2. Derived in part from Pavlov's work with dogs, behavioral theory suggests that internal responses can be changed by modifying behavior.
3. Classical conditioning results in automatic responses evoked by a stimulus.

C. Environmental consequences of behavior theory
1. Skinner's theory extends Pavlovian theory to human beings.
2. Learning is influenced by the effect of individuals' behaviors.
3. Behavior is shaped with positive and negative reinforcers, increasing or decreasing the likelihood that a given action will result or learning will occur (Skinner, 1953).

D. Interactional Model
1. K. Warner Schaie (1928–present) focused on development from young adulthood to older ages. The concept of goodness of fit (consonance) versus dissonance arises from situations and choices that are either in conflict or harmony with each other (Schaie, 1981).
2. Adult outcomes can be influenced by childhood events and adolescent experiences.
   a. Consonance involves having environmental demands and expectations in accord with one's capacity to respond.
   b. A sense of comfort or consonance makes optimal development possible.
   c. Progression from dependence to interdependence occurs throughout the developmental stages.
   d. Adaptation corresponds with the demands of a child's chronological age and particular interests.
      1) Dependency in infancy (0–1 year of age)
      2) Decreasing dependency in childhood (1–12 years of age)
      3) Dependency conflict in early adolescence, with a struggle toward independence in middle adolescence and independence achieved in late adolescence (i.e., older than 13 years of age)
      4) Interdependency achieved in adulthood (i.e., older than 21 years of age)

E. Dissonance Theories
1. Emotional discord or dissonance occurs when there is a situation that is in conflict with expectations (Gawronski, 2012). There is a mismatch between an individual's belief system and reality (or desired outcome). In other words, the heart and the mind do not agree.
2. Dissonance also occurs with two equally correct or valued choices, until an excuse for not selecting one of the choices is mentally composed and accepted. Emotional turmoil persists until a choice is made and rationalization is accepted.

3. Cooper (2007) suggests that mental steps are taken, consciously and unconsciously, during daily activities, for example, buying unhealthy food when grocery shopping with the self-promise of purchasing healthier food the next time.
4. Dissonance theory also relates to healthcare decisions.
   a. A type of mental arousal results when an individual acts responsibly, such as with self-reporting noncompliant behavior.
   b. Dissonance theory is applicable to family decisions, especially when there are opposing opinions about treatment or care.
   c. **Table 14-2** depicts dissonance about a life-changing decision from two different family-member perspectives.

F. Significance for Rehabilitation
1. Conditioning and learned behavior can be helpful when redirecting clients toward healthy behaviors.
2. Dissonance happens at many levels; for example, conflicts between rational and emotional reactions to stress.
3. Domains are applicable to cognitive behaviors and choices:
   a. 2.1: Decisions related to health-promotion activities require engagement in this choice.
   b. 2.2: Self-management is fostered by problem-solving behaviors.
   c. 2.3: Care transitions occur by selecting options that promote or maintain independence.

III. Cognitive Theories

A. Overview
1. Cognitive theories are closely related to learning and behavioral theories.
2. Constructivists such as John Dewey (1859–1952) believe learning occurs through exploration, whereas behaviorists believe concepts are learned from adults or teachers.
3. Piaget's and Vygotsky's theories of development share similarities, although Piaget's theory leans toward psychology, whereas Vygotsky's views are more sociocultural (Piaget, 1952; Vygotsky, 1978).

B. Piaget's Stages of Development
1. Jean Piaget (1896–1980) studied the development of children's understanding, including how children evolve ways of knowing and how they develop right and wrong answers.
2. He believed growth resulted from social and neurological maturity.
   a. Every child passes through stages of cognitive development in the same sequence, although not according to a given timetable.

Table 14-2. Combining the Nursing Process, Cognitive Dissonance Theory, and Domain 2.3
The Mother's Statements Logic: "I want to go to the nursing home." Value: "I love my daughter and must not ruin her life." Morals: "It would be wrong for me to go live with my daughter."
The Daughter's Statements Logic: "I can better care for Mom if she lives with me." Value: "I love my mother and want to help her now." Morals: "It would be wrong for me to send Mom away."
The Nursing Process The nurse collects subjective and objective data from the family. Factors such as finances and home environments are addressed by the family and the interdisciplinary team. The nurse continues to assess underlying beliefs and values. Love of family is a consistent theme between the mother and daughter. The statements of "wrong" imply that both mother and daughter will feel remorse if decisions are made that conflict with their perceived duties and desires. Although the mother has self-care issues, the nurse learns that the family's primary concern relates to their need to make a quick decision about living arrangements. In this scenario, a nursing diagnosis related to coping takes priority over the self-care deficit.
Cognitive Dissonance Theory Dissonance is a factor to consider when addressing discharge planning and the stress associated with a lifestyle change. As the family considers their moving plan, the nurse gathers additional resources and interventions for the mother and daughter, such as information on available respite care. The objective options (logistics of moving) are easier to identify than the subjective views (feelings) of family members. By using a cognitive dissonance framework, the value systems of both mother and daughter can be discovered and discussed.
Effective Care Transitions Although nurses are skilled at therapeutic communication, the analysis of belief systems is a more complex procedure. A process of recording that lists statements and responses is a good tool for deciphering and discussing the family's feelings underlying their verbalizations. A brief teaching session with clients to explain cognitive dissonance can be helpful. By listing the logic/value/moral aspects of a decision, family members can identify their common beliefs and work together for a united rationalization and effective transition.

   b. Every child develops strategies for interacting with the environment and knowing the environment's properties.
   c. A gradual progression takes place from one period of cognitive development to the next; acquisition of each new operation builds on existing ones.

d. Differentiation and complexity occur and are matched by increasing integration and co-ordination of schemata in this process of development.
e. Infants possess both fixed and flexible reflexes that enable them to develop abstract, intelligent behavior.
f. Children move through four general periods of cognitive development.
   1) Sensorimotor: Occurs from 0 to 2 years of age
      a) Development proceeds from reflex activity to representation and sensorimotor learning.
      b) Feelings and actions are inseparable.
      c) Sucking and touching actions by infants are innate at first.
      d) Infants begin to understand how personal behavior affects the world and become involved in trial-and-error actions.
   2) Preoperational: Occurs from 2 to 7 years of age
      a) Development proceeds from sensorimotor representation to prelogical thought.
      b) By maintaining stable and consistent images, children are able to create a representational world.
      c) Children begin to fantasize and use symbols to represent objects and feelings.
   3) Concrete operational: Occurs from 7 to 11 years of age
      a) Development proceeds from prelogical thought to logical, concrete thought.
      b) Rules are devised to govern behavior.
      c) Trial-and-error is replaced by the ability to problem solve.
   4) Formal operational: Occurs from 11 to 15 years of age
      a) Development proceeds from logical, concrete thought to logical solutions to all kinds of categories of problems.
      b) Reasoning and abstract conceptualizations are used to help guide future actions.
      c) The ability to "walk in another's shoes" is gained.
      d) Deductive logic is used (Piaget, 1952).

C. Vygotsky's Theoretical Framework
1. Lev Vygotsky (1896–1934) theorized that children build on previously learned experiences and ideas.
2. Social interaction provides the means for step-by-step changes in a child's thought process and behavior.
3. Development varies between cultures and worldviews.
4. The four basic principles of the Vygotskian sociocultural theory are as follows:
   a. Children construct their knowledge.
   b. Development cannot be separated from social context.
   c. Learning leads to development.
   d. Language has a major role in mental development.

D. Significance for Rehabilitation
1. Building on previously learned tasks and developmental achievements can facilitate progress (i.e., starting from a point of success or known ability).
2. Developmental guidelines assist with planning reasonable steps toward restoration.
3. Application of theories to domains related to growth and development
   a. 2.1: Prevention techniques vary depending on the developmental stage and associated risks.
   b. 2.2: Self-management is contingent on reasoning abilities and ongoing developmental achievements.
   c. 2.3: Transitions of care occur throughout periods of cognitive development.

IV. Moral Theories

A. Overview
1. Greek philosophers discussed moral issues in terms of happiness and harmony, whereas later theories concentrated on ethical/moral issues of right and wrong.
   a. Socrates: Virtue means knowing the meaning of good and evil.
   b. Plato: Virtue means all parts of the soul are in harmony.
   c. Aristotle: Good is that which is done for its own sake.
      1) The goal of all activities is happiness.
      2) Happiness means doing well; flourishing.
      3) The highest good is self-sufficiency, lacking nothing (Myers, 2007).
2. Kohlberg's and Gilligan's viewpoints of moral development are an expansion of Piaget's theories.
3. Focus of theories concerns moral development in adolescence; it can be applied to ethical situations. (See **Table 14-3** for a comparison of these theories.)

B. Levels of Moral Development
1. Lawrence Kohlberg (1927–1987) created three levels of moral development.

Table 14-3. A Comparison of Kohlberg's (1963, 1976) and Gilligan's (1982) Theories of Moral Development

	Kohlberg's Theory	Gilligan's Theory
Development of the self	Autonomy, individuality, independence	Connections with others, interdependence
Others	Objective concern for others; treats others fairly in terms of equality	Concern for others; helping, caring
Relationships	Reciprocity between separate individuals with a focus on fulfilling duties and obligations.	Responsiveness to others in the context of their situation and on their own terms.
Morality	Use of a "justice" approach: Moral problems are resolved by the use of impartial, abstract rules, principles, and standards of society, especially fairness.	Use of a "care" approach: Moral problems are resolved by reflecting or responding to the problem in the context of the individual; use of relativism and situational ethics; concern for maintaining relationships and interdependence.

Data from Gilligan, 1982; Kohlberg, 1963, 1976.

a. Preconventional morality (selfishness)
b. Conventional morality
c. Postconventional morality: principles higher than rules (Kohlberg, 1963, 1976)

2. Kohlberg's model is based on research and extends from childhood through adulthood.
   a. Kohlberg's theories are based on responses to hypothetical moral dilemmas.
   b. Women were not included in study samples.
3. Kohlberg outlined six stages within his three levels of moral development, as identified from his observations.
   a. Stage 1: A punishment and obedience orientation in children age 5–6 years, in which decisions are based on avoidance of punishment by an authority figure
   b. Stage 2: Instrumental/relativist orientation in children age 7–10 years, quid pro quo ("scratch my back, I'll scratch yours")
      1) Decisions are based on perceived benefits to self in return for agreeing to a rule.
      2) The focus is on reciprocity (i.e., the right action consists of satisfying one's own needs by seeking out rewards for good behavior).
   c. Stage 3: Good boy/nice girl orientation in early adolescence, in which decisions are based on seeking approval and on helping and pleasing others
   d. Stage 4: Law-and-order views in adolescence to young adulthood, in which decisions are based on adhering to rules for the sake of maintaining social order
   e. Stage 5: Social contract, legalistic orientation in adults
      1) Decisions are based on justice and fairness to others.
      2) The emphasis is on the possibility of changing laws to maintain social utility.
   f. Stage 6: A universal ethical principle orientation in adults, in which decisions are based on a person's self-chosen ethical principles, such as the universal principles of justice, equality of human rights; and respect for the individuality of human beings as people

C. Gender Studies

1. Carol Gilligan (1936–present) conducted research that included female participants.
2. Her study focused on female adolescents, which differed from Kohlberg's work based on all-male subjects.
   a. Consists of broad developmental patterns of orientation to care
   b. Does not address a stage hierarchy
3. Basic elements of moral judgment (Gilligan, 1982) include a definition and development of the self.
   a. Individuals define themselves in terms of their ability to form meaningful relationships or connections with others.
   b. They also define themselves in terms of their ability to care for others.
   c. A description of others is identified in relation to the self.
   d. The self's interdependence with others is crucial.
   e. Moral decision making is based on the context of the situation, although exceptions to rules are allowed. (See the comparison of Kohlberg's and Gilligan's theories in Table 14-3.)

D. Significance to Rehabilitation

1. Concepts of right, wrong, good, and bad highlight areas where clients and families might experience conflict.
2. Negative emotions, such as guilt, can be obviated or minimized when articulated and addressed.
3. Moral and ethical issues can be pertinent to choices of care and discussions of quality of life.
4. Application of domains involves the assessment of moral issues.
   a. 2.1: Health promotion requires deciding between right and wrong.

b. 2.2: Self-management goals can reflect levels of moral development as decisions are made, with a rationale given for these decisions.
c. 2.3: Care transitions reflect personal beliefs and values throughout the life span.

V. Personality Theories

A. Overview: Many theories address human behavior and thought processes that relate to emotional reactions. Several of these premises, such as how an event is explained (i.e., attribution theory) or how humans view themselves (i.e., self-perception and self-verification theories), are pertinent to mental health but are not reviewed in this section.

1. Personality is a branch of psychology that investigates human nature and individual differences. Many theories have an element of personality within their framework.
2. Early life experiences can be significant in terms of attitudes and actions, yet behaviors might not have any obvious connection or correlation with the theories that attempt to explain personality.
3. Personality types (e.g., introvert or extrovert) and personality traits (e.g., shy or creative) are defined differently.

B. Personality Assessment

1. Multiple personality tests have been developed, such as the Rorschach inkblot test, developed in 1921, and the Myers-Briggs Type Indicator, yet theories and debates abound concerning the roles of environment, heredity, DNA, social factors, birth order, and a host of other variables that fuel these debates (McGhee, Ehrler, & Buckhalt, 2008).
2. There is evidence that physical inactivity influences emotional and mental health. Immobility can also influence personality traits and delay personality development (Gallagher, Yancy, Denissen, Kuhnel, & Voils, 2013; Stephan, Sutin, & Terracciano, 2013).
3. Studies support the correlation between personality traits and patient care outcomes (Bunevicius et al., 2014; Israel & Moffitt, 2014).
4. Healthcare workers display personality traits that influence patient and worker outcomes (Montes-Berges & Augusto-Landa, 2014).
5. Hypotheses have been developed related to risk takers as well as those who prepare for worst-case scenarios. Studies identify potential survivor types, or a survivor IQ, that can predict who is most likely to live through catastrophic events (Sherwood, 2010).

C. Maslow's Hierarchy

1. Abraham Maslow (1908–1970) developed the idea of self-actualization.
2. A hierarchy of needs is listed in five layers, with the most important physiological human needs identified as air, water, food, and sex.
3. Safety and security needs are next in Maslow's hierarchy; they include concepts of shelter (home), job security, and monetary security (e.g., insurance and retirement plans).
4. Love and belonging follow safety and include family, work, and community belongingness; negativity can result in loneliness (Maslow, 1954).
5. Esteem needs include two types: (a) respect from others and (b) a sense of achievement and self-respect. If they are not achieved, inferiority complexes can develop.
6. Self-actualization allows people to achieve their potential, and homeostasis results (Maslow, 1971).

D. Fully Functioning Person: Carl Rogers (1902–1987) developed the fully functional person philosophy, with five basic categories that have elements of personality in each category.

1. Openness to experience: the antithesis of defensiveness
   a. Able to accept reality
   b. In touch with personal feelings and values
2. Existential living: living in the here and now
   a. Tendency to be balanced and not living in the past or future
   b. Sees dreams and memories for what they are, not what they should have been
3. Organismic trusting: self-trust with a tendency for self-actualization
4. Experiential freedom: People feel free to make available choices.
5. Creativity: People feel obligated to help others feel actualized.
   a. Joy in a job well done
   b. Similar concepts to Erikson's generativity philosophy (Rogers, 1980)

E. Multiple Intelligences

1. Howard Gardner (1943–present) conceptualized more than one IQ or intelligence in an individual.
2. Gardner's multiple intelligence categories include interpersonal/intrapersonal, kinesthetic, linguistic, logical/math, naturalist, musical, moral, and spatial.
3. His theory is similar to some learning theories; he suggests using different methods (such as a preferred learning approach) to capture the intelligence for maximum expertise and growth (Gardner, 1993).

F. Significance for Rehabilitation

1. The optimal treatment plans correlate client learning styles, personality traits, and innate abilities and preferences.
2. Client's responses are linked to their self-actualization issues and ability to focus on priorities.
3. Individual needs and expectations are housed within the scope of their personae and values of self.
4. Application of the domains to social functioning is relevant to self-actualization theories.
   a. 2.1: Safety is enhanced when intelligence and skills are used to prevent risks.
   b. 2.2: Self-management and the concept of being fully functional are similar premises.
   c. 2.3: Care transitions correlate to the hierarchy of needs as priorities are set in relationship to change.

VI. Family Development and Function Theories (Table 14-4)

A. Overview

1. The *family* is a group of people in varying stages of growth.
   a. Patterns of changes occur, and like the individual, the family unit progresses through stages of growth and development.
   b. Family life stages of development can be a useful frame of reference for rehabilitation nurses, who assess and intervene with families across the life span.
   c. Attachment theories provide a guide for assessing support systems and relationship risks (Becker, 1974; Bowlby, 1969).
2. The needs of the family can be anticipated, depending on the family's developmental stage (Anderson, 2000).

Table 14-4. Summary of Family Development and Function Theories

		Periods			
Theory	**Description**	**Stage 1**	**1–10 years**	**Stage 2**	
Duvall's (1977) Family Life Cycle	Family development is an 8-stage division that allows differentiation of the family's changes over time and an analysis of the relationship between the family and the individual's developmental tasks. These cycles begin with the establishment of the marital relationship and are based primarily on the age or school placement of the eldest child. Successful accomplishment of the tasks in each stage promotes growth and provides a basis for success in the next developmental stage. On the other hand, failure to successfully complete each stage's developmental tasks may result in unhappiness, societal disapproval, and difficulties in accomplishing the tasks in the next stage (Hogarth & Weeks, 1997; Youngblood, 1999).	Marriage and the joining of families	N/A	Families with infants	
Stevenson's (1977) Family Life Cycle	Four stages of family development are identified that are based on the couple's relationship over time. Success or failure of the family depends on the developmental tasks accomplished in each stage beginning in the first year of the relationship. The last stage ends with the death of one partner and the remaining partner grieving and continuing to grow (Hogarth & Weeks, 1997; Stevenson, 1977).	N/A	The emerging family	N/A	

Major Points

- *Family life cycle* is defined as the existence of a nuclear family unit (i.e., mother, father, child) from its inception to its dissolution.
- Family life cycle stages are viewed as the amount of time needed to complete each stage of family development.
- The family is a task-performance group that also has specific stage-related behaviors.
- A family evolves over time. The life history of a family is divided into expected stages of development.
- Each stage of development is characterized by relevant tasks and predictable crises associated with the achievement or nonachievement of specific developmental tasks.
- The life cycles defined by Duvall (1977) and Stevenson (1977) are based on a traditional nuclear family form. Neither theory reflects today's lifestyle changes and various types of families (e.g., divorce, alternative marriage, single parenting).
- Duvall's theory assumes that an intact family (i.e., marriage and children) has universal tasks as well as specific developmental tasks that must be accomplished by the family at eight different stages.
- Stevenson's four stages of family development are based on the length of the couple's relationship and specific developmental task completion throughout the relationshiop (Carter & McGoldrick, 1989; Youngblood, 1999).

B. Ruth Evelyn Millis Duvall (1906–1998) was a pioneer in applying developmental theories to the study of families.
   1. According to Duvall (1977), basic tasks of families occur during the family life cycle and include the following:
      a. Physical maintenance: keeping the family together
      b. Allocating resources: meeting the family's needs and allocating goods, facilities, space, and authority
      c. Division of labor: dividing chores within the family
      d. Socialization of family members: teaching family members active participation in society
      e. Providing for reproduction: recruitment and release of family members
      f. Maintaining order: keeping structure and organization within the family
      g. Placing family members into society
      h. Maintaining motivation and morale: giving encouragement and affection
         1) Meeting with personal and family crises
         2) Refining a philosophy of life and a sense of family loyalty through use of rituals
   2. Stages of family development
      a. Marriage and the joining of families
         1) Establishing an identity as a couple
         2) Establishing relationships with extended families
         3) Making decisions about parenthood
      b. Families with infants
         1) Maintaining the couple's relationship while bonding with and integrating the infant into the family
         2) Maintaining the couple's relationship while assuming the parenting role
      c. Families with preschool-age children
         1) Teaching socialization to children

	Periods								
	Stage 3	**Stage 4**	**Stage 5**	**Stage 6**	**11–25 years**	**Stage 7**	**26–40 years**	**Stage 8**	**More than 40 years**
	Families with pre-school-age children	Families with school-age children	Families with teenagers	Families as launching centers	N/A	Families of middle years (empty nesters)	N/A	Families in retirement (retirement to death)	N/A
	N/A	N/A	N/A	N/A	The crystallizing family	N/A	The integrating family	N/A	The actualizing family

2) Learning to adjust to the children being with babysitters or other adult caregivers

d. Families with school-age children

1) Helping the children develop peer relationships

2) Adjusting to longer periods of separation between parents and children

e. Families with teenagers

1) Adjusting to the children's increased autonomy, which is developing

2) Focusing on midlife issues

f. Families as launching centers

1) Adjusting to the children leaving home and becoming independent adults

2) Adjusting the couple's relationship as less parenting is required from them

g. Families of middle years ("empty nesters")

1) Adjusting to living alone again as a couple as the last child leaves home

2) Beginning to prepare for retirement

3) Developing new relationships with adult children and grandchildren

h. Families in retirement (from retirement to death)

1) Beginning to prepare for death of spouse

2) Adjusting to loss of family members and friends (Duvall, 1977)

C. Family Life Cycle Theory: Joan Stevenson-Hinde (1977) based this theory on the length of a couple's relationship.

1. The emerging family (years 1–10 of the relationship) involves the couple

a. Initiating work and career paths

b. Deciding to have/having children

2. The crystallizing family (years 11–24 of the relationship)

a. Dealing with adolescent children, a two-way relationship between parents and children

b. Launching children into independent status

c. Continuing to grow as a couple (parents)

d. Beginning participation in community life (the couple)

3. The integrating family (years 26–40 of the relationship)

a. The couple: renewing and enhancing their relationship

b. The couple: continuing work roles

c. The couple: developing leisure activities

d. The children: making adjustments to aging parents

4. The actualizing family (more than 40 years of a couple living together)

a. Continuing development

b. Dealing with aging, chronic illness, and disease; dying spouse or parents; and death

c. Grieving and continuing to grow if one partner dies (Stevenson-Hinde, 1977)

D. Attachment Theories

1. John Bowlby (1907–1990) developed a theory of attachment to explain infants' crying and distress when separated from their parents.

2. Adult attachment theories postulate adaptive and nonadaptive behaviors related to security and intimacy factors.

3. Three implications of adult attachment theory

a. Adult needs for attachment are similar to infant/caregiver relationships.

b. Romantic relationships are attachment relationships.

c. Early childhood experiences influence adult feelings of security and insecurity (Bowlby, 1969).

E. Significance for Rehabilitation

1. Theories such as Duvall's and Stevenson's, which describe family life stages, can be useful for those who study families and for practicing rehabilitation nurses, because the needs of the family can be anticipated depending on the stage of the family.

2. Because the life cycles defined by Duvall and Stevenson are based on the traditional nuclear family, caution is needed when rehabilitation nurses assess and assist nontraditional families.

3. Family function theories cannot be used to describe many of the families in today's society, which reflects different lifestyles and forms (e.g., divorce, alternative marriage, single parenting), yet the tasks may be similar (e.g., child rearing), and elements of these theories apply to rehabilitation.

4. Support from relationships can influence feelings of well-being when attachment promotes security.

5. Application of family theories to domains centers on social support.

a. 2.1: Family function and individual health risks are correlated.

b. 2.2: An aspect of self-management can involve family support.

c. 2.3: The concept of self does not imply that the self is alone, especially in terms of transitions throughout the life span.

VII. Nursing Theories and Conceptualizations

A. Overview

1. Nursing as a profession uses different categories to structure its discipline-specific knowledge.

2. The foundation (i.e., the metaparadigm) branches into grand and middle-range theories.

3. There are different ways to categorize conceptual models and theories, including an approach to earmark areas pertinent to rehabilitation nursing.
4. Since Nightingale's time, theories have emerged that relate to interactions, systems, and developmental concepts.

B. *Metaparadigms:* Generalized, global perspectives (e.g., the bio-psycho-social-spiritual or human-environment-wellness nursing models)
1. Metaparadigms and metatheories are abstract and difficult to research (Fawcett & Garity, 2009).
2. Grand, middle-range, and practice theories all can be part of a comprehensiveness paradigm.
3. Rehabilitation nurses use dimensions of person, environment, and nursing to provide restorative care.

C. *Philosophies:* Relate to beliefs and values about nursing
1. Nursing is generally believed to be an art and a science.
2. In rehabilitation, nurses value holistic care and develop interventions to meet the client's multiple needs (e.g., medical, vocational, educational, and interpersonal challenges).
3. Examples of early nurse philosophers are Virginia Henderson, Florence Nightingale, and Ernestine Weidenbach (Meleis, 2011).

D. *Conceptual Frameworks* (or models): Ideas rather than tested concepts
1. During the mid-1850s, Florence Nightingale presented her nursing views that provided a foundation for future nursing theories (Nightingale, 1860).
2. Conceptual models offer structure and a rationale for arranging concepts into consistent actions.
   a. Conceptual frameworks identify intuitive insights, expectations, and deductions.
   b. Conceptual frameworks are good tools for organizing areas of concern identified by rehabilitation clients and families.

E. Grand Nursing Theories: Less abstract but broad enough to provide a foundation for middle-range theories
1. *Grand theories* are those that offer traditional suppositions and congruent views to help focus nursing practice.
2. Because these theories are grand (i.e., inclusive), they are pertinent to most areas of nursing practice.
3. Holistic care is an example of how broad concepts are applied for the purpose of providing well-rounded care that promotes quality of life.
4. Well-known grand theorists include Myra Levine (conservation model), Betty Neuman (systems model), and Dorothea Orem (self-care model). Grand theories are particularly useful when planning nursing care for rehabilitation clients.
5. **Table 14-5** highlights early theorists and their relevance to restorative care.

F. Middle-Range Nursing Theories: Contain testable variables that have potential to contribute to evidence-based nursing practice
1. *Middle-range theories* are more concrete than grand theories and describe situations or phenomena.
   a. These theories explain relationships and commonalities between concepts.
   b. Middle-range theories are practical for research and practice applications.
2. Middle-range theories are particularly pertinent to rehabilitation nursing.
3. Commonly used theories include comfort theory (Katharine Kolcaba), health promotion theory (Nola Pender), and caring theory (Jean Watson).

G. Nursing Theory: Can be depicted as a tree, with roots and branches
1. The metaparadigm of person, environment, health, and nursing represents the roots.
2. Florence Nightingale's work forms the trunk.
3. The branches are shaped by three theory types: interactive, with Henderson and Peplau; systems, with Neuman and Roy; and development, with Rogers, Leininger, and Watson (Tourville & Ingalls, 2003).

H. Classification: Various theorists contribute to restorative concepts, although their classifications vary and can be difficult to identify.
1. Theories can be classified into multiple areas.
   a. Sister Roy's adaptation model can be both a grand theory and a middle-range theory, depending on its application.
   b. Margaret Newman's theory of health as expanding consciousness discusses the meaning of life, even when life changes—a theory that has been classified as both grand and middle range.
2. Various practice models can share dual classifications.
   a. Madeline Leininger's transcultural nursing model is both anthropological and caring.
   b. Humanistic models such as Patricia Benner's novice-to-expert theory have strong ties to social psychology theories.

Table 14-5. Selected Historical Views Significant to Rehabilitation

Nurse Theorists	Philosophies, Theories, and Models	Key Concepts	Applicability to Restorative Care
Abedellah, Faye (1919–Retired)	Philosophy: Nursing care tailored toward client problems	Three areas of nursing focus: Physical, social, and emotional; developed typology of outcomes	Nurses promote goals to maximize community resources.
Hall, Lydia (1926–1996)	Model: Care, core, and cure	Nurse-directed interventions to prevent fragmented care	Nurse as team leader; model initially used at Loeb rehabilitation center in New York
Henderson, Virginia (1897–1996)	Philosophy: Synopsis of nursing definition: To assist individual, sick or well, for health or its recovery	Nursing activities related to survival (e.g., air, food, sleep), clothing, hygiene, posture, play, work, worship, learn, communicate, safety	Substitutive nursing care (doing for), supplementary (helping), complementary (working with)
Johnson, Dorothy (1919–1999)	Behavior system model: Subsystems house motivation, predisposition, choice, and action components	Nursing diagnosis and treatment aimed at classifying and determining problem to evaluate balance	Nurses direct restoration and attainment of behavioral system balance and stability for clients.
Kenny, Elizabeth (1880–1952)	Philosophy: Unique interventions based on independent nursing assessments	Interdisciplinary model emerged from independent nursing care of people with polio	Kenny Institute in Minneapolis based on principles of muscle rehabilitation
King, Imogene (1923–2007)	Open system theory of adjustments to stressors; contributed to North American Nursing Diagnosis Association	Personal, interpersonal, and social systems are open and interacting; focus on goal attainment	Dynamic nurse-client dyad with mutual and purposeful goal setting
Leininger, Madeleine (1923–2007)	Model and theory: Transcultural nursing	Theory for providing culturally congruent nursing care; care is the essence of nursing	Caring is universal; nurses assess transcultural variables (i.e., values of self-care).
Levine, Myra (1920–1996)	Conceptual model of conservation; sought ways to teach nursing rather than theory development	Principles: Energy, structural integrity, personal integrity, social integrity; environments: perceptual, operational, conceptual	Conservation, redundancy, and therapeutic intention for promoting client integrity and holism
Neuman, Betty (1924–Retired)	Healthcare systems model: Prevention as an intervention	Optimal client stability; health is relative and remains in state of flux	Primary, secondary, and tertiary prevention practiced; help clients maximize their defenses
Nightingale, Florence (1820–1910)	Philosophy: Did not articulate a theory per se; writings described theory concepts	Emphasized clean and quiet environment, ventilation, warmth, and sunlight	Encouraged use of one's own powers; nurses help clients obtain the best condition possible so nature can cure
Orem, Dorothea (1914–2007)	Grand theory: Self-care and self-directed care	Wholly and partially compensatory; supportive	Nursing focus toward clients helping themselves; promotion of assistive devices and aids to obtain independence
Orlando, Ida Jean (1926–2007)	Nurse-client relationship	Nursing process followed to meet client's immediate needs	Nurses explore meanings behind client behaviors; determine nature of distress unique to the client
Peplau, Hildegard (1909–1999)	Psychodynamic nursing; nurse-client relationship	Client makes use of the nurse; four phases of relationship: orient, identify, exploit, and resolution	Nursing roles: Counselor, leader, resource person, teacher

continued

Table 14-5. Selected Historical Views Significant to Rehabilitation (continued)

Nurse Theorists	Philosophies, Theories, and Models	Key Concepts	Applicability to Restorative Care
Rogers, Martha (1914–1994)	Nursing focused on compassion; learned profession	Four-dimensional energy field; pattern and organization of characteristics and behaviors; knowledge of parts not predictive	Nurses promote change and facilitate order during rehabilitation of sick and disabled people.
Travelbee, Joyce (1926–1973)	Human-to-human relationship model; care of the whole person	Inductive theory; uses specific nursing situations to create ideas; humanistic approach	Positive nurse-client relationship brings favorable client outcomes
Weidenbach, Ernestine (1900–1996)	Philosophy: Clinical nursing is a helping art	Assess client's ability to resolve problems and identify when help is needed.	Concepts of maternal-child nursing are applicable to family units and their rehabilitation needs.

Data from Fawcett, 2005; Meleis, 2007.

c. Practice models by Rosemary Parse or by Josephine Paterson and Loretta Zderad share humanistic approaches.
d. Imogene King's framework fits into both interaction and system models.
e. Martha Roger's unitary theory (an energy field model) presents elements of growth and change, a theory that initially was considered radical and later described as nontraditional.

3. Rehabilitation nursing continues to be influenced by the expansion of theory-based practice and evidence-based research.
4. Multiple classifications of theories show versatility of application, which is especially important with respect to changes that occur during rehabilitation.
5. Age-specific nursing theories, such as Anne Casey's nursing model for children and families and Dorothea Orem's self-care model for adults, are helpful when practicing rehabilitation across the life span.
6. Theories can be shared by healthcare providers to promote restorative care, including long-used and improved theories from psychosocial disciplines, as previously reviewed.

I. Significance for Rehabilitation

1. Nursing theories are built on a wide range of interdisciplinary frameworks and models.
2. Nursing models and theories outline the needs of clients and family to promote recovery and quality of life.
3. Nurses use theory foundations based in history (perhaps more than is realized) on a daily basis.
4. Rehabilitation nursing continues to discover new theories.
5. The nursing profession continues to develop models and test associated theories to provide evidence-based care for optimal client outcomes (Schmidt & Brown, 2009).
6. A holistic approach to nursing care requires a Gestalt approach, through which the whole of the client, not just the parts, can be restored and rehabilitated.
7. **Table 14-6** shows the juxtaposition of theories and the nursing process for developing a plan of care for a rehabilitation client.
8. Application of nursing theories to Domains focuses on holism.
   a. 2.1: Health promotion often includes community interaction and interdisciplinary frameworks.
   b. 2.2: Various bio-psych-social-spiritual models are used to promote self-care.
   c. 2.3: Transitions occur within the subcultures of individuals, where humanistic and transcultural models work well.

VIII. Theory Application to Advanced Practice

A. Overview

1. Butts & Rich (2011) define theorizing or theoretical thinking as "the dynamic process of asking and answering specific types of questions" (p. 76).
2. For nurses, the ultimate result of applying and testing theories is to better promote healthy lifestyles and to assist with improved quality of life during rehabilitation.

B. Clinician

1. Uses developmental theories to link the determinants of health and illness across the life span (Hoeman, 2008; Jarvis, 2012)
   a. Provides a construct for interpreting how clients and families' experiences in their early years influence their later health and functioning

Table 14-6. A Gestalt Nursing Approach for Restorative Care

Case Synopsis	Nursing Process Examples	Theory-Based Considerations
Client T.S. had a bowel obstruction and spontaneous rupture that resulted in spillage of stool and barium (from her earlier gastrointestinal study) outside the intestines and throughout the abdomen. Two fistulas resulted, with openings that expelled feces from the intestinal area to colostomy bags attached to the outside of her abdomen.	FHP: Coping-stress tolerance S: "I can't believe this is happening." O: Open fistulas managed with ostomy bags ND: Coping, ineffective, denial NIC: Assess T.S.'s usual coping strategies, and explore the situation with T.S. NOC: T.S. identifies her own maladaptive coping behavior; acknowledges the situation, and verbalizes available support.	Coping challenges may occur across the lifespan. Coping mechanisms will vary, depending on developmental stage (i.e., Erikson). Multiple theories address defense mechanisms, such as denial and repression.
This health problem was a surprise to T.S., giving her little time to adjust to the situation. Fistula care resembled colostomy care, with wafers, bags, and emptying procedures. The intestinal obstruction and subsequent complications resulted in physical and emotional distress for T.S.	FHP: Self-perception S: "I have waste oozing from my abdomen; this is disgusting; it's worse than being a baby." ND: Disturbed body image. NIC: Encourage T.S. to express feelings; clarify any misconceptions (i.e., prognosis). NOC: T.S. demonstrates enhanced body image and self-esteem, as evidenced by her ability to look at and care for the altered body area and function with ostomy care.	Health issues related to elimination may have Freudian connotations. Fully functioning individuals (described by Carl Rogers) will accept reality and adjust. Dissonance (e.g., Schaie's theory) may occur when the person and the environment are not in sync.
Over 6 weeks, T.S. underwent three laparoscopies as surgeons tried to remove the barium and repair the fistulas. Her activity tolerance grew worse instead of better. T.S. was referred to rehabilitation.	FHP: Activity-exercise S: "I'm too weak to do anything for myself; this is so embarrassing." ND: Self-care deficit syndrome NIC: Assist T.S. in accepting the necessary amount of dependence; set realistic goals with T.S. NOC: Demonstrates total self-care by target date	Numerous variables may interrelate, such as dependency and self-perception issues when facing a rehabilitation challenge. Holistic care addresses diverse needs of clients and families. Physical needs may outweigh emotional needs, as outlined in Maslow's theory.
Apart from her general debilitation, T.S. exhibited anger and frustration, especially related to her ostomy care.	FHP: Cognitive-perceptual S: "I can't get these (curse word) bags to stop leaking. What can I do?" O: Stool on abdomen and bed; open areas on wafer ND: Knowledge, readiness for enhanced NIC: Support self-directed, self-designed learning; allow adequate time for integration; ensure that necessary supplies are available so the environment is conducive to learning. NOC: T.S. will demonstrate motivation to learn; will verbalize understanding and perform skill of ostomy self-care.	Cognitive and learning theories have implications for health education. Abilities vary, as do preferences and personalities for developing coping strategies. The multiple intelligence model (Gardner) is applicable as learning strategies are assessed and client strengths are identified. Formal health assessments may ask clients about their preferred learning style.
T.S. had recently moved to be near her elderly mother. T.S. became sick before she fully relocated, which resulted in her being unemployed. She did not want to move in with family, but medical bills had depleted her down payment for a home.	FHP: Coping-stress tolerance S: "I'm homeless and jobless, and I'm really mad and don't know what to do." ND: Resilience, impaired individual NIC: Emotional support; referral and counseling, if needed. Encourage client to evaluate options. NOC: Appraise support systems; relate available community resources.	Adaptation models help identify psychosocial problems and potential solutions. Nursing theories have elements of earlier philosophies of human growth and development. A combination of philosophies and interdisciplinary models provide a Gestalt approach to care.

Abbreviations. FHP, functional health pattern; ND, nursing diagnosis; NIC, nursing intervention classification; NOC, nursing outcomes classification; O, objective; S, subjective.

Data from Carpenito-Moyet, 2010; Doenges, Moorhouse, & Murr, 2010; Johnson, Bulechek, Dochterman, Maas, Moorhead, & Swanson, 2005.

b. Aids in understanding clients and families' health and well-being for nurses providing direct care

2. Applies developmental theories and tasks across the life span to provide paradigms for clinical issues
   a. Assesses and diagnoses healthcare needs
   b. Plans, implements, and evaluates proactively health and illness interventions when working with clients and families in various settings

C. Educator
1. Reviews developmental theories and tasks of clients and families when teaching
   a. Determines the most appropriate teaching strategy based on the developmental stage or point of life of the client and family
   b. Plans and implements educational interventions, such as choosing the best presentation method or teaching material to fit the needs of the client and family
   c. Evaluates formal and informal educational programs related to developmental needs of the client and family (Hamric, Spross, & Hanson, 2009)
2. Considers theories and tasks of clients and families when teaching professional and nonprofessional staff members
   a. Assesses client and family readiness for learning
   b. Plans and implements educational content, such as in-service offerings
   c. Evaluates informal and formal educational offerings

D. Leader and Consultant
1. Applies developmental theories and frameworks as a foundation for integrating child and adult health policies by emphasizing the potential for social and biological processes early in life to find clinical expression in adult-onset disease
2. Applies this knowledge to reduce the heavy human and economic costs of health care and to actively participate in healthcare policy making

E. Researcher
1. Identifies and expands theoretical frameworks to depict or explain relationships between concepts of interest in a study
2. Uses theories to form research designs or to participate in studies that nurse scientists develop and direct, such as the following:
   a. Improving the health and well-being of children
   b. Examining the effects of environmental influences on the health and development of children and adults
   c. Defining natural and human-made environmental factors that result in rehabilitation risks that can be prevented or minimized when identified by research data
      1) Biological and chemical factors
      2) Hazards in physical surroundings
      3) Social risk factors
      4) Risk-taking behaviors
3. Critically appraises and synthesizes evidence
   a. Analyzes how these elements interact with each other and the helpful or harmful effects they might have for clients across the life span
   b. Studies children and adults throughout their different phases of growth and development to better understand health and disease
   c. Contributes to best practices as determined by theory-based research (Barker, 2009; Derstine & Hargrove, 2001)
4. Uses assessment skills and critical thinking to apply diverse theories to rehabilitation
   a. The recovery model can be used for physical rehabilitation to show how a mental health theory assists patients with self-management skills (Bennett, Breeze & Neilson, 2014).
      1) The medical model aims at cure, but when the recovery theory is applied to rehabilitation nursing, the focus is on helping the client find purpose and empowerment.
      2) Self-efficacy and adaptation promote hope and individual goal setting for recovery.
      3) Clients identify a new functional baseline if a return to the previous health status is not possible.
   b. Self-management skills and informatics can be used to locate interventions and resources (Knight & Shea, 2014).
      1) Information literacy and the ability to locate reliable healthcare advice is particularly useful for those dealing with chronic illness.
      2) Technology provides a platform for helping patients prioritize and plan their care.

F. Significance for Rehabilitation
1. 2.1: Many different frameworks can be applied in concert with nursing tools to promote health **(Table 14-7)**
2. 2.2: Clients can be taught to locate and analyze multiple resources to facilitate their self-management.
3. 2.3: Ongoing research that addresses the care transitions of recovery and growth throughout the life span is needed.

ACKNOWLEDGMENT

Linda L. Pierce, PhD CNS RN CRRN FAHA, is acknowledged for her initial work on this chapter in previous editions.

Table 14-7 Combining the Nursing Process, Cognitive Dissonance Theory, and Domain 2.3
Scenario: An elderly mother and her adult daughter must make a decision between the mother moving to a long-term care facility or to her daughter's house. The mother states she wants to go to a nursing home, since she needs basic care assistance. Her daughter insists that she wants her mother to move in with her.
The Mother's Statements Logic: "I want to go to the nursing home." Value: "I love my daughter and must not ruin her life." Morals: "It would be wrong for me to go live with my daughter."
The Daughter's Statements Logic: "I can better care for mom if she lives with me." Value: "I love my mother and I want to help her now." Morals: "It would be wrong for me to send mom away."
The Nursing Process The nurse collects subjective and objective data from the family. Factors such as finances and home environments are addressed by the family and the interdisciplinary team. The nurse continues to assess underlying beliefs and values. Love-of-family is a consistent theme between the mother and daughter. The statements of "wrong" imply that both mother and daughter will feel remorse if decisions are made that conflict with their perceived duties and desires. Although the mother has self-care issues, the nurse learns that the family's primary concern relates to their need to make a quick decision about living arrangements. A *nursing diagnosis* related to coping is priority over self-care deficit in this scenario.
Cognitive Dissonance Theory Dissonance is a factor to consider when addressing discharge planning and the stress associated with a lifestyle change. As the family considers their moving plan, the nurse gathers additional resources and interventions for the mother and daughter, such as information on available respite care. The objective options (logistics of moving) are easier to identify than the subjective views (feelings) of family members. By using a cognitive *dissonance framework*, the value systems of both mother and daughter can be discovered and discussed.
Effective Care Transitions Although nurses are skilled at *therapeutic communication*, the analysis of belief systems is a more complex procedure. A process recording that lists statements and responses is a good tool for deciphering and discussing the family's feelings behind their verbalizations. A brief *teaching session* with clients to explain cognitive dissonance can be helpful. By listing the logic/value/moral aspects of a decision, family members can identify their common beliefs and work together for a united rationalization and effective transition.

References

Anderson, K. H. (2000). The family health system approach to family systems nursing. *Journal of Family Nursing, 6*(2), 103–117.

Association of Rehabilitation Nurses (ARN). (2014). ARN competency model for professional rehabilitation nursing. Retrieved from http://www.rehabnurse.org/uploads/files/education/ARN_Rehabilitation_Nursing_Competency _Model_FINAL_-_May_2014.pdf

Bandura, A. (1997). *Self-efficacy*. New York: W. H. Freeman.

Barker, A. M. (Ed.). (2009). *Advanced practice nursing: Essential knowledge for the profession*. Boston: Jones & Bartlett.

Barton, E. F. (1996). *Harry Stack Sullivan: Interpersonal theory and psychotherapy*. London: Routledge.

Becker, M. H. (Ed.). (1974). *The health belief model and personal health behavior*. Thorofare, NJ: Slock.

Bennett, B., Breeze, J., & Neilson, T. (2014). Applying the recovery model to physical rehabilitation. *Nursing Standard, 28*(23), 37–43.

Bowlby, J. (1969). *Attachment and loss*. New York: Basic Books.

Boyd, D., & Bee, H. (2006). *Lifespan development* (4th ed.). Upper Saddle River, NJ: Pearson.

Bradberry, T. (2007). *The personality code*. New York: Putnam.

Bunevicius, A., Brozaitiene, J., Staniute, M., Gelziniene, V., Duoneliene, I., Pop, V., . . . Dcnollet, J. (2014). Decreased physical effort, fatigue, and mental distress in patients with coronary artery disease: Importance of personality-related differences. *International Journal of Behavioral Medicine, 2*, 240–247.

Butts, J. B., & Rich, K. L. (2011). *Philosophies and theories for advanced nursing practice*. Sudbury, MA: Jones & Barlett Learning.

Carducci, B. J. (2009). *The psychology of personality*. Malden, MA: Wiley-Blackwell.

Carpenito-Moyet, L. J. (2010). *Handbook of nursing diagnosis* (13th ed.). Philadelphia: Lippincott Williams & Wilkins.

Carpenito-Moyet, L. J. (2012). *Handbook of nursing diagnosis* (14th ed.). Philadelphia: Lippincott Williams & Wilkins.

Carter, B., & McGoldrick, M. (1989) *The changing family life cycle: A framework for family therapy*. Needham Heights, MA: Allyn & Bacon.

Cooper, J. (2007). *Cognitive dissonance: Fifty years of a classic theory*. Los Angeles: Sage Publications.

Derstine, J. B., & Hargrove, S. D. (2001). *Comprehensive rehabilitation nursing*. Philadelphia: W. B. Saunders.

Doenges, M. E., Moorhouse, M. F., & Murr, A. C. (2010). *Nursing diagnosis manual: Planning, individualizing, and documenting client care* (3rd ed.). Philadelphia: F. A. Davis.

Doenges, M. E., Moorhouse, M. F., & Murr, A. C. (2013). *Nursing diagnosis manual: Planning, individualizing, and documenting client care* (4th ed.). Philadelphia: F. A. Davis.

Duvall, E. (1977). *Marriage and family development* (5th ed.). Philadelphia: Lippincott.

Ellis, W. D. (1938). *Source book of gestalt psychology*. New York: Harcourt, Brace & Company.

Erikson, E. (1963). *Childhood and society* (2nd ed.). New York: W. W. Norton.

Erikson, E. H., Erikson, J. M., & Kivnick, H. Q. (1986). *Vital involvement in old age*. New York: W. W. Norton.

Fawcett, J. (2005). *Contemporary nursing knowledge: Analysis and evaluation of nursing models and theories* (2nd ed.). Philadelphia: F. A. Davis.

Fawcett, J., & Garity, J. (2009). *Evaluating research for evidence-based nursing practice*. Philadelphia: F. A. Davis.

Festinger, L. (1957). *Theory of cognitive dissonance*. Stanford, CA: Stanford University Press.

Freud, S. (1959). Inhibitions, symptoms, and anxiety. In J. Strachey (Ed.), *The standard edition of the complete psychological works of Sigmund Freud* (Vol. 18, pp. 1–64). London: Hogarth.

Gallagher, P., Yancy, Jr., W. S., Denissen, J. A., Kuhnel, A., & Voils, C. I. (2013). Correlates to daily leisure-time physical activity in a community sample: Narrow personality traits and practical barriers. *Health Psychology, 32*, 1227–1235.

Gardner, H. (1993). *Multiple intelligences: The theory in practice*. New York: Basic Books.

Gardner, H. (2008). *Five minds for the future*. Boston: Harvard Business Press.

Gawronski, B. (2012). Back to the future of dissonance theory: Cognitive consistency as a core motive. *Social Cognition, 30*, 652–668.

Gay, P. (2006). *Freud: A life for our times*. New York: W. W. Norton.

Gilligan, C. (1982). *In a different voice: Psychological theory and women's development*. Cambridge, MA: Harvard University Press.

Glod, C. (1998). Developmental and psychological theories of mental illness. In C. Glod (Ed.). *Contemporary psychiatric-mental health nursing* (pp. 64–72). Philadelphia: F. A. Davis.

Goodman, C. J. (2009). *A history of modern psychology* (3rd ed.). Somerset, NJ: Wiley.

Hamric, A. B., Spross, J. A., & Hanson, C. M. (2009). *Advanced practice nursing: An integrative approach* (4th ed.). St. Louis: Saunders-Elsevier.

Hoeman, S. P. (2008). *Rehabilitation nursing: Prevention, intervention, and outcomes* (4th ed.). St. Louis: Mosby-Elsevier.

Israel, S., & Moffitt, T. E. (2014). Assessing conscientious personality in primary care: An opportunity for prevention and health promotion. *Developmental Psychology, 50*, 1475–1477.

Jarvis, C. (Ed.). (2012). *Physical examination & health assessment* (6th ed.). Philadelphia: W. B. Saunders.

Johnson, M., Bulelchek, G., Butcher, H., Dochterman, J. M., Maas, M., Moorhead, S. (2005). *NANDA, NOC, and NIC linkages*. St. Louis: Mosby.

Jung, C. G., & Wolfgang, P. (1955). *The interpretation of nature and psyche*. New York: Pantheon Books.

Kohlberg, L. (1963). Moral development and identification. In H. Stevenson (Ed.), *Child psychology*. Chicago: University of Chicago Press.

Kohlberg, L. (1976). Moral stages and moralization: The cognitive-developmental approach. In T. Lickona (Ed.), *Moral development and behavior: Theory, research and social issues*. New York: Holt, Rinehart & Winston.

Knight, E., & Shea, K. (2014). A patient-focused framework integrating self-management and Informatics. *Journal of Nursing Scholarship, 46*(2), 91 97.

Maslow, A. (1954). *Motivation and personality*. New York: Harper.

Maslow, A. (1971). *The farther reaches of human nature*. New York: Viking.

McGhee, R. L., Ehrler, D., & Buckhalt, J. (2008). *Manual for the five factor personality inventory*. Austin, TX: Pro Ed.

Meleis, A. I. (2007). *Theoretical nursing: Development and progress* (4th ed.). Philadelphia: Lippincott Williams & Wilkins.

Meleis, A. I. (2011). *Theoretical nursing: Development and progress* (5th ed.). Philadelphia: Lippincott Williams & Wilkins.

Montes-Berges, B., & Augusto-Landa, J. M. (2014). Emotional intelligence and affective intensity as life satisfaction and psychological well-being predictors on nursing professionals. *Journal of Professional Nursing, 30*(1), 80-88.

Myers, S. S. (2007). *Ancient ethics*. New York: Routledge.

Newman, B. M., & Newman, P. R. (2009). *Theories of human development*. Mahwah, NJ: Erlbaum.

Nightingale, F. (1860). *Nursing: What it is, and what it is not*. New York: D. Appleton.

O'Driscoll, D. (2014). The case for Dr. Freud. *Learning Disability Practice, 17*(3), 11.

Pavlov, I. (1927). *Conditioned reflexes: An investigation of the physiological activity of the cerebral cortex*. New York: Oxford University Press.

Piaget, J. (1952). *Origins of intelligence in children*. New York: International Universities Press.

Rogers, C. (1980). *A way of being*. Boston: Houghton Mifflin.

Schaie, K. (1981). Psychological changes from midlife to early old age: Implications for the maintenance of mental health. *American Journal of Orthopsychiatry, 51*(4), 199–218.

Schmidt, N. A., & Brown, J. M. (2009). *Evidence-based practice for nurses: Appraisal and application of research*. Sudbury, MA: Jones & Bartlett.

Shenk, J. W. (2009, June). What makes us happy? *Atlantic Monthly*, 36–54.

Sherwood, W. R. (2010). *The survivors club*. New York: Grand Central Publishing.

Sigelman, C. K., & Rider, E. A. (2011) *Lifespan human development* (7th ed.). Belmont, CA: Wadsworth Cengage Learning.

Skinner, B. F. (1953). *Science and human behavior*. New York: Macmillan.

Stephan, Y., Sutlin,A. R., & Terracciano, A. (2013). Physical activity and personality development across adulthood and old age: Evidence from two longitudinal studies. *Journal of Research in Personality, 49*, 1–7.

Stevenson-Hinde, J. (1977). *Issues and crises during middlescence*. New York: Appleton-Century-Crofts.

Sullivan, H. (1956). *Clinical studies in psychiatry*. New York: Norton.

Sullivan, H. (1971). *The fusion of psychiatry and social science*. New York: Norton.

Tauber, A. I. (2010). *Freud the reluctant philosopher*. Princeton, NJ: Princeton University Press.

Tourville, C., & Ingalls, K. (2003). The living tree of nursing theories. *Nursing Forum, 38*(3), 21–30, 36.

Townsend, M. C. (2014). *Essentials of psychiatric mental health nursing: Concepts of care in evidence-based practice* (8th ed.). New York: F. A. Davis.

Vygotsky, L. S. (1978). *Mind in society*. Cambridge, MA: Harvard University Press.

Whiting, S. (1997). Development of the person. In B. Johnson (Ed.), *Psychiatric mental health nursing: Adaptation and growth* (4th ed., pp. 357–373). Philadelphia: Lippincott Williams & Wilkins.

Youngblood, N. (1999). Family-centered care. In P. Edwards, D. Hertzberg, S. Hays, & N. Youngblood (Eds.), *Pediatric rehabilitation* (pp. 129–143). Philadelphia: W. B. Saunders.

Section III

Special Populations in the REHABILITATION SETTING

Chapter 15

Pediatric Rehabilitation Nursing

Deirdre F. Jackson, MSN RN APN CRRN CPN
Nicole C. Kelly, MSN RN CRRN CPN

LEARNING OUTCOMES

- Summarize the fundamental concepts in pediatric rehabilitation nursing.
- Identify the types of children who benefit from pediatric rehabilitation services.
- Formulate plans of care for clients with pediatric rehabilitation needs.
- Advocate for appropriate community services and supports for children and youth with disabilities.

KEY CHAPTER TOPICS

- Overview of pediatric rehabilitation nursing
- Traumatic and acquired conditions
- Birth defects and developmental disabilities
- Chronic illnesses
- Long-term planning: Community services for children and youths with disabilities
- Trends and future directions
- Advanced practice nurses in pediatric rehabilitation

PROFESSIONAL REHABILITATION NURSING DOMAINS AND COMPETENCIES

- Domain 1: Competencies 1.1, 1.2, 1.3, 1.4
- Domain 2: Competencies 2.1, 2.2
- Domain 3: Competency 3.4
- Domain 4: Competencies 4.2, 4.3 (Association of Rehabilitation Nurses [ARN], 2014)

Introduction

This chapter offers a unique body of knowledge specific to the care of children and adolescents with disabilities and chronic conditions, and to the support of their families. It provides a reference for nurses in a variety of settings across the continuum of care, from hospital to home and community. The emphasis is on the roles of the pediatric rehabilitation nurse in relation to care coordination and provision, health teaching and promotion, leadership, collaboration, advocacy, and professional practice.

I. Overview of Pediatric Rehabilitation Nursing

A. Definitions

1. *Pediatric rehabilitation nursing*: "Pediatric rehabilitation nursing is the specialty practice committed to improving the quality of life for children and adolescents with disabilities and their families. The mission is to provide, in collaboration with the interdisciplinary team, a continuum of nursing care from onset of injury or illness to productive adulthood. The goal of the rehabilitation process is for children, regardless of their disability or chronic illness, to function at their maximum potential and become contributing members of both their families and society" (ARN, 2007, para. 1).
2. *Habilitation*: Providing therapies for children with developmental disabilities and similar conditions to assist them in achieving function and skill never before acquired
3. *Rehabilitation:* Relearning or regaining skills and abilities after trauma or disease to meet age-related developmental expectations
4. *Children with special healthcare needs (CSHCN):* "Children with special health care needs are those who have or are at increased risk for a chronic physical, developmental, behavioral, or emotional condition and who also require health and related services of a type or amount beyond that required by children generally" (McPherson et al., 1998, p. 138).

B. Roles of the Pediatric Rehabilitation Nurse

1. Advocacy
2. Coordination of care
3. Leadership and consulting
4. Care provision
5. Health teaching and promotion
6. Team participation
7. Research
8. Professional practice, education, and evaluation (ARN, 2007)

C. Practice Settings

1. Pediatric rehabilitation hospitals (inpatient and outpatient)
2. Pediatric rehabilitation units in rehabilitation hospitals
3. Pediatric rehabilitation units in pediatric hospitals
4. Subacute and postacute rehabilitation units
5. Day treatment programs
6. Freestanding pediatric outpatient therapy centers
7. Outpatient primary care and specialty clinics
8. Health department outpatient services
9. State children's rehabilitation services
10. School or childcare centers
11. Home health agencies
12. Family homes

D. General Principles

1. *Patient- and family-centered care:* Patient- and family-centered care is an approach to the planning, delivery, and evaluation of health care that is grounded in mutually beneficial partnerships among healthcare providers, patients, and families. This philosophy recognizes the vital role that families play in ensuring the health and well-being of infants, children, and adolescents. It stresses the importance of emotional, social, and developmental support during health care.
   a. Core concepts include respect and dignity, information sharing, participation, and collaboration.
   b. All children are part of a family and within this concept, *family* refers to two or more persons who are related in any way—biologically, legally, or emotionally.
   c. An approach based on this concept leads to better health outcomes, wiser allocation of resources, and greater patient and family satisfaction (Institute for Patient-and Family-Centered Care, 2010).
2. *Community-based delivery systems:* Services that are delivered in the child's environment to promote community integration (e.g., day care, early intervention, school, medical home, pediatric outpatient therapy, home)
3. Medical home concept
   a. *Medical home:* A "family-centered medical home is not a building, house, hospital, or home healthcare service but rather an approach to providing comprehensive primary care" (American Academy of Pediatrics [AAP], 2010, para. 1). Pediatric healthcare professionals and parents act as partners in a medical home to identify and access all the medical and nonmedical services needed to help children and their families achieve the maximum potential for the child. This partnership forms a "mutually respectful relationship (i.e., one that honors diversity and is consistent with each family's cultural and religious beliefs)" (AAP, American Academy of Family Physicians [AAFP], & American College of Physicians [ACP], 2011, p. 187). A medical home for a child usually is part of a pediatric primary care office but can be part of a comprehensive outpatient program.
   b. The medical home includes three distinct care processes: preventive care, acute illness management, and chronic condition management (CCM).
   c. For CSHCN, the pediatric medical home concept also includes a registry of CSHCN in the primary care office, written care plans, care coordination, CCM visits in addition to health maintenance and acute illness management, more intense transition plans, and clearly defined roles for comanagement with medical subspecialties (AAP et al., 2011).
4. Human development: Pediatric rehabilitation nurses must have in-depth knowledge of developmental theories and normal development, related assessment skills, and knowledge of interventions that promote developmental milestones. (Refer to Chapter 15 for more information about developmental theories.)
5. Developmental levels: The child's developmental level should be considered in determining the rehabilitation plan and interventions.
   a. Infant and toddler (0–3 years old)
   b. Preschooler (3–5 years old)
   c. School-aged child (6–11 years old)
   d. Adolescent (12–21 years old)
6. Family development: Understanding family life stages of development is useful in assessing and planning interventions with children and families.
7. Prevention of secondary conditions: People with disabilities are at greater risk for preventable health problems or secondary conditions (Centers for Disease Control and Prevention National

Center on Birth Defects and Developmental Disabilities [CDC PNCBDDD], 2014c). Common secondary conditions in CSHCN include

a. Bowel and bladder problems
b. Injury
c. Overweight and obesity, which increases risk of hypertension, hyperlipidemia, type 2 diabetes, mobility problems, fatigue, pain, and pressure sores (Rimmer, Yamaki, Lowry, Wang, & Vogel, 2010).
d. Pain
e. Respiratory disorders
f. Joint contractures
g. Spasticity
h. Communication problems
i. Swallowing and feeding disorders and nutritional deficits
j. Emotional problems, depression, school problems, and social isolation

8. Interprofessional team approach: The team includes the child; family; nursing; medicine; physical, occupational, and speech therapy; nutrition; psychology; education; social work; therapeutic recreation; orthotics; medical subspecialties (e.g., dentistry, neurology, neurosurgery, ophthalmology, orthopedics,) and support services (e.g., audiology).
   a. The family plays a vital role in advocating for the child and is a core part of the rehabilitation team.
   b. Collaborate with team members to collect assessment data.
   c. Work collaboratively with other team members to promote optimal treatment outcomes, maximize potential and quality of life.
9. Assessment: Each child and family should be assessed in the following areas:
   a. Birth history
   b. Developmental history
   c. Current developmental level and expected level of development for the child's age
   d. The impact of the child's disability on his or her developmental level
   e. Health history
   f. Function level (i.e., WeeFIM II™ System, PEDI [Pediatric Evaluation of Disability Inventory™], MDS [Minimum Data Set]; refer to Chapter 15)
   g. Family functioning to determine strengths and areas for assistance or support
   h. Plans for important service system transitions, made according to age
      1) Neonatal intensive care unit to home in the case of congenital disability or prematurity
      2) Early intervention program to preschool
      3) Preschool to grade school, then middle school and high school
      4) High school to secondary school, vocational program, or independent living
      5) Pediatric medical home to adult care model
10. Interventions: Physical, emotional, social, cultural, educational, developmental, and spiritual dimensions all are considered in a holistic approach to care.
   a. Incorporate appropriate recreational activities, toys, and fun along with therapeutic interventions. Play, the means by which children learn about the world, is an integral part of the rehabilitation plan. Adaptive sports and recreational activities are important for quality of life (Hewitt-Taylor, 2010).
   b. Focus on helping the child meet his or her developmental milestones as much as possible.
   c. Investigate alternative ways to achieve tasks if developmental milestones cannot be met through therapy or assistive devices.
   d. Anticipate upcoming developmental challenges and plan ahead for age-appropriate interventions.
   e. Facilitate adaptation to the disability and treatment.
   f. Promote community integration.
11. Family interventions
   a. Provide family emotional support.
   b. Enhance parental self-efficacy and facilitate family adaption to the child's disability (Benzies, Trute, & Worthington, 2013; Greef, Vansteenwegen, & Gillard, 2012; Lucas, 2010).
   c. Educate family members about the child's disability and how to provide care or assist the child in achieving independence in his or her own care.
   d. Promote changes in family roles and responsibilities.
   e. Provide care management and resources (Sullivan-Bolyai, Knafl, Sadler, & Gilliss, 2004).
   f. Enable families to manage their child's care and to advocate for the child's needs.

E. Pediatric Rehabilitation Versus Adult Rehabilitation
   1. Wide variety of conditions: A defining characteristic of pediatric rehabilitation is the wide variety of different, and often rare, diagnoses and conditions that are managed in the pediatric rehabilitation setting. Although specific care needs vary and must be individualized, general principles

of pediatric rehabilitation are appropriate for all conditions.

2. Physiological and developmental immaturity: Children are not small adults; they are physiologically different from adults and are at various levels of developmental maturity. These differences apply irrespective of the child's diagnosis.
   a. Age- and growth-related vulnerabilities influence biomechanical response to injury (e.g., the amount of cartilage in children's bones often results in "greenstick"-type fractures; fractures involving the epiphyseal growth plate can cause lifelong deformity if not treated appropriately).
   b. Rapid changes in size of organs and in neurological development necessitate frequent monitoring in infants, toddlers, and preschoolers.
   c. Young children's renal and hepatic function is still developing, so they need adjustments in medication dosing until about 16 years of age.
   d. Rehabilitation goals are dynamic and need to be adjusted with respect to the ongoing growth and development of the child.
   e. The need to modify rehabilitation and adaptive equipment to meet current developmental level and growth (e.g., stroller to wheelchair; picture-based communication board to digital augmentative communication device; resized ankle-foot orthoses) is ongoing.
   f. Emergency equipment must be sized for the age of the child. Small airways are more vulnerable to injury with invasive procedures such as intubation.
   g. Independent mobility is essential for learning and socialization (Calhoun, Schottler, & Vogel, 2013).
   h. Age and developmentally appropriate safe passenger restraint systems must be provided (e.g., special needs car and booster seats). Safe wheelchair transportation must be considered for community and school activities.
   i. Special education services

II. Traumatic and Acquired Conditions

A. Traumatic Brain Injury

1. *Traumatic brain injury* (TBI) is "a nondegenerative, noncongenital insult to the brain from an external mechanical force, possibly leading to permanent or temporary impairment of cognitive, physical, and psychosocial functions, with an associated diminished or altered state of consciousness" (Dawodu, 2013). Children can experience deficits in physical, psychosocial, and cognitive functioning.
2. Incidence
   a. It is estimated that TBI in children from birth to 14 years of age results in 2,174 deaths, 35,136 hospitalizations, and 473,947 emergency department visits each year (Faul, Xu, Wald, & Coronado, 2010).
   b. In 2009, 248,418 children (age 19 years or younger) were treated for sports and recreation-related injuries that included a diagnosis of concussion or TBI (Centers for Disease Control and Prevention [CDC], 2011).
   c. Adolescents, young adults, and very young children are at the highest risk for TBI.
   d. As with adults, males are more likely to experience TBI than females.
3. Causes of injury: Causes of injury in children often differ based on age and developmental level. Infant brain injuries are often caused by abusive head trauma; in young children falls are common causes; in older children motor vehicle accidents are common causes; motor vehicle accidents, sports-related head injuries, and assault are more prevalent in adolescents and young adults (Geyer, Meller, Kulpan, & Mowery, 2013).
   a. Abusive head trauma (often referred to as "shaken baby syndrome") has become a leading cause of death in infants and toddlers. These children present with injuries requiring neurosurgical management and operative interventions. Nonaccidental injuries have greater rates of morbidity and mortality across all levels of injury. These children require intensive short- and long-term medical resources (Deans, Minneci, Lowell, & Groner, 2013).
   b. Mild TBI or concussion can range from no loss of consciousness, with only a brief change in mental status, to loss of consciousness for a few minutes with declining neurological status. Mild TBIs are often not considered serious, but some children can demonstrate an atypical clinical course with slow return to baseline functional status. Postinjury symptoms in children include headache, fatigue, balance, and sleep disturbances. Repeated mild TBIs that occur over an extended period can result in cumulative deficits. Similarly, repeated mild TBIs that occur within a short period (i.e., hours, days, or weeks) can be catastrophic or fatal (Blissitt, 2011).
4. TBI in children is different from TBI in adults.
   a. Response to injury, such as more diffuse cerebral edema after injury, makes acute management of elevated intracranial pressure

paramount. Management of intracranial pressure for sufficient cerebral perfusion provides more positive outcomes (Kochanek et al., 2012).

b. Characteristics of injury, such as those caused by delays in treatment, particularly in young children, can lead to increased ischemic injury.

c. The school system and special education are critical components in the rehabilitation of children with TBI.

5. Outcomes in children
   a. Children are more likely to survive TBI than adults.
   b. Predictors of outcomes in children and adolescents include the Glasgow Coma Scale rating, intracranial pressure, length of time in a coma, location of injury, and severity of injury (Fay et al., 2009; Kochanek et al., 2012; Krach, Gromly, & Ward, 2010).
   c. Other factors that are predictors of outcomes after TBI include preinjury intellectual ability, academic achievement, psychological symptoms, and lower socioeconomic status (Johnson, DeMatt, & Salorio, 2009).
   d. Children continue to grow and develop after TBI. Cognitive outcomes are affected in part by age at the time of injury. Children injured prior to late childhood are highly vulnerable to poor cognitive outcomes (Crowe, Catroppa, Babl, Rosenfeld, & Anderson, 2012). Children injured before 3 years of age demonstrate impaired development of attentional control skills; this puts them at an additional disadvantage with regard to future learning (Crowe, Catroppa, Babl, & Anderson, 2013). Sustained deficits in executive functions, attention, and memory, coupled with poor school performance are linked with decreased quality of life (Johnson et al., 2009).
   e. Impact on the family is even greater, because caregiving often is extended beyond childhood.
   f. The cost to family and society is higher, because a child with TBI generally has more years to live.
6. Assessment components. Perform assessments for common postinjury problems.
   a. Neurological deficit: Level of consciousness, intracranial pressure, seizure disorder, Glasgow Coma Scale
   b. Cognitive deficits: Use the Rancho Los Amigos Scale (Hagen, 1997). Assess executive function disorders, processing disorders, and memory deficits that would lead to a need for special education and school services.
   c. Behavioral problems: Impulsivity, secondary attention deficit disorder, aggression, and personality changes
   d. Motor and sensory deficits
   e. Vision (e.g., visual field and pupillary response changes) and hearing deficits
   f. Speech and language disorders
   g. Respiratory deficit: Adequate oxygenation. Some children need tracheostomy or mechanical ventilation initially; those with more severe injury could require long-term mechanical ventilation.
   h. Cardiovascular status: Hemodynamic instability
   i. Gastrointestinal and nutritional issues: Some children have dysphagia and feeding problems. They could need a nasogastric tube, a gastrostomy tube, or oral stimulation, and they could be at risk for choking, temporarily or in the long term (Morgan, 2010).
   j. Endocrine deficit: Syndrome of inappropriate antidiuretic hormone, diabetes insipidus, hyperglycemia
   k. Developmental level: Premorbid functioning
   l. Functional level: WeeFIM II™ System (Kramer et al., 2013; refer to Chapter 7, Figure 7-3)
   m. Family history and coping: Guilt, ability to care for child, financial concerns, sibling response
7. Rehabilitation issues
   a. Cognitive rehabilitation
   b. Behavioral and social problems, personality changes, need for close supervision
   c. Speech and language therapy
   d. Respiratory support: Proper positioning, tracheostomy care, ventilator weaning and/or management
   e. Dysphagia management
   f. Independence level appropriate for developmental level
   g. Prevention of further injury and complications: Identify safest, least restrictive environment throughout recovery (e.g., supervision, low beds, minimal restraint).
   h. Discharge planning: Daily care of child at home (including need for supervision), therapy and medical appointments, equipment and planning for an emergency, respite care, community resources
   i. Special education, integration into school, planning with school staff (Selekman & Vessey, 2010)

j. Community integration
k. Postconcussion care: "10%–20% of concussions in adolescents take longer than 1 month to heal" (Vidal, Goodman, Colin, Leddy, & Grady, 2012, p.1). Children with prolonged recovery from concussion benefit from targeted vestibular, aerobic, and speech therapies to manage ongoing symptoms (Vidal et al., 2012). All children with concussions need cognitive rest that keeps brain activity at a subsymptom level (e.g., no headache or fatigue) to prevent more severe deficits. Cognitive activity is gradually reintroduced from no activity to home school, to return to school, and finally to full activity. Physical activity is also gradually increased (Master, Gioia, Leddy, & Grady, 2012).

8. Family and child education topics
   a. Behavior modification strategies and appropriate supervision
   b. Use and care of equipment and assistive devices
   c. Medications
   d. Methods of promoting development and independence; "normalization"
   e. Prevention of further injury and use of protective equipment
   f. Service coordination and advocacy
   g. Teaching strategies that can include play therapy

B. Pediatric Stroke
1. *Stroke:* "A stroke occurs when a blood vessel is either blocked by a clot or bursts" (Engle & Ellis, 2012, p. e63).
2. Incidence: In the United States, approximately 2,000 children have a stroke each year (Engle & Ellis, 2012).
3. Causes: The most common cause of pediatric stroke is sickle cell disease. Other causes include congenital and acquired heart disease, trauma, infections, blood disorders, and arteriovenous malformations (AVMs).
   a. An AVM is a defect in the circulatory system, believed to arise during embryonic or fetal development or soon after birth. Approximately 2%–4% of all AVMs hemorrhage and result in hemorrhagic stroke (National Institute of Neurological Disorders and Stroke [NINDS], 2011).
4. Rehabilitation issues: Consequences and care needs for children with pediatric stroke are similar to those for TBI care in terms of assessment, rehabilitation issues, outcomes, and family and child education.
   a. Infants more often have hemiplegia and sensory and balance deficits. Older children can also have language disturbances and ataxia. All of these deficits can have a profound impact on future development, especially in the youngest children (Engle & Ellis, 2012).

C. Cerebral Hypoxia
1. *Cerebral hypoxia* is "a condition in which there is a decreased oxygen supply to the brain" (NINDS, 2014a, para. 1). Causes in children and adolescents include hypoxic-ischemic encephalopathy (HIE), near-drowning, choking, TBI, drug overdoses, cardiac arrest, status asthmaticus, or anesthesia complications.
2. Rehabilitation issues
   a. In mild cases, children require rehabilitation to address inattention, poor judgment, memory loss, and decrease in motor coordination.
   b. In more severe cases, children present in persistent coma and may have seizures. Comprehensive pediatric rehabilitation nursing care similar to care of patients with limited cognitive functioning as a result of TBI is indicated in these cases.

D. Spinal Cord Injury (SCI) (Refer to Chapter 23 for an in-depth discussion of SCI.)
1. Traumatic: SCI in children is typically caused by motor vehicle accidents. Falls, gunshot wounds, and sporting activities are other common etiologies. Violence-related SCIs have increased prevalence in adolescent and young-adult African-American males (Chen, Tang, Vogel, & DeVivio, 2013). Before puberty, young children have unique physical and developmental characteristics that predispose them to SCI from lap-belt injuries and injuries related to birth and child abuse.
2. Acquired
   a. *Transverse myelitis:* "A neurological disorder caused by inflammation across both sides of one level, or segment, of the spinal cord" (NINDS, 2014c, para. 1). At present, no effective treatment is available. One third of those affected fully recover, one third has partial recovery, and one third may have no recovery (NINDS, 2014c).
   b. Spinal cord tumor: Various tumor types can entwine themselves around the spinal cord and produce problems and care needs similar to those of other SCI types. In addition to basic SCI care, considerations include surgical treatments; effects of chemotherapy treatments (e.g., no rectal treatments should be given during the nadir [i.e., lowest point of white

and red blood cell count and platelet count after chemotherapy] due to risk of bleeding and infection); fatigue; palliative options; and child and family preferences. (See Section II. G., "Cancer," for more information.)

3. SCI in children is different from SCI in adults.
   a. SCI in children is relatively rare but can occur at all ages, including in utero, during delivery, and throughout childhood (Brand, 2006; Parent, Mac-Thiong, Roy-Beaudry, Sosa, & Labelle, 2011).
   b. Children, especially those younger than 8 years of age, are likely to have SCI without radiological abnormalities (SCIWORA). All children may have delayed onset of neurological deficits; high cervical injuries; and potential for additional common associated brain, chest, and limb injuries (Martin, Dykes, & Lecky, 2004; Nelson & Hornyak, 2010; Vogel, Hickey, Klaas, & Anderson, 2004).
   c. Neurological recovery in children with SCI is thought to be better than in the adult population.
   d. Scoliosis following SCI in children is a common complication, especially when the neurological insult occurs at a young age (Parent et al., 2011).
   e. Children injured before age 16 years have a reduced life expectancy (Shavelle, Strauss, & Brooks, 2013).
   f. Families and children experience a prolonged psychosocial impact, especially when the injury occurs during early childhood (Osorio, Reyes, & Massagli, 2014).
4. Assessment components
   a. Developmental level
   b. Cognitive levels
   c. Spinal stability
   d. Pain: Types of pain with SCI can be acute traumatic (postinjury), neuropathic, repetitive use (upper-limb discomfort from propelling a wheelchair), and related to muscles spasms (spasticity). (See Chapter 8 for more pain descriptions, assessment, and interventions.)
   e. Respiratory status (especially in tetraplegia and upper-level thoracic injury)
   f. Skin integrity
   g. Bladder and bowel function
   h. Functional level (i.e., using WeeFIM II™ System)
   i. Psychosocial issues
   j. Family history and coping
   k. Home environment accessibility
5. Rehabilitation issues
   a. Mobility: Immobilization and spine stabilization with bracing, functional-dependent to independent-mobility activities. Power and manual mobility for children as young as 1 year of age is encouraged. As children get older, increased reliance on a wheelchair helps them to keep up with their peers and should not be viewed as a failure (Calhoun et al., 2013).
   b. Risk for spasticity and contractures: Range of motion and splinting to help manage these issues
   c. Orthopedic complications: Scoliosis and hip instability is common. Scoliosis occurs in the majority of children who sustain SCI before skeletal maturity is complete (Calhoun et al., 2013; Nelson & Hornyak, 2010).
   d. Pain related to trauma, recovery, neuropathic pain: Use appropriate pain assessment tools, medication, and therapy approaches.
   e. Risk for autonomic dysreflexia (injuries at level T6 and above): Infants and young children likely are not able to describe their symptoms, so nurses must consider the possibility in any child with an injury at or above T6 who presents with sleepiness, irritability, crying, unexplained flushing, or facial sweating. Management is usually started at 15–20 mm Hg above baseline blood pressure (BP) in adolescents and 15 mm Hg above baseline BP in children. Medications (e.g., topical nitroglycerine) are used when systolic BP is greater than 120 mm Hg in children younger than 5, 130 mm Hg for children ages 6–12 years , and 140 mm Hg for adolescents (McGinnis et al., 2004). Because heart rate and BP baselines change with age, children with SCI should have baseline BPs documented annually (Osorio et al., 2014). Recommendation: The child should wear a medical alert bracelet, carry an autonomic dysreflexia information card, and keep care supplies in his or her travel backpack.
   f. Pulmonary function: Mechanical ventilation (if injury is at C3 and above). Infants and younger children with tetraplegia are at high risk for developing respiratory failure. Sleep studies are recommended when there is a history of excessive daytime sleepiness or prominent snoring (Nelson & Hornyak, 2010). Diaphragm pacing stimulation offers an option to mechanical ventilation for some children (Osorio et al., 2014).

g. Risk for deep vein thrombosis: Prophylactic treatment follows adult evidence-based practice guidelines.
h. Skin care: Adolescents can be at increased risk for pressure ulcers. The challenge of taking time to check skin, distraction by teen activities, and peer embarrassment increase their risk (Nelson & Hornyak, 2010).
i. Neurogenic bladder and bowel management
j. Risk for heterotopic ossification
k. Risk for osteopenia
l. Risk for hypercalcemia from immobility, especially common in boys (Nelson & Hornyak, 2010)
m. Latex sensitivity related to longevity of exposure. It is best to be in a latex-free environment to prevent development of latex sensitivity and allergy. Instruction in use of an epinephrine injection (EpiPen®) is indicated if an allergy develops (Nelson & Hornyak, 2010).
n. Risk for sexual dysfunction
o. Prevention of further injury
p. Plans for return to home, school, and community

6. Family and child education topics: Developmentally appropriate educational methods and an individualized educational SCI program are essential. Incorporate parental and child education adjustment from dependence to independence as the child grows into adulthood (Vogel et al., 2004).
   a. Autonomic dysreflexia (if injury is at T6 or above)
   b. Skin care
   c. Bladder and bowel program: Depending on fine-motor abilities and injury considerations, self-clean intermittent catheterization can be taught as early as 5 years of age. Bowel programs are initiated at about 3 years of age, transitioning to independence and directing caregivers at late school age to adolescence (Massagli, 2000; Vogel et al., 2004).
   d. Medications
   e. Sexuality: Effects on sexual function in children are similar to those in adults with SCI (e.g., pregnancy, fertility, erectile dysfunction, and ejaculation dysfunction). Education of parents and the child or adolescent is similar to that of children without SCI and as developmentally appropriate (Vogel et al., 2004).
   f. Emotional support: Proactive mental health interventions can support the well-being of teens with spinal cord injury (Klaas, Kelly, Anderson, & Vogel, 2014).
   g. Quality of life: Family-centered care and support to help the family system move toward their "new normal" is essential (Lucas, 2010).
   h. Community reintegration strategies

E. Burns
1. A *burn* is damage to any of the three layers of skin in which many of the affected cells die. Burns can be caused by fires; scalds (including immersion or splashing by hot liquids, grease, and steam); heat contact (touching a hot object or substance); chemicals; electricity; sunlight; or radiation. Cause of injury is closely related to the child's developmental stage and cognitive abilities. For example, infants and toddlers are often burned by scalds or nonaccidental trauma, and preschool and school-aged children are often burned playing with fire or matches, whereas school-aged children and adolescents can be burned by experimenting with flammable liquids or fireworks (Murphy et al., 2010).
2. Level of burn severity
   a. First degree or superficial
   b. Second degree or partial thickness
   c. Third degree or full thickness
   d. Some centers include a fourth degree, which includes muscles and bone (Weed & Berens, 2005).
3. Amount of body surface involved
   a. Use a standard chart such as the Lund-Browder burns assessment chart to estimate.
      1) Mild or minor: 10% of total body surface area (TBSA), partial thickness, and less than 2% full thickness, unless eyes, ears, face, or perineum is involved
      2) Moderate: 10%–20% TBSA regardless of depth, and 2%–10% TBSA full thickness, unless the eyes, ears, face, or perineum is involved
      3) Major: More than 20% TBSA, partial thickness; more than 10% TBSA, full thickness; all burns involving the face, eyes, ears, feet, and perineum; all burns that are electrical or involve inhalation injury; all burns with ancillary injury (e.g., fracture, tissue trauma) (Weed & Berens, 2005).
4. Assessment components
   a. Skin integrity: Use a skin risk-assessment scale (Gordon, Gottschlich, Helvig, Marvin, & Richard, 2004). Consider keeping a photo journal for documentation.

b. Respiratory condition: Preexisting conditions and comorbidities must be considered.
c. Mobility and functional levels (i.e., the WeeFIM II™ System)
d. Pain: Pain assessment tools must be chosen according to communication and developmental abilities. Evidence-based assessment tools include pain intensity self-report scales (e.g., 0–10 Numeric Pain Rating Scale, Wong-Baker Faces Pain Rating Scale, Faces Pain Scale-Revised, The Oucher, Poker Chip Tool; questionnaires and diaries) and behavioral observations (e.g., Observational Scale of Behavioral Distress; Children's Hospital of Eastern Ontario Pain Scale [CHEOPS]; Child Facial Coding System, Face, Legs, Activity, Cry, Consolability [FLACC]; COMFORT Scale; Pediatric Pain Profile) (Cohen et al., 2008; de Jong et al., 2010; Ely et al., 2012).
e. Nutrition
f. Sleep: Itching, splinting, and night terrors could interfere with rest.
g. Self-image
h. Developmental level (using Battelle Developmental Inventory)
i. Family history and coping

5. Rehabilitation issues: Children are more likely than adults to develop hypertrophic scars and keloids as a result of vigorous healing. Compliance can be challenged by uncomfortable and unsightly treatment modalities and extreme social pressure for acceptance by peers (Passaretti & Billmire, 2003).
   a. Risk for skin breakdown related to immobility, significant edema, nutrition alterations, injuries or operative procedures, moisture imbalance, splinting, and pressure garments. Consider a pressure-reducing mattress, frequent turning (more often than every 2 hours), nutrition support, skin emollients and protective moisture barriers, and skin checks with splint and pressure garment removal (Gordon et al., 2004). Skin graft sites, as well as new skin and scars, need to be monitored.
   b. Scar management: Options are based largely on clinical experience rather than evidence. Mainstays of management include silicone gel, silicone gel sheeting, pressure garments, and onion extract creams. Intralesional corticosteroid injections, laser therapy, and other options can be added for hypertrophic scars and keloids (Gold et al., 2014). Pressure garments must be worn constantly for an average of 6 to 24 months after acute burn (Passaretti & Billmire, 2003).
   c. Burn locations that are most challenging to functional ability: Axillae, neck, flexion areas, bottoms of feet
   d. Contracture management and surgeries for function or cosmesis: Scar contraction, joint contractures, muscle shortening, and growth restriction are issues for children. Physical and occupational therapy, splinting, massage, pressure garments, and surgical evaluation provide effective management during the child's growing years (Passaretti & Billmire, 2003; Vehmeyer-Heeman, Lommers, Van den Kerckhove, & Boeckx, 2005)
   e. Comfort level and pain management: Pharmacological (e.g., narcotic, nonnarcotic, anti-itch, and antianxiolytic formulations) treatment; moisturizers; topical corticosteroids; massage, pressure garments, silicone gel sheeting; cognitive/behavioral therapy; relaxation training; hypnosis; reassurance; parental support; guided imagery; biofeedback; distraction; therapeutic touch; and art, music, and play therapy can be considered (Gold et al., 2014; Habich et al., 2012).
   f. Nutrition deficit related to hypermetabolic state for as long as 1 year after burn injury. Enteral or parenteral nutrition for supplementation should be considered at a rate of 1.4 times resting energy expenditure in the pediatric population (Gordon et al., 2004; Pereira, Murphy, & Herndon, 2005; Przkora et al., 2006).
   g. Pulmonary function: Strength and exercise training to improve muscle strength and pulmonary function. Mild restrictive disease is often present after thermal burns. Exercise or activity improves pulmonary function (Suman, Mlcak, & Herndon, 2002).
   h. Elimination pattern: Toileting is complicated by difficult-to-remove pressure garments or splints. Decreased mobility and pain medications increase the risk of constipation.
   i. Risk for long bone fractures: Increased incidence in children younger than 3 years of age and with burns over more than 40% TBSA. Potential contributory factors: hormonal changes after burn, depressed vitamin D status, inadequate protein intake, decreased weight-bearing activity, opposition to physical therapy (Mayes, Gottschlich, Scanlon, & Warden, 2003)
   j. Medication management: Potential treatment of hypermetabolic state (in children with more

than 40% TBSA burns) with insulin, anabolic steroids, catecholamine antagonists, and anabolic and anticatabolic agents (Pereira et al., 2005)

   k. Restoration of self-image
   l. School reintegration: Potential compliance resistance necessitating assistance from school therapists for ongoing therapeutic management or a behavior-management program (Pidcock, Fauerback, Ober, & Carney, 2003)
6. Family and child education topics
   a. Signs and symptoms of infection
   b. Skin and wound care
   c. Personal care
   d. Care and use of pressure garments
   e. Importance of prevention of complications, contractures, loss of function, and ongoing exercise and therapy; include growth considerations
   f. Pain and itching management
   g. Nutrition
   h. Medications
   i. Psychosocial and behavioral interventions
   j. Home environment and safety as indicated; prevention of further injury
   k. Social reintegration strategies: School, community, camp opportunities

F. Limb Deficiency and Acquired Amputation
1. *Limb deficiency:*The absence of all or part of one or more limbs
2. Congenital limb deficiencies: Incidence is two to four per 10,000 births (CDC PNCBDDD, 2014b). Cause is unknown in most cases. Known causes include genetic syndromes, environmental toxins, medication, and vitamins. Other associated congenital anomalies including craniofacial, genitourinary, and cardiac defects are likely and have genetic causes (Gaebler-Spira & Lipschutz, 2010).
   a. Congenital limb deficiencies are classified as either transverse or longitudinal, according to the International Society for Prosthetics and Orthotics (the preferred classification system). The Frantz Classification system may still be used in some settings.
      1) *Transverse limb deficiency*, also referred to as *terminal deficiency*, is defined as the loss of all skeletal components distal to a particular transverse axis (e.g., transverse forearm or transverse radial limb deficiency) (Walsh, Bosker, & Santa Maria, 2010, Congenital amputation section, para. 2).
      2) *Longitudinal limb deficiency*, also referred to as *intercalary limb loss*, is defined as the loss (complete or partial) of one or more skeletal elements within the longitudinal axis of the limb, with preservation of some or all of the distal skeletal elements (Walsh et al., 2010, Congenital amputation section, para. 2).
3. Acquired amputations
   a. Trauma causes limb loss more often than disease. Common causes of traumatic limb loss are motor-vehicle accidents, burns, gunshot wounds, farm machinery accidents, lawnmower accidents, and high-tension wire injuries (Gaebler-Spira & Lipschutz, 2010).
   b. Cancer is the leading cause of disease-produced limb loss (Gaebler-Spira & Lipschutz, 2010) Severe infections (e.g., meningococcemia), and abnormal nerves and blood vessels are other causes.
      1) Van Ness rotationplasty: Generally used after osteosarcoma around the knee joint or congenital short femur, where the foot and ankle are preserved, rotated 180 degrees, and reattached to the distal femur, making a functional joint (Gupta, Alassaf, Harrop, & Kiefer, 2012).
   c. Acquired amputations are classified by extremity and location.
      1) Upper extremity
      2) Lower extremity
      3) Trans: Amputation across axis of long bone (e.g., transradial or below-elbow amputation, transfemoral or above-knee amputation)
      4) Disarticulation: Amputation through joint (e.g., hip disarticulation, knee disarticulation, or through-knee amputation)
      5) Partial: Amputation distal to the wrist or ankle joint (e.g., partial foot or partial hand amputation)
4. Assessment components
   a. Developmental level
   b. Musculoskeletal system
   c. Mobility: Ambulation and use of prosthesis
   d. Skin integrity or residual limb care
   e. Psychosocial adjustment
5. Rehabilitation issues
   a. Achieving appropriate developmental milestones and independence
   b. Prosthetics: Ongoing technological advances make it difficult to stay abreast of all available options. Selection of a prosthetic requires a team decision by a physical or occupational therapist and a prosthetist experienced in pediatric limb deficiencies, along with the family

and child, if age-appropriate (Gaebler-Spira & Lipschutz, 2010). Secure funding and long-term planning to allow frequent refittings and new prostheses related to growth.

1) Types of upper-extremity prostheses: Cosmetic or passive, body powered or conventional, externally powered or myoelectric, hybrid (with control cable system for myoelectric or body-power function)
2) Types of lower-extremity prostheses: Hip, above knee, through knee, below knee, special types of feet for various functions, customized shoes or orthotics (Walsh et al., 2010).

c. Prosthetic wear: Prosthetic wear and acceptance is a complex issue. It can be affected by the level of limb loss, other medical conditions, comfort of prosthesis, perceived usefulness of prosthesis, acceptance of limb deficiency by family, and child's age when prosthesis wear begins (Gaebler-Spira & Lipschutz, 2010).

1) Varying degrees of limb difference and function can occur with or without use of prostheses.
2) Upper-limb prosthesis wear is complicated by a lack of sensation, which is needed for functional use of the hand. Prostheses can be worn for cosmetic rather than functional reasons (Vasluian et al., 2013)
3) Lower-limb prostheses have a high acceptance rate and good functional outcomes.

d. Mobility: Ambulation and prosthesis introduction at developmentally appropriate milestones can lead to greater success with incorporating prosthesis into new tasks.

1) Upper extremity: Introduce a prosthesis when the child has developed sitting balance (at approximately 6 months of age) (Walsh et al., 2010).
2) Lower extremity: When the child has had an amputation before learning to ambulate, introduce the prosthesis during pulling to stand and beginning walking motions (at approximately 9–14 months of age) (Walsh et al., 2010).

e. Skin or residual limb management: Monitor for pressure areas on bony prominences, rashes from excessive moisture and heat (confinement in prosthesis), infection at surgical incisions for newer amputations, skin integrity of residual limb, and skin breakdown at amputation terminal ends related to bony overgrowth at the distal end of the residual limb (Walsh et al., 2010).

f. Pain management

1) The most common causes of and contributors to pain are postoperative surgical incision pain; anxiety; and bony overgrowth, or "spiking," at the end of the residual limb, which is most common in children who have had amputation through a long bone, especially in a lower extremity (Gaebler-Spira & Lipschutz, 2010).
2) Phantom pain: Historically, it was thought few children experience this phenomenon. However, recent studies and reviews identify phantom pain and treatment options, although limited (Walco, Dworkin, Krane, LeBel, & Treede, 2010).

g. Self-esteem and self-concept: Facilitate networking with other parents and their children with limb deficiencies or differences. Networking is often available through limb deficiency specialized outpatient clinics. Adaptations for activities and sports are critical for emotional, physical, self-esteem, and social development.

6. Family and child education topics
   a. Use and care of equipment or prosthesis
   b. Residual limb wrapping or "pull-sock" and skin care
   c. Pain management
   d. Safety and injury prevention
   e. Importance of weight control with lower-extremity prosthetics
   f. Loss of surface area with multiple limb loss can cause increased sweating and flushing of head and neck (Gaebler-Spira & Lipschutz, 2010).
   g. Therapy and prosthetic centers
   h. Community reintegration strategies, resources, and supports
   i. Coping: Body image, dealing with reactions, importance of parental support and peer-to-peer interactions (de Jong et al., 2012; Vasluian et al., 2013)
   j. For congenital deficiencies, genetic counseling for the parents or the child (Smith, 2006)

G. Cancer

1. Overview: Cancer is the second leading cause of death in children between 5 and 14 years of age (CDC National Center for Injury Prevention and Control [NCIPC], 2010). Treatment modalities have improved such that the 5-year survival rate is greater than 80% (better than in adults). The most common malignancies are acute lymphocytic leukemia, acute myeloid leukemia, brain tumors (the

most common of solid tumors in children), lymphomas, neuroblastomas, bone tumors, retinoblastomas, hepatic tumors, and Langerhans cell histiocytosis (American Cancer Society, 2014).

2. Assessment components
   a. Developmental level
   b. Functional ability related to disease progression
   c. Complications: Growth, endocrine, cardiopulmonary, renal, neuropsychological, secondary malignancies
   d. Monitor laboratory results for nadir and need for protective precautions
   e. Nutrition
   f. Family history and coping
   g. Community resources
3. Rehabilitation issues specific to brain tumors
   a. Behavioral and cognitive function impairments, short- and long-term memory problems, focal motor weaknesses and visual-perceptual impairments similar to those of acquired brain injury (Poggi et al., 2005; Vargo, Riutta, & Franklin, 2010)
   b. Dysphagia: Treatment is similar to that of stroke.
   c. Weakness and often gait disturbance
   d. Visual and perceptual impairment
   e. Increased incidence of seizures
4. Rehabilitation issues for all malignancies
   a. Pain management
   b. Disease progression
   c. Independence level related to developmental level
   d. Integration of rehabilitation, cancer treatment, and palliative care plan
   e. Skin integrity, especially with radiation
   f. Fatigue
   g. Self-image, especially with chemotherapy effects; amputation; scarring; alopecia
   h. Coping
5. Family and child education topics
   a. Use and care of equipment and assistive devices
   b. Medication regimen
   c. Pain-management techniques
   d. Energy conservation
   e. Community reintegration strategies

III. Birth Defects and Developmental Disabilities

A. Myelodysplasia or Myelomeningocele (Spina Bifida)

1. *Spina bifida* is a condition in which the neural tube fails to close during the first 3–4 weeks of fetal development, resulting in incomplete closure of the spinal column. The opening in the spine can be at any level, but thoracic and lumbar levels are the most common.
2. Types of spina bifida:
   a. Myelomeningocele: The most severe form. The spinal cord and meninges protrude from the opening in the spine; they can be covered with a sac or be open. Hydrocephalus occurs in about 80% of cases. Motor and sensory nerves below the level of the lesion are affected, resulting in paraplegia, neurogenic bowel and bladder, and lack of sensation.
   b. Meningocele: Meninges protrude from the open spine. Motor and sensory nerves below the level of the lesion can be affected.
   c. Closed neural tube defects: Spinal cord is marked by malformations of fat, bone, or meninges. Symptoms vary from none to incomplete paralysis with bowel and bladder dysfunction.
   d. Spina bifida occulta: An abnormal opening in the spinal column, without any nerve tissue protruding, and completely covered by skin. There can be a patch of hair covering the site but no unusual appearance. There usually is no disability (NINDS, 2013; Spina Bifida Association of America [SBAA], "What Is Spina Bifida?").
3. Incidence: In the United States, the incidence of spina bifida is 4.17 per 10,000 births in Hispanics; 3.22 per 10,000 births in Non-Hispanic Whites; and 2.64 per 10,000 births in African Americans (CDC PNCBDDD, 2011).
4. Causes and risk factors
   a. The exact cause is unknown but is thought to be multifactorial, involving genetics and environment.
   b. Folic acid supplementation in women of childbearing age significantly reduces the risk of a neural tube defect.
   c. Women who take valproic acid for seizures are more likely to have a child with a neural tube defect (Jentink et al., 2010).
5. Assessment components
   a. Motor and sensory deficits: Depend on the level of the spinal cord lesion and consequent functional level
   b. Developmental and cognitive level
      1) Children with hydrocephalus are more likely to be affected, with problems such as lower IQ and impaired learning, and memory and executive function deficits (Pico, Wilson, & Hass, 2010). Arnold-Chiari II malformation can also affect cognitive

functioning (Vinck, Maassen, Mullaart, & Rotteveel, 2006).

2) Depression, chronic pain, and anxiety are common but can also be signs of shunt malfunction or infection, so organic causes must be ruled out before beginning treatment (Bellin et al., 2010; Oddson, Clancy, & McGrath, 2006).

c. Neurological deficits: Neurological complications do not occur in every person, but they can significantly affect function and long-term outcomes.
   1) Spasticity
   2) Tethered spinal cord: The spinal cord is "caught" and cannot move as the child grows.
   3) Symptomatic Chiari malformation: A brain malformation associated with hydrocephalus that becomes symptomatic in about one third of children with spina bifida (Spina Bifida Association of America, "Symptomatic Chiari Malformation Health Info Sheet"; Vinck et al., 2006)

d. Signs of shunt malfunction: A ventriculoperitoneal shunt could be necessary to control hydrocephalus. Shunts can malfunction, become infected, or need revision because children grow.

e. Bladder function
   1) Neurogenic bladder related to level of injury, similar to effects from spinal cord injury
   2) At risk for urinary tract infection: Urinary tract infections are common and can damage ureters and kidneys.
   3) Infants are assessed at birth and regularly thereafter for reflux and kidney damage (Snodgrass & Gargollo, 2010).
   4) Child's readiness to begin self-care

f. Bowel function
   1) Neurogenic bowel related to level of cord involvement, similar to effects from spinal cord injury
   2) At risk for constipation
   3) Child's readiness to begin self-care

g. Skin integrity: Sensation is partially or completely lost below the level of the lesion. Sensory deficits increase risk for development of pressure ulcers.

h. Orthopedic concerns: Hip dysplasia, clubfoot, kyphosis, and scoliosis
   1) Preoperative and postoperative surgical repair
   2) Use of braces and mobility devices

i. Latex allergies: Latex allergy is common in people with spina bifida. Reactions to latex allergy range from mild to very severe (Pollart, Warniment, & Mori, 2009).

j. Visual perceptual deficits

k. Cardiopulmonary function: Can be compromised in children with high thoracic level lesions or with symptomatic Chiari malformation

l. Nutritional status: Adequate growth and development, prevention of overweight and obesity

m. Ability to perform activities of daily living (ADLs)

n. Self-concept and self-esteem

o. Family history and coping: Ability to care for child, stressors, support systems

6. Rehabilitation issues

a. Promotion of development and attainment of milestones as much as possible

b. Self-care and independence as appropriate for developmental level; ability to perform ADLs (Greenley, 2010). Motivation is a significant problem and stems in part from executive function deficits.

c. Promotion of mobility and upright position: Depending on the level of the lesion and the muscles affected, braces, crutches, a walker, or a wheelchair can be used. Children who are able to walk short distances with crutches and braces when they are small often move to wheelchair mobility in adolescence when they are older and heavier (Verhoef et al., 2006).

d. Bowel and bladder management
   1) Timed voiding, clean intermittent catheterization, and continent stomas that can be catheterized (e.g., the Mitrofanoff procedure) are some management methods. Social continence is a significant management challenge (Clayton & Brock, 2010).
   2) Bowel programs focus on preventing constipation and maintaining continence. Bowel programs are among the most frustrating tasks for children and parents (Sawin & Thompson, 2009).
   3) Use of the antegrade continence enema has contributed to increased continence in a flaccid bowel; however, it requires major abdominal surgery and placement of a *cecostomy*, an artificial opening to the intestine (Sawin & Thompson, 2009).

e. Skin care

f. Special education

g. Self-concept and self-esteem

h. Community inclusion

7. Family and child education topics
   a. Individualized bladder and bowel programs (Greenley, 2010; Mason, Tobias, Lutkenhoff, Stoops, & Ferguson, 2004)
   b. Skin care and pressure-relief techniques
   c. Shunt care and identification of malfunction (Greenley, Coakley, Holmbeck, Jandasek, & Wills, 2006)
   d. Use and care of equipment and orthoses
   e. Promotion of independence and ADLs at home and school
   f. Transfers and ambulation (if appropriate for level of lesion)
   g. Service coordination and advocacy

B. Neuromuscular Conditions

Most children with a progressive neuromuscular condition are cared for and followed in an outpatient setting. Inpatient rehabilitation services can be sought for postoperative endurance, after an acute respiratory deterioration, or for a condition unrelated to the child's neuromuscular condition (e.g., a car accident).

1. Types of diseases (Muscular Dystrophy Association [MDA], "Muscle Diseases")
   a. *Duchenne muscular dystrophy*: This is the most common. Its occurrence in males is caused by the absence of dystrophin. The age of recognition is at 2–6 years. This condition progresses rapidly and is X-linked recessive.
      1) Medical and mobility issues: Wheelchair use is often needed by age 9 years. Gross motor strength is significantly affected; able to do some fine motor independent skills with setup. Most often warrants surgical intervention for heel-cord releases, scoliosis corrective spine surgery, and respiratory support. Cardiomyopathy is common in the late teen years.
      2) Life span: Without intervention, patients may only live into their late teens or early 20s; often into 30s or longer with respiratory support and cardiac interventions
   b. *Becker muscular dystrophy:* A condition similar to but less severe than Duchenne. It is caused by insufficient production of dystrophin, and is X-linked recessive.
      1) Medical and mobility issues similar to Duchenne. Patients are often ambulatory through the teen years; can consider using a wheelchair for long distances.
      2) Life span: into late adulthood; could need cardiac intervention.
   c. *Congenital muscular dystrophy:* A group of genetic, degenerative diseases that affect voluntary muscles. This condition has onset at or near birth. Progression and disability vary. It is often seen as generalized muscle weakness; caused by autosomal recessive genes.
   d. *Myotonic dystrophy:* Affects generations and becomes progressively more involved with each generation; generalized weakness, muscle wasting, myotonia, and developmental disability appear in children; medical and mobility problems; often ambulatory into the late teens with wheelchair use for long distances; caused by a repeated section of DNA on chromosome 19; autosomal dominant.
   e. *Limb-girdle muscular dystrophy:* Presents as weakness and wasting of muscles around shoulders and hips; could present with functional challenges similar to Duchenne but is less severely progressive; mutation of different genes affecting proteins for muscle function; can be autosomal dominant or autosomal recessive.
   f. *Facioscapulohumeral muscular dystrophy:* Onset usually by age 20 years; weakness of eye and mouth muscles, shoulders, upper arms, and lower legs; missing area of chromosome 4; autosomal dominant.
   g. *Spinal muscular atrophy (SMA):* Deficiency of motor neuron protein SMN occurs on chromosome 5. Loss of motor neuron nerve cells in the spinal cord result in loss of voluntary muscle control. Mental, emotional, and sensory development are normal in SMA. All types are autosomal recessive (MDA, 2009).
      1) Type 1: Infantile (Werdnig-Hoffman Disease), onset birth to 6 months; rapid progression, often leading to death within the first 1–2 years of life. Increased longevity with respiratory ventilation and nutritional support
      2) Type 2: Intermediate, onset 6–18 months. Weakness occurs in central core muscles: shoulders, hips, thighs, upper back. Patients become wheelchair dependent and at risk for respiratory compromise. Life span can be into childhood, teens, or young adulthood.
      3) Type 3: Mild (Kugelberg-Welander Disease), onset after 18 months; often presents after the child has started walking; slower progression. Walking ability is often maintained at least until adolescence. Life span

is usually not affected, but respiratory function and spinal curvature should be assessed regularly.
4) Type 4: Adult-onset SMA; mildest type of SMA (NINDS, 2012).

h. *Charcot-Marie-Tooth (CMT):* Neurological damage to peripheral nerves; slowly progressive; muscle weakness often seen, along with wasting and loss of sensation in periphery; onset birth to adulthood; caused by defects in axons or genes for proteins found in myelin. Different forms of CMT: autosomal dominant, autosomal recessive, and X-linked.
i. *Friedreich's ataxia:* Genetic defect occurs in the frataxin protein. Diminishing energy production in mitochondria results in damage to peripheral nerves and cerebellum; affects all ages and can occur in patients as young as 2 years of age. Most cases are characterized by ataxia, loss of sensation, cardiac involvement, difficulty with speech and swallowing, and diabetes.
j. *Leukodystrophy* (NINDS, 2014b): There are different types; genetic related. Progressive degeneration of white matter of the brain is caused by decreased growth and development of myelin sheath. The prognosis varies, often quite debilitating and life limiting.

2. Assessment components
   a. Developmental level
   b. Respiratory status
   c. Cardiovascular
   d. Scoliosis
   e. Assistive, orthotic, or mobility devices
   f. Medication history, especially corticosteroid use
   g. Skin integrity
   h. Nutrition and fluid intake
   i. Seizures, in leukodystrophy
   j. Bladder and bowel function: Retained sensation, decreased motor control, and decreased motility as disease progresses
   k. Home environment accessibility
   l. Family genetics
   m. Family history and coping
3. Rehabilitation issues
   a. Pulmonary management and support
   b. Corticosteroid treatment, along with discussion of potential side effects (Angelini & Peterle, 2012)
   c. Maintenance of intact skin
   d. Toileting
   e. Assistance with ADLs, depending on severity and progression of condition
   f. Seizure management, as applicable
   g. Maintain independence as much as possible.
   h. Accessibility of home environment
4. Family and child education topics
   a. Pulmonary and cardiovascular maintenance and precautions
   b. Maintenance of skin integrity
   c. Range-of-motion exercises
   d. Use of assistive, orthotic, and mobility devices
   e. Nutrition and fluid intake
   f. Home environment modifications
   g. Medication management
   h. Mobility
   i. Community integration strategies

C. Joint and Orthopedic Conditions
1. *Legg-Calvé-Perthes disease:* A condition most common in males, in which the femoral head develops avascular necrosis
   a. Can occur at any age but usually occurs between 3 and 9 years of age.
   b. Cause is unknown, but various factors such as attention deficit hyperactivity disorder (ADHD), delayed skeletal age, metabolic factors, and mechanical dysfunction can play a role in its development.
   c. Treatment can be surgical or nonsurgical depending on severity of necrosis. Femoral osteotomy is the typical option for surgical management (Smith, 2014).
2. *Osteogenesis imperfecta (OI):* A metabolic bone and connective-tissue disease that results in brittle bones; it is commonly associated with fractures that can occur with normal movement and care of the child with this condition. Fractures that are characteristic of this condition can be mistaken for nonaccidental injury (Horner, 2012).
   a. The cause is a dominant genetic mutation.
   b. There are many different types of OI, ranging from very mild to lethal.
   c. OI is present from conception, but depending on the severity, it can be diagnosed at birth or later in life.
   d. Between 25,000 and 50,000 people in the United States have OI (Osteogenesis Imperfecta Foundation, n.d.).
   e. In most types, more fractures occur in childhood, and then become less frequent with age.
   f. Treatment varies with severity. Special handling techniques for children more significantly affected reduce the number of fractures. Frequent surgery could be needed to repair bone deformities (Osteogenesis Imperfecta Foundation, n.d.; Shapiro & Sponsellor, 2009).

3. *Leg length discrepancy:* Inequality of the leg lengths, usually more than 2 cm, can be the result of growth retardation (e.g., hip dysplasia, congenital malformations of the fibula, poliomyelitis, infections, trauma affecting the epiphyses, severe burns, tumors) or growth stimulation (e.g., vascular abnormalities, tumors) (Murphy et al., 2010).
   a. Minor discrepancies up to 3 cm can be treated using lifts in the shoe.
   b. In growing children, greater discrepancies between 3 and 6 cm can be treated with a surgical procedure to slow down the growth of the longer leg.
   c. Larger discrepancies (i.e., greater than 6 cm) can be treated with leg-lengthening surgery, often using an external fixator that extends the ends of the bone and soft tissues—about 3 months for each inch (Murphy et al., 2010).
4. *Juvenile idiopathic arthritis:* A chronic inflammation that involves the connective tissue, joints, and viscera and begins before the age of 16; formerly known as juvenile rheumatoid arthritis.
5. *Achondroplasia:* A skeletal dysplasia that causes short stature and bony deformities
   a. The cause is genetic, occurring in one out of 15,000–40,000 births (Defendi, 2014).
   b. Developmental delays, kyphosis, flexion contractures of joints, bowed legs, other hip and spine problems, and characteristic bowed forehead are associated with achondroplasia.
   c. Treatment includes human growth hormones, weight management, leg lengthening and other surgical treatment (Defendi, 2014; Murphy et al., 2010).
6. *Arthrogryposis multiplex congenital:* Congenital joint contractures, decreased fetal movement in utero related to a variety of reasons and conditions, most often associated with motor neuron involvement (i.e., amyoplasia). There is limited function of upper and lower extremities (Chen, 2013).
7. Assessment components
   a. Developmental level
   b. Level of disability related to diagnosis
   c. Pain assessment and management preoperatively and postoperatively
   d. Mobility, use, and care of equipment and assistive devices
   e. Ability to perform ADLs; self-care
   f. Family
      1) Medical history and genetics
      2) Coping and adaptive skills
      3) Ability to care for child
8. Rehabilitation issues
   a. Promotion of maximum independence level based on severity of the diagnosis
   b. Mobility
   c. Joint protection
   d. Pain management
   e. ADL modification
   f. Safety
   g. Preoperative and postoperative nursing care
   h. Psychological implications such as developmental regression, avoidance behavior, depression, social isolation (e.g., resulting from prolonged bed rest, disability, painful procedures)
   i. Community integration and school attendance
   j. Discharge planning, service coordination, and case management
9. Family and child education topics
   a. Medication regimen
   b. ADLs
   c. Safety
   d. Mobility versus joint protection
   e. Pain management
   f. Use and care of equipment and assistive devices
   g. Community resources

D. Cerebral Palsy
1. *Cerebral palsy* (CP) is a disorder of movement and posture caused by a nonprogressive lesion in an immature brain, occurring in utero, near the time of delivery or within the first 3 years of life. CP is the most common childhood disability.
2. Types of CP (CDC PNCBDDD, 2013b)
   a. Spastic: most common type. Hyperactive reflexes, increased muscle tone, muscle spasms, motor weakness, persistent reflexes. It is often described by the extremities involved: diplegia (legs affected more than arms), hemiplegia (one side of body; usually arm more than leg), quadriplegia (most severe; all four limbs, trunk, and face), monoplegia (one extremity; very rare).
   b. Dyskinetic: Abnormal involuntary movements, facial grimacing, dystonic movements, poor speech, distorted posturing
   c. Ataxia: Hypotonia, floppy muscle tone, impaired balance and coordination, unsteady gait
   d. Mixed: Combination of several types
3. Risk factors: The majority of CP (85%–90%) is congenital. In many cases, the specific cause is not known (CDC PNCBDDD, 2013a).
   a. Low birth weight
   b. Prematurity
   c. Multiple births

d. Assisted reproductive technology
e. Infections during pregnancy
f. Jaundice and kernicterus
g. Birth complications
4. Assessment components: Assessment must be highly individualized and reflect the child's age, level of involvement, and associated problems.
a. Developmental level
b. Cognitive level
c. Communication and speech
d. Ability to perform ADLs
e. Feeding pattern
f. Toileting
g. Muscle function
h. Ambulation
i. History of seizure disorders and other associated conditions
j. Vision and hearing
k. Skin integrity
l. Learning disability
5. Rehabilitation issues: Additional problems and symptoms can develop as the child progresses and grows (Horsman, Suto, Dudgeon, & Harris, 2010).
a. Neurodevelopmental and sensory therapies
b. Communication
c. Feeding problems
d. Positioning and therapeutic handling, depending on severity
e. Motor control
f. Spasticity management
g. Seizure management
h. Assistive technology
i. Surgery and nonsurgical procedures: Orthopedic procedures, intrathecal baclofen pump, selective dorsal rhizotomy (Yildiz & Demirkale, 2014)
j. Social and sexual relationships
k. Independent living skills
6. Family and child education topics
a. Skin assessment and care
b. Exercise and fitness programs
c. Medications
d. Spasticity management techniques
e. Self-care
f. Feeding and nutrition
g. Bowel and bladder management
h. Community integration strategies: School, leisure activities, transportation, independent living arrangements

E. Autism Spectrum Disorders
1. *Autism spectrum disorder* (ASD) is a developmental disability characterized by difficulties in social interaction, verbal and nonverbal communication, and repetitive behaviors in varying degrees. ASD diagnoses now include autistic disorder, pervasive developmental disorder not otherwise specified (PDD-NOS), and Asperger syndrome (CDC PNCBDDD, 2014a).
2. Incidence: About 1 child in 68 has been identified with autism spectrum disorder (ASD), according to estimates from the CDC's Autism and Developmental Disabilities Monitoring Network (CDC PNCBDDD, 2014a). Due to multiple factors, the number of people diagnosed with autism is increasing.
3. Cause: The specific cause is unknown, but there are likely many causes for multiple types of ASD, including environmental, biological, and genetic factors.
4. Rehabilitation issues: Treatment typically occurs in the outpatient setting. Early intensive behavioral intervention improves learning, communication, and social skills in young children.
a. Behavior and communication approaches
b. Dietary approaches
c. Medication
d. Complementary and alternative medicine (CDC PNCBDDD, 2014a)

IV. Chronic Illnesses

A. Bronchopulmonary Dysplasia
1. *Bronchopulmonary dysplasia* is a serious lung condition that occurs in preterm infants. It results from the infant's need for supplemental oxygen for at least the first 28 days of life. It has three grades of severity that are determined by the duration and level of supplemental oxygen needed at 36 weeks postmenstrual age (Jobe & Bancalari, 2001). Also known as chronic lung disease of infancy, it can last throughout childhood and into adulthood. Long-term outcomes can include chronic pulmonary disease with risk of respiratory failure in adolescence and adulthood and long-lasting cardiac disorders (Hayes et al., 2011; Kair, Leonard, & Anderson, 2012).
2. Incidence: Incidence is as low as 5% in premature infants weighing more than 1,500 g and as high as 75% in extremely low birth weight infants (McMorrow & Sweet, 2013). Changing epidemiology and varying definitions of the disorder make it difficult to determine incidence. The occurrence may be reduced by the use of antenatal steroids, various ventilatory measures, surfactant and caffeine administration, and adequate nutrition (Kugelman & Durand, 2011).
3. Causes and risk factors

   a. Prematurity: Born more than 10 weeks before the due date and weighing less than 2 pounds (about 1,000 grams) at birth.
   b. Mechanical ventilation and high levels of oxygen: Thought to be caused by exposure of the immature alveoli and microvasculature of the lungs to trauma from mechanical ventilation, high oxygen concentrations, and respiratory distress itself. The resulting decrease in oxygenation affects the lungs, heart, and brain (Kugelman & Durand, 2011).
   c. Infections
   d. Patent ductus arteriosus
   e. Possible genetic influences (Hadchouel et al., 2011; National Institutes of Health National Heart, Lung, and Blood Institute, 2012)
4. Assessment components
   a. Respiratory assessment: Adequacy of ventilation, function of assistive technology, patency of tracheostomy, early identification and treatment of infection, respiratory medications
   b. Growth and nutrition: Growth retardation and poor weight gain; evaluate for anemia and other deficiencies
   c. Gastroesophageal reflux and feeding disorders
   d. Cardiac conditions such as pulmonary arterial hypertension, systemic hypertension, and cor pulmonale (Poon, Edwards, & Kotecha, 2013)
   e. Renal calcification resulting from long-term use of diuretics
   f. Seizures
   g. Retinopathy of prematurity and other ophthalmic complications
   h. Developmental delays including cognitive disability, gross and fine motor deficits, speech and language problems, visual/motor integration disorders, ADHD, and behavioral problems (Anderson & Doyle, 2006)
   i. Family bonding, history, and coping
5. Rehabilitation issues
   a. Respiratory management with pulmonary specialists to ameliorate the impact of long-term ventilation or tracheostomy on development; chest physiotherapy; airway management
   b. Airway complications such as stenosis, granuloma, scarring, and tracheomalacia
   c. Frequent ear and sinus infections
   d. Oral feeding if possible; maintenance of gastrostomy tube and tube feedings; promotion of good nutrition; monitoring of growth and gastroesophageal reflux; administer medications as appropriate
   e. Skin care: Assess stomas for irritation, granulomatous tissue, and leakage
   f. Stoma care: Lack of patency of tracheostomy and gastrostomy tubes; inflammation and infection of stomas
   g. Health promotion and prevention: Immunizations; palivizumab (Synagis®) is needed to prevent respiratory syncytial virus (Parmigiani et al., 2009)
   h. Appropriate screenings: Vision, hearing, dental, and developmental
   i. Developmental interventions, including physical therapy, occupational therapy, speech therapy, and recreational therapy; promote attainment of developmental milestones. Assess self-care skills and ADLs in the older child. Promotion of independence as appropriate for age (Anderson & Doyle, 2006)
   j. Early intervention, special education, and school inclusion (Litt et al., 2012)
   k. Discharge planning
   l. Family stress and coping skills, ability to manage child's needs
6. Family and child education topics
   a. Management of technology in the home and community: Troubleshooting the ventilator, suctioning and changing the tracheostomy, administering tube feedings, changing the gastrostomy tube
   b. Medication management: Administration, side effects
   c. Prevention of complications and health maintenance
   d. Promoting independence in self-care in the child
   e. Negotiating with caregivers in the home, service coordination, school liaison
   f. Safety at home, at school, and in the community
   g. Maintenance of family equilibrium, dealing with siblings

B. Technology Dependence
1. *Technology dependence* refers to children who use "both a medical device to compensate for the loss of a vital bodily function and substantial and ongoing nursing care to avert death or further disability" (U.S. Congress, Office of Technology Assessment, 1987, p. 3).
   a. Examples include children with a tracheostomy or gastrostomy tube or who need home oxygen, mechanical ventilation, or other medical devices such as colostomies or intravenous

fluid pumps; they may need more than one device.
   b. These children need high-tech care from nurses, parents, or caregivers who have been specially trained.
   c. The number of children on long-term mechanical ventilation is increasing. Several studies estimate prevalence of this condition to be 6–14 children per 100,000 (Peterson-Carmichael & Cheifetz, 2012).
   d. Costs for inpatient hospitalization are high and increasingly supported by public rather than private funding (Peterson-Carmichael & Cheifetz, 2012).
2. Assessment components: child
   a. Developmental and cognitive level
   b. Language skills and communication methods
   c. Age-appropriate ability to perform ADLs and amount of assistance needed
   d. Frequent physiological assessment, particularly respiratory system, gastrointestinal system, genitourinary system, skin integrity, musculoskeletal system
   e. Ability to eat; nutrition
   f. Toileting and bowel and bladder management; signs of urinary tract infection, constipation
   g. Ambulation or form of mobility
   h. Psychosocial issues
   i. Hospital discharge planning
   j. Equipment and supplies: Appropriate for child, in good working order, and sufficient supply (e.g., suction catheters, gloves)
   k. Home assessment: Accessibility; enrichment of the environment (e.g., books, toys); cleanliness; safety; presence of an emergency backup plan for equipment or power failure; notification of emergency responders (e.g., for a child with a tracheostomy or using a ventilator); notification of public utility services (i.e., of the need for immediate attention to resumption of electrical service); availability of home nursing care, therapy, and medical care in the home community
   l. School assessment: Accessibility; plan for care while the child is in school; equipment and supplies; individualized educational plan; appropriate caregiver training (e.g., school nurse, licensed practical nurse, or designated caregiver (Hewitt-Taylor, 2010)
3. Assessment components: family
   a. Family stress and coping skills; sibling stress
   b. Ability to meet child's needs; confusion of parent role versus high-tech caregiver role
   c. Family and caregiver skill
   d. Financial stress
   e. Social isolation and depression (Toly, Musil, & Carl, 2012)
   f. Accessible transportation for medical services and recreational activities
   g. Fatigue and burnout
   h. Technology and nursing care in the home (Hewitt-Taylor, 2012)
4. Rehabilitation issues
   a. Plan for discharge
   b. Promote community integration and independence as appropriate for the child's developmental level and functional abilities (Earle, Rennick, Carnavale, & Davis, 2006).
   c. Ensure safety in the home, community, and school.
   d. Offer family support and referrals as needed and community resources.
5. Family and child education topics
   a. Operation and maintenance of assistive technology
   b. Clinical care of child
   c. Promotion of independence in self-care
   d. Need for increased vigilance and safety supervision
   e. Community integration
   f. Training of community service providers: Selection criteria for home care nurses include competence, caring, ability to partner with caregivers, and ability to fit in with family (Mendes, 2013).

C. Diabetes
1. In recent years, there has been an increase in type 2 diabetes in children and adolescents. Risk factors include sedentary lifestyle, obesity, family history, and hypertension. Diabetes is a complex medical condition that requires compliance with medical management as well as lifestyle changes. Noncompliance can be a significant issue for some children and families. Change in lifestyle to increase activity, promote weight loss, and make healthy nutritional choices are the primary preventive and corrective measures (Dabelea, et al., 2014; Wilson, 2013). A comprehensive program that incorporates educational, medical, physical, and psychological components can be effectively implemented in the pediatric rehabilitation setting.

V. Long-Term Planning: Community Services for Children and Youths with Disabilities

A. Philosophy of Inclusion

1. *Inclusion* is a philosophical viewpoint that asserts that children with disabilities are an integral part of the community and should participate with their peers in typical activities such as school.
2. Inclusion can occur in playgroups, school, recreation, social activities, and work.
3. *Inclusive education* means that children with disabilities receive educational services in a typical classroom, where other children, without disabilities, are schooled (Maryland Coalition for Inclusive Education, n.d.).

B. Special Education

1. The Individuals with Disabilities Education Act (IDEA Reauthorization 2004, final regulations published August 14, 2006) ensures that all children and youths ages 3–21 years receive a free, appropriate public education.
2. Education and special education services should be delivered in the least restrictive environment in settings that are as similar as possible to those for children without disabilities.
3. Children who need special education are entitled to receive an individualized education plan that is reviewed annually to best meet the child's educational needs.
4. Children with disabilities can also receive related services through school (e.g., physical therapy, occupational therapy, speech therapy, nutrition, other health-related services), as mandated by IDEA, if those services are necessary for learning.
5. Child Find is a system in place in each school district that identifies children who are eligible for special education services (U.S. Department of Education, n.d.b).
6. The No Child Left Behind (NCLB) legislation, passed in 2001, set high standards for the education of all children and requires accountability from schools in the areas of reading and math. Children are tested on a regular basis to determine whether their education meets standards. Children with disabilities that hinder learning can receive alternative testing or might be excluded from testing. Currently, some states have waivers for opting out of certain NCLB mandatory interventions (U.S. Department of Education, n.d.b).

C. Early Intervention

1. Part C of IDEA provides for early educational services for young children with or at risk for disabilities from birth to 3 years of age.
2. Eligible children and their families receive an individualized family service plan (IFSP) that includes interventions to eliminate or reduce the developmental delay or disability and offer family support.
3. Early intervention services can include those for speech and language, physical or occupational therapy, psychological services, service coordination, social work, vision screening, and medical services (U.S. Department of Education, n.d.a).

D. Other Legislation Affecting Children with Disabilities

1. Rehabilitation Act of 1973: Provides for supportive services in school for children with physical disabilities who do not qualify for special education
2. Title V of the Social Security Act was passed in 1935 and established the Maternal and Child Health Bureau to provide public health services for mothers and children, as well as disabled children (U.S. Department of Health and Human Services [U.S. DHHS], n.d.b).
3. The Children's Bureau was established in 1912 to promote child welfare. The Child Abuse Prevention and Treatment Act was passed in 1974 and reauthorized in 2003 (Child Welfare Information Gateway, 2011).
4. Americans with Disabilities Act of 1990 (refer to Chapter 1).
5. Vocational Rehabilitation Act (Section 504 of the Rehabilitation Act of 1973)

E. Home Health Care

1. Children who are technology dependent as a result of prematurity, illness, or injury often need skilled care at home and at school. Nearly 500,000 children are in need of home health services (Child and Adolescent Health Measurement Initiative, 2011).
2. Living at home is much better for the child's developmental, psychological, and social well-being than living in an institution.
3. Medicaid is the primary payer for home health care, with private health insurance covering only about 1% of costs. Medicaid's low reimbursement rate makes it difficult to locate qualified agencies to provide specialized pediatric care in the home (AAP Committee on Child Health Financing, Section on Home Care, 2006).
4. Although the assistance of home health is welcomed, the intrusiveness of strangers in the home on a daily basis and the need for role shift from care provider to mother or father can be stressful (Hewitt-Taylor, 2012; Mendes, 2013).
5. Many families' insurance does not cover home health care, and such families are forced to provide skilled nursing care without assistance, which can be extremely stressful for them. Caring for a

CSHCN creates a perceived financial burden for many families (Lindley & Mark, 2010).

a. In such cases, respite care, which gives families a break, can be very useful (Hewitt-Taylor, 2012).
b. Each state's division of developmental disabilities has respite care funding available.

F. Health Promotion and Prevention

1. According to Healthy People 2020, people with disabilities are more likely to
   a. Experience difficulties or delays in getting the health care they need.
   b. Not have annual dental visits.
   c. Not engage in fitness activities
   d. Use tobacco.
   e. Be overweight or obese.
   f. Have high blood pressure.
   g. Experience symptoms of psychological distress.
   h. Receive less social-emotional support.
   i. Have lower employment rates (U.S. DHHS, n.d.a)
2. Healthy People 2020 has set specific objectives for health promotion in children and adolescents that include reducing barriers to health care, increasing transition planning, increasing employment, and providing sufficient social and emotional support. As such, CSHCN need a medical home to provide family-centered, comprehensive, and coordinated systems (U.S. DHHS, n.d.a).
3. All children need to receive all universally recommended immunizations and health screenings, and CSHCN could need specific preventive activities such as prevention of secondary conditions (U.S. DHHS, n.d.a).
4. *Developmental screening* (identification of children who need in-depth assessment related to developmental delays) is the responsibility of the primary healthcare provider. Young children with an autism spectrum disorder or other developmental delays need to be screened, evaluated, and enrolled in early intervention services in a timely manner (U.S. DHHS, n.d.a)
5. Health promotion for CSHCN also includes good nutrition and physical activity. Although children and adolescents with disabilities are more likely to be inactive than those without disabilities, they should nevertheless participate in 60 minutes (1 hour) or more of physical activity, including aerobic and muscle-strengthening/bone-strengthening activities, daily as appropriate. These efforts will not only decrease the risk for health issues but also contribute to maintaining an appropriate body weight (U.S. DHHS, 2008).

G. Transition to Adulthood

1. *Transition* refers to the process of youths moving from child-centered systems to the world of adulthood. It includes transition in the areas of health care, education, decision making, and community services. "After the age of majority [age when individuals are legally considered capable of making their own decisions], all youth deserve to be treated as adults and to experience an adult model of care..." (AAP, AAFP, & ACP, 2011, p. 184). Some CSHCN need to change from pediatric to adult providers, whereas others need only to transition to an adult model of care with the same provider (e.g., family practice).
2. Limited progress: In 2002, a consensus statement was published by the American Academy of Pediatrics (AAP), American Academy of Family Physicians (AAPP), and American College of Physicians (ACP) supporting the importance of transitioning adolescents with special healthcare needs into adulthood (AAP, AAFP, ACP, & American Society of Internal Medicine, 2002). After more than 10 years, only limited progress has been made in the implementation of healthcare transitions, despite the desire expressed by CSHCN and their families. Some of the reasons cited include
   a. Lack of an identified person in pediatric practices to make it happen
   b. Insufficient knowledge of available community resources
   c. Financial barriers
   d. Anxiety on the part of pediatricians, parents, and youths about ending their professional relationship
   e. Lack of developmentally appropriate tools to assess readiness for transition
   f. Adult providers who are unprepared to care for young adults with complex chronic conditions due to lack of time, inadequate reimbursement, and insufficient training
   g. Difficulty locating adult providers (AAP, AAFP, & ACP, 2011; White & Hackett, 2009)
3. Transition planning: Transitioning is a process, not an event, and therefore it requires planning.
   a. "Transition planning should be a standard part of providing care for all youth and young adults, and every patient should have a transition plan regardless of his or her specific health care needs" (AAP, AAFP, & ACP, 2011, p.187).

b. All youths should be assessed for transition readiness during routine health maintenance visits.
c. Recommended timelines: Introduce the process of transition at 12 years of age during a health maintenance or chronic condition management visit. Initiate and individualize the transition plan at age 14 years. Review, revise, and update the plan annually. Transfer to an adult care provider between 18 and 21 years of age. Families of CSHCN might need to start the process earlier, given the additional complexity of needs (AAP, AAFP, & ACP, 2011).

4. Components of the transition plan: Plans need to be focused on the youth, not on his or her caregivers. Plans also should be individualized to meet the physical, developmental, behavioral, and cognitive needs of the CSHCN. Include the following:
   a. Difference between pediatric and adult models of care
   b. Development of skills to navigate adult health care (e.g., self-advocacy, explaining medical symptoms and history, making appointments); families need to gain comfort in transferring authority to the CSHCN
   c. Portable medical summary
   d. Emergency plan
   e. Health promotion and health education
   f. Educational goals
   g. Career/work goals
   h. Independence and transportation
   i. Identify adult care provider (White & Hackett, 2009).
5. Other transition issues
   a. Health insurance
   b. School-to-work transition services are provided by the school system, which links with vocational education, if appropriate (Betz, 2007).
   c. Legal issues (e.g., consent, confidentiality, guardianship, healthcare proxy/power of attorney)
   d. Culturally appropriate community services (White & Hackett, 2009).
6. Components of successful transition
   a. Self-determination
   b. Person-centered planning
   c. Preparation for adult health care
   d. Preparation for work
   e. Independence
   f. Inclusion in community life (White & Hackett, 2009)
7. Transition resources: A wide variety of tools are available to assist in the development, implementation, and evaluation of transition plans from Got Transition/Center for Health Care Transition, a cooperative agreement between the Maternal and Child Health Bureau and The National Alliance to Advance Adolescent Health, at www.GotTransition.org.

H. Vocational Rehabilitation and Higher Education
1. State and local vocational rehabilitation offices work closely with schools-in-transition programs and local employers.
2. Youths with disabilities who have academic capabilities could go on to higher education.
   a. Many city and community colleges and universities are reaching out to young adults with disabilities.
   b. Some vocational rehabilitation offices can provide assistive technology to aid youths in educational pursuits.
3. Although not all children have the potential to be working members of society, many are overlooked simply because they lack information about potential options (Thrall et al., 2012).

VI. Trends and Future Directions

A. Health Care
1. Healthcare reform legislation, the Patient Protection and Affordable Care Act, was enacted in March 2010. Implementation is ongoing and remains controversial. Currently, provisions that affect children with disabilities include the following:
   a. Mandate that nearly all people have coverage.
   b. Expand Medicaid and Child Health Plan eligibility and increase Medicaid payment for services to primary healthcare providers (e.g., family practice, pediatricians) to increase access to care for many children.
   c. Permit children to remain on their parent's insurance until age 26 years.
   d. Eliminate ability to exclude coverage based on preexisting conditions (e.g., children with disabilities).
   e. Improve coverage portability when families must change jobs or insurance.
   f. Prohibit health insurance plans from placing a lifetime limit on coverage. Currently, for example, premature infants with multiple medical complications often reach their lifetime limits on insurance funding before they are discharged to home for the first time.
   g. Improve funding of preventive care for children and youths.

h. Provide more funding for training of future and existing healthcare providers, particularly in chronic care (Henry J. Kaiser Family Foundation, 2013).

2. Technology is more readily available to preserve and improve life but at increasing expense. As a result, funding could become scarcer.
3. There will be a greater emphasis on quality and safety, with the impact of nursing care on outcomes being tracked.
4. Emphasis on research and evidence-based practice addresses new ideas and validates current practice.
5. With nursing shortages, there is a greater need for education in pediatrics and rehabilitation for nurses working with children and adolescents in a variety of settings.
6. Quality-of-life and end-of-life decision making that incorporate rehabilitation and developmental principles will be important, as will more nursing research to identify better treatment options.
7. Collaborative, interdisciplinary service models will continue to evolve, with growth in nonhospital settings.
8. The incidence of orthopedic and sports-related injuries will increase.
9. Genetics and stem-cell research will link diseases to certain genes, with the potential for new treatment options.
10. Continued work is needed on wider implementation of effective medical home models that provide cost-effective, patient- and family-centered care to the growing population of children with special healthcare needs (Golnik, Scal, Wey, & Gaillard, 2012; Hamilton, Lerner, Presson, & Klitzner, 2013).
11. More effective models of transition from pediatric medical home to adult care models need to be financed, supported, and developed (AAP, AAFP, & ACP, 2011).

B. Community
1. There will be less hospital-based care, with shorter stays and more outpatient, community, and home-based care.
2. There will be a greater need in schools and in the community for accommodations for children who are technology dependent.
3. There will be an increased need for home-care education and to train caregivers in various settings.
4. Foster parents will be more likely to accept medically fragile children if they have a good medical home.
5. Legislation and litigation will continue to be a means of providing services to the pediatric population at the state and federal levels.
6. As more children with special healthcare needs survive into adulthood, there will be a greater need for community supports to help them live independently (Thrall et al., 2012).

VII. Advanced Practice Nurses in Pediatric Rehabilitation

A. Qualifications
1. An advanced practice nurse (APN) has acquired the knowledge and practice experience for specialization, expansion, and advancement of pediatric rehabilitation nursing practice.

B. Characteristics of Graduate Nursing Education
1. Graduate nursing education prepares the APN to use critical thinking and decision-making skills to assess, plan, intervene, and evaluate the health and illness experiences of clients, families, and communities.
2. Essentials of practice include development of core competencies in the following areas:
   a. Scientific underpinnings for practice
   b. Organizational and systems leadership for quality
   c. Improvement and systems thinking
   d. Clinical scholarship and analytical methods for evidence-based practice
   e. Information systems/technology and patient care technology for the improvement and transformation of health care
   f. Policy for advocacy in health care
   g. Interprofessional collaboration for improving patient and population health outcomes
   h. Clinical prevention and population health for improving the nation's health
   i. Advanced nursing practice
   j. Additional competencies specific to specialty areas as delineated by national specialty nursing organization (American Association of Colleges of Nursing, 2006; Carter, 2011)

C. Variety of Titles and Settings
1. Clinical nurse specialists
   a. More likely to work in an acute care setting but can also work in community agencies such as health department programs for children with special needs
   b. Broad range of responsibilities, such as coordination of care, client education, and nursing education (Sparacino & Cartwright, 2009)
   c. Use nursing diagnosis to assess, plan, and intervene.
2. Nurse practitioners

a. Provide routine health care, preventive care, immunizations, minor illness care, and/or specialty nursing and medical care
b. Are prepared to diagnose and manage acute, episodic, and chronic illnesses
c. Can specialize, providing care alongside medical subspecialists such as neurologists
d. Provide care in community medical practices, ambulatory care, acute care, or long-term care settings.

D. Scope of Practice
1. Nurse practitioners have autonomous practice and ability to bill for services.
2. Advanced delivery of care in a specific specialty area (e.g., pediatric nurse practitioner, acute care clinical nurse specialist)
3. Complexity of situations or conditions managed
4. Leadership in the interprofessional team
5. In-depth understanding of interacting pathophysiological and psychosocial changes associated with chronicity and disability (American Association of Nurse Practitioners, 2013; American Medical Association, 2009)

E. Advanced Practice Roles
1. Clinician
a. Facilitates the design and implementation of the individualized plan of care and the transition from the hospital to home and community
b. Assesses health needs; develops diagnoses; plans, implements, and manages care; and evaluates outcomes of care
2. Educator
a. Provides health education for professionals and consumers about the needs of children with disabilities and their families
b. Bases teaching methods on developmental level, functional ability, learning needs and abilities, and sociocultural factors
3. Leader and consultant
a. Serves as a model for child, adolescent, and family advocacy through direct intervention
b. Promotes community and government knowledge of pediatric rehabilitation issues and works to influence policy-making bodies to improve care
c. Involves stakeholders in the decision-making process and considers factors related to safety, effectiveness, cost, and impact on practice
d. Provides consultation to influence the plan of care, enhances the practice of team members, and affects resource use
4. Researcher
a. Participates in research and quality-improvement projects and is responsible for providing evidence-based care
b. Critically evaluates current practice and uses scientific findings to improve client care outcomes
c. Identifies research questions and disseminates relevant research findings to various constituencies

References

American Academy of Pediatrics. (2010). Medical Home Fact Sheet. What Is a Family-Centered Medical Home? Retrieved from www.medicalhomeinfo.org/

American Academy of Pediatrics, American Academy of Family Physicians, American College of Physicians, & American Society of Internal Medicine. (2002). A consensus statement on health care transitions for young adults with special health care needs. *Pediatrics, 110*(6), 1304–1307. Retrieved from http://pediatrics.aappublications.org/content/110/Supplement_3/1304.full?sid=419ecf5b-dccf-4918-979a-7f71e76c7ce8

American Academy of Pediatrics, American Academy of Family Physicians, & American College of Physicians. (2011). Clinical report-Supporting the health care transition from adolescence to adulthood in the medical home. *Pediatrics, 128*(1), 182–200. doi:10.1542/peds.2011-0969

American Academy of Pediatrics Committee on Child Health Financing, Section on Home Care. (2006). Financing of pediatric home health care. *Pediatrics, 118*(2), 834–838. Retrieved from http://pediatrics.aappublications.org/content/118/2/834.full

American Association of Colleges of Nursing. (2006). The Essentials of Doctoral Education for Advanced Nursing Practice. Retrieved from http://www.aacn.nche.edu/publications/position/DNPEssentials.pdf

American Association of Nurse Practitioners. (2013). Standards of Practice for Nurse Practitioners. Retrieved from http://www.aanp.org/images/documents/publications/standardsofpractice.pdf

American Cancer Society. (2014). Cancer in children. Retrieved from http://www.cancer.org/acs/groups/cid/documents/webcontent/002287-pdf.pdf

American Medical Association. (2009). AMA Scope of Practice Data Series: A Resource Compendium for State Medical Associations and National Medical Societies: Nurse Practitioners. Retrieved from http://elephantcircle.net/wp-content/uploads/2011/01/08-0424-SOP-Nurse-Revised-10-09.pdf

Anderson, P. J., & Doyle, L. W. (2006). Neurodevelopmental outcome of bronchopulmonary dysplasia. *Seminars in Perinatology, 30*(4), 227–232. doi:10.1053/j.semperi.2006.05.010

Angelini, C., & Peterle, E. (2012). Old and new therapeutic developments in steroid treatment in Duchenne muscular dystrophy. *Acta Myologica, 31*(1), 9–15. Retrieved from http://www.ncbi.nlm.nih.gov/pmc/articles/PMC3440806/

Association of Rehabilitation Nurses (ARN). (2007). Role descriptions: Pediatric rehabilitation nurse. Retrieved from http://www.rehabnurse.org/pubs/role/Role-Pediatric-Rehab-Nurse.html

Association of Rehabilitation Nurses (ARN). (2014). ARN competency model for professional rehabilitation nursing. Retrieved from http://www.rehabnurse.org/uploads/files/education/ARN_Rehabilitation_Nursing_Competency _Model_FINAL_-_May_2014.pdf

Bellin, M. H., Zabel, T. A., Dicianno, B. E., Levey, E., Garver, K., Linroth, R., & Braun, P. (2010). Correlates of depressive and anxiety symptoms in young adults with spina bifida. *Journal of Pediatric Psychology, 35*(7), 778–789. doi:10.1093/jpepsy/jsp094

Benzies, K. M., Trute, B., & Worthington, C. (2013). Maternal self-efficacy and family adjustment in households with children with serious disability. *Journal of Family Studies, 19*(1), 35–43. doi:10.5172/jfs.2013.19.1.35

Betz, C. L. (2007). Facilitating the transition of adolescents with developmental disabilities: Nursing practice issues and care. *Journal of Pediatric Nursing, 22*(2), 103–115. doi:10.1016/j.pedn.2006.07.006

Blissitt, P. A. (Ed.) (2011). Care of the Patient with Mild Traumatic Brain Injury: AANN and ARN Clinical Practice Guideline Series. Retrieved from http://www.rehabnurse.org/uploads/AANN14_MildTBI.pdf

Brand, M. C. (2006). Focus on the physical series: Part 1. Recognizing neonatal spinal cord injury. *Advances in Neonatal Care, 6*(1), 15–24. doi:10.1016/j.adnc.2005.11.001

Calhoun, C. L., Schottler, J., & Vogel, L. C. (2013). Recommendations for mobility in children with spinal cord injury. *Topics in Spinal Cord Injury Rehabilitation, 19*(2), 142–151. doi:10.1310/sci1902-142

Carter, M.A. (2011). The impact of the essentials of doctoral education for advanced nursing practice. *Clinical Scholars Review, 4*(2), 68–70. doi:10.1891/1939-2095.4.2.68

Centers for Disease Control and Prevention (CDC). (2011). Nonfatal traumatic brain injuries related to sports and recreation activities among persons aged ≤19 years—United States, 2001–2009. *Morbidity and Mortality Weekly Report, 60*(39), 1337–1342. Retrieved from http://www.cdc.gov/mmwr/preview/mmwrhtml/mm6039a1.htm

Centers for Disease Control and Prevention National Center for Injury Prevention and Control. (2010). 10 Leading Causes of Death by Age Group, United States –2010. Retrieved from http://www.cdc.gov/injury/wisqars/pdf/10LCID_All_Deaths_By_Age_Group_2010-a.pdf

Centers for Disease Control and Prevention National Center on Birth Defects and Developmental Disabilities (CDC PNCBDDD). (2011). Spina bifida: Data and statistics. Retrieved from http://www.cdc.gov/ncbddd/spinabifida/data.html

Centers for Disease Control and Prevention National Center on Birth Defects and Developmental Disabilities (CDC PNCBDDD). (2013a). Causes and risk factors of cerebral palsy. Retrieved from http://www.cdc.gov/ncbddd/cp/causes.html

Centers for Disease Control and Prevention National Center on Birth Defects and Developmental Disabilities (CDC PNCBDDD). (2013b). Facts about cerebral palsy. Retrieved from http://www.cdc.gov/ncbddd/cp/facts.html

Centers for Disease Control and Prevention National Center on Birth Defects and Developmental Disabilities (CDC PNCBDDD). (2014a). Facts about ASD. Retrieved from http://www.cdc.gov/ncbddd/autism/facts.html

Centers for Disease Control and Prevention National Center on Birth Defects and Developmental Disabilities (CDC PNCBDDD). (2014b). Facts about upper and lower limb reduction defects. Retrieved from http://www.cdc.gov/ncbddd/birthdefects/ul-limbreductiondefects.html

Centers for Disease Control and Prevention National Center on Birth Defects and Developmental Disabilities (CDC PNCBDDD). (2014c). Related conditions. Retrieved from http://www.cdc.gov/ncbddd/disabilityandhealth/relatedconditions.html

Chen, H. (2013). Arthrogryposis. Retrieved from http://emedicine.medscape.com/article/941917-overview

Chen, Y., Tang, Y., Vogel, L. C., & DeVivo, M. J. (2013). Causes of spinal cord injury. *Topics in Spinal Cord Injury Rehabilitation, 19*(1), 1–8. doi:10.1310/sci1901-1

Child and Adolescent Health Measurement Initiative. (2011). National Survey of Children with Special Health Care Needs 2009-2010 [Data query]. Retrieved from http://www.childhealthdata.org/browse/survey/results?q=1677&r=1

Child Welfare Information Gateway. (2011). About CAPTA: A legislative history. Washington, DC: U.S. Department of Health and Human Services, Children's Bureau. Retrieved from https://www.childwelfare.gov/pubPDFs/about.pdf

Clayton, D. B., & Brock, J. W. (2010). Congenital anomalies. The urologist's role in the management of spina bifida: A continuum of care. *Urology, 76*(1), 32–38. doi:10.1016/j.urology.2009.12.063

Cohen, L. L., Lemanek, K., Blount, R. L., Dahlquist, L. M., Lim, C. S., Palermo, T. M.,...Weiss, K. E. (2008). Evidence-based assessment of pediatric pain. *Journal of Pediatric Psychology, 33*(9), 939–955. doi:10.1093/jpepsy/jsm103

Crowe, L. M., Catroppa, C., Babl, F. E., & Anderson, V. (2013). Executive function outcomes of children with traumatic brain injury sustained before three years. *Child Neuropsychology: A Journal on Normal and Abnormal Development in Childhood and Adolescence, 19*(2), 113–126. doi:10.1080/09297049.2011.651079

Crowe, L. M., Catroppa, C., Babl, F. E., Rosenfeld, J. V., & Anderson, V. (2012). Timing of traumatic brain injury in childhood and intellectual outcome. *Journal of Pediatric Psychology, 37*(7), 745–754. doi:10.1093/jpepsy/jss070

Dabelea, D., Mayer-Davis, E. J., Saydah, S., Imperatore, G., Linder, B., Divers, J.,...Hamman, R. F. (2014). Prevalence of type 1 and type 2 diabetes among children and adolescents from 2001 to 2009. *JAMA: Journal of The American Medical Association, 311*(17), 1778–1786. doi:10.1001/jama.2014.3201

Dawodu, S. T. (2013). Traumatic Brain Injury (TBI)-Definition, epidemiology, pathophysiology. Retrieved from http://emedicine.medscape.com/article/326510-overview

de Jong, A., Baartmans, M., Bremer, M., van Komen, R., Middelkoop, E., Tuinebreijer, W., & van Loey, N. (2010). Reliability, validity and clinical utility of three types of pain behavioural observation scales for young children with burns aged 0-5 years. *Pain, 150*(3), 561–567. doi:10.1016/j.pain.2010.06.016

de Jong, I. G. M., Reinders-Messelink, H. A., Janssen, W. G. M., Poelma, M. J., van Wijk, I., & van der Sluis, C. K. (2012). Mixed feelings of children and adolescents with unilateral congenital below elbow deficiency: An online focus group study. *PLoS ONE, 7*(6), e37099. doi:10.1371/journal.pone.0037099

Deans, K. J., Minneci, P. C., Lowell, W., & Groner, J. I. (2013). Increased morbidity and mortality of traumatic brain injury in victims of nonaccidental trauma. *Journal of Trauma and Acute Care Surgery, 75*(1), 157–160. doi:10.1097/TA.0b013e3182984acb

Defendi, G. L. (2014). Genetics of Achondroplasia. Retrieved from http://emedicine.medscape.com/article/941280-overview

Earle, R. J., Rennick, J. E., Carnavale, F. A., & Davis, G. M. (2006). "It's okay, it helps me to breathe": The experience of home ventilation from a child's perspective. *Journal of Child Health Care, 10*(4), 270–282. doi:10.1177/1367493506067868

Ely, E., Chen-Lim, M. L., Zarnowsky, C., Green, R., Shaffer, S., & Holtzer, B. (2012). Finding the evidence to change practice for assessing pain in children who are cognitively impaired. *Journal of Pediatric Nursing, 27*(4), 402–410. doi:10.1016/j.pedn.2011.05.009

Engle, R. & Ellis, C. (2012). Pediatric stroke in the U.S.: Estimates from the kids' inpatient database. *Journal of Allied Health, 41*(3), e63–e67. Retrieved from http://www.ncbi.nlm.nih.gov/pubmed/22968778

Faul, M., Xu, L., Wald, M. M., & Coronado, V. G. (2010). Traumatic brain injury in the United States: Emergency department visits, hospitalizations and deaths 2002 –2006. Retrieved from http://www.cdc.gov/traumaticbraininjury/pdf/tbi_blue_book_age.pdf

Fay, T. B., Yeates, K. O., Wade, S. L., Drotar, D., Stancin, T., & Taylor, H. G. (2009). Predicting longitudinal patterns of functional deficits in children with traumatic brain injury. *Neuropsychology, 23*(3), 271–282. doi:10.1037/a0014936

Gaebler-Spira, D. & Lipschutz, R. D. (2010). Pediatric limb deficiencies. In M. A. Alexander & D. J. Matthews (Eds.), *Pediatric rehabilitation: Principles and practice* (pp. 335–360). Retrieved from http://www.ipmr.kmu.edu.pk/sites/ipmr.kmu.edu.pk/files/Pediatric%20Rehabilitation%20Principles%20and%20Practice%204ed%20Michael%20A.%20Alexander.pdf

Geyer, K., Meller, K., Kulpan, C., & Mowery, B. D. (2013). Traumatic brain injury in children: Acute care management. *Pediatric Nursing, 39*(6), 283–289. Retrieved from http://www.highbeam.com/doc/1G1-355307165.html

Gold, M. H., McGuire, M., Mustoe, T. A., Pusic, A., Sachdev, M., Waibel, J.,...International Advisory Panel on Scar Management (2014). Updated international clinical recommendations on scar management: Part 2—Algorithms for scar prevention and treatment. *Dermatologic Surgery, 40*(8), 825–831. doi:10.1111/dsu.0000000000000050

Golnik, A., Scal, P., Wey, A., & Gaillard, P. (2012). Autism-specific primary care medical home intervention. *Journal of Autism and Developmental Disorders, 42*(6), 1087–1093. doi:10.1007/s10803-011-1351-5

Gordon, M. D., Gottschlich, M. M., Helvig, E. I., Marvin, J. A., & Richard, R. L. (2004). Review of evidence-based practice for the prevention of pressure sores in burn patients. *Journal of Burn Care & Rehabilitation, 25*(5), 388–410. doi:10.1097/01.BCR.0000138289.83335.F4

Greef, A. P., Vansteenwegen, A., & Gillard, J. (2012). Resilience in families living with a child with a physical disability. *Rehabilitation Nursing, 37*(3), 95–159. doi:10.1002/RNJ.00018

Greenley, R. N. (2010). Health professional expectations for self-care skill development in youth with spina bifida. *Pediatric Nursing, 36*(2), 98–102.

Greenley, R. N., Coakley, R. M., Holmbeck, G. N., Jandasek, B., & Wills, K. (2006). Condition-related knowledge among children with spina bifida: Longitudinal changes and predictors. *Journal of Pediatric Psychology, 31*(8), 828–839. Retrieved from http://jpepsy.oxfordjournals.org/content/31/8/828.full.pdf+html

Gupta, S. K., Alassaf, N., Harrop, A. R., & Kiefer, G. N. (2012). Principles of rotationplasty. *Journal of the American Academy of Orthopaedic Surgeons, 20*(10), 657–667. doi:10.5435/JAAOS-20-10-657

Habich, M., Wilson, D., Thielk, D., Melles, G. L., Crumlett, H. S., Masterton, J., & McGuire, J. (2012). Evaluating the effectiveness of pediatric pain management guidelines. *Journal of Pediatric Nursing, 27*(4), 336–345. doi:10.1016/j.pedn.2011.06.002

Hadchouel, A., Durrmeyer, X., Bouzigon, E., Incitti, R., Huusko, J., Jarreau, P. H.,...Delacourt, C. (2011). Identification of SPOCK2 as a susceptibility gene for bronchopulmonary dysplasia. *American Journal of Respiratory and Critical Care Medicine, 184*(10), 1164–1170. doi:10.1164/rccm.201103-0548OC

Hagen, C. (1997). Assessment Scales, Rancho Los Amigos—Revised Levels Of Cognitive Functioning. Retrieved from http://www.kean.edu/~mshulman/documents/Rancho%20Los%20Amigos.pdf

Hamilton, L. J., Lerner, C. F., Presson, A. P., & Klitzner, T. S. (2013). Effects of a medical home program for children with special health care needs on parental perceptions of care in an ethnically diverse patient population. *Maternal and Child Health Journal, 17*(3), 463–469. doi:10.1007/s10995-012-1018-7

Hayes, D., Meadows, J. T., Murphy, B. S., Feola, D. J., Shook, L. A., & Ballard, H. O. (2011). Pulmonary function outcomes in bronchopulmonary dysplasia through childhood and into adulthood: Implications for primary care. *Primary Care Respiratory Journal, 20*(2), 128–133. doi:10.4104/pcrj.2011.00002

Henry J. Kaiser Family Foundation. (2013). Summary of the Affordable Care Act. Retrieved from http://kaiserfamilyfoundation.files.wordpress.com/2011/04/8061-021.pdf

Hewitt-Taylor, J. (2010). Supporting children with complex health needs. *Nursing Standard, 24*(19), 50–56. doi:10.7748/ns2010.01.24.19.50.c7448

Hewitt-Taylor, J. (2012). Planning the transition of children with complex needs from hospital to home. *Nursing Children & Young People, 24*(10), 28–35. doi:10.7748/ncyp2012.12.24.10.28.c9464

Horner, G. (2012). Medical evaluation for child physical abuse: What the PNP needs to know. *Journal of Pediatric Health Care, 26*(3), 163–170. doi:10.1016/j.pedhc.2011.10.001

Horsman, M., Suto, M., Dudgeon, B. & Harris, S. R. (2010). Growing older with cerebral palsy: Insiders' perspectives. *Pediatric Physical Therapy, 22*, 296–303. doi:10.1097/PEP.0b013e3181eabc0f

Institute for Patient- and Family-Centered Care. (2010). Frequently Asked Questions. Retrieved from http://www.ipfcc.org/faq.html

Jentink, J., Loane, M. A., Dolk, H., Barisic, I., Garne, E., Morris, J. K., & de Jong-van den Berg, L. T. W. (2010). Valproic acid monotherapy in pregnancy and major congenital malformations. *New England Journal of Medicine, 362*(23), 2185–2193. doi:10.1056/NEJMoa0907328

Jobe, A. H., & Bancalari, E. (2001). Bronchopulmonary dysplasia. *American Journal of Respiratory and Critical Care Medicine,163*(7),1723–1729. Retrieved from http://www.atsjournals.org/doi/pdf/10.1164/ajrccm.163.7.2011060

Johnson, A. R., DeMatt, E., & Salorio, C. F. (2009). Predictors of outcome following acquired brain injury in children. *Developmental Disabilities Research Reviews, 15*(2), 124–132. doi:10.1002/ddrr.63

Kair, L. R., Leonard, D. T., & Anderson, J. M. (2012). Bronchopulmonary dysplasia. *Pediatrics in Review, 33*(6), 255–264. doi:10.1542/pir.33-6-255

Klaas, S. J., Kelly, E. H., Anderson, C. J., & Vogel, L. C. (2014). Depression and anxiety in adolescents with pediatric-onset spinal cord injury. *Topics in Spinal Cord Injury Rehabilitation, 20*(1), 13–22. doi:10.1310/sci2001-13

Kochanek, P. M., Carney, N., Adelson, P. D., Ashwal, S., Bell, M. J., Bratton, S.,...Warden, C. R. (2012). Chapter 3: Indications for intracranial pressure monitoring. *Pediatric Critical Care Medicine, 13*(Suppl. 1), S11–S17. doi:10.1097/PCC.0b013e31823f440c

Krach, L. E., Gromly, M. E., & Ward, M. (2010). Traumatic brain injury. In M.A. Alexander & D. J. Matthews (Eds.), *Pediatric rehabilitation: Principles and practice* (pp. 231–260). Retrieved from http://www.ipmr.kmu.edu.pk/sites/ipmr.kmu.edu.pk/files/Pediatric%20Rehabilitation%20Principles%20and%20Practice%204ed%20Michael%20A.%20Alexander.pdf

Kramer, M. E., Suskauer, S. J., Christensen, J. R., DeMatt, E. J., Trovato, M. K., Salorio, C. F., & Slomine, B. S. (2013). Examining acute rehabilitation outcomes for children with total functional dependence after traumatic brain injury: A pilot study. *Journal of Head Trauma Rehabilitation, 28*(5), 361–370. doi:10.1097/HTR.0b013e31824da031

Kugelman, A. & Durand, M. (2011). A comprehensive approach to the prevention of bronchopulmonary dysplasia. *Pediatric Pulmonology, 46*(12), 1153–1165. doi:10.1002/ppul.21508

Lindley, L. C. & Mark, B. A. (2010). Children with special health care needs: Impact of health care expenditures on family financial burden. *Journal of Child and Family Studies, 19*(1), 79–89. doi:10.1007/s10826-009-9286-6

Litt, J. S., Taylor, H. G., Margevicius, S., Schluchter, M., Andreias, L., & Hack, M. (2012). Academic achievement of adolescents born with extremely low birth weight. *Acta Paediatrica, 101*(12), 1240–1245. doi:10.1111/j.1651-2227.2012.02790.x

Lucas, L. E. (2010). Psychosocial aspects of pediatric rehabilitation. In M. A. Alexander & D. J. Matthews (Eds.), *Pediatric rehabilitation: Principles and practice* (pp. 493–500). Retrieved from http://www.ipmr.kmu.edu.pk/sites/ipmr.kmu.edu.pk/files/Pediatric%20Rehabilitation%20Principles%20and%20Practice%204ed%20Michael%20A.%20Alexander.pdf

Martin, B. W, Dykes, E., & Lecky, F. E. (2004). Patterns and risks in spinal trauma. *Archives of Diseases in Childhood, 89*(9), 860–865. doi:10.1136/adc.2003.029223

Maryland Coalition for Inclusive Education. (n.d.). What is inclusive education? Retrieved from http://www.mcie.org/pages/about-inclusive-education/what-is-inclusive-education

Mason, D., Tobias, N., Lutkenhoff, M., Stoops, M., & Ferguson, D. (2004). The APN's guide to pediatric constipation management. *The Nurse Practitioner: American Journal of Primary Health Care, 29*(7), 13–15, 19–23. doi:10.1097/00006205-200407000-00003

Massagli, T. L. (2000). Medical and rehabilitation issues in care of children with spinal cord injury. *Physical Medicine and Rehabilitation of North America, 11*(1), 169–182.

Master, C. L., Gioia, G. A., Leddy, J. J., & Grady, M. F. (2012). Importance of "return-to-learn" in pediatric and adolescent concussion. *Pediatric Annals, 41*(9), 1–6. doi:10.3928/00904481-20120827-09

Mayes, T., Gottschlich, M., Scanlon, J., & Warden, G. D. (2003). Four-year review of burns as an etiologic factor in the development of long bone fractures in pediatric patients. *Journal of Burn Care & Rehabilitation, 24*, 279–284. doi:10.1097/01.BCR.0000085844.84144.E0

McGinnis, K. B., Vogel, L. C., McDonald, C. M., Porth, S., Hickey, K. J., Davis, M.,...Jenkins, D. (2004). Recognition and management of autonomic dysreflexia in pediatric spinal cord injury. *Journal of Spinal Cord Medicine, 27*(Suppl. 1), S61–S74.

McMorrow, A., & Sweet, D. G. (2013). Bronchopulmonary dysplasia in 2013. *Infant, 9*(3), 80–84.

McPherson, M., Arango, P., Fox, H., Lauver, C., McManus, M., Newacheck, P. W.,...Strickland, B. (1998). A new definition of children with special health care needs. *Pediatrics, 102*(1, Pt. 1), 137–140. doi:10.1542/peds.102.1.137

Mendes, M. A. (2013). Parents' descriptions of ideal home nursing care for their technology-dependent children. *Pediatric Nursing, 39*(2), 91–96.

Morgan, A. T. (2010). Dysphagia in childhood traumatic brain injury: A reflection on the evidence and its implications for practice. *Developmental Neurorehabilitation, 13*(3), 192–203. doi:10.3109/17518420903289535

Murphy, K. P., Wunderlich, C. A., Pico, E. L., Driscoll, S. W., Moberg-Wolff, E., Rak, M., & Nelson, M. R. (2010). Orthopedics and musculoskeletal conditions. In M. A. Alexander & D. J. Matthews (Eds.), *Pediatric rehabilitation: Principles and practice* (pp. 361–423). Retrieved from http://www.ipmr.kmu.edu.pk/sites/ipmr.kmu.edu.pk/files/Pediatric%20Rehabilitation%20Principles%20and%20Practice%204ed%20Michael%20A.%20Alexander.pdf

Muscular Dystrophy Association (MDA). (2009). Facts About Spinal Muscular Atrophy. Retrieved from http://mdausa.org/sites/default/files/publications/Facts_SMA_P-181.pdf

Muscular Dystrophy Association (MDA). (n.d.). Muscle Diseases. Retrieved from www.mda.org/disease

National Institute of Neurological Disorders and Stroke (NINDS). (2011). Arteriovenous Malformations and Other Vascular Lesions of the Central Nervous System Fact Sheet. Retrieved from http://www.ninds.nih.gov/disorders/avms/detail_avms.htm

National Institute of Neurological Disorders and Stroke (NINDS). (2012). Spinal Muscular Atrophy Fact Sheet. Retrieved from www.ninds.nih.gov/disorders/sma/detail_sma.htm

National Institute of Neurological Disorders and Stroke (NINDS). (2013). Spina Bifida Fact Sheet. Retrieved from http://www.ninds.nih.gov/disorders/spina_bifida/detail_spina_bifida.htm

National Institute of Neurological Disorders and Stroke (NINDS). (2014a). NINDS Cerebral Hypoxia Information Page. Retrieved from http://www.ninds.nih.gov/disorders/anoxia/anoxia.htm

National Institute of Neurological Disorders and Stroke (NINDS). (2014b). NINDS Leukodystrophy Information Page. Retrieved from www.ninds.nih.gov/disorders/leukodystrophy/leukodystrophy.htm

National Institute of Neurological Disorders and Stroke (NINDS). (2014c). Transverse Myelitis Fact Sheet. Retrieved from http://www.ninds.nih.gov/disorders/transversemyelitis/detail_transversemyelitis.htm

National Institutes of Health National Heart Lung and Blood Institute. (2012). What Is Bronchopulmonary Dysplasia? Retrieved from http://www.nhlbi.nih.gov/health/health-topics/topics/bpd/

Nelson, V. S. & Hornyak, J. E. (2010). Spinal cord injuries. In M. A. Alexander & D. J. Matthews (Eds.), *Pediatric rehabilitation: Principles and practice* (pp. 261–276). Retrieved from http://www.ipmr.kmu.edu.pk/sites/ipmr.kmu.edu.pk/files/Pediatric%20Rehabilitation%20Principles%20and%20Practice%204ed%20Michael%20A.%20Alexander.pdf

Oddson, B. E., Clancy, C. A., & McGrath, P. J. (2006). The role of pain in reduced quality of life and depressive symptomology in children with spina bifida. *Clinical Journal of Pain, 22*(9), 784–789. doi:10.1097/01.ajp.0000210929.43192.5d

Osorio, M., Reyes, M. R., & Massagli, T. L. (2014). Pediatric spinal cord injury. *Current Physical Medicine and Rehabilitation Reports, 2*(3), 158-168. doi: 10.1007/s40141-014-0054-1

Osteogenesis Imperfecta Foundation. (n.d.). Facts About Osteogenesis Imperfecta. Retrieved http://www.oif.org/site/PageServer?pagename=AOI_Facts

Parent, S., Mac-Thiong, J. M., Roy-Beaudry, M., Sosa, J. F., & Labelle, H. (2011). Spinal cord injury in the pediatric population: A systematic review of the literature. *Journal of Neurotrauma, 28*(8), 1515–1524. doi:10.1089/neu.2009.1153Parmigiani, S., Pezzoni, S., Solari, E., Arena, V., De Martino, A., Allessandrini, C.,...Bevilacqua, G. (2009). Palivizumab for prophylaxis of RSV infection: Five epidemic seasons' experience on adverse effects (2002–2007). *Journal of Perinatal Medicine, 37*(3), 304–305. doi:10.1515/JPM.2009.079

Passaretti, D., & Billmire, D. A. (2003). Management of pediatric burns. *Journal of Craniofacial Surgery, 14*(5), 713–718. doi:10.1097/00001665-200309000-00021

Pereira, C. T., Murphy, K. D., & Herndon, D. N. (2005). Altering metabolism. *Journal of Burn Care & Rehabilitation, 26*(3), 194–199.

Peterson-Carmichael, S. L., & Cheifetz, I. M. (2012). The chronically critically ill patient: Pediatric considerations. *Respiratory Care, 57*(6), 993–1002. doi:10.4187/respcare.01738

Pico, E. L., Wilson, P. E., & Haas, R. (2010). Spina bifida. In M. A. Alexander & D. J. Matthews (Eds.), *Pediatric rehabilitation: Principles and practice* (pp. 199–230). Retrieved from http://www.ipmr.kmu.edu.pk/sites/ipmr.kmu.edu.pk/files/Pediatric%20Rehabilitation%20Principles%20and%20Practice%204ed%20Michael%20A.%20Alexander.pdf

Pidcock, F. S., Fauerbach, J. A., Ober, M., & Carney, J. (2003). The rehabilitation/school matrix: A model for accommodating the noncompliant child with severe burns. *Journal of Burn Care & Rehabilitation, 24*(5), 342–346. doi:10.1097/01.BCR.0000075848.03433.E9

Poggi, G., Liscio, M., Galbiati, S., Adduci, A., Massimino, M., Gandola, L.,...Castelli, E. (2005). Brain tumors in children and adolescents: Cognitive and psychological disorders at different ages. Psycho-Oncology, 14(5), 388–395. doi:10.1002/pon.855

Pollart, S. M., Warniment, C., & Mori, T. (2009). *Latex allergy. American Family Physician, 80*(12), 1413–1420. Retrieved from http://www.aafp.org/afp/2009/1215/p1413.html

Poon, C. Y., Edwards, M. O., & Kotecha, S. (2013). Long term cardiovascular consequences of chronic lung disease of prematurity. *Paediatric Respiratory Reviews, 14*(4), 242–249. doi:10.1016/j.prrv.2012.08.003

Przkora, R., Barrow, R. E., Jeschke, M. G., Suman, O. E., Celis, M., Sanford, A. P.,...Herndon, D. N. (2006). Body composition changes with time in pediatric burn patients. *Journal of Trauma Injury, Infections and Critical Care, 60*(5), 968–971. doi:10.1097/01.ta.0000214580.27501.19

Rimmer, J. H., Yamaki, K., Lowry, B. M., Wang, E., & Vogel, L. C. (2010). Obesity and obesity-related secondary conditions in adolescents with intellectual/developmental disabilities. *Journal of Intellectual Disability Research, 54*(Pt. 9), 787–794. doi:10.1111/j.1365-2788.2010.01305.x

Sawin, K. J., & Thompson, N. M. (2009). The experience of finding an effective bowel management program for children with spina bifida: The parent's perspective. *Journal of Pediatric Nursing, 24*(4), 280–291. doi:10.1016/j.pedn.2008.03.008

Selekman, J., & Vessey, J. A. (2010). School and the child with a chronic condition. In P. J. Allan, J. A. Vessey, & N. A. Schapiro (Eds.), *Primary care of the child with a chronic condition* (5th ed., pp. 42–59). St. Louis: Mosby/Elsevier.

Shapiro, J. R., & Sponsellor, P. D. (2009). Osteogenesis imperfecta: Questions and answers. *Current Opinion in Pediatrics, 21*(6), 709–716. doi:10.1097/MOP.0b013e328332c68f

Shavelle, R., Strauss, D., & Brooks, J. (2013). Discrepancies in the estimates of life expectancy after SCI. *Spinal Cord, 51*(12), 937. doi:10.1038/sc.2013.93

Smith, C. (2014). Increasing awareness of Legg-Calve-Perthes disease. *British Journal of School Nursing, 9*(1), 21–23. doi:10.12968/bjsn.2014.9.1.21

Smith, D. G. (2006). Congenital limb deficiencies and acquired amputation in childhood: Part 1. In Motion, 16(1). Retrieved from http://www.amputee-coalition.org/inmotion/jan_feb_06/congenital_limb_part1.html

Snodgrass, W. T., & Gargollo, P. C. (2010). Urologic care of the neurogenic bladder in children. *Urologic Clinics of North America, 37*(2), 207–214. doi:10.1016/j.ucl.2010.03.004

Sparacino, P. S., & Cartwright, C. C. (2009). The clinical nurse specialist. In A. B. Hamric, J. A. Spross, & C. M. Hanson (Eds.), *Advanced practice nursing: An integrative approach* (4th ed., pp. 349–374). St. Louis: Saunders.

Spina Bifida Association of America. (n.d.). Symptomatic Chiari Malformation Health Info Sheet. Retrieved from http://www.spinabifidaassociation.org/site/c.evKRI7OXIoJ8H/b.8031517/apps/s/content.asp?ct=12072853

Spina Bifida Association of America. (n.d.). What Is Spina Bifida? Retrieved from http://www.spinabifidaassociation.org/site/c.evKRI7OXIoJ8H/b.8277225/k.5A79/What_is_Spina_Bifida.htm

Sullivan-Bolyai, S., Knafl, K. A., Sadler, L., & Gilliss, C. L. (2004). Great expectations: A position description for parents as caregivers: Part II. *Pediatric Nursing, 30*(1), 52–56.

Suman, O. E., Mlcak, R. P., & Herndon, D. N. (2002). Effect of exercise training on pulmonary function in children with thermal injury. *Journal of Burn Care & Rehabilitation, 23*(4), 288–293. doi:10.1097/00004630-200207000-00013

Thrall, R. S., Blumberg, J. H., Beck, S., Bourgoin, M. D., Votto, J. J., & Barton, R. W. (2012). Beyond the medical home: Special Care Family Academy for children and youth. *Pediatric Nursing, 38*(6), 331–335.

Toly, V. B., Musil, C. M. & Carl, J. C. (2012). Families with children who are technology dependent: Normalization and family functioning. *Western Journal of Nursing Research, 34*(1), 52–71. doi:10.1177/0193945910389623

U.S. Congress, Office of Technology Assessment. (1987). Technology-Dependent Children: Hospital v. Home Care—A Technical Memorandum (Report No. OTA-TM-H-38). Retrieved from http://www.princeton.edu/~ota/disk2/1987/8728/8728.PDF

U.S. Department of Education. (n.d.a). Early Intervention Program for Infants and Toddlers with Disabilities. Retrieved from http://www2.ed.gov/programs/osepeip/index.html

U.S. Department of Education. (n.d.b). Office of Special Education Programs' (OSEP's) IDEA home page. Retrieved from http://idea.ed.gov/explore/home

U.S. Department of Health and Human Services (U.S. DHHS). (2008). 2008 Physical activity guidelines for Americans. Retrieved from http://www.health.gov/paguidelines/guidelines/

U.S. Department of Health and Human Services (U.S. DHHS). (n.d.a). Healthy People 2020: Disability and Health: Overview. Retrieved from http://www.healthypeople.gov/2020/topics-objectives/topic/disability-and-health

U.S. Department of Health and Human Services (U.S. DHHS). (n.d.b). Maternal and Child Health Bureau: About Us. Retrieved from http://mchb.hrsa.gov/about/index.html

Vargo, M. M., Riutta, J. C., & Franklin, D. J. (2010). Rehabilitation for patients with cancer diagnosis. In W. R. Frontera (Ed.), *DeLisa's physical medicine and rehabilitation: Principles and practice* (5th ed., pp. 1151–1178), Philadelphia: Lippincott Williams & Wilkins.

Vasluian, E., de Jong. I. G. M., Janssen, W. G. M., Poelma, M. J., van Wijk, I., Reinders-Messelink, H. A., & van der Sluis, C. K. (2013). Opinions of youngsters with congenital below-elbow deficiency, and those of their parents and professionals concerning prosthetic use and rehabilitation treatment. *PLoS ONE, 8*(6), e67101. doi:10.1371/journal.pone.0067101

Vehmeyer-Heeman, M., Lommers, B., Van den Kerckhove, E., & Boeckx, W. (2005). Axillary burns: Extended grafting and early splinting prevents contractures. *Journal of Burn Care & Rehabilitation, 26*(6), 539–542. doi:10.1097/01.bcr.0000185403.24519.ca

Verhoef, M., Barf, H. A., Post, M. W. M., van Asbeck, F. W. A., Gooskens, R. H. J. M., & Prevo, A. J. H. (2006). Functional independence among young adults with spina bifida in relation to hydrocephalus and level of lesion. *Developmental Medicine & Child Neurology, 48*(2), 114–119. doi:10.1017/S0012162206000259

Vidal, P. G., Goodman, A. M., Colin, A., Leddy, J. J., & Grady, M. F. (2012). Rehabilitation strategies for prolonged recovery in pediatric and adolescent concussion. *Pediatric Annals, 41*(9), 1–7. doi:10.3928/00904481-20120827-10

Vinck, A., Maassen, B., Mullaart, R., & Rotteveel, J. (2006). Arnold-Chiari II malformation and cognitive functioning in spina bifida. *Journal of Neurology, Neurosurgery & Psychiatry, 77*(9), 1083–1086. doi:10.1136/jnnp.2005.075887

Vogel, L. C., Hickey, K. J., Klaas, S. J., & Anderson, C. J. (2004). Unique issues in pediatric spinal cord injury. *Orthopedic Nursing, 23*(5), 300–308. doi:10.1097/00006416-200409000-00004

Walco, G. A., Dworkin, R. H., Krane, E. J., LeBel, A. A., & Treede, R. D. (2010). Neuropathic pain in children: Special considerations. *Mayo Clinic Proceedings, 85*(Suppl. 3), S33–S41. doi:10.4065/mcp.2009.0647

Walsh, N. E., Bosker, G. & Santa Maria, D. (2010). Upper and lower extremity prosthetics. In W. R. Frontera (Ed.), *DeLisa's physical medicine and rehabilitation: Principles and practice* (5th ed., pp. 2017–2050). Philadelphia: Lippincott Williams & Wilkins.

Weed, R. O., & Berens, D. E. (2005). Basics of burn injury: Implication for case management and life care planning. *Lippincott's Case Management, 10*(1), 22–29. doi:10.1097/00129234-200501000-00004

White, P. H., & Hackett, P. (2009). On the threshold to the adult medical home: Care coordination in transition. *Pediatric Annals, 38*(9), 513–520. doi:10.3928/00904481-20090820-11

Wilson, V. (2013). Type 2 diabetes: An epidemic in children. *Nursing Children and Young People, 25*(2), 14–17. doi:10.7748/ncyp2013.03.25.2.14.e136

Yildiz, C. & Demirkale, I. (2014). Hip problems in cerebral palsy: Screening, diagnosis and treatment. *Current Opinion in Pediatrics, 26*(1), 85–92. doi:10.1097/MOP.0000000000000040

Suggested Resources

Amputee Coalition of America: http://www.amputee-coalition.org/

Autism: http://www.autismspeaks.org/

Brain Injury Association of America: http://www.biausa.org/brain-injury-children.htm

Center for Parent Information and Resources (legacy NICHCY resources): http://www.parentcenterhub.org/resources/

Disabled Sports USA: http://www.disabledsportsusa.org/

Families of Spinal Muscle Atrophy: www.fsma.org.

Got Transition/Center for Health Care Transition: http://www.gottransition.org/

I-Can International Child Amputee Network: http://child-amputee.net/

Institute for Patient-and Family-Centered Care: http://www.ipfcc.org/

Muscular Dystrophy Association: http://mda.org/

National Amputation Foundation: http://www.nationalamputation.org/

National Ataxia Foundation: http://www.ataxia.org/

National Center for Injury Prevention and Control: http://www.cdc.gov/injury/index.html

National Center for Medical Home Implementation: http://medicalhomeinfo.org/

National Center for Learning Disabilities: http://www.ncld.org/

National Center on Birth Defects and Developmental Disabilities: http://www.cdc.gov/ncbddd/index.html

National Institute of Neurological Disorders and Stroke: http://www.ninds.nih.gov/

The National Spinal Cord Injury Association Pediatric Spinal Cord Injury and Disease Page: http://www.spinalcord.org/resource-center/askus/index.php?pg=kb.book&id=23

National Sports Center for Disabled: http://www.nscd.org/

New England Disabled Sports: http://nedisabledsports.org/default.aspx

Office of Special Education and Rehabilitative Services: http://www2.ed.gov/about/offices/list/osers/index.html

Spina Bifida Association: http://www.spinabifidaassociation.org/site/c.evKRI7OXIoJ8H/b.8028963/k.BE67/Home.htm

United Cerebral Palsy: http://ucp.org/

Chapter 16

Gerontological Rehabilitation Nursing

Kristen L. Mauk, PhD DNP RN CRRN GCNS-BC GNP-BC FAAN
Maria Radwanski, MSN RN CRRN

LEARNING OUTCOMES

- Review the normal aging process.
- Identify rehabilitation nursing interventions for those with common congenital disabilities.
- Recognize standards of rehabilitation nursing practice in the care of older adults with acquired disability.
- Discuss the impact of major geriatric syndromes on the rehabilitation process.

KEY CHAPTER TOPICS

- Aging
- Gerontological rehabilitation nursing
- Lifespan
- Normal aging
- Acquired disability

PROFESSIONAL REHABILITATION NURSING DOMAINS AND COMPETENCIES

- Domain 1: Competencies 1.2, 1.3, 1.4
- Domain 2: Competencies 2.1, 2.2
- Domain 4: Competency 4.2 (Association of Rehabilitation Nurses [ARN], 2014)

Introduction

The rapid growth in the older adult population is beginning to have a major impact on the healthcare delivery system. Currently, one in every eight Americans is older than 65 years of age. The population age 65 years and older accounted for 41.4 million people in 2011 (Administration on Aging, U.S. Department of Health and Human Services, 2012). Experts predict this number will increase to 55 million by 2020 (a 36% increase for that decade) (Greenberg, 2009); this increase reflects the aging of the Baby Boomer generation and increases in life expectancy. The oldest old, those older than 85 years, are the fastest-growing age group in the country. As a person's age increases, so does the likelihood of chronic illness and functional limitations. In light of these statistics, rehabilitation nurses must be prepared to meet the demands of an aging society. They can do so only through special knowledge and training in gerontology and rehabilitation.

I. Theories of Aging

A. Biological (Lange & Grossman, 2014)

1. Genes or biological clock: Each person has a genetic program that helps predetermine life expectancy.
2. Wear and tear: The length of life is inversely related to the rate of living (i.e., the more wear and tear placed on the body, the faster one ages).
3. Lipofuscin and connective tissue: This lipoprotein byproduct of metabolism increases with age, resulting in visible signs of aging.
4. Free radicals: Unstable molecules damage cells, causing injury and signs of aging. Examples include tobacco smoke, herbicides and pesticides, radiation, and ozone.
5. Stress: Aging is related to or influenced by life stress.
6. Orgel's hypothesis: Errors in protein synthesis occur with aging, causing genes to mutate.
7. Autoimmune or immunological: The body perceives old, irregular cells as hostile agents and begins to attack itself; the immune system becomes less effective with age.
8. Nutritional: Length of life and age-related changes can be either positively or negatively influenced by nutritional intake.
9. Environmental: Pollutants in one's surroundings, such as air and noise pollution

or radiation, adversely affect health and cause signs of aging.

B. Psychological
  1. Human needs (Maslow, 1954)
    a. Hierarchy of five basic needs that motivate human behavior
      1) Physiologic
      2) Safety and security
      3) Love and belonging
      4) Self-esteem
      5) Self-actualization
    b. Failure in self-growth may lead to feelings of failure and depression (Lange & Grossman, 2014).
  2. Individualism (Jung, 1960)
    a. Lifespan view of development versus need attainment
    b. Older adults engage in an inner search to evaluate their lives.
    c. Successful aging includes accepting the past and coping positively with changes.
  3. Lifespan development paradigm (Buhler, 1933)
    a. Life occurs in stages.
    b. Life satisfaction is related to goal achievement.
    c. Successful adaptation to changes in life may include a reevaluation of the older person's beliefs relative to societal expectations.
  4. Selective optimization with compensation (Baltes, 1987)
    a. Emerged from Buhler's work
    b. Successful aging comes from learning to cope with losses of aging through choices.
    c. Selective optimization with compensation suggests that as people age they choose activities and roles that provide the most satisfaction, which facilitates successful aging (Baltes & Baltes, 1990).

C. Sociological
  1. Activity theory: Older adults should remain active, occupied, and contributing to society to age positively and avoid the negative effects of advanced age (Havighurst, Neugarten, & Tobin, 1963).
    a. Research has shown a direct relationship between life satisfaction and activity in older adults (Lemon, Bengston, & Peterson, 1972).
    b. Informal activities such as gathering with friends, having hobbies, and engaging in group activities provide more life satisfaction than solitary activities, and meaningful activities have also been correlated with successful aging and life satisfaction (Harlow & Cantor, 1996; Schroots, 1996; Vaillant, 2002).
  2. Disengagement: Society and older adults mutually withdraw from one another as one ages; disengagement is thought to maintain social equilibrium (Cumming & Henry, 1961).
    a. This theory has been and continues to be challenged by numerous studies that support activity theory.
    b. The Harvard Aging Study, which followed three cohorts of more than 800 people each for more than 50 years, provides evidence that happiness in later life is more related to individual lifestyle choices than genetics, wealth, race, or other largely uncontrollable factors (Vaillant, 2002), raising questions about the validity of disengagement theory.
  3. Continuity: Older adults continue with the same personality and behavior patterns they developed throughout their lives (Havighurst, Neugarten, & Tobin, 1968). There are four personality types of older adults:
    a. *Integrated*: Well adjusted, actively engaged
    b. *Armored/defended*: Continue activities and roles from middle age
    c. *Passive/dependent*: Uninterested or dependent on others
    d. *Unintegrated*: Fails to cope successfully with aging
    e. A study by Agahi, Ahacic, and Parker (2006) showed that active participation tends to decline over time and that previous life patterns predict involvement in activities in later life.
  4. Gerotranscendence: Older adults move toward oneness with the universe by maintaining close relationships, accepting impending death, and remaining connected with people of other generations (Tornstam, 1994).
    a. Three main elements
      1) The cosmic level (Tornstam, 2011)
      2) The self
      3) Social and individual relations
    b. A study investigating whether staff could recognize signs of gerotranscendence revealed that an interpretive framework for use in settings such as nursing homes would be of assistance in acceptance of these behaviors as a normal part of aging (Wadensten & Carlsson, 2001).

II. Review of Normal Aging

A. Cardiac and Circulatory System
  1. Decreased cardiac output
  2. Valvular changes that may result in stenosis (Pugh & Wei, 2001) or heart murmurs (Jett, 2008)
  3. Decreased ability to adapt to increased demands

4. Age-associated changes across time may vary between individuals (Heineman, Hamrick-King, & Scaglione Sewell, 2014).
5. Increased incidence of varicose veins
6. Increased thickness of heart and arterial walls (Ferrari, Radaelli, & Centola, 2003)
7. Elevated systolic blood pressure (Heineman et al., 2014)
8. Electrophysiological dysfunction increases with age (Soares-Miranda et al., 2014).
9. Normal changes in an electrocardiogram include slightly elevated PR, QRS, and Q–T intervals (Jett, 2008).

B. Respiratory System
1. Decreased elasticity of the lungs
2. Impaired gas exchange over time, caused by a loss of elasticity and decreased surface area of alveoli
3. Increased carbon dioxide retention, caused by a less efficient system
4. Less useful oxygen with each breath
5. Reduced pulmonary functional reserve (Smith & Cotter, 2012), reduced vital capacity but no change in total lung capacity (Krauss Whitbourne, 2002)
6. Decreased blood oxygen level
7. Diminished ciliary and macrophage activity (Smith & Cotter, 2012)
8. Drier mucus membranes (Smith & Cotter, 2012)
9. Decreased cough reflex (Smith & Cotter, 2012).

C. Musculoskeletal System
1. Decreased muscle mass, sarcopenia, and related loss of muscle strength (Benton, Whyte, & Dyal, 2011)
2. Changes in range of motion in joints (Monda, Goldberg, Smitham, Thornton, & McCarthy, 2013).
3. Untreated postmenopausal osteoporosis increases risk for fragility fractures (Cohen-Mansfield, Thein, Marx, & Dakheel-Ali, 2014) and decreased overall height caused by compression of vertebrae over time (Smith & Cotter, 2012)
4. Decreased bone density, leading to increased risk for fractures (Smith & Cotter, 2012).
5. Decreased cartilage surface of joints, leading to possible limitations in range of motion (Antonelli & Starz, 2012)

D. Genitourinary System
1. In women
   a. Decreased estrogen with perimenopause and menopause (Hall, 2004)
   b. Average age for menopause, defined as occurring 1 year after the final menstrual period, is about 51 years (Hall, 2007)
   c. Ovaries atrophy, vagina shortens and narrows, uterus decreases in size, and supporting ligaments weaken (Digiovanna, 2000)
   d. Decreased vaginal lubrication, often leading to pain during sexual intercourse
   e. Stress incontinence (common but treatable)
   f. Other types of incontinence (common but not a normal part of aging)
2. In men
   a. Testes decrease in size and weight, penis shows fibrous changes in erectile tissues by age 55 or 60 years (Digiovanna, 2000).
   b. No significant changes in sexual libido or previous patterns of behavior
   c. Longer refractory times during phases of sexual intercourse
   d. Fewer complete erections and less frequent orgasms
   e. Enlarged prostate, resulting in clinical benign prostatic hyperplasia in 13% of men by age 60 years and 23% by age 85 years (Hafez & Hafez, 2004; Smith & Cotter, 2012)
3. In both men and women
   a. Decreased bladder capacity, caused by bladder shrinkage and changes in capacity and contractility (Digiovanna, 2000; Smith & Cotter, 2012)
   b. Increase in urinary frequency and nocturia (Asplund, 2004), which can affect sleep quality
   c. Decreased kidney mass, blood flow, and glomerular filtration rate (Smith & Cotter, 2012)

E. Neurological System (Heineman, Hamrick-King, & Scaglione Sewell, 2014)
1. Brain decreases in size and weight
2. Loss of 10% of functioning neurons over lifespan in both genders, but neuron loss may be less than previously thought (Peters, 2002)
3. Cognition
   a. Some memory loss is common but should be distinguished from abnormalities such as those that occur with Alzheimer's disease.
   b. Intelligence and ability to learn are not affected (Wilson et al., 2013).
4. Proprioception (awareness of body position in space) may decrease with age, which can result in less coordination and balance, leading to falls.
5. Slower voluntary reflexes (Smith & Cotter, 2012)
6. Deep tendon reflexes still responsive
7. More difficulty responding to multiple stimuli
8. Decreased kinesthetic sense
9. Complaints of feeling tired (even if staying in bed longer) caused by sleep pattern changes such as a decrease in stage IV, rapid eye movement sleep

10. Decreased dopamine levels, which may contribute to Parkinsonian features such as abnormal gait
11. Spinal cord cells begin to decline around age 60 years (Beers & Berkow, n.d.), and the spine may narrow, causing pressure on the spinal cord that over time can cause changes in sensation.

F. Sensory System
1. Vision
   a. Presbyopia: Farsightedness or trouble focusing on near objects, caused by age-related changes in the shape of the eye that begin around age 40 years (Digiovanna, 2000) and is considered a normal change in aging (Cacchione, 2014).
   b. Decreased peripheral vision
   c. The most common age-related eye diseases are cataracts (extremely common but highly treatable with surgery and intraocular lens implants), glaucoma, macular degeneration, and diabetic retinopathy (Jackson & Owsley, 2003).
   d. Decreased tear production, which increases susceptibility to infections
   e. Changes in depth perception
2. Hearing
   a. Presbycusis: Most common sensory deficit in older adults (Adams-Wendling, Pimple, Adams, & Titler, 2008)
   b. Decrease in hearing acuity, especially the ability to detect high-frequency tones and discern speech (Rees, Duckert, & Carey, 1999)
   c. Impacted wax: Hair fibers in ear canal less able to help with earwax removal and protect canal (NICHE, 2012a)
   d. Need for hearing aids, which may amplify extraneous noises
   e. Eardrum thickens (NICHE, 2012a)
3. Smell: General decrease in acuity (Seiberling & Conley, 2004)
4. Taste: Atrophied taste buds, slight decrease in taste around age 60 years, and more exaggerated past age 70 years (Seiberling & Conley, 2004)
5. Touch: Decreased ability to distinguish sensations and textures (Digiovanna, 2000)
6. Pain
   a. Pain in the absence of disease is not a normal part of aging (Hanks-Bell, Halvey, Paice, 2004).
   b. Increased tolerance for pain
   c. General decreased sensitivity to light touch
   d. Increased pain threshold

G. Endocrine System
1. Changes in sex hormones
2. Decreased efficiency of the entire system
3. Changes in thyroid hormone production and glucose tolerance, which may warrant treatment (e.g., thyroid changes may lower the metabolic rate)

H. Hematological System
1. Anemia is common in 8%–44% of older adults (Hardin, 2010; Nilsson-Ehle, Jagenburg, Landahl, & Svanborg, 2000), particularly iron deficiency and pernicious types.
2. Hypoalbuminemia
   a. Serum albumin has been shown to predict geriatric rehabilitation outcomes (Aptaker, Roth, Reichhardt, Duerden, & Levy, 1994).
   b. Albumin less than 3.5 g/dL may place a person at risk for poor outcomes, including pressure ulcers (Aptaker et al., 1994).

I. Immune System
1. Generally less efficient; immunosenescence is the aging of the immune system.
2. Less effective T cells
3. Possibly less resistant to infections
4. Possible absence of typical symptoms of illness (e.g., elevated temperature with pneumonia)

J. Integumentary System
1. Skin (Heineman et al., 2014)
   a. Becomes more wrinkled, thinner
   b. Loses elasticity
   c. Is dry, which may lead to itching
   d. Has greater potential for tears and bruising
   e. Decreased number of sweat glands, which may lead to impaired thermoregulation
2. Hair
   a. Pigment loss, resulting in gray or white hair
   b. Development of facial hair (in women)
   c. Thinning, balding (in men)
3. Nails: More brittle, changes in color and texture
4. Fat: Distributed more on the trunk and less on the arms and legs

K. Gastrointestinal System: Intestinal problems are common among older adults (McKay, Fravel, & Scanlon, 2012; Heineman et al., 2014).
1. Slowed absorption in intestines
2. Decreased digestive enzymes
3. Decreased saliva production
4. Decreased esophageal and intestinal peristalsis
5. Constipation
6. Weaker gag reflex or delayed swallowing, which can increase the risk of aspiration
7. Impaired sensation to defecate (NICHE, 2012a)
8. Loss of rectal elasticity and thicker anal sphincter (NICHE, 2012a)
9. Atrophy of protective mucosa (NICHE, 2012a)
10. Weakening of large intestinal wall (NICHE, 2012a)

L. Renal System
1. The kidneys shrink, with a potential loss of up to half of functioning nephrons (Minaker, 2004).
2. Decreased glomerular filtration rate, related in part to changes in blood flow (Digiovanna, 2000)
3. There is less effective filtration of wastes, which may allow medications to stay in the body longer and increase the risk of side effects.

III. Aging and Disability: Acquiring a Disability at an Advanced Age

There are two distinct ways in which disability can affect older adults: acquiring a disability at an advanced age and aging with an early-onset disability. The effects of age and aging can differ in each case.

A. Factors Affecting Rehabilitation Potential
1. Age
   a. Scivoletto, Morganti, Ditunno, Ditunno, and Molinari (2003) found that adults older than age 50 years with new spinal cord injury (SCI) have less favorable outcomes than younger people with the same injuries in regard to walking and bladder and bowel independence and tend to have more associated medical problems.
   b. Bagg, Pombo, and Hopman (2002) reported that the Functional Independence Measure (FIM™) score at admission is a better predictor than FIM™ score at discharge in older adults with stroke and recommended that age not be a factor in the decision to admit a client to rehabilitation.
   c. Yu (2005) found that an age of 80 years or older and admission function affected functional gains and rehabilitation efficiency in an outpatient rehabilitation program.
2. Frailty
   a. One definition of *frailty* is unintentional weight loss, exhaustion, low energy expenditure, slow walking speed, and weakness in the older adult (Fried, Ferrucci, Darer, Williamson, & Anderson, 2004).
   b. Another research-based definition of *frailty* is an accumulation of deficits, which include symptoms, signs, diseases, and disabilities. The more deficits, the more frail (Rockwood, Mitniski, Song, Steen, & Skoog, 2006).
   c. Overall, frailty is the outcome of declines at the molecular, cellular, and physiologic system levels (Bandeen-Roche et al., 2006).
   d. Frailty involves "visible changes such as weight loss, decreased physical activity, fatigue, weakness, and impaired mobility, as well as the accumulation of health conditions and deficits" (Nelson, 2014, pp. 226–227).
   e. Frail older adults are at higher risk for morbidity, disability, and mortality. Between 10% and 25% of people age 65 years and older are considered frail (Ostir, Ottenbacher, & Markides, 2004).
   f. Positive psychological factors, including positive affect, reduce the risk of frailty (Ostir et al., 2004).
   g. Frailty is associated with increased risk of hospitalization, poor outcomes, and decreased lifespan (U.S. Preventive Services Task Force [USPSTF], 2012).
3. Effects of normal aging: Reductions in endurance, strength, and function affect the speed of and potential for recovery.
   a. Exercise tolerance: Pulmonary, cardiac, and muscle effects of aging affect exercise tolerance.
   b. Strength is reduced by a decrease in muscle mass and endurance.
   c. Balance is affected by comorbidities and the side effects of multiple medications.
   d. Mobility is changed by vision impairments, side effects of medications, weight changes, unsteady gait, foot problems.
4. Effects of chronic diseases: Chronic disease significantly compromises physical function and adversely affects the rehabilitation potential of the client after injury or trauma. In addition to the knowledge about the disease, an understanding of the client's functional expectations is essential during restorative management because rehabilitation depends on active participation in the program.
   a. Diabetes
      1) Glucose control: Poor glycemic control leads to deficits in cognitive function (memory and processing) and increases the risk of vascular disease (Awad, Gagnon, & Messier, 2004).
      2) Peripheral neuropathy reduces sensations, increases risk of falls and injury, and also alters mobility if there are foot problems.
      3) Gastroparesis
      4) Blurred vision is common in clients with poor glycemic control. Glaucoma, blindness, and retinopathy are also noted. They can pose an extra challenge to rehabilitation efforts.

5) Skin changes at the cellular level increase the risk of infection and lead to poor healing.
6) Vascular disease: Loss of elasticity and hardening of arteries, risk of neuropathy
7) Amputation after injury of lower extremities: More than 60% of nontraumatic amputation occurs in clients with diabetes (Centers for Disease Control and Prevention [CDC], 2011).

b. Heart disease: Severity of disease and comorbidity reduce the potential for rehabilitation.
1) Exercise tolerance is reduced.
2) Ejection fraction is affected by damaged heart muscle, reducing the client's ability to meet the demands of rehabilitation.
3) Fluid balance: Overload may worsen functioning and increase dependency.
4) Angina symptoms may be masked by reduced sensory perception.
5) Edema affects the ability to participate in activity and build endurance.

c. Vascular disease
1) Wounds heal poorly; risk is increased by poor circulation.
2) Amputation is 15 times more common in people with diabetes.
3) Pain sensation is reduced by neuropathy.
4) Mobility is impaired in Charcot foot.
5) Exercise tolerance is reduced.

d. Lung disease
1) Exercise tolerance is reduced.
2) Oxygenation is reduced.

e. Parkinson's disease (National Institute of Neurological Disorders and Stroke [NINDS], 2015)
1) Cognition: More time is needed to process information.
2) Mobility: Slow, stiff, poor coordination, shuffling gait (bradykinesia and rigidity are major problems)
3) Balance unsteady; tendency toward retropulsion
4) Tremors: Increase in purposeful tremors
5) "Despite the benefits of dopaminergic therapies, improvement of signs and symptoms is temporary in the setting of progressive disabilities such as cognitive impairment, psychosis, postural instability, failing speech/swallowing" (NINDS, 2014, p. 3).

f. Dementia
1) The ability to learn varies depending on the area affected and level of injury.
2) Memory impairments
3) Behavior is unpredictable.
4) Behavioral and psychological symptoms of dementia (BPSD) may include disturbed perception, thought content, mood, and behaviors such as aggression, agitation, wandering, hoarding, verbal aggression, anxiety, depression, hallucination, delusions, and paranoia (Schwartzkopf & Twigg, 2014).

g. Depression: Prevalence is 1.8%–8.9% among older adults residing in the community and 25% among older adults residing in nursing homes (Menzel, 2008).
1) Ability to learn
2) Cognitive status
3) Motivation
4) Higher rate of suicide among older adults, particularly older White men (Lochner & Byrd, 2014)

h. Anemia: A study conducted by Witkos, Uttaburanont, Lang, and Haddad (2009) showed that clients treated for anemia had better functional outcomes on discharge than untreated clients. Anemia affects the blood supply to the body, which is directly correlated with the following:
1) Exercise tolerance (affecting rehabilitation outcome)
2) Healing of injury and recovery outcomes
3) Postural hypotension (reduced oxygenation and volume)

i. Human Immunodeficiency Virus (HIV) and Acquired Immune Deficiency Syndrome (AIDS)
1) Exercise tolerance is reduced by a cachectic state.
2) Healing is poor because of comorbidity and poor nutrition.
3) Nutritional status is poor, leading to fatigue, muscle wasting, and higher risk of infection.

j. Cancer
1) Pain varies.
2) Exercise tolerance decreases.
3) Mobility deteriorates with advancing stages.

k. Patrick, Knoefel, Gaskowsk, and Rexrath (2001) found that the severity of medical comorbidity was a significant predictor of rehabilitation efficiency (gains in functional independence divided by length of stay) in older adults with various disabilities.

l. Yu (2005) reported that the number of medical comorbidities and age affected length of stay in an outpatient rehabilitation program for older adults.

5. Baseline functional status: Yu (2005) found that age of 80 years or more and admission function affected functional gains and rehabilitation efficiency in an outpatient rehabilitation program.
6. Higher vital capacity and higher albumin are predictors of survival among older adults 2 years after rehabilitation (Nicosia et al., 2012).
7. Baseline cognitive status is needed to predict outcomes and develop a plan of care.
   a. Ability to learn
   b. Memory
   c. Motivation
   d. Mast, MacNeill, and Lichtenberg (1999) reported that 34.7% of people with stroke and 27.8% of those with lower-extremity fracture in their study met the criteria for dementia. Also, 33.3% of people with stroke and 25.1% of those with lower-extremity fracture scored as depressed on the Geriatric Depression Scale. They noted that older adults with stroke and lower-extremity fracture need treatment not only for the stroke or fracture but also for geriatric-specific problems such as depression, dementia, and multiple comorbidities.
   e. Hershkovitz, Kalandariov, Hermush, Weiss, and Brill (2007) reported that cognitive function, nutritional status, and depression were important prognostic factors affecting success of rehabilitation outcome in older adults with proximal hip fracture.
8. Polypharmacy
   a. *Polypharmacy* is defined as the concurrent use of multiple medications (Antimisiaris & Cheek, 2014). It is also defined as the prescription, administration, or use of more medications than are clinically indicated in a given client (Charles & Lehman, 2006).
   b. The risks of polypharmacy include increased likelihood of drug–drug or drug–disease interactions, adverse drug events, and client nonadherence to the medication plan (Charles & Lehman, 2006).
   c. Home health nurses in one study reported that up to 21% of older adults did not understand their medications on discharge from hospital, 78% took five or more drugs, 11% had limited cognitive ability, and 9% had medications ordered by more than one provider (Ellenbecker, Frazier, & Verney, 2004).
   d. Ostwald, Wasserman, and Davis (2006) reported that stroke survivors in their study were discharged home with an average of 11.3 medications from five different drug classifications. The number of medications prescribed correlated with the number of stroke-related comorbidities. Receipt of medication from several different drug categories was also correlated with having more stroke-related comorbidities and more complications. The authors of this study reported that the average cost for a stroke survivor taking 10 commonly prescribed poststroke medications was $724.29 per month.
   e. Of people older than age 65 years, about 30% of hospital admissions are for medication-related problems (Marcum et al., 2012).
9. Social supports
   a. Family and significant others can have a positive impact on recovery time.
   b. Sources of income
      1) Social Security
      2) Pension
   c. Funding for healthcare
      1) Medicare
      2) Medicaid
      3) Private insurance
   d. Housing
      1) Members of the household can assist in care or provide moral support.
      2) The physical layout of the home environment determines the client's ability to be independent with activities of daily living (ADLs). Features such as stairs, ramps (if wheelchair use is warranted), safety devices (e.g., rails in shower), and countertops at a convenient work level influence discharge goals and length of stay.
   e. Transportation: Access to and availability of public and private transportation affect follow-up visits and health maintenance.
      1) Medical visits
      2) Grocery store
      3) Shopping
      4) Church and social groups
   f. Beaupre and colleagues (2005) demonstrated that functional status in a population age 65 years and older was lower in clients with hip fracture and poor social supports than in those with good social supports. Subjects with poor social supports were also more likely to be living in an institution 6 months after discharge from rehabilitation than those with better social support.
10. Commonly acquired disability in older adults

a. Stroke
   1) Stroke is a leading cause of long-term disability in the United States.
   2) Onset is secondary to cardiovascular disease, high blood pressure, diabetes, smoking, high cholesterol, obesity, and family history.
   3) On average, one person in the United States has a stroke every 40 seconds.
   4) 88% of stroke deaths occur in people age 65 years and older.
   5) 88% of strokes are ischemic, 9% intracranial hemorrhage, and 3% subarachnoid hemorrhage.
   6) Nearly 75% of strokes occur in those over age 65 years (The Internet Stroke Center, 2014).

b. Head injury
   1) "Those aged 75 and older have the highest rates of traumatic brain injury–related hospitalization and death due to falls" (Alzheimer's Association, 2014).
   2) Traumatic brain injuries (TBIs) in older adults account for 80,000 emergency department visits per year, 75% of which result in hospitalization (Menzel, 2008).
   3) Brenner, Homaifar, and Schultheis (2008) reported that 60% of brain injury survivors experience increased fatigue, especially mental fatigue and physical fatigue. Contributing factors are cognitive disturbances, sleeping problems, anxiety, depression, and alterations in endocrine neurotransmitters.
   4) Older women are more likely to be hospitalized after injury than older men.
   5) The rate of TBI in the general population is 60.6 per 100,000 people; after age 65 years, it increases to 155.9 per 100,000.
   6) Some research has shown that older adults with a history of moderate TBI had a 2.3 times greater risk of developing Alzheimer's than older adults without TBI. People with history of severe TBI had a 4.5 times greater risk. Other research studies have been inconclusive on this point (Alzheimer's Association, 2014).
   7) Older age is recognized as an independent predictor for worse outcomes from TBI (CDC, 2003; Thompson, McCormick, & Kagan, 2006).
   8) The risk of developing seizures after TBI increases after age 65 years (LeBlanc, de Guise, Gosselin, & Feyz, 2006).
   9) Older adults have poor cognitive functioning after TBI, necessitating increased family involvement and increased use of community services or nursing homes.

c. Falls with fracture
   1) Secondary to muscle weakness, impaired balance, osteoporosis, sensory loss, impaired gait, reduced muscle strength, poor vision, and use of psychoactive medication (Sherrington et al., 2008)
   2) One-third of falls in older adults are caused by environmental hazards in the home (**Figure 16-1**).

Figure 16-1. Potential Environmental Risk Factors for Falls

- Flooring, such as throw rugs, high-pile carpeting, or slippery or wet tile
- Outdoor walkways that are wet or have leaves, snow, or ice on them
- Small children and pets
- Stairs and steps (especially those without handrails and those not clearly marked)
- Clutter in walkways and around the bedroom and bathroom areas
- Lack of handrails in the bathroom
- Adaptive equipment such as rolling walkers, canes, or splints
- Poor lighting in rooms or walkways
- Lack of a system to call for help (e.g., whistle, bell)
- Long cords such as those for phones or supplemental oxygen tanks
- Poor arrangement of living space, which requires a person to reach or move in ways that upset balance

   3) Hip fractures cause the most deaths and disability in older adults.
   4) More than 95% of hip fractures are due to falls (CDC, 2013b).
   5) Up to one third of previously independent community-dwelling older adults experiencing hip fractures from falls remain institutionalized after 1 year (CDC, 2013b).

d. Deconditioning: Often a result of the enforced immobility of acute hospitalization superimposed on the normal changes of aging. Between 25% and 60% of hospitalized older adults risk the loss of function during hospitalization. Prolonged hospitalization leads to nursing home placement and death (Francis, 2005).
   1) Loss of strength
   2) Reduction of muscle mass
   3) Weakness
   4) Increased risk of falls

e. Contributing factors
   1) Lack of awareness by staff about importance of functional impairment on quality of life
   2) Organizational structure and process that limits knowledge about the client's baseline functional capacity

B. Geriatric Syndromes that Can Affect Rehabilitation

1. Delirium
   a. Defined as acute onset of confusion; fluctuates during the course of the day; short attention span, impaired memory, and usually an identifiable and treatable cause
   b. The prevalence of delirium is thought to range from 10% to 80%, with those at greater risk being the very medically ill, the terminally ill, those who have undergone cardiac surgery (Uguz et al., 2010), and older adults in intensive care. Long-term care facilities may have an incidence as high as 40% (Rose, 2014).
   c. Multiple causative factors and risk factors (Inouye, 2006; Tullmann, Fletcher, & Foreman, 2012)
      1) Advanced age
      2) Dementia
      3) Acute illness or infection
      4) Polypharmacy
      5) Substance abuse
      6) Untreated pain
      7) Electrolyte imbalance
      8) Change in surroundings
      9) Male gender (NICHE, 2012a)
      10) Depression (NICHE, 2012a)
      11) Dehydration (NICHE, 2012a)
      12) Sensory impairment (NICHE, 2012a)
      13) Malnourishment (NICHE, 2012a
   d. Delirium has several forms: hyperactive, hypoactive, and mixed (Rose, 2014).
      1) *Hyperactive*: Increased psychomotor activity, rapid speech, irritability, and restlessness
      2) *Hypoactive*: Lethargy, slowed speech, decreased alertness, apathy; patients are not disruptive, may go undiagnosed or be misdiagnosed as depressed.
      3) *Mixed*: Shift between hyperactive and hypoactive states. Shifts may cause incorrect assumption that condition has improved (NICHE, 2012a).
   e. Nurses often do not recognize the symptoms of delirium (Inouye, Foreman, Mion, Katz, & Cooney, 2001).
   f. Delirium is associated with negative outcomes (Tullmann et al., 2012)
      1) Increased cost
      2) Long-term disability
      3) Increased length of stay during hospitalization
      4) Increased mortality
      5) Increased complications
   g. General nursing interventions
      1) Identify and minimize risk factors when possible.
      2) Review medications.
      3) Provide a therapeutic environment.
      4) Monitor lab values.
      5) Treat signs and symptoms of delirium promptly.
      6) Work with the geriatric clinical nurse specialist (GCNS) or gerontological nurse practitioner (GNP) to monitor and treat.

2. Falls
   a. More than one third of older adults fall each year (Gray-Micelli, 2008).
   b. There are multiple causative factors.
   c. Falls are the leading cause of death and disability among older adults and the most common cause of nonfatal injuries (CDC, 2013a).
   d. The highest fall incidence occurs in nursing homes, where 50%–75% of clients fall annually (Gray-Micelli, 2008).
   e. Of those who fall, 20%–30% sustain moderate to severe injuries that reduce independence and mobility.
   f. For people age 75 years and older, those who fall are four to five times more likely to be admitted to a long-term care facility for a year or longer.
   g. Falls are a leading cause of TBI and fractures in older adults (CDC, 2013a).
   h. Fear of falling has been shown to cause older adults to limit their activities, leading to reduced mobility and fitness and increased risk of falls (CDC, 2013a).
   i. Risk factors
      1) Prior falls
      2) Advanced age
      3) Impaired gait
      4) Functional disability
      5) Physical restraints
      6) Polypharmacy
   j. General nursing interventions (Gray-Micelli, 2008)
      1) Assess fall risk upon admission and frequently thereafter (using a tool is recommended).
      2) Document and communicate findings with the rest of the team.

3) Implement and monitor safety measures including general precautions.
4) Incorporate fall prevention into the interdisciplinary plan of care.

3. Dizziness
   a. Multiple causative factors (Mauk, Hanson, & Hain, 2014)
   b. Four major types
      1) Vertigo
      2) Presyncope (lightheadedness)
      3) Disequilibrium (related to balance)
      4) Poorly defined (does not fit other categories)
   c. The most common types of dizziness in older adults are Ménière's syndrome and benign paroxysmal positional vertigo (BPPV).
   d. Tinetti, Williams, and Gill (2000) reported that 24% of people 72 years and older reported dizziness, 74% reported several triggering factors, and 56% of the dizzy subjects reported differing sensations. Associated factors included anxiety, depression, impaired hearing, polypharmacy, postural hypotension, impaired balance, and past myocardial infarction. The risk of dizziness increased with each added characteristic.
   e. General nursing interventions
      1) Determine the cause.
      2) Work with the GCNS, GNP, or physician to rule out BPPV if medications for vertigo are not effective.
      3) Educate the client and family about the type of vertigo and its treatment.
4. Urinary incontinence (UI)
   a. Multiple causative factors (Dowling-Castronovo & Spiro, 2013)
   b. Risk factors
      1) Immobility
      2) Decreased fluid intake
      3) Cognitive impairment
      4) Medications
      5) Constipation
      6) Environmental barriers
      7) Urinary tract infections
      8) Diabetes
      9) Stroke
      10) Obesity
      11) Smoking
   c. Consequences include falls, depression, pressure ulcers, and social isolation (Dugger & Cochran, 2014).
   d. General nursing interventions (Dowling-Castronovo & Bradway, 2008; Dugger & Cochran, 2014)
      1) Identify the type of UI.
      2) Implement interventions specific to the type of UI (e.g., stress incontinence improves with pelvic floor muscle exercises).
      3) Monitor fluid intake and urine output.
      4) Keep an incontinence diary.
      5) Limit bladder irritants.
      6) Modify the environment to promote successful toileting.
      7) Avoid indwelling urinary catheters when possible.
      8) Evaluate for any contributing medications.
      9) Educate the client and family about prevention of UI episodes.
5. Malnutrition
   a. Multiple causative factors, with dysphagia a major cause that is underrecognized and undertreated (Crogan, 2014).
   b. Major risk factor for complications and delayed recovery
   c. Often caused by disease or functional impairments
   d. Natural progression of end-stage dementia; supplemental, invasive feeding in clients with dementia is an ethical concern.
   e. Includes both obese and underweight people
   f. Malnutrition increases risk of complications and death.
   g. 40%–60% of hospitalized older adults have been found to be malnourished (Institute of Medicine, 2000), and 40%–60% of people in nursing home have dysphagia (Crogan, 2014).
   h. General nursing interventions (DiMaria-Ghalili, 2008)
      1) Check serum albumin or prealbumin.
      2) Consult with the dietitian.
      3) Alleviate dry mouth.
      4) Encourage oral intake.
      5) Make food appealing by controlling the environment.
      6) Provide oral supplements throughout the day.
6. Dehydration
   a. Multiple causative factors, including decreased thirst, reduced total body water in proportion to weight, body composition changes, impaired renal conservation of water, decreased effectiveness of vasopressin, and multiple comorbidities
   b. Risk factors for dehydration

1) Age greater than 85 years
2) Decreased mobility
3) Decreased ability to perform ADLs
4) More than four chronic conditions
5) More than four medications
6) Poor oral intake (which may be related to decreased thirst mechanism that occurs with age)
7) Communication difficulties
8) Fever
9) Few opportunities to drink

c. Atypical presentation in older adults: Confusion, falls, change in level of consciousness, weakness, fatigue (Rose, 2014)

d. General nursing interventions are similar to those for malnutrition, particularly increasing fluid intake (Mentes & Kang, 2013).

7. Functional loss
   a. 22% of people 85 years and older need assistance with personal care.
   b. 20%–40% of older adults experience functional decline during hospitalization.
   c. Risk factors
      1) Acute illness
      2) Exacerbation of chronic illness
      3) Injuries
      4) Medications
      5) Depression
      6) Malnutrition
      7) Decreased mobility
      8) Restraints
   d. Complications include loss of independence, falls, incontinence, malnutrition, depression, decreased socialization, and increased risk for institutionalization (Kresevic, 2012)
   e. In a systematic review of 66 studies, researchers found that "regular aerobic activity and short-term exercise programmes confer a reduced risk of functional limitations and disability in older age" (Paterson & Warburton, 2010, paragraph 6).
   f. General nursing interventions are those for immobility, including physical and occupational therapy as needed. (See Chapter 19 for more information.)

8. Polypharmacy
   a. 25%–40% of all prescriptions in the United States are written for older adults (Antimisiaris & Cheek, 2014).
   b. 5%–15% of all hospitalizations are medication related.
   c. 40%–50% of all over-the-counter medications are consumed by older adults. 90% of older adults take over-the-counter medications (NICHE, 2012b).
   d. In the United States, 106,000 fatal adverse drug events occur annually.
   e. On average, the number of prescriptions per person increases with age (Stagnitti, 2009).
   f. Community-dwelling adults average six medications daily.
   g. Symptoms of problems with medications include mental status changes, weight loss, dehydration, agitation, anorexia, urinary retention, and decline in functional status (Antimisiaris & Cheek, 2014).
   h. General nursing interventions (Antimisiaris & Cheek, 2014)
      1) Obtain a thorough history of medication use, including over-the-counter medications.
      2) Be familiar with the medications that are problematic for older adults.
      3) Participate in medication reconciliation within the hospital system.
      4) Monitor clients' serum blood urea nitrogen and creatinine.
      5) Understand and recognize normal aging changes and the effect on absorption, metabolism, and excretion of medications in the aging body.
      6) Use the Cockcroft–Gault formula for creatinine clearance as a more accurate measure than serum creatinine alone (because it accounts for age, ideal body weight, and gender).
      7) Be alert to recent dosage changes.
      8) Educate clients and families about the side effects of medications.
      9) Consider nonpharmacologic approaches to treatment.

C. Rehabilitation Nursing Interventions to Promote Successful Aging (**Figure 16-2**)
   1. Primary prevention (Haber, 2014)
      a. Young age groups without disability: Prevention of chronic disease through promotion of healthy lifestyles
         1) Nutrition: Maintaining balanced diet, healthy diet in moderation
         2) Exercise: Daily exercise to maintain health and wellness
         3) Weight management: To prevent side effects of obesity (hypertension, diabetes)
         4) Smoking prevention or cessation
         5) Safety awareness: Preventing avoidable injuries, driving within limits, wearing helmets,

Figure 16-2. Suggestions for Teaching Older Adults
Visual
Use bright, direct lighting unless contraindicated because of visual disturbances (such as recent cataract surgery).
Do not stand by a window; avoid glare.
When using visual aids, use large, well-spaced letters (black on white is best).
Keep clients close to the speaker, or, if in a large room, be certain that the audience can see and hear the speaker.
For individual teaching, make sure that the client's glasses are clean.
Auditory
Limit distractions: Eliminate extraneous noise, close doors, turn off television or radio, limit interruptions.
Face the audience; speak directly to the individual in a one-to-one setting.
Never cover your mouth when speaking (many older adults rely on lip reading to compensate for hearing deficits).
Speak slowly and clearly. If appropriate, wear bright lipstick to help elderly people who lip read.
Before proceeding, ask whether the client can hear you.
Use assistive devices as needed (make certain that hearing aids and microphones are turned on and that batteries are working).
General Teaching and Learning Suggestions
Keep teaching sessions short and to the point.
Design handouts to be simple and clear.
Relate the relevance of the topic to adult experiences within the group.
Use the principles of adult learning when planning an educational session.
Pace the presentation to reflect the unique needs and understanding of the group or individual.
Avoid the temptation to overload with too much information.
Remember that adults need a motivation to learn.
Provide immediate feedback to questions and comments.
Give an overview of the material to be covered and explain its relevance.
Keep information simple and specific; avoid technical jargon.
Use a variety of teaching modalities such as videotapes, hands-on experiences, samples of products, group discussion, overheads, pamphlets, and handouts.
Emphasize the client's learning responsibility.
Be enthusiastic about the subject; if the teacher isn't, the learner will not be.
Summarize important points.
Teach a procedure close to the time it will take place.
When teaching skills, allow time for practice, return demonstrations, questions, and review sessions.
Stick to the essentials needed to maintain life and prevent complications but be prepared to address additional questions.
Keep the environment conducive to learning; for group sessions, the room temperature should be comfortable for the majority, potentially noxious stimuli (such as cigarette smoke) should be avoided, seats must be easily accessible.
Use a large enough room to accommodate those with wheelchairs, walkers, and other assistive devices. Make certain exits are not blocked. Have additional nursing personnel available should needs arise (such as toileting).
Be thoroughly familiar with resources available in the community and the individual facility.
From *Gerontological rehabilitation nursing: Competencies for care* (p. 143), by K. L. Mauk, 2014, Burlington, MA: Jones & Bartlett. Reprinted with Permission.

following safety recommendations at home and work

b. Early education about potential problems of aging and how to prevent them
   1) In the rehabilitation setting, demonstrate cultural competency without language barriers. Teach the client, caregiver, and family. Provide adequate educational material in an understandable language, accommodating the needs of impaired clients and following principles of adult learning.
   2) Provide education during the maintenance (stable) phase of disability, when perception and client readiness are highest.
c. Older adults with or without disability: Prevent new chronic disease or disability through

promotion of healthy lifestyles. Many aspects of mortality are modifiable through behavior change. Therefore, the U.S. Preventive Services Task Force and the Surgeon General have set some guidelines for screening and counseling for adults (Spalding & Sebesta, 2008).

1) Nutrition: Diets rich in healthy fats, fruits, and vegetables; nutrition counseling for clients with diabetes, hypertension, and risk for coronary heart disease (CHD)
2) Daily exercise reduces the risk of death and prevents osteoporosis and obesity. The U.S. Surgeon General recommends aerobic exercise 30 minutes three times per week and strengthening exercise twice a week.
3) Weight management reduces the risk of diabetes and CHD.
4) Smoking prevention or cessation: A 3-minute counseling session with or without a pharmacological aid (Chantix, Wellbutrin, or nicotine patch) is recommended.
5) Safety awareness: Falls are a major cause of TBI and fractures. Maintaining a safe environment can reduce the risk of falls.
   a) Home environment: Keep the home free of barriers and obstacles that restrict mobility and increase risk of falls.
   b) Home safety evaluation: Identify unsafe conditions and measures to increase safety; educate family and caregivers on steps to prevent falls and injury.
6) Medication management
   a) Polypharmacy simulates symptoms produced by disease (delirium, hypotension, pseudoparkinsonism). A national initiative is under way to reduce the number of medications used.
   b) Risk factors: Age, sex, living arrangements, number of medications taken (Farrell, Hill, Hawkins, Newman, & Learned, 2003)
   c) Psychoactive medications should not be used to control behavioral problems.
7) Driving skills must be reassessed because decline in cognition and visual and auditory changes can affect response time, decision making, and judgment.
8) Fall prevention: Addressing physical impairments leading to falls is the major goal (Muché & McCarty, 2009).
9) Vision correction is recommended because poor vision can lead to social isolation, decline in ability to perform ADLs, depression, and altered self-image (Muché & McCarty, 2009).
10) Hearing correction will prevent deterioration of social function, depression, and falls.
11) Seat belts: Seat belt use can reduce secondary injury.
12) Limit alcohol intake to two drinks per day for men, one drink per day for women.
13) Social supports
14) Aspirin therapy for clients at risk for CHD
15) Aggressive statin therapy for clients with high cholesterol levels and established cardiovascular disease or risk for CHD
16) Cancer screening: Depends on type of cancer screening, comorbidity, functional status, and life expectancy; colorectal screening is recommended for clients 50 years and older (Nelson, 2014; Spalding & Sebesta, 2008).
17) Pneumonia vaccine for those older than 65 years and other high-risk clients; revaccinate every 5 years.
18) Influenza vaccine yearly
19) Zoster: People age 60 years and older (see CDC recommendations for adult vaccination)
20) Tetanus: After 5 years for wound management in clients older than age 65 years (CDC, 2009); tetanus/diphtheria/pertussis once every 10 years
21) Varicella: Two doses for adults who have not had varicella

2. Secondary prevention for all age groups, with and without disability
   a. Smoking cessation: A 3-minute counseling session with or without pharmacological aid (Chantix, Wellbutrin, or nicotine patch) is recommended (Spalding & Sebesta, 2008).
   b. Pneumonia vaccine: Follow CDC (2014) recommendations.
   c. Flu vaccine yearly: 60% of seasonal flu hospitalizations are for patients older than 65 years (CDC, 2014).
   d. Zoster: People age 60 years and older (see CDC recommendations for adult vaccination)
   e. Tetanus: After 5 years for wound management in clients older than age 65 years (CDC, 2014); tetanus/diphtheria/pertussis once every 10 years
   f. Varicella: Two doses for adults who have not had varicella
3. Tertiary prevention in older adults without disability

a. Chronic disease management
b. Health maintenance
c. Educating the older adult about:
1) The disease process
2) How to prevent disease progression
3) Recognition of complications and what to do
4) Treatment compliance

4. Societal level
a. Redesign of cars
b. Redesign of roadways
c. License renewal restrictions
d. Special transportation services

5. CDC programs to promote healthy aging
a. Web-based educational resources and tools related to aging issues
b. Outreach services for older adults on disease prevention, advance directives, and end-of-life issues

6. Senior-friendly website to educate seniors: An easy-to-use website that reads content aloud to the viewer, developed by the National Institute on Aging and National Library of Medicine, is available at www.nihseniorhealth.gov.

IV. Aging and Disability: Aging with an Early-Onset Disability

A. Longevity: People with early-onset disability are living longer. An estimated 12 million people are currently living into middle and late life with an early-onset disability.
1. Antibiotics and other medication advances
2. Advances in technology
3. Improvements in public health
4. Improved medical care (Kemp & Mosqueda, 2004)

B. Aging as an Uncharted Course
1. Atypical aging seems to be the norm. Unanticipated changes occur in midlife (Kemp & Mosqueda, 2004).
2. Research gaps in understanding aging with disability have been identified (Freedman, 2014).
3. Higher rates of medical and functional problems often occur 20–25 years earlier than in those without disability. Disability often occurs in those who have been most active, and changes occur in the amount of assistance needed (Kailes, 2002; Kemp & Mosqueda, 2004).
4. This population has three to four times as many secondary health problems as age-matched peers (Jensen et al., 2012; Kailes, 2002).
5. Accelerated aging is aging related to the disability itself at the cellular or organ level (Kailes, 2002).
6. Wear and tear refers to increased stress on the body from living with disability over time (Kailes, 2002).
7. Results of rehabilitation depend on the era of onset: People disabled 30, 40, or 50 years ago received rehabilitation in a different era. Many factors have changed over time. People who are disabled today may not have the same outcomes in 20, 30, or 40 years (Kailes, 2002; Jensen et al, 2012;Molton et al., 2014).
8. Latent illness: An impairment such as polio or cerebral palsy (CP) can start a cascade of events that cause illnesses in later life (Kailes, 2002).
9. Contributing factors
a. Environment
1) Limited accessibility exacerbates the effects of disability and aging.
2) Modifications in the home and community can increase safety and accessibility and facilitate health maintenance.
3) Nonaccommodating environments may increase stress on the body (Kailes, 2002).
b. Equipment: Manual equipment may increase stress on joints and limbs over time (Fattal et al., 2014).
c. Medications: Long-term use of medications may affect the aging and health of body systems.
d. Sedentary lifestyle: Increases the risk of cardiovascular disease and disuse syndromes.
e. Preventive service use: Many people with disabilities do not maintain preventive services (e.g., vaccinations, cancer screening) because of a lack of knowledge, funding, or available and accessible services (LaPlante, 2014).

C. Unexpected Medical, Functional, and Psychosocial Problems (Kailes, 2002; Jensen et al., 2012)
1. Loss of strength, endurance, and range of motion (Fattal, 2014; Molton et al., 2014)
2. Pain: Chronic pain, physical and emotional pain, limited coping strategies and training (Molton et al., 2014).
3. Employment difficulties: Ageism, changing work environment (Johnson, Brown, & Knaster, 2010)
4. Decreased quality of life: Decreased income, unpredictable financial resources
5. Family stress: Lack of support, loss of loved one, caregiver role, grandparenting role (Miyamoto, Tachimori, & Ito, 2010; Watkins, 2014)

D. Late Life Syndrome: Disability-specific changes with aging are common, superimposed on normal changes of aging.
1. Polio

a. Postpolio syndrome (PPS) (Amtmann, Bamer, Verrall, Salem, & Borson, 2013)
    1) 440,000 people are at risk for PPS; 25%–60% of polio survivors may develop PPS.
    2) Signs and symptoms appear 30–40 years after original onset of polio (Laffont et al., 2010).
    3) The exact cause is unknown, but it is thought to be a degeneration of overworked nerve terminals in motor units that remain after initial illness.
    4) Slow, stepwise, unpredictable course
    5) Decreased strength, fatigue (Jensen et al., 2011)
        a) In muscles previously affected by polio and in muscles not previously affected by polio
        b) Muscle atrophy occurs in some cases.
        c) PPS fatigue affects more than 1.63 million American polio survivors (Bruno, Cohen, Galski, & Frick, n.d.).
    6) Decreased respiratory efficiency: Pneumonia (Laffont et al., 2010)
    7) Dysphagia: Aspiration pneumonia
    8) Joint pain (Laffont et al., 2010)
    9) Muscle pain, cramping reported by 90% of clients (Jensen et al., 2011)
    10) Gait disturbance
    11) Autonomic dysfunction
    12) Sleep apnea (Laffont et al., 2010)
    13) Flat back syndrome (Muñiz, 2011)
    14) Decreased function
    15) Depression
    16) Restless leg syndrome (Laffont et al., 2010)
b. The severity of PPS is predicted by the severity of initial residual disability after polio (Klingbiel, Baer, & Wilson, 2004; NINDS, 2006b).

2. CP
    a. 65%–90% of children with CP live into adulthood.
    b. Organ systems (heart, lungs) age prematurely.
    c. Postimpairment syndrome includes pain, weakness, and fatigue (Morgan & McGinley, 2014; Riquelme, Cifre, & Montoya, 2011).
    d. Decline in functional status (Morgan & McGinley, 2014)
        1) Walking
        2) Self-care
    e. Increased falls
    f. Contractures, especially lower extremities in nonambulators
    g. Progressive deformity
    h. Pulmonary changes impair breathing, making speech inaudible, and motor impairment in later life can cause difficulty in phonation and sentence production.
    i. Kyphoscoliosis
        1) Pneumonia, right-sided heart failure, hypoxemia, decreased vital capacity
        2) Problems with positioning, seating
    j. Increased bowel and bladder dysfunction
        1) Urinary tract infections
        2) Incontinence
    k. Osteoporosis, osteopenia, and fractures: Genetically low bone mass density results in increased fracture rate with mobility (Jasien, Daimon, Maudsley, Shapiro, & Martin, 2012)
    l. Oral motor and dental disorders
        1) Increased difficulty chewing, eating, and swallowing
        2) Increased risk of aspiration, malnutrition, and dental decay
        3) More common in those with dyskinesias or spastic CP
    m. Arthritis: Association between presence of pain in weight-bearing joints and a cessation of ambulation around age 45 years
    n. Spasticity is increased.
    o. Pain
        1) Often related to musculoskeletal dysfunction, degenerative arthritis, and overuse syndromes
        2) Common sites include hip, knee, ankle, and lumbar and cervical spine
    p. Spinal stenosis (Klingbiel et al., 2004; NINDS, 2006a)
    q. Life expectancy is lower for those with severe impairment and poor mobility (De Vivo, 2004).
    r. Strauss, Ojdana, Shavelle, and Rosenbloom (2004) found a marked decline in ambulation with aging for those with CP who were mobile when they became adults. There was a greater need for assistance with ADLs as age increased, greater need for residence in nursing facilities, and poorer survival among those who lost mobility. People with the most severe disability did not live to age 60 years.
        1) Premature sarcopenia, obesity, and sedentary behavior lead to increased chronic disease risk and associated decline in function and mobility (Peterson, Gordon, & Hurvitz, 2013)
        2) Biomechanical overuse, compounded by an injured nervous system, results in

accelerated physiologic aging (Peterson et al., 2013).

3. Spina bifida
   a. Overuse syndrome
      1) Wheelchair users: Shoulders, wrists, hands; carpal tunnel syndrome; rotator cuff injuries (Fattal, 2014)
      2) Ambulators: Hip and knee pain
   b. Reduced muscle strength and endurance lead to decreased mobility and ability to ambulate and transfer.
   c. Reduced nerve function reduces sensations and circulation.
   d. Shunt malfunction
   e. Tethered cord syndrome (Brei & Merkens, 2003)
      1) Chiari problem: Apnea
      2) Syrinx
   f. Knee pain
   g. Osteoporosis: Increased risk for fractures; uneven pressure on joints causes arthritis and pain
   h. Kyphosis and scoliosis
   i. Charcot joints
   j. Skin changes: Pressure ulcers, abrasions
   k. Increased incidence and severity of latex allergy
   l. Obesity from decreased mobility
   m. Renal system changes
      1) Renal damage leading to renal failure
      2) Bladder cancer associated with neurogenic bladder
      3) Changes in bladder control
   n. Increased risk of latex allergies (Klingbiel et al., 2004)
   o. Bowel function: Constipation, need for bowel evacuations and high-fiber diet
   p. Need for braces and equipment due to poor balance and increasing need for ADL assistance
   q. Reduced socialization leads to isolation
   r. Depression
   s. Different levels of need for ADL assistance depending on cognitive level (Brei & Merkens, 2003)
   t. Accelerated cognitive aging with impaired memory may occur (Dennis, Nelson, Jewell, & Fletcher, 2010), with executive dysfunction (Liptak, Garver, & Dosa, 2013)
4. Down syndrome
   a. 50% of infants who survive to age 1 year can be expected to live past 50 years of age.
   b. Show signs of aging 20–30 years ahead of others in the general population
      1) Accelerated deterioration in later life after stressful event, depression, underactive thyroid; visual and hearing impairments are common.
      2) Depression
      3) Hypothyroidism
      4) Hearing and visual impairment
      5) Vascular disease
      6) Graying hair
      7) Glucose intolerance and degenerative bone disease
      8) High rates of cancer
      9) Cognitive losses
   c. Early-onset dementia
      1) Typically around age 40–50, as many as 75% of people with Down syndrome exhibit signs of mild cognitive impairment and onset of Alzheimer's-type dementia (Krinsky-McHale & Silverman, 2013).
      2) Atypical signs and symptoms
         a) Seizures
         b) Changes in ADL ability
   d. Accelerated rate of functional losses after age 45 years
      1) Need the same health promotion programs at an earlier age as nondisabled people age 50–80 years (Chen, 2006; Merck Manuals Online Medical Library, 2003)
      2) Menopause may occur 5–6 years earlier than in the general population (Holland & Benton, 2004).
   e. Quality of life (Brown, Taylor, & Matthews, 2001)
      1) The majority report being happy.
      2) Privacy is important.
      3) Reminiscence may be helpful.
      4) Tidiness and cleanliness of surroundings are valued.
5. SCI
   a. Menter and Hudson's model of aging that develops functional decline identifies three post-SCI phases (Winkler, 2008).
      1) Acute restoration phase (first 2 years after SCI): Maximal function regained within limitations of SCI
      2) Maintenance phase
         a) Stable level of function over time
         b) Stable time varies
      3) Decline phase
         a) Degenerative effects of SCI
         b) Aging

b. Functional decline begins 10–20 years after injury.
   1) Depends on genetics, lifestyle, age at the time of injury (Wirz & Dietz, 2012), current age (Rodakowski et al., 2014), level of injury, weight, health history, comorbidities (van der Woude et al., 2013), available social support
   2) Children with SCI may have 20 years of stable functioning after injury, whereas adults older than age 50 may have just 5–7 years before decline begins (Hitzig, Eng, Miller, Sakakibara, & SCIRE Research Team, 2011).
c. Overuse syndrome
   1) Pain
      a) Incidence of pain increases from 41% 1 year after injury to about 80% more than 5 years after injury.
      b) More than 70% of people with SCI report upper extremity pain (Fattal, 2014).
      c) Nearly two thirds of people with SCI have compressive neuropathies in the upper extremities.
   2) The most common overuse syndromes are degenerative joint disease, rotator cuff tears, rotator cuff tendinitis, subacromial bursitis, and capsulitis (Fattal et al., 2014; Winkler, 2008).
d. Osteoporosis and fractures
   1) 6% of people with SCI have a lower extremity fracture, most commonly femur; fracture potential is reached 1–9 years after SCI (Dolbow et al., 2011). Functional electrical stimulation and muscle contraction stresses bones and reduces risk of osteoporosis.
   2) As many as 10% of these fractures result in nonunion (Dolbow et al., 2011).
e. Scoliosis
   1) Nearly 97% of children and adolescents with SCI develop scoliosis.
   2) Nearly 50% of adults with SCI develop scoliosis.
f. Cardiovascular function (Jensen et al., 2012)
   1) Incidence of cardiovascular disease is more than 200% higher than in the noninjured population.
   2) Hypertension is twice as common in people with paraplegia as in the general population.
   3) Stroke risk is higher in aging adults with SCI than in the general population (Lavela et al., 2012).
g. Gastrointestinal tract: Complications and dysfunction increase with age. 74% develop hemorrhoids, 43% develop abdominal distention, and 20% develop difficulty in bowel evacuation. Fewer older adults with SCI are independent with bowel care than younger adults (Furusawa et al., 2012).
h. Genitourinary tract
   1) Incidence of bladder cancer increases from 0.2% in the first 10 years after injury to 9% after 30 years.
   2) Urinary tract infections remain a prevalent risk (Eves & Rivera, 2010).
i. Skin: Soft tissue changes and thinning of subcutaneous fat lead to risk of skin tears, breakdown, and poor healing.
   1) Susceptibility to pressure ulcers increases with age.
   2) Sitting tolerance may decrease with age because of the loss of adipose tissue.
   3) The incidence of pressure ulcers increases with age; 15%–30% of people with SCI develop pressure ulcers.
j. Decreased immunity
   1) Frequency of urinary tract infections, increased risk of falls
   2) Pneumonia risk increases as a function of underlying comorbidities and decreased mobility.
k. Decreased pulmonary function; restrictive pulmonary disease can accelerate decline. There is a higher incidence of sleep apnea (Winkler, 2008).
l. Insulin resistance risk increases fourfold after SCI (LaVela et al., 2012).
m. Hardware breakdown: Spinal rods
n. Social isolation (Menter, 1998; Winkler, 2008)
o. Bowel function: The ability to manage neurogenic bowel decreases after age 60 years when the injury is 30 or more years old. There is an increased risk of colorectal cancer.
p. ADLs: The need for ADL assistance increases with age. Reasons for needing assistance include the following:
   1) Increased weakness
   2) Increased weight gain
   3) Increased pain
q. ADLs most affected are
   1) Bathing
   2) Transfer
   3) Dressing

r. Instrumental ADLs with which most SCI-injured people need assistance include the following:
   1) Household chores
   2) Shopping
   3) Meal preparation

6. TBI: Overwhelming behavioral changes and personality changes can make TBI frightening to the family and the client. A recent study of 286 survivors of moderate to severe TBI revealed the following chronic health conditions an average of 14.2 years after injury:
   a. Nervousness and tension
   b. Headaches
   c. Dizziness
   d. Sensitivity to noise and light
   e. Personality changes
   f. Arthritis
   g. Sleep disturbances
   h. Vision changes
   i. Hearing changes
   j. Allergies
   k. Potential for seizures
   l. Breathing problems (Colantonio, Ratcliff, Chase, & Vernich, 2004)
   m. Studies have shown an increased rate of social isolation.
   n. Memory problems, including slower processing, difficulty processing

7. Multiple sclerosis (MS)
   a. People older than 65 years have greater disability.
   b. Disease course and length of time after diagnosis are stronger predictors of current status than current age and other demographics (DeVivo, 2004).
   c. Finlayson, Van Denend, and Hudson (2004) found that women aging with MS perceived that they had less freedom and needed more assistance than peers without MS. They shared concerns about unmet needs in the areas of personal care, housework, support groups, assistive technology, travel, and socialization.

E. Rehabilitation Nursing Interventions to Promote Successful Aging in Those with Early-Onset Disability. (See Section III.C in this chapter for guidelines for primary prevention for young age groups and older adults, and ongoing secondary prevention for all age groups with disability.)

V. Psychosocial Issues

A. Grief and Loss
   1. Life changes with age
      a. Retirement
      b. Death of a spouse, children, friends
      c. Possible decline in health, including chronic illness and disability
      d. Menopause
      e. Possible change in economic status
      f. Possible social isolation
      g. Possible change in living arrangements
   2. Role changes with age
      a. Widowhood
      b. Caregiver role reversal (i.e., the person who has provided care becomes the person who is being cared for)

B. Stress and Coping
   1. The ability to deal well with stress and adopt positive coping mechanisms is associated with successful aging (Vaillant, 2002).
   2. Assess coping strategies in relation to the amount of stress the person is experiencing and promote the use of positive coping strategies.
      a. Increased social support
      b. Activity and exercise
      c. Faith, hope, and spirituality
      d. Involvement in leisure activities the client enjoys

C. Depression and Anxiety
   1. Depression
      a. It is estimated that 6 million older adults experience depression in some form (Geriatric Mental Health Foundation, 2014).
      b. Risk factors (Kurlowicz & Harvath, 2008)
         1) Incontinence
         2) History of substance abuse
         3) Social isolation
         4) Chronic pain or illness
         5) Being a caregiver
         6) Living alone (especially widow or widower)
         7) Functional disability
         8) Poor social support
      c. Signs and symptoms
         1) Insomnia
         2) Memory impairment
         3) Feelings of worthlessness or powerlessness
         4) Fatigue
         5) Vague physical complaints
      d. Results of depression (Lochner & Byrd, 2014)
         1) Decreased quality of life
         2) Associated anxiety
         3) Higher mortality rates from other conditions
         4) Higher risk for cancer
         5) Poorer outcomes after surgery
         6) Higher rate of suicide

e. Nursing interventions (Kurlowicz & Havath, 2008; Lochner & Byrd, 2014)
   1) Psychotherapy or counseling
   2) Medications, especially tricyclic antidepressants, selective serotonin reuptake inhibitors, and antipsychotics (monoamine oxidase inhibitors used less because of side effects)
   3) Encourage participation in social activities.
   4) Promote a healthy lifestyle, including proper nutrition, good sleeping habits, and a daily routine.
   5) Enhance coping strategies.
   6) Connect to community resources.
   7) Enhance social support systems.
   8) Inspire hope.
   9) Be alert to suicidal ideations.
   10) Provide a nonjudgmental atmosphere.

2. Anxiety
   a. Anxiety should be treated in conjunction with depression for best outcomes.
   b. Most older adults with major depression also have anxiety.
   c. Anxiety is not well understood or studied in older adults.
   d. Assess for risk factors such as certain medical conditions and medications that exacerbate anxiety (Lochner & Byrd, 2014).
   e. Selective serotonin reuptake inhibitors (used to treat depression) are medications of choice (Anxiety Disorders Association of America, 2006).
   f. Also treated with cognitive–behavioral therapy
   g. Nursing interventions are similar to those for depression; in addition, the rehabilitation nurse should develop a trusting relationship with the primary healthcare provider.

D. Life Review and Reminiscence
1. Older adults may be undertaking an end-of-life review.
2. They may experience anticipatory grieving.
3. Erikson's development stage for older age, ego integrity versus despair, suggests that older adults need to feel that their life has purpose and meaning. (See Chapter 16 for more information on developmental stages.)
4. Rehabilitation nurses can use reminiscence therapy to help older adults recall positive memories that can be shared and discussed (Lochner & Byrd, 2014).

E. Suicide (Merck Manual, 2008)
1. Older White men are at highest risk for suicide.
2. Older men tend to use more lethal means of suicide (e.g., firearms, hanging), whereas older women use less lethal means such as pills.
3. Suicide is associated with alcoholism, diagnosis of a terminal disease, depression, presence of a chronic disease, being unmarried and living alone, having few support systems, drug abuse, bereavement, intractable pain, and social isolation; depression is the most notable associated condition.
4. 15% of older adults with untreated depression end their life by suicide (Merck Manual, 2008).
5. Up to 75% of those committing suicide visited their primary care physician within a month beforehand (National Institute of Mental Health [NIMH], 2006).
6. The risk can be lessened by strengthening social supports, treating depression, increasing involvement in social activities, and taking definitive action when suicidal ideations are expressed (Merck Manual, 2008).

F. Rehabilitation of Clients Who Are Terminally Ill
1. Nurses should explore their own feelings about the rehabilitation of those who are at the end of life.
2. There are many potential examples of situations that involve rehabilitating older adults with terminal illnesses.
   a. Late-stage cancer, including melanoma
   b. Rapidly growing, inoperable tumors
   c. End-stage renal disease
   d. Last stages of AIDS
   e. Other incurable diseases
3. Explore with the client and family the goals of rehabilitation therapy.
   a. Increase the quality of life.
   b. Increase independence enough to go home to die rather than remaining in a facility.
4. Discuss the purposes of palliative care and hospice (Warring & Krieger-Blake, 2014).
   a. Hospice helps clients "live until they die."
   b. Hospice provides bereavement services for the family after the death.
   c. Hospice provides pain management.
   d. Hospice provides symptom control at the end of life.
   e. Palliative care can occur in many settings, and clients do not have to be terminally ill to benefit from palliative care.

VI. General Aging Issues

A. Preventive Services for Older Adults
1. Primary
   a. Activities for health promotion and disease prevention

1) Increasing leisure time activity
2) Increasing walking time activity (Soares-Miranda et al., 2014)

b. Immunizations to prevent illness; those recommended by the CDC for adults older than 65 years and those at high risk include the following (CDC,2015):
1) Annual flu vaccine
2) Pneumococcal vaccine once after age 65 years and one-time revaccination for those older than age 75 years
3) Zoster (shingles) one dose
4) Tetanus and diphtheria vaccine every 10 years

2. Secondary
a. Follow recommendations of *Healthy People 2010* (www.healthypeople.gov/).
b. Screenings for clients at risk
c. Screenings recommended by the U.S. Preventive Services Task Force with sufficient evidence to support (Nelson, 2014)
1) Tobacco use
2) Depression
3) Hyperlipidemia
4) Hypertension
5) Osteoporosis for women older than 65 years
6) Vision and hearing for older adults
7) Mammography every 1–2 years for women
8) Colorectal cancer screening by fecal occult blood test or sigmoidoscopy
9) Physical and dental checkup (Lau & Kirby, 2009)

3. Tertiary
a. Rehabilitation of chronic health alterations as discussed throughout this core curriculum
b. Focus on prevention of complications and maintenance of function

B. End of Life
1. Patients who have end-of-life discussions with loved ones and healthcare professionals receive hospice services more often, but palliative care often remains an add-on rather than planned (Potera & Pfeifer, 2014).
2. Hospice or end-of-life care is focused on the dying process. It is prescribed by a physician for clients who are terminally ill and have less than 6 months to live (Pace, Burke, & Glass, 2006).
a. More than 75% of hospice clients die at home (National Hospice and Palliative Care Organization, 2004).
b. Hospice care provides support for people in the last phase of terminal illness.
c. Promotes the concept of "living until you die"
d. Hospice recognizes dying as a normal part of living.
e. Focuses on maintaining quality of life until death
f. Grief and bereavement support for client and family
g. Pain management is a priority.
h. Services provided include the following:
1) Nursing care
2) Psychological counseling
3) Spiritual care
4) Grief counseling
5) Social service support
6) ADL care
7) Household chores
8) Respite services for caregivers (Pace et al., 2006)

3. Palliative care
a. Palliative care is comprehensive care for the discomfort, symptoms, and stress of serious illness (DiBello & Coyne, 2014). It also helps provide relief from pain, shortness of breath (Pastor & Moore, 2013), fatigue, constipation, nausea, loss of appetite, and sleep disorders. It can help with the side effects of medical treatment. Palliative care has three operational components (Mahon, 2010) to provide timely and effective management of physical, emotional, and spiritual care and education about disease processes and treatment options. The patient and caregiver can make informed decisions about their healthcare consistent with their values and beliefs (Labson, Sacco, Weissman, Gornet, & Stuart, 2013).
1) Aggressive symptom management
2) Assistance with decision making
3) Interventions of interdisciplinary team can reduce rehospitalizations in the last years of life (Center for Home Care Policy and Research, 2009).
4) End-of-life care when appropriate; this is comfort based, not curative.

b. Clients can receive treatment for conditions and still receive palliative care; pursuing treatment does not exclude clients from palliative care.
c. Based on an interdisciplinary team model
d. Funded by Medicare, Medicaid, and private insurance (DiBello & Coyne, 2014)
e. Provides emotional support for the client and family
f. Rehabilitation nurses can assist clients in the process of dying well because there is potential

for self-growth even in the dying process (Byock, 1997).

4. Nursing interventions
   a. Advance directives
   b. Patient Self-Determination Act requires that healthcare institutions that receive government subsidies provide patients with information about their legal rights to participate in making medical decisions, including the right to accept or refuse medical treatment and to formalize their wishes about medical treatments in a written document, the advance directive. The advance directive is important at any stage of life (Center for Home Care Policy and Research, 2009).
      1) Living will
         a) Important at any stage of life (Center for Home Care Policy and Research, 2009)
         b) Designates proxy to make health decisions (Center for Home Care Policy and Research, 2009)
         c) Is used in cases of terminal illness
         d) Makes the client's wishes known in advance when death is imminent, as certified by a physician
      2) Declaration document of life-prolonging procedures
         a) Describes steps to take to prolong life
         b) Is determined by the client
      3) Durable power of attorney for health care
         a) Allows another person to make decisions on behalf of the client
         b) Can encompass health, financial, property, and other issues
      4) Healthcare representative: Allows a healthcare professional to make decisions at the client's behest regarding health-related issues
      5) Five wishes (Aging with Dignity, 2011)
         a) Not legally recognized in all states
         b) In the states where this is recognized, people may complete the forms, available online, without the use of an attorney.
         c) Cost effective and easy to use
         d) A nontraditional type of advance directive that answers these five items according to a person's wishes
            (i) Who makes healthcare decisions when the person is unable
            (ii) What kind of medical treatment is wanted or not wanted
            (iii) Comfort measures the person wants
            (iv) How people should treat the person
            (v) What he or she wants loved ones to know
      6) Allow natural death (Meyer, 2001; Warring & Krieger-Blake, 2014): More descriptive and positive than a do-not-resuscitate order
   c. Intervening with common problems at the end of life
      1) Dyspnea
         a) Opioid therapy such as morphine can reduce shortness of breath.
         b) Elevate head of the bed 30–45 degrees.
         c) Provide a fan to move air in the room.
         d) Cool, humidified air
         e) Control oral secretions.
      2) Anxiety can be worsened by fear of suffering; antianxiety agents such as lorazepam given orally, sublingually, or rectally can help (McKinnis, 2002).
      3) Constipation
         a) Immobility, lack of exercise, decreased food and fluids, and use of pain medications contribute to constipation.
         b) Use a stool softener and stimulant combination.
      4) Nausea and vomiting
         a) Treatment depends on the cause.
         b) A combination of medications may be indicated.
         c) Prepare foods away from client's room.
         d) Eliminate noxious stimuli.
         e) Ice chips may help in eliminating aftertaste and dryness of mouth.
      5) Poor appetite
         a) Narcotic use reduces desire to eat.
         b) Eat as desired.
         c) Maintain a clean, tidy environment.
         d) There is a natural decrease in desire for food at the end of life.
         e) Artificial hydration may prolong suffering and increase edema through fluid overload (End of Life Nursing Education Consortium, 2004).
         f) Provide meticulous mouth care as fluid intake decreases.
      6) Pain
         a) Typically undertreated in older adults. Clinicians should discuss pain to maximize quality of life (Hawkins et al., 2013).

b) Identify and treat the type of pain.
c) Fear of addiction should not be a factor.
d) Cancer pain treatment generally follows a three-step ladder (World Health Organization, 1990) of nonsteroidal anti-inflammatory drugs, opioids, and analgesic adjuvants in combinations.
e) Be aware of cultural variations in tolerance to pain and expression of pain.
f) Offer effective pain interventions.
g) Use nonpharmacological methods such as music and aroma therapy.

d. Educating families about what to expect at the end of life
   1) Signs of impending death (Marrone, 1997)
      a) Decreased urine output
      b) Changes in breathing patterns
      c) Increasing periods of unresponsiveness
      d) Mottling of extremities
      e) Changes in vital signs
   2) Ask about specific cultural or spiritual practices at end of life and death.

e. Ethical and moral dilemmas
   1) Withholding treatment: Not beginning treatment (advance directives make the client's wishes explicit)
   2) Withdrawing treatment: Removing life-sustaining interventions after they have been implemented (e.g., disconnecting a ventilator from a person who is unable to breathe independently, discontinuing nutritional interventions for a person who cannot otherwise eat or drink independently)
   3) Assisted suicide
      a) Defined as helping a person to terminate his or her own life
      b) Illegal in most states
      c) Legal in Oregon for a terminally ill client to be prescribed a lethal dose of medication by the physician; must be taken willingly by the client
   4) Euthanasia
      a) Purposefully hastening the death of another person (Pereira, 2012)
      b) An outside person may play a more active role in hastening the death of another with the purpose of ending his or her suffering.

C. Use of Physical and Chemical Restraints

1. Approximately 15% of nursing home residents are restrained for some portion of the day (Beers & Berkow, n.d.). Some side effects of restraint use include:
   a. Falls while attempting to free oneself from the restraint
   b. Confusion caused by forceful restrictions of movement, inability to position, and reduced stimulation
   c. Death from choking and entrapment
   d. Pressure ulcers caused by immobility, damage to skin from friction, and shear forces in attempts to free oneself
   e. Pneumonia aspiration, fluid accumulation from reduced attempts to deep breathe and cough
   f. Urinary tract infections, reduced fluid intake, withholding urge due to lack of access and immobility caused by restraints, incomplete emptying
2. The use of physical restraints must be assessed, justified, and documented every day and as recommended by regulatory agencies.
3. Physical restraints should be used only when the person is a danger to himself or herself or others.
4. The routine use of chemical restraints is inappropriate except in the most extreme circumstances for client safety.
5. Alternatives to restraints exist and should be explored (Dean, Harrison, & Zwicker, 2014).
   a. The National Partnership to Improve Dementia Care was launched in 2012 to address inappropriate use of medications in people with dementia (Fitzsimmons, Barba, Stump, & Bonner, 2014).
   b. Provide nonpharmacological strategies and interventions based on the specific needs, preferences, and functional abilities of the resident (Cohen-Mansfield et al., 2012).
   c. Companions or close supervision
   d. Modifying the environment to reduce barriers and provide easy access
   e. Reality orientation
   f. Activities for diversion (Waszynski et al., 2013)
   g. Increasing physical activities
6. Restraint use increases the likelihood of injury in many instances.
7. A physician order is required for restraint use and must include documentation of the medical condition necessitating restraint, the type of restraint, the length of time for use, and guidelines for release and repositioning (according to Omnibus Budget Reconciliation Act 1987 guidelines) (Dean, Harrison, & Zwicker, 2014)

D. Abuse or Mistreatment of Older Adults

1. Violation of human rights and a significant cause of illness, injury, loss of productivity, isolation, and despair (World Health Organization, 2011).
2. May take many forms, including neglect, financial exploitation, and passive or active physical, emotional, and sexual abuse
3. Elder abuse is difficult to obtain statistics on and difficult to research (National Center on Elder Abuse, 2006).
   a. Often not reported or underreported by victims
   b. As many as 5 million victims of financial abuse
   c. Between 700,000 and 1.2 million older adults may be victims of abuse and neglect each year (Bond & Butler, 2013).
   d. Between 1 and 2 million older Americans may have been victimized in some way by those they depended on.
4. Characteristics of abusers
   a. May have been victims of abuse themselves
   b. May be men or women
   c. May be family members or caregivers
   d. May have social and emotional problems or a history of psychological problems
   e. May abuse drugs or alcohol
   f. May have a high level of stress or frustration, minimal coping abilities, and lack of knowledge
5. Characteristics of victims (DeCalmer & Glendenning, 1993; Pritchard, 1995, 1996): Many rehabilitation clients are at risk because of the following factors:
   a. Social isolation
   b. Advanced age
   c. Poor health
   d. Widowhood
   e. Significant physical limitations
   f. Gender (women are victims more often)
   g. Dependence on others
   h. History of family violence
   i. African Americans are at greater risk of financial and environmental neglect (Burnett et al., 2014).
6. Possible signs and symptoms of abuse or mistreatment
   a. Poor physical hygiene
   b. Dehydration or malnutrition
   c. Multiple bruises of different colors (indicating different stages of healing)
   d. A withdrawn, cowering, fearful, anxious, depressed, or hopeless demeanor
   e. Presence of burns, skin tears, broken bones, or severe rashes that, when explained, do not fit the injury or trauma
   f. Poor eye contact, communicates with short answers
7. Nursing interventions (**Figure 16-3**)

Figure 16-3. Nursing Indications for the Prevention of Elder Abuse

- Establish a trusting relationship with the elderly person.
- Be able to refer families to resources available in the community.
- Strengthen social supports.
- Encourage regular respite for the caregiver.
- Identify caregivers who are at the highest risk of being abusers and target interventions to prevent stress from caregiver burden.
- Be aware of risk factors and contributing factors.
- Perform a thorough physical assessment and carefully document findings, including the client's appearance, nutritional state, skin condition, mental attitude and awareness, and the need for aids to enhance sensory perception.
- If abuse is suspected, interview the caregiver and other possible informants to confirm or refute suspicions.
- Know the laws governing the reporting of abuse.

From *Gerontological rehabilitation nursing: Competencies for care* (p. 819), by K. L. Mauk, 2014, Burlington, MA: Jones & Bartlett. Reprinted with permission.

   a. Perform a complete history and physical assessment.
   b. Make certain the explanation fits the injury, realizing that rehabilitating older adults may experience falls as they increase their level of independence.
   c. Be alert to possible signs and symptoms of abuse or neglect.
   d. Interview the suspected abuser and the victim separately.
   e. Consult with available resources as needed (e.g., psychologist, social worker).
   f. Report any suspected case of abuse. This can be done anonymously to an adult protective services office.
   g. Do not alienate the suspected perpetrator.
   h. Take the necessary steps to protect the client.
   i. Maintain confidentiality of conversation and develop client trust.
   j. Home visitation and respite programs may help families develop counseling, support, and social skills for caregivers (Daly, 2010).

E. Polypharmacy
   1. *Polypharmacy* involves the use of multiple medications (e.g., more than five medications) or an inappropriate use of medication (e.g., using

multiple medications to treat the same condition, simultaneous use of medications that cause drug interactions, inappropriate dosage, and medications used to counteract the side effects of other medications.)

a. Older adults commonly take many medications, which can increase the risk of adverse reactions for many reasons (Riker & Setter, 2013).
   1) Drugs are excreted more slowly by the kidneys.
   2) Absorption in the intestines is slower.
   3) Metabolism slows with age.
   4) Physiological changes and multiple comorbidities increase risk for drug reactions and drug–drug interactions (Riker & Setter, 2012).

b. Older adults consume 34% of prescription medications and about 40% of nonprescription medications (American Society of Consultant Pharmacists, 2000). 39% of older adults take five or more medications, and 90% take over-the-counter medications (NICHE, 2012b).

c. The aforementioned factors cause the drugs to remain present in the body for a longer time.

d. Adverse drug reactions may occur at any time, or at a later time than expected with younger adults.

e. Older adults may use over-the-counter medications or herbal therapies they do not consider "drugs," but these substances may interact with other medications.

f. Incidence of polypharmacy is thought to increase with age.

g. Those older than age 85 years are at higher risk because they typically take more medications.

h. Polypharmacy is associated with:
   1) Number and severity of illnesses
   2) Hospitalization
   3) Number of physicians seen
   4) Number of pharmacies used
   5) Advanced client age
   6) May lead to a decreased quality of life (Riker & Setter, 2013).

i. In long-term care facilities, psychotherapeutics are often misused.

j. Interventions to avoid polypharmacy have not been well researched or documented.

2. Nursing interventions

a. Complete medication reconciliation to identify potential medication-related problems including medication errors; identify high-risk medications and adverse events (Pincus, 2013).

b. Avoid unnecessary polypharmacy.
   1) Teach clients and families to use a primary care provider to coordinate care.
   2) Obtain a list of all physicians and pharmacies used.
   3) Check for duplication of medications.
   4) Encourage use of one pharmacy.
   5) Be sure all physicians are informed of all medications prescribed by other physicians.
   6) Use Beer's criteria to review potentially inappropriate medication (Zwicker & Fulmer, 2008).
      a) List of medications to avoid for older adults
      b) Medications should not be taken under certain conditions.
      c) Review the medication list with every visit.
      d) Avoid duplications.
   7) Use the brown bag method of self-reporting to evaluate medication use.
      a) Encourage patient at admission to bring all medications from home.
      b) Document medication types, instructions, dates, and duration of use.
      c) Helps identify multiple prescribers and pharmacies.
      d) Include prescription medications, over-the-counter drugs, herbal remedies, supplements, alcohol, and nicotine use (NICHE, 2012b).
   8) Encourage practitioners to assess the need for every medication. Consider a drug holiday if possible.
   9) Ask about alternative medications and over-the-counter medications.
   10) Encourage the client to use the same source for refills.

c. Avoid negative effects of polypharmacy.
   1) Obtain a comprehensive medication history.
   2) Monitor blood urea nitrogen, creatinine, and creatinine clearance to check kidney function.
   3) Consider the possibility of adverse drug reactions when new symptoms appear (Dean, Harrison, & Zwicker, 2014).
   4) Use or consider use of nonpharmacologic treatment when possible.
   5) Simplify the medication regimen.
   6) Review dietary habits.
   7) Consider effects and interactions of food and medication.

8) Educate family and clients to be informed consumers.
d. Family and client education regarding medication errors
   1) Include the client and the family or caregiver.
   2) Follow the principles of teaching and learning with family members and with the client.
   3) Allow time for demonstration and return demonstration.
   4) Teach more than one family member whenever possible.
   5) Use medication boxes to assist with organization of medications and promote independence of the client when appropriate.
   6) Use large and simple medication lists that are readily accessible.
   7) Use pictures of medications on the list to assist with recognition.
   8) Be sure the client and family understand the purpose of the medication, time to be taken, amount, and route.
   9) Provide written discharge instructions in simple language (fourth-grade level).
   10) Encourage the client to carry a medication list with dosages in his or her wallet.
   11) Encourage the family and client to know medications by name and not by color or size of the medication.
e. Use of medication boxes
   1) Organizes the client's medications
   2) Provides a system to decrease the risk of making medication errors at home
   3) Allows family members to help monitor or set up the client's medications
f. Evaluate the client's ability to self-medicate using the Drug Regimen Unassisted Grading Scale (DRUGS) before discharge from the hospital and periodically.

F. Caregiver Issues

1. Aging caregivers
   a. Many caregivers of older adults are older themselves.
   b. When the caregiver's health is poor, caregiver stress is likely to be higher; older caregivers are more likely to have more chronic illnesses because of their age (Wong & Wallhagen, 2014).
   c. Caregiving may also fill a need for the caregiver (Krieger-Blake, 2006).
2. Caregiver stress: A Japanese study revealed that behavioral, psychological, and functional symptoms of dementia in the form of aggression, screaming, and impaired ability to perform ADLs increase the burden of caregivers (Miyamoto et al., 2010).
   a. Caregiver stress is defined as the emotional burden of caregiving.
   b. The level of dependency on the caregiver increases the amount of stress.
   c. Lack of family support adds to the burden of stress.
   d. The burden of caring can lead to depression, anxiety, difficulty coping, and problems with physical health of the caregiver.
   e. Women are more prone to this problem.
   f. Signs of caregiver stress include the following (U.S. Department of Health and Human Services, 2006):
      1) Sleeping problems
      2) Weight loss or gain
      3) Fatigue
      4) Irritability
      5) Withdrawal
      6) Headaches, stomach upset, or frequent vague physical symptoms
      7) Anxiety
   g. Interventions for reducing caregiver stress and improving quality of life
      1) Obtain respite care as needed.
      2) Get assistance in the home.
      3) Take care of one's own health through diet, daily exercise, and relaxation.
      4) Use community resources (e.g., National Family Caregiver Support Program).
      5) Use faith-based resources if possible.
      6) Attend support groups.
      7) Obtain caregiver training (McCullagh, Brigstocke, Donaldson, & Kalra, 2005).
      8) Caregiver resources: American Association of Retired Persons (AARP) caregiver website, Alzheimer's Association, Administration on Aging website, Red Cross.

G. Postrehabilitation Care

1. Settings for care
   a. Long-term care facilities
      1) Provide a variety of levels of care
      2) May range from independent living to nursing home or skilled care
      3) Costs vary widely but depend largely on geographic location and nature of services needed.
   b. Independent living
      1) Senior living apartment
      2) Private home
      3) Apartment within a long-term care facility

c. Assisted living and personal care
  1) Freestanding facilities
  2) Within a long-term care facility
  3) Group or foster homes
  4) Other community-based homes
  5) Adult day care services (for daytime only, not 24-hour supervision)
d. Nonmedical home care services
  1) Services vary according to the agency.
  2) Private pay for services unless the client financially qualifies for state waiver program.
  3) Many agencies provide companion services that include light housekeeping, meal preparation, and assistance with personal care and ADLs.
  4) If additional in-home therapy or nursing services are needed, investigate the exact nature of services that each agency will render and how expenses are billed.

2. Assist clients and families with postrehabilitation placement.
   a. Address cultural influences.
   b. Realize that people with some cultural backgrounds consider placement in a nursing home to be unacceptable and that other resources must be explored.
   c. Explore cultural norms and influences with the family and client.
3. Help select a facility
   a. Know the options available in the community that coincide with the patient's functional abilities and safety needs.
   b. Obtain information through industry organizations such as the American Health Care Association.
   c. Access facilities' survey histories from the Centers for Medicare & Medicaid Services (formerly the Health Care Financing Administration) or from state health departments.
4. Assist family members with placement decisions. Use appropriate resources such as social services to assist with placement, transfers, and finances.
   a. Provide the family with viable options and lists of community resources.
   b. Use mutual goal-setting techniques.
   c. Consult with the client's case manager or social worker for specific information on area facilities.
   d. Refer the family to information checklists available in the facility or through agencies such as the AARP or the United Way.

H. Funding: Public programs for long-term care needs

1. See Chapter 13 for a discussion of funding and insurance.
2. Medicare Parts A and B (Beam & O'Hare, 2003)
   a. A social insurance program for people age 65 years and older and certain younger people with disabilities and people of all ages with end-stage renal disease (www.longtermcare.gov)
   b. Part A
      1) Hospital insurance
      2) Funds hospital care, skilled nursing facility, hospice, and home healthcare, including mental healthcare (www.medicare.gov)
   c. Part B
      1) Medical insurance
      2) Fees for physicians, surgeons, other healthcare providers, outpatient therapy services
      3) Medical equipment rental
      4) Medical procedures, labs, diagnostics, X-rays, radiation, certain screenings
      5) Monthly premium is paid; usually covers 80% of the Medicare-approved amount
   d. Medicare does not provide for custodial care unless skilled nursing or rehabilitation is also needed.
3. Medicare Part C (Medicare.gov, 2010)
4. Medicare Part D (Medicare.gov, 2006)
   a. Available to anyone with Medicare
   b. Income does not matter.
   c. A prescription drug plan through the federal government
   d. Private companies issue plans through Medicare.
   e. Many different plans in each state
   f. Many different categories from which plans must offer at least two prescription drugs in each category, but plans do not cover all drugs
   g. Nurses can educate older adults to choose the best plan for them.
   h. A monthly premium is paid for the drug plan.
   i. Most plans have an annual deductible before Medicare pays.
   j. Costs to the person range from paying 100% out of pocket for those with low annual drug costs to 5% for those with high costs (e.g., more than $5,100, although this varies by plan).
   k. Financial assistance is available for those with low income; this is called "extra help."
   l. There is no cost containment for these drugs.
5. Medicare Advantage Plan, purchased by individuals to get Medicare benefits through private

companies or groups approved by Medicare; also includes prescription drug coverage
6. Medicaid (Beam & O'Hare, 2003). Medicaid laws change frequently, so these are general guidelines.
   a. State-run program
   b. Largest source of medical care payments for low-income people
   c. Largest payer for nursing home services
   d. About 30 states offer optional personal care services for people to remain in the home.
   e. Individual income must be lower than a designated dollar amount to qualify.
   f. Applicants must pass an asset limitation test (i.e., assets must be spent down).
   g. State may adopt a medically needy program, which may include children younger than 18 years, pregnant women, older adults, or people who are blind or disabled.
7. Veteran's benefits (Beam & O'Hare, 2003)
   a. A potential source of long-term care benefits from a government source
   b. Veterans who satisfy a means test that looks at income and assets may be eligible.
   c. Care is generally provided in Veterans Administration facilities.
   d. Basic health benefits of the Veterans Administration
      1) Prevention and screenings
      2) Primary health care
      3) Diagnosis and treatment
      4) Surgery
      5) Mental health and substance abuse treatment
      6) Urgent care
      7) Medications
      8) Hospice and palliative care
      9) Limited other services such as certain nursing homes and adult day care in some programs
      10) Attendant care program provides personal care services, including bathing, assistance with ADLs, and light housekeeping for veterans who qualify
8. The Older Americans Act is a federal program designed to organize, coordinate, and provide home- and community-based services to older adults and their families to help clients remain in the community as independently as possible.
9. Long-term care insurance
   a. For cost coverage outside a hospital
   b. May cover any or all of the following services (Beam & O'Hare, 2003):
      1) Nursing home
      2) Assisted living
      3) Hospice
      4) Home health
      5) Adult day care
      6) Respite
      7) Caregiver training
      8) Home health coordinators
   c. Premiums (at age 65 years) range from $1,000 to $2,650 per year.
   d. Premiums increase with age.
   e. Benefits include peace of mind, more choices, and preservation of assets (Mauk & Mauk, 2010).
   f. Nurses should always ask whether clients have this type of coverage.

VII. Role of the Advanced Practice Nurse (APN)

A. Clinician
1. According to the American Nurses Credentialing Center (ANCC, 2005), gerontological clinical nurse specialists:
   a. Provide, direct, and influence care of older adults and their families
   b. Work in a variety of settings
   c. Have in-depth knowledge of aging
   d. Have intervention skills focused on health promotion and management of health alterations
   e. Provide comprehensive gerontological services
   f. Engage in practice, research, theory use, collaboration, consultation, and administration
   g. Certification through the ANCC (2010a) earns the gerontological clinical nurse specialist (GCNS-BC) credential
2. Gerontological nurse practitioners (ANCC, 2005)
   a. Are experts in healthcare provision to older adults
   b. Work in a variety of settings, particularly primary care
   c. Practice independently and collaboratively with other healthcare professionals
   d. Maximize clients' functional abilities
   e. Promote, maintain, and restore health
   f. Prevent or minimize disabilities
   g. Promote death with dignity
   h. Engage in case management, education, consultation, research, administration, and advocacy for older adults
   i. Certification through the ANCC (2010b) earns the gerontological nurse practitioner (GNP-BC) credential.
3. Both the GNP-BC and the GCNS-BC credentials and exams are being phased out in favor of adult gerontology certifications and curricula (ANCC, 2014)

4. The certifications being made available now combine adult gerontology and include (ANCC, 2014)
   a. Adult gerontology CNS
   b. Adult gerontology primary NP
   c. Adult gerontology acute NP

B. Educator: The APN in the educator role may work in a variety of settings related to gerontological rehabilitation nursing.
   1. Settings
      a. Rehabilitation unit in acute care hospital
      b. Freestanding rehabilitation facility
      c. Primary care practice in collaboration with physicians
      d. Outpatient clinic
      e. Academic setting or joint appointment collaborative agreement
      f. Private practice as consultant or seminar leader
   2. Target audience
      a. Clients and families
      b. Interdisciplinary staff
      c. Physicians or other APNs
      d. Rehabilitation nurses
         1) Locally
         2) Regionally or nationally as an educational consultant
      e. Nursing students or other students in an academic setting

C. Leader
   1. As a leader, the gerontological rehabilitation nurse may be involved in a variety of organizations relating to both specialties or in organizations dedicated to the advancement of the nursing profession through research.
      a. ARN
      b. American Gerontological Society (interdisciplinary)
      c. The Gerontological Society of America
      d. Association for Geriatrics in Higher Education (interdisciplinary)
      e. National Gerontological Nursing Association
      f. John A. Hartford Institute for Geriatric Nursing (devoted to education of nurses in excellent care of older adults)
      g. Sigma Theta Tau International (international nursing honor society)
   2. As a leader, the gerontological rehabilitation nurse in an advanced practice role may engage in the following activities:
      a. Membership in interdisciplinary care teams
      b. Developing standards of care for the specialty and professions
      c. Developing clinical guidelines
      d. Writing and advocating for certain healthcare policies
      e. Educating and mentoring colleagues in gerontological rehabilitation nursing
      f. Participating in research related to gerontological rehabilitation
      g. Membership in professional organizations

D. Consultant
   1. Legal
      a. Expert opinion
      b. Expert testimony or expert witness
      c. Types of cases commonly include the following:
         1) Elder abuse or neglect
         2) Wrongful death
         3) Malpractice
         4) Other cases related to practice below the appropriate standard of care
      d. Employment as a regular part of a law office
      e. Life care planning (Mauk & Mauk, 2010)
   2. Educational
      a. Through rehabilitation facilities, giving presentations in various locations
      b. Self-employed
      c. Working for others to develop online courses for continuing education, academic credit, or instructional materials for purchase
   3. Clinical
      a. May be combined with other types of consulting, including legal and educational
      b. The expert clinician may be highly sought after as an educator in a variety of settings.
      c. May develop subspecialty in other areas such as wound care or incontinence related to older adults with disabilities
   4. Other (Mauk & Mauk, 2010)
      a. Life care planning
      b. Advocacy
      c. Guardianship

E. Researcher
   1. As researcher, the APN may participate in the following activities:
      a. Clinical expert on an interdisciplinary team
      b. Link to clinical setting for collaborative research with academics
      c. Advocate for using evidence-based practice in long-term care and rehabilitation facilities
      d. Helping develop research agendas for professional organizations
   2. Those prepared at the DNP level also focus on:
      a. Designing and conducting evidence-based practice projects

b. Using existing research to facilitate change on unit and within organizations
c. Acting as a change agent to promote evidence-based practice for populations
d. Publishing and disseminating clinical findings

3. Those prepared at the PhD level also focus on
   a. Designing and conducting original research
   b. Contributing to the development of nursing theory in gerontological rehabilitation
   c. Obtaining funding for research in the field
   d. Publishing findings to be used by others
   e. Disseminating findings through presentations at conferences

References

Adams-Wendling, L., Pimple, C., Adams, S., & Titler, M. (2008). Nursing management of hearing impairment in nursing facility residents. *Journal of Gerontological Nursing 34*(11), 9–17.

Administration on Aging, Department of Health and Human Services. (2012). *A profile of older Americans 2012.* Washington, DC: Author.

Agahi, N., Ahacic, K., & Parker, M. S. (2006). Continuity of leisure participation from middle age to old age. *The Journal of Gerontology, 61B*(6), S340–S346.

Aging with Dignity. (2011). *Five wishes.* Retrieved from www.agingwithdignity.org/five-wishes.php

Alzheimer's Association. (2014). Traumatic brain injury. Retrieved from www.alz.org/dementia/traumatic-brain-injury-head-trauma-symptoms.asp

American Nurses Credentialing Center (ANCC). (2005). Gerontological nurse: Application for ANCC. Retrieved from www.nursingworld.org/ancc

American Nurses Credentialing Center (ANCC). (2010a). Clinical nurse specialist in gerontology. Retrieved from www.nursecredentialing.org/NurseSpecialties/GerontologicalCNS.aspx

American Nurses Credentialing Center (ANCC). (2010b). Gerontological nurse practitioner. Retrieved from www.nursecredentialing.org/NurseSpecialties/GerontologicalNP.aspx

American Nurses Credentialing Center (ANCC). (2014). Certification. Retrieved from www.nursecredentialing.org/GerontologicalNursing

American Society of Consultant Pharmacists. (2000). Senior care pharmacy: The statistics. *Consultant Pharmacist, 15,* 310.

Amtmann, D., Bamer, A. M., Verrall, A., Salem, R., & Borson, S. (2013). Symptom profiles in individuals aging with post-polio syndrome. *Journal of the American Geriatrics Society, 61*(10), 1813–1815.

Antimisiaris, D., & Cheek, D. (2014). Polypharmacy. In K. Mauk (Ed.), *Gerontological nursing: Competencies for care* (pp. 416–454). Burlington, MA: Jones & Bartlett.

Antonelli, M. C., & Starz, T. (2012). Assessing for risk and progression of osteoarthritis: The nurse's role. *American Journal of Nursing, 112*(3), S26–S31.

Anxiety Disorders Association of America. (2006). Anxiety in the elderly. Retrieved from www.adaa.org/GettingHelp/AnxietyDisorders/Elderly.asp

Aptaker, R. L., Roth, E. J., Reichhardt, G., Duerden, M. E., & Levy, C. E. (1994). Serum albumin level as a predictor of geriatric stroke rehabilitation outcome. *Archives of Physical Medicine and Rehabilitation, 75*(1), 80–84.

Asplund, R. (2004). Nocturia, nocturnal polyuria, and sleep quality in the elderly. *Journal of Psychosomatic Research, 56*(5), 511–525.

Association of Rehabilitation Nurses (ARN). (2014). ARN competency model for professional rehabilitation nursing. Retrieved from http://www.rehabnurse.org/uploads/files/education/ARN_Rehabilitation_Nursing_Competency _Model_FINAL_-_May_2014.pdf

Awad, N., Gagnon, M., & Messier, C. (2004). The relationship between impaired glucose tolerance, Type 2 diabetes and cognitive function. *Journal of Clinical and Experimental Neuropsychology, 8,* 1044–1080.

Bagg, S., Pombo, A. P., & Hopman, W. (2002). Effect of age on functional outcomes after stroke rehabilitation. *Stroke, 33,* 179–185.

Baltes, P. B. (1987). Theoretical propositions of life-span developmental psychology: On the dynamics between growth and decline. *Developmental Psychology, 23,* 611–626.

Baltes, P. B., & Baltes, M. M. (1990). Psychological perspectives on successful aging: The model of selective optimization with compensation. In P. B. Baltes & M. M. Baltes (Eds.), *Successful aging: Perspectives from the behavioral sciences* (pp. 1–34). New York: Cambridge University Press.

Bandeen-Roche, K., Xue, Q. L., Ferrucci, L., Walston, J., Guralnik, J. M., Chaves, P., . . . Fired, L. P. (2006). Phenotype of frailty: Characterization in the Women's Health and Aging Studies. *Journals of Gerontology Series A: Biological Sciences and Medical Sciences, 61,* 262–266.

Beam, B. T., & O'Hare, T. P. (2003). *Meeting the financial need of long-term care.* Bryn Mawr, PA: The American College.

Beaupre, L. A., Cinats, J. G., Senthilselvan, A., Scharfenberger, A., Johnston, D. W., & Saunders, L. D. (2005). Does standardized rehabilitation and discharge planning improve functional recovery in elderly patients with hip fracture? *Archives of Physical Medicine and Rehabilitation, 86,* 2231–2239.

Beers, M., & Berkow, R. (Eds.). (n.d.). *The Merck manual of geriatrics* (Internet ed.). Whitehouse Station, NJ: Merck & Company, Inc. and Medical Services USMEDSA, USHH. Retrieved from www.merck.com/mrkshared/mm_geriatrics/home.jsp

Benton, M., Whyte, M., & Dyal, B. (2011). Sarcopenic obesity: Strategies for management. *American Journal of Nursing, 111*(12), 38–44.

Blais, K., & Ballinger, N. (2014). Teaching older adults and their families. In K.L. Mauk. (Ed.), *Gerontological nursing: Competencies for care* (pp. 123–148). Burlington, MA: Jones & Bartlett.

Bond, M. C., & Butler, K. H. (2013). Elder abuse and neglect: Definitions, epidemiology, and approaches to emergency department screening. *Clinics of Geriatric Medicine, 29*(1), 257–273.

Brei, T., & Merkens, M. (2003). Challenging issues in care for adolescence and adults living with spina bifida. Retrieved from www.spinabifidasupport.com/adultsbhealthcare.htm

Brenner, L. A., Homaifar, B. Y., & Schultheis, M. (2008). Driving, aging and traumatic brain injury: Integrating findings from the literature. *Rehabilitation Psychology, 53*(1), 18–27.

Brown, R., Taylor, J., & Matthews, B. (2001). Quality of life: Ageing and Down syndrome. *Down Syndrome Research and Practices, 6*(3), 111–116.

Bruno, R. L., Cohen, J. M., Galski, T., & Frick, N. M. (n.d.). The neuroanatomy of post-polio fatigue. Retrieved from www.ott.zynet.co.uk/polio/lincolnshire/library.html

Buhler, C. (1933). *Der menschliche Lebenslauf als psychologisches Problem* [Human life as a psychological problem]. Oxford, England: Hirzel.

Burnett, J., Carmel, B., Halphen, J. M., Achenbaum, W. A., Green, C. E. , Booker, J. G., & Diamond, P. M. (2014). Four subtypes of self-neglect in older adults: Results of a latent class analysis. *Journal of the American Geriatrics Society, 62*(6), 1127–1132.

Byock, I. (1997). *Dying well.* New York: Free Press.

Cacchione, P. (2014). Sensory impairment: A new research imperative. *Journal of Gerontological Nursing, 40*(4), 3–5.

Center for Home Care Policy and Research. (2009). *Palliative care and advanced illness management: Evidence brief, CHAMP—Advancing home health care excellence for older people.* April 2009, Series C, Report 7, pp. 1–8.

Centers for Disease Control and Prevention (CDC). (2003). Public health and aging: Non-fatal fall-related traumatic brain injury among older adults: California 1996–1999. *MMWR Weekly, 52,* 276–278.

Centers for Disease Control and Prevention (CDC). (2009). Caregiving resources. Retrieved from www.cdc.gov/aging/caregiving/resources.htm

Centers for Disease Control and Prevention (CDC). (2011). National diabetes fact sheet, *2011.* Retrieved from www.cdc.gov/diabetes/pubs/pdf/ndfs_2011.pdf

Centers for Disease Control and Prevention (CDC). (2013a). Falls among older adults: An overview. Retrieved from www.cdc.gov/homeandrecreationalsafety/falls/adultfalls.html

Centers for Disease Control and Prevention (CDC). (2013b). Hip fractures among older adults. Retrieved from www.cdc.gov/homeandrecreationalsafety/falls/adulthipfx.html

Centers for Disease Control and Prevention (CDC). (2014). What vaccinations are for you? Retrieved from www.cdc.gov/vaccines/adults/rec-vac/

Centers for Disease Control and Prevention (CDC). (2015). *Recommended immunizations for adults: By age.* Retrieved from http://www.cdc.gov/vaccines/schedules/downloads/adult/adult-schedule-easy-read.pdf

Charles, C. V., & Lehman, C. A. (2006). Medications and laboratory values. In K. Mauk (Ed.), *Gerontological nursing: Competencies for care* (pp. 293–320). Sudbury, MA: Jones & Bartlett.

Chen, H. (2006). *Down syndrome.* Retrieved from www.emedicine.com/ped/topic615.htm

Cohen-Mansfield, J., Thein, K., Marx, M. S., & Dakheel-Ali, M. (2012). What are the barriers to performing non-pharmacological interventions for behavioral symptoms in the nursing home? *Journal of the American Medical Directors Association, 3,* 400–405.

Cohen-Mansfield, J., Thien, K., Marx, M. S., & Dakheel-Ali, M. (2014). Recognition and treatment of post-menopausal osteoporosis. *Journal of Gerontological Nursing, 40*(3), 10–14.

Colantonio, A., Ratcliff, G., Chase, S., & Vernich, L. (2004). Aging with traumatic brain injury: Long-term health conditions. *International Journal of Rehabilitation Research, 27*(3), 209–214.

Crogan, N. L. (2014). Dysphagia and malnutrition. In K. Mauk (Ed.), *Gerontological nursing: Competencies for care* (pp. 620–646). Burlington, MA: Jones & Bartlett.

Cumming, E., & Henry, W. (1961). *Growing old.* New York: Basic Books.

Daly, J. M. (2010). Evidence-based practice guidelines: Elder abuse prevention. *Journal of Gerontological Nursing, 37*(11), 11–17.

Dean, M., Harrison, B., & Zwicker, D. (2014). Falls in older adults. In K. L. Mauk (Ed.) *Gerontological Nursing: Competencies for Care* (pp. 456–480). Burlington, MA: Jones and Bartlett.

DeCalmer, P., & Glendenning, F. (Eds.). (1993). *The mistreatment of the elderly people.* London: Sage.

Dennis, M., Nelson, R., Jewell, D., & Fletcher, J. M. (2010). Prospective memory in adults with spina bifida. *Child's Nervous System, 26*(12), 749–755.

DeVivo, M. J. (2004). Aging with a neurodisability: Morbidity and life expectancy issues. *NeuroRehabilitation, 19,* 1–2.

DiBello, K., & Coyne, N. (2014). Palliative care hits a triple win: Access, quality, and cost. *Home Healthcare Nurse, 32*(3), 183–190.

Digiovanna, A. G. (2000). *Human aging: Biological perspectives* (3rd ed.). Boston: McGraw-Hill.

DiMaria-Ghalili, R. A. (2008). Nursing standard of practice protocol: Nutrition in aging. Retrieved from http://consultgerirn.org/topics/nutrition_in_the_elderly/want_to_know_more

Dolbow, D. R., Gorgey, A. S., Daniels, J. A., Adler, R. A., Moore, J. R., & Gater, D. R. (2011). The effects of spinal cord injury and exercise on bone mass: A literature review. *Neurorehabilitation, 29*(3), 261–269.

Dowling-Castronovo, A., & Bradway, C. (2008). Nursing standard of practice protocol: Urinary incontinence (UI) in older adults admitted to acute care. Retrieved from http://consultgerirn.org/topics/urinary_incontinence/want_to_know_more

Dowling-Castronovo, A., & Spiro, E. L. (2013). Urinary incontinence assessment in older adults. Retrieved from http://consultgerirn.org/uploads/File/trythis/try_this_11_2.pdf

Dugger, B. R., & Cochran, A. (2014). Urinary incontinence. In K. Mauk (Ed.), *Gerontological nursing: Competencies for care* (pp. 544–579). Burlington, MA: Jones & Bartlett.

Ellenbecker, C. H., Frazier, S. C., & Verney, S. (2004). Nurses' observations and experiences of problems and adverse effects of medication management in home care. *Geriatric Nursing, 25*(3), 164–170.

End of Life Nursing Education Consortium. (2004). *ELNEC curriculum.* Princeton, NJ: Robert Woods Johnson Foundation and City of Hope.

Eves, F., & Rivera, N. (2010). Prevention of UTIs in SCI in home health. *Home Healthcare Nurse, 28*(4), 230–241.

Farrell, V. M., Hill, V. L., Hawkins, J. B., Newman, L. M., & Learned, R. E., Jr. (2003). Clinic for identifying and addressing polypharmacy. *American Journal of Health-System Pharmacy, 60*(18), 1834–1835.

Fattal, C. (2014). Rotator cuff surgery in persons with spinal cord injury: relevance of a multidisciplinary approach. *Journal of Shoulder Elbow Surgery, 23,*1263-71.

Ferrari, A., Radaelli, A., & Centola, M. (2003). Invited review: Aging and the cardiovascular system. *Journal of Applied Physiology, 95*(6), 2591–2597.

Finlayson, M., Van Denend, T., & Hudson, E. (2004). Aging with multiple sclerosis. *Journal of Neuroscience Nursing, 26,* 245–248.

Fitzsimmons, S., Barba, B., Stump, M., & Bonner, A. (2014). Non-pharmacological interventions in long term care feasibility and recent trends. *Journal of Gerontological Nursing, 40*(5), 10–14.

Frances, D. (2005). Iatrogenesis. Retrieved from http://consultgerirn.org/topics/iatrogenesis/want_to_know_more

Freedman, V. A. (2014). Research gaps in the demography of aging with disability. *Disability Health Journal, 7*(1 Suppl), S60–S63.

Fried, L. P., Ferrucci, L., Darer, J., Williamson, J. D., & Anderson, G. (2004). Untangling the concepts of disability, frailty, and comorbidity: Implications for improved targeting and care. *Journals of Gerontology. Series A, Biological Sciences and Medical Sciences, 59A,* 255–263.

Furusawa, K., Tokuhiro, A., Tajima, F., Uchida, R., Tominaga, T., Tamaka, H., . . . Sumida, M. (2011). Effect of age of bowel management in traumatic central cord syndrome. *Spinal Cord, 50*(1), 51–56.

Geriatric Mental Health Foundation. (2014). Late life depression. Retrieved from www.gmhfonline.org/gmhf/consumer/factsheets/depression_factsheet.html

Gray-Micelli, D. (2008). Falls: Nursing standard of practice protocol: Fall prevention. Retrieved from http://consultgerirn.org/topics/falls/want_to_know_more

Greenberg, S. (2009). *A profile of older Americans: 2009.* Washington, DC: Administration on Aging, U.S. Department of Health and Human Services.

Haber, D. (2014). Promoting healthy aging. In K. Mauk (Ed.), *Gerontological nursing: Competencies for care* (pp. 187–222). Burlington, MA: Jones & Bartlett.

Hafez, B., & Hafez, E. (2004). Andropause: Endocrinology, erectile dysfunction, and prostate pathophysiology. *Archives of Andrology, 50,* 45–68.

Hall, J. (2004). Neuroendocrine physiology of the early and late menopause. *Endocrinology and Metabolism Clinics of North America, 33*(4), 637–659.

Hall, J. (2007). Neuroendocrine changes with reproductive aging in women. *Seminars in Reproductive Medicine, 25,* 344–356.

Hanks-Bell, M., Halvey, K., & Paice, J. (2004). Pain assessment and management in aging. *Online Journal of Issues in Nursing, 40*(4), 3–5.

Hardin, S. (2010). Anemia of chronic disease, older adults, and medicine. *Journal of Gerontological Nursing, 36*(10), 3–4.

Harlow, R. E., & Cantor, N. (1996). Still participating after all these years: A study of life task participation in later life. *Journal of Personality and Social Psychology, 71,* 1235–1249.

Havighurst, R. J., Neugarten, B. L., & Tobin, S. S. (1963). Disengagement, personality and life satisfaction in the later years. In P. Hansen (Ed.), *Age with a future* (pp. 419–425). Copenhagen, Denmark: Munksgaard.

Havighurst, R. J., Neugarten, B. L., & Tobin, S. S. (1968). Disengagement and patterns of aging. In B. L. Neugarten (Ed.), *Middle age and aging* (pp. 67–71). Chicago: University Press.

Hawkins, K., Musich, S., Bottone, F. G. Jr., Ozminkowski, R. J., Cheng, Y., Rush, S., . . . Yeh, C. S. (2013). Impact of pain on physical and mental quality of life in adults 65 and older. *Journal of Gerontological Nursing, 39*(6), 32–44.

Heineman, J. M., Hamrick-King, J., & Scaglione Sewell, B. (2014). Review of the aging of physiological systems. In K. Mauk (Ed.), *Gerontological nursing: Competencies for care* (e-chapter). Burlington, MA: Jones & Bartlett.

Hershkovitz, A., Kalandariov, Z., Hermush, V., Weiss, R., & Brill, S. (2007). Factors affecting short-term rehabilitation outcomes of disabled elderly patients with proximal hip fracture. *Archives of Physical Medicine and Rehabilitation, 88*(7), 916–921.

Hitzig, S. L., Eng, J. J., Miller, W. C., Sakakibara, B. M., & SCIRE Research Team. (2011). An evidence-based review of aging of the body systems following spinal cord injury. *Spinal Cord, 49*(6), 684–701.

Holland, T., & Benton, M. (2004). Ageing and its consequences for people with Down's syndrome: A guide for parents and carers. Retrieved from www.downs-syndrome.org.uk/component/content/article/28-medical-and-health/250-ageing-and-its-consequences-for-people-with-downs-syndrome.html

Inouye, S. K. (2006). Delirium in older persons. *New England Journal of Medicine, 354,* 1157–1165.

Inouye, S. K., Foreman, M. D., Mion, L. C., Katz, K. H., & Cooney, L. M. (2001). Nurses' recognition of delirium and its symptoms: Comparison of nurse and researcher ratings. *Archives of Internal Medicine, 161*(20), 2467–2473.

Institute of Medicine. (2000). Overview: Nutritional health in the older person. In *The role of nutrition in maintaining health in the nation's elderly: Evaluating coverage of nutrition services for the Medicare population.* Retrieved from http://fermat.nap.edu/books/0309068460/html/46.html

The Internet Stroke Center. (2014). *Stroke statistics.* Retrieved from www.strokecenter.org/patients/about-stroke/stroke-statistics/

Jackson, G., & Owsley, C. (2003). Visual dysfunction, neurodegenerative diseases, and aging. *Neurology Clinics of North America, 21,* 709–728.

Jasien, J., Daimon, C. M., Maudsley, S., Shapiro, B. K., & Martin, B. (2012). Aging and bone health in individuals with developmental disabilities. *International Journal of Endocrinology, 2012*(2012).

Jensen, M. P., Alschuler, K. W., Smith, A. E., Verrall, A. M., Goetz, M. C., & Molton, I. R. (2011). Pain and fatigue in persons with post-polio syndrome: Independent effects on functioning. *Archives of Physical Medicine and Rehabilitation, 92*(11), 1796–1801.

Jensen, M. P., Molton, I. R., Grouh, S. L., Campbell, M. L., Charliful, S., Chiodo, A., . . . Tate, D. (2012). Secondary health conditions in individuals aging with SCI: Terminology, concepts, and analytic approach. *Spinal Cord, 50*(5), 373–378.

Jett, K. (2008). Physiological changes with aging. In P. Ebersole, P. Hess, T. Touhy, K. Jett, & A. Luggen (Eds.), *Toward healthy aging: Human needs and nursing response* (7th ed., pp. 65–87). St. Louis: Mosby Elsevier.

Johnson, K. L., Brown, P. A., & Knaster, E. S. (2010). Aging with disability in the workplace. *Physical Medicine and Rehabilitation Clinics of North America, 21*(2), 267–279.

Jung, C. G. (1960). The structure and dynamics of the psyche. In *Collected works* (Vol. VIII). Oxford, England: Pantheon.

Kailes, J. I. (2002). *Aging with disability.* Retrieved from www.jik.com/awdrtcawd.html

Kemp, B. J., & Mosqueda, L. (2004). Introduction. In *Aging with a disability: What the clinician needs to know.* Baltimore: Johns Hopkins University Press.

Klingbiel, H., Baer, H. R., & Wilson, P. E. (2004). Aging with a disability. *Archives of Physical Medicine and Rehabilitation, 85*(93), S68–S73.

Krauss Whitbourne, S. (2002). *The aging individual: Physical and psychological perspectives* (2nd ed.). New York: Springer.

Kresevic, D. M. (2012). Function: Nursing standard of practice protocol: Assessment of function in acute care. Retrieved from http://consultgerirn.org/topics/function/want_to_know_ Krieger-Blake, L. S. (2006). Changes that affect independence in later life. In K. Mauk (Ed.), *Gerontological nursing: Competencies for care* (pp. 321–354). Sudbury, MA: Jones & Bartlett.

Krinsky-McHale, S. J., & Silverman, W. (2013). Dementia and mild cognitive impairment in adults with intellectual disability issues of diagnosis. *Developmental Disability Research Review, 18*(1), 31–42.

Kurlowicz, L. H., & Harvath, T. A. (2008). *Nursing standard of practice protocol: Depression.* Retrieved from http://consultgerirn.org/topics/depression/want_to_know_more

Labson, M., Sacco, M., Weissman, D., Gornet, E., & Stuart, B. (2013). Innovative models of home-based palliative care. *Cleveland Clinic Journal of Medicine, 80*(electronic suppl 1), eS30–eS35.

Laffont, I., Julia, M., Tiffreau, V., Yelnik, A., Herisson, C., & Pelissier, J. (2010). Aging and sequelae of poliomyelitis. *Annals of Physical Medicine, 53*(1), 24–33.

Lange, J., & Grossman, S. (2014). Theories of aging. In K. L. Mauk (Ed.), *Gerontological nursing: Competencies for care* (pp. 62–94). Burlington, MA: Jones & Bartlett.

LaPlante, M. P. (2014). Key goals and indicators for successful aging of adults with early-onset disability. *Disability Health Journal, 7*(1 suppl), S44–S50.

Lau, D. T., & Kirby, J. B. (2009). The relation between living arrangement and preventive care among community dwelling elderly person. *American Journal of Public Health, 99*(7), 1315–1321.

LaVela, S. L., Evans, C. T., Prohaska, T. R., Miskevics, S., Ganesh, S. P., & Weaver, F. M. (2012). Males aging with a spinal cord injury: Prevalence of cardiovascular and metabolic conditions. *Archives of Physical Medicine and Rehabilitation, 23*(1), 90–95.

LeBlanc, J., de Guise, E., Gosselin, N., & Feyz, M. (2006). Comparison of functional outcome following acute care in young, middle-aged and elderly patients with traumatic brain injury. *Brain Injury, 20*(8), 779–790.

Lemon, B. W., Bengston, V. L., & Peterson, J. A. (1972). An exploration of the activity theory of aging: Activity types and life satisfaction among in-movers to a retirement community. *Journal of Gerontology, 27,* 511–523.

Liptak, G. S., Garver, K., & Dosa, N. P. (2013). Spina bifida grown up. *Journal of Developmental Behavioral Pediatrics, 34*(3), 206–215.

Lochner, M., & Byrd, L. (2014). Anxiety & depression in the older adult. In K. Mauk (Ed.), *Gerontological nursing: Competencies for care* (pp. 512–542). Burlington, MA: Jones & Bartlett.

Mahon, M. M. (2010). Advance care decision making: Asking the right people the right question. *Journal of Psychosocial Nursing, 48,* 7.

Marcum, Z. A., Amuan, M. E., Hanlon, J. T., Aspinall, S. L. Handler, S. M., Ruby, C. M. M., & Pugh, M. J. (2012). Prevalence of unplanned hospitalizations caused by adverse drug reactions in older veterans. *Journal of the American Geriatric Society, 60*(1), 34–41.

Marrone, R. (1997). *Death, mourning & caring.* Philadelphia: Wadsworth.

Maslow, A. H. (1954). *Motivation and personality.* New York: Harper & Row.

Mast, B. T., MacNeill, S. E., & Lichtenberg, P. A. (1999). Gero-psychological problems in medical rehabilitation: Dementia and depression among stroke and lower extremity fracture patients. *Journals of Gerontology: Biological Sciences and Medical Sciences, 54,* M607–M612.

Mauk, J. M., & Mauk, K. L. (2010). Future trends in gerontological nursing. In K. Mauk (Ed.), *Gerontological nursing: Competencies for care* (pp. 782–795). Sudbury, MA: Jones & Bartlett.

Mauk, K. L., & Urban, K. (2014) Abuse and mistreatment of older adults. In K. L. Mauk, (Ed.) *Gerontological nursing: Competencies for care* (pp. 811–830). Burlington, MA: Jones & Bartlett.

Mauk, K. L., Hanson, P., & Hain, J. (2014). Management of common illnesses, diseases, and health conditions. In K. L. Mauk (Ed.), *Gerontological nursing: Competencies for care* (pp. 270–376). Burlington, MA: Jones & Bartlett.

McCullagh, E., Brigstocke, G., Donaldson, N., & Kalra, L. (2005). Determinants of caregiving burden and quality of life in caregivers of stroke patients. *Stroke, 36,* 2181. Retrieved from http://stroke.ahajournals.org/cgi/content/abstract/strokeaha;36/10/2181

McKay, S., Fravel, M., & Scanlon, C. (2012). Management of constipation. *Journal of Gerontological Nursing, 38*(7), 9–15.

McKinnis, E. A. (2002). Dyspnea and other respiratory symptoms. In B. M. Kingbrunner, J. J. Weinreb, & J. S. Pliczer (Eds.), *Twenty common problems in end-of-life care* (pp. 147–162). New York: McGraw-Hill.

Medicare.gov. (2006). Medicare prescription drug coverage. Retrieved from www.medicare.gov/publications/pub/pdf/11109.pdf

Medicare.gov. (2010). Medicare Advantage (Part C). Retrieved from www.medicare.gov/navigation/medicare-basics/medicare-benefits/part-c.aspx

Menter, R. (1998). Aging with spinal cord injury. Retrieved from www.thecni.org/reviews/09-1-p16-menter.htm

Mentes, J., & Kang, S. (2013). Hydration management. *Journal of Gerontological Nursing, 39*(2), 11–19.

Menzel, J. C. (2008). Depression in the elderly after traumatic brain injury: A systematic review. *Brain Injury, 22*(5), 375–380.

Merck Manuals Online Medical Library. (2003). Aging body. Retrieved from www.merckmanuals.com/home/sec26/ch327/ch327a.html

Merck Manual: Home Health Handbook. (2008). Suicidal behavior. Retrieved from www.merckmanuals.com/home/mental_health_disorder/suicidal_behavior/suicidal_behavior.html

Meyer, C. (2001). Allow natural death: An alternative to DNR? Retrieved from www.hospicepatients.org/and.html

Minaker, K. (2004). Common clinical sequelae of aging. In L. Goldman & D. Ausiello (Eds.), *Cecil textbook of medicine* (22nd ed., pp. 105–111). Philadelphia: W. B. Saunders.

Miyamoto, Y., Tachimori, H., & Ito, H. (2010). Formal caregiver burden in dementia: Impact of behavior and psychological symptoms of dementia and activities of daily living. *Geriatric Nursing, 31*(4), 246–253.

Molton, I. R., Terrill, A. L., Smith, A. E., Yorkston, K. M., Alschuler, K. N., Ehde, D. M., & Jensen, M. P. (2014). Modeling secondary health conditions in adults aging with physical disability. *Journal of Aging Health, 26*(3), 335–359. doi: 10.1177/0898264313516166. Epub 2014 Jan 3.

Monda, M. K., Goldberg, A., Smitham, P., Thornton, M., & McCarthy, I. (2013). Use of inertial measurement units to assess age-related changes in gait kinematics in an active population. *Journal of Aging and Physical Activity, 21*(4).

Morgan, P., & McGinley, J. (2014). Gait function and decline in adults with cerebral palsy: A systematic review. *Disability Rehabilitation, 36*(1), 1–9.

Muché, J. A., & McCarty, S. (2009). Geriatric rehabilitation. Retrieved from http://emedicine.medscape.com/article/318521-overview

Muñiz, F. M. (2011). Postpolio syndrome. Retrieved from http://emedicine.medscape.com/article/306920-overview#showall

National Center on Elder Abuse. (2006). *Elder abuse prevalence and incidence.* Fact sheet. Washington, DC: Author.

National Hospice and Palliative Care Organization. (2004). *Keys to quality care.* Retrieved from http://nhpco.org/i4a/pages/index.cfm?pageid=3303

National Institute of Mental Health (NIMH). (2006). Depression and suicide facts. Retrieved from www.nimh.nih.gov/publicat/elderlydepsuicide.cfm

National Institute of Neurological Disorders and Stroke (NINDS). (2006a). Cerebral palsy: Hope through research. Retrieved from www.ninds.nih.gov/disorders/cerebral_palsy/detail_cerebral_palsy.htm

National Institute of Neurological Disorders and Stroke (NINDS). (2006b). *Post-polio syndrome fact sheet.* Retrieved from www.ninds.nih.gov/disorders/post_polio/detail_post_polio.htm

National Institute of Neurological Disorders and Stroke (NINDS). (2014). *NINDS Parkinson's disease 2014 research recommendations.* Retrieved from www.ninds.nih.gov/research/parkinsonsweb/PD2014/2014-NINDS-PD-Recommendations.htm

National Institute of Neurological Disorders and Stroke (NINDS). (2015). *NINDS Parkinson's disease information page.* Retrieved from http://www.ninds.nih.gov/disorders/parkinsons_disease/parkinsons_disease.htm

Nelson, J. M. (2014). Identifying and preventing common risk factors in the elderly. In K. Mauk (Ed.), *Gerontological nursing: Competencies for care* (pp. 222–265). Burlington, MA: Jones & Bartlett.

Nicosia, F. B., Bonnetti, F., Ghisla, M. K., Cossi, S., Romanelli, G., & Marengoni, A. (2012). Predictors of survival within 2 years of inpatient rehabilitation among older adults. *European Journal of Internal Medicine, 23*(6), 519–523.

Nilsson-Ehle, H., Jagenburg, R., Landahl, S., & Svanborg, A. (2000). Blood haemoglobin declines in the elderly: Implications for reference intervals from age 70 to 88. *European Journal of Haematology, 65*(5), 297–305.

Nurses Improving Care for Healthsystem Elders (NICHE). (2012a). Geriatric resource nurse module 2: Age related changes in health. NICHE GRN core curriculum. (4th ed.)Retrieved from http://elearningcenter.nicheprogram.org.

Nurses Improving Care for Healthsystem Elders (NICHE). (2012b). Geriatric resource nurse module 8: Medications. NICHE GRN core curriculum. (4th ed.) Retrieved from http://elearningcenter.nicheprogram.org.

Ostir, G. V., Ottenbacher, K. J., & Markides, K. S. (2004). Onset of frailty in older adults and the protective role of positive affect. *Psychology and Aging.* Retrieved from www.apa.org/pubs/journals/releases/pag-193402.pdf

Ostwald, S., Wasserman, J., & Davis, S. (2006). Medications, comorbidities and complications in stroke survivors: The CAReS study. *Rehabilitation Nursing, 31,* 10–14.

Pace, B., Burke, A. E., & Glass, R. M. (2006). *JAMA* patient page. Hospice care. *JAMA, 295*(6), 712.

Pastor, D., & Moore, G. (2013). Uncertainties of the heart: Palliative care and adult heart failure. *Home Healthcare Nurse, 31*(1), 29–36.

Paterson, D. H., & Warburton, D. E. R. (2010). Physical activity and functional limitations in older adults: A systematic review related to Canada's Physical Activity Guidelines. *International Journal of Behavioral Nutrition and Physical Activity, 7*(38). doi:10.1186/1479-5868-7-38

Patrick, L., Knoefel, F., Gaskowsk, P., & Rexrath, D. (2001). Medical comorbidity and rehabilitation efficiency in geriatric patients. *Journal of the American Geriatrics Society, 49,* 1471–1477.

Pereira, A. (2012). Legalizing euthanasia or assisted suicide: The illusion of safeguards and controls. *Current Oncology 19*(3), e227.

Peters, A. (2002). The effects of normal aging on myelin and nerve fibers: A review. *Journal of Neurocytology, 31,* 581–593.

Peterson, M. D., Gordon, P. M., & Hurvitz, E. A. (2013). Chronic disease risk among adults with sarcopenia, obesity, and sedentary behavior. *Obesity Review, 14*(2), 171–182.

Pincus, K. (2013). Transitional care management services: Optimizing medication reconciliation to improve the care of older adults. *Journal of Gerontological Nursing, 39*(10), 10–15.

Potera, C., & Pfeifer, G. (2014). Newscap: Nurses are still using physical restraints to ensure safety in elder care. *American Journal of Nursing, 114*(1), 15.

Pritchard, J. (1995). *The abuse of older people: A training manual for detection and prevention.* London: Jessica Kingsley Publishers.

Pritchard, J. (1996). Darkness visible: Elder abuse. *Nursing Times, 92*(42), 26–31.

Pugh, K., & Wei, J. (2001). Clinical implications of physiological changes in the aging heart. *Drugs & Aging, 18*(4), 263–276.

Rees, T., Duckert, L., & Carey, J. (1999). Auditory and vestibular dysfunction. In W. Hazzard, J. Blass, W. Ettinger Jr., J. Halter, & J. Ouslander (Eds.), *Principles of geriatric medicine and gerontology* (4th ed., pp. 617–632). New York: McGraw-Hill.

Riker, G., & Setter, S. (2012). Polypharmacy in older adults at home: What it is and what to do about it. Implications for home healthcare and hospice: Part 1. *Home Healthcare Nurse, 30*(8), 474–485.

Riker, G., & Setter, S. (2013). Polypharmacy in older adults at home: What it is and what to do about it. Implications for home healthcare and hospice: Part 2. *Home Healthcare Nurse, 31*(2), 77–79.

Rincus, K. (2013). Transitional care management services: Optimizing medication reconciliation to improve the care of older adults. *Journal of Gerontological Nursing, 39*(10), 10–15.

Riquelme, I., Cifre, I., & Montoya, P. (2011). Age-related changes in pain experience in cerebral palsy and healthy individuals. *Pain Medicine, 12*(4), 535–545.

Rockwood, K., Mitniski, A., Song, X., Steen, B., & Skoog, I. (2006). Long-term risks of death and institutionalization of elderly people in relation to deficit accumulation at age 70. *Journal of the American Geriatrics Society, 54,* 975–979.

Rodakowski, J., Skidmore, E. R., Anderson, S. J., Begley, A., Jensen, M. P., Buhule, O. D., & Boninger, M. L. (2014). Additive effects of age on disability for individuals with spinal cord injuries. *Archives of Physical Medicine and Rehabilitation, 95*(6), 1076–1082.

Rose, S. S. (2014). Delirium. In K. Mauk (Ed.), *Gerontological nursing: Competencies for care* (pp. 482–511). Burlington, MA: Jones & Bartlett.

Schroots, J. J. F. (1996). Theoretical developments in the psychology of aging. *Gerontologist, 36,* 742–748.

Schwartzkopf, C. E., & Twigg, P. (2014). Nursing management of dementia. In K. Mauk (Ed.), *Gerontological nursing: Competencies for care* (pp. 376–454). Burlington, MA: Jones & Bartlett.

Scivoletto, G., Morganti, B., Ditunno, P., Ditunno, J. F., & Molinari, M. (2003). Effects of age on spinal cord lesion patients' rehabilitation. *Spinal Cord, 41,* 457–464.

Seiberling, K., & Conley, D. (2004). Aging and olfactory and taste function. *Otolaryngologic Clinics of North America, 37*(6), 1209–1228.

Sherrington, C., Whitney, J. C., Lord, S. R., Herbert, P. D., Cummings, R. E., & Close, J. C. (2008). Effective exercise for the prevention of falls: A systematic review and meta-analysis. *Journal of the American Geriatrics Society, 56*(12), 2234–2243.

Smith, C., & Cotter, V. (2012). *Geriatric nursing protocol: Age-related changes in health.* New York: Hartford Institute for Geriatric Nursing. Retrieved from http://consultgerirn.org/

Soares-Miranda, L., Sattelmair, J., Chaves, P., Duncan, G. E., Siscovick, D. S., Stein, P. K., & Mozaffarian, D. (2014). Physical activity and heart rate variability in older adults: The cardiovascular health study. *Circulation, 129*(27), 2100–2010.

Spalding, M. C., & Sebesta, S. C. (2008). Geriatric screening and preventive care. *American Family Physician, 78*(2), 206–215.

Stagnetti, M. N. (2009). Average number of total and unique prescription by select person characteristics, 2006. Retrieved from http://meps.ahrq.gov/mepsweb/data_files/publications/st245/stat245.pdf

Strauss, D., Ojdana, K., Shavelle, R., & Rosenbloom, L. (2004). Decline in function and life expectancy of older persons with cerebral palsy. *Neurorehabilitation, 19,* 69–78.

Strax, T. E., Luciano, L., Dunn, A. M., & Guevedo, J. P. (2010). Aging and developmental disability. *Physical Medicine and Rehabilitation Clinics of North America, 21*(2), 419–427.

Thompson, H. J., McCormick, W. C., & Kagan, S. H. (2006). Traumatic brain injury in older adults: Epidemiology, outcomes and future implications. *Journal of the American Geriatrics Society, 54,* 1590–1595.

Tinetti, M. E., Williams, C. S., & Gill, T. M. (2000). Dizziness among older adults: A possible geriatric syndrome. *Annals of Internal Medicine, 132,* 337–344.

Tornstam, L. (1994). Gerotranscendence: A theoretical and empirical exploration. In L. E. Thomas & S. A. Eisenhandler (Eds.), *Aging and the religious dimension* (pp. 203–226). Westport, CT: Greenwood.

Tornstam, L. (2011). Maturing into gerotranscendence. *Journal of Transpersonal Psychology, 43*(2), 166–180.

Tullmann, D. F., Fletcher, K., & Foreman, M. D. (2012). Delirium nursing standard of practice protocol: Delirium: Prevention, early recognition, and treatment. Retrieved from http://consultgerirn.org/topics/delirium/want_to_know_more

Uguz, F., Kayurak, M., Cicek, E., Kayhan, F., Ari, H., & Altunbas, G. (2010). Delirium following acute myocardial infarction: Incidence, clinical profiles, and predictors. *Perspectives in Psychiatric Care, 46*(2), 135–142.

U.S. Department of Health and Human Services. (2006). Caregiver stress. Retrieved from www.womenshealth.gov/publications/our-publications/fact-sheet/caregiver-stress.cfm

U.S. Preventive Services Task Force (USPSTF). (2012). Focus on older adults. Retrieved from www.uspreventiveservicestaskforce.org/tfolderfocus.htm

Vaillant, G. (2002). *Aging well.* Boston: Little, Brown.

van der Woude, L. H., deGroot, S., Postema, K., Bussman, J. B., Janssen, T. W., ALLRISC, POST MW. (2013). Active lifestyle rehabilitation interventions in aging spinal cord injury (ALLRISC): Multicenter research program. *Disability Rehabilitation, 35*(13), 1097–1103.

Wadensten, B., & Carlsson, M. (2001). A qualitative study of nursing staff members' interpretations of signs of gerotranscendence. *Journal of Advanced Nursing, 36,* 635–642.

Warring, P., & Krieger-Blake, L. S. (2014). End of life care. In K. Mauk (Ed.), *Gerontological nursing: Competencies for care* (pp. 881–930). Burlington, MA: Jones & Bartlett.

Waszynski, C., Veronneau, P., Therrien, K., Brousseau, M., Massa, A., & Levick, S. (2013). Decreasing patient agitation using individualized therapeutic activities. *American Journal of Nursing, 113*(10), 32–39.

Watkins, T. (2014). Decreasing informal caregiver burden with social media. *Improving Family Caregiver Support, 32*(5), 304–308.

Wilson, R., Boyle, P., Yu, L., Barnes, L., Schneider, J., & Bennett, D. (2013). Life-span cognitive activity. *Neurology, 11*(4), 314–321.

Winkler, T. (2008). Spinal cord injury and aging. Retrieved from www.emedicine.com/pmr/topic185.htm

Wirz, M., & Dietz, V. (2012). Concepts of aging with paralysis: Implications for recovery and treatment. *Handbook of Clinical Neurology, 109,* 77–84.

Witkos, M., Uttaburanont, M., Lang, C., & Haddad, R. (2009). Effects of anemia on rehabilitation outcomes in elderly patients in the post-acute care setting. *Topics in Geriatric Rehabilitation, 25*(3), 222–230.

Wong, C., & Wallhagen, M. (2014). Family caregivers of value of emotion-focused coping strategies when dealing with behavioral symptoms in individuals with fronto-temporal dementia. *Journal of Gerontological Nursing, 40*(1), 30–40.

World Health Organization. (1990). *Cancer pain relief and palliative care.* Geneva, Switzerland: Author.

World Health Organization. (2011). *Elder maltreatment.* Fact sheet no. 357. Retrieved from www.who.int/mediacentre/factsheets/fs3571/en/

Yu, F. (2005). Factors affecting outpatient rehabilitation outcomes in elders. *Journal of Nursing Scholarship, 27*(3), 229–236.

Zwicker, D., & Fulmer, T. (2008). *Medication. Nursing standard of practice protocol: Reducing adverse drug events.* New York: Hartford Institute of Geriatric Nursing. Retrieved from http://consultgerirn.org/topics/medication/want_to_know_more#Wrap

Suggested Resources

American Geriatrics Society: http://www.americangeriatrics.org/

Depression and Bipolar Support Alliance: www.dbsalliance.org

Hartford Institute for Geriatric Nursing: http://consultgerirn.org

Mental Health America: www.nmha.org

National Alliance for the Mentally Ill: www.nami.org

Nurses Improving Care for Healthsystem Elders: http://www.nicheprogram.org/

National Institutes of Health SeniorHealth: www.nihseniorhealth.gov

Signs of depression: http://www.webmd.com/depression/guide/depression-symptoms-and-types

USPSTF 2014 http://www.ahrq.gov/professionals/clinicians-providers/guidelines-recommendations/guide/cpsguide.pdf

Chapter 17

Military Considerations in Rehabilitation Nursing

Mary Sue Biggins, MBA BSN CRRN
Brenda R. French, MSN RN-BC CRRN CBIS
Paul Mittelsteadt, MSN LTC AN U.S. Army (Ret)

LEARNING OUTCOMES

- Review rehabilitation issues that are unique to the military population.
- Describe the military polytrauma system of care.
- Discuss rehabilitation for medical issues that are found in both the military and civilian populations, particularly posttraumatic stress syndrome (PTSD) and burns.

KEY CHAPTER TOPICS

- Polytrauma system of care
- Veterans Administration and Department of Defense coordination of care
- Pain management issues
- Posttraumatic stress syndrome
- Burn care

PROFESSIONAL REHABILITATION NURSING DOMAINS AND COMPETENCIES

- Domain 1: Competencies 1.1, 1.2, 1.3, 1.4
- Domain 2: Competencies 2.1, 2.2, 2.3
- Domain 4: Competencies 4.1, 4.2 (Association of Rehabilitation Nurses [ARN], 2014)

Introduction

After the terrorist attacks on September 11, 2001, the United States became engaged in the global war on terrorism (GWOT), resulting in combat engagements in Afghanistan (Operation Enduring Freedom [OEF]) and Iraq (Operation Iraqi Freedom [OIF] and Operation New Dawn [OND]). As of mid-2014, it seems likely that our military engagement in the GWOT will continue and could even escalate. The manner of combat today is different from that of past generations and has dictated changes in the care we give to combat service members and veterans.

The unprecedented survival rates from OEF, OIF, and OND—more than 95% of seriously wounded service members (Cifu & Blake, 2011)—have already significantly affected rehabilitation nursing. The complexity of the wounds seen in the rehabilitation facilities that serve this population include traumatic brain injury (TBI) (mild, moderate, and severe); limb amputations; spinal cord injuries and burns; combat-related stress; visual and auditory impairment; fractures and musculoskeletal pain; and, in many instances, multiple types of injury (i.e., polytrauma) (Cifu & Blake, 2011; U.S. Department of Veterans Affairs [U.S. DVA], n.d.).

Polytrauma is defined as complex, serious injuries to more than one body system that occur in a single incident. Multiple body parts or organ systems are involved, and physical, cognitive, psychological, psychosocial, and functional impairments and disabilities can result (Biggins, Engstrom, Jackson, Sommers, & Thorne-Odem, 2013; Kerns & Dobscha, 2009). Rehabilitation nursing for some of these injuries is discussed in other chapters of this book, but a closer look is warranted to understand how these injuries occur, in addition to military interventions, the roles and responsibilities of the U.S. Department of Defense (DoD) and the Veterans Health Administration (VHA), the implications of comorbid PTSD, and the role of the family or caregiver.

The rehabilitation process for service members and veterans is best facilitated when nurses have an understanding of military culture, including the "hidden wounds of war" (Cifu & Blake, 2011), the significant role of family and caregivers in this young cohort of wounded, the changes in patterns of wounds that have resulted from the terrorist element of these wars, and improved body armor. The purpose of this chapter is to share information with rehabilitation nurses who encounter service members and veterans in their practice.

I. Background

A. Our troops have been engaged in the longest combined wars in U.S. history with the engagements in Afghanistan and Iraq.
   1. OEF/OIF/OND have accounted for the deployment

of more than 2.5 million troops (Biggins et al., 2013; Cifu & Blake, 2011).
2. The lengthy, repetitive deployments (sometimes as many as five to six for an individual) and the need for constant vigilance because of the lack of a safe zone are elements that contribute to the hidden wounds of war such as PTSD and mild traumatic brain injury (mTBI) (Biggins et al., 2013; Cifu & Blake, 2011).
3. The battlefield includes urban warfare and the weapons of choice of today's enemies, such as improvised explosive devices in the form of roadside and car bombs and rocket-propelled grenades.
4. The enemy wears no specific uniform and is indistinguishable from the common populace, a fact that creates unprecedented hazards for soldiers who find it difficult to identify who the enemy is.
5. Women and children are frequently used as bomb carriers, a previously unheard of and emotionally traumatic situation for our troops.

B. Aspects of Military Care Related to the U.S. DoD
1. Advances in body armor allow better protection of vital organs.
    a. Changed pattern of wounds extends to extremities, head, and neck (Cifu & Blake, 2011)
    b. Increased survival rates result in complex, polytraumatic injuries
2. Improved combat medicine training of all U.S. military personnel saves lives.
    a. Basic lifesaving skills, airway management, and tourniquet application (Kent, Upp, & Buckenmaier, 2011)
    b. Rapid onsite battlefield treatment, stabilization, and evacuation (Cifu & Blake, 2011)
    c. Stabilization surgery at local facilities
    d. Air transport to Landstuhl Army Medical Center, Germany; military treatment facility (MTF) (U.S. DVA, n.d.)
        1) Transport via air ambulance
        2) Critical care team
        3) Surgery, further stabilization
        4) Restorative/reconstructive care
            a) Possible presence of family
    e. Air transport to stateside MTF—Walter Reed Army Medical Center, San Antonio Military Medical Center, and National Naval Medical Center (U.S. DVA, n.d.)
        1) Intensive care
        2) Inpatient stay of months to years
        3) Frequent presence of family

C. Aspects of Military Medical Care Related to Veteran Affairs (VA)
1. Transfer to VA rehabilitation
    a. Shared resources VA/DoD
        1) Case management (VA/DoD)
        2) High-tech team communication hand-off from DoD to VA
        3) Video teleconference
        4) Telephone consulting
        5) Shared electronic record, remote data access
            a) VA/DoD transfer summary with medical history, treatment, goals
            b) Patient/family involvement in plan of care
2. Air or ambulance transport to polytrauma rehabilitation center (PRC)
    a. Five PRCs in the VA system (**Figure 17-1**)
        1) Richmond, VA
        2) Tampa, FL
        3) San Antonio, TX
        4) Palo Alto, CA
        5) Minneapolis, MN
    b. Premier state-of-the-art inpatient rehabilitation for OEF/OIF/OND service members and veterans
        1) Complex polytrauma injuries
        2) TBI from combat/noncombat (Lamberty et al., 2014; U.S. DVA 2013, U.S. DVA, n.d.)

D. VA Polytrauma System of Care (PSC)
1. Complex national model of care
2. Addresses severe nature of injuries seen
3. Bidirectional system movement between DoD and VA
    a. VA/DoD nurse liaison at MTFs
        1) Oversee placement and transfer process
        2) Problem solve transfer issues
        3) Bridge two systems of DoD and VA
    b. Case management (CM) coordinator
        1) CM assignment to each veteran
        2) CM at all levels of care
        3) Lifelong CM for severely injured veterans
4. Geographic movement nationally to meet veterans' needs
    a. Definitive hand-off process for smooth, safe transitions
        1) Electronically shared DoD/VA transfer summary
        2) Video teleconference between MTF and VA by interdisciplinary team (IDT)
        3) VA PRC/PNS site visits by family
        4) Electronic access across systems to medical record
5. Veterans benefits administration counselors
6. Rural access to services via telehealth
7. Specialized rehabilitative services by IDT

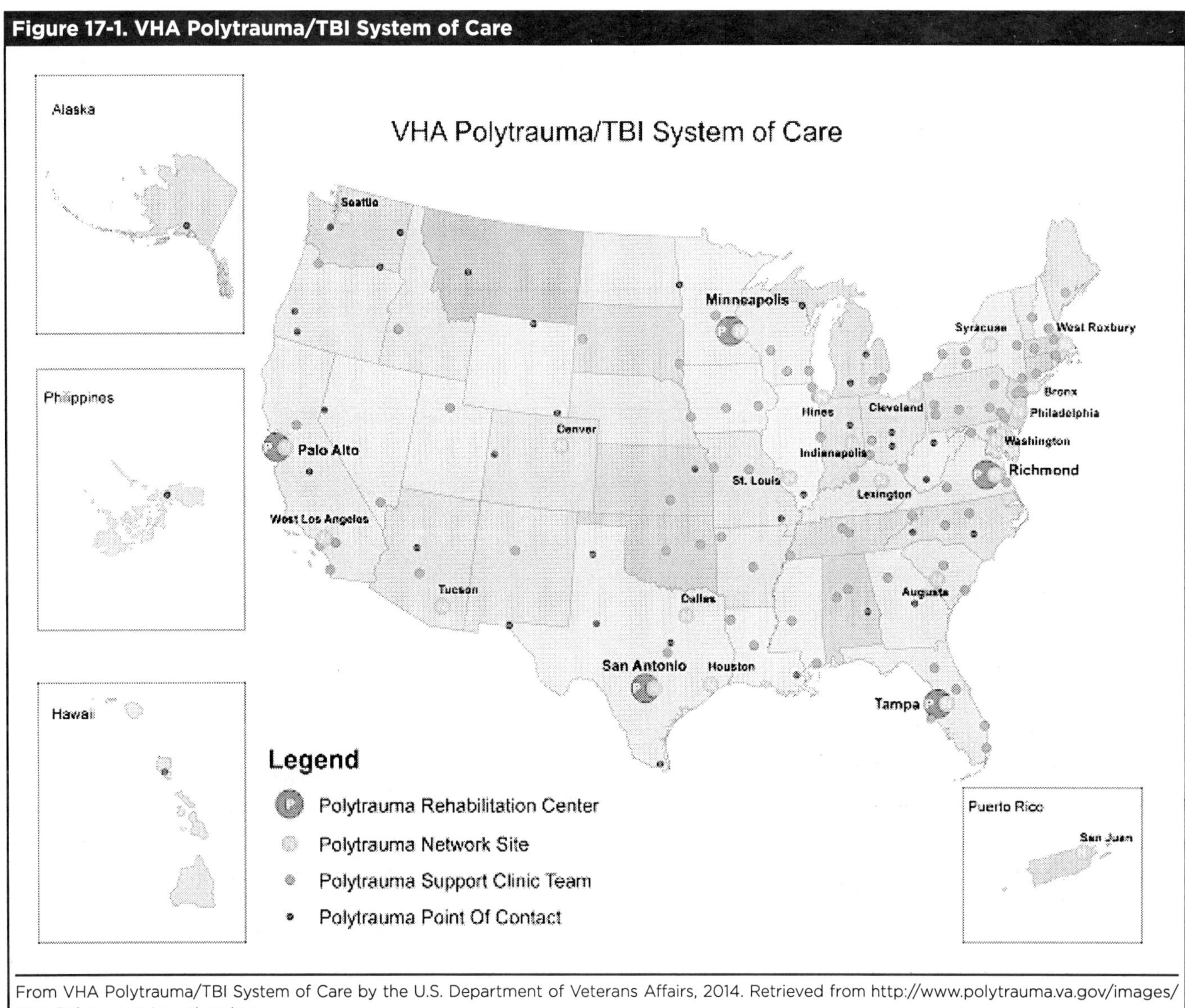

Figure 17-1. VHA Polytrauma/TBI System of Care

From VHA Polytrauma/TBI System of Care by the U.S. Department of Veterans Affairs, 2014. Retrieved from http://www.polytrauma.va.gov/images/Map-Polytrauma-Locations.jpg

a. Staff at all levels of the PSC demonstrate rehabilitation clinical expertise through education, training, and potential certification (U.S. DVA, n.d., 2013)

8. Integrated national network
   a. Polytrauma rehabilitation centers (PRCs = 5)
      1) State-of-the-art coordinated care
      2) Accredited by the Commission on Accreditation of Rehabilitation Facilities (CARF)
      3) Comprehensive inpatient acute rehabilitation, outpatient, and TBI services
      4) IDT
      5) Specialty consultants related to polytrauma
      6) Serve as consultants to others in PSC
         a) Provide clinical leadership
         b) Perform collaborative research
         c) Educate veterans, families, caregivers, and clinicians
         d) Collaborate with DoD and academic facilities to promote best practices
         e) Serve on national committees as advocates of rehabilitation care
      7) Veteran-centered care
      8) Veteran/family/significant other: core part of IDT
         a) Individualized treatment/follow-up process
         b) Family support, counseling, training
         c) Family care map process (**Figure 17-2**)
      9) Emerging consciousness programs
      10) Assistive technology labs
      11) Polytrauma telerehabilitation
      12) Vocational services
      13) Community reentry program
         a) Ability to resume age, gender, and culture-appropriate roles

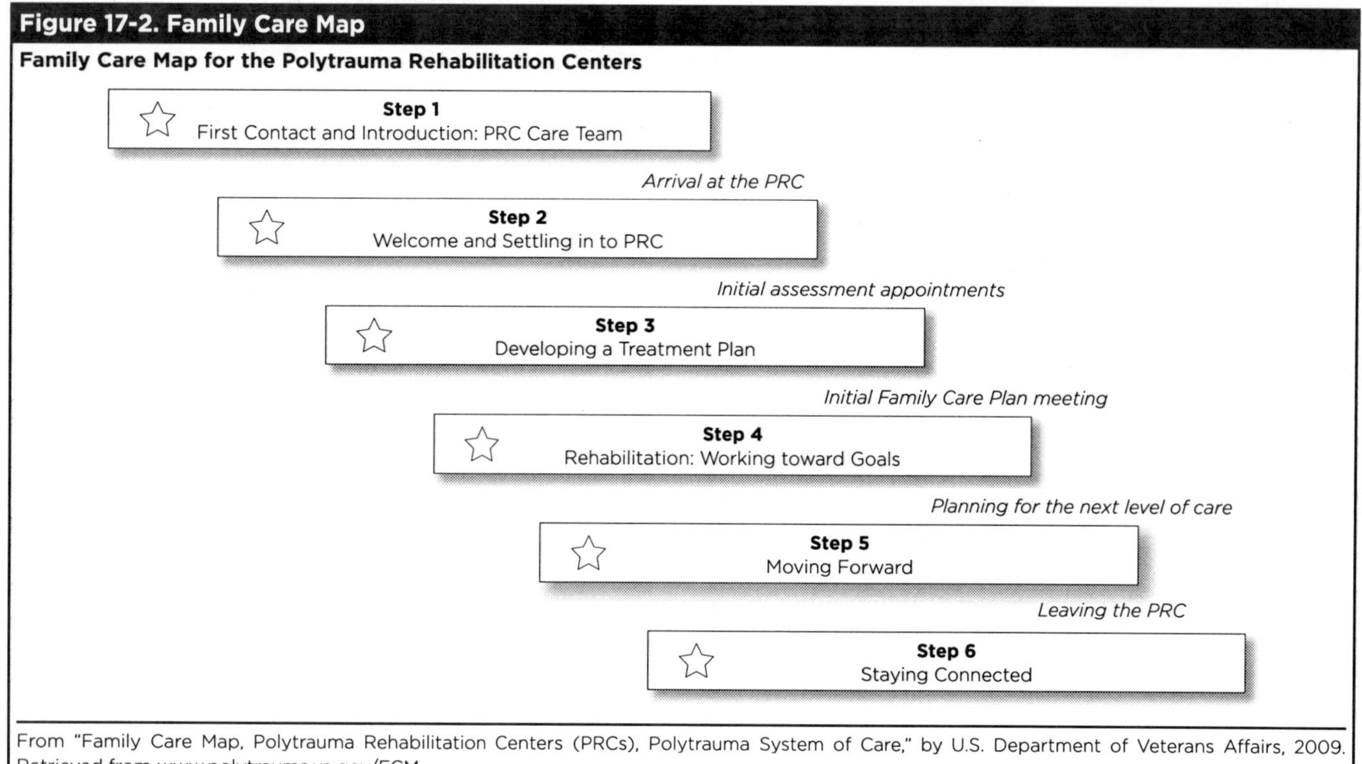

Figure 17-2. Family Care Map

From "Family Care Map, Polytrauma Rehabilitation Centers (PRCs), Polytrauma System of Care," by U.S. Department of Veterans Affairs, 2009. Retrieved from www.polytrauma.va.gov/FCM.

b) Include veteran, family, and peers to achieve functional competence in natural setting
c) Achieve skills and adaptations to resume roles in home, school, work, and community
d) Ongoing assessment of progress and modification of goals

14) Military liaison to address service issues
15) Polytrauma transitional rehabilitation program
  a) Goal-oriented residential rehabilitation
  b) Partner with veteran or service member
  c) Improve ability to function for community reintegration (U.S. DVA, n.d., 2013)

b. Polytrauma network sites (PNS = 23)
  1) Specialized postacute rehabilitation
  2) Interdisciplinary team led by physiatrist
  3) Consultation with PRCs and specialists
  4) Veteran and family education and training
  5) Clinical leadership for geographical area
  6) Education and training to staff on polytrauma/TBI
    a) Polytrauma support clinic teams
    b) Polytrauma points of contact
    c) Facility staff and community-based outpatient clinics
    d) Community organizations
  7) Proactive CM
    a) Identify existing and emerging conditions
    b) Identify local VA and non-VA resources
    c) Maximize resource utilization and access to services
    d) Promote veteran-driven quality care
    e) Coordinate services across agencies
    f) Communicate with veteran, family, caregiver, and IDT to meet needs
    g) Implement the VHA Individualized Rehabilitation and Community Reintegration Plan of Care
      (i) Identify veteran's needs based on assessment
      (ii) Coordinate strategies to address needs
      (iii) Collaborate with veteran, family, and IDT for measurable, realistic goals and ongoing planning
      (iv) Set timeline for goal achievement
      (v) Identify and access available resources
      (vi) Document interactions with veteran and progress
      (vii) Track progress with the Mayo-Portland Adaptability Inventory (M2PI) (U.S. DVA, n.d., 2013)

c. Polytrauma support clinic teams (PSCTs = 87)
  1) Located closer to veterans' homes

2) Interdisciplinary in structure
3) Rehabilitation providers for follow-up services
4) Consult with regional and network specialists at PRC and PNS
5) Manage long-term effects of polytrauma
6) Direct care, consultation, and telerehabilitation (U.S. DVA, n.d., 2013)

d. Polytrauma points of contact (PPOC = 39)
1) Provide basic screening
2) Refer to closest PNS or PSCT as needed
a) Comprehensive evaluation
b) Treatment (U.S. DVA, n.d., 2013)

e. Family care and involvement
1) Family and veteran included as focal point of IDT for treatment and care
a) Family provides history, values, and support for veteran
b) Critical component in the rehabilitation process
2) Education and training on care at all levels of the PSC
3) Ongoing assessment and interventions to support family
a) Offer resources in VA and DoD for housing, financial, counseling, and mental health support
b) Provide community resources
c) Solicit active participation in the rehabilitation/treatment process
d) Include in development of plan of care (U.S. DVA, n.d.)
4) Caregivers and veterans: Omnibus Health Services Act of 2010
a) Education/training for family caregiver (CG)
b) Respite care
c) Optional health insurance
d) Mental health services and counseling
e) Peer outreach
f) Readjustment services
g) CG website with social media
h) CG support coordinator at each VA hospital
i) CG support group
j) Stipend for CG service: www.caregiver.va.gov
5) Family care map at PRCs (Figure 17-2)
a) Available services at PRCs
b) Rehabilitation IDT with names/contacts
c) Rehabilitation process/plan of care
d) Family care map: www.polytrauma.va.gov/FCM
6) Fisher House at VA facilities
a) Complimentary "home-away-from-home" support for family
(i) Privately funded
b) Located on major military and VA hospital grounds (U.S. DVA, n.d.)

f. Unprecedented collaboration
1) Between DoD and VA
2) Private and academic healthcare providers (Cifu & Blake, 2011)
3) Joining forces
a) Launched April 2012 by Michelle Obama and Jill Biden
b) Collaborative education effort between the American Academy of the Colleges of Nursing (AACN) and VA Office of Nursing service (Biggins et al., 2013)
c) Joining Forces Initiative toolkit developed: Enhancing Veterans' Care Toolkit
(i) Nursing faculty resource for teaching care of veterans
(ii) VA, military, and community resource websites
(iii) Curriculum options from schools of nursing
(iv) Enhancing Veterans' Care Toolkit: http://www.aacn.nche.edu/downloads/joining-forces-tool-kit (Biggins et al., 2013)
4) Development of centers of excellence
a) Defense and Veterans Brain Injury Center (DVBIC)
b) Vision Center of Excellence (VCoE)
c) Center for the Intrepid (CFI)

g. Extensive increase in research
1) Prosthetics
2) Adaptive devices
3) Effects of blast injury and mTBI
4) Comorbid results of pain, TBI, and PTSD (Cifu & Blake, 2011)

h. Assistive technology (AT)
1) Enhances the ability of veterans and active duty service members with disabilities to fulfill their life goals. All PRCs have AT programs and provide the following services:
2) Consultations, evaluations, and training on AT devices and software
a) Offer education and caregiver training
b) Educate and train staff
c) Provide rehabilitation engineering services
d) Offer AT telehealth services
3) Devices

a) Augmentative and alternative communication
b) Adaptive computer access
c) Adaptive driving
d) Adaptive sports
e) Electronic aides to daily living
f) Electronic cognitive devices
g) Powered mobility and seating

4) Members of the AT team include
a) Physiatrist
b) Occupational therapist
c) Physical therapist
d) Speech-language pathologists
e) Rehabilitation engineer
f) Rehabilitation engineering technician
g) Recreation therapist (adaptive sports specialist)
h) Kinesiotherapist (driving specialist)

II. Specific Medical and Rehabilitation Issues Confronting Service Members and Veterans

A. Pain

1. Pain implications for OEF/OIF/OND service members and veterans
   a. Includes neuropathic, chronic widespread pain, musculoskeletal/joint pain, and pain from spinal cord injury
   b. Study gender, ethnic, and racial differences in prevalence and care (Kent, Upp, & Buckenmaier, 2011)
   c. Pain is the most frequently reported symptom of returning combat veterans
      1) Prevalence is high for headaches and joint, muscle, back, and abdominal pain
      2) Risk is greater for OEF/OIF/OND military due to blasts, gunshot wounds, and motor vehicle accidents
      3) The high numbers of older-aged reservists and National Guard soldiers serving in combat increases the risk factor for pain
      4) Lengthy and repeated deployments increase the risk for pain issues. (Gironda, Clark, Massengale, & Walker, 2006)
   d. Viewed as pathophysiological process by U.S. military
   e. Early battlefield pain management has been shown to decrease rates of PTSD
   f. Multimodal approach to pain management
   g. Minimize pain, optimize functionality during rehabilitation
   h. Aggressive treatment of acute pain close to point of injury improves immediate and future functional outcomes and comorbidities
   i. Pain management task force established in 2009 by army surgeon general
      1) Develop holistic, multidisciplinary, multimodal pain plan
      2) Improve integrated clinical pain medicine
      3) Enhance pain education for providers and patients
      4) Develop an objective pain tool to be utilized by the DoD and VA
         a) Validated 11-point scale
         b) Functional language coincides with each number of the scale
         c) Evaluate the biopsychosocial impact of pain
            (i) Pain impact on general activity
            (ii) Impact of pain on the mind
            (iii) Level of stress
            (iv) Impact on sleep
         d) Improve the evaluation of pain treatment goals and treatment plan of care
      5) Invest in pain research
      6) Implemented September 2010: U.S. Army Medical Command (MEDCOM) Comprehensive Pain Management Campaign Plan (Kent, Kuhl, & Kupfer, 2011)

B. PTSD

1. Overview
   a. *PTSD* is classified as a trauma- and stressor-related disorder in the *Diagnostic Statistical Manual of Mental Disorders*, 5th edition (*DSM-5*) (Reiger et al., 2013).
   b. Definitions include
      1) A mental health condition that is triggered by a terrifying event
         a) Symptoms can include flashbacks, nightmares, severe anxiety, and uncontrollable thoughts about the event (see http://www.mayoclinic.org/diseases-conditions/post-traumatic-stress-disorder/basics/definition/con-20022540).
      2) An anxiety problem that develops in some people after an extremely traumatic event such as combat, crime, an accident, or a natural disaster (see http://www.apa.org/topics/ptsd/)
   c. PTSD was recognized as early as the third century B. C. (Nayback, 2009).
      1) References to PTSD occur in Homer's *Iliad* and Shakespeare's *Henry IV* (Nayback, 2009).
      2) In 19th-century Great Britain, PTSD was recognized among postal workers and

railway workers who witnessed railway crashes.

a) Symptoms included sleep disorders, nightmares, intolerance to railway travel, and chronic pain.

b) Called "railway spine" or "accident neurosis" (Nayback, 2009)

d. Also recognized in the 19th century by military physicians describing soldiers' responses to combat

1) Called "soldiers heart," "DeCosta's syndrome," and "effort syndrome"

2) Attributed to cardiovascular compromise secondary to combat stress (Nayback, 2009)

e. Named "shell shock" by a British psychiatrist in 1915

1) Symptoms noted included inability to move or speak, unresponsiveness, memory loss, loss of capacity to feel, weeping, and screaming

2) Symptoms attributed to microtears in the brain secondary to exploding shells (Nayback, 2009)

f. Called "war neurosis" during World War II

1) 1944: Military focused on prevention and treatment

2) Front-line psychiatry emerged; soldiers were treated close to the battlefield and returned to combat.

3) Impact of environment and relationships was recognized (Nayback, 2009).

g. PTSD was included as a psychiatric diagnosis in the third edition of the *DSM* and an anxiety disorder in the fourth edition. Both editions indicated it was fear based. Dysphoria (sadness) or anhedonia (loss of interest in usually pleasurable activities) are prominent signs.

h. PTSD is now classified under a new category, trauma and stressor-related disorders, in which the onset of each occurrence has been preceded by exposure to a traumatic or otherwise adverse environmental event (see http://www.ptsd.va.gov/profesional/PTSD-overview/ptsd-overview.asp).

i. The month of June has been designated PTSD Awareness Month.

2. Epidemiology and incidence

a. Sixty percent of men and 50% of women experience at least one trauma during their lives.

1) Women are more likely to experience sexual assault and child sexual abuse. Men are more likely to experience accidents, physical assault, combat, and disaster, or to witness death or injury.

b. U.S. statistics

1) Seven percent to 8% of the population will have PTSD at some point in their lives.

2) An estimated 5.2 million adults have PTSD during a given year.

3) Women are more likely than men to develop PTSD. Ten percent of women develop PTSD at some time during their lives, compared with 5% of men.

4) PTSD in the military

a) Is found in about 11%–20% of veterans of the Iraq and Afghanistan Wars, in as many as 10% of veterans of the Gulf War (Desert Storm), and in about 30% of veterans of the Vietnam War (see http://www.ptsd.va.gov/public/PTSD-overview/basics/how-common-is-ptsd.asp)

3. Types

a. *Acute stress reaction (ASR)*: onset with trauma; lasts hours to days after the event

b. *Combat and operational stress reaction (COSR):* reflects acute reactions to a high-stress or combat-related event. ASR/COSR can present with a broad group of physical, mental, and emotional symptoms and signs (e.g., depression, fatigue, anxiety, decreased concentration/memory, and hyperarousal, among others). The diagnosis of ASR/COSR applies to stress reactions that do not resolve within 4 days after the event, after other disorders have been ruled out (U.S. DVA & U.S. Department of Defense [U.S. DoD], 2010)

c. *Acute stress disorder (ASD)*: The above mentioned symptoms last more than 2 days after the traumatic event but less than a month (if symptoms last longer than 1 month, the person could develop PTSD). Reexperiencing the event, as well as avoidance, increased arousal, and at least three out of five dissociative symptoms, are exhibited.

4. Symptoms

a. Dissociative symptoms, which include

1) Being unaware of one's surroundings

2) The feeling that one is outside one's body

3) The feeling that "this is really not happening to me."

4) Not being able to remember important things about the traumatic event

5) Believing that "I can't feel"

6) Feelings of detachment

b. PTSD
1) Symptoms last more than 1 month after exposure to event and causes distress or impairment in social, occupational, or other important areas of functioning. In addition, the onset can be delayed for up to 6 months. Patients can exhibit
a) Persistent symptoms of reexperiencing the traumatic event
b) Persistent avoidance of stimuli associated with the event
c) Numbing of general responsiveness
d) Persistent symptoms of heightened arousal
2) Acute PTSD: Symptoms last more than 1 month but less than 3
3) Chronic PTSD: Symptoms last more than 3 months

5. Etiology
a. PTSD trigger: Exposure to actual or threatened death, serious injury, or sexual violation
b. The exposure must result from one or more of the following scenarios:
1) Directly experiencing the traumatic event
2) Witnessing the traumatic event
3) Learning that the traumatic event occurred to a close family member or close friend (with the actual or threatened death being violent or accidental)
4) Experiencing first-hand repeated or extreme exposure to aversive details of the traumatic event

6. Risk factors
a. Risk of PTSD increases if a person
1) Was exposed to the traumatic event as a victim or a witness
2) Was seriously injured during the trauma
3) Experienced a trauma that was long lasting or very severe
4) Perceived himself or herself or a family member to be in imminent danger
5) Had a severe negative reaction during the event, such as a feeling of detachment from his or her surroundings, or a panic attack
6) Felt helpless during the trauma and was unable to help self or a loved one (U.S. DVA, 2010a)
7) Experienced an interpersonal trauma such as rape or assault
b. Trauma-related risk factors
1) Nature, severity, and duration of the trauma exposure
2) Previous trauma exposure (U.S. DVA & U.S. DoD, 2004)
c. Pretrauma risk factors: Adverse childhood events, younger age, female gender, minority race, and low socioeconomic or educational status (U.S. DVA & U.S. DoD, 2004)
d. Posttrauma risk factors: Poor social support and life stress (U.S. DVA & U.S. DoD, 2004)

7. *DSM-5* focus on behavioral symptoms
a. *Reexperiencing*: spontaneous memories of the traumatic event, recurrent dreams related to it, flashbacks, or other intense or prolonged psychological distress (American Psychiatric Association [APA], 2013)
b. *Avoidance*: dodging distressing memories, thoughts, feelings, or extreme reminders of the event (APA, 2013)
c. *Negative cognition and mood*: represents myriad feelings, including a persistent, distorted blaming of self or others; estrangement from others; markedly diminished interest in activities; and an inability to remember key aspects of the event (APA, 2013)
d. *Arousal*: marked by aggressive, reckless, or self-destructive behavior, sleep disturbances, hypervigilance, or related problems. *DSM-4* and *DSM-5* emphasize the fight-or-flight response often observed in PTSD (APA, 2013)

8. Pathophysiology
a. Several key psychobiological mechanisms that enable humans to cope successfully with stressful situations function abnormally in clients with PTSD.
1) Fight-or-flight response (sympathetic nervous system [SNS] activation)
2) Abnormal increases in SNS reactivity
3) Hypothalamic-pituitary-adrenocortical mobilization
a) Lower urinary cortisol levels
b) Elevated lymphocyte glucocorticoid receptor levels
c) Dexamethasone super-suppression
4) Exaggerated acoustic startle response
5) *Fear conditioning*: Neutral cues associated with a traumatic event acquire the capacity to evoke a conditioned emotional (i.e., fearful) response in the absence of the aversive stimulus known as the Pavlovian response (Friedman, 2000).
6) *Appraisal*: Capacity to evaluate the situation as benign or dangerous is impaired (Friedman, 2000)

b. Physical abnormalities (structure and function)
   1) Reduced hippocampal volume
   2) Changes in regional cerebral blood flow to limbic and paralimbic areas (Friedman, 2000)
c. Effects of PTSD on health
   1) Increased vulnerability to hypertension and atherosclerotic heart disease
   2) Abnormalities in thyroid and hormone function
   3) Increased susceptibility to infection
   4) Problems perceiving or tolerating pain
d. Behavioral health risks associated with PTSD
   1) Smoking
   2) Substance abuse
   3) Poor nutrition
   4) Conflict, violence
   5) Anger, hostility

9. Management options
   a. Nonpharmacological
      1) Psychotherapy for PTSD to include individual, group, couple, and family
         a) Exposure-based therapies emphasize in vivo, imaginal, and narrative (i.e., oral and/or written) exposure but also generally include elements of cognitive restructuring (e.g., evaluating the accuracy of beliefs about danger), as well as relaxation techniques and self-monitoring of anxiety. Examples of therapies that include a focus on exposure include prolonged exposure therapy, brief eclectic psychotherapy, narrative therapy, written-exposure therapy, and many of the cognitive therapy packages that incorporate in vivo and imaginal/narrative exposure.
         b) Cognitive-based therapies emphasize cognitive restructuring (i.e., challenging automatic or acquired beliefs connected to the traumatic event, such as beliefs about safety or trust) but also include relaxation techniques and discussion/narration of the traumatic event, either orally and/or through writing. Examples include cognitive processing therapy and various cognitive therapy packages tested in RCTs.
         c) Stress inoculation training (the specific anxiety management package most extensively studied in the PTSD literature) places more emphasis on breathing retraining and muscle relaxation but also includes cognitive elements (e.g., self-dialogue, thought stopping, role playing) and often exposure techniques (e.g., in vivo exposure, narration of traumatic event).
         d) Eye movement desensitization and reprocessing (EMDR) (extensively studied in a large number of RCTs) closely resembles other cognitive behavioral therapy modalities in that an exposure component (e.g., talking about the traumatic event and/or holding on to distressing traumatic memories without verbalizing them) exists, along with a cognitive component (e.g., identifying a negative cognition and an alternative positive cognition, and assessing the validity of the cognition), and relaxation/self-monitoring techniques (e.g., breathing, "body scan"). Alternating eye movements are part of the classic EMDR technique (and the name of this type of treatment); however, comparable effect sizes have been achieved with and without eye movements or other forms of distraction or kinesthetic stimulation. Although the mechanisms of effectiveness in EMDR have yet to be determined, it is likely that they are similar to other trauma-focused exposure and cognitive-based therapies (U.S. DVA & U.S. DoD, 2010).
   b. Pharmacological
      1) Although found to be helpful in relieving some symptoms, pharmacological treatment of PTSD is not a cure-all.
      2) The following medications have had positive results, according to research studies to date:
         a) Selective serotonin reuptake inhibitors (SSRIs)
            (i) First-line pharmacological treatment
            (ii) Serotonin is important in mood regulation, anxiety relief, stress modulation, appetite regulation, and sleep.
            (iii) Reduces symptoms of reexperiencing, hyperarousal, avoidance, and emotional numbing
            (iv) Paroxetine, fluoxetine, sertraline

b) Selective serotonin/norepinephrine uptake inhibitors (SNRIs)
   (i) Effects similar to SSRIs
   (ii) Venlafaxine
c) Atypical antipsychotics
   (i) Act on dopamine and serotonin systems
   (ii) Can best help if used to augment SSRIs
   (iii) Can elevate glucose and cholesterol levels
   (iv) Risk of tardive dyskinesia and extrapyramidal side effects
   (v) Olanzapine, risperidone, quetiapine
d) Antiepileptics: Valproate
e) Beta-adrenergic antagonist
   (i) Reduces intrusive recollections, reactivity to traumatic stimuli, hyperreactivity
   (ii) Limited research trials
   (iii) Propranolol
f) Antiadrenergic: Prazosin for nightmares and insomnia (U.S. DVA & U.S. DoD, 2010).

10. Rehabilitation issues
   a. Screening, recognition, and provision of treatment for PTSD
   b. Family structure and processes
   c. Client and family education
   d. Symptom management
      1) Behavior
         a) Impatience
         b) Anger
         c) Agitation
         d) Violence
         e) Hypervigilance
         f) Elevated startle reflex
      2) Sleep and rest
      3) Lack of concentration
      4) Substance abuse
   e. Safety of self and others
      1) Suicidal ideation
      2) Anger, acting out
   f. Inability to join group activities
      1) Trust
      2) Startle
      3) Anger
   g. Comorbidities that either exacerbate or mask symptoms of PTSD
      1) TBI
      2) Depression
      3) Anxiety

11. Nursing process: assessment
   a. Presence of PTSD
      1) Recognition of risk
      2) Screening with a validated, reliable instrument: primary-care PTSD screen
      3) Communication with other providers
      4) Knowledge of trauma history
   b. Sleep and rest
      1) Erratic sleep patterns
      2) Nightmares
      3) Recurrent dreams
      4) Difficulty falling and staying asleep
      5) Hypersomnia
   c. Cardiac and pulmonary
      1) Hypertension
      2) Episodes of tachycardia and palpitations
      3) Episodes of tachypnea, breathlessness
      4) Perspiration, hot and cold spells
   d. Psychological
      1) Behaviors
         a) Self-report
         b) Significant-other report
         c) Observation
      2) Concentration
      3) Hypervigilance
      4) Fear
      5) Flashbacks
      6) Anger
      7) Impulse control
      8) Risk of self-harm
         a) Suicidal ideation
         b) Past suicide attempts
      9) Risk of harm to others
      10) Coping measures
         a) Usual
         b) Current
            (i) Isolation
            (ii) Illicit drugs
            (iii) Alcohol
            (iv) Cigarettes
   e. Pain
   f. Social interactions
      1) Avoidance
      2) Disinterest
   g. Medications
   h. Therapy received

12. Plan
   a. Reduce psychological distress and the effects of secondary stressors.
   b. Treat specific symptoms when they interfere with normal healing processes.
   c. Assist the normal healing process by supporting the client and family.

d. Protect the client from further exposure to stress.
e. Encourage the client to verbalize and express painful emotions as able.
f. Encourage the client to be with other people.
g. Educate the client and family about PTSD, interventions, and expected outcomes.
h. Coordinate care with other providers.

13. Interventions
a. Provide safety for the client and family.
b. Help the client improve self-esteem and regain a sense of control over feelings and actions.
c. Encourage the development of assertive, rather than aggressive, behaviors.
d. Promote an understanding that the outcome of the present situation can be significantly affected by one's own actions.
e. Help the client and family to learn healthy ways to deal with and realistically adapt to changes and events that have occurred.
f. Provide active listening and support for the client and family.

14. Evaluation
a. Safety
1) Client
2) Significant others
b. Management of PTSD symptoms
1) Sleep and rest disturbances
2) Hypervigilance
3) Anger, agitation
4) Fear
c. Community reintegration
d. In fiscal year 2011, 476,515 veterans with a primary or secondary diagnosis of PTSD received treatment at DVA medical centers and clinics. All veterans who come to the DVA for the first time are screened for the presence of symptoms of PTSD and depression (U.S. DVA, 2014a).

C. Burns: The military healthcare system is a known leader in burn care. Burn units at major military centers, such as the Institute for Surgical Research at Fort Sam Houston in San Antonio, TX, care for both military and civilian burn patients. Burns are included in this section because of military leadership in the area of burn care, but the content that follows certainly applies to both military and civilian populations.

1. Burns and armed conflict
a. Overview
1) Burn injuries have occurred in every armed conflict (Atiyeh, Nayek, & Gunn, 2005).
2) Weapons development increases risk of burns (Galbraith, 2001).
3) Burns require extensive hospitalization and rehabilitation and tie up military resources. Weapons producing burns can have strategic level effects.
4) Secondary effects of terror and loss of morale cannot be understated.
5) Burns and trauma (e.g., blasts, penetrating and blunt) are common, as is polytrauma.

b. Epidemiology and incidence
1) Seventy-eight percent of casualties in the Iraq and Afghanistan Wars involved an explosion-related injury (Owens et al., 2008).
2) United Kingdom epidemiological studies detail similar statistics (Foster, Moledina, & Jeffery, 2001).
3) From 2003 to 2007, 540 casualties were evacuated to military burn centers (Renz et al., 2008).
a) Young (19–52 years of age)
b) Male (96%)
c) Fifty-one percent sustained polytraumatic injuries; orthopedics
d) Sixty-two percent sustained combat-related injuries
e) Kauver, Cancio, Wolf, Wade, & Holcomb (2006) reported an inhalation injury rate of 16.4% among combat casualties, compared with 5.9% among noncombat wounded.
f) Mortality has decreased significantly, from 8% (Vietnam War) to 4% (current wars in Iraq and Afghanistan).
(i) "Mortality does not differ between civilians evacuated locally and military personnel injured in distant austere environments treated at the same center" (Wolf et al., 2006 p. 786).
(ii) Well-conditioned and young casualties
(iii) Advances in personnel protection: body armor and flame-retardant uniforms
(iv) Advances in medical treatments
(v) Rapid evacuation (movement) from point of injury to dedicated U.S. DoD Burn Center
(1) Military aircraft equipped as flying intensive care units
(2) Specially trained military medical burn flight teams
(3) The United States Army Burn Center treated more than 895

military burn casualties from 2003 to 2013 (Renz et al., 2012).

(a) More than 365 of these casualties were air transported by teams.

(b) Essential to have dedicated burn center and rehabilitation team to care for multiextremity amputation and patients with burns for an extended period

(c) Rapid air transport of military burn casualties facilitates this care.

c. Etiology

1) Head and hands most frequently burned (Wolf et al., 2006)

a) Hand burns difficult to treat, but treatment is essential for function (Hedman et al., 2008).

b) Even patients with small full-thickness hand burns are evacuated for evaluation.

c) According to Kauver and collagues (2006), burn sizes averaged 52% of the hands and 45% of the face.

2) Modern vehicular combat (land, air, and sea) increases risk.

a) Confined spaces are related to an increase in inhalation injuries and the risk of polytrauma.

b) Exposure to burning fuels or combustibles

c) Injuries from exploding ammunition or munitions

d) Improvised explosive devices or shaped charges

3) Infantry-type walking patrols characterized by "dismounted injuries" (Valerio, Sabino, Mundinger, & Kumar, 2014)

a) Greater exposure to direct blast

b) Greater incidence of concurrent traumatic amputations

c) Foreign debris in wounds from surrounding environment; infections

4) Combat-related burns comprise 5%–10% of all casualty types (Roeder & Schulman, 2010).

a) Mortality rate of 5% versus mortality rate of 2% for noncombat-related burns (Kauver et al., 2006)

5) Noncombat-related burns, defined as *unintentional burns* by Kauver and colleagues (2009), occurred at a higher rate in the deployed setting compared with a similar civilian cohort.

a) Use of burn pits and burning waste products

b) Accidents involving fuel products

c) Accidents related to handling munitions

d) Accident rate decreased over observed period

d. Mitigating risks and facilitating rehabilitation

1) The DoD's Joint Trauma System (JTS) was developed to address historical and evolving risks (U.S. Army Institute of Surgical Research, 2014a).

a) The mission of the JTS is to improve trauma care delivery and patient outcomes across the continuum of care.

b) JTS utilizes continuous performance improvement and evidence-based medicine driven by the concurrent collection and analysis of data maintained in the DoD Trauma Registry.

c) JTS defines *continuum of care* as an integrated system of all events, phases, levels, and intensities of trauma patient care across the DoD, including but not limited to prevention, point of injury, prehospital, patient movement, medical treatment facility (acute and subacute), chronic care, and lifelong rehabilitation.

d) The JTS vision is to expand globally as a resource.

e) The JTS is located at the United States Army Institute of Surgical Research, Fort Sam Houston, San Antonio, TX.

2) JTS applications for rehabilitation (U.S. Army Institute of Surgical Research, 2014b)

a) As an integral component of the DoD's JTS, rehabilitation services in acute care facilities and dedicated rehabilitation centers provide coordinated care for combat casualties who have sustained severe or catastrophic injuries that result in long-standing or permanent impairments.

b) Patients with less severe injuries also can benefit from rehabilitative programs that enhance recovery and speed return to function and productivity.

c) The goal of rehabilitative interventions is to allow the patient to return to the highest level of function, reduce disability, and avoid handicap whenever possible.

d) In the combat environment, some basic rehabilitation services are provided; however, patients who require extensive rehabilitation are usually evacuated from the combat theater and receive rehabilitation at a higher level of care. This could potentially include the facilities in the VA system.

e) The rehabilitation process should begin in the acute care MTF as soon as possible, ideally within the first 24 hours after an injury occurs. Both inpatient and outpatient rehabilitation services should be available.

f) Rehabilitation specialists should be members of the multidisciplinary advisory committee to ensure that rehabilitation issues are integrated into the trauma system plan.

g) The trauma system should demonstrate strong links and transfer agreements between stateside MTFs and their referral rehabilitation facilities.

h) Plans for repatriation of military patients should be part of rehabilitation system planning.

i) Feedback on functional outcomes after rehabilitation should be made available to the MTFs.

j) The JTS ensures that adequate rehabilitation facilities have been integrated into the trauma system and that these resources are made available to all populations that require them.

k) The JTS has incorporated, within the trauma system plan and the MTF standards, requirements for rehabilitation services, including interfacility transfer of combat casualties to rehabilitation centers.

l) Rehabilitation centers and outpatient rehabilitation services provide data on combat casualties to the MTF that transferred the patient to them and to the Department of Defense Trauma Registry. These data include final disposition, functional outcome, and rehabilitation costs. The rehabilitation centers also participate in performance-improvement processes.

m) A resource assessment for the rehabilitation needs of the JTS has been completed and is regularly updated.

n) The trauma system has reviewed a comprehensive system status inventory that identifies the availability and distribution of current rehabilitation capabilities and resources.

e. Military burn center rehabilitation (U.S. Army Institute of Surgical Research, 2014c)

1) The U.S. Army Institute of Surgical Research Burn Center serves as the sole facility caring for combat burn casualties, beneficiaries, and civilian emergencies within the DoD.

a) The Burn Center provides interdisciplinary care by a team of approximately 300 medical professionals.

b) State-of-the-art scientific care is coupled with combat casualty care research focused on the priorities of the Burn Center to improve battlefield care for our combat wounded.

c) Prevention and mitigation of severe thermal injury is another important aspect of the Burn Center's ongoing mission.

2) Integrated rehabilitation

a) The Burn Center's rehabilitation staff continues to provide physical and occupational therapy designed to maximize the return to duty of the thermal injury soldier and the long-term functional outcomes of soldiers who have been most severely injured by burns.

(i) Provide advanced, timely, and research-based burn rehabilitation to all patients.

(ii) Develop individualized treatment plans for each patient with the input of the patient and his or her family or caregiver.

(iii) Prevent and correct burn scar contracture and deformity to maximize functional outcomes and promote patient independence. Actively pursue clinical research to improve the care of burn patients.

b) The rehabilitation team continues to evaluate and improve methods of therapy to improve range of motion (ROM) and functional outcome and has performed studies to ensure that the most effective therapies are implemented as early as possible during the recovery process.

(i) Restore patient mobility, activities of daily living (ADLs), ROM, and strength.
(ii) Promote scar tissue modeling, and control scar formation.
(iii) Prevent contractures and deformity; maintain functional position of joints.
(iv) Protect burns, skin grafts, skin substitutes, and orthopedic injuries.
(v) Prepare patient to maximize prosthetic use when required.
(vi) Minimize and prevent negative effects of bed rest.
(vii) Adapt environment or patient equipment for enhanced independence.
(viii) Maximize functional outcomes and return to work, school, and leisure activities.
(ix) Maximize patient and family education and participation.
(x) Assist patient and family with psychosocial adjustment.
(xi) Actively participate in interdisciplinary discharge planning.
(xii) Actively pursue clinical research to improve the care of burn patients.

f. The Center for the Intrepid (CFI) (Brooke Army Medical Center, 2014)
  1) Mission
    a) Provide rehabilitation (outpatient) for OIF/OEF casualties who have sustained amputation, burns, or functional limb loss.
    b) Provide education to DoD and DVA professionals on cutting-edge rehabilitation modalities.
    c) Promote research in the fields of orthopedics, prosthetics, and physical/occupational rehabilitation.
    d) The staff and equipment for the CFI building were selected to provide the full spectrum of amputee and advanced outpatient rehabilitation for burn victims and limb salvage for patients with residual functional loss.
  2) Vision
    a) Multidisciplinary team collaboration
    b) Provide state-of-the-art amputee care.
    c) Assist patients as they return to the highest levels of physical, psychological, and emotional function.
  3) History
    a) Arnold Fisher and the Intrepid Fallen Heroes Board of Directors proffered a rehabilitation facility in 2005.
    b) Secretary of The Army Harvey accepted the proffer, and funds for the facility were received from more than 600,000 Americans.
    c) Ground was broken for the CFI, a four-story, 65,000-square-foot outpatient rehabilitation facility and two new, 21-handicap-accessible suites (i.e., the Fisher Houses) on September 22, 2005.
    d) Patient care in the facility began on February 15, 2007.
    e) The CFI is an outpatient facility under the command and control of the BAMC, and specifically, the department of orthopedics and rehabilitation.
    f) The CFI is staffed by active-duty army medical staff, Department of the Army civilians, contract providers, and nine full-time DVA employees.
    g) Together, the staff works to maximize the patients' rehabilitative potential and to facilitate reintegration whether they remain on active duty or return to civilian life.
  4) Capabilities
    a) The capabilities of the CFI include state-of-the-art technologies designed to be used for rehabilitation, research, education, and training.
    b) Patients are challenged by state-of-the-art physical and occupational therapy, demanding and challenging sports equipment, and virtual reality systems.
    c) Patients benefit from individualized case management, access to behavioral medicine services, and in-house prosthetic fitting and fabrication.
    d) The computer-assisted rehabilitation environment provides virtual-reality training.
    e) The motion analysis lab allows specialists to detect gait deviations not discernable to the naked eye.

f) The firearms training simulator reacquaints patients with their military weapons systems.

g) The FlowRider® surf machine integrates balance, core-strength training, and excitement into the rehabilitation process.

h) Services are presented to patients using an interdisciplinary approach and include physical medicine, case management, behavioral medicine, occupational therapy, physical therapy, wound care, and prosthetic fitting and fabrication.

i) During a typical week, 140–145 patients are seen and account for 550–650 patient visits. During the first year of operation, more than 28,000 patient visits were documented at the CFI.

2. Burn care

a. Overview

1) Burns are injuries to tissues caused by heat, friction, electricity, sunlight, nuclear radiation, or chemicals.

2) Fires and burns are the seventh leading cause of unintentional injury and death in the United States for people 1–85 years of age (Centers for Disease Control and Prevention [CDC], 2010).

3) In the United States in 2008, someone was injured by burns every 30 minutes on average (Karter, 2011).

4) Death rates from serious burns have declined because of advances in fluid resuscitation, nutritional support, skin replacement, topical antimicrobials to prevent infection, early surgical interventions, and improvement in the management of inhalation injury and hypermetabolism (National Institutes of Health, 2010).

5) Rehabilitation of the client with burns requires interdisciplinary teamwork to achieve restoration of function and reintegration into the community.

6) Rehabilitation nurses must be knowledgeable in wound management and healing and in the pathophysiological and psychological aspects of burn injuries.

7) The majority of the U.S. population lives within 2 hours of a burn center, yet only 40% of all burn patients are treated at a burn center (American College of Surgeons Health Policy Institute, 2011; Ortiz-Pujols et al., 2011).

a) Ground ambulance transfer is feasible.

b) Studies show better outcomes when patients are treated at a burn center.

b. Skin

1) The skin is the largest organ of the body.

2) The skin's major functions are to protect internal organs from infection and trauma, prevent fluid loss, and regulate body temperature. Body image is an important concept related to function.

3) Exposure to heat more than 120 degrees can result in burns.

c. Epidemiology

1) More than 450,000 burns warrant medical assistance in the United States each year, and approximately 40,000 of these warrant hospitalization (American Burn Association, 2013).

2) Approximately 20,000 of these burns are major burns that involve at least 25% of the total body surface.

3) Children, older adults, and people with disabilities are the highest-risk groups for burn injuries. Other high-risk groups include African Americans and Native Americans, those living in rural areas, the poor, and those living in substandard housing (CDC, 2009).

4) Survival rate: 96.6%

a) Gender: 69% male, 31% female

b) Ethnicity: 59% White, 20% African American, 14% Hispanic, 7% other

c) Admission cause: 43% fire/flame, 34% scald, 9% contact, 4% electrical, 3% chemical, 7% other

d) Place of occurrence: 72% home, 9% occupational, 5% street/highway, 5% recreational/sport, 9% other

5) Cooking equipment is the leading cause of home structure fires and fire injuries (Ahrens, 2010).

d. Etiology

1) Thermal

a) Flame (e.g., house fire, burning leaves)

b) Scald (stream of hot liquid [e.g., boiling water])

c) Flash (e.g., flame burn associated with explosion)

2) Contact (e.g., hot metal or tar)

3) Chemical: Strong acids or alkalis (e.g., common household cleaning agents) can be ingested or inhaled or come in contact with skin or mucous membranes. The amount of damage depends on the concentration and

quantity of the agent, duration of skin contact, and degree of penetration into the tissue (Lewis, Heitkemper, & Dirkson, 2004).

4) Electrical: The amount of damage caused by exposure to electrical current depends on the type of circuit, voltage and amperage, pathway of the current through the body, and duration of contact.
   a) Exposed or faulty wiring
   b) High-voltage power lines
   c) Lightning strikes
   d) Flash burns without direct contact secondary to arcing effects
5) Radiation
   a) Sunburn
   b) Therapeutic radiation for cancer treatment
   c) Nuclear radiation incidents
6) Smoke and inhalation: Directly inhaled smoke, hot air, or flames damage the tissues of the respiratory tract and can contain chemicals, such as carbon monoxide, that poison the body's cells.
   a) Super-heated steam inhalation injuries associated with commercial operations are devastating (Still, Friedman, Law, Orlet, & Craft-Coffman, 2001).
   b) Combination of super-heated water vapor and blast pressure results in deep respiratory tract injury.
   c) Chlorine or ammonia gases from commercial accidents or potential terrorist acts are current concerns.

e. Pathophysiology
   1) Primary injury results from tissue necrosis at the center of the burn from exposure to electricity, chemicals, or heat (Singer, Brebbia, & Soroff, 2007).
   2) The extent of a burn depends on the temperature and duration of exposure, skin thickness, and vascular supply (Singer, Brebbia, & Soroff, 2007).
   3) Burns consist of three zones: necrotic center, ischemic zone (can be reversible), and zone of hyperemia.
   4) Burns are classified according to depth and surface area.
      a) Degree of burn (**Figure 17-3**) (Singer, Brebbia, & Soroff, 2007)
         (i) First degree
            (1) Epidural layer, pain, erythema
            (2) Dry, pink skin
            (3) Usually heals within several days without scarring
         (ii) Second degree
            (1) Entire epidermis and part of underlying dermis
            (2) Superficial partial thickness
               (a) Erythema, blisters, weeping
               (b) Painful
               (c) Usually heals within 2 weeks with minimal scarring
            (3) Deep partial thickness
               (a) Deeper, can convert to third degree
               (b) Nonelastic white or red layer on top of burn, does not blanch with pressure
               (c) Takes up to 3 weeks to heal
               (d) Potential for scarring and contractures
         (iii) Third degree
            (1) Entire epidermis and dermis
            (2) White, brown, or tan; leathery
            (3) Not sensitive to touch, does not blanch
            (4) Warrants excision and grafting
      b) Extent of burn
         (i) Measured as a percentage of total body surface area (TBSA)

Figure 17-3. Levels of Burn Severity

First Degree (partial thickness)
• Does not extend below the epidermis • Is dry and very painful • Heals in a matter of days
Second Degree
• Involves the epidermis and part of the dermis • May be superficial (moist, painful, blisters) or deep thickness (less painful); may have a white or red base • Superficial burns heal in 1–2 weeks; deep thickness burns heal in 3 weeks or more.
Third Degree (full thickness)
• Extends into dermis • Is dry and involves no pain because sensory nerves are damaged; can be any color (e.g., white, black, yellow, brown) • Autograft is the usual form of treatment.
Fourth Degree
• Extends beyond fat and into the muscle and bone • Involves no pain and has variable color • Amputation of extremity is often necessary; autografting is the primary method for healing.

(ii) Rule of 9: This is a formula that divides the body into anatomical sections, each representing 9% or a multiple of 9% (i.e., head and neck = 9%, arms = 9% each, anterior trunk = 18%, posterior trunk = 18%, legs = 18% each, and perineum = 1%). Calculations are modified for infants and children younger than 10 years of age because of their larger head and smaller body size.

c) American Burn Association (ABA) Burn Center Referral Criteria (American Burn Association [ABA], 2006)

(i) A patient of any age who presents with the following should be referred and, if necessary, transferred to the closest burn center:

(1) Partial thickness burns greater than 10% TBSA
(2) Burns that involve the face, hands, feet, genitalia, perineum, or major joints
(3) Third-degree burns in any age group
(4) Electrical burns, including lightning injury
(5) Chemical burns
(6) Inhalation injury
(7) Burn injury in patients with preexisting medical disorders that could complicate management, prolong recovery, or affect mortality
(8) Any patients with burns and concomitant trauma (such as fractures) in which the burn injury poses the greatest risk of morbidity or mortality. In such cases, if the trauma poses the greater immediate risk, the patient can be initially stabilized in a trauma center before being transferred to a burn unit. Physician judgment is necessary in such situations and should be in concert with the regional medical control plan and triage protocols.
(9) Burned children in hospitals without qualified personnel or equipment for the care of children
(10) Burn injury in patients who will require special social, emotional, or long-term rehabilitative intervention

5) Clinical manifestations

a) Local: Capillaries of the injured tissue become leaky

(i) Increased capillary permeability results in plasma loss, drawing water with it, resulting in edema of the involved tissue and pain.

Figure 17-4. Systemic Responses to Burn Injury

Vascular Alterations

- Vasoconstriction results from exposure to heat and from stress response, resulting in decreased blood flow.
- Dilation of adjacent vessels and capillaries and increased capillary permeability occur after the initial vasoconstriction.
- Sodium pump is disturbed.
- Fluid shifts from the vascular space into the extracellular space, resulting in edema. If edema is not corrected, ischemia in the underlying tissues can occur.
- Cardiac output is decreased as a result of hypovolemia.
- Fluid resuscitation must be initiated to prevent cell shock and to maintain cardiac output and renal and tissue perfusion. Adults with burns of a total body surface area greater than 15% need fluid resuscitation.

Pulmonary Alterations

- Obstruction can occur when damage around the neck area becomes tight or when superheated air, steam, gases, flames, or smoke is inhaled.
- Depending on the severity, treatment can range from humidified air to mechanical ventilation.

Hematologic Alterations

Destruction of red blood cells in the burned area results in anemia.

Hematocrit level increases and blood flow decreases as the fluid shifts to the extravascular space, resulting in possible ischemia of underlying tissue and thrombosis.

Immune Response

- Immune responses decrease because of damage of the protective skin layer, stress, protein and caloric malnutrition and side effects of immunosuppressant medication and steroids.
- The individual is highly susceptible to infection.

Gastrointestinal Alterations

- Ileus is due to vasoconstriction.
- Parenteral route is used if an ileus is present.

Nutritional Alterations

- The metabolic rate increases, resulting in increased caloric need of about two times normal (Wilson, 1996).
- The metabolic rate will slowly return to normal when the wound is healed (Wilson, 1996).
- Blood glucose rises.
- Nutritional support may include oral supplements, tube feeding, intravenous supplements, or total parenteral nutrition.

b) Systemic responses: A major burn can affect all body systems and can cause serious complications through excessive fluid loss and tissue damage (i.e., systemic inflammatory response) (**Figure 17-4**).

c) Complications from burn surface

(i) Pain related to exposed nerve endings in partial-thickness burns and donor sites (ABA, 2009)

(ii) Scars

(1) Hypertrophic scars are red, thick, and raised above the level of normal skin but are within the boundaries of the burn wound and result from an imbalance between collagen synthesis and collagen lysis.

(2) Keloid scars are thick, nodular, and ridged scar tissue that grows beyond the site of injury; they can become binding and limit mobility if they are extensive (Burn Survivor Resource Center, n.d.).

(3) Scar tissue affects thermal regulation. Shivering is not possible with a full-thickness scar with extensive grafting. Ability to sweat is greatly reduced due to loss of sweat glands.

(iii) *Contractures*: Tightening and shortening of the tendons and muscles, resulting in immobility and decreased ROM. Prevention is the most effective treatment (e.g., splinting, exercising, positioning, using pressure garments). Surgery could be needed depending on the severity and location of contractures.

(iv) *Heterotopic ossification:* Abnormal deposit of new bone in soft tissue surrounding a joint that does not normally ossify. Surgical intervention could be needed if mobility is limited.

(v) *Altered sensation:* Diminished or absent response to sharp/dull and hot/cold; caution is needed to avoid further injury

(vi) *Pruritus:* Itching as the wound heals (ABA, 2009)

f. Management options

1) Prevention (Burn Prevention Network, 2010; CDC, 2009a)

a) House fires

(i) Use a smoke detector on each floor (one must be outside your bedroom door), replace batteries at least once a year, and test them monthly.

(ii) Keep emergency numbers by your phone.

(iii) Have a fire extinguisher in the kitchen.

(iv) Use a cooking timer with a loud alarm.

(v) Install a sprinkler system.

(vi) Place firefighting decals on the windows of children's bedrooms.

(vii) Make sure an address is clearly visible on the outside of your house.

b) Hotels and workplace

(i) Keep matches and lighters out of the reach of children.

(ii) Have a fire escape plan, know two ways out of every room, and practice fire drills and meeting at a designated space (a safe distance outside, away from the house).

(iii) Keep fire escape routes free of clutter.

b) Hotels and workplace

(i) Become familiar with exits and the posted evacuation plan.

(ii) Learn the location of building exits.

(iii) Respond to every alarm as if it were a real fire.

(iv) Keep a flashlight and room key on the table near the bed for easy access.

c) Hot water

(i) Do not exceed 120 degrees.

(ii) Turn handles of pots and pans inward while cooking.

(iii) Place cold water in the bathtub first, then add hot water to an appropriate temperature.

d) Chemical: Lock all flammable and caustic substances out of reach of children.

e) Electrical

(i) Cover outlets with childproof protectors.
(ii) Do not use appliances with frayed or worn cords.
(iii) Avoid overloading outlets.
(iv) Keep electrical appliances and cords away from water.

f) Ultraviolet sun rays
(i) Avoid extended exposure to sun.
(ii) Wear hats and sunblock with a minimum sun protection factor of 15.

g) Static electricity
(i) Leave your cell phone inside your vehicle or turn it off during refueling.
(ii) Do not reenter a vehicle during refueling.
(iii) If you need to reenter your vehicle during refueling, close the door after getting out, and make contact with metal before pulling out the nozzle to discharge static electricity from your body.

h) Precautions for those with disabilities
(i) Keep a wheelchair or assistive device close to the bed.
(ii) Keep a whistle nearby to alert rescuers of your location.
(iii) Place a firefighting decal on your bedroom window.
(iv) Do not smoke if using oxygen.

2) Acute phase: Airway management, fluid resuscitation, wound care, pain management, nutritional therapy, and psychosocial care

3) Management of burn surface (Singer et al., 2007)

a) Burn location and severity determine treatment. Wound care should focus on cleaning the wound and removing debris until healthy tissue is present.

b) Wound management includes moist dressing, infection control, debridement of necrotic tissue (i.e., removal of dead tissue), or surgical care.

c) Wound care goals (to permanently cover the wound) are to reduce pain and contamination, prevent infection, and minimize scarring.

d) Nonsurgical care (Singer et al., 2007)
(i) Keep blisters intact if possible.
(ii) First-degree wounds
(1) No specific therapy
(2) Superficial partial thickness
(3) Topical antimicrobial, synthetic, or biological occlusive dressing
(4) Specific treatments depend on infection and amount of exudate.
(iii) Deep-partial-thickness and third-degree burns are managed by a burn specialist with referral to a burn center.

e) Common topical antimicrobials
(i) Silver sulfadiazine, silver nitrate
(ii) Bacitracin, pupuricin
(iii) Mafenide acetate

f) Burn dressings
(i) Silver (nanocrystalline) (Acticoat®) (coated with silver)
(ii) Hydrocolloid wound dressing (Duoderm®) (donor sites)
(iii) Molnlycke mepitel tendra (Mepitel®) (silicone mesh)
(iv) Biological dressings
(1) Ferrous fumarate/polysaccharide iron complex/vitamin c/ vitamin b3 (Integra®), human fibroblast-derived dermal substitute (TransCyte®), allogeneic cultured keratinocytes and fibroblasts in bovine collagen (Apligraf®)
(2) Surgical debridement needed first

g) Minor burn care (Singer et al., 2007)
(i) Scene safety; protect yourself
(ii) Treat associated injuries.
(iii) Cool the burn with cool water.
(iv) Manage pain.
(v) Irrigate with soap and water.
(vi) Leave blisters intact.
(vii) Debride as needed.
(viii) Apply occlusive dressing or topical antimicrobial and absorptive dressing.
(ix) Update tetanus vaccine.

h) Surgical care (major burns)
(i) Change dressings one to three times daily (American Burn Association, 2009)
(ii) Keep graft and donor sites clean, moist, and covered (American Burn Association, 2009)

(iii) Surgical excision of damaged tissue (eschar)
(iv) Surgical debridement (American Burn Association, 2009)
(v) *Escharotomy:* Cutting through the burned tissue until healthy tissue is reached to relieve pressure from circumferential wounds that extend around the whole chest, leg, arm, or digits
(vi) *Dermabrasion:* Smoothing scar tissue by shaving or scraping off the top layers of the skin to minimize scars, restore function, and correct disfigurement resulting from an injury
(vii) Grafting to close deep partial- or full-thickness wounds and protect the skin as it heals on its own
   (1) *Autograft:* Use of the client's own skin from another site
      (a) The donor site is the harvested area of the client's own skin.
      (b) Partial-thickness wounds require an absorbent dressing because of excessive drainage.
      (c) Vacuum-assisted closure devices manage drainage, promote healing, and reduce infection, and can allow increased mobility with portable units (Low, Chong, & Tan, 2013).
   (2) *Cultured epithelium:* Take a small piece of unburned skin from the client, and grow skin under special tissue-culture conditions until it forms confluent sheets that can be used as skin graft.
   (3) Cadaver skin: Obtained through a graft bank
   (4) Allograft: From another living or dead person
   (5) *Xenograft:* Usually from pigs because their skin is most similar to human skin
   (6) *Skin substitutes:* Tissue bioengineering advances allow temporary-to-permanent burn-wound coverage (Murphy & Evans, 2012).
      (a) Reduced risk of infection or tissue rejection
      (b) Large quantities can be generated to cover large burn wounds
      (c) Expense of products can limit use

4) Management of complications
   a) Begin positioning and splinting immediately on admission to maintain the functional position of joints and prevent contractures. After the graft is stable, the splint should be worn continuously for at least 3 months.
   b) Use pressure garments against the skin to reduce scar formation and deformities for 23 hours per day for 1–2 years until the scar is fully mature, removing for bathing and cleaning of garments only (Burn Survivor Resource Center, n.d.).
   c) Use topical scar treatment gel and massage therapy to limit scar tissue formation.
   d) Manage pain by administering over-the-counter analgesics, nonsteroidal anti-inflammatory drugs, and narcotics and using diversional activities (e.g., music, imagery, relaxation techniques) during dressing changes.
   e) Infection control: Apply topical antimicrobial cream and employ strict infection control procedures.
   f) Nutritional therapy: Increase protein and calories; add vitamin supplements.

5) Nursing process
   a) Assessment
      (i) Begin with a history.
      (ii) Note the cause of the burn and any contributing factors.
      (iii) Assess pain (e.g., location, quality, duration, intensity).
      (iv) Assess function, including ROM.
      (v) Evaluate diet.
      (vi) Perform a psychosocial evaluation (e.g., support systems, coping strategies).
      (vii) Perform a complete physical and functional assessment, including the amount of burn area involved

and the depth, severity, and any complications from the injury.
   - (viii) Use a body diagram to document the location and appearance of burns, grafted areas, and donor sites.
- b) Plan of care
   - (i) Pain management
   - (ii) Nutritional intake to meet caloric needs
   - (iii) Skin and wound care
   - (iv) Interventions to attain and maintain function
   - (v) Psychological support
- c) Nursing diagnoses
   - (i) Alteration in comfort related to pain and itching
   - (ii) Self-care deficit related to burn, contracture, wound care, splitting, or pressure garment
   - (iii) Impaired skin integrity related to burn injury
   - (iv) Impaired physical mobility related to burn injury, contracture, wound care, splitting, or pressure garment
   - (v) Risk of infection related to loss of skin integrity
   - (vi) Inadequate nutrition related to diuresis, metabolic response to burn injury, inactivity, and self-care deficit (inability to self-feed)
   - (vii) Anxiety related to treatment regimen
   - (viii) Body image disturbance related to burn injuries, contractures, and scarring
   - (ix) Ineffective coping related to burn injury, pain, prognosis, and long-term outcomes
   - (x) Knowledge deficit related to burn process, treatment regimen, and signs and symptoms of complications
- d) Goals
   - (i) Report pain relief as a result of pain management interventions.
   - (ii) Maintain independence or demonstrate progression toward independence in performing ADLs.
   - (iii) Show signs of adequate wound healing.
   - (iv) Maintain full ROM and return, at a minimum, to baseline.
   - (v) Remain free of complications caused by burn injuries such as extensive scarring or contracture.
   - (vi) Remain free of signs and symptoms of infection.
   - (vii) Maintain present weight and maintain fluid hydration.
   - (viii) Verbalize feelings about change in appearance, and develop a realistic body image.
   - (ix) Develop effective coping strategies to adjust to burn injury.
   - (x) Verbalize understanding about the healing process, treatment options, and signs and symptoms of complications.
- e) Interventions
   - (i) Provide pain relief with prescribed analgesics, especially before wound care; elevate legs; and use nonpharmacological methods of pain control (e.g., imagery, distraction, relaxation, music).
   - (ii) Use therapeutic positioning, splints, and ROM exercises to maintain proper position and prevent contractures.
   - (iii) Provide assistive devices for use in performing ADLs.
   - (iv) Provide care for the wound and the development of healing tissue.
   - (v) Use a pressure garment to prevent or minimize scarring.
   - (vi) Prevent infection by applying topical antimicrobials as ordered, adhering to strict handwashing protocols, maintaining aseptic technique, and monitoring for signs and symptoms of infection.
   - (vii) Ensure adequate hydration and nutrition (e.g,, high protein, high calories, and vitamin supplements for wound healing).
   - (viii) Provide psychological support and health education regarding health status, treatments, nutritional needs, prevention of infections, and support groups.

(ix) Provide education on the healing process, treatment options, pain-relief measures, and complications.

f) Evaluation: Modify care according to the client's response to nursing interventions.

References

Ahrens, M. (2010). Home structure fires. Quincy, MA: National Fire Protection Association. Retrieved from http://www.nfpa.org/assets/files/PDF/OS.Homes.pdf

American Burn Association (2006). Burn center referral criteria. Retrieved from http://www.ameriburn.org/BurnCenterReferralCriteria.pdf

American Burn Association. (2009). White paper: Surgical management of the burn wound and use of skin substitutes. Retrieved from http://ameriburn.org/WhitePaperFinal.pdf?PHPSESSID=238c889e2b37ed68288f844717ba3447

American Burn Association. (2013). 2013 National Burn Repository report of data from 2003-21012. Retrieved from http://www.ameriburn.org/2013NBRAnnualReport.pdf

American Burn Association. (2014). Burn center referral criteria. Retrieved from http://www.ameriburn.org/

American College of Surgeons, Health Policy Research Institute. (2011). Retrieved from http://www.acshpri.org/documents/ACSHPRI_FS9.pdf

American Psychiatric Association (2013). *Posttraumatic stress disorder. DSM 5 collection*. Arlington, VA: Author.

Association of Rehabilitation Nurses (ARN). (2014). ARN competency model for professional rehabilitation nursing. Retrieved from http://www.rehabnurse.org/uploads/files/education/ARN_Rehabilitation_Nursing_Competency_Model_FINAL_-_May_2014.pdf

Atiyeh, B. S., Nayek, S. N., & Gunn, S. W. A. (2005). Armed conflict and burn injuries: A brief review. *Annals of Burns and Fire Disasters, 18*, 45–46.

Biggins, M. S., Engstrom, C., Jackson, P., Sommers, E. T., & Thorne-Odem, S. (2013). Transforming nursing care for veterans, personalized, proactive, and patient-driven healthcare. *Nurse Leader, 11*(5), 28–36.

Brooke Army Medical Center (2014). Center for the Intrepid. Retrieved from http://www.bamc.amedd.army.mil/departments/orthopaedic/cfi/

Burn Prevention Network. (2010). Resources. Retrieved August 11, 2010, from www.burnprevention.org/site/resources/

Burn Survivor Resource Center. (n.d.). Medical care guide: Types of scars. Retrieved August 10, 2010, from www.burnsurvivor.com/scar_types.html

Centers for Disease Control and Prevention. (2009). Fire deaths and injuries. Retrieved from www.cdc.gov/homeandrecreationalsafety/Fire-prevention/fires-factsheet.html

Centers for Disease Control and Prevention. (2010). WISQARS leading causes of death. Retrieved from http://webappa.cdc.gov/sasweb/ncipc/leadcaus10.html

Cifu, D.X., & Blake, C. (2011). Post-deployment syndrome: The illness of war. Military and veteran health care systems: A traditional approach. In N. Henson (Ed.), *Overcoming post-deployment syndrome: A six-step mission to health* (pp. 15–17, 37–40). New York: Demos Medical Publishing.

Foster, M. A., Moledina, J., & Jeffery, S. L. (2001). Epidemiology of U. K. military burns. *Journal of Burn Care & Research, 32*(3), 415–420.

Friedman, M. A. (2000). Posttraumatic Stress Disorder. Retrieved from www.acnp.org/g4/GN401000111/CH109.html

Galbraith, K.A. (2001). Combat casualties in the first decade of the 21st century: New and emerging weapons systems. *Journal of the Royal Army Medical Corps, 147*(1), 80–86.

Gironda, R. J., Clark, M. E., Massengale, J. P., & Walker, R. L. (2006). Pain among veterans of operations Enduring Freedom and Iraqi Freedom. *American Academy of Pain Medicine, 7*(4), 339–343.

Hedman, T. L., Renz, M., Richard, R. L., Quick, C. D., Dewey, W. S., Barillo, D. J.,...Holcomb, J. B. (2008). Incidence and severity of combat hand burns after all army activity message. *The Journal of Trauma; Injury, Infection, and Critical Care, 64*(2) (Suppl.), S169–S173.

Karter, M. J., Jr. (2010). Fire loss in the United States 2008. Retrieved from http://www.nfpa.org/assets/files/PDF/OS.fireloss.pdf

Kauver, D. S., Cancio, L. C., Wolf, S. E., Wade, C. E., & Holcomb, J. B. (2006). Comparison of combat and non-combat burns from ongoing U.S. military operations. *Journal of Surgical Research, 132*, 195–200.

Kauver, D. S., Wade, C. E., & Baer, D. G. (2009). Burn hazards of the deployed environment in wartime: Epidemiology of noncombat burns from ongoing United States military operations. *Journal of the American College of Surgeons, 209*(4), 453–460.

Kent, M. L., Upp, J. J., & Buckenmaier, C.C. (2011). Acute pain on and off the battlefield: What we do, what we know, and future directions. *International Anesthesiology Clinics, 49*(3), 10–32.

Kerns, R. D., & Dobscha, S. K. (Eds.). (2009). Pain among veterans returning from deployment in Iraq and Afghanistan: Update on the veterans health administration pain research program. *American Academy of Pain Medicine, 10*(7), 1161–1164. doi:10.1111/j. 1526-4637.2009.00722.x

Lamberty, G. J., Nakase-Richardson, R., Farrell-Carnahan, L., McGarity, S., Bidelspach, D., Harrison-Felix, C., & Cifu, D. X. (2014). Development of a traumatic brain injury model system within the Department of Veterans Affairs polytrauma system of care. *Journal of Head Trauma Rehabilitation, 29*(3), E1–E7. doi:10.1097/HTR.0b013e31829a64d1

Lewis, S. M., Heitkemper, M. M., & Dirkson, S. R. (2004). Medical-surgical nursing: Assessment and management of clinical problems (6th ed.). St. Louis,: Mosby.

Low, O., Chong, S. J., & Tan, B. (2013). The enhanced total body wrap—The new frontier in dressing care for burns. *Burns, 39*(7), 1420–1422. Retrieved from http://www.sciencedirect.com/science/article/pii/S0305417913000843

National Center for PTSD. (2010). What is PTSD? Retrieved from www.ptsd.va.gov/public/pages/what-is-ptsd.asp

Murphey, P. S., & Evans, G. R.D, (2012). Advances in wound healing: a review of current wound healing products. Plastic Surgery International. Retrieved from http://www.ncbi.nlm.nih.gov/pmc/articles/PMC3335515/ . Doi: 10.1155/2012/190436

Nayback, A. M. (2009). Posttraumatic stress: A concept analysis. *Archives of Psychiatric Nursing, 23*(3), 210–219.

National Institutes of Health. (2010, September). Fact sheet: Burns and traumatic injury. Retrieved from www.nih.gov/about/researchresultsforthepublic/BurnsandTraumaticInjury.pdf

Ortiz-Pujols, S. M., Thompson, K., Sheldon, G. F., Fraher, E. P., Ricketts, T. C., & Cairns, B. A. (2011). Burn care: Are there sufficient providers and facilities? Chapel Hill, NC: American College of Surgeons Health policy Research Institute. Retrieved from http://www.acshpri.org/

Owens, B. D., Kragh, J. F., Jr., Wenke, J. C., Macaitis, J, Wade, C. E., & Holcomb, J. B (2008). Combat wounds in Operation Iraqi Freedom and Operation Enduring Freedom. *The Journal of Trauma, 64*, 295–299.

Reiger, D. A., Kuhl, E. A., & Kupfer, D. J. (2013). The DMS-5: Classification and criteria changes. *World Psychiatry, 12*(2), 92–98. doi:10.1002/wps/20050 PMCID: MMC3683251

Renz, E. M., Cancio, L. C., Barillo, D. J., White, C. E., Albrecht, M. C., Thompson C. K.,…Holcomb, J. B. (2008). Long range transport of war-related burn casualties. *The Journal of Trauma, 64*(2), (Suppl. 2), S136–S144.

Renz, E. M., King, B. T., Chung, K. K., White, C. E., Lundy, J. B., Lairet, K. F., & Blackbourne, L. H. (2012). The US Army Burn Center: Professional service during 10 years of war. *Journal of Trauma and Acute Care Surgery, 73*(6) (Suppl. 5), S409–S416.

Roeder, R. A., & Schulman, C. L. (2010). An overview of war-related thermal injuries. *Journal of Craniofacial Surgery, 21*(4), 971–975.

Singer, A. J., Brebbia, J., & Soroff, H. H. (2007). Management of local burn wounds in the ED. *American Journal of Emergency Medicine, 25*, 666–671.

Still, J., Friedman, B., Law, E., Orlet, H. & Craft-Coffman, B. (2001). Burns due to exposure to steam. *Burns, 27*, 379–381.

U.S. Army Institute of Surgical Research (2014a). Joint trauma system. Retrieved from http://www.usaisr.amedd.army.mil/10_jts.html

U.S. Army Institute of Surgical Research (2014b). Joint trauma system development, conceptual framework and optimal elements. Retrieved from http://www.usaisr.amedd.army.mil/pdfs/Joint_Trauma_System_final_clean2.pdf

U.S. Army Institute of Surgical Research (2014c). Burn center general information. Retrieved from http://www.usaisr.amedd.army.mil/burn_center.html

U.S. Department of Veterans Affairs (n.d.). Polytrauma system of care. Rebuilding lives through excellence in rehabilitation. *Employee Education System*, 1–17.

U.S. Department of Veterans Affairs (2009). Family Care Map, Polytrauma Rehabilitation Center (PRC), polytrauma system of care. Retrieved from http://www.polytrauma.va.gov/FCM

U.S. Department of Veterans Affairs (2010a). National center for PTSD. Retrieved from www.ptsd.va.gov/professional/index.asp

U.S. Department of Veterans Affairs (2010b). Polytrauma/TBI system of care. Definitions. Retrieved from http://www.polytrauma.va.gov/definitions.asp#polytrauma

U.S. Department of Veterans Affairs (2013). Polytrauma system of care, VHA Handbook 1172.01. *Physical Medicine and Rehabilitation Service*, 1–56.

U.S. Department of Veterans Affairs (2014a). Veterans Posttraumatic Stress Disorder (PTSD). Retrieved from http://www.va.gov/opa/issues/ptsd.asp

U.S. Department of Veterans Affairs (2014b). VHA Polytrauma/TBI system of care. Retrieved from www.polytrauma.va.gov

U.S. Department of Veterans Affairs & U.S. Department of Defense (2010). Clinical practice guideline for the management of post-traumatic stress. Retrieved from http://www.healthquality.va.gov/ptsd/CPG_Summary_FINAL_MgmtofPTSDfinal.pdf

Valerio, I., Sabino, J., Mundinger, G. S., & Kumar, A. (2014). From battleside to stateside: The reconstructive journey of our wounded warriors. *Annals of Plastic Surgery 72*(5) (Suppl. 1), S38–345.

Wolf, S. E., Kauvar, D. S., Wade, C. E., Cancio, L. C., Renz, E. M., Horvath, E. E.,…Holcomb, J. B. (2006). Comparison between civilian burns and combat burns from Operation Iraqi Freedom and Operation Enduring Freedom. *Annals of Surgery, 243*(6), 786–792, discussion 792–785.

Suggested Resources

PTSD

American Psychological Association. Post-traumatic Stress Disorder: http://www.apa.org/topics/ptsd/

Gateway to PTSD Information: www.ptsdinfo.org

Mayo Clinic. PTSD: http://www.mayoclinic.org/diseases-conditions/post-traumatic-stress-disorder/basics/definition/con-20022540

National Center for PTSD: www.ptsd.va.gov

National Institutes of Mental Health: www.nimh.nih.gov/health/topics/post-traumatic-stress-disorder-ptsd/index.shtml

National Institutes of Mental Health: http://www.nimh.nih.gov/health/topics/post-traumatic-stress-disorder-ptsd/index.shtml

U.S. DVA/DoD Clinical Practice Guideline: Posttraumatic Stress Disorder: www.healthquality.va.gov/ptsd/ptsd_full.pdf

U.S. DVA PTSD Screening Guidelines for PTSD: www.ptsd.va.gov/professional/pages/screening-and-referral.asp

For service members, veterans, and providers

About Face: http://www.ptsd.va.gov/apps/aboutface/

After Deployment: www.afterdeployment.org

Center for the Study of Traumatic Stress: www.centerforthestudyoftraumaticstress.org

Military OneSource: www.militaryonesource.com

My HealtheVet: www.myhealth.va.gov

National Center for PTSD: www.ptsd.va.gov

Our Military: www.ourmilitary.mil

Real Warriors: www.realwarriors.net

RESPECT: www.Milpdhealth.mil

VA Military Sexual Trauma Counseling: www.vetcenter.va.gov

VAs Make the Connection: www.maketheconnection.net

PTSD Tools

Make the Connection http://maketheconnection.net/conditions/ptsd?gclid=CISwqfvE774CFYhAMgodNgYAzg

PTSD coach app available free of charge. Download on iPhone or Android devices.

Strong at the Broken Places: http://www.blogs.va.gov/strongatbrokenplaces/

Burns

http://www.usaisr.amedd.army.mil/default.html

http://www.history.army.mil/books/Green-Ramp/POPEC.HTM

Section IV

Functional
HEALTHCARE PATTERNS

Chapter 18

Health Maintenance and Management of Therapeutic Regimens

Kristen L. Mauk, PhD DNP RN CRRN GCNS-BC GNP-BC FAAN
Maria Radwanski, MSN RN CRRN

LEARNING OUTCOMES

- Understand the meaning of a family-centered plan of care.
- Recognize models for community-based care.
- Define the role of the rehabilitation nurse in health maintenance and restorative activities.
- List rehabilitation nursing interventions to prevent risk for injury, especially falls.
- Consider the role of the rehabilitation nurse in disaster planning for people with disability.

KEY CHAPTER TOPICS

- Health maintenance
- Health models
- Health and wellness
- Fall prevention
- Risk for injury
- Ineffective therapeutic regimen
- Disability and natural disasters

PROFESSIONAL REHABILITATION NURSING DOMAINS AND COMPETENCIES

- Domain 1: Competencies 1.3, 1.4
- Domain 2: Competencies 2.2, 2.3
- Domain 3: Competencies 3.2, 3.3, 3.4
- Domain 4: Competency 4.3 (Association of Rehabilitation Nurses [ARN], 2014)

Introduction

The purpose of this chapter is to provide the rehabilitation nurse with the theoretical structure necessary to develop and implement a family-centered plan of care so that a person with a disability can successfully maintain and manage his or her therapeutic regimens in the community.

"Rehabilitation nursing is a specialty practice that offers a unique, holistic perspective to the care of clients with disabilities and chronic health problems" (Jacelon, 2011, p. 1). Rehabilitation clients must use effective health management strategies to achieve and maintain an optimal quality of life. People with disabilities are living longer and need long-term health promotion interventions. Maintenance of optimal health includes both the prevention of further loss of function and the prevention of secondary conditions such as cardiovascular, cardiopulmonary, and psychosocial disorders. In addition, the impact of falls and injuries on both clients and their families exacerbates the challenge of successful health maintenance and management. "A rehabilitative focus on the body has expanded to consider the impact of physiological impairment on individuals' lives that includes the environment and society" (Kearney, Pryor, & Lever, 2012, p. 28). Therefore, successful rehabilitation nursing includes the transfer of knowledge and accountability for healthcare needs from nurses to clients and their families and significant others in a manner that promotes health and wellness for the person with a disability (Viggiani, 2000). Strategies are best conceived when developed in a nursing theory framework that provides education and training to address weaknesses and maximize strengths to meet the needs of clients and families and to promote health in the community.

I. Background

Current Status of Disabilities in the United States: The 2012 Disability Status Report (Erickson & Von Schrader, 2014) provides the rehabilitation nursing community with a summary of the most recent demographic and economic statistics: 6 million noninstitutionalized people with disabilities. This report focuses primarily on the working-age population because "employment is a key factor in the social integration and economic self-sufficiency of working-age people with disabilities" (Erickson & Von Schrader, p. 1). The statistics selected were chosen based on their value in the development of a home- and community-based plan of care. An overall description of the state of disability in the United States is represented by the following statistics (Erickson & Von Schrader, 2014).

A. Age: In the United States in 2012, the prevalence of disability across the lifespan was
  1. 12.1% for people of all ages
  2. 0.8% for people age 4 years and younger
  3. 5.3% for people age 5–15 years
  4. 5.5% for people age 16–20 years
  5. 10.4% for people age 18–64 years
  6. 25% for people age 65–74 years
  7. 50% for people age 75 years and older.

B. Race: In the United States in 2012, the prevalence of disability for working-age people (age 21–64 years) was
  1. 10.2% among Whites
  2. 14.2% among African Americans
  3. 4.3% among Asians
  4. 17.6% among Native Americans
  5. 9.9% among people of other races.

C. Education: In the United States in 2012, the percentage of working-age people with disabilities with
  1. Only a high school diploma or equivalent was 13.6%
  2. Only some college or an associate degree was 10.0%
  3. A bachelor's degree or more was 4.4%.

D. Employment, Poverty, Education, and Health Insurance Coverage: In 2012, the employment rate of working-age people (ages 21–64 years) with disabilities in the United States was 33.5%, with another 10.8% looking for work. The poverty rate for working-age people with disabilities was 28.4%, and 82.8% of working-age people with disabilities had health insurance.

E. Legislation: The Americans with Disabilities Act (ADA, 2010) protects the 54 million Americans with physical or mental impairments that substantially limit daily activities. These activities include working, walking, talking, seeing, hearing, or caring for oneself. Its five titles oversee legislation in the areas of employment (Title I), public services (Title II), public accommodations and services operated by private entities (Title III), telecommunications (Title IV), and miscellaneous provision (Title V).

II. Conceptual Framework

The use of a conceptual framework provides structure within which to organize thinking, provide rationales for chosen interventions, and explain choices and options to others. Rehabilitation nurses create conceptual frameworks using nursing theories, various viewpoints of health, and knowledge of community settings to create a family-centered plan of care.

A. Viewpoints of Health
  1. Health: "Health is a state of complete physical, mental, and social well-being and not merely the absence of disease or infirmity" (World Health Organization, 1948, p. 100). "Optimal health is a dynamic balance of physical, emotional, social, spiritual, and intellectual health" (O'Donnell, 2009, p. iv). Health within illness may reflect the experience of many who live with chronic illness and disability (Kearney, Pryor, & Lever, 2012).
  2. Wellness
     a. Wellness is often viewed on a continuum from health to illness with every dynamic in between.
     b. "Wellness is first and foremost a choice to assume responsibility for the quality of your life. It begins with a conscious decision to shape a healthy lifestyle. Wellness is a mind set, a predisposition to adopt a series of key principles in varied life areas that lead to high levels of well-being and life satisfaction" (Ardell, n.d.).
  3. Health promotion
     a. "Health promotion is the process of enabling people to increase control over, and to improve, their health. To reach a state of complete physical, mental, and social well-being, an individual or group must be able to identify and to realize aspirations, to satisfy needs, and to change or cope with the environment. Health is, therefore, seen as a resource for everyday life, not the objective of living. Health is a positive concept emphasizing social and personal resources, as well as physical capacities. Therefore, health promotion is not just the responsibility of the health sector, but goes beyond healthy life-styles to well-being" (World Health Organization, 1986).
     b. "Health promotion is the art and science of helping people discover the synergies between their core passions and optimal health, enhancing their motivation to strive for optimal health, and supporting them in changing their lifestyle to move toward a state of optimal health" (O'Donnell, 2009, p. iv).
     c. "The Disability and Health objectives (2020) highlight areas for improvement and opportunities for people with disabilities to:
        1) Be included in public health activities.

2) Receive well-timed interventions and services. Interact with their environment without barriers.
3) Participate in everyday life activities" (Healthy People.gov, 2014, para 2).

B. Settings and Models of Community-Based Care: The settings for the provision of community-based rehabilitation nursing concepts include residential institutions, such as long-term care facilities and subacute care centers, outpatient programs, community and faith-based organizations, and private homes (**Table 18-1**).

1. Outpatient rehabilitation clinics: Nurses in outpatient rehabilitation clinics focus on integrating rehabilitation principles into the community.
2. Assisted living: Nurses in assisted living environments focus on promoting health in a structured community living setting that is accessible for people with disabilities and provided adaptations for the aged.
3. Home: Home healthcare nurses provide hands-on nursing care in the client's home. Advanced practice nurses providing services in the home focus on comprehensive assessment, diagnosis, and treatment to help patients age in place.

Table 18-1. Settings, Models, and Programs Where Community-Based Rehabilitation Is Used

Setting	Purpose	Types of Clients	Delivery System	Nursing Roles
Home health care	To provide health care to individuals and families in their place of residence for the purpose of prompting or restoring health, maximizing independence, and minimizing the effects of disability (Hankwitz, 1993)	All age levels; Common conditions: • Fractures • Degenerative joint disease • Multiple sclerosis • Parkinson's disease • Cancer • Alterations in function secondary to neuropathy or myopathy • Amputations • Burns	Primary care Case management	Partner Teacher Resource manager Clinician (Neal, 1998)
Subacute care	To serve clients whose medical treatment does not allow for participation in acute rehabilitation programs or who are classified as slow to progress or who cannot qualify for a standard rehabilitation program (Mumma & Nelson, 1996)	Typically older than age 16, although specialty pediatric facilities are available; Common conditions: • Closed-head injury with quadriparesis • Anoxic encephalopathy secondary to cardiac arrest • Strokes • Aneurysms	Team nursing: • Primary care delivered by nursing assistants • Licensed vocational nurses (LVNs) provide unit supervision and treatments • RNs serve in the case management and coordination role	Planner Coordinator Evaluator of client outcomes Client advocate
Long-term care	To serve clients who are unable to live independently and meet their self-care needs	Primarily the geriatric population, as well as an unknown number of younger people with chronic disabilities; Common conditions: • Joint fractures • Strokes • Closed-head injury • Anoxia • Rheumatoid arthritis	Team nursing: • Primary care delivered by LVNs and nursing assistants • RNs serve the case coordination and management role	Planner Coordinator Evaluator of client outcomes Client advocate
Independent living	To serve individuals who want to take control of their lives, participate in decision making, and achieve the highest level of independence possible	Primarily adults; Common conditions: • Spinal cord injury • Closed-head injury	Care provided by personal care attendants RN serves as care manager	Partner Educator Client advocate

4. School: School nurses provide education, counseling, and referral services for health promotion and disease prevention and for meeting the needs of children with disabilities.
5. Congregation: Parish nurses act as health counselors, educators, and referral sources; use a holistic focus with a foundation based on spiritual health; and usually provide counseling and advocacy within a faith community.
6. Case managers: Case managers act as liaisons, health educators, health promoters, and referral sources. They facilitate return to work for workers with injuries and integrate workers with catastrophic injuries back into the community.

C. Roles of Rehabilitation Nurses in Health Maintenance and Health Restoration Activities

1. Coach or physical caregiver: Clients and families have become more educated as consumers and take responsibility for making healthcare choices, resulting in a shift of the nurse–client relationship to one of collaboration. The client assumes primary responsibility for setting the goals, and the nurse's role varies depending on the client's degree of independence.
2. Teacher
   a. The most important goal of teaching in community-based rehabilitation is to help the client and family achieve the following possible outcomes:
      1) Improvements in care
      2) Facilitation of health promotion
      3) Reduction of complications
      4) Resumption of functional activities
   b. Sharing knowledge about healthcare improves client and family satisfaction (Kim & Moon, 2007). Education increases the client's and family's sense of control by encouraging mutual participation in care planning.
3. Resource or care manager: In this role, the nurse maintains responsibility for tracking and directing the client's care and progress throughout the healthcare system. The nurse oversees the client's primary needs:
   a. Assesses the client appropriately
   b. Establishes the plan of care
   c. Delegates specific nursing care tasks to other qualified personnel
   d. Initiates interventions
   e. Coordinates and collaborates with the healthcare team
   f. Acts as a care facilitator or navigator with the patient and the healthcare system (ARN, 2013)
   g. Evaluates outcomes: Collaboration and care coordination are vital to the implementation of this role because rehabilitation clients and families interact with many healthcare professionals who have different areas of expertise and training. The care manager facilitates the client's treatment plan to ensure that it is consistent with the client's needs and is achieved in a timely manner. In addition, the nurse in this role must have an effective understanding of the cultural norms of the client's community and their influence on the client's behavior.
4. Advocate
   a. An advocate defends the cause of another person. In nursing, advocacy involves empowering clients, families, and client populations through knowledge (**Figure 18-1**).
   b. Works to change the system, collaborating with other professionals, role modeling, and maximizing the use of community resources
   c. Coordinates referrals to not-for-profit and private home care agencies

Figure 18-1. Keys to Developing Advocacy Skills

Understanding and Knowledge of Self Personally and Professionally
- Knowledge of oneself: Awareness of personal goals and how these goals affect relationships with clients
- Realistic self-concept: Awareness of own limitations and abilities that will affect client care
- Value clarification: Awareness of personal bias and prejudices, moral and ethical values; knowledge of personal perceptions concerning what is fair and acceptable and how these perceptions may affect relationships with clients

Knowledge of Treatment and Intervention Options
- Development of a strong knowledge base about interventions and outcomes
- Awareness of rationale for interventions

Knowledge of the Healthcare System
- Awareness of how the healthcare system relates to clients, families, and the community
- Awareness of specific aspects of community (e.g., politics, economy) and how these factors affect the healthcare system

Knowledge of How to Put Advocacy into Action
- Assessment
  - What does the client identify as the problem?
  - What support or resources does the client already have?
  - What knowledge does the client have about health services and treatment options?
  - In what areas does the client feel a need for more personal control?
- Planning: Mobilizing resources, consulting, collaborating with the healthcare team
- Implementation: Educating and empowering the client (the nurse helps the client assert control over variables affecting the client's life)

d. Identifies agencies that provide free care or sliding-scale fees for services based on income and the duration of needed services
e. Arranges for social work services to help gain access to community systems that can provide subsidized housing, Medicaid applications, Supplemental Security Income and Social Security Disability Insurance, counseling services, advocacy assistance, equipment, and transportation and that can help find organizations that provide services
f. Contacts the local department of human services about services available for rehabilitation care
g. Evaluates outcomes of care to evaluate individual goal achievement and aggregate data to evaluate service quality
h. Contacts legislators (via phone, letter, e-mail, or in person) to support funding for transferring clients to independent living centers and for training care attendants and supplemental funding that allows people with disabilities to work without a drastic reduction in or termination of medical benefits
i. Attends public hearings on issues that affect people with disabilities
j. Acts as a community advocate to increase environmental accessibility, decrease architectural barriers, increase access to public transportation, decrease cost of services to older and disabled adults on fixed incomes, and increase access to healthcare services
k. Makes referrals to rehabilitation counselors, peer counselors, and those providing psychological services
l. Contacts state disability offices, commissions, or departments for assistance
m. Promotes the education of healthcare providers and caregivers within facilities and the community
n. Provides in-service education
o. Consults one-on-one with providers regarding healthcare issues, ways to manage individual clients' healthcare needs, and ways to promote access to healthcare services
p. Encourages family involvement early in the rehabilitation process and teaches family members about equipment, procedures, medications, and ways to manage emergencies
q. Coordinates a home visit by the rehabilitation team to evaluate the need for modifications, equipment, and safety improvements
r. Promotes interagency communication about rehabilitation needs, follow-up teaching needs, and previous nursing interventions in the event of a transfer to a different environment
s. Periodically reassesses and evaluates the client's ability to perform activities of daily living, changes in levels of independence, healthcare needs, and barriers to necessary services
t. Contacts healthcare providers in the community to determine access to buildings, cost of services, insurance coverage, ways to modify the office environment, and availability of transportation
u. Speaks at service club meetings
v. Actively participates in professional organizations that support legislation and advocacy activities for people with disabilities
w. Promotes the appointment of people with disabilities to public office and commissions and to private sector industry and business boards
x. Helps clients with disabilities prepare testimony for legislative hearings
y. Participates in health planning endeavors and advocates for services that meet the needs of children and adults

III. Nursing Challenges: Ineffective Health Maintenance

A higher percentage of adults with disabilities (40%) report fair or poor health than do adults without disabilities (10%). Among adults with disabilities, African Americans, Hispanics, and Native Americans report fair or poor health at disproportionately higher rates than Whites and Asian Americans. Finally, adults with disabilities are more likely than adults without disabilities to smoke, to be obese, and to be physically inactive (Centers for Disease Control and Prevention [CDC], n.d.).

A. Definition of Problem: The North American Nursing Diagnosis Association (NANDA) defined ineffective health maintenance as the "inability to identify, manage, and/or seek out help to maintain health" (Ackley & Ladwig, 2014, p. 412).
B. Defining Characteristics
   1. Demonstrated lack of adaptive behaviors to environmental changes
   2. Demonstrated lack of knowledge about basic health practices
   3. History of lack of health-seeking behavior
   4. Impairment of personal support systems
   5. Inability to take responsibility for meeting basic health practices
   6. Lack of expressed interest in improving health behaviors (Ackley & Ladwig, 2014).
C. Related Factors
   1. Cognitive impairment

2. Complicated grieving
3. Deficient communication skills
4. Diminished fine motor skills
5. Diminished gross motor skills
6. Inability to make appropriate judgments
7. Ineffective family coping
8. Ineffective individual coping
9. Insufficient resources (e.g., equipment, finances)
10. Perceptual impairment
11. Spiritual distress
12. Unachieved developmental tasks

D. Nursing Outcomes Classification (NOC): Suggested outcomes include improving health-seeking behavior and supporting health promotion behaviors.

E. Assessment

1. Client's self-management abilities and knowledge
   a. Assess the client's feelings, values, and reasons for not following the prescribed plan of care.
   b. What is the client's coping status regarding responsibility for and access to health care?
   c. Assess family patterns, economic issues, and cultural patterns that influence compliance with a given medical regimen.
   d. Consider the client's health and lifestyle before the injury or illness.
   e. Assess the client's perception of health.
   f. Assess for use of and reasons for not using health services.
   g. Does the client's health insurance plan cover ongoing telephone disease management by nurses?
   h. Is the client interested in a health management program?
   i. What is the client's ability and motivation to take responsibility for health, including knowledge of nutritional needs?
   j. Does the client have access to healthcare providers and facilities?
   k. What is the client's knowledge of prescribed medications and their effects?
   l. What is the client's knowledge of his or her medical status and related treatment program, such as written action plans developed collaboratively by the client and primary care practitioner (e.g., physician, nurse practitioner, physician assistant, or clinical specialist)?
2. Client's emotional and spiritual state
   a. What stage of grief is the patient experiencing related to the injury or disease?
   b. What methods of coping does the client use?
   c. Assess the effect of fatalism on the client's ability to modify health behavior.
   d. Is there evidence of chemical dependency? Self-neglect? Self-mutilation?
   e. What are the client's sources of hope and strength?
   f. Does the client believe in God or another deity?
   g. What is the client's perceived relationship between spiritual beliefs and health?
   h. Does the client observe religious practices?
3. Client's social support system: Five categories of caregivers can make up a client's social support system: family, friends, social service organizations or churches, agencies, and private pay services. What is the frequency, amount, kind, and level of support provided to the client by each category? Who are the contacts within each category? How does the client manage this information? Is there a plan in place in case support from one or more sources is temporarily or permanently unavailable?

F. Nursing Interventions Classifications (NIC)

1. Educate the client at his or her learning level using age-specific adult learning principles to facilitate health maintenance.
2. Determine readiness to learn.
3. Assess knowledge of self-care.
4. Controlled stimulation may be needed to help the client focus on the learning task.
5. Use teaching tools (e.g., written materials, audiotapes or videotapes, lectures, models).
6. Use demonstrations and return demonstrations.
7. Use memory aids (e.g., written reminders [large print when necessary], medication dispensers, and consistent location of supplies).
8. Provide progressive sequential learning experiences that build on skills without overwhelming the learner (e.g., help the client take on progressive responsibility for bladder management).
9. Design a physical environment that minimizes dependency and the sick role by maximizing all opportunities to create a feeling of home.
10. Encourage the client and healthcare providers to wear street clothes.
11. Encourage the client to eat meals with others and follow the family's pattern of eating as much as possible.
12. Help the client identify and begin to resume family role responsibilities.
13. Provide privacy when the client is performing physical care and interacting with others and allow time for the client to be alone.

14. Introduce the client to role models (e.g., other clients who competently manage their health and wellness).
15. Encourage the client to set realistic and achievable goals with the help of healthcare providers.
16. Encourage the client to become involved in all phases of care planning; promote the client's control of the process.
17. Provide information that supports informed decision making.
18. Negotiate to simplify or alter client behaviors and outcomes; adapt program methods or schedules to the client's preferred routine.
19. Avoid assuming a "powerful other" role that reinforces eternal control.
20. Create a contract with the client to define agreed-upon responsibilities, conditions, and goals for program participation.
21. Help the client and caregivers manage desired health practices and promote wellness.
22. Provide anticipatory guidance to maintain and manage effective health practices during periods of wellness.
23. Identify adaptation strategies to use when progressive illness or long-term health problems occur.
24. Monitor adherence to a prescribed medical regimen and evaluate side effects and treatment outcomes.
25 Help the client and family develop stress management skills.
26. Identify ways to adapt an exercise program to meet the client's changing needs, abilities, and environmental concerns.
27. Educate the client about the symptoms of life-threatening illness, such as myocardial infarction or cerebrovascular accident and the need for timeliness in seeking care.
28. Provide culturally targeted education and healthcare services.
29. Provide nurse-led case management.
30. Include a health promotion focus for the client with disabilities, with the goals of reducing secondary conditions (e.g., obesity, hypertension, pressure sores), maintaining functional independence, providing opportunities for leisure and enjoyment, and enhancing overall quality of life.
31. Provide support and individual training for care.

IV. **Nursing Challenges: Ineffective Therapeutic Regimen Management**

A. Definition of Problem: NANDA defined *ineffective therapeutic regimen management* as a "pattern of regulating and integrating into family processes a program for treatment of illness and sequelae of illness that is unsatisfactory for meeting specific health goals" (Grosiran, 2012).

B. Defining Characteristics (Grosiran, 2012, para 2)
1. Choices of daily living are ineffective for meeting the goals of a treatment or prevention program.
2. Client did not take action to reduce risk factors for progression of illness and sequelae.
3. Client verbalizes little or no desire to manage the treatment of illness and prevention of sequelae.
4. Client verbalizes difficulty with regulation of one or more prescribed regimens for prevention of complications and treatment of illness or its effects.
5. Client did not take action to include treatment regimens in daily routines.

C. Causes or Related Factors (Grosiran, 2012, para 3)
1. Perceived barriers
2. Social support deficits
3. Powerlessness
4. Perceived susceptibility
5. Perceived benefits
6. Mistrust of regimen or healthcare personnel
7. Knowledge deficit
8. Family patterns of health care
9. Family conflict
10. Excessive demands made on individual or family
11. Economic difficulties
12. Decisional conflicts
13. Complexity of therapeutic regimen
14. Complexity of healthcare system
15. Perceived seriousness
16. Inadequate number and types of cues to action

D. Nursing Outcomes Classification (NOC)
1. The middle-range theory of caregiver stress was developed from Roy's Adaptation Model. There are four assumptions in the caregiver stress theory:
   a. "Caregivers can respond to environmental change.
   b. Caregivers' perceptions determine how caregivers respond to environmental stimuli.
   c. Caregivers' adaption is a function of their environmental stimuli and adaptation level.
   d. Caregivers' effectors (e.g., physical function, self-esteem and mastery, role enjoyment, and marital satisfaction) are results of chronic caregiving" (Tsai, 2003, p. 139).
2. The symptoms of dementia related to aggression and decreased ability to perform activities of daily living (ADLs) are thought to increase caregiver burden (Miyamoto, Tachimori, & Ito, 2010).

3. Hanks, Rapport, and Vangel (2007) found a modest to strong relationship between caregivers' perceived social support and caregiver assessment of family functioning.
4. Health-seeking behavior
5. Knowledge of treatment regimen
6. Participation in healthcare decisions

E. Nursing Interventions Classification (NIC)
1. Determine the types of equipment, supplies, and services that are lacking for an adequate health state to be maintained safely.
2. Identify who in the client's support system is willing to develop the strategies necessary to improve management of the therapeutic regimen.
3. Foster the client's advocate as he or she assumes responsibility in promoting the client's wellness and health management.
4. Encourage the client's advocate to use reliable electronic sources when searching for health-related information (**Table 18-2**).
5. Educate the client and the client's primary advocate on their learning level using age-specific adult learning principles and native language to facilitate health maintenance.

V. Nursing Challenge: Ineffective Community Coping

NANDA defined ineffective community coping as a "pattern of activities for adaptation and problem solving that is unsatisfactory for meeting the demands or needs of the community" (Ackley & Ladwig, 2014, p. 272).

A. Defining Characteristics
1. Community does not meet its own expectations.
2. Deficits in community participation
3. Excessive community conflicts
4. Expressed community powerlessness
5. Expressed vulnerability
6. High illness rates
7. Increased social problems
8. Stressors perceived as excessive (Ackley & Ladwig, 2014, pp. 272–275)

B. NOC
1. Community competence
2. Community health status
3. Community violence level

C. NIC
1. Participate with the community in the identification of stressors and assessment of distress.
2. Identify the health services and information resources that are currently available in the community.
3. Provide support to the community and help community members identify and mobilize additional supports.
4. Advocate for the community in multiple arenas and government agencies.
5. Write grant proposals to help community members obtain funds for programs that reduce stress or improve coping.
6. Work with members of the community to identify and develop coping strategies that promote a sense of power.
7. Work with members of the community to prioritize and target health goals specific to the community.
8. Establish and sustain partnerships with key individuals within communities when developing and implementing programs (Ackley & Ladwig, 2014, pp. 272–275).

D. Accessibility
1. Accessibility means more than transportation (**Figure 18-2**).
   a. There are more than 56.7 million Americans with disabilities who need care associated with their disability as well as primary care services (U.S. Census Bureau, 2012).
      1) Are there the outpatient and community services available that the client needs?
      2) Are there funding sources available in adequate amounts to support acquisition of the services?
      3) Can the client get in and out of his or her home?
      4) What are geographic barriers (rural, urban, metropolitan) that influence access to services?
   b. In addition, accessibility related to transportation means more than transportation to healthcare services or access to social services.
   c. There remains a high prevalence of unmet needs for home and- community-based services among people with disabilities.
   d. There is need for improved access to information about services and benefits and access to in-home supports (Mitra, Bogen, Long-Bellil, & Heaphy, 2011).
   e. The dynamic interplay of real-world factors (violence, street activity, street conditions) is an important determinant of whether those with disabilities have positive social and interpersonal interactions to obtain preventive healthcare or participate in civic duties such as voting in government elections (Clarke, Ailshire, Nieuwenheijsen, & deKleijnde Vrankrijiker, 2011).

Table 18-2. Use of Websites for Health Information	
Accuracy	Is the information accurate, reliable, and free from error?
Authority	Is the author identified? Are the author's credentials presented? Is the publisher identified? Is contact information, such as a phone number or e-mail address, provided? What is the domain (e.g., .gov, .edu, .com, .org)?
Objectivity	What is the goal of the site? Is there bias? Is the information trying to sway opinion?
Currency	Is a date provided for publication or updates? Is the site updated regularly?
Coverage	Is a special browser or payment of a fee required for complete viewing? Are the topics explored in depth? Are the links relevant?

Figure 18-2. Gaining Access to Community Resources

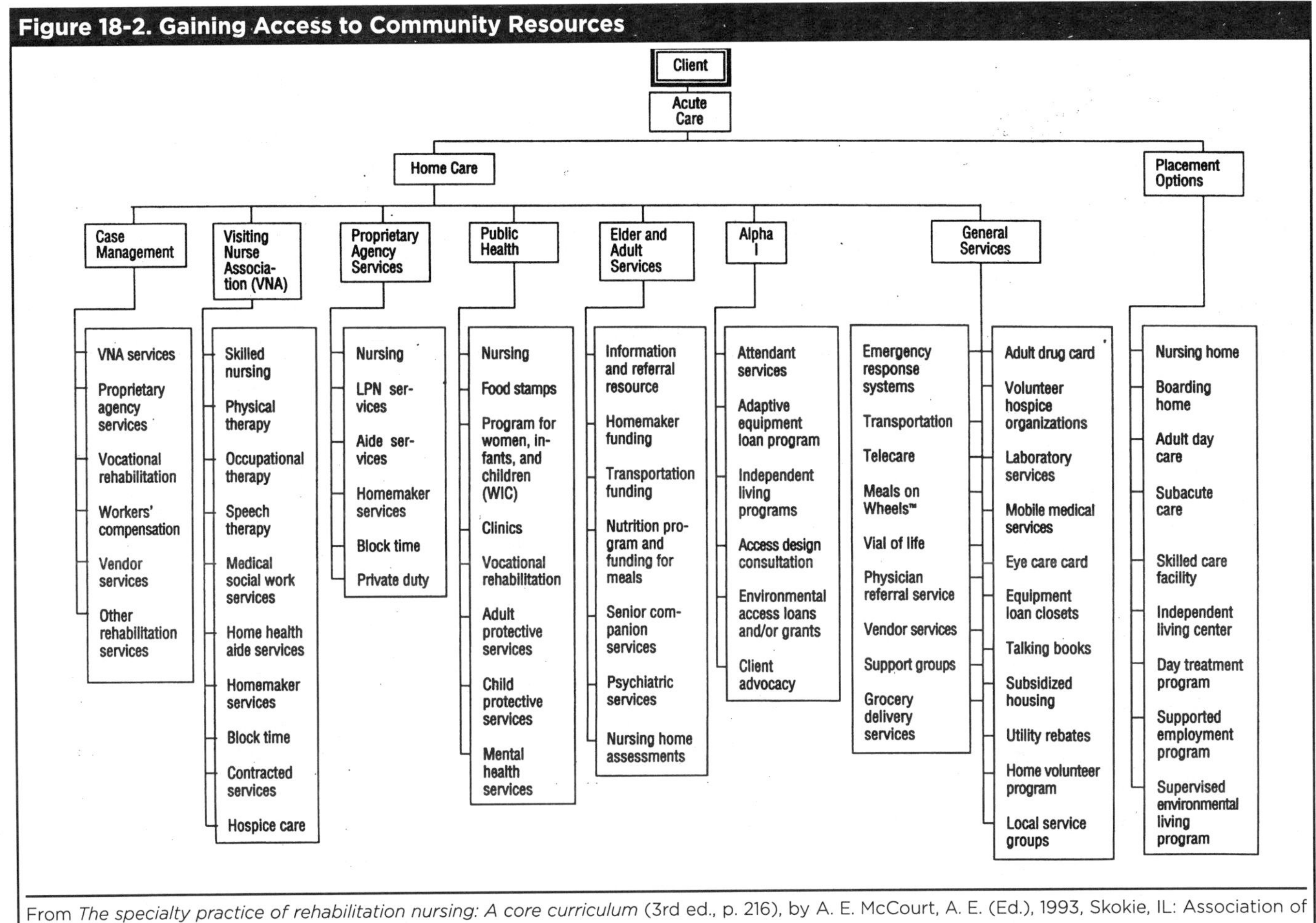

From *The specialty practice of rehabilitation nursing: A core curriculum* (3rd ed., p. 216), by A. E. McCourt, A. E. (Ed.), 1993, Skokie, IL: Association of Rehabilitation Nurses. Copyright 1993 by the Association of Rehabilitation Nurses.

f. Transportation is necessary for grocery shopping, filling prescriptions, or simply enjoying the pleasures of a public park.
   1) People with spinal cord injury face environmental barriers to many types of community participation (Newman, 2010).
   2) One can become easily overwhelmed by the multitude of community barriers.

g. The most prevalent unmet need is for information on disability-related services, legal rights, and needs for primary, specialty, and mental health care, case management, and instrumental activities of daily living services (Mitra et al., 2011).

h. People with functional limitations who live in communities with more barriers felt more limited in ability to perform ADLs even when they did not perform ADLs any less frequently (Keysor et al., 2010).

2. However, it is essential for the rehabilitation team to be familiar with the limitations of the home and community setting to which the client is returning because that setting may not be an appropriate option for discharge.
   a. Additionally, one aspect of the rehabilitation nursing role is to facilitate the health and wellness of the community, and identifying

accessibility deficits is a first step in helping the community develop a corrective plan of action.

1) Transportation: Adults with disabilities are twice as likely as those without disabilities to have inadequate transportation (31% versus 13%; CDC, n.d.). Determine the availability and the costs of clients accessing transportation services, including the following:
   a) Service to clients living in rural areas
   b) Vehicle modifications or purchase of a modified vehicle
   c) Designated parking
   d) Private transportation services
   e) Reduced-rate bus passes
   f) Paratransit services
   g) Parking stickers
2) Funding for attendant care: Funding is typically tied to eligibility for income assistance, and the waiting period can be as long as 2 years. Challenges include minimal reimbursement for care attendants, which makes it difficult to recruit and retain qualified people. Funding levels fluctuate by age group, so the adolescent who is able to procure services at 17 years may have to compete at age 18 years for a sharply reduced pot of funds as a member of a broader age range (e.g., 18–55 years). The use of novel funding approaches (e.g., prelitigation funding, letter of protection) can provide many families with relief from the burden of care, allowing patients to remain comfortably in their own home and avoiding nursing home placement (Romano, 2014, pp. 265–266). Nursing home use increases when there are perceived home environmental barriers and the patient lives alone (Stineman et al., 2012).
3) Funding for independent living arrangements (residential and nonresidential models): Although funding is mandated by the Rehabilitation, Comprehensive Services, and Developmental Disabilities Amendments of 1978, the amendment is not formula driven but rather funded based on voted amounts. States may be able to provide some attendant assistance and community support services through Medicaid Title XIX funding. Most states provide an Internet database identifying licensed residential and nonresidential service providers by county. These government websites are valuable resources for identifying legitimate providers for home- and community-based services, healthcare services, medical care, and long-term and day care.
4) Potentials barriers to medical services.
   a) Pharr and Chino (2013) found that structural barriers in clinic sites were most prevalent where practice administrators had limited knowledge of the ADA law.
   b) Harrington, Hirsch, Hammond, Norton, and Bockenek (2009) conducted an assessment of people with disabilities and their perceived barriers to primary care services. Results revealed that most people participating in the survey have a primary care physician and receive routine screening and health maintenance examination. The prevalent barrier was lack of primary care physician knowledge related to the disability rather than physical barriers to care. The physical barriers reported included examination rooms too small to negotiate in a wheelchair, lack of transfer assistance to an examination table, and the inability of women with a disability to maintain correct positioning for Pap smears and mammograms. The sample was made up of people receiving treatment at a rehabilitation clinic; therefore, the viewpoint of people who lack transportation or are homebound were not captured.
   c) A study of the barriers to mammography by women with disabilities (Barr, Giannotti, Van Hoof, Mongoven, & Curry, 2008) revealed difficulty accessing care sites, lack of transportation, nonadjustable equipment, communication challenges, and fears, both of the examination and of being touched by strangers.
   d) More nurse practitioners are used to provide services to the disadvantaged, including those with a disability (DesRoches et al., 2013).
   e) Under the Affordable Care Act, some states have opted out of the federal Medicaid expansion, and the Medicaid benefits of disabled people in those states may be affected. Such funding cuts may occur with outpatient therapy

services, dental care, podiatry care, and hospice; some people may even remain uninsured (Kaplan, 2012).

5) Funding for consumable and durable medical supplies: Assess a client's ability to obtain needed equipment, supplies, and medications. This assessment should include availability of delivery, availability of all necessary medications, delivery costs, deductibles, and coverage limits.
6) Accessible housing
   a) Architectural modification of a client's living environment takes time, and projects often are completed long after discharge. Determine whether the client's home is accessible, taking into consideration the equipment needed after discharge. Checklists are available from a variety of academic and government sources that rehabilitation teams and families can use to assess the appropriateness of the home environment (**Figure 18-3**).
   b) If a client wants to modify his or her home, is there technical assistance available for the development, design, and building of the modifications? Are there building loans available for the specialized modifications? Federal programs are available for housing modification.
   c) The U.S. Department of Veterans Affairs Specially Adapted Housing Grant provides not more than 50% of the costs, up to $67,555 maximum (in 2014; changes each fiscal year). Eligible veterans have a service-connected disability due to military service and have lost at least one lower extremity and have other disabilities. The grant will not modify vehicles, and any veteran 18 years and older may qualify. There is no time limit for use of the grant monies. Veterans should contact a local VA office, and more information is available at www.benefits.va.gov/homeloans/sah.asp.
   d) The U.S. Department of Agriculture (USDA) provides grants (maximum $7,500) and loans ($20,000) to help very-low-income applicants remove health and safety hazards or repair their homes. The applicants must be in a rural area with a population of 10,000 or less, and the loan homeowner must be 18 years of age or older and the grant homeowner 62 years of age or older. The monies may not be used to modify vehicles. Interested applicants should contact the local USDA office, and more information is available at www.rurdev.usda.gov/rhs/common/indiv_intro.htm.
7) Employment: Twice as many adults with disabilities live in poverty, with annual household incomes below $15,000, compared with those without disability (28.4% versus 12.4%; Erickson & Von Schrader, 2012). Federal legislation prohibits discriminatory hiring, compensation, and training practices. The U.S. Equal Employment Opportunity Commission enforces the federal laws related to employment discrimination against a person with a disability.
   a) Title I and Title V of the ADA of 1990, as amended, prohibit employment discrimination against qualified people with disabilities in the private sector and in state and local governments.
   b) Sections 501 and 505 of the Rehabilitation Act of 1973 prohibit discrimination against qualified people with disabilities who work in the federal government.
   c) Title VII of the Civil Rights Act of 1964 (Title VII) prohibits employment discrimination based on race, color, religion, sex, or national origin.
   d) The National AgrAbility Project was created to assist people with disabilities employed in agriculture. The project links the cooperative extension services at a land grant university with a private nonprofit disability service organization to provide practical education and assistance that promotes independence in agricultural production and rural living. The AgrAbility Project assists people involved in production agriculture who work on both small and large operations. State projects may be located at www.agrabilityproject.org.
   e) The Job Accommodation Network (2009) has conducted an ongoing study since 2004 of 1,182 employers. The study results have consistently shown that employers want to provide accommodations so they can retain valued and qualified employees. The majority of employers, 56%, reported that the

Figure 18-3. Home Safety Checklist

1. **Entry to Home**
    - ❑ Adequate lighting surrounding driveway, walkway, garage, doors, and trash receptacles
    - ❑ Sturdy handrails on both sides; condition of steps, risers, and treads
    - ❑ Condition of walkway and driveway; curb cuts with adequate transitions between surfaces; need for ramp
    - ❑ Garage pathway clear and accessible
    - ❑ Working doorbell
    - ❑ House number visible

2. **Entry, Interior Doors, and Landings**
    - ❑ Landings wide and deep enough to safely open doors
    - ❑ Nonskid contrasting floor rugs and floor surfaces
    - ❑ Doors with easily turning knobs
    - ❑ Doors open and close slowly and easily
    - ❑ Floor level changes?
    - ❑ Stair rail condition, right and left side; condition of stair risers and treads, free of clutter
    - ❑ Adequate lighting in stairway

3. **Hallways and Living Spaces**
    - ❑ Hall width and pathways adequate for walker or wheelchair and clear of obstacles
    - ❑ Thresholds minimal, rugs with nonslip grips or rug tape, bare floors slip resistant
    - ❑ Chairs available with arm rests
    - ❑ Ability to turn on light and TV; access telephone from bed, chair, and sofa

4. **Bathroom**
    - ❑ Grab bars and tub bench available in tub, shower, and toilet
    - ❑ Toilet height appropriate for sitting and standing
    - ❑ Ability to step in and out of bath and shower
    - ❑ Toiletries easily reached, handheld shower head, faucets easy to reach and use
    - ❑ Nonskid surface in tub and shower
    - ❑ Water temperature regulated, hot water pipes covered

Figure 18-3. Home Safety Checklist

5. Kitchen

- ❑ Frequently used items are easily visible and reached in cabinets and refrigerator
- ❑ Burners and control knobs clearly labeled and easy to use
- ❑ Clear resting space for hot items coming out of oven
- ❑ Microwave easy to read, reach, and operate
- ❑ Overhead and task lighting adequate
- ❑ Adequate counter space to prepare food

6. Laundry

- ❑ Safe access to washer and dryer
- ❑ Adequate lighting
- ❑ Route to laundry room safe
- ❑ Control knobs easy to access, read, and operate
- ❑ Laundry supplies easy and safe to reach
- ❑ Nonslip floor surface, floor free of tripping hazards

7. Bedrooms

- ❑ Lighting adequate, light reachable from the bed
- ❑ Bed height allows for sitting and standing
- ❑ TV control and telephone easy to reach from bed
- ❑ Clear, unobstructed path wide enough to navigate with wheelchair or walker
- ❑ Closet and bureau accessible, easy to open, and easy to access clothing

8. General Home Safety

- ❑ Carbon monoxide, smoke alarms, and fire extinguisher present and operable
- ❑ Thermostat easily accessible, readable, and adjustable
- ❑ Able to open/close windows, doors, drapes, blinds, and curtains
- ❑ Sufficient and accessible electrical outlets, light switches accessible at entrance of each room
- ❑ Medications and cleaning supplies out of reach of children

accommodations cost nothing, another 37% experienced a one-time cost, and only 5% stated that the accommodation resulted in an ongoing, annual cost. The typical one-time expenditure was $600.

f) Employers are expected to make reasonable accommodations for employees with disabilities. The costs associated with those accommodations are often nominal. The Job Accommodation Network conducted a survey that found that 71% of accommodations made by small businesses cost less than $500.

g) Employers may want to offer employment to people with disabilities but need financial assistance to make the necessary accommodations. The IRS offers tax incentives to businesses that hire people with disabilities and incentives for businesses that must make accommodations. Examples include the Disabled Access Credit, Barrier Removal Tax Deduction, and Work Opportunity Credit. Information on the Tax Incentives Packet of the ADA may be located at http://www.ada.gov/archive/taxpack.htm.

8) Recreation: Recreation activities and sports inspire confidence and restore dignity while helping people with disabilities deal with challenge and change (Disabled Sports USA, n.d.)

a) The U.S. National Park Service offers free lifetime park passes to people with disabilities. The ADA published guidelines for accessibility to recreation facilities in the Federal Register on September 3, 2002; however, they have not been incorporated into the Department of Justice accessibility standards and are therefore unenforceable (Disability.gov, n.d.).

b) Disability.gov refers readers seeking information on disability travel and recreation resources to http://www.makoa.org/travel.htm. The website includes travel planning, travel companies, and destinations. Many parks and recreation divisions across the United States have information on their websites on special programs and activities and their level of accessibility and available equipment.

9) Resources: The federal website Disability.gov and the website www.makoa.org have a plethora of Web links and information for professionals, consumers, and family members on a wide number of subjects. Topics are easy to navigate on one side of the page and include employment, housing, recreation, emergency preparedness, and technology, to name a few. A primary advantage to using federal and state websites and databases is that the sites are frequently updated and maintained by reputable sources. Because not all websites contain accurate information or are not from reputable sources, rehabilitation nurses, clients, and family members should assess websites before using their contents (see Table 18-2).

VI. Nursing Challenges: Risk for Injury

A. Injury Prevention

1. Public health experts and epidemiologists identify three levels of injury prevention that are defined by the timing of an injury. For every injury event, there is a primary (pre-event), secondary (event), and tertiary (postevent) period. Another way to present the three levels of injury prevention is to consider injury as the result of disease or a negative health state.
2. Primary prevention consists of activities that decrease the opportunity for illness or injury. Secondary prevention includes early diagnosis and treatment of a condition to lessen its severity, and tertiary prevention is the restoration to one's optimum function (Murray, Zentner, Pangman, & Pangman, 2006).
3. When a rehabilitation nurse is planning prevention strategies for a particular type of injury occurrence, the strategy should include actions that can be taken at all three levels (Indian Health Services, n.d.).

B. Secondary Conditions

1. Adults with physical disabilities are at risk for a variety of secondary conditions that may reduce their health and independence. The American Association on Health and Disability (2009) defined secondary conditions as "a condition that results from a specific type of primary disability, birth defect or medical condition. Examples of secondary conditions are pressure sores, bowel/bladder challenges, depression."
2. A secondary condition differs from a comorbidity in that a comorbidity is an additional disease that occurs after diagnosis of the primary disabling condition.

3. The term *secondary conditions* adds three dimensions not captured by the term *comorbidity*: nonmedical events (such as isolation), conditions that affect the general population (such as obesity), and problems that arise at any time during the lifespan.
4. The public health goal is to prevent and reduce secondary conditions associated with unnecessary activity limitations, health costs, lost wages, reduced participation, and reduced quality of life (CDC, 2014b).
5. Strategies or interventions that will reduce the likelihood of secondary conditions include the following:
   a. Available and accessible medical facilities, private offices, fitness centers, shelters, mobile units, and transportation
   b. Modified equipment in those facilities
   c. Websites with approved accessibility features
   d. Policies that facilitate postsecondary education, hiring, and purchase of the best technology (CDC, 2014b).

C. Definition: NANDA defined risk for injury as "a result of the interaction of environmental conditions interacting with the individual's adaptive and defensive resources" (Ackley & Ladwig, 2014, p. 430).

D. Risk Factors: This is a broad label that includes both external and internal risk factors. This nursing diagnosis should be used only for people who are at unusually high risk for this problem because most people are at some degree of risk for injury and should take precautions.
1. External: Biological (e.g., the percentage of the community vaccinated for influenza), chemical (e.g., exposure to contaminated water, foods), human (e.g., hospital-acquired infections), mode of transport, nutritional, physical
2. Internal: Abnormal blood profile, developmental age, autoimmune dysfunction, and physical, psychological, or sensory dysfunction or malnutrition (Ackley & Ladwig, 2014)

E. NOC
1. Risk control: Actions that will eliminate or reduce actual, personal, and modifiable health threats, including the following:
   a. Monitoring environmental and personal behavior risk factors
   b. Developing and following selected risk control strategies
   c. Modifying lifestyle to reduce risk
2. Safety behavior: Client or caregiver actions to minimize environmental factors that might cause physical harm or injury in the home.
3. Clients and caregivers manipulate the physical environment to promote safety.
4. Safety behavior: Client or caregiver efforts to control behaviors that might cause physical injury, such as the following:
   a. Identify risks that increase susceptibility to injury.
   b. Avoid physical injury.
5. Safety status: Fall occurrence (number of falls in the past week)
6. Safety status: Physical injury (severity of injuries from accidents and trauma)

F. NIC
1. Assessment
   a. Identify factors that affect safety needs, such as changes in mental status, fatigue, medications, and motor or sensory deficits (e.g., with gait, balance).
   b. Identify environmental factors that create risk for falls.
   c. Check the client for presence of constrictive clothing, cuts, burns, or bruises.
2. Exemplars: People with disabilities are susceptible to physical conditions and injuries. Collaboration with professionals in sports medicine, recreation therapy, and physical therapy provides rehabilitation nurses with valuable insight on a client's risk for injury because people with disabilities increasingly participate in recreational and competitive sports.
   a. People with cerebral palsy are at high risk for orthopedic conditions such as contractures, physical deformities, and hip dislocations, which can develop over time and decrease the person's range of motion, cause pain, negatively affect posture, and increase the risk of overuse injuries (Naugle, Stopka, & Brennan, 2006a). In addition, people with cerebral palsy commonly experience incontinence and drooling, which can lead to dehydration during activities if not monitored and treated.
   b. People born with spina bifida are predisposed to hip dislocation and fracture, which they may not notice because of the lack of sensation in the lower extremities (Naugle, Stopka, & Brennan, 2007).
   c. There are nearly 2 million people living in the United States with limb loss (Amputee Coalition, 2014), either congenital or acquired. Many of these people participate in athletics. They are susceptible to blisters, pressure ulcers, "choke syndrome" (i.e., tissue swelling caused by an obstruction in the venous outflow due to

constriction in the prosthetic socket), dermatitis, folliculitis, and muscle contractures (Naugle, Stopka, & Brennan, 2006b).

d. Hyperthermia and hypothermia are potential problems for people with spinal cord injuries participating in recreation events. There is impaired sweating below the lesion level and lack of heat loss by convection and radiation because of venous pooling in the lower limbs (Patel & Greydanus, 2010). In addition, because they do not shiver below the level of injury, people participating in water sports such as swimming are at higher risk for hypothermia. People with spinal cord injuries using a wheelchair are at higher risk for skin breakdown because their knees often are higher than their buttocks, placing additional pressure over the sacrum (Patel & Greydanus, 2010).

3. Interventions
   a. Specify the techniques the client and family must learn to prevent injury after discharge.
   b. Use heating devices with caution to prevent burns in clients with sensory deficit.
   c. If appropriate, use an alarm to alert the caregiver when a client is getting out of bed or leaving the room.
   d. Place a bell or call light within reach of dependent clients at all times.
   e. Instruct clients to call for assistance with movement, as appropriate.
   f. Remove environmental hazards.
   g. Make no unnecessary changes in the physical environment.
   h. Refer to interventions for fall prevention as appropriate.

VII. Nursing Challenge: Risk for Falls

NANDA defines risk for falls as "increased susceptibility to falling that may cause physical harm" (Ackley & Ladwig, 2014, p. 334).

A. Risk Factors
1. Age: Adults age 65 years and older
2. History of falls
3. Lower limb prosthesis
4. Use of assistive devices
5. Impaired sensation or perception, which may increase the risk of falls: temperature (neuropathies), touch (neuropathies), positive sense (proprioception), vision, and hearing
6. Unmet elimination need or urinary incontinence
7. Use of chemical or physical restraints
8. Environmental hazards
9. Lack of knowledge related to safety
10. Impaired mobility
11. Cognitive deficits
12. Clutter, inadequate lighting, and safety hazards (e.g., throw rugs, tub mats) in the home (Ackley & Ladwig, 2014)

B. NOC
1. *Fall prevention behavior:* Personal or family caregiver actions to minimize risk factors that might precipitate falls
2. *Fall occurrence:* Number of times a client falls (specify number per period of time) and situation
3. Knowledge, personal safety: Extent of client's understanding about prevention of unintentional injuries

C. NIC
1. Falls
   a. "In 2011, emergency departments treated 2.4 million nonfatal fall injuries among older adults; more than 689,000 of these patients had to be hospitalized" (CDC, 2014a).
   b. The consequences of falls are both emotional and physical. They include morbidity and mortality, hip fractures, decreased quality of life, and the emotional fear of a repeat fall, and they can lead clients to self-impose restrictions on independence and mobility (CDC, 2014a).
   c. In 2010, falls in the older adult population in the United States cost the healthcare system more than $30 billion in direct costs (CDC, 2014a). Fall prevention and management strategies must take a multifactorial approach that includes assessing intrinsic and extrinsic fall risks and developing personalized muscle strengthening and balance retraining and health and environment risk factor screening and intervention (Dite, Connor, & Curtis, 2007; Gates, Fisher, Cooke, Carter, & Lamb, 2008).
   d. Joint Commission standards require facilities to assess patient risk and have a plan of action for interventions to prevent falls (DecisionHealth, 2013).
2. Assessment
   a. Monitor gait, balance, and fatigue level with ambulation.
   b. Determine risk or presence of altered gait, orthostatic hypotension, dizziness, or altered mental status associated with prescribed medications.
   c. "Carpet flooring, vertigo, being an amputee, confusion, cognitive impairment, stroke, sleep disturbance, anticonvulsants, tranquilizers and antihypertensive medications, age between 71 and 80, previous falls, and need for transfer

assistance are risk factors for geriatric patient falls in rehabilitation hospital settings" (Vieira, Freund-Heritage, & da Costa, 2011, p. 799).

3. Interventions for use in institutions are listed in **Figure 18-4**. For use in the home and community:
   a. Evaluate the degree of risk by using a home safety assessment tool.
   b. Assess the clients and family's knowledge of safety needs and injury prevention and motivation to prevent injury in home, community, and work settings.
   c. Assess socioeconomic status and availability and use of resources.

Figure 18-4. Fall-Prevention Behavior

Domain: Health Knowledge and Behavior — Care Recipient:
Class-Risk Control and Safety (T) — Data Source:
Scales(s): Never demonstrated to Consistently demonstrated (m)
Definition: Personal or family caregiver actions to minimize risk factors that might precipitate falls in the personal environment
Outcome Target Rating: Maintain at__________ Increase to __________

Fall Prevention Behavior Overall Rating		Never demonstrated 1	Rarely demonstrated 2	Sometimes demonstrated 3	Often demonstrated 4	Consistently demonstrated 5	
Indicators:							
190903	Places barriers to prevent falls	1	2	3	4	5	N/A
190905	Uses handrails as needed	1	2	3	4	5	N/A
190915	Uses grab bars as needed	1	2	3	4	5	N/A
190914	Uses rubber mats in tub/shower	1	2	3	4	5	N/A
190910	Uses well-fitting tied shoes	1	2	3	4	5	N/A
190901	Uses assistive devices correctly	1	2	3	4	5	N/A
190918	Uses vision-correcting devices	1	2	3	4	5	N/A
190902	Provides assistance with mobility	1	2	3	4	5	N/A
190919	Uses safe transfer procedure	1	2	3	4	5	N/A
190922	Provides adequate lighting	1	2	3	4	5	N/A
190909	Uses stools/ladders appropriately	1	2	3	4	5	N/A
190906	Eliminates clutter, spills, glare from floors	1	2	3	4	5	N/A
190907	Removes rugs	1	2	3	4	5	N/A
190908	Arranges for removal of snow and ice from walking surfaces	1	2	3	4	5	N/A
190911	Adjusts toilet height as needed	1	2	3	4	5	N/A
190912	Adjusts chair height as needed	1	2	3	4	5	N/A
190913	Adjusts bed height as needed	1	2	3	4	5	N/A
190916	Controls agitation and restlessness	1	2	3	4	5	N/A
190917	Uses precautions when taking medications that increase risk for falls	1	2	3	4	5	N/A

From *Nursing outcomes classification (NOC)*, 3rd edition, by S. Moorhead, M. Johnson, and M. Maas, p. 268, 2003, St. Louis: Mosby Elsevier.

d. Identify interventions and safety devices to promote a safe physical environment and individual safety. Make referrals to occupational or physical therapists as appropriate.
e. If it is covered by the client's health insurance plan, arrange a home safety evaluation by a home health agency. Teach the client and family to monitor environmental hazards and recommend changes to promote the highest level of safety.
f. Install secured grab bars or handrails.
g. Use mobility devices as appropriate.
h. Unclutter the floors (e.g., have a clear walking path, remove throw rugs).
i. Place frequently used items in easily accessible places (e.g., small kitchen appliances, pots, and pans). Ensure adequate lighting, especially at night; most falls occur at night en route to the bathroom.
j. Place the bed in a low position. Use a floor mat if appropriate for patients who tend to roll out of bed at night.
k. Help the client meet self-care needs until independence can be achieved or until the care attendant or caregiver has received appropriate education.
l. Teach the client, family, and significant others about the potential side effects of medications and alcohol. Monitor the effects of medications that could cause dizziness or poor balance.
m. Ensure safety for the client who has deficits in cognitive or thought processes by changing the environment to meet safety needs.
n. Provide methods to communicate with caregivers.
o. Establish a toileting program.
p. Install door locks or an escape alarm.
q. Provide an organized, consistent, uncluttered environment.
r. Install a large bell on the door of a room where entrance is restricted; the noise may stop the client and alert others to wandering (Joint Commission on Accreditation of Healthcare Organizations [JCAHO], 2003).
s. Install bright yellow tape strips on the floor in front of doors (JCAHO, 2003).
t. Place a traffic stop sign on exit doors or restricted areas to prevent wandering and falls (JCAHO, 2003).
u. Teach ways to compensate for sensory-perceptual deficits.
v. Test water before bathing.
w. Use compensatory strategies for visual field deficits.
x. Prevent burns, frostbite, and skin integrity penetrations.
y. Teach the client and family the signs and symptoms of seizure activity and ways to maintain safety during and after a seizure.
z. Teach safety factors associated with transfer techniques, gait training, and mobility devices.
aa. Provide proper, well-maintained footwear with an adequate toe box and keep the client from going barefoot. Ensure that the toileting program is adequate to meet nighttime needs.
bb. Teach the client and family how to decrease the effects of orthostatic hypotension (e.g., sit on the edge of the bed for several seconds before transferring).
cc. Provide appropriate information on community resources (e.g., emergency call devices for outside assistance when the client is alone).
dd. Use distraction, redirection, humor, and quiet areas to decrease agitated behavior and avoid the use of restraints.
ee. If available, put the telephone within easy reach.

D. Restraints

1. The use of restraints in facilities is declining because they have proven to be counterproductive and lead to falls and injuries (Dunn, 2001).
2. In response to both research results and consumer awareness, regulatory bodies have defined with greater specificity the use of restraints in client care. Centers for Medicare & Medicaid Services (CMS, 2013) implemented revised regulations outlining the use of restraints and seclusion for behavior management. CMS provided guidelines listing critical elements for the use of physical restraints. A physical restraint "includes all devices and practices used by the facility that restrict freedom of movement and normal access to one's body" (CMS, 2013, p. 1).
3. The following list of nursing measures, provided by Cindy Gatens, RN CRRN-A (2007), allows the rehabilitation nurse to predict and anticipate behaviors that increase a client's injury risk and to individualize the client's plan of care.
   a. Avoid medications that can aggravate acute confusion in older adults (e.g., hypnotics, sedatives, antianxiety agents, tricyclic antidepressants, other medications with anticholinergic side effects).

b. Look for other medical conditions that could cause confusion, such as infection, dehydration, and pain.
c. Potential restraint-free interventions for managing clients with confusion include maximizing structure and consistency (e.g., memory book, calendar, consistent routines), frequent reorientation, a room near the nursing station, opportunities for exercise and ambulation, toileting schedules, lower bedrails (or use of half rails if ambulatory), implementation of wheelchair and bed exit alarms, discontinuation of lines and tubes if possible, low bed, abdominal binder, and long-sleeved clothing (or knit sleeve to limit access to lines and tubes).
d. Use exit alarms that signal an attempted elopement and continuous observation or recommend family staying with client, if appropriate.
e. Restraint-free interventions for impulsivity include cuing the client to stop, think, and act.
f. Verbally review steps before beginning an activity, have the client rehearse the steps to complete a task, and intervene immediately when impulsive behaviors occur.
g. Review and rehearse how to appropriately engage in a behavior.
h. Complete frequent checks, activating and explaining the bed and wheelchair exit alarms.
i. Use a low bed, if appropriate, place the client in a common area where staff can frequently visualize client and behaviors, arrange for constant observation, or ask the family to stay with the client, if appropriate.
j. Document activities and behaviors that may trigger agitation and aggression.
k. Modify behavior by moving and speaking quietly, slowly, and directly; staying relaxed; safely positioning self; redirecting the client to a less stimulating or frustrating activity; discontinuing an activity; not arguing with a client about behavior; being flexible; and modifying treatment interventions.
l. Modify the environment to minimize stimulation (e.g., lights, noise, visitors).
m. Maximize consistency; provide safe motion, activity, and verbalization; provide clear expectations of interactions and treatment; schedule rest periods; facilitate safety by removing items that could cause injury; and arrange for constant observation or involve family (if calming and reassuring to the client).

VIII. Disaster Management

A. Disasters such as severe storms (rain, snow, earthquake, hurricanes, flooding) require special community preparation to ensure the safety and health of people with disabilities.
B. There are known preexisting inequalities in disaster outcomes, with children, older adults, women, racial minorities, the poor, immigrants, and people with physical or mental disabilities being especially vulnerable to the harmful impacts of disaster (Peek & Stough, 2010).
C. The National Organization on Disability noted that between 21.3% and 27.1% of persons affected by Hurricane Katrina were people with disabilities (Stough, Sharp, Decker, & Wilker, 2010).
D. Research has shown that people with disabilities are least likely to evacuate in response to disaster warnings and evacuation orders. Reasons given include lack of adequate warning for the blind and or deaf, lack of transportation and accessible shelter, and being less likely to have prior evacuation plans (Peek & Sough, 2010).
E. Disasters often involve displacement before or after the event, with loss of or changes to previously familiar environments. Unfamiliar environments can trigger delirium, illness, and falls in susceptible older adults.
F. Ensuring adequate services can be challenging for people with disabilities and chronic illness during and after disaster.
   1. Physical evacuation from site of disaster
   2. Special diets
   3. Accessible environments
   4. Housing
   5. Transportation
   6. Appropriate supplies and equipment
   7. Medications
   8. Specialty services such as dialysis
   9. Specialty medical or nursing care
   10. Schools and employment
   11. Caregiver respite
   12. Service animals
   13. Pets
   14. Financial support
G. Children are especially prone to separation from parents and other skilled caregivers. In particular, it has been found that children separated from caregivers are more likely to experience illness and disease, malnutrition, and abuse.
H. Some studies have identified increased mortality in the aftermath of disaster, especially among older adults (Sastry & Gregory, 2012).

I. During Hurricane Katrina, as many as 40% of deaths were due to drowning, 25% to injury and trauma, and 19% to "Katrina-related causes" (Sastry & Gregory, 2012). Morbidity has also been found to increase during and after disasters, including psychological states such as posttraumatic stress disorder and depression.

J. Barriers identified by case managers for people with disabilities to successfully recover from Hurricane Katrina included housing, public transportation availability, and the ability to navigate social systems of relief and aid (Stough et al., 2010).

K. Disaster case management is one method of decreasing the effects of disasters on people with disabilities.

L. Rehabilitation nurses are especially appropriate for case management for the disabled population in times of emergency. Suggestions for rehabilitation nurses include

1. Becoming involved in local government to help with disaster planning for disabled citizens of your community
2. Advocating for adequate disaster planning for disabled citizens in your community through interaction with state and federal senators and representatives.
3. Educating your community on disaster planning for people with disabilities through interaction with church groups, social clubs, and written contributions to your local newspaper.
4. Educating local case managers on disaster planning for people with disabilities.
5. Examining your own place of employment for disaster planning for people with disabilities.
   a. Become familiar with your facility's disaster plan and ask yourself, "Will this work for a person with a disability?"
   b. Short-term evacuation processes versus staying in place
   c. During- and after-care plans
   d. Equipment for evacuation without electricity, especially from upper floors
   e. Plans for delivering care without water, heating, cooling, or electricity
   f. Ethical and legal issues
6. Reading a nonfiction account of disaster affecting nurses: *5 Days at Memorial: Life and Death in a Storm-Ravaged Hospital* by Sheri Fink (2013, Crown Publishers).

References

Ackley, B., & Ladwig, G. (2014). *Nursing diagnosis handbook: An evidence-based guide to planning care* (10th ed.). St. Louis: Mosby.

American Association on Health and Disability. (2009). Secondary conditions. Retrieved from www.aahd.us/page.php?pname=about

Americans with Disabilities Act. (2010). ADA National Network: Information, guidance, and training on the Americans with Disabilities Act. Retrieved from http://adaanniversary.org

Amputee Coalition. (2014). Limb loss. Retrieved from www.amputee-coalition.org/limb-loss-resource-center/resources-by-topic/limb-loss-statistics/limb-loss-statistics/index.html

Ardell, D. (n.d.). Seek wellness. Retrieved from www.seekwellness.com/wellness/articles/what_is_wellness.htm

Association of Rehabilitation Nurses (ARN). (2013). *The essential role of the rehabilitation nurse in facilitating care transitions.* Chicago: Author.

Association of Rehabilitation Nurses (ARN). (2014). *ARN competency model for rehabilitation nursing.* Retrieved from http://www.rehabnurse.org/uploads/files/education/ARN_Rehabilitation_Nursing_Competency _Model_FINAL_-_May_2014.pdf

Barr, J., Giannotti, T., Van Hoof, T., Mongoven, J., & Curry, M. (2008). Understanding barriers to participation in mammography by women with disabilities. *The Journal of Health Promotion, 22*(6), 381–385.

Centers for Disease Control and Prevention (CDC). (2014a). Costs of falls among older adults. Retrieved from www.cdc.gov/HomeandRecreationalSafety/Falls/fallcost.html

Centers for Disease Control and Prevention (CDC). (2014b). Disability and health: Related conditions. Retrieved from www.cdc.gov/ncbddd/disabilityandhealth/relatedconditions.html

Centers for Disease Control and Prevention (CDC). (n.d.). CDC promoting the health of people with disabilities. Retrieved from www.cdc.gov/ncbddd/disabilityandhealth/pdf/PromotingHealth508.pdf

Centers for Medicare & Medicaid Services (CMS). (2007). Medicare and Medicaid programs; Hospital conditions of participation: Patients' rights: Final rule. (Federal Register 42 CFR Part 482). Retrieved from www.cms.gov/CFCsAndCoPs/downloads/finalpatientrightsrule.pdf

Centers for Medicare and Medicaid Services (CMS). (2013). Stage 2 critical elements for the use of physical restraints. Retrieved from www.cms.gov/Medicare/Provider-Enrollment-and-Certification/SurveyCertificationGenInfo/Downloads/CMS-20077-Critcal-Elements-Physical-Restraints.pdf

Clarke, P. J., Ailshire, J. A., Nieuwenheijsen, E. R., & deKleijnde Vrankrijiker, M. W. (2011). Participation among adults with disability: The role of the urban environment. *Social Science Medicine, 12*(10), 1674–1684.

DecisionHealth. (2013). Inside the Joint Commission. Retrieved from https://www.ecri.org/Documents/Reprints/Aggressively_Assess_Patient_Risk_for_Falls_to_Save_Money_Meet_Future_CMS_Criteria(Inside_the_Joint_Commission).pdf

DesRoches, C. M., Gaudet, J., Perloff, J., Donelan, K., Lezzoni, L. I., & Buerhaus, P. (2013). Using Medicare data to assess nurse practitioner–provided care. *Nursing Outlook, 61*(6), 400–407.

Disability.gov. (n.d.). Accessibility guidelines for recreation facilities. Retrieved from www.disability.gov/clickTrack/

Disabled Sports USA. (n.d.). Retrieved from www.dsusa.org/about-overview.html

Dite, W., Connor, H., & Curtis, H. (2007). Clinical identification of multiple fall risk early after unilateral transtibial amputation. *Archives of Physical Medicine Rehabilitation, 88*(1), 109–114.

Dunn, K. (2001). The effects of physical restraints on fall rates in older adults who are institutionalized. *Journal of Gerontological Nursing, 27*(1), 40–48.

Erickson, W., & Von Schrader, S. (2014). *Disability statistics from the 2012 American Community Survey (ACS).* Ithaca, NY: Cornell University Employment and Disability Institute (EDI).

Gatens, C. (2007, October/November). Restraints and alternatives. *Association of Rehabilitation Nursing Network*, p. 8.

Gates, S., Fisher, J., Cooke, M., Carter, Y., & Lamb, S. (2008). Multifactorial assessment and targeted intervention for preventing falls and injuries among older people in community and emergency care settings: Systematic review and meta-analysis. *British Medical Journal, 336*(7636), 130–133.

Grosiran, B. (2012). Ineffective therapeutic regimen. Retrieved from http://nanda-nic-noc.blogspot.nl/2013/03/ineffective-therapeutic-regimen.html

Hanks, R., Rapport, L., & Vangel, S. (2007). Caregiving appraisal after traumatic brain injury: The effects of functional status, coping style, social support and family functioning. *NeuroRehabilitation, 22*(1), 43–52.

Hankwitz, P. E. (1993). Role of the physician in home care. In B. J. May (Ed.), *Home health and rehabilitation concepts of care* (pp. 1–23). Philadelphia: F. A. Davis.

Harrington, A., Hirsch, M., Hammond, F., Norton, H., & Bockenek, W. (2009). Assessment of primary care services and perceived barriers to care in persons with disabilities. *American Journal of Physical Medicine and Rehabilitation, 88*(10), 852–863.

Healthy People.gov. (2014). Disability and health. Retrieved from www.healthypeople.gov/2020/topicsobjectives2020/overview.aspx?topicid=9

Indian Health Services. (n.d.). The 5 public health principles. Retrieved from www.ihs.gov/medicalprograms/portlandinjury/worddocs/getting%20started/publichealthprinciples.pdf

Jacelon, C. S. (2011). Health care, rehabilitation, and rehabilitation nursing. In C. Jacelon (Ed.), *The specialty practice of rehabilitation nursing: A core curriculum* (5th ed., pp 1–13). Glenview, IL: Association of Rehabilitation Nurses.

Job Accommodation Network. (2009). *Workplace accommodations: Low cost, high impact.* Retrieved from http://askjan.org/ENews/2009/Enews-V7-I4.htm#5

Joint Commission on Accreditation of Healthcare Organizations (JCAHO). (2003). Alternatives to restraint and seclusion. In *Complying with Joint Commission standards* (Chapter 3). Oak Brook, IL: Joint Commission Resources.

Kaplan, L. (2012). Advocacy in practice: A primer on Medicaid and its expansion in 2014. *The Nurse Practitioner: The American Journal of Primary Health Care, 37*(12), 7–8.

Kearny, P. M., Pryor, J., & Lever, S. (2012). Theories, models, and frameworks for chronic illness, disability, adaptation, and coping. In K. L. Mauk (Ed.), *Rehabilitation nursing: A contemporary approach to practice* (pp. 28–50). Burlington, MA: Jones & Bartlett.

Keysor, J., Jette, A., LaValley, M., Lewis, C., Torner, J., Nevitt, M., & Felson, D. (2010). Community environmental factors are associated with disability in older adults with functional limitations: The MOST Study. *Journal of Gerontology, 65*(4), 393–399.

Kim, J. W., & Moon, S. S. (2007). Needs of family caregivers caring for stroke patients: Based on the rehabilitation treatment phase and the treatment setting. *Social Work in Health Care, 45*(1), 81–97.

McCourt, A. E. (Ed.). (1993). *The specialty practice of rehabilitation nursing: A core curriculum* (3rd ed., p. 216). Skokie, IL: The Rehabilitation Nursing Foundation of the Association of Rehabilitation Nurses.

Mitra, M., Bogen, K., Long-Bellil, L. M., & Heaphy, D. (2011). High prevalence of unmet needs for home and community-based services among persons with disabilities in Massachusetts. *Disability Health Journal, 4*(October 4), 219–228.

Miyamoto, Y., Tachimori, H., & Ito, H. (2010). Formal caregiver burden in dementia: Impact of behavior and psychological symptoms of dementia and activities of daily living. *Geriatric Nursing, 31*(4), 246–253.

Moorhead, S., Johnson, M., & Maas, M. (2004). *Nursing outcomes classification (NOC)*. St. Louis: Mosby.

Mumma, C., & Nelson, A. (1996). Models for theory-based practice of rehabilitation nursing. In S. P. Hoeman (Ed.), *Rehabilitation nursing: Process and application* (2nd ed., pp. 21–33). St. Louis: Mosby.

Murray, R., Zentner, J., Pangman, V., & Pangman, C. (2006). *Health promotion strategies through the life span*. Toronto, ON: Prentice Hall.

Naugle, K., Stopka, C., & Brennan, J. (2006a). Disability and special needs: Medical conditions to know about when working with athletes with cerebral palsy. *Athletic Therapy Today, 11*(5), 44–45.

Naugle, K., Stopka, C., & Brennan, J. (2006b). Medical conditions of athletes with amputations. *Athletic Therapy Today, 11*(4), 39–41.

Naugle, K., Stopka, C., & Brennan, J. (2007). Common medical conditions in athletes with spina bifida. *Athletic Therapy Today, 12*(1), 18–20.

Neal, L. (1998). *Rehabilitation nursing in the home health setting*. Glenview, IL: Association of Rehabilitation Nurses.

Newman, S. (2010). Evidence-based advocacy using photovoice to identify barriers and facilitators to community participation after spinal cord injury. *Rehabilitation Nursing, 35*(2), 47–59.

O'Donnell, M. (2009). Definition of health promotion: Embracing passion, enhancing motivation, recognizing dynamic balance, and creating opportunities. *American Journal of Health Promotion, 24*(1), iv.

Patel, D., & Greydanus, P. (2010). Sport participation by physically and cognitively challenged young athletes. *Pediatric Clinics of North America, 57*(3), 795–813.

Peek, L., & Stough, L. M. (2010). Children with disabilities in the context of disaster: A social vulnerabilities perspective. *Child Development, 81*(4), 1260–1270.

Pharr, J., Chino, M. (2013). Predicting barriers to primary care for patients with disabilities: A mixed methods study of practice administrators. *Disability and Health Journal, 6*(2), 116–123.

Romano, J. (2014). Discharge planning difficulties for patients with traumatic brain injury: Unique funding options. *Journal of Head Trauma Rehabilitation, 29*(3), 265–266.

Sastry, N., & Gregory, J. (2012). The effect of Hurricane Katrina on the prevalence of health impairments and disability among adults in New Orleans: Differences by age, race and sex. *Social Science and Medicine, 80*(2013), 121–129.

Stineman, M. G., Xie, D., Streim, J. E., Pan, Q., Kurichi, J. E., Henry-Sanchez, J. T., . . . Salibu, D. (2012). Home accessibility, living circumstances, stages of activity limitation, and nursing home use. *Archives of Physical Medicine and Rehabilitation, 93*(9), 1609–1212.

Stough, L. M., Sharp, A. N., Decker, C., & Wilker, N. (2010). Disaster case management and individuals with disability. *Rehabilitation Psychology, 35*(3), 211–220.

Tsai, P. (2003). A middle-range theory of caregiver stress. *Nursing Sciences Quarterly, 16*(2), 137–145.

U.S. Census Bureau (2012). Americans with disabilities: 2010. Household Economic Studies. Retrieved from www.census.gov/prod/2012pubs/p70-131.pdf

Vieira, E. R., Freund-Heritage, R., & da Costa, B. R. (2011). Risk factors for geriatric patient falls in rehabilitation hospital settings: A systematic review. *Clinical Rehabilitation, 25*(9), 788–799. doi:10.1177/02692155114000639

Viggiani, K. (2000). Health maintenance and management of therapeutic regimen. In P. Edwards (Ed.), *The specialty practice of rehabilitation nursing* (pp. 80–101). Glenview, IL: Association of Rehabilitation Nurses.

World Health Organization. (1948). Preamble to the Constitution of the World Health Organization as adopted by the International Health Conference, New York, 19–22 June, 1946; signed on 22 July 1946 by the representatives of 61 States (Official Records of the World Health Organization, no. 2, p. 100) and entered into force on 7 April 1948. Retrieved from www.searo.who.int/EN/Section898/Section1441.htm

World Health Organization. (1986). *The Ottawa Charter for Health Promotion. First International Conference on Health Promotion.* Retrieved from www.who.int/healthpromotion/conferences/previous/ottawa/en/

Suggested Resources

Access to Disability Data: www.infouse.com/disabilitydata/home/index.php

American Association on Health and Disability: www.aahd.us

BlazeSports America: www.blazesports.org

Bureau of Labor Statistics: Employment Status of People with Disabilities: www.bls.gov/cps/cpsdisability.htm

CaregiverNJ: www.adrcnj.org

disABILITY Information and Resources: www.makoa.org/

Disability.gov: www.disability.gov

Disabled Sports USA: www.dsusa.org

Fall Prevention Clinics of America: www.fallpreventionclinics.com/

Minnesota Safety Council: www.minnesotasafetycouncil.org/seniorsafe/fallcheck.pdf

National Guideline Clearinghouse: www.guideline.gov

Online Resource for U.S. Disability Statistics: www.disabilitystatistics.org

Special Olympics International: www.specialolympics.org

Tax Benefits for Businesses Who Have Employees with Disabilities: www.irs.gov/Businesses/Small-Businesses-&-Self-Employed/Tax-Benefits-for-Businesses-Who-Have-Employees-with-Disabilities

Temple University Institute on Disabilities: www.temple.edu/instituteondisabilities/

Texas Agrilife Extension Service: AgriLife.org

U.S. Association of Blind Athletes: www.usaba.org

U.S. Census Bureau American Fact Finder: http://factfinder.census.gov/faces/nav/jsf/pages/index.xhtml

U.S. Census Bureau Disability Statistics Home Page: www.census.gov/people/disability/

U.S. Department of Labor: Finding Facts and Figures: Disability Data Resources: www.dol.gov/odep/pubs/fact/data.htm

U.S. Paralympics: www.usparalympics.org

USA Deaf Sports Federation: www.usadsf.org

Wheelchair Sports USA: www.wsusa.org

Chapter 19

Physical Healthcare Patterns and Nursing Interventions

Jill Rye, MA RN CRRN CNL
Mary Pat Murphy, MSN CRRN CBIST

LEARNING OUTCOMES

- Discuss implications of physical healthcare patterns in the care of patients with disability and chronic illness.
- Identify appropriate nursing interventions for variances in physical healthcare patterns.
- Appreciate the level of evidence associated with specific interventions.

KEY CHAPTER TOPICS

- Nutrition and swallowing
- Skin integrity and impairment
- Bowel and bladder function
- Sleep and rest
- Mobility and immobility
- Disuse
- Self-care and activities of daily living
- Sexuality and reproduction

PROFESSIONAL REHABILITATION NURSING DOMAINS AND COMPETENCIES

- Domain 1: Competencies 1.1, 1.2, 1.3, 1.4
- Domain 2: Competencies 2.1, 2.2 (Association of Rehabilitation Nurses [ARN], 2014)

Introduction

Changes in the physical patterns of health form the basis of rehabilitation nursing. Nutrition, elimination, sleep, rest, activity, exercise, and sexual and reproductive patterns all are affected by the major illnesses, impairments, and disabilities seen in rehabilitation practice. Rehabilitation nurses must be experts in identifying actual and potential problems resulting from the disruption of these health patterns. In collaboration with clients and their families or caregivers, rehabilitation nurses set realistic, appropriate goals and must be astute when selecting interventions to reach these goals in a timely and cost-effective manner.

The nursing process provides a working framework, functional health patterns provide substance, and the nurse's professional philosophy and emerging evidence-based guidelines all influence nursing practice. The nursing process begins with an understanding of what the client needs, expects, or wants, followed by a thorough assessment of the client's current health status. When planning care, nurses address identified needs (or nursing diagnoses [NDs]) (North American Nursing Diagnosis Association International [NANDA-I], 2012–2014) using thoughtfully selected interventions from the Nursing Interventions Classification [NIC] (Johnson et al., 2011) in a stepwise fashion as short-term goals are or are not met. The process concludes with ultimate goals (expected outcomes, or nursing outcomes classification [NOC]) (Johnson et al., 2011) that promote optimal restoration of client health, independence, family function, interaction with others, and self-actualization. Nurses must integrate nursing practice into the interdisciplinary team's work of restoration and rehabilitation. Although all rehabilitation professionals work together to provide interdisciplinary care, rehabilitation nurses and case managers coordinate care, interact with family and community supports, and advocate for the client across disciplines whenever services must be added, adapted, or revised.

As the nursing profession evolves toward evidence-based practice (EBP), existing facility clinical pathways, protocols, policies, and procedures will be challenged by emerging science. Nursing interventions are being scrutinized for efficacy, efficiency, and economy. What was once accepted as tried and true is now being put to the test. The electronic age is here, and access to resources for international nursing knowledge and science is ever expanding. EBP emphasizes conscientious and judicious decision making based on current research and consideration of the client's goals and wishes (Ehrlich-Jones, O'Dwyer, Stevens, & Deutsch, 2008). Combining best evidence with the client's goals and wishes is the art of rehabilitation nursing (Kautz, 2010). Rehabilitation nurses are stretching beyond their comfort zone to keep current with best practice guidelines and recommendations.

We have focused our efforts to provide the most current clinical guidelines available for each topic in this chapter to provide a level of evidence (LOE) for the major interventions listed. Nurses are encouraged to obtain these guidelines for more detailed information and to view the original sources. Many studies lacked sufficient numbers of subjects or the scientific rigor needed for meaningful conclusions. Many of the interventions recommended have not been systematically tested for their effectiveness. Rehabilitation nurses need to be at the forefront of research to test the efficacy of these interventions. LOEs are defined as follows:

- LOE 1: Evidence obtained from meta-analysis or systematic review of randomized controlled trials
- LOE 2: Evidence obtained from controlled studies or randomized controlled trials
- LOE 3: Evidence obtained from quasi-experimental or descriptive studies
- LOE 4: Evidence obtained from expert committee reports or respected authorities

I. Nutrition: Eating, Swallowing, and Feeding

A. Overview

1. Adequate nutrition is of particular importance for people with disabilities, chronic illness, or developmental difficulties.
2. Malnutrition is a major contributor to increased morbidity and mortality, decreased function and quality of life, increased frequency and length of hospitalization, and greater healthcare costs. Individuals who lack adequate calories and nutrients for tissue maintenance and repair experience malnutrition. This is a primary concern for clients in acute, chronic, and transitional care settings (Jenson, 2011; White et al., 2012).
3. Adequate nutrition and hydration provide the energy, strength, and endurance clients need to participate in therapeutic exercises and relearn daily activities.
4. Inadequate or excessive intake of food or fluid for body demands places the client at significant risk for multiple complications.
5. Although poor oral care and periodontal disease are no longer thought to cause heart disease, stroke, or poor glycemic control, they are likely to be risk factors exacerbating these systemic diseases. However, there is a correlation between oropharyngeal bacterial colonization secondary to poor oral hygiene, particularly in high-risk populations (e.g., patients in an intensive care unit, elderly patients, medically compromised patients), and lower-respiratory pneumonia with aspiration (Ameet, Avneesh, Babita, & Pramod, 2013; Kuo, Poison, & Kang, 2008). Rehabilitation nurses must promote or assist with good mouth care and promote regular dental care whenever possible.
6. Impaired swallowing and risk for aspiration, often seen in people with neurological illness or injury, warrants prompt and accurate identification to minimize the risk of aspiration and its associated complications. These individuals may require support and strategies for safe eating and are at higher risk for nutritional issues.
7. Rehabilitation nurses must assess nutritional adequacy and select appropriate interventions to restore nutritional health.

B. Nutritional Needs

The body needs more than 40 nutrients and micronutrients each day, including carbohydrates, fats, proteins, vitamins, minerals, and water. Dietary preferences vary widely, and cultural food items, medically prescribed diets, and religious restrictions must be respected when helping clients achieve the appropriate balance of nutrients during both health and illness. Factors that affect nutritional status include psychosocial factors, mobility, medication regimens, dietary supplements and herbs, physical disorders, occupation, eating habits, substance abuse, home environment, education, social support, financial resources, and access to nutritional food. The goal for rehabilitation clients is to have adequate nutritional intake to support healing and meet metabolic demands, and to modify the diet as needed during acute and chronic illness or disability.

1. Nursing assessment of nutritional status and adequacy includes the following (Mueller, Compher, Druyan, & American Society for Parenteral and Enteral Nutrition, 2009):
   a. Body weight and height
   b. Food/nutrient intake through estimated calorie counts; recent and remote dietary history, preferences, and cultural and religious patterns
   c. Health history and clinical diagnoses including presence or absence of inflammation, dentition status, dysphagia, colitis, fluid retention, loss of muscle or fat, constipation, and substance abuse or chemical dependency, including recent and remote past
   d. Recent and remote dietary history, preferences, and cultural and religious patterns
   e. Functional assessment of hand-grip strength
   f. Ability to purchase, select, store, and prepare food properly (i.e., mobility and economic, cognitive, and access factors)
   g. Apparent muscle wasting and absence of body fat stores (i.e., as assessed by triceps measurement)

1) Acute illness
2) Comorbidities
3) Depression
4) Eating disorders (e.g., anorexia, bulimia), malabsorption syndromes
5) Substance abuse

h. Presence of excessive body fat stores: The client who is morbidly obese could have severe underlying nutritional deficiencies.
1) Energy demands of body weight
2) Inactivity
3) Greater reliance for energy on fats, simple carbohydrates, and glucose
4) Lower dietary fiber intake

i. Diagnostic laboratory data
1) Serum albumin indicates available protein stores.
2) Hemoglobin indicates the ability to transport oxygen.
3) Glycohemoglobin (hemoglobin A1c) indicates average blood glucose during the past 3 months.
4) Prealbumin level indicates nutritional status, protein synthesis, and catabolism.
5) Lab measures of inflammation including elevated C reactive protein, erythrocyte sedimentation rate, and elevation of white blood cell count

j. Review of home medications, over-the-counter medications, supplements, and herbs for potential nutritional implications and drug interactions (e.g., Ritalin®, Adderal® Provigil®, steroids)

k. Aging process
1) Impaired mastication due to poor dentition or dentures
2) Decreased esophageal peristalsis
3) Decreased production of salivary secretions and digestive enzymes

2. NDs related to fluid and nutritional status (NANDA-I, 2012–2014)
a. Deficient (hypertonic or hypotonic) fluid volume
b. Deficient (isotonic) fluid volume
c. Excess fluid volume
d. Risk for electrolyte imbalance
e. Risk for deficient fluid volume
f. Risk for imbalanced fluid volume
g. Risk for unstable blood glucose
h. Risk for impaired liver function
i. Readiness for enhanced fluid balance
j. Imbalanced nutrition, less than body requirements
k. Imbalanced nutrition, more than body requirements
l. Imbalanced nutrition, risk for more than body requirements
m. Readiness for enhanced nutrition
n. Adult failure to thrive
o. Impaired oral mucous membrane
p. Impaired swallowing
q. Nausea
r. Impaired dentition

3. NDs related to eating, dietary choices, and dietary and fluid intake (NANDA-I, 2012–2014)
a. Fatigue
b. Anxiety
c. Grieving
d. Hopelessness
e. Ineffective coping
f. Ineffective denial
g. Chronic or situational low self-esteem
h. Disturbed personal identity
i. Disturbed body image
j. Dysfunctional family process
k. Ineffective family therapeutic regimen management
l. Noncompliance (adherence, ineffective)
m. Deficient knowledge
n. Bowel incontinence
o. Perceived constipation
p. Diarrhea
q. Dysfunctional gastrointestinal motility
r. Urge urinary incontinence
s. Urinary retention (acute or chronic)
t. Disturbed sensory perception (specify: visual, auditory, kinesthetic, gustatory, tactile, or olfactory)
u. Impaired comfort
v. Hyperthermia
w. Impaired physical mobility
x. Impaired spontaneous ventilation
y. Impaired verbal communication
z. Risk for aspiration

4. Nursing interventions (NIC) to promote nutritional adequacy (See the U.S. Department of Health and Human Services and U.S. Department of Agriculture's *Dietary Guidelines for Americans* [2005] and LOE 1 and 2.)
a. Teach daily recommended intake of essential nutrients, and help the client select balanced meals. All food selections should be based on the following three overarching guidelines:
1) Maintain calorie balance over time to achieve and sustain a healthy weight by decreasing calories and increasing physical

activity. For substantial health benefit and balancing calories, it is suggested adults exercise at least 75 minutes of moderate intensity per week.

2) Focus on consuming nutrient-dense foods and beverages including vegetables, fruits, whole grains, fat-free or reduced-fat milk and milk products, seafood, lean meat, poultry, eggs, beans, soy products, and unsalted nuts and seeds.

3) Limit intake of saturated and trans fats, cholesterol (less than 300 mg per day) and saturated fatty acids (less than 10% of calories); avoid added sugars, salt, and alcohol.

b. With the client's help, maintain prescribed restrictions and adaptations appropriate to client condition (e.g., calories, carbohydrates, fats, protein, sodium, uric acid, allergies, intolerances, pregnancy, age).

c. Monitor actual intake at mealtime for quantity and nutrient value. Note estimated calorie counts and postmeal plate waste.

d. Pay attention to possible food–drug interactions.

e. Encourage and support efforts to improve intake for desired weight loss, gain, or maintenance.

f. Monitor weight, albumin levels, and hemoglobin levels.

g. Use nutritional supplements, vitamins, and fluids as needed or prescribed.

h. Institute small, frequent meals to meet caloric needs when indicated.

i. Encourage sufficient fiber intake to promote bowel peristalsis.

j. Ensure adequate fluid intake for nutritional balance and elimination. Fluid restrictions may be appropriate for those with heart failure and renal disease.

k. Adjust food consistency for ease of chewing, for client safety, and to compensate for swallowing impairment.

l. Teach the client to read food labels.

m. Teach the client about correct and adequate portion control.

n. Assess the need for medications to stimulate appetite, such as oxandrolone (Oxandrin®) or megestrol (Megace®).

o. For clients with diabetes, see the standards for medical care in diabetes (American Diabetes Association, 2014) for guidelines on glucose monitoring, A1C, glycemic goals, and diabetes self-management, as well as recommendations for nutrition and physical activity.

p. For clients with complex needs, consider referral to a registered clinical dietitian.

q. Provide a pleasant environment with limited distractions, particularly for individuals with swallowing issues or distractibility.

r. Provide training for professional and family caregivers who are hand feeding clients. When feeding a client, follow the nursing interventions for dysphagia in section I.E. Dependence for feeding, not dysphagia, is the strongest predictor of aspiration pneumonia (Langmore et al., 1998).

C. Swallowing Disorders (Dysphagia)

1. Swallowing disorders can occur throughout the different phases of the swallowing process. The symptom can be caused by functional or structural abnormalities of the oral cavity, pharynx, or esophagus.

a. Causes of dysphagia may be the result of neurological disorders including stroke, brain injury, multiple sclerosis, amyotrophic lateral sclerosis, Parkinson's disease, dementia, spinal cord injury, muscular dystrophy, or cerebral palsy. Other causes may include radiation; problems of the head and neck including cancer, injury or surgery to neck; changes in dentition; reflux; esophageal disease; or, in hospitalized patients, "high risk co-morbid conditions such as older age, dehydration, malnutrition… cardiac disease and the need for rehabilitation" (Altman, Yu, & Schaefer, 2011, p. 789; American Speech Language Hearing Association, 2014)

b. Clinical manifestations that indicate a high risk of aspiration and the need for a swallowing evaluation by a Speech Language Pathologist (SLP) include coughing during or right after drinking or eating, difficulty with chewing or swallowing, food leaking or pocketed in the mouth, need for oral pharyngeal suctioning, dysarthria (slurred, slow speech), dysphonia (impairment of the voice), weak voluntary cough, drooling, wet voice or nasal regurgitation after water bolus, presence of a nasogastric tube, tracheal intubation, shortness of breath, reflux, or vomiting.

c. Dysphagia can predispose clients to aspiration, malnutrition, and dehydration.

d. Dysphagia and potential aspiration consumes hospital resources, affects discharge planning, and is linked to increased hospital length of stay and mortality (Altman, Yu, & Schaefer, 2011).

e. The swallowing process
   1) Swallowing (deglutition) is a series of complex physiologic activities that require both voluntary and involuntary actions.
   2) The cerebral cortex controls voluntary movements, and the brain stem controls involuntary movements needed for swallowing.
   3) Several cranial nerves affect nutrition and swallowing (**Table 19-1**).

Table 19-1. Cranial Nerve Functions Related to Swallowing and Nutrition

Cranial Nerve	Major Functions Related to Swallowing and Nutrition
CN I: Olfactory	Transmits sensation of smell to olfactory area of the cerebral cortex
CN V: Trigeminal	Innervates muscles of mastication and facial expression Sensory impulses from teeth, gums, and lips
CN VII: Facial	Receives sense of taste from anterior two-thirds of tongue Sensation of oropharynx
CN IX: Glossopharyngeal	Motor impulses to the muscles of the pharynx used in swallowing Sensory impulses from taste buds of posterior one-third of tongue
CN X: Vagus	Contractions of muscles of pharynx (swallowing) and larynx (phonation)
CN XI: Spinal accessory	Innervates the skeletal muscles of the soft palate, pharynx, and larynx, which contract reflexively during swallowing
CN XII: Hypoglossal	Motor innervations of the muscles of the tongue, allowing for coordinated contraction of the tongue muscles necessary for food manipulation, swallowing, and speech

2. Normal anatomy and physiology of swallowing (**Figure 19-1**): There are four phases (stages) of swallowing, although some texts combine the oral preparatory and oral phases.
   a. Oral preparatory phase
      1) Food is prepared, food is smelled, salivation occurs, food is put into the mouth.
      2) Food is manipulated in the mouth to form a bolus and is pushed posteriorly toward the oropharynx.
      3) Voluntary event
   b. Oral phase
      1) The tongue is elevated to the roof of the mouth (palate).
      2) Lips close to contain oral contents.
      3) Buccal and facial tone are necessary for chewing.
      4) Voluntary event
   c. Pharyngeal phase
      1) The bolus is carried by the swallowing reflex through the pharynx.
      2) The soft palate and uvula are elevated to close the nasal pharynx.
      3) The hyoid and larynx are elevated so that food is less likely to enter the trachea.
      4) An involuntary event is elicited by stimulation of sensory receptors located at the opening of the oral pharynx. This phase takes less than 1 second.
   d. Esophageal phase
      1) The bolus enters the stomach via peristalsis and gravity.
      2) The lower esophageal sphincter opens.
      3) Takes 5–8 seconds for solid foods
      4) Involuntary event
3. Dysphagia screening, clinical swallowing evaluation, and nursing assessment
   a. Bedside assessment/clinical evaluation: a thorough assessment of oral phase disorders and possible pharyngeal disorders characterized by weak lip closure, poor tongue control, or difficulty swallowing or chewing food; coughing or choking
   b. Identifies whether the individual is at risk during swallowing; as it is a pass/fail test; if person fails, they remain in a nothing by mouth (NPO) status until clinical swallow evaluation by the SLP is completed (Donovan et al., 2013).
   c. The bedside assessment can be completed by the SLP or nurse who is experienced in the selected screening tool.
   d. Many good dysphagia screening tools are available that have varying degrees of complexity, sensitivity, validity and reliability:
      1) 3-oz water swallow test (Suiter & Leder, 2008)
      2) Modified Mann: (Antonios et al., 2010)
      3) The Toronto Bedside Swallowing Screening Test (Tor-BSST) (Martino et al., 2009)
      4) EAT-10 (Eating Assessment Tool-10) (Courtney & Flier, 2009)
   e. If the individual fails screening, they should remain NPO until the the SLP completes a clinical swallowing evaluation (described in j. of this section) (Donovan et. al., 2013).

Figure 19-1. Normal Swallow

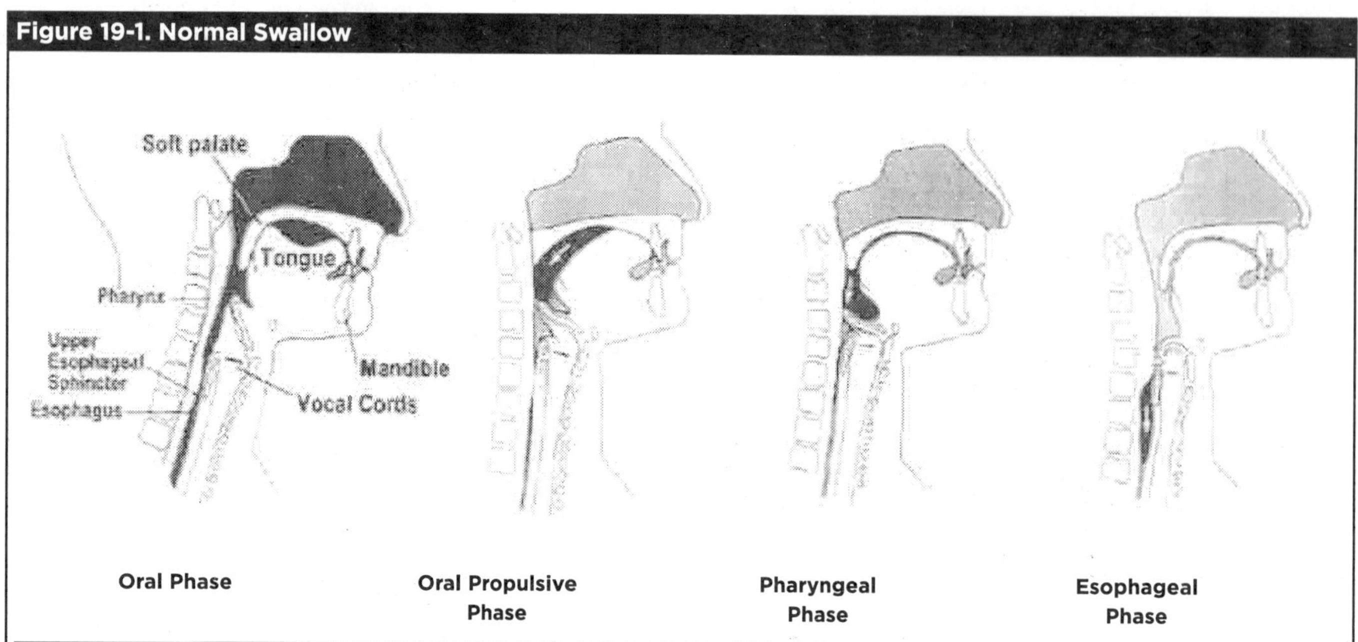

From "Cough and aspiration of foods and liquids due to oral-pharyngeal dysphagia: ACCP evidence-based clinical practice guidelines," by C. A. Smith Hammond and L. Goldstein, 2006, *Chest, 129*, 156S. Copyright 2006 by the American College of Chest Physicians. Reprinted with permission.

f. In addition to the bedside evaluation, the nursing assessment should include the medical history to identify the presence of neurologic diagnoses, with possible dysphagia sequelae, poor medical health, tracheostomy, dehydration, loss of weight, or frequent aspiration pneumonias. Dentition should also be noted.

g. When asked, clients may report that they have difficulty swallowing, or that they choke or cough while eating or drinking. Staff may report that clients eats too quickly, their food is poorly chewed or left in their mouth, or they take bites of food that are too big.

h. Other symptoms to note include voice changes characterized by dysarthria; wet, gurgled sounds; or a weak and breathy sound. Also to note are poor lip closure, affected tongue movement or drooling, leakage of food while eating or drinking, or pocketing food. Missing teeth can also affect swallowing.

i. Silent aspirators show no sign of dysphagia.
   1) Nursing should complete a bedside screening for aspiration for certain diagnostic categories; namely, patients with neurologic disorders including stroke, traumatic brain injury (TBI), multiple sclerosis (MS), amyotrophic lateral sclerosis (ALS), dementia, gastroesophageal reflux disease, radiation treatment, or debilitated
   2) During the bedside nursing assessment, history, and clinical screening, if there is suspicion of possible aspiration, have the client remain NPO until an SLP evaluation is completed.

j. When it is determined the client has dysphagia, a clinical swallowing evaluation is completed by the SLP.
   1) It is a behavioral assessment of swallowing function that consists of an extensive cranial nerve evaluation and direct examination of swallowing, using food and liquids of various textures and consistencies. Instrumental dysphagia studies, such as videofluoroscopy or fiber optic endoscopic evaluation of swallowing (FEES), could also be recommended. These tests
      a) Identify the swallowing impairment
      b) Show the effects of compensatory strategies during assessment (e.g., chin tuck, thickened liquids)

k. Instrumental tests: (See http://www.asha.org/policy/gl2004-00059/ for information on the role of the SLP in FEEs and and videofluoroscopic swallowing studies guidelines) Combined with the SLP's clinical swallowing evaluation, these tests help the therapist to determine methods for supporting hydration and nutrition, including consistency and/or volume of oral intake, use of compensatory techniques, and positioning and staff supervision. It also allows the team to better plan techniques to improve swallowing.
   1) FEES

a) Indication: patients with neurodegenerative diseases, neurological injury; following head and neck treatment for cancer, tracheostomy
b) The FEES is performed by an SLP or an ear, nose, and throat specialist and can be performed at bedside or in a physician's office. A small endoscope with a light on the end is passed through the nose; it records information before and after a swallow. The tip of the endoscope sits above the larynx.
c) The FEES assesses the lift of the soft palate and the movement of the tongue and larynx. The purpose of the study is to assess normal and abnormal anatomy of swallow, integrity of airway protection, and effectiveness of bolus modifications as it proceeds to the esophagus.

2) Videofluoroscopic swallowing studies or modified barium swallow study
a) Indication: patients with neurodegenerative diseases and neurological injury or also after head and neck treatment for cancer. Documents minute aspiration. It does not document before and after the swallow.
b) Completed with SLP and radiologist in a radiology department
c) The test assesses the swallowing process and examines the protective mechanism of the airway, and the progression and changes of the bolus.
d) Using videofluoroscopy and barium, one can view all phases of swallow; early and late oral, pharyngeal, and lower two thirds of the esophagus. It documents penetration or aspiration of barium as well as before and after the swallow.

l. The clinical swallowing evaluation provides recommendations for diet and hydration level (e.g., food textures, liquids, and quantities), strategies, positions, staff level of support, and remediation techniques. The National Dysphagia Diet (NDD) provides guidelines for progressive diets for those with dysphagia (Garcia & Chambers, 2010). Diets must be individualized and reassessed as the client's condition or skills change.

D. The NDD provides guidelines for progressive diets for those with dysphagia (Garcia & Chambers, 2010). Diets must be individualized and reassessed as the client's condition or skills change.

1. NDD level 1: Dysphagia-pureed
   a. Puddinglike consistencies
   b. No chunks
   c. Avoid lumpy foods and small pieces.
2. NDD level 2: Dysphagia-mechanically altered
   a. Soft, moist foods
   b. Ground meats, soft vegetables
   c. No bread, peas, or corn
   d. Avoid skins and seeds.
   e. Mechanical soft (same as a through d but can have bread, cakes, rice)
3. NDD level 3: Dysphagia-advanced
   a. Regular foods except very hard, sticky, or crunchy foods
   b. Avoid hard fruits and vegetables, corn, skins, nuts, and seeds.
4. Liquid consistencies (viscosities) are described as spoon thick, honeylike, nectarlike, or thin. Some facilities use the descriptors pudding, applesauce, honey, syrup, and thin. Several studies have noted variability in the viscosity of thickened liquid consistencies, even among SLPs. Emerging studies detail various methods for measuring and standardizing the interpretation of these terms.

E. Water Protocols for Clients with Dysphagia or While NPO: Rehabilitation nurses are encouraged to work with SLPs in their own facility when implementing a water protocol. Information about both protocols can be obtained from the American Speech Language Hearing Association's website (www.asha.org).

1. The Frazier Rehabilitation Institute (Louisville, KY) developed the Frazier Free Water Protocol, allowing clients with dysphagia or NPO to drink water between meals (Panther, 2008; Suiter, 2005). The rationale is that small amounts of water, even when aspirated, do not contribute to aspiration pneumonia, provided the client practices good oral hygiene. This protocol has been used for more than 20 years at the Frazier Rehabilitation Institute and is gaining popularity across the country. The Frazier protocol balances safety, hydration, and quality of life. Good oral hygiene is the foundation of the protocol. This protocol is described as follows:
   a. All clients are first screened with 3 ounces of water at the bedside. Videofluoroscopic swallowing evaluation is recommended to identify silent aspirators. Impulsive clients or those with excessive coughing and discomfort are restricted to drinking water only under supervision. The physical stress of coughing could prevent oral intake of water in patients with extreme coughing.

b. For clients on oral diets, water is permitted after oral care, before meals, and starting 30 minutes after meals, once again after oral care. The 30-minute time frame allows the client to swallow completely and clear the oral cavity of food residue.
c. Medications are administered whole or crushed with a spoonful of applesauce, pudding, yogurt, or thickened liquid—never with water.
d. Staff, clients, and families are educated on the rationale for encouraging water between meals, the guidelines for the intake of free water, and any restrictions. In some facilities, clients on the protocol wear armbands that state "No thin liquids except water between meals, after oral care."
e. In all cases, the SLP's recommendations for safe swallowing in each client should be followed. Additional compensatory measures may be recommended, such as chin tuck, head turn, or fluids by spoon or cup only.

F. Nursing Interventions Classification (NIC) for Dysphagia: Rehabilitation nurses are encouraged to obtain the Smith Hammond and Goldstein (2006) evidence-based guidelines developed by the American College of Chest Physicians Medical Specialty Society. They were current as of June 2010. Unless otherwise noted, LOEs for interventions in this section were determined by Smith Hammond and Goldstein (2006). Nurses are also encouraged to review guidelines available on the American Speech Language Hearing Association's website (http://www.asha.org/Members/ebp/compendium/guidelines/Cough-and-Aspiration-of-Food-and-Liquids-Due-to-Oral-Pharyngeal-Dysphagia--ACCP-Evidence-Based-Clinical-Practice-Guidelines.htm).

1. Clients with a reduced level of consciousness should not be fed orally until consciousness has improved (LOE 2).
2. Clients with cough and a high risk of aspiration should be observed drinking 3 ounces of water. If the client coughs or shows clinical manifestations of aspiration, refer to an SLP for further evaluation before further oral intake (LOE 2).
3. Clients with dysphagia are best managed by an interdisciplinary team, including an SLP, nurse, physician, dietitian, and physical and occupational therapists (LOE 2).
4. Clients with intractable aspiration may be considered for surgical intervention (e.g., an endogastric or percutaneous endoscopic gastrostomy tube).
5. Abnormal lung radiographs of the right lower lobe, right upper lobe, and left lower lobe, and auscultated rales and rhonchi are typical findings in true aspiration pneumonia. Lung assessment before and after a meal is essential in suspected "silent aspiration" (Sievers, 2008).
   a. Although ongoing pulmonary assessment is indicated in the rehabilitation setting, silent aspiration is most likely to be identified only after videofluoroscopic evaluation or the development of physical signs such as abnormal breath sounds, cough, fever, elevated white blood cell count, and changes on an X ray indicating pneumonia.
6. Clients could have difficulty swallowing medications. (See Wright, 2009, for a consensus guideline for these clients.)
7. The best way to position a patient to eat is fully upright with the pelvis tipped slightly forward.
   a. This position facilitates the best function of the muscles used when swallowing, encourages alertness, reduces the risk of reflux, and optimizes efforts to clear the airway with coughing.
   b. Remove the armrests, if necessary, so that the patient can get close to the table.
   c. Place both forearms on the table in a weight-bearing position, while ensuring that the head and neck are upright and midline.
   d. Feet should be properly supporting this position and may require support with a footrest, low stool, or other device.
   e. Adaptive cushions and supports in a wheelchair can be used to support centered, balanced, upright postures. Some patients can eat better using a full lap tray rather than a table (Avery, 2011).
8. Minimize distractions. Provide a quiet environment with no television, and discourage talking during meals. After being given strategies for safe swallowing, the individual should be evaluated for supervision and cueing to ensure adherence to the strategies.
9. Select foods of appropriate consistency and texture.
   a. Progress gradually from pureed to ground to solid food.
   b. With ground food, gradually add food that fragments easily.
   c. Stay with one food and texture at a time.
   d. Do not mix solids and liquids.
10. Progress liquid intake from pudding thick, to honey thick, to nectar or syrup thick, to thin. Use

a commercial thickener to achieve the appropriate consistency as needed.

11. The SLP may recommend placing food on the unaffected side of the mouth and taking small mouthfuls; encourage the client to turn his or her head to the unaffected side to bring food into the midline.
12. Teach the client to concentrate fully on chewing each small mouthful, forming a food bolus, and swallowing it before taking another mouthful or speaking.
13. Use the chin-tuck method to protect the airway.
    a. Encourage the client to do a tongue sweep of the mouth to self-check for food pocketing.
    b. Use compensatory strategies such as a double swallow between mouthfuls to prevent aspiration.
    c. Instruct the client to take small sips of water between mouthfuls or to alternate liquid and solid mouthfuls as appropriate.
14. Visually inspect the oral cavity for pocketing and use wide-mouth drinking vessels to allow visualization of progress of liquids into the oral cavity.
    a. A cutout cup can also be recommended to reduce head tipping when drinking.
15. Provide a calm, unhurried atmosphere and appropriate supervision. Do not allow the client to eat unattended or unobserved.
    a. Use adaptive devices for self-feeding and independence.
    b. Give clients with impulsivity one item of food or drink at a time and limit distractions.
        1) A quiet room with a single caregiver, and the door closed and the TV off, may be needed to limit distractions and improve safe intake.
        2) Allow ample time for distractible patients.
16. Give cues for strategies; follow the speech and occupational therapist's recommendations.
17. Ensure that the client remains upright for 20–30 minutes after eating a meal.
18. Before discharge, instruct family and caregivers in dysphagia precautions, the current dysphagia diet, use of thickeners if necessary, signs of aspiration, and the Heimlich maneuver. Suggest enrollment in a cardiopulmonary resuscitation course (Sievers, 2008).
    a. Observe caregiver/family member assisting with feeding the patient to ensure adequate learning has taken place.

G. Administration of Specialized Nutritional Support

1. Rehabilitation nurses could care for clients who need enteral (i.e., feeding tube) or parental (i.e., intravenous) nutritional support. The American Society for Parenteral and Enteral Nutrition (2009) regularly updates its clinical guidelines for assessing clients in need of specialized nutritional support, access devices, and administration of nutritional supplements through the enteral and parenteral routes. The recommendation for clients with acute TBI is to attain full caloric replacement feeding by day 7 after injury to avoid nitrogen wasting (LOE 2) (Brain Trauma Foundation, 2007).
2. Clients are fed by gastrostomy tube to provide temporary or permanent access to the gut when oral intake is not possible. Aspiration pneumonia is a lethal complication of tube feeding.
    a. Ensure adequate fluid intake by frequently assessing hydration status.
    b. Monitor body weight and serum albumin.
    c. Regularly check tube placement and aspirate gastric contents for residuals before instillations.
    d. Maintain head-of-bed position at 30 degrees or higher during feeding, and do not lay the client flat for at least 30 minutes after meals (LOE 2). Minimize nighttime feedings. Never add blue dye to enteral formula.
    e. Time feedings so that they are either continuous or bolus. If caloric needs can be met, bolus is preferred, with a gradual return to normal patterns of intake.
    f. Assess lungs for rales and rhonchi often.
    g. Sterile water is preferred for flushes and hydration purposes in immunocompromised and critically ill clients (LOE 4). Flushes of 30 ml water should be provided every 4 hours during continuous feedings and before and after intermittent feedings, aspirations for residuals, and medication administrations (LOE 2).
    h. Medications should be diluted in water before administration. Each medication should be administered individually to prevent physical and chemical incompatibilities and tube obstruction (LOE 2). Liquid dosage forms are preferred. Do not crush enteric-coated, time-release, or extended-release tablets. Flush with at least 15 ml sterile water between medications. Do not add medications directly into the formula.
    i. Acceptable hang times of enteral formula for adults are 8 hours for open systems using decanted formula and 24–48 hours in closed systems per the manufacturer's guideline. Administration sets for open systems should be

changed at least every 24 hours (LOE 2). Maintain aseptic technique with tubing changes.

j. Use portable equipment to allow participation in the therapy regimen.

k. Protect the gastrostomy site with skin shields and routine skin cleansing.

l. Encourage client and family participation in feeding and medication administration as soon as possible. Before discharge with a gastric tube in place, teach auscultation for tube placement, aspiration for gastric contents, skin care at the insertion site, cleansing of equipment, preparation and administration of medication, and storage and measurement of formula and water boluses.

3. Clients are fed by hyperalimentation via central intravenous catheters when use of the gut is not possible. All aspects of facility policies and procedures regarding hyperalimentation and central venous access devices should be reviewed annually for compliance with current best practice.

   a. Provide special care for the access site, tubing, and solution.

   b. Ensure adequate caloric intake through periodic use of lipid solutions.

   c. Regularly monitor body chemistries to help in the adjustment of solution electrolytes and lipids.

   d. Gradually introduce oral intake and taper hyperalimentation.

H. Expected Outcomes (NOC)

1. The client achieves and maintains a healthful weight (body mass index between 18.5 and 24.9).
2. Laboratory measures of albumin, prealbumin, hemoglobin A1c, hemoglobin, hematocrit, blood urea nitrogen, protein, and creatinine are all within normal limits.
3. The client experiences no complications related to dysphagia, parenteral alimentation, or hyperalimentation.

II. Skin Integrity, Impairments, and Interventions

A. Overview

1. Rehabilitation clients present with multiple risk factors for skin injury and breakdown. Clients at highest risk are those who have been hospitalized longer than 1 week, those who have been residents of long-term care facilities for longer than 4 weeks, clients older than 65 years of age, children younger than age 5, neonates, and those with spinal cord injury. "Adult inpatient hospital stays with a diagnosis of pressure ulcers totaled $11 billion in 2006" (Wound, Ostomy and Continence Nurses Society, 2010, p. 1). Pressure ulcers significantly increase the length of hospital stay from the usual 3–5 days to 13 or 14 days, and clients are three times more likely to be discharged to long-term care facilities (Wound, Ostomy and Continence Nurses Society, 2010).
2. Client and family education about prevention of skin breakdown is extremely important during care and must be a component of the interdisciplinary plan of care.
3. Several groups have published practice guidelines based on extensive critiques of research literature and expert reviews on the prevention and treatment of pressure ulcers. The major resources and guidelines for this section are from the Wound, Ostomy and Continence Nurses Society (2010), the National Pressure Ulcer Advisory Panel and the European Pressure Ulcer Advisory Panel (NPUAP & EPUAP) (2009), and the Registered Nurses Association of Ontario (2005). The Registered Nurses Association of Ontario guideline was used to provide the LOEs for many of the interventions listed here.
4. Rehabilitation nurses need to be skilled in maintaining intact skin and identifying, documenting, and aggressively treating pressure ulcers upon initial discovery. In addition, skillful identification and treatment of vascular ulcers, neuropathic ulcers, surgical incisions, skin tears, and burns is extremely important because these lesions are commonly encountered in rehabilitation practice.
5. Rehabilitation nurses should immediately institute appropriate interventions to prevent, identify, and treat skin breakdown due to maceration (e.g., moisture from incontinence or intertriginous skin folds) and fungal, bacterial, or viral skin infections.
6. The nursing priorities for skin care are to prevent and heal wounds. All wounds should be treated with appropriate techniques and dressings that protect the wound and facilitate healing.

B. Anatomy and Function of the Skin (DuVivier, 1993; Porth & Matfin, 2008)

The major functions of skin are protection, immunity, thermoregulation, sensation, metabolism, and communication. The skin is the largest organ, covering almost 2 square meters in the average adult, weighing about 6 pounds, and receiving one third of the body's circulating blood. Adult skin varies in thickness from 0.5 mm to 6 mm (Bryant & Nix, 2012) (**Figure 19-2**).

1. *Epidermis*: The outermost layer, made of five thin layers. It lacks a blood supply, contains melanin and keratin to protect deeper layers of the skin, and is constantly replaced by newer cells from

Figure 19-2. Normal Skin

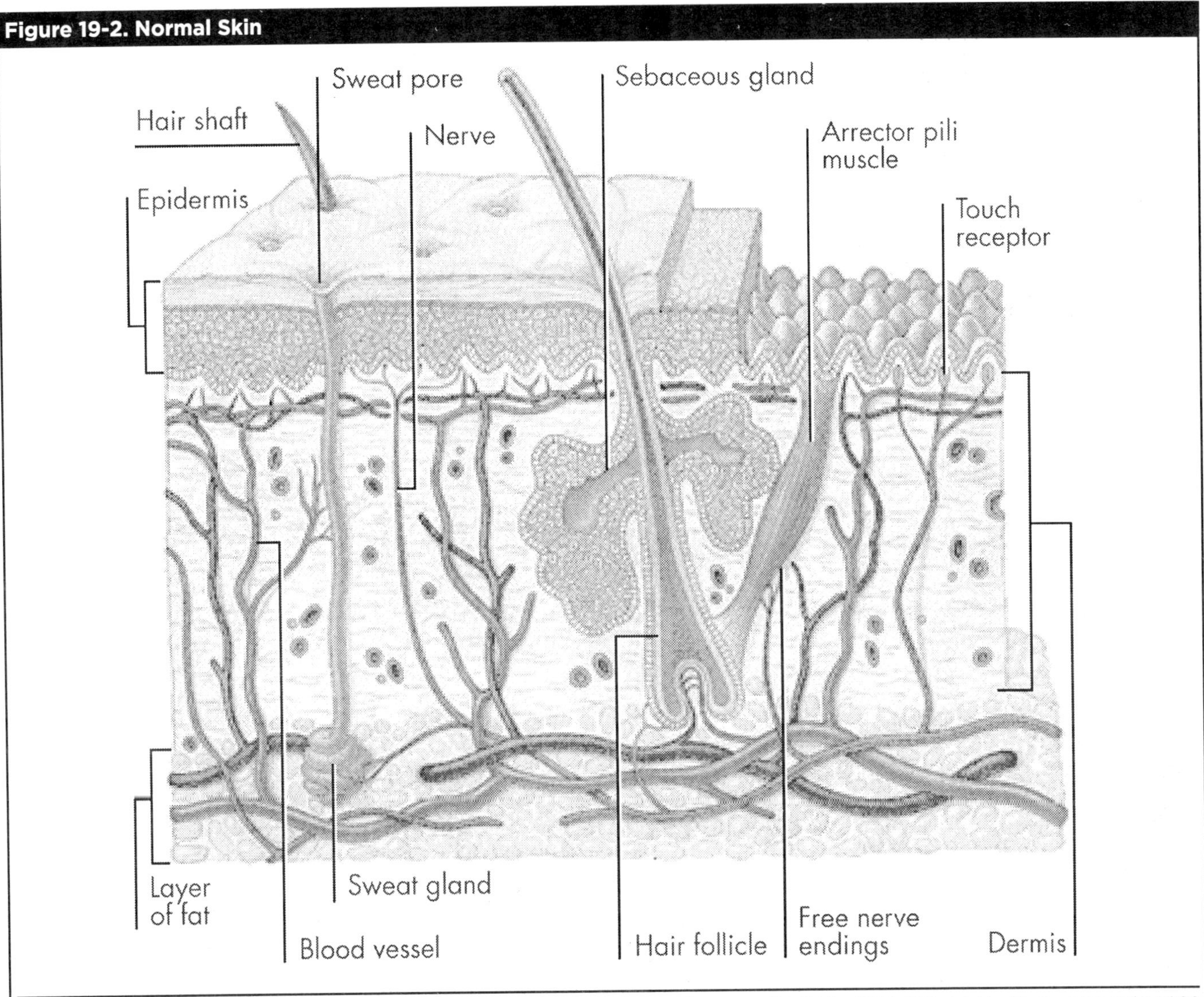

From *Acute and chronic wounds: Current management concepts* (3rd ed.), by R. A. Bryant and D. P. Nix, 2006, Philadelphia: Mosby. Copyright 2006 by Mosby. Reprinted with permission.

the dermis every 45–75 days, or about every 2 months. Mucous membranes are a modified form of very thin epidermis that lacks tough keratin layers.

a. Protects against ultraviolet radiation
b. Protects against environmental antigens
c. Protects the body from injury
d. Retains moisture
e. Excretes waste products
f. Assists in regulating body temperature

2. *Dermal layer*: Fibrous connective tissue, thicker than epidermis; contains blood supply, lymphatic vessels, nerves, glands, hair follicles, and nail beds
   a. Allows elasticity of skin
   b. Permits motion
   c. Supports healing
   d. Contains sweat glands, oil glands, and hair follicles
   e. Contains neuron receptors for touch, pain, and vasomotor response
   f. Provides nutritional support, immune surveillance, thermal regulation, hemostasis, and antiinflammatory responses
3. *Subcutaneous layer*: Forms a continuous layer of connective tissue over muscles, tendons, ligaments, and bones; sometimes called the fatty insulation layer, with the upper portion being fatty and the lower layer being thin elastic tissue; varies in thickness with little or no tissue at heels, bridge of nose, scalp, and behind ears
4. *Fascia*: The fibrous connective tissue membrane that covers and separates muscles, ligaments, and tendons
   a. Contains fat, collagen, sweat glands, and tissue fluids
   b. Varies in thickness and composition depending on body location

5. Circulation
   a. Provides nutrients, oxygenation, and moisture
   b. Promotes healing through increased blood supply, phagocytosis, and tissue rebuilding
   c. Provides support and healing in response to tissue load damage
6. Nerve supply: Provides response to environment and supports homeostasis

C. Normal Skin Changes with Aging
1. Epidermis and dermis become thinner, fat in subcutaneous layer decreases, fine hair on limbs and face decreases, and cohesion of the dermal and epidermal layers decreases (i.e., flattening of the junction layer).
2. Blood vessels become more prominent.
3. Production of basal cells, mast cells, collagen, melanin, elastin, and Langerhans cells decreases.
4. Physiologic functions such as hair and nail growth, glandular secretions, immune surveillance, vascular supply, vitamin D synthesis, inflammatory response, and tissue repair decrease.
5. Surface becomes pale, wrinkled, dry, and less stretchable; brownish spots appear on the face and hands.
6. Reduced sensation, especially pain receptors
7. Itching is common.
8. Sensitivity to fabrics, soaps, deodorants, and cosmetics increases.
9. Difficulty regulating body temperature due to reduced fatty insulation of the subcutaneous layer, more prone to hypothermia and heat stroke
10. Increased vulnerability to minor trauma (e.g., skin tears, hematomas, bruises, abrasions, and lacerations)

D. Risk Factors for Loss of Skin Integrity
1. Physiological factors
   a. Altered metabolic states that increase the body's need for nutrients, indicated by low serum protein, albumin, prealbumin, and hemoglobin, which impair the body's cellular rebuilding ability
   b. Underlying acute or chronic medical conditions (e.g., diabetes, cardiopulmonary or renal disease) or disease treatment (e.g., high-dose steroids after spinal cord injury, radiation)
   c. Impaired circulation as a result of peripheral neuropathies, anemia, atherosclerosis, hypertension, or smoking, which causes vasoconstriction and impairs the vascular bed
   d. Prolonged pressure and immobility, leading to pressure ulcer formation
   e. Neurological injuries that result in impaired sensations of proprioception, temperature, and touch, the consequence of which is the inability to perceive the need to move the body
   f. Immunosuppressant medications
   g. Poor nutrition, especially inadequate intake of protein, vitamin C, thiamine, and zinc
   h. Bladder and bowel incontinence
   i. Advanced age: Older adults have less effective skin protection because of changes in the epidermis, diminished glandular secretions and vascular supply, thinning of the dermis, reduced numbers of elastin fibers, reduced tactile sensitivity, and slowed inflammatory response, all of which contribute to delayed wound healing. Older adults also have a higher incidence of skin disorders (e.g., stasis dermatitis, seborrheic dermatitis and keratoses, comedones, benign tumors, dermatophytosis, xerosis, cherry and spider angiomas, eczema, psoriasis, lichen planus, nevi, skin tags, lentigo, ringworm, rosacea, tinea pedis and cruris, varicosities, and neoplasms) and are more likely to have comorbidities and mobility problems (Balin, 1990).
2. Mechanical factors
   a. *Sustained pressure*: Resting surfaces that are hard and unyielding and maintain constant pressure in one direction, particularly over bony prominences when repositioning is infrequent
   b. *Shearing*: The movement of muscle, subcutaneous, and fat tissues downward and compression against the bony skeleton while the epidermis does not slide (as occurs when the client is sitting up in bed and slides down in response to gravity)
   c. *Friction*: Rubbing of tissue across a rough surface (as occurs with incomplete lifting or dragging of a client to pull him or her up in bed) and ill-fitting prostheses, braces, orthoses, or shoes, especially in the presence of neuropathy
   d. *Body moisture*: Incontinence, diuresis, or sweating, especially in the skin folds of an obese client; drainage associated with stomas (e.g., gastrostomy tube, tracheostomy, colostomy, ileostomy, and urostomy)
3. Psychosocial factors
   a. Noncompliance with recommended healthcare practices
   b. Substance abuse that impairs judgment, nutrition, mobility, or sensation
   c. Impaired cognitive or intellectual ability
   d. Depression

e. Social isolation, particularly when the client needs assistance in daily care

E. Assessment of Clients at Risk for Impaired Skin Integrity: Assess all of the following on admission to a rehabilitation facility and daily for those identified as at risk for skin breakdown (LOE 4) (Registered Nurses Association of Ontario, 2005). Many facilities now require documentation of skin risk assessments at every shift.

1. General assessment components
   a. Underlying medical conditions
   b. Nutritional status: Protein, albumin and prealbumin, hemoglobin, transferrin, and white blood cell count; hemoglobin A1c if diabetic, appetite, and recent unintentional weight loss or gain
   c. Hydration status
   d. Circulatory support
   e. Presence of neurological injury
   f. Exposure to moisture: Incontinence of bladder or bowel, body moisture
   g. Sensory-perceptual ability
   h. Mobility, activity and exercise, body positioning
   i. Pressure, shearing, and friction, which can occur during the course of bedside care
   j. Age: Older adults are at particular risk for developing pressure ulcers, because they are most likely to have problems in all of these categories.
2. Assessment scales: Assessment scales are routinely used in all inpatient care settings. However, only one study, from Brazil, was located that demonstrated good predictive validity of the Braden Scale in older long-term care facility residents (Tosta de Souza, Conciecao de Gouveia Santos, Iri, & Oguri, 2010). The Braden Scale is the most popular in the United States and internationally. Other assessment scales exist (e.g., Performance Palliation Scale, Karnofsky Performance Scale, Neonatal Skin Risk Assessment Scale, Neonatal Skin Condition Score, and Starkid Skin Scale), but data to support their reliability and validity are limited. Rehabilitation nurses need to gather data to show whether completing a risk assessment scale actually triggers specific interventions that prevent skin breakdown.
   a. The Braden Scale for pressure ulcer risk was developed in 1987 and is used internationally. Its reliability and validity have been tested with evidence-based interventions. It contains six weighted elements—sensory perception, moisture, activity, mobility, nutrition (each of which is graded from 1 [very poor or very limited] to 4 [excellent, normal]), and friction/shear (which is scored from 1 to 3). Grades are summed across all elements for a total risk status score (**Figure 19-3**). The subscales for activity and friction/shear alone have shown higher predictive value than other subscales on the tool. Scores of 15–18 indicate mild risk, 13–14 indicate moderate risk, 10–12 indicate high risk, and scores of 9 or below are very high risk. The Braden Q Scale was developed later and adapted for pediatric populations.
   b. Norton scale: Developed in 1961, it contains a simpler list of five weighted elements—physical condition, mental condition, activity, mobility, and incontinence—that are scored from 1 (immobile or poor) to 4 (excellent) and summed for a total risk status score. Scores of 14 or higher indicate mild risk, 13 indicates moderate risk, and 12 or below indicates high risk.
   c. For both scoring systems, low scores prompt specific interventions to decrease risk and maintain or restore skin integrity. Skin risk scores over time can be reviewed to demonstrate improvement.

F. Nursing Diagnoses Related to Skin Integrity and Associated Risk Factors (NANDA-I, 2012–2014)

1. Impaired bed and impaired wheelchair mobility
2. Impaired transfer ability
3. Activity intolerance
4. Impaired physical mobility
5. Ineffective peripheral tissue perfusion
6. Acute and chronic pain
7. Posttrauma syndrome
8. Bowel incontinence
9. Diarrhea
10. Urinary incontinence (functional, overflow, reflex, stress, urge)
11. Imbalanced nutrition, less than body requirements
12. Imbalanced nutrition, more than body requirements
13. Impaired oral mucous membrane
14. Impaired swallowing
15. Self-neglect
16. Unilateral neglect
17. Risk for peripheral neurovascular dysfunction
18. Disturbed sensory perception (kinesthetic, tactile)
19. Deficient fluid volume
20. Noncompliance (ineffective adherence) with preventive interventions (e.g., weight shifts, turning

Figure 19-3. Braden Scale for Predicting Pressure Sore Risk

Patient's Name ______ Evaluator's Name ______ Date of Assessment ______

SENSORY PERCEPTION Ability to respond meaningfully to pressure-related discomfort	**1. Completely Limited** Unresponsive (does not moan, flinch, or grasp) to painful stimuli due to diminished level of consciousness or sedation. OR Limited ability to feel pain over most of the body	**2. Very Limited** Responds only to painful stimuli; cannot communicate discomfort except by moaning or restlessness OR Has a sensory impairment that limits the ability to feel pain or discomfort over $1/2$ of body.	**3. Slightly Limited** Responds to verbal commands but cannot always communicate discomfort or the need to be turned. OR Has some sensory impairment that limits ability to feel pain or discomfort in one or two extremities.	**4. No Impairment** Responds to verbal commands; has no sensory deficit that would limit ability to feel or voice pain or discomfort.				
MOISTURE Degree to which skin is exposed to moisture	**1. Constantly Moist** Skin is kept moist almost constantly by perspiration, urine, etc. Dampness is detected every time a patient is moved or turned.	**2. Very Moist** Skin is often, but not always, moist. Linen must be changed at least once a shift.	**3. Occasionally Moist** Skin is occasionally moist, requiring an extra linen change approximately once a day.	**4. Rarely Moist** Skin is usually dry; linen only requires changing at routine intervals.				
ACTIVITY Degree of physical activity	**1. Bedfast** Confined to bed	**2. Chairfast** Ability to walk is severely limited or nonexistent. Cannot bear own weight and/or must be assisted into a chair or wheelchair.	**3. Walks Occasionally** Walks occasionally during the day but for very short distances, with or without assistance. Spends majority of each shift in bed or chair.	**4. Walks Frequently** Walks outside the room at least twice a day and inside the room at least once every two hours during waking hours				
MOBILITY Ability to change and control body position	**1. Completely Immobile** Does not make even slight changes in body or extremity position without assistance	**2. Very Limited** Makes occasional slight changes in body or extremity position but is unable to make frequent or significant changes independently.	**3. Slightly Limited** Makes frequent though slight changes in body or extremity position independently.	**4. No Limitation** Makes major and frequent changes in position without assistance.				

continued

Figure 19-3. Braden Scale for Predicting Pressure Sore Risk (continued)

NUTRITION Usual food intake pattern	**1. Very Poor** Never eats a complete meal. Rarely eats more than 1/3 of any food offered. Eats two servings or less of protein (meat or dairy products) per day. Takes fluids poorly. Does not take a liquid dietary supplement OR Is NPO and/or maintained on clear liquids or IV for more than 5 days.	**2. Probably Inadequate** Rarely eats a complete meal and generally eats only about 1/2 of any food offered. Protein intake includes only three servings of meat or dairy products per day. Occasionally will take a dietary supplement. OR Receives less than optimum amount of liquid diet or tube feeding	**3. Adequate** Eats over half of most meals. Eats a total of four servings of protein (meat, dairy products) per day. Occasionally will refuse a meal, but will usually take a supplement when offered OR Is on a tube feeding or total parenteral nutrition regimen which probably meets most of nutritional needs	**4. Excellent** Eats most of every meal. Never refuses a meal. Usually eats a total of 4 or more servings of meat and dairy products. Occasionally eats between meals. Does not require supplementation.				
FRICTION AND SHEAR	**1. Problem** Requires moderate to maximum assistance in moving. Complete lifting without sliding against sheets is impossible. Frequently slides down in bed or chair, requiring frequent repositioning with maximum assistance. Spasticity, contractures or agitation leads to almost constant friction	**2. Potential Problem** Moves feebly or requires minimum assistance. During a move skin probably slides to some extent against sheets, chairs, restraints, or other devices. Maintains relatively good position in a chair or bed most of the time but occasionally slides down.	**3. No Apparent Problem** Moves in bed and in chair independently and has sufficient muscle strength to lift up completely during a move. Maintains good position in a bed or chair.					
				Total Score				

in bed, management of incontinence, daily skin checks, disease management, dietary restrictions)

21. Contamination (of lesions, wounds, or incisions)
22. Impaired environmental interpretation syndrome
23. Hyperthermia
24. Hypothermia
25. Impaired verbal communication
26. Disturbed personal identity
27. Impaired skin integrity
28. Risk for impaired skin integrity
29. Impaired tissue integrity
30. Ineffective thermoregulation
31. Ineffective health self-management
32. Deficient knowledge (of self-care, skin care, hygiene, foot care)
33. Ineffective therapeutic regimen management
34. Ineffective family therapeutic regimen management

G. NIC to Maintain Skin Integrity: Unless indicated otherwise, the LOE is 4 for all of the following interventions (NPUAP & EPUAP, 2009; Registered Nurses Association of Ontario, 2005; Wound, Ostomy and Continence Nurses Society, 2010).

1. Ensure good nutritional support; use supplements if needed. Protein or calorie malnutrition inhibits wound healing by reducing fibroblast and collagen synthesis.
2. Manage tissue loads.
   a. Turn and reposition the client frequently.
      1) Every 2 hours in bed, even if using a pressure-reducing mattress
      2) Every hour in a chair
      3) Weight shift every 15 minutes in a chair if independent
   b. Use good lifting, transfer, and turning techniques. Consult an occupational or physical therapist as needed.
   c. Cushion bony prominences.
   d. Protect skin against friction and shearing. Elevate heels off the mattress with pillows or pressure-relieving boots. Use turn sheets to reposition or lift the client. Maintain the head of bed at or below 30 degrees unless contraindicated by the condition; position at 30 degrees or less lateral incline for side lying.
   e. Position the client with adequate support; avoid placing the client on an existing ulcer.
   f. Increase the client's efforts toward mobility and activity. An overhead trapeze may be appropriate for some clients.
   g. Provide a pressure redistribution mattress (i.e., low-air-loss or air-fluidized mattress for stage III or IV [LOE 1]) and a wheelchair cushion for high-risk clients. Gel or air cushions are more effective than foam in preventing ischial pressure ulcers (LOE 1).
   h. Involve the interdisciplinary team.
   i. Avoid foam rings, donuts, and sheepskin. These can provide temporary comfort but do not provide pressure relief; they transfer pressure to surrounding tissue and may contribute to friction or shear (NPUAP & EPUAP, 2009).
3. Routine daily skin care:
   a. Inspect skin daily and pay special attention to all bony prominences.
   b. Cleanse skin at regular intervals, and use a mild cleansing agent to preserve the neutral pH of the skin.
   c. Apply nonsensitizing, pH-balanced emollients to help maintain skin moisture (LOE 3).
   d. Avoid massaging bony prominences to prevent tissue damage (LOE 2).
   e. Minimize exposure to incontinence, perspiration, or wound drainage (LOE 4).
      1) Use wicking materials to draw moisture away from the skin (e.g., underpads, diapers, or briefs).
      2) Use topical agents as protective barriers.
      3) Institute bladder and bowel training regimens for incontinence management. Consider short-term use of indwelling or external catheters while the client is extremely immobile. Consider a pouch or collection device for urine, stool, or draining wounds.
      4) Change wet or soiled absorbent briefs immediately. Cleanse gently and dry the skin thoroughly. Avoid the use of absorbent briefs and propping urinals for long periods through the night. Remove bedpans promptly after use. A bedside commode is preferable to a bedpan at night as soon as the client is able to transfer safely and maintain sitting balance.
4. Teach clients and caregivers about the importance of self-efficacy in nutrition, management of tissue loads, skin inspection, and general skin care (LOE 3).

H. Essential Elements for Planning Wound Care and Expected Client Outcomes (NOC)

1. Nutritional assessment and support: Nutritional support provides sufficient protein to produce serum albumin values of at least 3.5, and the client's weight will be more than 80% of ideal. Several weeks of intensive therapy are needed to increase serum albumin. Prealbumin testing shows a rise in 3–5 days.

2. Management of tissue loads: Resting surfaces and positioning provide adequate protection for tissue load to encourage healing and prevent further breakdown (LOE 4).
3. Wound care: Wound-specific care promotes wound cleansing and healing. Response to treatment could be slow because of underlying vascular damage, comorbidities, and immobility.

I. NIC for Wounds and Pressure Ulcers

1. Promote increased protein intake, vitamin supplementation, and adequate hydration. Correct any nutritional deficiencies (LOE 4). Ensure that the client's diet provides 30–40 kcal per kilogram body weight per day and total protein of 1.25–1.5 g protein per kilogram body weight (NPUAP & EPUAP, 2009). Consult a dietitian for appropriate supplementation, especially if a client with a pressure ulcer is underweight or losing weight (NPUAP & EPUAP, 2009). Small studies have demonstrated improved healing rates in high-risk clients who are given supplemental protein, arginine, zinc, and vitamin C for 3 weeks (Wound, Ostomy and Continence Nurses Society, 2010).
2. Keep the client off the wound as much as possible (LOE 3).
3. Turn and reposition the client at least every 2 hours while in bed, every hour in a chair, using sheets to lift (not drag) the client; if possible, use an over-the-bed trapeze to encourage the client to assist with lifting (LOE 3).
4. Use positioning pillows and blocks to maintain pressure relief; consider using pressure-reducing devices (e.g., air mattresses, specialty foam surfaces, gel pads, low-air-loss mattresses, and wheelchair cushions). Float heels off the bed using pillows, foam, or sheepskin-lined boots or other flotation devices (LOE 3).
5. Manage pain. Encourage mobility (LOE 3).
6. Assess circulatory status. Wounds must receive adequate circulation to heal (LOE 4).
7. Keep the skin clean, dry, and lubricated; do not massage reddened bony prominences, because this can cause capillary destruction (LOE 3).
8. Manage incontinence. Initiate toileting and bladder and bowel training programs. Change linens promptly and clean the skin after any episodes of bladder or bowel incontinence; remove wrinkles in linens to prevent further pressure. Apply a moisture barrier (e.g., ointment, paste, lotion, or film-forming spray) to exposed skin for further protection (LOE 3).
9. Provide consistent, timely treatments and document progress (LOE 3). Spray cleanse the wound with isotonic saline, Vulnopur (saline, aloe vera, silver chloride, and decyl glucoside), a commercial wound cleanser, or sterile water. Recent studies found no statistical difference in wound healing when saline was compared with water, but there was a significant improvement for wounds cleansed with Vulnopur (Moore & Cowman, 2005).
10. Focus treatment approaches on the whole person and the environment; pressure ulcers tend to be multivariate in cause (LOE 4).
11. Assess and reassess pressure ulcers using standard staging guidelines. Pressure ulcers are staged according to depth, characteristics of the wound bed, and potential involvement of deep fascia (**Figure 19-4**). In some states, inpatient healthcare facilities are required to report all stage III and stage IV pressure ulcers. Therefore, some facilities allow only specially trained nurses to document the stage of ulcers.

J. Wound-Specific Nursing Interventions for Pressure Ulcers (**Table 19-2**)

K. Phases of Wound Healing

1. Vascular supply and wound stabilization (i.e., the wound bleeds and then clots)
2. Inflammation of the tissues with influx of lymphocytes, macrophages, and granulocytes, concurrently while phagocytes remove dead tissue (inflammatory phase)
3. Proliferation of fibrin and formation of a loose matrix within the wound, which supports additional tissue formation and retention (granulation and epithelialization)
4. Maturation of the fibrin matrix into intact skin (remodeling)

L. Documentation of Wound Healing (LOE 4)

1. Stage and document the wound upon first discovery. Describe the location and measure (in centimeters) length (head to toe), width (side to side), and depth of the wound; use transparent grids for accuracy in measurement if needed. Measure wounds each week to determine effectiveness of treatments and healing.
2. Describe the wound base and tissue type (e.g., color, presence or absence of moisture, epithelialization, granulation, hypergranulation, slough, eschar).
3. Evaluate undermining or sinus tract or tunneling formation by gently probing the wound with sterile gauze swabs to determine the depth of pockets, tunnels, or tracts. Use the clock method to describe the location of the undermine or tract (e.g., "2-cm tunnel at 2 o'clock").

Figure 19-4. Stages of Pressure Ulcers

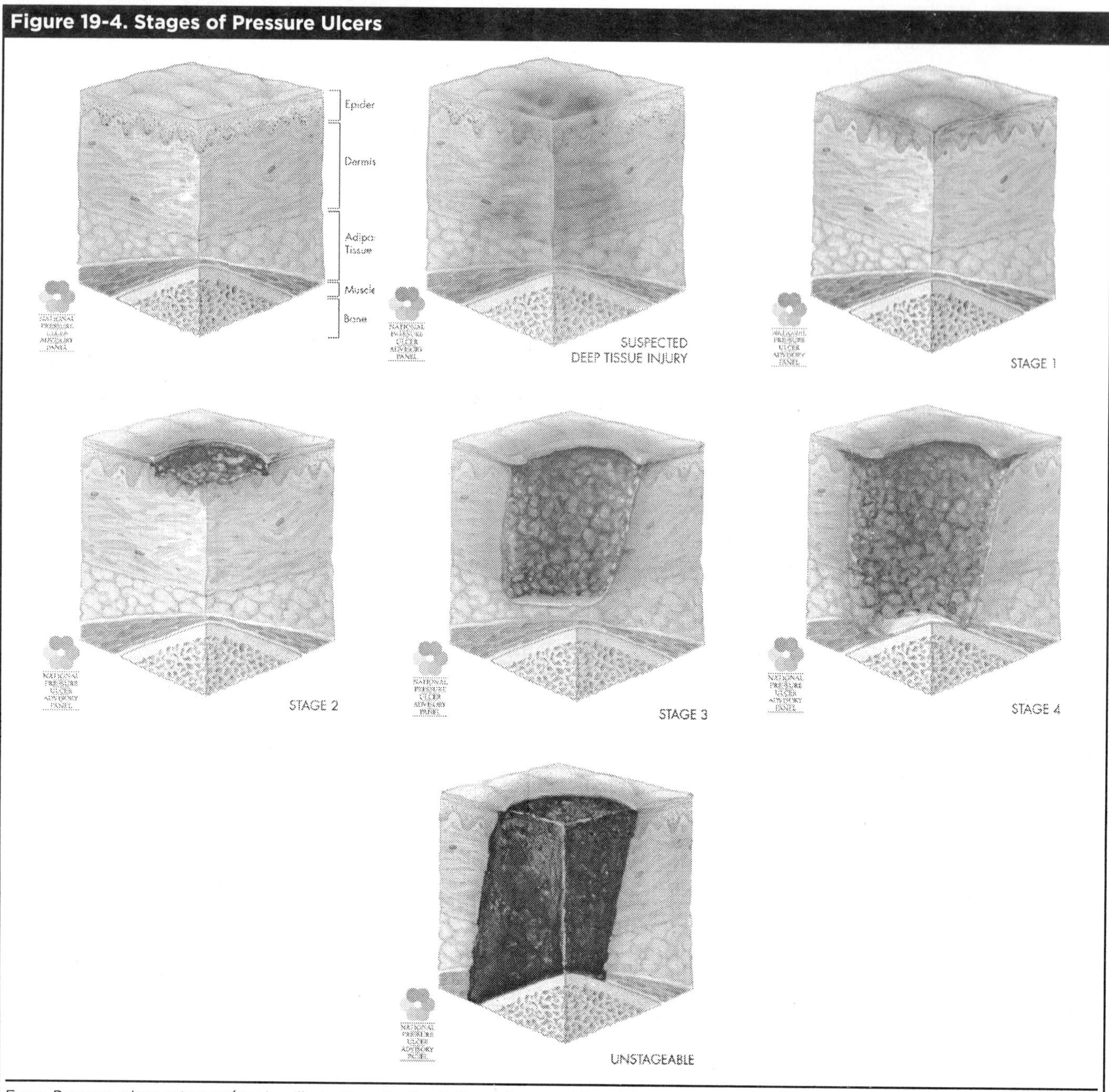

From *Pressure ulcer category/staging illustrations*, by the National Pressure Ulcer Advisory Panel. (n.d.), Retrieved from http://npuap.org/resources.htm/educational-and-clinical-resources/pressure-ulcer-categorystaging-illustrations. Copyright by National Pressure Ulcer Advisory Panel. Reprinted with permission.

4. Evaluate the amount and type of drainage. Note any odor from the wound.
5. Evaluate the periwound skin. Note any erythema, maceration, or callus formation. Evaluate for infection (presence or absence) and wound edges (open, attached, closed, or rolled).
6. Note evidence of pain, induration, or inflammation, and remember that redness, hardness, or discoloration around pressure areas that have poor blood supply (e.g., heels, sacrum) can mask major tissue necrosis underneath apparently intact skin.
7. Include the present and planned treatment regimen.
8. Photograph the wound for baseline reference and repeat at periodic intervals (generally every week) until the wound is healed. This is a helpful visual measure to document the effectiveness of therapy. Obtain written client consent before taking pictures.
9. Document pressure wounds that are healing by retaining the label of the original stage, adding the descriptor "healing"; do not revert to lesser staging as the wound heals. Exception: The Minimum

Table 19-2. Nursing Interventions for Pressure Ulcers	
Wound cleansing	Wear gloves, gown, mask, and eyewear or face shield as appropriate to anticipate potential for overspray of contaminated matter. Minimize trauma to the wound. Cleanse the periwound area and the wound to reduce the bacterial count. Appropriate solutions include the following: • Water: Tap, distilled or cooled boiled; use sterile water if client is immunosuppressed or if tap water is of poor quality • Saline: No statistical benefit over water Avoid antiseptics and products designed for use on intact skin or for removal of fecal material because these may be toxic to the wound bed.
Techniques	Irrigation, swabbing, showering, or bathing Whirlpool has been shown to have no statistical benefit since 2005. For heavy exudate, use a commercial wound cleanser containing surfactant. Use nonabrasive, light scrubbing with a cloth or sponge, minimizing trauma to the wound bed. Use high-pressure irrigation of 4–15 psi to remove slough or necrotic tissue. A 35-ml syringe with a 19-gauge needle or angiocatheter yields 8 psi.
Signs of infection or colonization	New or increased pain, delayed healing, friable granulation tissue, discoloration of the wound bed, change in odor, increased serous exudate, induration, pocketing, tunneling, or bridging Infection is defined as bacteria >105 CFU/cm^2 or presence of beta-hemolytic streptococcus (NPUAP & EPUAP, 2009; LOE 3).
Treatments	Topical antibiotics for 14 days for wounds that show poor healing or have had purulent exudate for more than 2 weeks of routine care Silver or honey dressings for wounds with multiple organisms on culture, in combination with alginate or foam dressing (WOCN, 2010). Silver dressings speed healing, decrease odor and exudate, and allow longer wear time. Honey dressings have shown increasing evidence of efficacy for chronic wounds taking more than 5 weeks to heal. However, randomized trials are lacking. Antiseptics are used in the short term to control bacteria and reduce inflammation in wounds that are not expected to heal. Systemic antibiotics are used in the presence of bacteremia, sepsis, advancing cellulitis, or osteomyelitis. These antibiotics do not reach ischemic or granulation tissue. Therefore, topical antibiotics are applied directly to the wound.
Debridement	Surgical is recommended for wounds with extensive tunneling, undermining, or necrosis. Conservative sharp. Mechanical, as in saline wet-to-dry. High-pressure fluid irrigation. Ultrasonic mist reduces purulent drainage, but evidence of effectiveness for debridement is insufficient. Autolysis, either chemical or enzymatic using collagenase Larval using maggots has limited evidence of effectiveness Dry eschar must be scored or cross-hatched before application of collagenase. Hard, dry eschar on ischemic limbs or feet should not be debrided.
Stage I	Keep skin clean and dry. Use barrier lotion or spray to protect from abrasion or maceration. Use pressure redistribution devices, padding, or elevation off hard surfaces at sites of reddened, intact skin and bony prominences. Keep head of bed at or below 30 degrees, use good turning techniques to prevent friction and shearing.

continued

Table 19-2. Nursing Interventions for Pressure Ulcers (continued)	
Stage II	Cleanse wound at each dressing change (see "Wound Cleansing" items). If necessary, irrigate gently to remove nonadherent particles. Keep wound moist and clean. Use foam, hydrocolloids, hydrogels, hydrofiber, or transparent absorbent acrylic dressings. Adjust frequency of dressing change to allow assessment, but avoid disturbing fibroblastic action and possible introduction of pathogens. Initially, change dressings every 2–3 days. As healing progresses, reduce frequency.
Stage III	Cleanse and irrigate the wound at each dressing change. Assess for slough, exudate, tunnels, and undermining. Select dressing type based on appearance of the wound bed. For shallow wounds with granulation, use hydrocolloid or transparent absorbent acrylic dressing. For wounds with slough, use a targeted enzymatic debridement product and a secondary dressing. If tunneling is noted, pack dead spaces with an appropriate absorbent wicking product (e.g., foam, alginate tape) and cover with a secondary dressing (e.g., antimicrobials, gauze, or foam). Adjust the frequency of dressing changes according to the amount of drainage. Apply a barrier wipe or spray to the periwound intact skin to protect from moisture and provide a surface allowing adhesives to adhere well. Vacuum-assisted closure may be appropriate for particular wounds. Debridement of eschar and slough as described in "Debridement."
Stage IV	Cleanse as indicated for stage III. Vacuum-assisted closure, surgical closure, grafts, or flaps may ultimately be selected after clean margins are established. Electrical stimulation may be helpful for stages II, III, and IV. Cytokines may be prescribed for use on stage II, III, and IV wounds.

Data from National Pressure Ulcer Advisory Panel & European Pressure Ulcer Advisory Panel. 2009; Wound, Ostomy and Continence Nurses Society, 2010.

Data Set and Inpatient Rehabilitation Facility Patient Assessment Instrument both require staff to revert to lesser staging.

M. Expected Client Outcomes (NOC) Related to Potential or Impaired Skin Integrity
1. Expect signs of healing within 14 days (LOE 2).
2. Intact skin
3. The client performs appropriate self-efficacy measures in the maintenance of skin integrity.
4. No new areas of skin breakdown

III. Elimination: Bladder and Bowel Function

A. Overview
1. The human body eliminates the waste of metabolism through urine and stool.
2. Requirements for normal function include the following:
   a. Anatomical integrity
   b. Intact neurological components for both voluntary control and synergistic emptying
   c. A predictable pattern of waste production
   d. Physical and mental ability and the willingness to carry out toileting-related tasks
3. Clients in rehabilitation facilities often need treatment for constipation, urinary or bowel incontinence, or management of neurogenic bowel and bladder.
4. Bowel and bladder disorders are major barriers to community living, employment, and social activity.
5. Rehabilitation nurses must be knowledgeable about the normal physiology of bladder and bowel function, clinically astute in identifying disruptions that produce incontinence and dysfunction, and expert in selecting interventions that will help the client develop predictable, effective elimination patterns.
6. Management of bowel and bladder function is a key aspect of rehabilitation nursing; however, bowel and bladder goals are best achieved with an interdisciplinary team approach because cognitive ability, communication ability, hand function, level of independence in activities of daily living (ADL), and transfers are key factors in the choice of appropriate bowel and bladder management strategies.
7. Desired outcomes (NOC) of bladder management are to remain continent, preserve renal function by emptying the bladder completely; minimize the

risk of other conditions associated with the bladder, including urinary tract infections (UTIs) and bladder stones; and to optimize the individual's quality of life (Ginsberg, 2013b).

8. Desired outcomes (NOC) of bowel management are to remain continent; have a formed bowel movement on a regular schedule; prevent diarrhea and constipation; and prevent complications such as hemorrhoids, abdominal distention, autonomic dysreflexia, and fecal impaction.

B. Physiology of Bladder Elimination (Doughty, 2006; Keyock & Newman, 2011, Mauk, 2012)

1. The purpose of the bladder is to store and control the elimination of urine.
2. The bladder wall is made of smooth muscle (the detrusor muscle) that communicates with the parasympathetic fibers of the autonomic system.
3. Once the bladder is full (about 300–500 ml), nerve impulses are sent to the brain. Bladder filling control originates in the T10–L2 segments of the spinal cord.
4. When ready to void, the detrusor muscle contracts, forcing urine through the bladder neck; the internal and external sphincters relax via parasympathetic signals from S2–S4. The external sphincter relaxes with somatic voluntary control via the pudendal nerve.
5. Inhibition or facilitation of urination is controlled by spinal cord reflex centers, the micturition center in the pons, and cortical and subcortical centers in the brain.
6. Skeletal muscle in the external sphincter and pelvic muscles that support the bladder are controlled by the pudendal nerve, which exits the spinal cord from the S2–S4 segments.

C. Urinary Incontinence (UI): *Urinary incontinence* is the involuntary loss of urine resulting from pathological, anatomical, or physiological factors. The International Incontinence Society (Abrams et.al, 2002, p. 167) provides a subjective definition: "the complaint of any involuntary leakage." There are two types of incontinence: persistent or chronic, and reversible or acute (transient). When the underlying cause is addressed, the transient incontinence resolves. Persistent urinary incontinence continues over time and is not related to an acute process. Refer all clients who dribble or leak urine for diagnosis and treatment. Treatment decisions are best made after completing a detailed client history, physical exam, and diagnostic tests including a voiding diary, postvoid residual bladder scan, urodynamic testing, and urological workup by a physician, advanced practice nurse, or specialty nurse trained to manage urinary incontinence.

1. Types of urinary incontinence related to lower urinary tract function (Newman, 2009b)
   a. Stress UI: Complaint of involuntary loss of urine on effort or physical exertion (e.g. sporting activities), or sneezing or coughing; sphincter dysfunction due to relaxation and weakness of the pelvic floor muscle and reduction in urethral resistance. Some risk factors include age, vaginal delivery and parity, smoking, obesity, prostate cancer treatment such as radical prostatectomy, menopause, and exercise.
   b. Urgency UI: Complaint of involuntary loss of urine accompanied or immediately preceded by urgency. Overactive bladder (urgency/frequency) syndrome is defined as urinary urgency, usually accompanied by frequency and nocturia, with or without urgency urinary incontinence, in the absence of UTI or other obvious pathology; bladder pressure exceeds urethral pressure and causes urine loss. Bladder contractions are the result of detrusor activity associated with neurological conditions such as MS, stroke, or Parkinson's disease.
   c. Mixed UI: Complaint of involuntary loss of urine associated with urgency and also with effort or physical exertion, sneezing or coughing; combination of bladder and urethral dysfunction causing stress and urge incontinence
   d. Continuous UI is the complaint of continuous leakage.
   e. Overflow incontinence (incontinence with high postvoid residuals): sudden overflow of urine when pressure inside the bladder exceeds the pressure of a urethral obstruction. Symptoms include small, frequent voiding; postvoid dribbling; hesitance; and straining to void. This term is not a symptom or condition; the International Continence Society believes it to be misleading and suggests the use of "urgency UI," "stress UI," or "mixed UI with high postvoid residual."
2. Other types of incontinence (Doughty, 2006; Newman, 2009)
   a. Transient incontinence is caused by reversible factors such as delirium, infection, atrophic vaginitis, pharmaceuticals, psychological conditions, conditions resulting in excess urine production, restricted mobility, and stool impaction.
   b. Functional incontinence is a type of UI unrelated to the urinary tract. The Agency for Healthcare Policy and Research (1996)

guidelines define it as "urinary leakage associated with chronic impairments of a physical and/or cognitive functioning." It also refers to urine loss as the result of an inability to reach the bathroom due to physical or psychological disabilities that do not allow for self-toileting.

3. Assessment data (Keyock & Newman, 2011)
   a. Screen for type of lower tract (bladder) urinary dysfunction with key questions including: Do you get a sudden feeling you need to go to the bathroom? Do you experience a loss of urine when you sneeze, cough, or laugh? How often do you go the bathroom? Is it more than 8 times in a day? How often at night? (Newman, 2009b).
   b. While obtaining the history, question the onset, duration, and characteristics of UI including frequency of urination day and night, frequency and amount of leakage, type of incontinence, difficulty starting stream, and pain with urination. The Three Incontinence Questions (3IQ) is an easy-to-use tool with good sensitivity and reliability. The tool is available at http://www.fpnotebook.com/Uro/Exam/ThrIncntncQstns.htm.
   c. Other items as part of the history should include acquired or congenital neurological conditions; neurological symptoms including onset, evolution, and treatment; spasticity and autonomic dysreflexia; mobility and sensation; mental status; prior surgeries; pregnancy history; medications; mobility; and hand function (Stohrer et al., 2009).
   d. Fluid-intake volume and pattern or voiding diary: a recording of strict intake and output monitoring for 3 days, including times of day
   e. Age and activity level
   f. Prior history of bladder problems: Onset, frequency, urgency, stress incontinence, retention, infections, childbirth, prolapse of uterus or bladder, enlarged prostate, prostate surgery, bladder surgery
   g. Mobility impairments, prescribed restrictions, braces, splints, immobilizers
   h. Neuromuscular status, including anal wink and bulbocavernosis reflex
   i. Communication impairments
   j. Sensory and motor status
   k. Environment: accessibility, privacy
   l. Adaptive equipment use, current needs
      1) Current medications, drug allergies, comorbidities
      2) Postvoid residual volumes per ultrasound scan
   m. Urine analysis, microscopic examination and culture
      1) Presence or absence of indwelling catheter upon admission (LOE 4)
   n. Collaborate with other team members to determine whether incontinence is transient, established, or both; document type and duration (LOE 1).
   o. Collaborate with team members to identify and document possible etiologies of incontinence (LOE 1).
4. Nursing diagnoses related to urinary incontinence and neurogenic bladder (NANDA-I, 2012–2014)
   a. Impaired urinary elimination
   b. Urgency to urinate
   c. Readiness for enhanced urinary elimination
   d. UI (functional, overflow, reflex, risk for urge, stress, urge)
   e. Urinary retention (acute or chronic)
   f. Associated diagnoses: mobility impairments, ego integrity items, deficient or excess fluid volume, self-care deficit in toileting, self-neglect, disturbed sensory perception, pain, communication impairment, and social isolation
   g. Risk for autonomic dysreflexia
5. General bladder training NIC for all types of incontinence: The Cochrane Collaboration published an exhaustive review of literature between 1980 and 2005, compiled by Wallace, Roe, Williams, and Palmer (2009), that compared randomized and quasi-randomized studies of bladder training with variables that included no treatment, biofeedback, behavioral treatment (specified), pharmacological treatment (specified), psychological treatment (specified), surgical intervention (specified), and specified medical devices. In addition, combinations of bladder training with these same variables were compared. Both short- and long-term outcomes were examined, along with client perception of cure and quality of life. Results and conclusions were disappointing. Wallace et al.'s (2009) conclusions and implications for practice are as follows:

   > *There is inconclusive evidence to judge the effects of bladder training in both the short and long term. The results of the trials reviewed tended to favor bladder training (with no evidence of adverse effect) but there were too few data to assess this reliably. The data that were available were from trials of variable quality and small size. There are*

resource implications but the magnitude of these is not clear from the trials. The data are also too few to provide any guidance on the choice among bladder training, drug treatment, or other conservative approaches, or on whether adding bladder training to another treatment enhances any effect. (p. 18)

LOEs for the interventions listed were retrieved from Milne (2008) and Stevens (2008).

a. Adequate fluid intake: Monitor intake and output; individuals with UI symptoms often limit their intake. Individuals with urge incontinence with high fluid intake may show reduction in symptoms and voiding frequency by lowering their fluid intake. Limit fluids after the evening meal to minimize nocturia, and consider a scheduled fluid program of 240–300 ml eight times a day (Keyock & Newman, 2011).
b. Toileting self-care assistance: Ensure a clear pathway and assist to toilet. Use a bedside commode at night. Evaluate needs for assistive devices. Modify the environment to facilitate continence (LOE 1).
c. Bladder training: This is a specific program designed to increase bladder capacity and reduce urinary frequency. It is targeted for individuals with symptoms of overactive bladder urge, stress, mixed, and functional incontinence. Focuses on strategies for controlling urgency and delaying voiding (Doughty, 2006). Initiate a timed (scheduled) toileting program. Help the client sit on the toilet, bedpan, or commode for at least 5 minutes, at 2-hour intervals. As continence improves, gradually reduce toileting to every 3 hours, especially before and after meals and before bedtime. Enlist the cooperation and assistance of therapy staff to provide opportunities to toilet between therapies. In addition, teach pelvic floor muscle training (e.g., Kegel exercises) to increase success.
d. Assess for urinary retention: Perform at least two postvoid residual bladder scans within 20 minutes after voiding to assess bladder emptying. The usual measurement of concern is a repeated measurement of greater than 100–200 ml (Doughty, 2006).
e. Nighttime incontinence care: Initially, disposable diapers can be used day and night. As continence improves, discontinue diapers at night; instead, use absorbent underpads. Consider condom catheters for men who sleep so soundly that they do not awaken with incontinent episodes. Do not prop urinals or leave the client on a bedpan for long periods. Remove bedpans promptly after use. Discontinue bedpans as soon as the client is mobile enough to use a bedside commode at night. Perform a skin check and provide perineal hygiene in conjunction with a timed toileting program.
f. Avoid indwelling catheters whenever possible to avoid risk of urinary tract infection (LOE 1).
g. Immediately cleanse the skin after incontinent episodes, and apply barrier ointments to prevent skin breakdown (LOE 1).

6. Specific interventions (i.e., NIC) for incontinence (**Table 19-3**). The following interventions are also listed:
   a. Stress incontinence interventions range from behavioral approaches to surgery.
      1) Teach pelvic floor muscle or Kegel exercises. According to the literature, the recommended duration of the prescribed regimen varies widely, with 3 months being most frequently recommended. A trial of supervised (with continence nurse specialists or physical therapists) pelvic floor exercises for a minimum of 3 months, as a first-line treatment for urinary incontinence, is widely suggested because it has demonstrated up to 70% improvement of symptoms in females (Keyock & Newman, 2011; National Institute for Health & Clinical Excellence, 2012) (LOEs 1 and 2).
      2) Clients can consciously use pelvic floor muscle exercises to occlude the urethra during activities that precipitate leakage (e.g., coughing or sneezing); one of these exercises is the Knack, or quick-squeeze, maneuver.
      3) Self-monitoring (bladder diary); lifestyle changes such as weight loss and fluid and diet management are also helpful.
      4) Voiding regimens including scheduled voiding and delayed voiding or urge-suppression strategies.
      5) Refer to other team members for biofeedback or pharmacological or surgical therapy.
   b. Urge incontinence (Gormley et al., 2014; Newman, 2009a)
      1) Self-monitoring with bladder diary for 3 to 7 days before initiating behavioral therapy can be useful; document each void,

Table 19-3. Management of Bladder Dysfunctions

Impairment	Symptoms	Etiology	Management
Stress incontinence	Small loss of urine occurring with increased abdominal pressure as with coughing, sneezing, laughing, and exercising	Weak external sphincter, weak pelvic floor musculature, and secondary effects of smoking and obesity	Dietary modifications: Avoid caffeine, carbonated beverages, alcohol, chocolate, artificial sweeteners, tomato, citrus, and spicy foods. Adjust fluid intake: Achieve 2,000-3.000 ml daily in increments of 250-300 ml 8–10 times a day. Limit fluids after 8 pm. Kegel exercises: Ten contractions then 30 seconds of rest five times daily. Timed voiding program: Every 2 hours while awake, every 3–4 hours at night; assist as needed. Slowly extend intervals to every 3 or 4 hours. Biofeedback, electronic stimulation
Urge incontinence/ overactive bladder	Urgency, frequency, nocturia	Detrusor hyperreflexia, uninhibited bladder contractions, suprapontine lesions	Urge suppression training; Crede; condoms catheter at night; surgery (bladder augmentation, diversion); weight loss; smoking cessation; use of oxybutynin, tolterodine, flavoxate, and imipramine
Spastic bladder	Unable to store urine	Upper motor neuron injury	
Mixed stress and urge incontinence			
Overflow	Frequent small voids	Reflex or neurogenic components, external sphincter dyssynergy, weak detrusor	Pessary, trigger void, double void, Foley or suprapubic catheter followed by bladder retraining, botox injection of sphincter, use of Flomax or alpha blockers, surgery (stent, TURP, sphincterotomy)
Flaccid bladder	Unable to empty urine	Lower motor neuron injury	
Functional incontinence	Incontinence in route to toilet	Mobility, coordination or cognitive impairments interfere with allowing adequate time to get to the toilet	Timed or prompted voiding program with helper assist as need; modify environment to reduce obstacles
Neurogenic-retention	Episodic large voids	Destrusor-sphincter dyssynergia	Intermittent catheterization at 4- or 6-hour intervals for bladder scan volumes greater than 400 ml

circumstance, and volume for clinician to plan and monitor treatment.

2) Implement bladder training, time voiding, and delayed voiding.
3) If the client is cognitively intact and motivated, teach urge inhibition (LOE 4).
4) Combine bladder training with pelvic floor muscle exercises (LOE 3) "The Cochrane review concluded PFMT was more likely to improve stress incontinence than urge even for those with mixed bladder" (Myer, 2014, p. 5).
5) Collaborate with prescribing team members if pharmacological therapy is warranted.
6) Initiate referrals for a further diagnostic workup if the client does not improve.

c. Overflow incontinence
   1) Self-monitoring with bladder diary; document each void to determine fluid balance
   2) Allow sufficient time for voiding.
   3) Determine postvoid residuals (LOE 4).
   4) Provide the client with education about double voiding.
   5) Consider potential causes to include constipation and inadequate fluid intake.
   6) If catheterization is needed, sterile intermittent is preferable to indwelling (LOE 2).
   7) Refer clients needing pharmacological or surgical intervention.

d. Mixed incontinence (Keyock & Newman, 2011; Meyers, 2014)
   1) Fluid management/reduce fluid intake; spread intake throughout the day with no fluid intake 3 to 4 hours before bed (LOE 2)
   2) Avoid foods that affect bladder function such as caffeine products and alcohol.
   3) Avoid constipation.

4) Time voids with increasing increments between voiding; conscious pelvic floor muscle contractions should be done as needed.
5) Weight loss (LOE 1)
6) Referral to other team members for pharmacological therapy (for urge component) or surgical therapy.

e. Functional incontinence
1) Modify the environment to be conducive to maintaining independence with continence (LOEs 1 and 4)
2) Provide individualized scheduled or prompted voiding (LOEs 1 and 4).
3) Provide adequate fluid intake.
4) Refer for occupational and physical therapy as indicated.

6. The Quality of Care Act (1991; Suppl. 2005) regulations require that
a. Residents entering a facility without an indwelling urinary catheter not receive one unless medically necessary
b. Residents with UI receive appropriate services and treatment to prevent urinary tract infections and restore as much bladder control as possible.
c. Catheter-associated UTI, a common and potentially preventable complication of hospitalization, is one of the hospital-acquired complications chosen by the Centers for Medicare and Medicaid Services for which hospitals no longer receive additional payment. The 2009 Centers for Disease Control and Prevention Guideline for Prevention of Catheter-Associated Urinary Tract Infections (http://www.cdc.gov/hicpac/pdf/CAUTI/CAUTIguideline2009final.pdf) is an excellent resource, as it provides evidence-based recommendations on catheter-associated UTI prevention for patients who require an indwelling urinary catheter. Indications for a Foley catheter include acute urinary retention or urethral obstruction; need for accurate urinary output measurements in patients who may have hemodynamic or blood pressure instability; perioperative use for selected surgical procedures to include urologic or other surgeries on the genitourinary tract; anticipated prolonged surgery duration; and, if catheter is inserted, it should be removed in the postanesthsia care unit (PACU); operative patients with UI; need for intraoperative hemodynamic monitoring; and patients who receive large-volume infusions or diuretics during surgery

D. Neurogenic Bladder and Its Management
1. Classifications of neurogenic bladder disorders (there is a variety of classifications to describe neurogenic lower urinary tract dysfunction based on urodynamic findings, neurourological criteria, or lower urinary tract function) (Stohrer et al., 2009).
a. *Reflex urinary incontinence* (Doughty, 2006; Mauk, 2014; Stohrer, 2009), as defined by the International Incontinence Society, is uncontrolled urine loss occurring as a result of neurogenic disorders and caused by neurogenic detrusor overactivity; leakage occurs in the absence of a desire to void. Defining characteristics include absence of sensory awareness to void, urinary retention, and large residuals of urine. There is an interruption to the ascending sensory tract above the S2–S4 level.
1) Present in traumatic and nontraumatic disorders, cerebral palsy, MS, Gullain-Barré syndrome. Physiological changes could include detrusor overactivity, detrusor/sphincter dyssynergia, and autonomic dysreflexia.
2) Complications can include urinary calculi, UTI and polynephritis, and autonomic dysreflexia.
b. Flaccid bladder or atonic bladder: the bladder is areflexic and acontractile. The bladder fails to empty urine, resulting in urinary retention; it is often associated with lower motor neuron spinal cord injuries or spinal shock (Mauk, 2012).
c. Overactive bladder or detrusor hyperreflexia without detrusor sphincter dyssynergia, often seen with suprapontine lesions from other cerebrovascular diseases
2. Specific neurogenic bladder management strategies: The Consortium for Spinal Cord Medicine (2006), Ginsberg (2010), and Stohrer et al. (2009) presented the indications, contraindications, advantages, disadvantages, and nursing considerations for the most common bladder management strategies. The Consortium noted that there is no strong evidence that one method is superior to another. The goals of any bladder management program are to prevent upper urinary tract damage, minimize lower urinary tract complications (e.g., stones, fistulas, chronic effects of infections), and be compatible with client and caregiver lifestyles. When choosing a management strategy, a urologic evaluation is necessary to detect and manage spinal shock, uninhibited

bladder contractions, autonomic dysreflexia, or detrusor-external sphincter dyssynergia during the acute phase of rehabilitation. Head injury can accompany spinal cord injury, complicating bladder function and choice of bladder management strategy. Under debate in the literature is the use of sterile or clean technique for intermittent self-catheterization during hospitalization. Small studies have revealed insignificant or minimal increased incidence of UTI among clients using clean technique for several days before discharge. Some contend that this reduces client and caregiver confusion during the transition back to the home environment. Others point out the increased risk for hospital-acquired infection. Large, carefully controlled studies are needed to determine best practice.

a. Intermittent catheterization (IC) provides regular emptying of the bladder. The individual or caregiver is taught using sterile, asceptic, or clean technique. Compared with clean technique, asceptic technique provides a significant benefit in reducing contamination.
   1) IC may be effective for those who have sufficient manual dexterity or a caregiver willing to perform intermittent catheterization (LOE 3).
   2) Paralyzed Veterans of America recommends keeping bladder volumes below 500 ml by catheterizing every 4–6 hours to prevent overdistention of the bladder. The client may need to wake during the night for catheterization. Keeping bladder volumes below 400 ml has been recommended in the past by many sources (LOE 4).
   3) Catheterization frequency and avoidance of bladder overfilling are key measures to prevent infection. Fluid management and recording of output can be important.
   4) Train the client or caregiver and institute clean intermittent catheterization before discharge (LOE 3). See the ARN website at www.rehabnurse.org for client education materials.
   5) Consider sterile catheterization in those with recurring symptomatic infections (LOE 3).
   6) Treat urine leakage between catheterizations with anticholinergic medication and limit fluid intake (LOE 3). (Note: Botulinum toxin injections have been used experimentally as nerve blocks in the urinary sphincter with good short-term results. However, this is currently an off-label use not approved by the U.S. Food and Drug Administration.)
   7) Catheter selection depends on economic considerations and latex sensitivity.
   8) Hands are cleansed with soap and water or aseptic wipes both before and after catheterization.
   9) Ideally, single-use, sterile catheter kits are used in the outpatient environment. Many medical supply companies have disposable kits containing sterile catheters of various materials and lengths, with or without urine collection bags.

b. For areflexic bladder management, the goal is to empty the bladder to avoid distention caused by the intermittent catheterization procedure. The Credé and Valsalva maneuvers are not recommended, because they can potentially cause reflux (Stohrer et al., 2009).

c. Indwelling catheters: Urethral or suprapubic catheters are used for those with high fluid intake, poor manual dexterity, cognitive impairment, active substance abuse, elevated detrusor pressures managed with anticholinergic drugs, vesicoureteral reflux, lack of success with less invasive methods, or limited assistance from a caregiver (LOE 3). See ARN's website at www.rehabnurse.org for client education materials. Long-term use is associated with many potential complications including urethral erosion, urinary tract infections, and bladder cancer (Doughty, 2006).
   1) Suprapubic catheterization has several benefits over urethral catheterization and is especially preferred by those with quadriplegia or complete spinal cord injury. Suprapubic catheters are recommended for those with urethral abnormalities, bladder or urethral trauma, small bladder capacity, recurrent catheter obstruction, urethral incompetence, prostatitis, or epididymitis and those who want improved sexual genital function (Mauk, 2012).
   2) Surveillance for urinary tract infections and bladder stones is recommended.
   3) Urethral catheters (14–16 Fr) with a balloon filled with 5–10 ml sterile water are replaced every 2–4 weeks or weekly in those prone to catheter encrustation or bladder stones.
   4) Suprapubic catheters (22–24 Fr) are changed every 4 weeks by a trained

healthcare provider, and more often in those with catheter encrustation or stones.

5) Anchor the catheter with a belt, tape, or other device to the abdomen or thigh. To prevent urethral trauma alternate legs for the tubing anchor point daily.
6) Daily irrigation is not recommended. Irrigation is used only to clear clots or obstructions.
7) If daytime and nighttime collection devices are reused, clean daily with a 1:10 bleach solution or 1:3 vinegar solution.
8) Maintenance of a closed drainage system has been found to be a key element in prevention of catheter-associated urinary tract infections. Disconnection invites bacterial invasion.
9) Urine for culture and sensitivity should be obtained only from a newly inserted catheter and drainage bag to avoid culturing the system (i.e., the catheter and drainage bag) rather than the urine.

d. Reflex voiding with a condom catheter is appropriate for men who have adequate hand skills, poor compliance with fluid restriction, and small bladder capacity (LOE 4). See ARN's website at www.rehabnurse.org for client educational materials.

1) Apply the condom catheter securely to avoid constriction and leakage for 24 hours.
2) To avoid skin breakdown, wash the glans daily when the condom is changed and air-dry skin for 20–30 minutes. Anchor the tubing on the alternate leg each day to prevent skin breakdown.
3) Clean urinary collection bags and tubing daily with a 1:10 bleach solution.
4) Choose the appropriate size and length of self-adhesive condom catheter. Those with allergies to the adhesive can use nonadhesive condoms. Those with latex allergy can use nonlatex condom catheters.

e. Additional management strategies: The Consortium guideline outlines recommendations for these additional bladder management strategies and provides advisory information about application in clients who might benefit from each strategy, potential complications, and nursing considerations for each strategy.

1) Alpha blockers
2) Botulinum toxin injection
3) Urethral stents
4) Transurethral sphincterotomy
5) Electrical stimulation and posterior sacral rhizotomy
6) Bladder augmentation
7) Continent urinary diversion
8) Urinary diversion
9) Cutaneous ileovesicostomy

f. Potential long-term complications of indwelling catheters include the following:

1) Bladder stones
2) Kidney stones
3) Urethral erosions
4) Epididymitis
5) Recurrent infection
6) Incontinence
7) Pyelonephritis
8) Hydronephrosis due to fibrosis or thickening of the bladder wall
9) Bladder cancer

E. FIM™ Scoring: Rehabilitation nurses must enter scores for bladder function on the FIM™ tool daily (**Table 19-4**).

F. Bowel Function

1. Normal anatomy and physiology of bowel elimination

a. Peristalsis moves the stool along the gut. Haustral contractions roll and mix fecal materials.
b. The small intestine and ascending colon absorb nutrients from liquid stool (chyme).
c. The transverse colon absorbs some of the fluid, and stool begins to be more formed. Mass movements propel stool toward the descending colon—occurring up to three times daily, usually after a meal—and generally lasting up to 30 minutes.
d. The descending, sigmoid, and rectal portions of the colon absorb additional water and electrolytes. Kidney waste is added. Stool is compacted into a more solid form. The moisture content of stool depends on the length of time stool rested in the distal colon.
e. The internal sphincter retains stool in the rectum.
f. The external sphincter expands to allow the passage of stool from the rectum.
g. Abdominal wall musculature assists with evacuation.
h. Bowel function continues with cerebral or spinal cord impairment.

1) Voluntary and involuntary innervations occur at the reflex, segmental, and cortical levels.

Table 19-4. Functional Independence Measure (FIM™) Scoring—Bladder
Part 1: Level of Assistance
7 = Complete independence—Client does not require helper, assistive device or medication, does not void (dialysis)
6 = Modified independence—Requires assistive device or medications, performs intermittent self-cath, applies/removes condom cath, Foley, ileostomy or suprapubic cath, urinal, bedpan elevated or bedside commode, peripad or adult diaper. Independently manages device and discards urine, changes appliances, empties collection bags. Medications: Detrol, Ditropan, Flomax, Sudafed (pseudoephedrine) urecholine, Cardura. Must score as 6 even if the client uses the toilet during the day and only uses the urinal, commode, or condom cath at night.
5 = Supervision or set-up—Nursing empties the urinal, sets out equipment or supplies, client requires cues to maintain clean or sterile technique or to maintain an intermittent cath or voiding schedule, client discards the peripad or diaper properly.
4 = Minimal assistance—Client participates in >75% of bladder management tasks, requires touching to assist to place equipment in hand.
3 = Moderate assistance—Client participates 50%–75%, performs only one or two tasks, consistently tells helper of urge to void, full bladder, requires assistant to place urinal, bedpan, apply gloves, open packages and hand supplies to client.
2 = Maximum assistance—Client participates in 25%–50% of tasks, inconsistently tells helper of urge to void, bladder fullness, may participate in changing diaper or peripad, may tell helper leg bag needs emptying but cannot participate in the task.
1 = Total assistance—Client participates less than 25%. Helper changes diapers, peripads, maintains Foley or condom cath, performs intermittent cath, cleans patient, and changes clothing and linens after incontinent episodes.
0 = This score is not valid for bladder.
Part 2: Frequency of Accidents
7 = 100% continent, never has accidents, does not void due to dialysis
6 = 100% continent but uses an assistive device or medication to maintain bladder control
5 = 1 episode incontinence, urinal or bedpan spill in the past 7 days AND patient cleans self and soiled linens
4 = 2 episodes incontinence/spills in the past 7 days AND patient cleans self and soiled linens/clothing
3 = 3 episodes incontinence in the past 7 days AND cleans self and linens
2 = 4 episodes incontinence in the past 7 days AND cleans self, linens, changes clothes
1 = 5 episodes or helper must clean patient, linens, and clothing
0 = Not a valid score for bladder.
Note: Admission score includes events of the past 3 days, enter the lowest scores.
Score Part 1, score Part 2, enter lowest score on Uniform Data System Inpatient Rehabilitation Facility Patient Assessment Instrument (UDS IRF-PAI). The form is used by inpatient rehabilitation facilities to submit data to the national data base in Buffalo, NY.
Functional Independence Measure © Copyright 1997 by Uniform Data System for Medical Rehabilitation (UDSMR), a division of UB Foundation Activities, Inc. All rights reserved. Reprinted with permission of UDSMR.

2) Parasympathetic and sympathetic innervations occur from the autonomic nervous system.
3) The enteric nervous system influences the intrinsic neural control of the mobility, absorption, and secretion activities of the gut; it is independent of but influenced by the autonomic nervous system.
4) Like the bladder, the bowel is capable of emptying at a reflex level when stretch fibers in the descending large colon stimulate the reflex arc.

2. Requirements for stool formation and normal bowel function
   a. Adequate fiber in the diet to produce bulk and trap water in the stool; adequate solid matter for peristalsis to move the stool and allow the body to defecate in an organized, effective manner
   b. Adequate fluid intake to limit the amount of liquid reabsorbed from the descending colon
   c. General activity and mobility to support and enhance peristalsis
   d. Upright posture to allow gravity to assist in stool formation and passage
3. Patterns of defecation throughout the life span
   a. Infants: The gut functions at the reflex level.
   b. Children: As the child matures, he or she develops cortical control over the time and place of defecation.
   c. Adults: Middle age is a time of intense activity and relative regularity, which can vary slightly with diet changes, infrequent bouts of illness, or activity; however, the bowel generally responds to simple interventions.
   d. Older adults
      1) Changes occur in striated and smooth muscle strength.
      2) Activity gradually lessens.

3) Older adults generally consume less roughage and have poorer dentition.
4) Self-limiting hydration may be present secondary to concerns about urinary incontinence or nocturia.
5) Comorbidities may begin, along with increased medication use. These give rise to problems of constipation and help explain the focus on bowel regularity by many older adults.

G. Bowel Impairment (Mauk, 2012)

1. Constipation: Infrequent, small, hard, dry stool less than three times per week or none at all in several days, accompanied by straining and sensations of abdominal bloating or fullness
   a. Acute constipation: Recent onset of symptoms, a large amount of stool in the rectal ampulla, colon, or rectum
   b. Chronic constipation: Symptoms lasting longer than 3 months; enlarges the descending colon and produces dependency on laxatives, cathartics, or enemas
   c. Severe constipation and impaction cause sympathetic systemic problems (e.g., sweating, nausea, irritability, acute abdominal discomfort, and elevated blood pressure)
2. Diarrhea: Highly frequent liquid stool with accompanying cramping
   a. May be explosive, generally related to excessive caffeine ingestion, infection, irritability of the gut, or possible food poisoning
   b. May be associated with ulcerative colitis if not self-limiting
3. Sensory paralytic (afferent nerve root loss or damage)
   a. Occurs subsequent to diabetes or tabes dorsalis
   b. Produces diminished or absent ability to distinguish the need or time of defecation but rarely produces incontinence, because the motor function of the rectum is intact
4. Motor paralytic (efferent nerve root loss or damage)
   a. Occurs subsequent to poliomyelitis, intervertebral disc disease, tumor, or trauma
   b. Results in the inability to assist with defecation
   c. Associated with incontinence only if there is widespread disease due to the innervation of the intestines
5. Colostomies and ileostomies: Artificial openings on the abdominal wall to provide an exit for stool. (To obtain the current guidelines on ostomy care, consult the Wound, Ostomy and Continence Nurses Society's website at www.wocn.org.)
   a. Used when the colon has become obstructed and the rectum cannot be used (malignant tumors)
   b. Used when the gut is irritated beyond repair (ulcerative colitis)
   c. Used when it is necessary to rest the colon while it repairs (major abdominal resections)
   d. Can be an option for bowel management with chronic autonomic dysreflexia with a regular bowel program
6. Neurogenic bowel disorders associated with spinal cord injury
   a. Reflexic neurogenic bowel (upper motor neuron)
      1) The bowel is capable of reflexive emptying of the rectum without cortical awareness of the need to defecate.
      2) Associated with spinal cord injury above T12–S1 or damage to the cerebral cortex
      3) Because of the innervation of the sympathetic nervous system, the client may be aware of defecation and nervous system activity but have no conscious control over it.
   b. Autonomous, areflexic, flaccid, or atonal bowel (lower motor neuron)
      1) Subsequent to spinal cord damage at or below T12–S1
      2) No cortical control
      3) Lack of tone in the internal and external sphincters with frequent oozing of stool, caused by damage to the reflex arc

H. Nursing Assessment of Bowel Function

1. Prior level of function, past bowel habits, usual time of day, frequency of stool, past reliance on laxatives, dietary measures, exercise, or other aids
2. Age and activity level
3. Usual diet and fluid intake pattern
4. Prior history of incontinence, frequent diarrhea, constipation, hemorrhoids, diverticulitis, or bowel surgery
5. Present bowel status and pattern, including time and characteristics of last stool
6. Oozing or small hard stool alternating with watery discharge, which may indicate impaction
7. Abdominal palpation to determine abdominal discomfort or palpable obstruction; rectal exam (with anal wink testing and bulbocavernosis reflex testing)
8. Medications that can affect bowel function (e.g., sedatives, opioids, diuretics, antihistamines)
9. Infection, trauma, or stress that can affect stool formation
10. Malodorous breath, dentition status

11. Problems that can affect selection of interventions
    a. Neuromuscular dysfunction related to current diagnosis
    b. Cardiac conditions, which would preclude the use of digital stimulation or the Valsalva maneuver
    c. Renal impairment, which would preclude the use of milk of magnesia
    d. Mobility restrictions related to current diagnosis
    e. Communication abilities
    f. Sensory and motor status
    g. Current medications and drug allergies
    h. Tube feeding schedule
    i. Cognitive deficits, dementia, psychosis

I. NDs Related to Bowel Impairments (NANDA-I, 2012–2014)
1. Activity intolerance
2. Impaired bed mobility
3. Impaired transfer ability
4. Risk for autonomic dysreflexia
5. Bowel incontinence
6. Perceived risk for constipation
7. Diarrhea
8. Dysfunctional gastrointestinal motility
9. Nausea
10. Imbalanced nutrition, less than body requirements
11. Toileting self-care deficit
12. Self-neglect
13. Anorexia
14. Confusion (acute, chronic)
15. Pain (acute, chronic)
16. Impaired comfort
17. Impaired physical mobility
18. Impaired sensory perception
19. Impaired verbal communication
20. Social isolation
21. Delayed growth and development

J. NIC for Bowel Impairments: It is possible to use existing neural pathways to establish a regular bowel pattern; therefore, interventions for impaired bowel elimination are similar, although clients can have different clinical pictures.
1. Prevention of constipation (adapted from Rehabilitation Nursing Foundation [RNF], 2002 and Mauk, 2012): Rehabilitation nurses need to conduct initial trials to determine the true effectiveness of these standards of practice.
    a. Toileting habits should include a nurse promptly responding to the client's urge to defecate and providing a consistent time for defecation and privacy (LOE 4).
    b. Use an upright position if possible. If the client is unable to sit, a left-side-lying position is recommended (LOE 4). The left-side-lying position is recommended to receive an enema or suppository because this promotes absorption. Right-side lying promotes evacuation of stool. Position the client with knees against the chest to help open the pelvic floor. Abdominal massage right to left may promote evacuation.
    c. Use a toilet or commode with a backrest and side rails for defecation. Avoid use of bedpans (LOE 4).
    d. Provide the client with 20–35 g fiber per day and 2 L fluid per day.
    e. An exercise program should be a component of plans to prevent or treat constipation.
    f. Pharmacological treatment of constipation should be short term. Stool softeners and bulking agents are administered once or twice daily until bowel patterns are reestablished, then only as needed.
2. Neurogenic bowel management (adapted from Consortium for Spinal Cord Medicine, 2010a, and RNF, 2002). Those with neurogenic bowel also need to follow the guidelines for preventing constipation.
    a. Reflexic bowel: Use an appropriate chemical suppository or mechanical rectal stimulant, a consistent personalized schedule (preferably after a meal), and appropriate adaptive equipment (LOE 4).
    b. Areflexic bowel management includes manual evacuation, a consistent personalized schedule, and appropriate adaptive equipment (LOE 4).

K. NOC Related to Bowel Elimination
1. Establishment of a regular bowel regimen with complete emptying of soft stool from the rectum every 1–3 days using as little medication as possible
2. Maintenance of a consistent habit and time
3. No incontinent episodes
4. Absence of complications: Hemorrhoids, abdominal distention, autonomic dysreflexia, or fecal impaction

L. FIM™ Scoring: Rehabilitation nurses must enter scores for bowel function on the FIM™ tool daily (**Table 19-5**).

IV. Sleep and Rest

A. Overview
1. Adequate and restful sleep is essential to maintaining health, strength, endurance, and cognitive functioning.

Table 19-5. Functional Independence Measure (FIM™) Scoring—Bowel
Part I: Level of Assistance
7 = Complete independence—Does not require a helper, medication, or assistive device to maintain a normal stooling pattern.
6 = Modified independence—Requires an assistive device or medication to manage bowel function; is independent in using and maintaining the device or equipment; may use a bedpan, commode, colostomy, ileostomy, suppository, stool softener, or prunes; but client applies, empties, and cleans equipment independently, inserts own suppository and is never incontinent.
5 = Supervision or set-up—Client performs more than 75% of tasks; requires cues, set-up, or supervision from helper; helper hands supplies or a suppository to the client; helper empties the commode or bedpan.
4 = Minimum assistance—Client performs more than 75% of tasks but requires touching assistance, helper disposes of or empties the stool-collection device, client cannot place suppository.
3 = Moderate assistance—Client performs 50%-74% of tasks and requires touching assistance to perform more than one task in bowel management.
2 = Maximum assistance—Client performs 25%-50% of tasks, helper handles most equipment and supplies, client participates in applying or emptying the appliance, but requires touching assistance to do so.
1 = Total assistance—Client performs less than 25% of tasks; is dependent on a helper to apply, maintain, and clean assistive device, empty appliance, and change diaper; helper places suppository, cleans client, changes client clothing and linens after incontinent episodes.
0 = Not a valid score for bowel.
Part 2: Frequency of Accidents
7 = Complete independence—Does not require an assistive device or medication to maintain normal stooling pattern; is never incontinent.
6 = Modified independence—Is never incontinent and uses medication or an assistive device (e.g., elevated toilet, commode, bedpan, colostomy, or ileostomy) but completely manages, maintains, empties, and cleans the appliance or assistive device independently. Client manages medications independently, including stool softeners, suppositories, bowel stimulants, fiber supplements, enemas, or prunes.
5 = 1 accident in the past week and client cleans up independently.
4 = 2 accidents in the past week, cleans up independently.
3 = 3 accidents in the past week, cleans up independently.
2 = 4 accidents in the past week, cleans up independently.
1 = 5 or more accidents in the past week OR helper is required to clean the client, linens, and change the client's clothing following an incontinent episode.
0 = Not a valid score for bowel function.
Admission score includes the events of the past 3 days, enter the lowest score.
Score Part 1, score Part 2, enter the lowest score on the UDS IRF-PAI form.
Functional Independence Measure © Copyright 1997 by Uniform Data System for Medical Rehabilitation (UDSMR), a division of UB Foundation Activities, Inc. All rights reserved. Reprinted with permission of UDSMR.

2. Illness, particularly neurological injury, deep pain, the effects of medications such as sedatives and hypnotics, the comorbidities of aging, and recent intensive care hospitalization all affect sleep patterns.
3. Illness and disability can also contribute to fatigue (Crosby, Munshi, Karat, Worthington, & Lincoln, 2012; Englander, Bushnik, Oggins, & Katznelson, 2010, Gervasoni, Cattaneo, Montesano, & Jonsdotti, 2012; Kluger, Krupp, & Enoka, 2013).
4. The comorbidities of aging and recent intensive care hospitalization further affect sleep patterns.
5. Hospital/institutional environments are known to have higher levels of noise, light, and interruptions that can disturb sleep. Individual perceptions of a loss of control further interfere with sleep (Adachi et al., 2013).
6. Rehabilitation nurses often care for people who have experienced major illnesses and subsequent disruption of normal sleep cycles.
7. To promote healing and endurance, rehabilitation nurses should assess disruptions in clients' sleep, and apply specific interventions to restore restful sleep patterns.
8. There is a great need for nursing research to identify level-1 evidence for effective nursing interventions to promote sleep for clients admitted to rehabilitation facilities.

B. Normal Sleep Patterns (adapted from Porth & Matfin, 2008): Normal sleep patterns are a middle-range theory.
   1. Sleep is part of the sleep-wake cycle. The inactivity that is part of sleep appears to restore mental and physical function. Melatonin, a hormone

produced by the pineal gland, is generally believed to have a role in regulating the sleep-wake cycle.

2. There are two types of sleep: rapid eye movement (REM) sleep and nonREM sleep.
   a. REM sleep is characterized by rapid eye movements, a lack of muscle movement, and vivid dreaming. The person is responding to internal auditory and visual sensory circuits.
   b. NonREM sleep is characterized as quiet sleep, with a fully regulating brain and fully movable but inactive body. NonREM sleep is divided into four stages, each one deeper than the stage before.
      1) Stage 1: Brief transitional stage, occurs at the onset of sleep. The person appears asleep but is easily aroused and if asked later may deny having been asleep.
      2) Stage 2: Deeper sleep, lasts 10–25 minutes. Slowed respiration and heart rate, metabolic rate, and muscle tone continue into stages 3 and 4.
      3) Stages 3 and 4: Deep sleep. Muscles of the body relax, and gastrointestinal activity is slowed.
3. The sleep-wake cycle is integrated into a 24-hour circadian rhythm, controlled by the hypothalamus (hypothalamic suprachiasmatic nuclei) and influenced by melatonin synthesis.

C. Changes in Sleep Patterns Throughout the Life Span (adapted from Porth & Matfin, 2008)
1. In the newborn, REM sleep occurs at sleep onset, and periods of sleep and waking are distributed throughout the day.
2. By 8 months of age, an infant sleeps an average of 13 hours a day, and REM is approximately one third of that time.
3. At 12–15 years of age, sleep is approximately 8 hours a day, and REM is one quarter of that time.
4. Children usually do not complain of sleep disorders; common complaints of parents about their children include irregular sleep habits, too little or too much sleep, nightmares, sleep terrors, sleepwalking, and bedwetting.
5. Sleep changes in aging include circadian rhythm disturbance, fragmented sleep, shorter duration of stages 3 and 4 sleep, reduced REM sleep, and increased likelihood of periodic leg movement in sleep and apnea (Neukrug & Ancoli-Israel, 2010). Older adults are also likely to have health problems and take medications that interfere with sleep. Research is inconclusive regarding older adults requiring less sleep (Bliwise, Ansari, Straight, & Parker, 2005).

D. Disruptions in Sleep Patterns Related to Illness and Disability: Managing the clinical manifestations of these illnesses and disabilities will assist in restoring the sleep-wake cycle.
1. TBI and stroke: Between 30% and 80% of these patients report sleep disruption (Mathias & Alvaro, 2012). Sleep-wake disturbance and initial reversal of day-night cycles are usually temporary. Insomnia; hypersomnia; and excessive daytime sleepiness, narcolepsy, and periodic limb movement in sleep (PLMS) (Castriotta et al., 2007). Sleep-disordered breathing, which can be caused by immobilization, hypoxia, pain, incontinence, and depression (Mauk, 2012)
2. Myasthenia gravis: Sleep apnea caused by skeletal muscle weakness
3. MS, spinal cord injury, and uremia caused by renal disease: Muscle twitching (clonus) or restless legs syndrome (RLS)/PLMS
4. Rheumatoid arthritis: Stiff, aching joints that make comfortable positioning difficult and frequent repositioning necessary. Sleep disturbance can also exacerbate perceived pain (Lee et al., 2013).
5. Cardiac disease: Treatment with diuretics, necessitating nighttime toileting and disruption of sleep
6. Pulmonary disease: Orthopnea, dyspnea, disrupted ability to breathe deeply
7. Increased body mass index: Associated with sleep disturbance (Castriotta et al., 2007; Verma et al., 2007)
8. Morbid obesity: Potentially partially occluded trachea caused by the compressing effect on the neck and jaw from facial and neck fat when supine
9. Permanent lifestyle changes resulting from injury and body image disruption: Depression that causes disruption of adequate restful sleep and affects other family members and caregivers
10. Medications (particularly sedatives, hypnotics, tranquilizers, and antidepressants): Disrupted normal sleep, primarily through depression of delta wave sleep. Barbiturates depress delta and REM sleep, decrease consolidated sleep, and leave the person feeling less rested.
11. Medications that are poorly timed or create the need to urinate can disrupt sleep.

E. Fatigue
1. According to Aaronson and colleagues (1999), fatigue is "the awareness of a decreased capacity for physical and/or mental activity due to an imbalance in the availability, utilization, and/or restoration of resources needed to perform activity" (p. 46).

2. Causes can be physical (e.g., disease or injury) or secondary (e.g., the result of depression, sleep disturbance, anxiety).
3. Measured by
   a. Visual Analogue Scale for Fatigue
   b. Fatigue Severity Scale
   c. Barrow Neurological Institute Fatigue Scale
   d. Global Fatigue Index
   e. Causes of Fatigue Questionnaire
4. Associated with greater motor deficits and potential hormonal changes, especially growth hormone deficiency (Englander et al., 2010)
5. Negatively affects quality of life and employability, and leads to a greater confinement to home

F. NDs Related to Sleep (NANDA-I, 2012–2014)
1. Insomnia
2. Readiness for enhanced sleep
3. Sleep deprivation
4. Disturbed sleep pattern

The following sections on sleep are summarized and adapted from Chasens, Williams, and Umlauf (2011).

G. Interdisciplinary Management of Chronic Primary Insomnia or Excessive Sleepiness
1. Clients in acute rehabilitation settings are likely to have difficulty sleeping because of noise, being awakened during the night for procedures, and a disruption of their usual sleep routines. Young, Bougeois, Hilty, and Hardin (2009) outlined strategies to optimize sleep in the hospital. Sleep restriction-sleep compression therapy and multicomponent cognitive behavioral therapy have been demonstrated to help in older adults. Evidence-based guidelines for promoting sleep of inpatients were not found. This is a key area for rehabilitation nursing research. (Allen, Coon, Uriri-Glover, & Grando, 2013). After the client is discharged home, clinical manifestations of his or her disability or chronic illness can continue to impair sleep. If so, the nursing interventions recommended in section H could be effective if implemented.
2. If nursing interventions do not correct these sleeping problems, the client may need a comprehensive evaluation by sleep medicine specialists, including the following (adapted from Chasens et al., 2011 [LOE 1]):
   a. Sleep history (LOE 1)
   b. Clinical measures to assess excessive sleepiness
      1) Epworth Sleepiness Scale (LOE 2)
      2) Avidan (2005) (LOE 1)
      3) Multivariable Apnea Prediction Index
      4) Functional Outcomes of Sleep Questionnaire
      5) Pittsburgh Sleep Quality Scale
   c. Overnight sleep studies (polysomnography; LOE 1)
   d. Evaluation of the client's knowledge and use of sleep hygiene measures (LOE 1)
   e. Assessment for clinical manifestations of disorders causing excessive sleepiness, including obstructive sleep apnea (OSA), insomnia, RLS, PLMS, and narcolepsy (LOE 1)

H. Interdisciplinary Interventions (LOE 1)
1. Adjust medications that cause drowsiness and sleep impairment.
2. Ensure that positive airway pressure devices are being used appropriately; educate the client and family as needed.
3. Weight loss, regular exercise, and long-term diabetes control (LOE 1)

I. NIC to Promote Sleep in Those with Chronic Insomnia or Excessive Sleepiness (adapted from Chasens et al., 2011; Schutte-Rodin, Broch, Buysse, Dorsey, & Sateia, 2008) (LOE 1)
1. Manage problems that interfere with sleep (see section D).
2. Refer the client to a sleep specialist for OSA and RLS.
3. Help the client implement sleep hygiene measures.

J. Sleep Hygiene Measures (LOE 1) (adapted from Chasens et al., 2011): Sleep hygiene measures are effective only when OSA, RLS, and other sleep disorders have been treated.
1. Use the bed and bedroom only for sleeping and sex.
2. Adopt consistent and rest-promoting bedtime routines, including maintaining the same bedtime and waking time every day.
3. Get out of bed slowly upon awakening.
4. If awakening during the night, avoid looking at the clock, because this heightens anxiety and makes sleep onset more difficult. For those with insomnia, remove clocks from the bedroom.
5. Avoid naps entirely or limit naps to 10–15 minutes.
6. Sleep in a quiet, cool, and dark environment. Sleep with earplugs or a mask if necessary.
7. If unable to fall asleep after 15–20 minutes, get up, go to another room, and read or do a quiet activity using dim lighting until sleepy again. Do not watch television, which emits too much bright light. Low-impact activities, including board games and gentle stretching, have been shown to improve daytime performance and sleep quality.
8. Before bedtime avoid the following:
   a. Tobacco, stimulants, caffeine, or alcohol 4–6 hours before bedtime

b. Large meals or exercise 3–4 hours before bedtime
c. Emotionally charged, upsetting, unpleasant, or stimulating activities right before bedtime

9. If sleeping with pets or another person contributes to sleeping problems, moving to another bed or couch for a few nights or keeping pets from sharing the bed can be helpful.

K. Short-Term Use of Medications to Treat Insomnia in Clients Admitted to Rehabilitation Units
The following recommendations are based on a review of literature for management of insomnia in hospitalized clients by Young and colleagues (2009). Nurses are encouraged to consult this source:
1. Nonpharmacological approaches are the first line of treatment. If they are ineffective, short-term use of the following agents may be effective:
   a. Intermediate-acting benzodiazepines (e.g., estazolam, temazepam) are good first-line agents.
   b. Eszopiclone, zaleplon, zolpidem, and zopoiclone improve sleep outcomes and decrease sleep latency and number of awakenings (Fisher & Valente, 2009).
2. Note that clients taking medications for sleep are at higher risk of falls.

L. Nonpharmacological Nursing Interventions for Clients Admitted to Rehabilitation Units (These are common practices that cannot cause harm; however, the authors have not identified sources that establish the LOE for these interventions.)
1. Use aspects of the client's prior bedtime routines (e.g., unwinding, relaxing activities).
2. Play low music with gentle rhythm patterns (e.g., classical or chamber music).
3. Provide milk or herbal decaffeinated teas and low-sugar snacks.
4. Provide skin care or massage, especially backrubs or lotions.
5. Ensure toileting before lights out.
6. Provide warmth (e.g., light blanket, bath blanket, socks).
7. Use comfort measures (e.g., hand holding, touch therapy, prayer, guided imagery, relaxation).
8. Ensure a quiet environment.
9. Ensure low levels of light, sound, and voices during the night.
10. Provide pain medication if indicated.
11. Use sleep medication only as a last resort, because it produces artificial sleep.
12. Use available waking time, whenever that occurs, to consolidate nursing activities (e.g., repositioning, toileting, skin care, medications, vital signs) in ways that encourage returning to sleep.
13. Maintain an unhurried demeanor that calms the client; keep the lights low and voices hushed unless doing otherwise is absolutely necessary.
14. Express confidence that sleep will come if the client rests calmly.
15. Improve staff knowledge of sleep hygiene techniques (LaRue-Evans, Nesbitt, & Oka, 2013).

M. NIC for Common Sleep-Related Problems
These are common practices that do not cause harm; however, the authors have not identified sources that establish the LOE for these interventions.
1. Nightmares and night terrors: Use low lights to reorient the person, offer reassurance, and reestablish sleep-inducing interventions.
2. Snoring and sleep apnea: Reposition the person to a side-lying position and use pillows to maintain that position.
3. Restlessness and irritability: Provide the person with a quiet, private opportunity to discuss what is troubling him or her, offer comfort and reassurance, and then redirect to sleep.
4. Sleepwalking: Gently guide the person back to bed; it is not necessary to wake the client.
5. Loud talking in sleep: Reposition the client; it is not necessary to wake the client.

N. NOC Related to Sleep Patterns
1. An established pattern that provides high-quality sleep and restoration of energy and comfort
2. Knowledge of effective sleep-enhancing modalities
3. NOC: Sleep

V. Mobility and Immobility

A. Overview (Mauk, 2014)
1. The desire to maximize mobility and independence in ADL through physical and occupational therapy is the key reason clients are admitted for rehabilitation. Nurses have a key role in ensuring that clients are able to participate in therapy and that they follow through with goals on the inpatient unit and at home.
2. Mobility allows clients to care for themselves, to interact with the environment, and to carry out purposeful activities.
3. Balance, strength, and endurance are all components of mobility.
4. Mobility can be lost suddenly through disease or trauma or more gradually through inactivity or illness.
5. Prolonged immobility produces marked diminution of all body functions and places clients in a

life-threatening situation. Adverse effects of immobility include decreased cardiac output; orthostatic hypotension and inability to sit or stand; dehydration; and increased risk of deep vein thrombosis, pneumonia, renal calculi, pressure ulcers, sensory deprivation, and impaired thought processes (Porth & Matfin, 2008).

6. Strength, flexibility, and endurance decline with aging. Strength training activities can help prevent progressive functional limitations and maintain flexibility to prevent falls and subsequent injuries (Seco et al., 2013).
7. Rehabilitation nurses identify problems of impaired mobility; set realistic goals; and collaborate with clients, families, and therapy team members to achieve these goals.
8. People aging with chronic diseases can be limited in their ability to maintain mobility (Seco et al., 2013). Cultural and ethnic diversities play a role in attitudes toward physical activity, diet, weight, and disease-management behaviors. Sensitivity to these considerations is important when working with clients and their support systems (Gallant, Spitze, & Grove, 2010).

B. Nursing Assessment for Mobility (See Chapter 12 for more information on equipment.)

1. Assessment of functional mobility traditionally includes four major areas.
   a. Bed mobility
   b. Transfers, including toilet transfers
   c. Wheelchair mobility
   d. Ambulation
2. All interdisciplinary team members evaluate levels of assistance by using rankings and descriptive tools that are reliable and valid. These tools identify the amount of help or supervision needed or a device the person needs to perform a specific activity safely, over the required distance, and in a timely fashion. The FIM™ instrument, for use with adults, and the WeeFIM™, for pediatric populations, are the most common instruments used in rehabilitation facilities. To subscribe to the Uniform Data System for Medical Rehabilitation (UDSMR), FIM™ System, or WeeFIM™ system and for the most current versions of the FIM™ and WeeFIM™, instructions in their use, and other related topics, go to www.udsmr.org.
   a. The FIM™ instrument (Uniform Data System for Medical Rehabilitation [UDSMR], 1997a) is scored as follows for 18 domains (e.g., eating; grooming; dressing, upper; dressing, lower; bathing):
      1) 7 = Independent
      2) 6 = Modified independence (device)
      3) 5 = Supervision or setup
      4) 4 = Minimal assistance (patient is able to do 75% or more of task)
      5) 3 = Moderate assistance (patient is able to do 50%–74% of task)
      6) 2 = Maximal assistance (patient is able to do 25%–49% of task)
      7) 1 = Total assistance (patient is able to do less than 25% of task)
   b. The FIM™ is required in acute rehabilitation facilities by prospective payment systems.
   c. WeeFIM™ (UDSMR, 1997b): The FIM™ instrument, adapted for pediatric populations, is scored as follows for three domains (16 motor, 14 cognitive, 6 behavioral):
      1) 0 = Never
      2) 1 = Rarely
      3) 2 = Sometimes
      4) 3 = Usually
   d. Other functional scales (e.g., Barthel, Katz, NANDA) are available.
   e. The Continuity Assessment Record and Evaluation tool has been demonstrated to be a valid and reliable tool to measure individual function from acute care to postacute care sites (U.S. Department of Health & Centers for Medicare and Medicaid Services, 2012).
3. Nurses assess the components of mobility.
   a. Range of motion (ROM): Evaluate the range of unassisted active motion of both sides (**Figure 19-5**) and distinguish between active, assisted, and passive ROM. Rehabilitation nurses who use these ROM terms will be better able to communicate with physical therapists, occupational therapists, and physiatrists when discussing the client's mobility goals.
   b. Balance: Sitting, standing, moving, amount of assistance needed, and distance involved
   c. Bed mobility: Ability to turn side to side, move up in bed, move to the side of the bed, sit up in the bed, and bridge (i.e., raise hips while in the supine position)
   d. Transfer ability: Ability to move between wheelchair and bed, toilet, bath bench or shower chair, standard seating (or automobile)
   e. Wheelchair mobility
   f. Ambulation
   g. Neuromuscular problems (e.g., spasticity, rigidity, resting tremors, intention tremors, flaccidity)
   h. Coordination and proprioception
   i. Ability to follow and remember instructions

Figure 19-5. Range of Motion

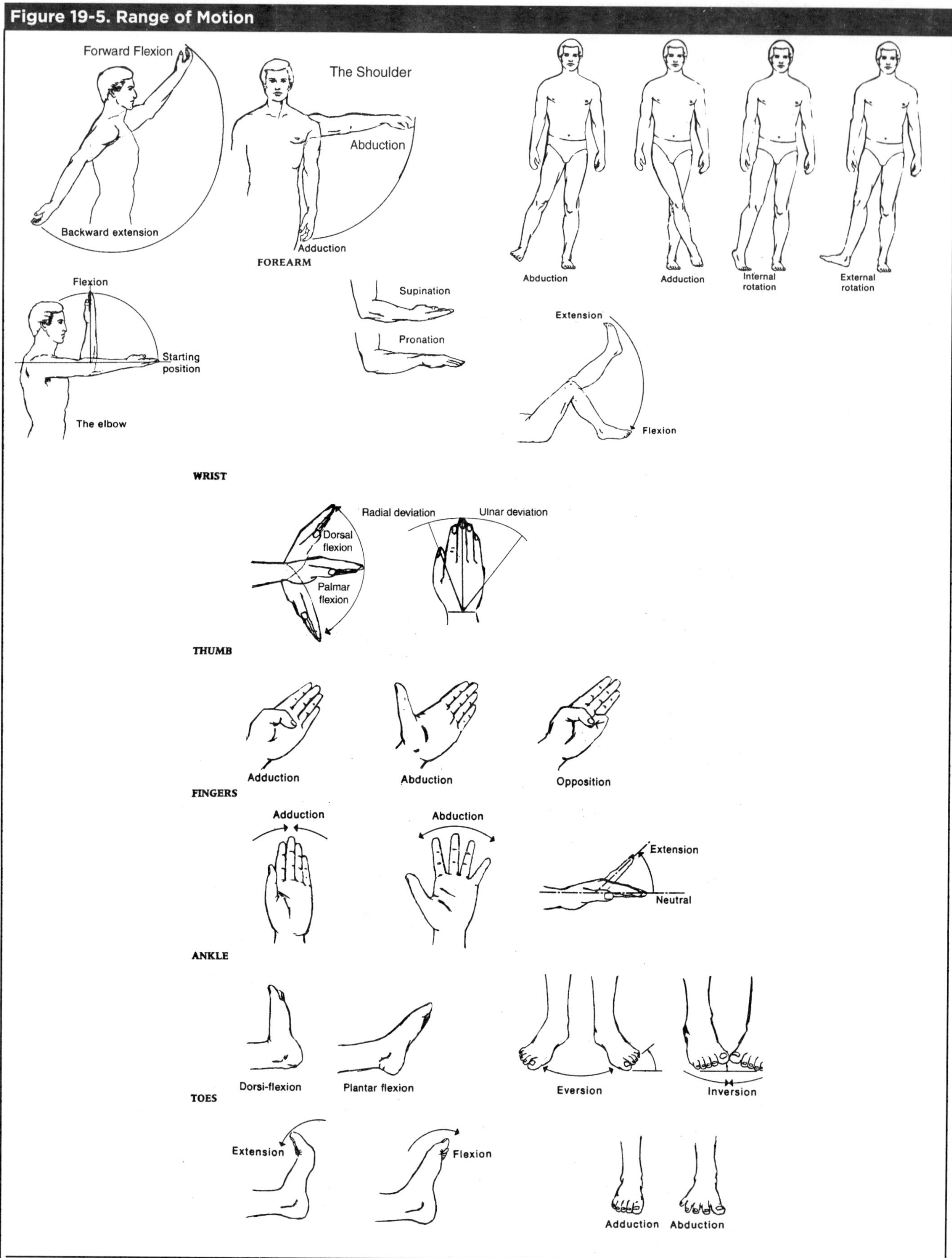

From *Lippincott manual of nursing practice* (8th ed.), by S. M. Nettina, 2006, Philadelphia: Lippincott Williams & Wilkins. Copyright 2006 by Lippincott Williams & Wilkins. Reprinted with permission.

j. Client's expectations and past level of mobility, both recent and remote
k. Age-appropriate growth and development and behaviors
l. Comorbidities and general endurance

C. Expected Patient Outcomes Related to Impaired mobility
1. Attain optimal functional mobility using the simplest level of assistance possible.
2. Demonstrate the safe use of any needed device.

D. Injury Prevention: Nurses are at risk for injury when transferring clients, assisting clients with ADL, and helping clients ambulate (Meyeda-Letourneau, 2014).

E. Nursing Interventions (at the time of publication no guidelines were available to determine LOEs for the following interventions; rehabilitation nurses need to develop evidence-based practice guidelines for all these interventions):
1. For bed mobility
   a. Provide adequate changes in position and encourage the client's active participation.
   b. Use assistive devices (e.g., side rails, trapeze, overhead frame).
2. For transfers
   a. Provide the amount of assistance needed using a consistent approach and verbal cues.
   b. Use assistive devices (e.g., slide board, sit-to-stand lift, total or mechanical lift).
   c. Make adaptations for impaired transfer mobility.
      1) For impaired weight-bearing mobility of one side of the body (e.g., hemiplegia, total hip precautions, fractures of the leg, unilateral leg amputation): The client's physical therapist may make recommendations other than the following for helping clients transfer. Follow the therapist's recommendations.
         a) The nurse places the wheelchair on the client's strong or unaffected side (the nearest armrest may need to be removed if the client is unable to come to a standing position), locks the brakes, and moves foot pedals out of the way.
         b) The client comes to a standing position and places the strong or unaffected foot forward toward the chair.
         c) The client places his or her unaffected arm on the armrest of the opposite side of the chair.
         d) The client rotates his or her body on the ball of the unaffected foot so the body is square to the chair.
         e) The client lowers himself or herself into the chair.
         f) When another person helps the client, the nurse explains the planned moves and encourages the client to take sufficient time to complete each move and maintain as much weight over his or her own feet as possible. The helper should stand in front of the client and use his or her own knees to control the client's descent into the chair seat while keeping one foot in front of the client's feet to guard against slipping.
      2) For impaired weight-bearing mobility of both legs (e.g., paraplegia, bilateral amputation)
         a) The nurse places the wheelchair perpendicular to the middle of the bed in the locked position.
         b) The client raises himself or herself to sit on the bed with legs and back to the chair.
         c) The client lifts his or her trunk by pushing down on the mattress and hitching the trunk backward.
         d) The client grasps the arms of the wheelchair and lifts himself or herself into the chair.
      3) For impaired weight-bearing mobility due to poor balance or low strength (using a slide board)
         a) The nurse places the wheelchair next to the bed in the locked position and removes the armrest nearest to the bed.
         b) The client comes to a sitting position at the side of the bed.
         c) The nurse places one end of the slide board just under the client's buttocks and the other end on the chair.
         d) The client hitches himself or herself toward the chair along the board by pushing down with the arms and raising the trunk, or by pulling on the armrest of the wheelchair. The legs and feet follow.
         e) Once in the chair, the client tilts away from the bed so the slide board can be removed.
      4) For impaired weight-bearing mobility due to poor balance or low strength (e.g., sliding board, sit-to-stand lift, or total or mechanical lift)

a) The nurse positions slings under the client either in one piece or under the arms and the thighs.
b) The nurse positions the lift over the client and lowers it so the crossbar is accessible.
c) The nurse uses the chains to attach the slings to the crossbar, ensuring that there is equal length on each side and that the hooks are facing away from the client.
d) With a second person available to guide the legs and torso, the nurse pumps up the lift until the client's body clears the bed.
e) The nurse slowly moves the lift away from the bed and over the wheelchair, which is in the locked position.
f) The nurse slowly releases the lift, allowing the client to descend into the wheelchair.
g) The nurse removes the chains and may leave the slings in place for ease in returning the client to bed.

3. For impaired ability to ambulate
   a. Requirements for ambulation: Balance, strength, endurance, and ability to navigate various walking surfaces (e.g., floor, carpet, stairs, grass, pavement, uneven surfaces, hills)
   b. Components of a normal gait: Erect balance, foot lift, push off with alternate foot, heel strike, ride-over, and heel strike of opposite foot; contralateral arms may swing to provide stability and balance
   c. Protective assistance (e.g., gait belt, hands-on supervision, verbal cues)
   d. Quadriceps strengthening exercises for knee and hip strength (e.g., isometric tightening of the knee and gluteus muscles, holding the contraction for 3–5 seconds and then relaxing; repeated in sets of 5–10 and increasing in frequency as strength returns), bicep and tricep exercises for crutch weight bearing
4. Advances in improving functional mobility to aide in ADLs
   a. Use of robotic technology to promote walking in patients with stroke and spinal cord injury (Tefertiller, Pharo, Evans, & Winchester, 2011)
   b. Treadmill training can promote improvements in gait patterns for some patients with Parkinson's disease and patients poststroke (Earhart & Williams, 2012; Tyrell, Roos, Rudolph, & Reisman, 2011).
   c. Functional electrical stimulation to restore or preserve function in patients, improve truncal stability, and improve bone and muscle health after spinal cord injury (Gater, Dolbow, Tsui, & Gorgey, 2011).
5. For all clients
   a. Encourage functioning at a maximally safe independent level.
   b. Use verbal cues, reinforce learning, provide sufficient rest periods, and encourage adequate nutrition.

VI. Disuse

A. Review

1. Skeletal muscle atrophy can occur after prolonged bed rest or as a result of medications, injury, starvation, extremity immobilization, and aging. Although they are often poorly defined, several mechanisms contribute to muscle atrophy, including mitochondrial-mediated apoptosis and iron accumulation (Marzetti et al., 2011).
2. Immobility also causes muscle fibers to break down due to reduced muscle protein synthesis and breakdown (Marimuthu, Murton, & Greenhaff, 2011; Powers, Wiggs, Duarte, Zergeroglu, & Demirel, 2012).
   a. A manual muscle test can be conducted by a physical therapist to determine the strength of muscle groups. Muscle strength is graded on a 0-to-5 scale. Grade 5 is normal strength and grade 0 is no movement (Mauk, 2014). A copy of the Muscle Strength Grading Scale can be found at http://nursing.advanceweb.com/SharedResources/Downloads/2002/070102/NP/npp24table5.pdf.
3. Immobility affects all body systems, not just limbs affected by disease.
   a. Decreased cardiac output
   b. Orthostatic intolerance
   c. Dehydration
   d. Thrombophlebitis
   e. Muscle atrophy from disuse, especially in quadriceps
   f. Bone demineralization from decreased stress on bones
   g. Pneumonia from lowered tidal volume and decreased ability to clear bronchial secretions
   h. Formation of renal calculi, urinary retention, and urinary reflux
   i. Skin breakdown and the development of pressure ulcers from compromised circulation and pressure
   j. Bowel constipation from lowered peristalsis and inactivity

k. Sensory deprivation
l. Impaired thought processes, feelings of isolation, and depression
4. Expected client outcomes related to actual or potential hazards of immobility
a. Prevention of as many of the sequelae of immobility as possible
b. Early identification of impairments related to disuse
c. Self-advocacy regarding the need to include preventive measures in daily self-care
5. Nursing interventions to prevent or limit the effects of disuse
a. Provide frequent turning and skin care to relieve pressure and restore circulation.
b. Use pressure redistribution surfaces (e.g., air mattresses, seat cushions).
c. Pay careful attention to skin to ensure early recognition of reddened areas, wash skin gently with neutral pH soap, use lotions to lubricate skin and protect from moisture.
d. Pay attention to episodes of incontinence; provide frequent checks, thorough cleaning, and protective barrier creams; and adjust bowel and bladder training regimens.
e. Encourage adequate fluid intake by mouth, by gastrostomy tube, or intravenously; monitor regularly for symptoms of dehydration.
f. Establish an effective bowel program without creating long-term dependence on laxatives, cathartics, or enemas.
g. Monitor lung sounds and encourage frequent deep breathing and coughing to move and clear bronchial secretions.
h. Provide regular gentle exercise such as ROM exercises (e.g., quadriceps-setting exercises).
i. Ensure early identification of venous thrombus (e.g., fever, pain).
j. Implement strategies for postural hypotension (e.g., quadriceps-setting exercises, elastic stockings, sitting before standing).
k. Use weight-bearing exercises to encourage retention of calcium in bones (e.g., stand aid, supported transfers).
l. Use recreational and diversional therapy to stimulate social interaction.

VII. Self-Care and Activities of Daily Living

A. Overview (Mauk, 2014)
1. The functional pattern of activity and exercise includes the basic elements of self-care (e.g., feeding, toileting).
a. ADLs include eating, bathing, dressing, and grooming.
b. Instrumental activities of daily living (IADLs), or more complex aspects of independence: includes meal preparation, household management, finances, transportation, and outdoor and community-based activities
2. Payer sources play a major role in determining the extent of services provided and the setting in which these services are provided.
3. Rehabilitation nurses are the link between therapies, expected outcomes, and the realities of returning to community living.
4. Self-care is an important component of promoting health, preventing disease, and seeking health-screening opportunities. It is an essential component for individuals aging with chronic illnesses. Self-care is essential to overall health (Lubkin & Larsen, 2009).
5. Maintaining self-care support for children and young people to maintain their independence, provide a sense of community, and promote confidence throughout their lives (Kirk, Beatty, Callery, Milnes, & Pryjmachuk, 2012).

B. Nursing Assessment of Self-Care Ability
1. Assess ability to independently perform basic ADLs (e.g., bathing, dressing, grooming, and eating); IADLs (e.g., meal preparation, shopping, and housework) and social activities, and determine the assistance needed to accomplish these tasks.
2. Use rating scales to measure the level of independence or burden of care.
a. FIM™ and WeeFIM™ systems.
b. NANDA-I (2012–2014) scores for self-care and mobility: 0 = fully independent, 4 = dependent and unable (note that scoring is the opposite of FIM™ scoring).
c. Mini-mental state exam: A short test of cognitive functions including orientation, registration, recall, calculation, language, and visual constructs
3. Assess specific motor impairments.
a. Spasticity; paralysis; flaccidity; tremors (e.g., constant, resting, intention); rigidity; contractures
b. Energy, endurance, strength, and safety
c. Balance while sitting and standing and the ability to self-correct alone or if pushed gently
4. Assess specific sensory impairments.
a. Visual field and acuity: Diminished or lost visual field and acuity, hemianopia, peripheral field loss, macular degeneration, use of corrective lenses

b. Tactile loss: Paresthesia, proprioception, temperature discrimination (needed for bathing and meal preparation)
c. Hearing: Diminished or lost hearing, use of hearing aids
5. Assess cognitive ability, which can affect the ability to perform ADLs.
6. Assess level of pain, which can interfere with learning and create additional body splinting.
a. Assess location, intensity, and possible causes of pain.
b. Treat pain before planned therapy.

C. Expected Client Outcomes Related to Impaired Self-Care Ability
1. Complete basic self-care activities as safely and independently as possible, with or without devices as appropriate.
2. Demonstrate the ability to use and care for assistive devices if appropriate.
3. Perform IADLs as independently as possible.
4. Demonstrate the ability to direct self-care when unable to perform independently.

D. Nursing Interventions for Impaired Self-Care Ability
1. Use general teaching strategies.
a. Use the client's preferred method of learning as much as possible.
b. Begin with simple tasks that are familiar and meaningful to the client.
c. Repeat sequential tasks consistently.
d. Use demonstration, hand-over-hand, verbal, and written instruction.
e. Select the time of day at which the client's attention span and energy are highest.
f. Collaborate in teaching with other disciplines so the client receives consistent, reinforcing instruction.
2. Use available devices for specific losses.
a. Feeding: Plate guards, rocker knives, hand braces for utensils, nonskid place mats for stability, drinking cups with weighted bases and wide mouths
b. Bathing and hygiene: Face cloths, mitts, soap-on-a-rope, long-handled sponges, nailbrushes with suction cups, hand braces for toothbrush, freestanding mirrors, shower mats, grab bars, shower seats
c. Dressing: Long-handled shoehorns, reachers, Velcro® closures for clothes, elastic shoelaces, devices that help to don socks
d. Grooming: Long-handled combs, adapted holders for razors, long-handled mirrors for skin inspection
e. Toileting: Raised toilet seats, transfer bars
3. Adapt care to manage impaired energy and endurance.
a. Teach pacing techniques.
b. Provide work simplification strategies.
c. Ensure changes in the workplace environment to accommodate height and sitting needs.
d. Recruit assistance for the client.
e. Gradually increase tasks when the client's skills and strength begin to return.
4. Provide strategies for household management and use of community resources.

VIII. Sexuality and Reproduction

People with disability or chronic illness are unique and their expressions of sexuality vary greatly. Healthcare professionals often avoid discussing sexual concerns with clients because of fear, embarrassment, or lack of knowledge (Mauk, 2014). Addressing sexuality and relationships with people with disabilities in the context of their gender roles, identities, and expressions of sexuality are important for rehabilitation nurses (Higgins, 2010, Moreno, Lasprilla, Gan, & McKerral, M. 2013).

A. Overview
1. Sexuality and reproduction are important issues for rehabilitation clients.
2. Disability and major illnesses affect sexual function, self-esteem, body image, and social relationships. It is likely that all clients with new disabilities will have sexual changes. Some will want information on coping with these changes; others will not care. However, it is best to ask all clients whether they have questions.
3. Rehabilitation nurses play a major role in educating clients about the effects of injury or illness on sexual function and reproduction.
4. To promote an atmosphere of permission and acceptance when discussing sexuality, rehabilitation nurses should keep their own values and attitudes separate to address the issue objectively.
5. Rehabilitation nurses should know about available methods and aids to enhance sexual expression and conception after disability. A key intervention is to provide clients and their partners with educational materials. To find information for clients and their partners on specific chronic illnesses or disabilities, use a search engine and type in "sex and arthritis" or "sex and head injury," for example. For more information on sex after stroke, see Kautz (2007) and the resources listed in **Table 19-6**.

B. Kaplan's (1990) Stages and Descriptions of Human Sexual Response Cycle: common problems, changes with aging, and recommendations (**Table 19-7**)

Table 19-6. Sex Education Resources for Clients and Their Partners

The Web addresses and publications listed in this table were active and available at the time of publication; however, titles of publications and Web addresses often change.

Resources for Information and Comfortable Positions for Intercourse	Sex Education Websites
Being Close: COPD and Intimacy: http://lungline.njc.org Chronic Low Back Pain and How It May Affect Sexuality: http://ukhealthcare.uky.edu/patiented/booklets.htm Sex and Arthritis: www.orthop.washington.edu Sex After Stroke: Our Guide to Intimacy After Stroke: www.strokeassociation.org Sex and Cancer (several Web articles by the American Cancer Society): www.cancer.org Intimacy and Diabetes: www.netdoctor.co.uk Diabetes and Men's Sexual Health and Diabetes and Women's Sexual Health: www.diabetes.org	The following are professional websites that are highly recommended for those with chronic illness and disabilities. These are legitimate sex education websites, not pornography sites. • www.womenshealth.org • www.erectile-dysfunction-impotence.org • http://marriage.about.com • www.4woman.gov (sexuality and disability for women)

Table 19-7. Stages of Human Sexual Response and Common Sexual Problems

Building on early work by Masters and Johnson, Kaplan (1990) identified a triphasic model of human sexual response. The three phases are desire, excitement, and orgasm. Kaplan's model is more useful to the rehabilitation nurse than Masters and Johnson's because it helps the nurse understand why neurological impairment leads to sexual problems. Most sexual problems can be classified as desire, excitement, or orgasm phase disorders, or combinations of the three. For decades, changes in sexual response have been considered normal consequences of aging.

Phase and Physiological Response	Neurological Control	Common Problems in All Adults	Changes with Aging
The desire phase includes the sensations that move one to seek sexual pleasures. Love is a powerful stimulus to sexual desire.	Sexual desire is probably stimulated by endorphins, and the pleasure centers in the brain are stimulated by sex; pain inhibits sexual desire.	Fatigue from work, family, and home responsibilities often interferes with desire.	Desire may or may not change with aging; levels of desire may remain the same throughout life.
The excitement phase consists primarily of myotonia, or increased muscle tone and vasodilation of the genital blood vessels. In men the penis becomes erect. In women the vagina becomes lubricated, the clitoris and vagina become longer and wider, and the labia minora extend outward.	Sexual excitement is controlled by the sympathetic nervous system; fear inhibits sexual excitement.	Occasional difficulty in achieving an erection or vaginal lubrication occurs in most adults throughout the lifespan.	Erections may require more direct stimulation and may be softer. Vaginal lubrication may be decreased and require more direct stimulation.
The orgasm phase is a climatic release of the genital vasodilation and myotonia of the excitement phase.	Orgasm is an automatic spinal reflex response.	Premature ejaculation is common in men. Anorgasmia is common in women.	Ejaculation may not be as forceful. Women's orgasms may feel different.

C. Normal Physiology of Sexual Response

1. Men
   a. The penis is innervated by sympathetic (T10–L2), parasympathetic (S2–S4), and somatic (pudendal nerve) fibers.
   b. Erection is under parasympathetic, sympathetic, and somatic control.
   c. Psychogenic response is initiated by cortical input, including visual and tactile senses, and mediated by sympathetic pathways (T10–L2).
   d. Reflex is initiated by internal or external tactile stimulation and mediated by the sacral spinal reflex (S2–S4).
   e. Emission is under sympathetic control (T10–L2), and ejaculation is under sympathetic and somatic control (S2–S4).
   f. Fertility depends on endocrine regulation, ejaculatory ability, and semen quality.

2. Women
    a. Genitalia are innervated by sympathetic (pudendal and perineal) and parasympathetic (splanchnic) nerve fibers.
    b. Orgasm is thought to be under parasympathetic (S2–S4) and somatic control.
    c. Fertility depends on endocrine regulation of ovulation cycles.

D. NOC Related to Sexual Function
1. Personal satisfaction with sexual function
2. Avoidance of sexually transmitted diseases
3. Pregnancy, if desired and possible; avoidance of pregnancy if not desired
4. Ability to plan and carry out parenting roles if appropriate

E. PLISSIT Model for Sexual Counseling (Annon, 1976)
1. *Permission*: Process of allowing questions or fears to be raised and giving permission to talk about the subject
2. *Limited information*: Providing some specific information related to questions raised or concerns expressed and allowing the person to pursue the issue further if he or she is comfortable
3. *Specific suggestions*: Assisting people with problem identification, providing specific suggestions to resolve a problem (e.g., suggestions to deal with erectile dysfunction, bowel and bladder concerns, positioning, contraception). Ginsberg (2010) provided additional information on erectile dysfunction.
4. *Intensive therapy*: Providing expert assistance for intensive discussion and interventions (e.g., psychotherapy for marriage and relationship counseling, medical management of impotence, infertility, childbirth)

F. Common Classes of Medications and Their Effects on Sexual Functioning (**Table 19-8**)

G. Functional Problems and Their Potential Effects on Sexual Relationships (**Table 19-9**)

H. Sex and Intimacy Problems with Chronic Illnesses and Disability (**Table 19-10**)

I. Comfortable Intercourse Positions for Those with Chronic Illness or Disability: Finding a comfortable position for sex can be very difficult for those who have chronic obstructive pulmonary disease or back, hip, or knee pain, or who are hemiparetic after a head injury or stroke (**Figure 19-6**).

J. Additional Issues Surrounding Reproduction
1. Contraception: The method should be based on the client's physical ability, cognitive ability to comply, potential medical risks of oral contraceptive use, and personal preferences. An excellent source for information on contraception and chronic illness is Greydanus and Matytsina (2010).
2. Pregnancy, childbirth, and parenting: Options vary according to the disability, available resources, and medical issues.
3. Fertility
    a. Causes of infertility in men: Erectile dysfunction, anejaculation, poor semen quality, and altered endocrine function are a result of spinal cord injury and other chronic diseases. Fertility can also be affected. The Male Fertility Research Program of the Miami Project to Cure Paralysis provides resources in the field of male infertility after spinal injury (Brackett, Ibrahim, & Lynne, 2011; Kautz, 2010).
    b. For men with spinal cord injury, see the Consortium for Spinal Cord Medicine's *Sexuality and Reproductive Health in Adults with Spinal Cord Injury* (2010b).

K. Safety Issues Related to Sexuality
1. Sexually transmitted diseases
    a. Syphilis, gonorrhea
    b. AIDS
    c. Hepatitis
    d. Herpes
2. Sexual abuse

L. Age-Specific Iissues
1. Pediatric: Injury and congenital disorders
2. Adolescence: Concerns about acceptance, roles, and relationships. The American Academy of Pediatrics Committee on Adolescence (2013) published a position statement that addresses the needs of youths dealing with lesbian, gay, bisexual, and transgender issues. These youths require comprehensive, confidential, and developmentally appropriate assessment for sexual risk factors that could require monitoring or intervention.
3. Adults: Concerns about fertility, biological parenthood, pregnancy, and parenting Older adults: Consideration of the normal effects of aging and their relationship to disability or availability of a partner. It is the responsibility of the healthcare team to respond appropriately to the expression of sexuality in older adults in all settings, including long-term care (Othman & Engkasan, 2011).

Table 19-8. Medications and Sexual Functioning
The following groups of medications have been shown to contribute to sexual dysfunction by decreasing sexual desire in men and women, promoting vaginal dryness in women or erectile dysfunction in men, or delaying or preventing orgasm in men or women. These sexual side effects may lessen 6–8 weeks after the medication is started. If the sexual dysfunction persists, a general recommendation for those experiencing sexual dysfunction is to contact the healthcare provider who prescribed the medication and ask whether a different medication from the same class or another class can be prescribed. Sometimes, despite changing medications, the side effects persist and the person taking the medication will need to seek treatment for the sexual dysfunction (Bostwick, 2010; Ginsberg, 2010; Krychman & Kellogg-Spadt, 2009; Mintzer, 2010).
Antidepressants, including tricyclics, monoamine oxidase inhibitors, and selective serotonin reuptake inhibitors, can decrease sexual desire in women and delay or prevent orgasm in both men and women.
Antihypertensives, especially thiazide diuretics and beta blockers. Centrally acting alpha receptor blockers and peripherally acting antiadrenergics may also cause problems.
Anticholinergics: Probanthine and atropine.
Anticonvulsants: Phenytoin, phenobarbital, carbamazepine.
Histamine 2 blocking agents: Cimetidine, ranitidine
Lipid-lowering agents: Niacin, clofibrate
Digoxin
Opioids

Table 19-9. Functional Problems and Their Potential Effects on Sexual Relationships

Functional Problem	Potential Effect	Suggestion
Sensory/Perception		
Vision	Decreased ability to appreciate visual stimuli, difficulties with depth perception	If unilateral, uninjured partner should lie on unaffected side; use other senses (e.g., verbal, touch)
Sensation	Increased sensitivity or decreased or absent tactile sensation	Define areas of tactile loss, modify stimuli to that part, modify touch to areas of hypersensitivity
Proprioception (position sense)	Injured partner may not know where body parts are without visualizing, making sexual play clumsy or uncomfortable	Allow enough light for visualization; use positioning supports for comfort
Right-left discrimination	Injured partner may not be able to follow through with directions from partner	Direct injured partner by using terms other than right or left; use hand-over-hand guidance
Neglect or denial of deficits	Injured partner may have difficulty recognizing limitation and overstate abilities; may cause embarrassment for both partners if overstated abilities are acted out	Uninjured partner take more active role and gently redirects partner; use positioning with pillows; alternate positions
Communication		
Aphasia or dysarthria	Injured partner may have difficulty correctly interpreting affect of partner or expressing own desires	Use nonverbal communication (touching, gestures).
Concrete thinking	Injured partner may miss subtle cues; sexual play may be concretely focused and one sided	Uninjured partner may need to be very direct with sexual communication and give more specific directions to focus on mutual pleasure
Disinhibition or impulse control	Injured partner may make inappropriate or offending statement to partner; may increase number of sexual partners as a result of impulse control; may show inappropriate public display of sexual impulses or activity	Uninjured partner should give feedback to partner about responses and provide suggestions for better alternatives; enforce privacy and a consistent routine; do not reinforce inappropriate behaviors; may need to implement social skill retraining in matters related to sexual behaviors with the opposite sex

continued

Table 19-9. Functional Problems and Their Potential Effects on Sexual Relationships (continued)		
Functional Problem	**Potential Effect**	**Suggestion**
Cognition		
Attention or concentration	Injured partner may be restless, unable to focus on sexual play; may affect ability to sustain an erection	Decrease external distractions during sexual play; use relaxation, imagery, or guided fantasy by uninjured partner
Memory or judgment	If short-term memory is impaired, injured partner may persevere on a sexual activity or request or pressure partner for frequent sex; contraceptive use should not rely on memory of injured partner	Log sexual activity; discuss contraceptive options with physician; uninjured partner may need to take responsibility for contraception
Initiative	Injured partner may lack ability to take active role in creating a supportive environment	Uninjured partner may need to initiate, provide romantic environment, encourage
Mobility Impairment		
Paralysis	Inability to move body or a body part to position self or to respond to moves by the uninjured partner	Use pillows, alternate positioning strategies; uninjured partner may need to take more active role
Spasticity	Involuntary muscle contractions of affected parts of body; may interfere with attempts to position or reposition	Use positions that place less stress on muscles that tend to spasm; select positions so that if spasms occur, they will not disrupt activity; use reminders to tend to bowel and bladder needs before initiating foreplay; be aware that pain in another part of the body may set off spasms; pay attention to positioning
Elimination		
Bladder dysfunction	Bladder accidents decrease the appeal of sexual activity; presence of Foley catheter may hinder sexual activity; presence of urostomy may hinder sexual enjoyment	Restrict fluids before sexual activity; complete toileting; keep towel or urinal nearby for potential accidents; if Foley catheter present, can be taped to the side (for women to the thigh, for men to the abdomen or place a condom over the shaft of penis); avoid positions that place pressure on the bladder; cover urostomy or tape to abdomen
Bowel dysfunction	Bowel accidents decrease the appeal of sexual activity; presence of colostomy or ileostomy may hinder sexual activity	Complete bowel regime before sexual activity; avoid positions that place pressure on the bowels; cover ostomy, tape to the side or remove and use an ostomy cap over stoma
Erectile Dysfunction or Anorgasm		
Man is unable to establish or maintain an erection	Decreased ability for penile-vaginal intercourse	Explore alternative forms of sexual satisfaction, stuffing method, exploration of erogenous zones; seek psychological counseling; get referrals for erectile dysfunction assessment; use impotence treatments and medications (e.g., topical, intraurethral, oral, injectable); use external vacuum therapy; use penile implants (e.g., semirigid, inflatable).
Woman is unable to achieve orgasm	Decreased ability to reach climax	Explore alternative forms of sexual satisfaction; seek psychological counseling; educate about potential to have orgasm; encourage use of clitoral stimulation.

Data from Rehabilitation Nursing Foundation, 1995; Sipski & Alexander, 1998.

Table 19-10. Sex and Intimacy Problems with Chronic Illnesses

Chronic Illness	Common Changes in Sex and Intimacy	Recommendations for Overcoming the Problems
Heart disease Hypertension Peripheral vascular disease	Atherosclerosis and some medications may lead to erectile dysfunction in men and vaginal dryness (dyspareunia) in women. Both men and women may have fear of chest pain during sex. Fatigue may interfere with desire and lead to sexual dysfunction.	Smoking cessation, weight loss, and a consistent exercise program may increase genital circulation and reverse sexual dysfunction. Encourage couples to walk together to increase intimacy and endurance. If medications are leading to vaginal dryness or erectile dysfunction, ask the physician to switch to a different medication in the same drug class.
Diabetes	Peripheral and autonomic neuropathy cause decreased genital sensation, erectile dysfunction, and vaginal dryness. Gastroparesis leads to flatulence. Ketosis leads to bad breath. Fatigue may lead to sexual dysfunction.	Smoking cessation, weight loss, and exercise all may assist in overcoming problems. Keeping the hemoglobin A1c below 7 may reverse clinical manifestations of neuropathy, atherosclerosis, gastroparesis, and ketosis. Explain that clinical manifestations vary over time.
Chronic lung disease	Loss of stamina, fatigue, and chronic cough all may lead to decreased desire and sexual dysfunction. Chronic cough often leads to stress incontinence in older women.	Smoking cessation, weight loss, and exercise all may improve breathing, reduce fatigue, and increase desire and sexual function. Adopt positions that prevent shortness of breath (see Figure 19-6). Wear oxygen cannula during sexual activity.
Arthritis (degenerative joint disease, rheumatoid arthritis, gout)	Impaired mobility and joint pain may limit sexual activity. Chronic pain will decrease sexual desire.	Plan for sex at a time of day when pain is less, often mid morning when pain medications are at peak effect. Adopt sexual positions that don't cause pain (see Figure 19-6). Plan time for intimacy to combat feelings of worthlessness and depression.

Figure 19-6. Comfortable Intercourse Positions for Those with Chronic Illness or Disability

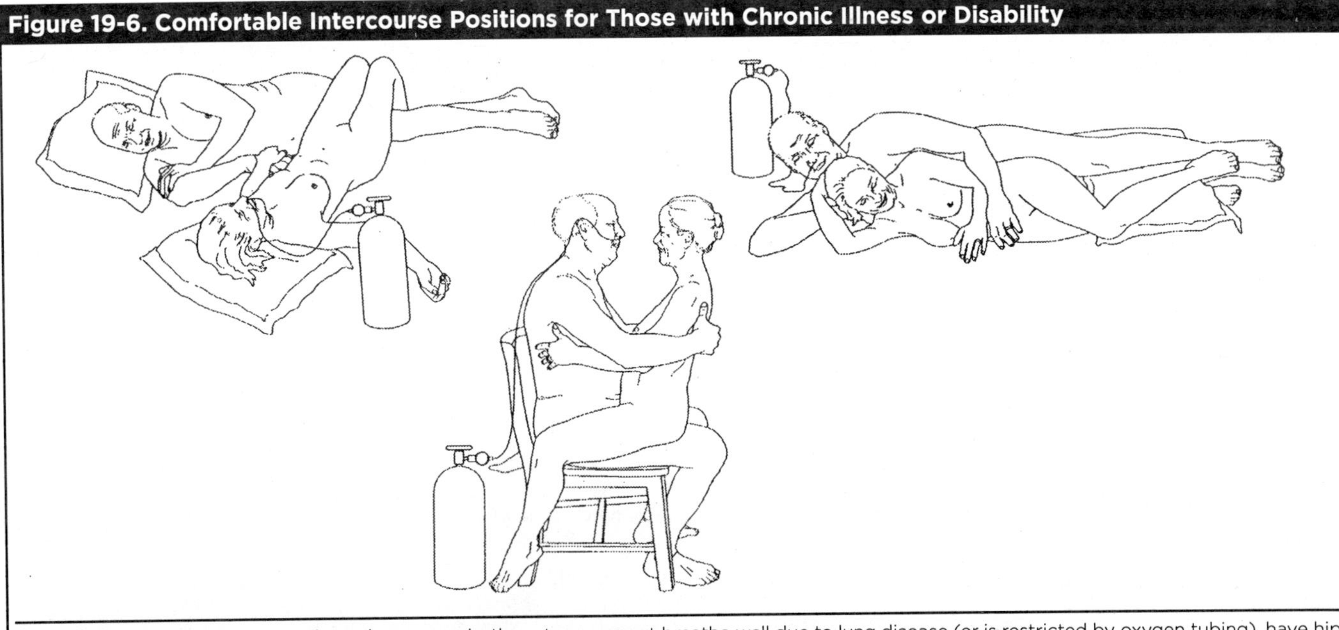

Note. These positions are appropriate when one or both partners cannot breathe well due to lung disease (or is restricted by oxygen tubing), have hip or knee pain due to arthritis, have back pain, or have limitations after a hip or knee replacement. These positions also work well if one or both partners have hemiparesis after a stroke. When side lying, lie on the affected side.

From *Gerontological nursing: Competencies for care* (2nd ed., p. 621), by K. L. Mauk (Ed.), 2010, Sudbury, MA: Jones & Bartlett. Copyright 2010 by Jones & Bartlett. Reprinted with permission.

References

Aaronson, L. S., Teel, C. S., Cassmeyer, V., Neuberger, G. C., Pallikkathayil, L., Pierce, J.,...Wingate, A. (1999). Defining and measuring fatigue. *Image—The Journal of Nursing Scholarship, 31*, 45–50.

Abrams, P., Cardozo, L., Fall, M., Griffiths, D., Rosier, P., Ulmsten, U.,...Weiin, A. (2002). The standardization of terminology of lower urinary tract function. *Neurourology and Urodynamics 21*, 167–178.

Ackley, B., & Ladwig, G. (2013). *Nursing diagnoses handbook: 2012-2014*. St. Louis: Elsevier.

Adachi, M., Staisiunas, P. G., Knutson, K. L., Beveridge, C., Meltzer, D. O., & Arora, V. M. (2013). Perceived control and sleep in hospitalized older adults: A sound hypothesis? *Journal of Hospital Medicine, 8*, 4.

Agency for Health Care Policy and Research. (1996). Identifying and Evaluating Urinary Incontinence. AHCPR Clinical Practice Guidelines, 2. Retrieved from http://www.ncbi.nlm.nih.gov/books/NBK52164/

Allen, A. M., Coon, D. W., Uriri-Glover, J., & Grando, V. (2013). Factors associated with sleep disturbance among older adults in inpatient rehabilitation facilities. *Rehabilitation Nursing, 38*(5), 221–230.

Altman, K., Yu, G., & Schaefer, S. (2011). Consequences of dysphagia in the hospitalized patient. *Archives of Otolaryngology—Head & Neck Surgery, 136*(8) 784–789.

Ameet, M., Avneesh, T., Babita, P., & Pramod, M. (2013). The relationship between periodontitis and systemic diseases: Hype or hope? *Journal of Clinical and Diagnostic Research 7*(4), 758–762.

American Academy of Pediatrics Committee on Adolescence. (2013). Policy statement: Office-based care for lesbian, gay, bisexual, transgender, and questioning youth. *Pediatrics, 132*, 198–203. doi:10.1542/peds.2013-1282 20140615172156316856742

American Diabetes Association. (2014). Standards of medical care in diabetes. *Diabetes Care, 37*(1), 14–80.

American Society for Parenteral and Enteral Nutrition (2009). ASPEN enteral nutrition practice recommendations. *Journal of Parenteral and Enteral Nutrition, 33*(2), 122–167.

American Speech-Language-Hearing Association. (2003). Role of the speech language pathologist in performance and interpretation of endoscopic evaluation of swallowing: *Guidelines*. Retrieved from www.asha.org/policy/GL2004-00059/

American Speech-Language-Hearing Association. (2014). Guidelines for speech language pathologists performing videofluorscopic swallowing studies. Retrieved from www.asha.org/policy/GL2004-00050/

American Speech-Language-Hearing Association. (2014). Swallowing disorders (dysphagia) in adults. Retrieved from www.asha.org/public/speech/swallowing/Swallowing-Disorders-in-Adults

Annon, J. S. (1976). The PLISSIT model: A proposed conceptual scheme for behavioral treatment of sexual problems. *Journal of Sex Education Therapy, 2*, 1–15.

Antonios, N., Mann, G., Crary, M., Miller, L., Hubbard, H., Hood, K.,...Silliman S. (2010). Analysis of a physician tool for evaluation of dysphagia on an inpatient stroke unit: The Modifed Mann Assessment of Swallowing Ability. *Journal of Stroke and Cerebrovascular Diseases, 19*(1): 49–57.

Association of Rehabilitation Nurses (ARN). (2014). ARN competency model for professional rehabilitation nursing. Retrieved from http://www.rehabnurse.org/uploads/files/education/ARN_Rehabilitation_Nursing_Competency _Model_FINAL_-_May_2014.pdf

Avidan, A. Y. (2005). Sleep disorders in the older patient. *Primary Care, 32*, 563–583.

Avery, W. (2011). Dysphagia. In G. Gillen (Ed.). *Stroke rehabilitation: A function-based approach* (3rd ed., pp. 629–647). New York: Elsevier Mosby.

Balin, A. K. (1990). Aging of human skin. In W. R. Hazzard, R. Andres, E. L. Bierman, & J. P. Blass (Eds.), *Principles of geriatric medicine and gerontology* (2nd ed., pp. 383–412). New York: McGraw-Hill.

Bliwise, D. L., Ansari, F. P., Straight, L. B., & Parker, K. P. (2005). Age changes in timing and 24-hour distribution of self-reported sleep. *The American Journal of Geriatric Psychiatry, 13*(12), 1077–1082.

Bostwick, J. M. (2010). A generalist's guide to treating patients with depression with an emphasis on using side effects to tailor antidepressant therapy. *Mayo Clinic Proceedings, 85*, 538–550.

Brackett, N. L., Ibrahim, E., & Lynne, C. M. (2011). The Miami project to cure paralysis. Retrieved from http://www.themiamiproject.org/page.aspx?pid=183

Brain Trauma Foundation (2007). Management of severe traumatic brain injury. *Journal of Neurotrauma, 24*(1), S1–S95.

Bryant, R. A., & Nix, D. P. (2012). *Acute and chronic wounds: Current management concepts* (4th ed.). St. Louis, MO: Mosby.

Castriotta, R. J., Wilde, M. C., Lai, J. M., Atanasov, S., Masel, B. E., & Kuna, S. T. (2007). Prevalence and consequences of sleep disorders in traumatic brain injury. *Journal of Clinical Sleep Medicine: JCSM: Official Publication of the American Academy of Sleep Medicine, 3*(4), 349.

Chasens, E. R., Williams, L. L., & Umlauf, M. G. (2011). Excessive sleepiness. In M. Boltz, E. Capezuti, T. Fulmer, D. Zwicker, & A. O'Meara (Eds.). *Evidence-based geriatric nursing protocols for best practice* (4th ed., pp. 459–476). New York: Springer.

Consortium for Spinal Cord Medicine (2006). *Bladder management for adults with spinal cord injury: A clinical practice guideline for health care providers*. Washington, DC: Paralyzed Veterans of America.

Consortium for Spinal Cord Medicine (2010a). *Neurogenic bowel management in adults with spinal cord injury*. Washington, DC: Paralyzed Veterans of America.

Consortium for Spinal Cord Medicine (2010b). *Sexuality and reproductive health in adults with spinal cord injury*. Washington, DC: Paralyzed Veterans of America.

Courtney B., & Flier, L. (2009). RN dysphagia screening: A stepwise approach. *Journal of Neuroscience Nursing, 41*(1), 28–38.

Crosby, G. A., Munshi, S., Karat, A. S., Worthington, E., & Lincoln, N. B. (2012). Fatigue after stroke: Frequency and effect on daily life. *Disability and Rehabilitation, 34*(8), 633–637.

Donovan, N., Daniels, S., Edmiaston, J., Weinhardt, J., Summers, D., & Mitchell, P. (2013). Invitational conference proceeding from the state of the art nursing symposium, international stroke conference 2012. *Stroke, 44*, 24–31.

Doughty, D. B. (2006). *Urinary and fecal incontinence: Current management concepts* (3rd ed.). St. Louis: Mosby.

Dumoulin, C., Hay-Smith, E. J., & Mac Habée-Séguin, G. (2014). Pelvic floor muscle training versus no treatment, or inactive control treatments, for urinary incontinence in women. Cochrane Database System Review, 2014(5):CD005654. doi: 10.1002/14651858.CD005654.pub3

DuVivier, A. (1993). *Atlas of clinical dermatology* (2nd ed.). London, England: Times Mirror International.

Earhart, G. M., & Williams, A. J. (2012). Treadmill training for individuals with Parkinson's disease. *Physical Therapy, 92*(7), 893–896.

Ehrlich-Jones, L., O'Dwyer, L., Stevens, K., & Deutsch, A. (2008). Searching the literature for evidence. *Rehabilitation Nursing, 33*(4), 163–169.

Elias, J., & Ryan, A. (2011). A review and commentary on the factors that influence expressions of sexuality by older people in care homes. *Journal of Clinical Nursing, 20,* 1668–1676. doi:10.1111/j.1365-2702.2010.03409.x

Englander, J., Bushnik, T., Oggins, J., & Katznelson, L. (2010). Fatigue after traumatic brain injury: Association with neuroendocrine, sleep, depression and other factors. *Brain Injury, 24*(12), 1379–1388.

Fisher, D., & Valente, S. (2009). Evaluating and managing insomnia. *The Nurse Practitioner, 34*(8), 20–26.

Gallant, M. P., Spitze, G., & Grove, J. G. (2010). Chronic illness self-care and the family lives of older adults: A synthetic review across four ethnic groups. *Journal of Cross Cultural Gerontology, 25*(1), 21–43. doi:10.1007/s10823-010-9112-z 201406121942301788444996 20140612200002817853331

Garcia, J. M., & Chambers, E. IV. (2010). Managing dysphagia through diet modification: Evidence-based help for patients with impaired swallowing. *American Journal of Nursing, 110*(10), 26–33.

Gater, D. R., Jr., Dolbow, D., Tsui, B., & Gorgey, A. S. (2011). Functional electrical stimulation therapies after spinal cord injury. *NeuroRehabilitation, 28,* 231–248. doi:10.3233/NRE-2011-0652

Gervasoni, E., Cattaneo, D., Montesano, A., & Jonsdottir, J. (2012). Effects of fatigue on balance and mobility in subjects with multiple sclerosis: A brief report. *ISRN Neurology,* (2012) Article ID 316097). doi: 10.55402/2012/316097

Ginsberg, D. (2013a). The epidemiology and pathophysiology of neurogenic bladder. *The American Journal of Managed Care, 19*(10) 191–196.

Ginsberg, D. (2013b). Optimizing therapy and management of neurogenic bladder. *The American Journal of Managed Care, 19*(10) 197–204.

Ginsberg, T. B. (2010). Male sexuality. *Clinics in Geriatric Medicine, 26,* 185–195.

Gormley, E. A., Lightner, D. J., Burgio, K. L., Chai, T. C., Clemens, J. Q., Culkin, D. J.,…Vasavada, S. P. (2014). *Diagnosis and treatment of overactive bladder (non-neurogenic) in adults: AUA/SUFU guideline.* Linthicum, MD: American Urological Association.

Greydanus, D. E., & Matytsina, L. A. (2010). Contraception in adolescent females with chronic illness: A clinical review. *International Journal of Child and Adolescent Health, 3,* 39–52.

Higgins, D. (2010). Sexuality, human rights and safety for people with disabilities: The challenge of intersecting identities. *Sexuality and Relationship Therapy, 25*(3), 245–257. doi:10.1080/14681994.2010.489545 20140612201008750842929

Jenson, G., Mirtallo, J., Compher, C., Dhaliwal, R., Forbes, A., Figueredo, R., …Waitzberg, D. (2010). Adult starvation and disease-related malnutrition: a proposal for etiology based diagnoses in the clinical practice setting from the International Consensus Guidelines Committee. *Journal of Clinical Nutrition,* 1-3. doi:10.1016/jclnu2009.11.010

Johnson, M., Moorhead, S., Bulechek, G. M., Butcher, H. K., Maas, M. L., & Swanson, E. (2011). *NOC and NIC linkages to NANDA-I and clinical conditions: Supporting critical reasoning and quality care (NANDA, NOC, and NIC linkages)* (3rd ed.). St. Louis: Mosby.

Kaplan, H. S. (1990). Sex, intimacy, and the aging process. *Journal of the American Academy of Psychoanalysis, 18,* 185–205.

Kautz, D. D. (2007). Hope for love: Practical advice for intimacy and sex after stroke. *Rehabilitation Nursing, 32*(3), 95–103.

Kautz, D. D. (2010). Great rehabilitation nurses combine art and science to create magic. *Rehabilitation Nursing, 36*(1), 13–15.

Keyock, K., & Newman, D. (2011). Understanding stress urinary incontinence. *The Nurse Practitioner. 36*(10) 25–36.

Kirk, S., Beatty, S., Callery, P., Milnes, L., & Pryjmachuk, P. (2012). Perceptions of effective self-care support for children and young people with long-term conditions. *Journal of Clinical Nursing, 21,* 1974–1987. doi:10.1111/j.1365-2702.2011.04027.x

Kluger, B. M., Krupp, L. B., & Enoka, R. M. (2013). Fatigue and fatigability in neurologic illnesses Proposal for a unified taxonomy. *Neurology, 80*(4), 409–416.

Krychman, M. L., & Kellogg-Spadt, S. (2009). Female sexual dysfunction: Working toward new understanding. *Women's Health Care: A Practical Journal for Nurse Practitioners, 8*(5), 37–48.

Kuo, L., Poison, A., & Kang, T. (2008). Associations between periodontal diseases and systemic diseases: A review of inter-relationships and interactions with diabetes, respiratory diseases, cardiovascular diseases and osteoporosis. *Public Health, 122*(4), 417–433.

Langmore, S. E., Terpenning, M. S., Schork, A., Chen, Y., Murray, J. T., Lopatin, D., & Loesche, W. J. (1998). Predictors of aspiration pneumonia: How important is dysphagia? *Dysphagia, 13*(2), 68–81. doi:201406130943311322014213

La Rue-Evans, D., Nesbitt, K., & Oka, R. K. (2013). Sleep hygiene program implementation in patients with traumatic brain injury. *Rehabilitation Nursing, 38*(1), 2–10.

Lee, Y. C., Lu, B., Edwards, R. R., Wasan, A. D., Nassikas, N. J., Clauw, D. J.,...Karlson, E. W. (2013). The role of sleep problems in central pain processing in rheumatoid arthritis. *Arthritis & Rheumatism, 65*(1), 59–68.

Lew-Starowicz, M., & Rola, R. (2013). Prevalence of sexual dysfunctions among women with multiple sclerosis. *Sexuality and Disability,*1-26. doi:10.1007/s11195-013-9293-9201406121953221921214819

Lubkin, I. M., & Larsen, P. D. (2009). *Chronic illness* (7th ed.). Sudbury, MA: Jones & Bartlett.

Marimuthu, K., Murton, A. J., & Greenhaff, P. L. (2011). Mechanisms regulating muscle mass during disuse atrophy and rehabilitation in humans. *Journal of Applied Physiology, 110,* 555–560. doi:10.1152/japplphysiol.00962.2010 201406131228001503563881

Martino, R., Silver, F., Reasell, R., Bayley, M., Nicholson, F., Streiner, D., & Diamant, N. (2009) The Toronto bedside swallowing screening test. *Stroke, 40,* 555 –561.

Marzetti, S., Hwang, J. C., Lees, H. A., Wohlgemuth, S. E., Dupont-Versteegden, E. E., Carter, C. S.,...Leeuwenburgh, C. (2011). Mitochondrial death effectors: Relavance to sarcopenia and disuse muscle atrophy. *Biochimica et Biophysica Acta, 1800*(3), 235–244. doi:10.1016/j.bbagen.2009.05.007 201406131223571160084844 20140612193800492232561

Mathias, J. L., & Alvaro, P. K. (2012). Prevalence of sleep disturbances, disorders, and problems following traumatic brain injury: A meta-analysis. *Sleep Medicine, 13*(7), 898–905.

Mauk, K. L. (Ed.). (2010). *Gerontological nursing: Competencies for care.* Sudbury, MA: Jones & Bartlett.

Mauk, K. L. (2012). *Rehabilitation nursing: A contemporary approach to care.* Sudbury, MA: Jones & Bartlett.

Mauk, K. L. (Ed.). (2014). *Gerontological nursing: Competencies for care* (3rd ed.). Burlington, MA: Jones & Bartlett.

Meyeda-Letourneau, J. (2014). Safe patient handling and movement: A literature review. *Rehabilitation Nursing, 39*(3), 123–129. doi:10.1002/rnj.133 20140612193941584635377

Meyers, D. (2014) Female mixed urinary incontinence a clinical review. *JAMA, 311*(19), 2007–2014.

Milne, J. L. (2008). Behavioral therapies for overactive bladder: Making sense of the evidence. *Journal of Wound, Ostomy, and Continence Nursing, 35*(1), 93–101.

Mintzer, S. (2010). Metabolic consequences of antiepileptic drugs. *Current Opinion in Neurology, 23,* 164–169.

Moore, Z. E. H., & Cowman, S. (2005). Wound cleansing for pressure ulcers. *Cochrane Database of Systematic Reviews,* Article CD004983. doi:10.1002/14651858

Moreno, J. A., Lasprilla, J. C., Gan, C., & McKerral, M. (2013). Sexuality after traumatic brain injury: A critical review. *NeuroRehabilitation, 32,* 69–85. doi:10.3233/NRE-130824 20140612200758837525844

Mueller, C., Compher, C., Druyan, M. E., & American Society of Parenteral and Enteral Nutrition Board of Directors (2011). ASPEN clinical guidelines: Nutrition screening, assessment, and intervention in adults. *Journal of Parenteral and Enteral Nutrition, 35*(1), 16–24.

Myer, D. (2014). Female mixed urinary incontinence: A clinical review. *Journal of the American Medical Association, 311*(19) 2007–2014.

National Institute for Health & Clinical Excellence. (2012). Urinary incontinence in neurological disease. NICE clinical guidelines. Retrieved from www.guidance.nice.org.uk/cg148.

National Pressure Ulcer Advisory Panel. (n.d.). *Pressure ulcer category/staging illustrations.* Washington, DC: Author.

National Pressure Ulcer Advisory Panel & European Pressure Ulcer Advisory Panel. (2009). *Prevention and treatment of pressure ulcers: Clinical practice guideline.* Washington, DC: National Pressure Ulcer Advisory Panel.

Neukrug, A., & Ancoli-Israel, S. (2010). Sleep disorders in the older adult—A mini-review. Gerontology, 56(2), 181–189.

Newman, D. (2009a). Talking to patients about bladder control problems. *The Nurse Practitioner, 34*(12), 33–45.

Newman, D. (2009b). *Causes of incontinence and identification of risk factors in managing and treating urinary incontinence* (2nd ed.). Baltimore, MD: Health Professions Press.

North American Nursing Diagnosis Association International. (2012–2014). Nursing diagnoses: Definitions & classification: 2012-2014. Retrieved from www.nanda.org/Marketplace/NANDAIPublications/20092011TaxonomyPrint.aspx.

Othman, A., & Engkasan, J. P. (2011). Sexual dysfunction following spinal cord injury: The experiences of Malaysian women. *Sexuality and Disability, 29*(4), 329–337. doi:10.1007/s11195-011-9207-7 201406122003001261123896

Panther, K. (2008). *Frazier water protocol: Safety, hydration, and quality of life.* Rockville, MD: ASHA Product Sales.

Porth, C. M., & Matfin, G. (2008). *Pathophysiology: Concepts of altered health states* (8th ed.). Philadelphia: Lippincott Wilkins & Williams.

Powers, S. W., Wiggs, M. P., Duarte, J. A., Zergeroglu, A. M., & Demirel, H. A. (2012). Mitochondrial signaling contributes to disuse muscle atrophy. *American Journal of Physiology, Endocrinology and Metabolism, 303,* E31–E39. doi:10.1152/ajpendo.00609.2011 201406131216191139079809

Quality of Care Act, 42 C.F.R. §483.25d (1991 & Supp. 2005). Retrieved from www.cms.hhs.gov/transmittals/downloads/R8SOM.pdf

Registered Nurses Association of Ontario (RNAO). (2005). Risk assessment and prevention of pressure ulcers. Toronto, ON, Canada: Author. Retrieved from www.rnao.org/Storage/12/638_BPG_Pressure_Ulcers_v2.pdf.

Rehabilitation Nursing Foundation. (1995). *Rehabilitation nursing: Directions for practice—A basic nursing rehabilitation course* (3rd ed., pp. 164–170). Glenview, IL: Author.

Rehabilitation Nursing Foundation. (2002). *Practice guidelines for the management of constipation in adults.* Glenview, IL: Author.

Saint, S., Meddings, J., Calfee, D., Kowalski, C., & Krein, S. (2009). Catheter associated UTI and the Medicare rule change. *Annals of Internal Medicine. 150*(12) 877–884.

Schutte-Rodin, S., Broch, L., Buysse, D., Dorsey, C., & Sateia, M. (2008). Clinical guideline for the evaluation and management of chronic insomnia in adults. *Journal of Clinical Sleep Medicine, 4,* 487–504.

Seco, J., Abecia, L. C., Echevarria, E., Barbero, I., Torres-Unda, J., Rodriquez, V., & Calvo, J. I. (2013). Balance in older adults. A long-term physical activity training program increases strength and flexibility and improves balance in older adults. *Rehabilitation Nursing, 38*(1), 37–47. doi:10.1002/rnj.64 201406121947221433272243

Sievers, A. E. F. (2008). Nursing evaluation and care of the patient with dysphagia. In R. Leonard & K. Kendall (Eds.), *Dysphagia assessment and treatment planning: A team approach* (2nd ed.). San Diego, CA: Plural Publishing.

Sipski, M. L., & Alexander, C. J. (1998). Sexuality and disability. In J. A. DeLisa & B. M. Gans (Eds.), *Rehabilitation medicine: Principles and practice* (3rd ed.). Philadelphia: Lippincott-Raven.

Smith Hammond, C. A., & Goldstein, L. (2006). Cough and aspiration of foods and liquids due to oral-pharyngeal dysphagia: ACCP evidence-based clinical practice guidelines. *Chest, 129,* 154–168.

Stevens, K. A. (2008). Urinary elimination and continence. In S. P. Hoeman (Ed.), *Rehabilitation nursing: Prevention, intervention & outcomes* (4th ed., pp. 334–368). St. Louis: Mosby Elsevier.

Stohrer, M., Blok, B., Castro-Diaz, D., Chartier-Kastler, E., Del Popolo, G., Kramer, G.,...Wyndaele, J. (2009). EAU Guidelines on neurogenic lower urinary tract dysfunction. *European Urology, 56,* 81–88.

Suiter, D. (Ed.). (2005). Frazier free water protocol: Evidence and ethics. Retrieved from www.asha.org.

Suiter D., & Leder, S. (2008). Clinical utility of the 3-ounce water swallow test. *Dysphagia, 23,* 244–250.

Sussman, C., & Bates-Jensen, B. (2007). Wound healing physiology: Acute and chronic. In C. Sussman, & B. Bates-Jensen (Eds.), *Wound care: A collaborative practice manual for health professionals* (3rd ed., pp. 21–51). Baltimore, MD: Lippincott Williams & Wilkins.

Tefertiller, C., Pharo, B., Evans, N., & Winchester, P. (2011). Efficacy of rehabilitation robotics for walking training in neurological disorders: A review. *Journal of Rehabilitation Research & Development, 48*(4), 387–416. doi:201406131117431496836305

Tosta de Souza, D. M. S., Conceicao de Gouveia Santos, V. L., Iri, H. K., & Oguri, M. Y. S. (2010). Predictive validity of the Braden scale for pressure ulcer risk in elderly residents of long-term care facilities. *Geriatric Nursing, 31*(2), 95–104.

Tyrell, C. M., Roos, M. A., Rudolph, K. S., & Reisman, D. S. (2011). Influence of systematic increases in treadmill walking speed on gait kinematics after stroke. *Physical Therapy, 91*(3), 392–403. doi:20140613111540881148577

Uniform Data System for Medical Rehabilitation. (1997a). *Functional independence measure.* Buffalo, NY: University of Buffalo.

Uniform Data System for Medical Rehabilitation. (1997b). *Functional independence measure for children.* Buffalo, NY: University of Buffalo.

U.S. Department of Health and Human Services & Centers for Medicare and Medicaid Services. (2012). *Report to Congress: Post acute care payment reform demonstration (PAC-PRD).* Retrieved from http://www.cms.gov/Research-Statistics-Data-and-Systems/Statistics-Trends-and-Reports/Reports/downloads/Flood_PACPRD_RTC_CMS_Report_Jan_2012.pdf

U.S. Department of Health and Human Services & U.S. Department of Agriculture. (2005). *Dietary guidelines for Americans, 2005.* Retrieved from www.health.gov/dietaryguidelines/dga2005/document/default.htm

Verma, A., Anand, V., & Verma, N. P. (2007). Sleep disorders in chronic traumatic brain injury. *Journal of clinical sleep medicine, 3*(4), 357.

Wallace, S. A., Roe, B., Williams, K., & Palmer, M. (2009). Bladder training for urinary incontinence in adults (review). *Cochrane Database of Systematic Reviews, 2004*(1), CD001308.

White, J., Guenter, P., Jensen, G., Malone, A., Schofield, M., Academy Malnutrition Work Group,...ASPEN Board of Directors. (2012). Consensus statement of the Academy of Nutrition and Dietetics/American Society of Parenteral and Enteral Nutrition: Characteristics recommended for the identification and documentation of adult malnutrition (undernutrition). *Journal of the Academy of Nutrition and Dietetics, 112*(5), 730–738.

Wound, Ostomy and Continence Nurses Society. (2010). Guideline for prevention and management of pressure ulcers. Retrieved from www.guideline.gov/content.aspx?id=23868.

Wright, K. J. (2009). Administering medication to adult patients with dysphagia. *Nursing Standard, 23*(29), 61–68.

Young, J. S., Bougeois, J. A., Hilty, D. M., & Hardin, K. A. (2009). Sleep in hospitalized medical patients, part 2: Behavioral and pharmacological management of sleep disturbances. *Journal of Hospital Medicine, 4,* 50–59.

Chapter 20

Psychosocial Healthcare Patterns and Nursing Interventions

Margit B. Gerardi, PhD WHCNP PMHNP-BC

LEARNING OUTCOMES

- Identify cognitive influences on psychosocial health.
- Describe barriers and facilitators to psychosocial health.
- List roles and relationships related to psychosocial health.
- Discuss unique aspects of psychosocial health related to the rehabilitation patient.
- Compare acute and chronic psychosocial disorders that might be seen in the rehabilitation patient.
- Identify the role of the rehabilitation nurse in caring for the patient with a psychosocial disorder.

KEY CHAPTER TOPICS

- Cognitive influences including cognition, orientation, attention, judgment, problem solving, and motivation
- Barriers and facilitators including self-concept, self-esteem, body image, grief, stigma, hope, and powerlessness
- Roles and relationships including family type, social support, independence, dependence and helplessness
- Coping and stress tolerance
- Anxiety disorder, depressive disorder, bipolar disorder, substance abuse disorders, and PTSD

PROFESSIONAL REHABILITATION NURSING DOMAINS AND COMPETENCIES

- Domain 1: Competencies 1.2, 1.3, 1.4
- Domain 2: Competencies 2.1, 2.2 (Association of Rehabilitation Nurses [ARN] 2014)

Introduction

Rehabilitation nurses will be better able to care for their clients if they understand relevant concepts of psychosocial health, which involve the influences of psychological processes and social interactions on behavior. Theories of self-perception, roles and relationships, coping and stress tolerance, values, and beliefs, and concepts such as hope and dignity, support psychosocial healthcare patterns. Specific psychosocial disorders that influence rehabilitation nursing care are highlighted to help rehabilitation nurses provide relevant, evidenced-based interventions.

I. Cognitive Influences on Psychosocial Health

A. Cognition

1. Description
    a. *Cognition* is defined as the process of knowing and consists of awareness, perception, and reasoning (Gazzaniga, Ivry, & Mangun, 2013). Cognitive deficits arise can involve one or more of these components.
    b. Cognitive development allows the processing of information through decoding, encoding, transferring, combining, storage, and retrieval (Bennett, Motes, Rao, & Rypma, 2012).
    c. Cognition depends on sensory input, prior experiences, learning, and recall and memory.
    d. Normal aging, as well as injury to the cortex of the brain or the neural pathways, interferes with sensory input, cognitive integration, and planning of appropriate responses (Bennett & Madden, 2014).
    e. The cerebral cortex, internal nuclei, basal ganglia, and the cerebellum process and integrate

sensory input and motor planning (**Table 20-1**).

f. Recovery depends on the extent, quality (e.g., edema versus destruction), and area of the injury (Bennett & Madden, 2014).

2. Assessment
   a. Conduct initial and ongoing cognitive assessment.
   b. Evaluate the client's ability to determine pertinent and irrelevant stimuli, to learn, to understand situations or conversations, to problem solve, and to follow a plan of action.
   c. Obtain a symptom history from the person and family.
   d. Review the medical history and current medications, including alternative medications and treatments.
   e. Assess the ability to perform activities of daily living (ADLs) (Knopman & Petersen, 2014).
   f. For clients with brain injury, use the Rancho Los Amigos Levels of Cognitive Function Scale as an assessment tool (Flannery, 1998).
   g. Assess attention abilities, short- and long-term memory for processing information, recall and retrieval, and problem solving (Knopman & Petersen, 2014).
3. Nursing interventions
   a. Holistic consideration for structuring the environment, caregiver education and support, adaptive communication, and simplification of tasks to address unmet needs and environmental overload (Kales, Gitlin, Lyketsos, & the Detroit Expert Panel on the Management of the Neuropsychiatric Symptoms of Dementia, 2014).
   b. Use helpful cues (e.g., the client's name, pictures of familiar people or pets) to help the client identify locations.
   c. Encourage the client to use daily logs, written schedules, and patterns for ADLs.
   d. Use sensory stimulation programs (e.g., visual, auditory, olfactory, cutaneous, taste, motion) that focus on short-term interventions several times a day to increase cognition.
   e. Make materials meaningful for each person.
   f. Use optimal timing; perform interventions when the person is not tired, rushed, hungry, or distracted.
   g. Simplify the situation and repeat it to help ensure understanding.
   h. Ensure a consistent schedule, staff, and environment.
   i. Recommend a power of attorney for financial and health decisions.
4. Research study findings
   a. Children with acquired brain injury often experience cognitive, motor, and psychosocial deficits that affect participation in everyday activities. In one study, children's behavior improved with coaching, although their problem solving did not (Missiuna et al., 2010).
   b. Present neuropsychological tests or global functional assessments might not capture the range of cognitive deficits associated with traumatic brain injury (TBI). Care must be taken to assess social communication and emotional function, because these cognitive constructs have a significant influence on successful recovery (Donovan, 2011).

Table 20-1. Cognitive Functions Affected by Brain Injury

Area of the Brain	Function	Results of Injury
Frontal lobe	Controls higher intellectual and social processing	Loss of intellect and inappropriate social behaviors
Temporal lobe	Controls new memory and learning	Impaired learning
Temporal lobe (hippocampus)	—	Temporary memory loss, lack of contralateral orientation, distractibility, hyperactivity, attention deficits, perseveration
Right hemisphere	Controls recognition of geometric patterns, faces, environmental sounds, a second language, music, sense of direction, and memory for pictures	Learning impairments, memory impairments
Left hemisphere	Controls memory for language, letters, works, verbal memory (e.g., reading, writing, speech), arithmetic	Deficits with math and communication
Limbic lobe of the right and left hemispheres	Controls attention that affects socialization	Deficits with socialization

B. Orientation
1. Definition: *Orientation* is the ability to know about oneself (e.g., name, age, date of birth, address), the time (e.g., current date, month, year), and facts about the environment
2. Assessment
a. Conduct an initial and ongoing assessment of orientation.
b. Distinguish between confusion, disorientation, physical conditions (e.g., electrolyte imbalance, medications, fluid imbalance, fatigue) and sensory deficits (Knopman & Petersen, 2014).
c. Use the Mini-Mental State Examination (MMSE) (Folstein, Folstein, & McHugh, 1975).
3. Nursing interventions
a. Use cues to orient the client (e.g., familiar photographs of the client, family, or pets; familiar furniture; calendars; holiday decorations; clocks with large, clear numbers; schedules of daily events).
b. Clearly identify family, relatives, friends, and staff when interacting with the client.
c. Ensure that the client uses intact, functional sensory aids.
d. Provide a consistent environment and staff.
4. Research study findings
a. To determine how altered orientation influences rehabilitation outcomes in people with stroke and how decreased orientation 6 months after stroke influences ADLs and social activities, Pedersen, Jorgensen, Nakayama, Raaschou, and Olsen (1996) analyzed the independent influence of orientation in acute stroke on rehabilitation. The level of orientation influences basic ADLs, higher-level instrumental ADLs, and social activities in acute and chronic stroke. This finding suggests that rehabilitation of memory and attention might be important in people with stroke and impaired orientation.

C. Attention
1. Definition: *Attention* is the ability to respond to and prioritize relevant information and to ignore or put aside irrelevant information
a. Older adults are vulnerable for attentional fatigue caused by age-related physiological changes in vision, hearing, touch, and taste.
b. Attentional capacity is influenced by the capacity to direct attention, attentional demands, attentional fatigue, and restorative activities.
c. Attention works through global neural inhibitory mechanisms that allow the focusing that is needed for prolonged or intense directed attention (Gazzaniga, Ivry, & Mangun, 2013).
2. Assessment
a. Assess short-term memory, planning, problem solving, incidence of accidents, irritability, impulsiveness, and frustration (Wilson, 2013).
b. Use standard questions to assess attention.
1) Inquire about home activities that require more or new effort (e.g., physical or environmental factors).
2) Discern the feelings that the client experiences most often.
3) Identify times the client would like to but cannot express feelings and share experiences.
c. Assess changes in the person's feelings, emotions, anger, and frustration, which can accompany loss of motivation (Kales et al., 2014).
3. Nursing interventions
a. Use conservation and restoration measures to reduce neurological fatigue.
1) Conservation measures: Reduce or limit the extent and number of attentional demands in the internal and external environments; help the client complete necessary and desired activities in a controlled, stable environment (Ponsford et al., 2014).
2) Restoration measures: Allow rest and recovery by changing activities (e.g., taking a walk in a park, gardening, bird watching).
b. Prioritize activities for attention and break the task into parts, focusing on step-by-step instructions.
c. Screen sleep patterns and treat sleep-wake disorders (Ponsford et al., 2014).
d. Encourage daily physical activity.
e. Advise the client to avoid alcohol and drugs.
f. Individualize music selections and avoid stressful selections.
g. Modify expectations to fit the reality of the client's status.
h. Provide growth and development opportunities.
i. Allow for variance in the client's attention throughout the day.
j. Identify triggers (e.g., situations, people, places, events) that contribute to intellectual or emotional conflict.
k. Provide client and family education.
l. Avoid denial, devaluation, or demeaning of the client.
m. Participate in group therapy (Stuart, 2013).

n. Allow rest to recover from the overwhelming fatigue of dealing with loss of cognitive abilities (Stuart, 2013).

4. Research study findings: Findings from a study of 40 individuals with a recent history of moderate to severe TBI demonstrated that they had a slowed speed of information processing and difficulties sustaining attention, performing two or more tasks simultaneously, and ignoring distractions. These problems affected their ability to concentrate and process thoughts when compared with 40 healthy controls (Willmott, Ponsford, Hocking, & Schönberger, 2009).

D. Judgment

1. Definition: *Judgment* is remembering, planning, foresight, abstraction, transference of information, and evaluating the appropriateness of an action.
2. Assessment
   a. Evaluate the client's ability to comprehend physical and cognitive limitations and maintain recommended safety precautions.
   b. Observe the client's accuracy with managing money, learning new skills, applying old knowledge in new situations, solving problems, and creating and following through with realistic plans.
   c. Periodically reassess the client's judgment deficits to meet his or her increasing or decreasing needs.
3. Nursing interventions: Tailor interventions to match the client's level of cognition.
   a. For clients with high cognitive functioning, coordinate counseling, education, crisis management, vocational assessment and planning, and individualized self-care.
   b. For clients with moderate cognitive functioning, provide or coordinate scheduled routines, a structured environment, counseling, individualized education, and vocational assessment and planning.
   c. For clients with lower cognitive functioning, help coordinate supervised living situations, a protective environment, sheltered vocational opportunities, case management, and legal guardians.
4. Research study findings
   a. An autoethnographic exploration of one woman's illness narrative provides an in-depth understanding of her lived experience of rehabilitation after a TBI and polytrauma. The narrative confirms the importance of providing people with self-determined choice as a primary component of rehabilitation. The voices and values of clients are integral to professional judgment. This narrative supports clients' personal choice and freedom during the rehabilitation process as a means of increasing their sense of self-determination and empowerment while improving overall health outcomes (Lawson, Delamere, & Hutchinson, 2008).

E. Problem Solving

1. Definition: *Problem solving* is a high-level cognitive function that involves considering, recalling, and analyzing factors and selecting appropriate choices from various alternatives.
2. Assessment
   a. Assess the ability to problem solve initially and in an ongoing manner.
   b. Assess the ability to plan and organize thoughts and behaviors.
   c. Assess the ability to formulate alternative solutions for a problem.
   d. Assess the ability to comprehend potential consequences of choices.
3. Nursing interventions
   a. Help the client approach problems by taking one step at a time.
   b. Encourage the client to differentiate between solutions to a problem and examine the consequences of solutions.
   c. Encourage successful problem-solving plans and build on successes.
   d. Examine unsuccessful problem-solving plans, and discuss ways to select positive action plans.
   e. Plan family and caregiver education with a focus on brain function and strategies for dealing with the client's lack of decision-making skills after a stroke or head injury (Williams & Dahl, 2002).
   f. Involve the family and caregivers in discharge planning decisions for the client after a stroke or head injury.
4. Research study findings
   a. As part of a larger study designed to evaluate social communication abilities after TBI, participants completed measures of executive functioning, affect perception, perceived communication ability, and functional outcome (Struchen et al., 2008). Executive functioning performance accounted for 13.3% of the variance in occupational functioning and 16% of explained variance in social integration. These results provide evidence of the value of executive functioning and social communication

measures in the prediction of functional outcomes.

F. Motivation

1. Description
   a. *Motivation* is the external, internal, or combined forces that influence behavior to satisfy needs and achieve goals.
   b. Motivation can be influenced by needs and wants, the cost and rewards of participating in an activity, and personal beliefs about the ability to participate and succeed (Bandura, 1977).
2. Assessment
   a. Assess the amount and persistence of the client's activities toward achieving goals.
   b. Assess the barriers to client motivation (e.g., memory impairment, problem-solving deficits, cultural barriers).
   c. Use the Apathy Evaluation Scale, an 18-item instrument that measures a person's thoughts, actions, and emotions during the previous month. This instrument helps determine motivation that affects discharge function and functional levels after rehabilitation (Resnick, Zimmerman, Magaziner, & Adelman, 1998).
3. Nursing interventions
   a. Help the client establish immediate and long-term goals.
   b. Help the client and family set a realistic plan to achieve goals.
   c. Break long-term goals into small, attainable goals.
   d. Reward successes with family and peer recognition.
   e. Provide resources that lead to the successful achievement of goals.
4. Research study findings
   a. When compared with the dominant English-speaking culture in Australia, people from cultural and linguistic minority groups displayed differences in outcome and levels of distress over role changes after TBI, independent of socioeconomic background and access to rehabilitation (Saltapidas & Ponsford, 2007).

II. Barriers to and Facilitators of Psychosocial Health

A. Self-Concept and Self-Perception

1. Description: *Self-concept* is the way one thinks about oneself. It is a clear sense of who a person is with respect to others, a sense of being a separate person with strengths and weaknesses. People with strong self-concept acknowledge their emotions and find constructive ways to bring meaning into life. The person with a healthy self-concept views others realistically and is able to relate to them in a satisfying manner, which includes the capacity for intimacy and love. The person with a healthy self-concept handles life's realities and problems with appropriate coping behaviors (Craven & Hirnle, 2009). Self-concept is a person's perception of himself or herself in relation to others and the environment. It addresses all aspects of the person.
2. Middle-range theory: People change over time, particularly after incurring a disability. The person's environment also changes over time. These changes affect the person-environment interaction. This framework includes four components of the person's identity (e.g., nondisabled, disabled, identity project, and identity imputed by others) and four components of the environment (e.g., the given, the reactive during interaction, modified after interaction, and internalized). The praxis of rehabilitation can be enhanced by taking into account the relationships between these subsets of personal identity and environment in program planning; for instance, in the matching of person and assistive technology or home support services. This framework can build a theory of person–environment interaction in disability that is compatible with interaction in other forms of difference between individuals (Jahiel & Scherer, 2010).
3. Assessment
   a. Observe for self-concept adjustment (e.g., positive thinking, satisfaction at small successes, interest in appearance).
   b. Observe for self-criticism (e.g., negative thinking, expectations of failure).
   c. Observe for self-diminution (e.g., avoiding, neglecting, or refusing to recognize personal assets) (Stuart, 2013).
4. Nursing interventions
   a. Encourage activity in community-based social integration programs to develop social skills (Barry, Clarke, Jenkins, & Patel, 2013).
   b. Encourage the client to approach life with open, realistic expectations.
   c. Encourage and reinforce the client's evaluations of his or her personal assets.
   d. Encourage the client to interact with family and friends.
   e. Reinforce success, which can academically and vocationally increase self-concept (Stuart, 2013).

f. Participation in artistic activities can contribute to positive self-identification (Geue et al., 2010).
5. Research study findings
a. Soyupek, Aktepe, Savas, and Askin (2010) compared the self-concept of children with cerebral palsy (CP) with that of children without disability to investigate predictive variables that could affect self-concept and quality of life (QOL). Significant differences in mean scores favoring the control group were found for the Piers-Harris Self-Concept Scale; the Physical Scale of Peds QOL report was a significant predictor of self-concept. Self-concept and QOL of the children with CP were lower than for the children without CP. With the presence of incontinence, the self-concept rating and Gross Motor Function Classification System level were important for predicting domains of QOL.

B. Self-Esteem
1. Definition: *Self-esteem* is an attitude or feeling of pride in oneself and self-concept represented by behavior. It the person's sense of personal value and ability to consider himself or herself with dignity, love, and reality.
a. Self-esteem affects the inner person and the person's relationships with others.
b. Positive self-esteem is fostered by integrity, honesty, responsibility, compassion, and competence.
c. Self-esteem is based on a personal evaluation of self-worth, perceived successes, and competence (Sadock, Sadock, & Ruiz, 2014).
d. A person with low self-esteem and self-worth often has a "victim mentality" and expects deprecation.
2. Middle-range theory
a. Schreuer and colleagues incorporated variables from the cognitive coping model (i.e., self-esteem, appraisal, and social support) and the occupational performance model (i.e., engagement in activities, involvement in work or study, time of typing performance, and environmental adaptations) to explore adjustment to disability in 90 adults with severe physical disabilities. Subjects were tested with respect to their adjustment to severe disabilities in their adapted computerized work environment 1 year after occupational therapy consultation. Findings indicated that self-esteem and time of performance were core variables connecting cognitive and functional variables. Age and ADLs were the only background variables that contributed to the model (Schreuer, Rimmerman, & Sachs, 2006).
3. Assessment
a. Observe for feelings of defeat, failure, worthlessness (Satir, 1988), weakness, helplessness, hopelessness, fright, vulnerability, fragility, incompleteness, and inadequacy (Stuart, 2013).
b. Assess the client to identify a personal situation in which mastery was achieved through positive coping with disability effects.
4. Nursing interventions
a. Allow time for relaxation.
b. Help the client realize what is occurring and his or her reaction to the situation.
c. Encourage the client to communicate with family and supportive persons to share experiences (Wu, 2011).
d. Encourage the client to listen to others and try to reflect on how both parties perceive the communication.
e. Foster relaxed, flexible family expectations.
f. Encourage the client to declare, "I am unique," "I can love myself," and "I am okay" (Satir, 1988).
g. Encourage family and friends to express that the client is a person of value (Zhang et al., 2014).
h. Prepare the client to perform to personally identified standards for life functions and roles (Stuart, 2013).
i. Encourage spirituality as a basis for self-concept, which has been related to positive rehabilitation outcomes (Vespa, Jacobsen, Spazzafumo, & Balducci, 2011).
5. Research study findings
a. Development of self-esteem and self-efficacy in adolescents with chronic physical illness with and without psychological symptoms was measured for 1 year after a medical inpatient rehabilitation treatment of 4 to 6 weeks. Gender- and diagnosis-related differences were analyzed. A total of 243 chronically ill adolescents were interviewed at the beginning of their rehabilitation treatment and 1 year later. Therapy for chronically ill adolescents in medical rehabilitation affects their self-esteem positively, with differences in self-esteem found between adolescents who show clinically relevant psychological symptoms and those who do not. Only minor changes were noticed in ratings of self-efficacy at school and other social contexts.

Gender- and diagnosis-related differences have not been found (Kiera, Stachow, Petermann, & Tiedjen, 2010).

b. To explore the effect of self-esteem level, self-esteem stability, and admission functional status on discharge depressive symptoms in acute stroke rehabilitation, 120 survivors serially completed a measure of state self-esteem during inpatient rehabilitation and a measure of depressive symptoms at discharge. Functional status was rated at admission using the Functional Independence Measure™ (FIM™). After potential moderating variables were controlled for, self-esteem level interacted with FIM™ self-care and cognitive functioning to predict discharge depressive symptoms, such that survivors with lower self-rated self-esteem and poorer functional status indicated higher levels of depressive symptoms. Self-esteem stability interacted with FIM™ mobility functioning, such that self-esteem instability in the presence of lower mobility functioning at admission was related to higher levels of depressive symptoms at discharge (Vickery, Evans, Sepehri, Jabeen, & Gayden, 2009).

C. Body Image

1. Definition: *Body image*: A person's subjective picture of his or her own appearance that is based on observations, comparisons, and reactions by others.
2. Middle-range theory
   a. A multidisciplinary, integrated review approach was used to identify the basic elements and the underlying theoretical framework of mirror interventions. Qualitative and quantitative strategies for reviewing evidence were used, and a narrative synthesis approach was used to guide the comprehensive synthesis. Underlying theoretical models were identified, and five elements of mirror interventions (i.e., self-knowledge, therapeutic intervention, repetition, homework, and imagery or relaxation) were synthesized from the literature (Freysteinson, 2009).
3. Assessment
   a. Observe for grooming and hygiene status.
   b. Observe for initiation of self-care activities.
   c. Observe the functional abilities for self-care and ADLs.
   d. Observe the effect of the client's appearance on family, friends, and the community.
4. Nursing interventions
   a. Provide for independent or assisted grooming.
   b. Ensure that the client has appropriate street clothing for activities.
   c. Coordinate barber and hairdressing services.
   d. Encourage the use of prosthetics.
   e. Reinforce occupational therapy.
   f. Provide recreational therapy and community reentry activities.
   g. Encourage the client to recognize successful people with disabilities (e.g., athletes who use wheelchairs).
   h. Promote positive public images of people with disabilities in business, politics, and the media.
   i. Incorporate people with disabilities into play therapy (e.g., childhood books that include characters with disabilities, dolls in wheelchairs, cartoons with positive images of people with disabilities).
   j. Encourage the client to attend support groups for people with disabilities.
5. Research study findings
   a. A qualitative, retrospective, cross-sectional, descriptive study based on interview data from 15 women with spinal cord injury (SCI) was undertaken to explore consumer values important to rehabilitation practice. Four specific values are discussed: genuine interest and respect for the person, fostering autonomy, valuing lay knowledge and expertise, and promoting hopefulness (Yoshida et al., 2009).

D. Grief Associated with Disability

1. Definition: "*Grief* is the normal but bewildering cluster of ordinary human emotions arising in response to significant loss, intensified and complicated by the relationship to the person or the object lost" (Anderson, 2010, p. 128). Additionally, "grief is not only normative but also dynamic, pervasive, and individual" (Olson & Dossey, 2013, p. 463). Grief can vary in temporal quality from a brief response to a prolonged or complicated grief.
2. Middle-range theory
   a. Yalom's (1980, 1986) model is used as a foundation to explore the four existential issues of death, freedom and responsibility, loneliness, and meaninglessness. This model is applied to communication disorders based on the work of D. Lutterman (1984, 2001). These four existential issues are juxtaposed with K. Moses's (1989) model of the grief response, which includes denial, anxiety, fear, depression, anger, and guilt. Suggestions for responding within one's scope of practice are provided. When combined, existential and grieving models can offer clinicians new insight into clients' loss

resolution work. This inner work constitutes a spiritual journey that can parallel the journey through therapy and rehabilitation. The case has been made that attending to these issues can enhance long-term outcomes of treatment (Spillers, 2007).

b. A systematic review of the literature on predictors of complicated grief (CG) was undertaken. Predictors of CG before the death include previous loss, exposure to trauma, a previous psychiatric history, attachment style, and the relationship to the deceased. Factors associated with the death include violent death, the quality of the caregiving or dying experience, close kinship relationship to the deceased, marital closeness and dependency, and lack of preparation for the death. Perceived social support played a key role after the death, along with cognitive appraisals and great distress at the time of the death (Lobb et al., 2010).

3. Assessment
   a. Observe for appetite loss, fatigue, apathy, lack of socialization, somatic complaints, and decreased activities.
   b. Observe the client's emotions (e.g., feelings of emptiness and numbness, low self-esteem, sadness, guilt) (Stuart, 2013).
   c. Observe the client's level of willingness to participate in rehabilitation.
4. Nursing interventions
   a. Encourage family and friends to reassure the client that he or she is loved for himself or herself, not for his or her appearance, physical abilities, or work capacity.
   b. Foster peer modeling and mentoring (Kent et al., 2013).
   c. Encourage the client and family to seek psychological counseling.
   d. Help the client build a social, cultural, and economic network of support.
   e. Help the client cultivate a positive and realistic outlook (Tyrrell, Levack, Ritchie, & Keeling, 2012).
   f. Allow time for adjustment because clients often do not internalize the entire impact of a disability until the rehabilitation phase of treatment.
   g. Refer the client for interpersonal psychotherapy, which focuses on grief, interpersonal role disputes, and role transitions (Wyman-Chick, 2012).
5. Research study findings
   a. Focusing beyond survival, the priority of modern burn care is an optimal quality of life. The aim of one study, which was informed by phenomenology, was to describe and identify invariant meanings in the experience of life after major burn injury. Fourteen adults who had sustained a major burn were interviewed, on average, 14 months after injury, and asked about their experience of important aspects of life. The accident meant facing an extreme situation that demanded vigilance, appropriate action, and the need for assistance. The aftermath of the burn injury and treatment included having to put significant effort into creating coherence in their disrupted personal life stories. Continuing life meant accepting the unchangeable, including going through recurrent processes of enduring grief, fatalism, comparisons with others, and new feelings of gratefulness. Furthermore, a continuous struggle to change what was changeable and to achieve personal goals, independence, relationships with others, and a meaningful life were all efforts to regain freedom, aiming for a life as it was before—and sometimes even better (Moi & Gjengedal, 2008).
   b. Despite its popularity, few attempts have been made to empirically test the stage theory of grief. This study aimed to replicate and extend the findings of Maciejewski, Zhang, Block, and Prigerson (2007), who found that different states of grieving can peak in a sequence that is consistent with stage theory. The association between time since loss and five grief indicators (focusing on disbelief, anger, yearning, depression, and acceptance) among an ethnically diverse sample of young adults who had been bereaved by natural ($n = 441$) and violent ($n = 173$) causes was explored. In general, limited support was found for stage theory, alongside some evidence of an "anniversary reaction" marked by heightened distress and reduced acceptance for participants approaching the second anniversary of the death. Overall, sense making emerged as a much stronger predictor of grief indicators than time since the loss, highlighting the relevance of a meaning-oriented perspective (Holland & Neimeyer, 2010).

E. Stigma
1. Definition: *Stigma* is the application of set attitudes about and stereotypes of people with disabilities. Stigma begins in the attitudes of others but can be internalized by the person with a

disability and eventually influence that person's behaviors (Goffman, 1974). Goodman (2014, p. 203) described stigma as arising from "ignorance (lacking the relevant knowledge), prejudices (attitudes that people hold), and discrimination (behaviors)."

2. Middle-range theory: The Framework Integrating Normative Influences on Stigma (FINIS) brings together theoretical insights from micro-, meso-, and macro-level research, including the understanding that stigma occurs in social relationships. All social interactions take place in a context in which organizations, media, and larger cultures structure normative expectations, which creates the possibility of marking difference. FINIS offers the potential to build a broad-based scientific foundation based on an understanding of the effects of stigma on the lives of people with mental illness and disability, the resources devoted to the organizations and families who care for them, and policies and programs designed to combat stigma (Pescosolido, Martin, Lang, & Olafsdottir, 2008).
3. Assessment
   a. Observe for statements of self-deprecation.
   b. Observe for self-isolating behaviors.
   c. Observe alienation and hostility by others.
   d. Note family and friends' attitudes toward people with disabilities.
4. Nursing interventions
   a. Encourage the client to reevaluate the importance of physique.
   b. Encourage a realistic appraisal of the difficulties of dealing with disability.
   c. Encourage the evaluation of personal assets and abilities.
   d. Encourage the client and family to focus on the total person, not just the disability.
   e. Provide counseling on dealing with stigma in the community.
   f. Encourage positive images of those with disabilities in the media, business, academia, athletics, and music.
   g. Ensure that children and adults with disabilities are mainstreamed into educational and recreational activities.
5. Research study findings
   a. The author used phenomenological (i.e., interpretive) ethnography to investigate the experience of physical disability and its attached meanings in relation to self, world, and other for adolescents born with spina bifida. In-depth interviews were conducted with 11 late-stage adolescents (18–24 years of age), and analysis revealed the theme "experiencing self as dissimilar other." Findings implied that adolescents born with spina bifida face biological, psychological, and social challenges that might interfere with normative developmental tasks of adolescence, including identity formation. Greater emphasis must be directed toward humanizing and emancipating the physical and social environment for young people with physical disabilities to maximize developmental opportunities and potential while fostering positive identity (Kinavey, 2007).

F. Hope and Hopelessness

1. Definitions
   a. *Hope*: Key dimensions "include (i) time, both past experience as well as the important future reference of hope; (ii) broad and specific goals; (iii) control, which may be internal (personal activity) and/or external (environmental and contextual factors); (iv) relations, such as partnerships and spirituality or a sense of purpose in life; and (v) personal characteristics such as inner strength, motivation and energy to pursue one's goals. The concept includes a (vi) reality reference, in that the desired outcomes or goals are subjectively perceived as being possible, and (vii) it allows for hope to arise both from a negative as well as a positive starting point, i.e., as a desire for the improvement of an undesirable or an already satisfactory situation" (Schrank, Hayward, Stanghellini, & Davidson, 2011, pp. 229–230).
   b. *Hopelessness*: A sustained subjective emotional state in which a person sees no alternatives or personal choices available to solve problems or to achieve what is desired and cannot mobilize energy on his or her own behalf to establish goals (Carpenito-Moyet, 2010)
      1) Associated feelings of hopelessness include powerlessness, despair, helplessness, and apathy.
2. Middle-range theory
   a. The aim of this longitudinal study was to deepen the understanding of the phenomenon of hope and develop a theoretical framework of hope in a context of SCI. Findings revealed nine themes: universal hope, uncertain hope, hope as a turning point, the power of hope, boundless creative and flexible hope, enduring hope, despairing hope, body-related hope, and existential hope. The conceptual model was derived from these themes, illustrated as the battle between hoping and suffering and the

road of hope. The interpretations also revealed a distinction between being in hope and having hope, and having a hope of improvements was the main focus at the early stage of rehabilitation, whereas being in hope as being just fine was the main focus after 3–4 years of rehabilitation (Lohne, 2008).

3. Assessment
   a. Observe for the characteristics of powerlessness, despair, and apathy.
   b. Observe for the lack of initiative for self-help.
   c. Observe for depression.
4. Nursing interventions
   a. Enhance the client's sense of power, which precedes hopefulness.
   b. Establish short- and long-term goals with the client and family.
   c. Encourage family and social support.
   d. Encourage spiritual empowerment and strength.
   e. Encourage use of the word *hope*, characterized by active responsibility, rather than the word *hopeful*, which is more passive (Kautz, 2006, October).
5. Research study findings
   a. Lohne and Severinsson (2006) conducted a qualitative study to examine the experience of hope for those with SCI. The findings indicated that hope was important because it provided the energy and power to achieve progress and personal development after injury.

G. Powerlessness

1. Definition: *Powerlessness* is the inability to use personal energy to initiate and guide personal behavior. When patients are hindered in participating or taking responsibility in their care in a treatment or rehabilitation setting, they can feel powerless (Berglund, Westin, Svanström, & Sundler, 2012). In addition, powerlessness can be heightened when a patient feels he or she has low outcome expectancy related to wound or disease status, is not able to change health outcomes, and has personal habits or behaviors that can negatively affect health, such as substance abuse (Sheridan et al., 2012).
   a. The lack of personal power makes a person powerless, which is destructive to the self (Satir, 1988).
   b. Powerlessness can be learned through negative reinforcement of dependency.
   c. Powerlessness as a reaction to threats can lead to patterns of impotence, withdrawal, and passiveness.
2. Middle-range theory
   a. This review provides the foundations on which to construct a framework of power and powerlessness. Current frameworks, such as antioppressive practice, could be insufficient in identifying the range and complexity of power relationships that can be enacted within a social situation. A framework for analyzing the operation of different forms of power, one that acknowledges the potential of power to be both damaging and productive, is presented. There is an exploration of how the framework can provide a useful tool for underpinning emancipatory practice (Tew, 2006).
3. Assessment
   a. Note a lack of initiative in goal planning and achievement.
   b. Note passivity.
   c. Note withdrawal from family, social, and vocational decisions and interactions.
   d. Assess apprehension and fear.
4. Nursing interventions (Stuart, 2013)
   a. Encourage the client and family to maintain control in decision making, and promote environmental predictability and emotional support.
   b. Help the client realize that although the injury or illness that led to the disability cannot be changed, his or her response to the disability is a personal choice.
   c. Enable the client and family to recognize and mobilize their strengths and resources, feel confident, and use effective coping skills.
   d. Encourage the client to achieve self-direction and self-determination.
   e. Encourage the client and family to seek spiritual support.
   f. Encourage and value the client and family's involvement as participants in the interdisciplinary team.
   g. Encourage the client's involvement with group and community support systems.
   h. Provide follow-up rehabilitation care in the home setting if applicable.
5. Research study findings
   a. Clinical example: Injury or illness leading to disability can destroy a person's normal level of life control and predictability. Relocation stress experienced during the recovery and rehabilitation process and powerlessness are influenced by a decrease in biopsychosocial status, anxiety, depression, apprehension, guilt,

denial, and lowered self-esteem (Nypaver, Titus, & Brugler, 1996).

b. Aujoulat, Luminet, and Deccache (2007) explored situations and feelings of powerlessness from which a process of empowerment might evolve. They conducted 40 interviews of people with various chronic conditions and looked for the commonalities in their experiences. Powerlessness extends well beyond medical- and treatment-related issues and can include distressing feelings of insecurity and a threat to social and personal identities (Aujoulat et al., 2007).

c. Berglund and colleagues (2012) noted in their phenomenological analysis of participants across the life span that support and knowledge were key means of increasing power and enhancing influence when patients enter healthcare settings. These needs were often unmet after interaction with healthcare professionals, as patients' uncertainty or fears were not addressed.

H. Self-Efficacy

1. Definition: *Self-efficacy* is a sense of control that consists of coping with, appraising, and managing one's life and leads to the conviction that the person can determine behaviors that lead to desired outcomes (Bandura, 1977).

2. Middle-range theory

a. Self-efficacy, a core construct of Bandura's social cognitive theory, has wide appeal and usefulness in the health and social sciences. Self-efficacy is frequently used across disciplines to assess a person's beliefs about his or her likelihood to engage in a certain behavior. Several factors contribute to inaccurate or inappropriate assessment, measurement, interpretation, and application of this important construct; numerous scales used to measure efficacy, various contexts, related constructs, and moderating effects of efficacy make it difficult to achieve best use of efficacy measurement and application. A study by O'Sullivan & Strauser (2009) outlined the theory of self-efficacy, distinguished its closely related constructs, summarized common moderating effects, and provided important considerations for clinical practice and research.

3. Assessment

a. Investigate the client and family's short- and long-term goals.

b. Identify fears of and barriers to self-efficacy.

c. Identify learning needs associated with self-efficacy.

d. Identify resources needed for self-efficacy.

e. Identify the client's ability to provide or direct self-care.

f. Identify the client's ability to manage the vocational and recreational aspects of life.

4. Nursing interventions

a. Individualize self-care education for the client and family.

b. Encourage the client to choose activities.

c. Encourage opportunities for self-responsibility.

d. Encourage behaviors and activities that lead to self-assurance.

e. Encourage alternative solutions for problem solving.

f. Provide opportunities to practice and direct self-care.

g. Provide resources for education and vocational development.

h. Provide opportunities for recreation and socialization.

i. Provide resources for goal achievement.

j. Encourage the client to evaluate the situation completely.

k. Plan with goal setting and identification of resources.

5. Research study findings

a. Exercise adherence after cardiac rehabilitation (CR) is problematic. Effects of an intervention targeting self-efficacy, outcome expectations, and adherence to upper-body resistance exercise after CR were explored. Clients in cardiac rehabilitation ($N = 40$) were randomly allocated to receive either standard exercise recommendations (wait-list control) or an intervention involving a theory-based instructional manual and Thera-Band resistive bands for upper-body resistance exercise. Self-efficacy and outcome expectations were assessed at baseline and 4 weeks later. Participation in resistance exercise was measured 4 weeks after baseline and at 3-month follow-up. The intervention group reported higher levels of self-efficacy, outcome expectations, and resistance exercise volume compared with the control group at the 4-week follow-up. Adherence differences were sustained at 3-month follow-up, with some evidence that self-efficacy for adhering to resistance training mediated the effects of the intervention on follow-up exercise training frequency (Millen & Bray, 2009).

b. Using a pretest-posttest design, Hartley, Vance, Elliott, Cuckler, and Berry (2008) tested the relationships between hope, self-efficacy for rehabilitation, depression, and functional ability reported by people undergoing joint replacement surgery. One hundred community-dwelling older adults were administered measures of hope, self-efficacy for rehabilitation, pain, depression, body mass index, and mental status 1 month before and 6 weeks after joint replacement surgery. Demographic, health information, and functional outcome measures were also obtained. Hope was significantly predictive of presurgery depression, but it was not predictive of depression or functional ability after surgery. Higher levels of self-efficacy were predictive of lower postsurgery depression scores. Results imply that social cognitive constructs could have utility in the prediction of emotional adjustment before and after joint surgery, but they could have limited value in anticipating functional abilities after these surgeries. Theoretical and clinical implications are discussed.

I. Suicidal Behavior

1. Definitions
   a. *Suicidal behavior* exists on a continuum from ideation to completion.
   b. *Suicidal ideation* encompasses feelings and thoughts related to death wishes and potential suicide.
   c. *Suicide attempt* is a sequence of behaviors that are initiated by the client, who expects that this set of actions will lead to her or his own death.
   d. *Suicide* is the term now used for cases in which a suicide attempt leads to death. Lethality is also sometimes used as a descriptor. Terms such as *successful suicide* are no longer used (Van Orden et al., 2010).
      1) Risk for suicide increases with the presence of chronic medical illnesses as well as chronic pain (Gray, 2013). It is believed that the cause for this is multifactorial. Acute brain injuries can lead to disinhibition and increased impulsivity. Depression or psychosis secondary to chronic medical illness can also lead to increased risk. In addition, chronic pain or altered self-image could be overwhelming for some clients, heightening the risk for suicide. Other risk factors for suicide include a previous suicide attempt, access to lethal weapons such as firearms, being single or widowed, sexual orientation (i.e., lesbian, gay, bisexual, or transgender); family history of suicide, history of childhood abuse, and the presence of personal risk factors such as hopelessness. Males are more likely to complete a suicide than females and may use more lethal means. Lastly, 90% of those who complete suicide had been diagnosed (or were diagnosable) with a psychiatric disorder at the time of their death. A common myth some nurses believe is that asking about suicide will increase their clients' risk of suicidal behavior; however, that is not true.
2. Assessment
   a. Lethality assessment can be completed when a client expresses suicidal ideation. According to the American Association of Suicidology (2012), the assessment includes inquiry, documentation, and follow-up of the following components:
      1) An estimation of immediate risk of life-threatening behavior (e.g., cutting)
      2) Directly asking "Are you thinking of suicide?"
      3) An assessment of suicidal ideation, intent, and plan to include the means, such as access to a firearm or other weapon, and whether an attempt is in progress
      4) Previous suicide attempts and lethality of any attempts
      5) Depth or level of depressed mood
      6) Prior psychiatric or mental health history
      7) Substance use and current status
      8) Stressors (e.g., loss, financial, chronic medical conditions, chronic pain)
      9) Degree of hopelessness and helplessness
      10) Use and availability of family, community, and other support resources
   b. SADPERSONS scale (Sex, Age, Depression, Previous attempt, Ethanol abuse, Rational thinking loss, Social supports lacking, Organized plan, No spouse, and Sickness)
3. Nursing interventions (Gray, 2013)
   a. Take time to establish rapport, appear unrushed, and provide privacy.
   b. Start with open-ended and general questions, then move to more specific questions such as: "Do you ever think you would be better off dead?"
   c. Assess for frequency, duration, and intensity of suicidal thoughts and feelings, as well as hopelessness and future orientation (i.e., negativity regarding the future)

d. Plan for continued care or disposition with appropriate follow-up. Remove access to firearms or other means for suicide. Provide contact numbers for crisis hotlines and support services. Involve family as much as possible with specific and direct information regarding warning signs and symptoms as well as need for return/follow-up.

4. Research study findings
   a. Suicide contracts are no longer used, because evidence-based practice does not support their efficacy. A brief crisis intervention to reduce suicidal risk could be completed using the Crisis Response Plan model (Stanley & Brown, 2012). Safety planning can be completed with the client and their family and involves reviewing five components, including personal warning signs; self-management strategies such as internal coping strategies and reasons for living; social support such as friends, family, or support groups; and contact information for crisis management including clinician names/numbers and information about the crisis hotline. One strategy that has been used is to have the client write down this information on a 3 x 5 or similar-sized card and carry it with him or her to enhance self-efficacy and recovery.

III. Roles and Relationships Related to Psychosocial Health

A. Types of Families

1. Description (refer to Chapter 18 for additional information on family roles and theories)
   a. The family unit is an active, operating system.
   b. The person with disability is not in isolation but is considered in the context of family.
   c. Family relationships are the living links that bind the family together.
   d. As a system, the family assigns roles and rules that are established for each member.
   e. Functions of the family include acquiring the means to provide for the necessities of daily life.
   f. The family is essential for dealing with internal change and external disruptions.
2. Nurturing families
   a. Characteristics include a sense of aliveness, affection, genuineness, honesty, open communication, and love.
   b. Nurturing families make plans, adjust plans, problem solve without panic, and accept change as part of life.
3. Troubled families
   a. Characteristics include coldness, rigidity, control, guarded communication; tolerance rather than love; and secrecy.
   b. Adjustment and problem solving are difficult because family members rigidly hold on to assigned roles and responsibilities (Satir, 1988).
4. The effect of disability on a family
   a. Any family member's disability can cause permanent disruptions in family patterns.
   b. Established roles and responsibilities of the family change.
   c. Life patterns continue to change as children mature, siblings marry, members move away, parents grow older, health status changes within the family, and family members die.
   d. Problem solving and adapting to change are necessary skills for positive family life.
5. Middle-range theory
   a. The concept of family-centered care was introduced to the public more than 4 decades ago, stressing the importance of the family in a child's well-being. Since then, family-centered values and practices have been widely implemented in child and adult health care. Bamm and Rosenbaum (2008) offer an overview of the development and evolution of family-centered theory as an underlying conceptual foundation for contemporary health services. The focus includes key concepts, accepted definitions, barriers, and supports that can influence successful implementation and discussion of the valid quantitative measures of family-centeredness currently available to evaluate service delivery. They also provide the foundation and propose questions for future research (Bamm & Rosenbaum, 2008).
   b. Military personnel returning from war with TBI present with a complex array of stressors encountered during combat and on reentry, often with additional physical and mental health comorbidities. Family-focused therapy is uniquely suited to address the complex issues presented by returning military personnel. The adaptation of an existing family intervention for a chronic condition that focuses on enhancing both individual and family functioning is a useful for working with veterans and others with TBI (Dausch & Saliman, 2009).
6. Assessment
   a. Observe family members' communication patterns.
   b. Observe the family's cohesiveness during change.

c. Examine the family's planning strategies.
d. Examine the family's actions, behaviors, and roles.

7. Nursing interventions
   a. Encourage family therapy with a focus on the entire family. This should include information about the injury or illness, strategies for handling emotional distress, assistive services, opportunities to share concerns, and assistance with coping (Butcher, 1994).
   b. Provide training in communication skills (e.g., structured marriage-enrichment programs, effective listening, self-awareness, conflict resolution) (Captain, 1995).
   c. Provide the means for lifetime planning for continued care (costs of long-term needs, costs of care and rehabilitation) (Deutsch, Allison, & Cimino-Ferguson, 2005).
   d. Help the client and family identify and cope with changes in roles and responsibilities caused by disability (Paterson & Stewart, 2002).
8. Research study findings
   a. The disability of one family member who needs inpatient rehabilitation care can negatively affect all family members and ultimately disrupt family integrity. Current research findings indicate that rehabilitation nurses are in a key position to promote hope and family integrity by facilitating open communication between family members, fostering a tone of togetherness within and between families, and helping families resolve feelings of guilt and move toward forgiveness. Kautz and Van Horn (2009) presented a review of research to support these activities and offered practical suggestions for rehabilitation nurses to incorporate these strategies into their daily practice with clients and their families.

B. Social Support
1. Definition: *Social support* is a multifaceted concept that includes instrumental support (e.g., equipment, services); affective support (e.g., concern, being loved, feeling important, supportive presence); and cognitive support (e.g., education, advice, information, role modeling, counseling) (Rintala, Young, Spencer, & Bates, 1996).
2. Middle-range theory
   a. Through in-depth interviews, the process of recovery after total hip replacement (THR) surgery from the perspective of the older adult was explored. In-depth interviews were conducted with 10 people older than 65 years old who had been discharged from the hospital for a period of 4–6 months after THR surgery. Findings showed that three distinct but interrelated processes constitute the physical, psychological, and social recovery process: reclaiming physical ability, re-establishing roles and relationships, and refocusing self. Intervening conditions that affect the recovery process include comorbid conditions, the personal outlook of the client, clients' relationships, and social support. The recovery process can lead to changes in personal and social functioning that clients might not anticipate (Grant, St. John, & Patterson, 2009).
3. Assessment
   a. Observe for barriers in socialization (e.g., fatigue, multiple problems, isolation, lack of self-confidence, apathy) (Abjornsson, Orbaek, & Hagstadius, 1998).
   b. Observe the frequency of contact with family and friends and leisure and physical activities.
   c. Use the Life Satisfaction Index (Diener, 1984).
   d. Use the Sickness Impact Profile (De Bruin, Diederiks, De Witte, Stevens, & Philipsen, 1994).
   e. Use the Community Integration Questionnaire (Willer, Ottenbacher, & Coad, 1994).
   f. Use the Quality of Social Support instrument (Bethoux, Calmels, Gautheron, & Minaire, 1996).
   g. Observe the client's patterns of behaviors such as alcohol use after injury. Increased consumption of alcohol is associated with lower levels of social support (Boraz & Heinemann, 1996).
4. Nursing interventions
   a. Encourage the client to use problem- and emotion-focused coping skills.
   b. Encourage social networking (Cormier-Daigle & Stewart, 1997).
   c. Involve the spouse with instrumental (i.e., task-oriented) and emotional support.
   d. Encourage the client to engage in meaningful, rewarding activities.
   e. Encourage social roles for identity, power, and family position (Nir, Wallhagen, Doolittle, & Galinsky, 1997).
   f. Encourage the client to attend support groups.
   g. Provide crisis therapy and stress management.
   h. Encourage cognitive activation and memory training (Abjornsson et al., 1998).
   i. Encourage the use of support groups using computer-based systems. This is especially helpful for those in rural areas or with

fewer transportation resources (Hill, Schillo, & Weinert, 2004).

j. Provide access for social support to promote participation in life situations (Lund, Nordlund, Nygard, Lexell, & Bernspang, 2005).

k. Encourage the peer mentoring experience as a complement to social support (Sherman, Sperling, & DeVinney, 2004).

l. Encourage emotion-focused coping to promote social reintegration. Other pertinent factors for social reintegration include family support, information, and removal of social barriers (Song, 2005).

5. Research study findings

a. Isaksson, Skar, and Lexell (2005) conducted a qualitative study among women with SCI to investigate perceptions of social networking. Data analysis indicated that the subjects needed the social support to function in their occupations. The subjects also reported that they established new relationships with other people who had disabilities.

b. The Multidimensional Scale of Perceived Social Support instrument was used to measure self-reported adequacy of social support (family, friends, and significant others) with 560 coronary artery disease patients who were enrolled in a cardiac rehabilitation program (Staniute, Brozaitiene, & Bunevicius, 2013). Stressful life events and social support had an independent effect on health related quality of life. For women, lower scores in psychological domains of health-related quality of life were found in those who believed they lacked social support. Researchers suggest that nursing interventions could need to target those who experience high levels of health-status–related stress and report low social support in rehabilitation settings.

c. Ferguson, Richie, and Gomez (2004) conducted a qualitative study to investigate the psychological factors contributing to recovery for those with traumatic amputations. Results of the study indicated that acceptance of the loss and level of psychological recovery were greatly influenced by social support and societal attitudes toward the disabled.

C. Independence and Dependence

1. Independence can be fostered when people with disabilities have responsibility for self-care and are expected to participate in family roles.

2. Dependence can result when clients are not encouraged to take control of their situations.

3. Middle-range theory

a. Self-responsibility and self-control are meaningful values in the activities and decisions of everyday life. Dignity and being respected as an individual are closely connected to the ability to manage on one's own and remain independent of others' help. Including other people into one's life situation can be an important sign of self-management. However, the critical interpretation shows that it is the view of the human being that determines whether help from others and managing on one's own can be combined. With a relational view of the human being (i.e., the basic condition that people always enter into relationships of dependence), there is no contradiction between independence and dependence. The objective of the interview study was to highlight themes in the clients' views of health and illness related to their chronic condition and the significance of these views for their mastery of everyday life (Delmar et al., 2006).

4. Assessment

a. Observe for initiation of ADLs.

b. Assess the client's level of functional abilities.

c. Assess the client's cognitive abilities.

d. Use the FIM™ instrument to assess cognitive and functional abilities and the need for supervision, especially for clients with TBI (Smith & Schwirian, 1998).

e. Observe participation in academic and vocational activities.

f. Assess for initiation of recreational activities.

g. Assess for perceptions of poor health and emotional distress, which are often associated with increased dependency (Janssen, 2011).

h. Use the FAMTOOL (a family health assessment tool) to evaluate communication; shared beliefs; shared work and play; value connectedness; and effort toward physical, emotional, social, and spiritual health (Weeks & O'Connor, 1997).

i. Assess role expectations from the different viewpoints of family members, especially those related to pressures, demands, personal resources, and family structure (Satir, 1988).

j. Use the QOL Scale (Ferrans, 1996).

5. Nursing interventions

a. Encourage independence within the family unit.

b. Provide more intensive family support during transitional periods (e.g., moving from acute

care to rehabilitation, rehabilitation to home, home to independence).
   c. Eliminate environmental barriers.
   d. Provide resources for adaptive housing, equipment, and attendant care (Brillhart & Johnson, 1997).
   e. Encourage thoughts such as "I have control of my life," "I can do things," "I feel close to others," and "Others understand me" to promote independence (Secrest, 2006).
   f. Encourage family counseling
      1) Appropriate support for the client
      2) Education about the client's discomfort with being a unilateral receiver and burden rather than a bidirectional receiver and giver
      3) The appropriate help needed by the client
   g. Encourage the family to reestablish life trajectories, meet developmental needs, and reintegrate the survivor into the family (Brzuzy & Speziale, 1997).
6. Research study findings
   a. Elfstrom, Ryden, Kreuter, Taft, and Sullivan (2005) investigated the relationship between coping strategies and QOL among 256 people with SCI. The findings of this study indicated that revaluation of life values (acceptance) and fewer dependency behaviors (social reliance) were positively related to QOL.
   b. Stephens and Yoshida (1999) examined issues of autonomy and independence in the lives of people with rheumatoid arthritis. The subjective experiences of the informants were examined using qualitative interviews. The data show that the personal meanings people give to being independent or dependent involve issues of autonomy. Autonomy issues are manifested in restricted choice and control regarding one's body and disease, everyday tasks and routines (and related use of assistance and aids), lifestyle patterns, and major life decisions. Although independence and autonomy are interrelated concepts, the connection has not received much attention in the rehabilitation literature because of the dominance of the ADL perspective. The authors argued that attention to everyday autonomy furthers our understanding of the personal and social impact of a disabling condition.

D. Helplessness
1. Definition: *Helplessness* is the belief that a person is dependent on others for support for a situation that seems impossible to change. The person could perceive that events are beyond his or her control.
2. Middle-range theory
   a. Faulkner (2001) investigated the relevance of learned helplessness (LH) and learned mastery (LM) theories in the respective development of dependence and independence in older hospitalized people. Participants exposed to the LH-inducing strategy demonstrated LH effects within both the meal and psychomotor tasks. These effects were alleviated through exposing participants to the LM-inducing intervention. Exposing older hospitalized people to uncontrollable or disempowering circumstances can potentially lead them to develop an LH-induced dependence. This can be alleviated by increasing the client's expectation of control, leading to the development of LM.
3. Assessment
   a. Observe for inactivity and nonparticipation in rehabilitation.
   b. Observe for self-isolation and withdrawal.
   c. Observe for general behaviors (e.g., slow movements, low voice tones, sitting alone quietly).
   d. Observe for disturbances in motivation, cognition, and emotion.
   e. Observe for the absence of voluntary response to a situation.
   f. Observe for learned dependence (i.e., the inability to act and make decisions).
   g. Observe for fear and depression.
   h. Observe for suicidal ideation and behaviors.
4. Nursing interventions
   a. Foster voluntary responses and independence.
   b. Encourage learning and reinforce successes.
   c. Form the expectation of independence for the client and family.
   d. Encourage the client to evaluate his or her personal assets and affirm his or her feelings or expressions of hope.
   e. Encourage memory and increased coping abilities (Davidhizar, 1997).
   f. Refer the client for psychotherapy as necessary.
5. Research study findings
   a. The outcome expectation for exercise (OEE), helplessness, and literacy on arthritis outcomes in two community-based, randomized controlled trials were examined. Findings indicated that disability after intervention was not predicted by helplessness, literacy, or OEE. Helplessness predicted pain, fatigue, and

stiffness (Bhat, DeWalt, Zimmer, Fried, & Callahan, 2010).

IV. Coping and Stress Tolerance

A. Coping

1. Description
   a. *Coping* is defined as cognitive and behavioral efforts directed toward managing demanding and stressful situations.
      1) Problem-focused coping efforts are directed toward decreasing or eliminating threats.
      2) Emotion-focused coping efforts are directed toward decreasing negative emotions.
   b. Personal competence with coping includes many factors (Satir, 1988) such as
      1) The components of relationships (being content with self and others)
      2) Differentiation (distinguishing between self and others)
      3) Autonomy (relying on self, separately and distinctly from others)
      4) Self-esteem (feeling worthy about self)
      5) Power (using energy to initiate and guide behaviors)
      6) Productivity (manifesting competence)
      7) Love (being compassionate, accepting, and giving as well as receiving affection)
   c. The antecedents of stress require coping skills, including
      1) Personal and environmental demands that exceed resources
      2) Ambiguity and uncertainty
      3) Loss of control
      4) Loss of social support
   d. Many variables influence coping efforts, such as
      1) Developmental age
      2) Severity of disability
      3) Visibility of disability
      4) Threat of chronicity
      5) Sense of control
      6) Prior coping abilities
      7) Self-esteem
      8) Values
      9) Perceived social support
2. Middle-range theory
   a. Factors associated with the development and persistence of work disability can be related to the worker, work environment, compensation policies, healthcare system, and insurance system. Workers' understanding and representations of their disability are associated with coping behaviors aimed at helping them adapt to or solve their health problem. Theories from anthropology, sociology, and psychology are analyzed to gain a better understanding of their application to people with work-related injuries. The identified models are mainly descriptive. Integrating unique perspectives and taking social interactions into account can enhance understanding of workers' representations and the behaviors they adopt to manage their musculoskeletal-disorder–related disability (Coutu, Baril, Durand, Côté, & Rouleau, 2007).
3. Assessment
   a. Assess the level and sources of stress expressed by the client and family.
   b. Assess the client's ability to solve problems.
   c. Note changes in the client and family's abilities to meet their needs.
   d. Note changes in communication patterns that reflect frustration (e.g., verbal manipulation, hostility).
   e. Note inappropriate behavior, activity, and responses that reflect frustration.
   f. Use the Assessment Instrument of Problem-Focused Coping, a self-report instrument that focuses on a person's own assessment of competence in coping with ADLs, personal problems, and level of satisfaction with ADLs (Tollen & Ahlstrom, 1998).
   g. Use the Multidimensional Acceptance of Loss Scale, developed by Ferrin (2002), which evaluates the ability to enlarge the scope of values, contain the disability, subordinate the physique, and change comparative status values to asset values.
   h. Assess the continuing impact of chronic illness and exacerbation of symptoms (Stuifbergen, 2005).
   i. Assess spirituality as a factor in QOL (Vespa, Jacobsen, Spazzafumo, & Balducci, 2011).
4. Nursing interventions
   a. Provide rehabilitation and education, and locate resources beyond personal care and independence, which can allow people with disability to expand their leisure and productive roles and promote socioeconomic integration (Forhan & Backman, 2010).
   b. Explore the meaning of illness for the client and family, which can lead to understanding their behaviors and responses.
      1) The meaning the client or family associates with illness can have a profound effect on coping and adjustment and can influence relationships with the healthcare team.

2) The meaning of illness is influenced by cultural beliefs, religion, values, life philosophy, and past experiences (Howell, 1998).

c. Encourage purposeful and meaningful time expenditure, which contributes to an improved QOL even more than the ability to be independent with ADLs (Cardol, Elvers, Oostendorp, Brandsma, & deGroot, 1996).

d. Understand the unique experience of the person with disability as influenced by his or her psychological, emotional, and spiritual needs, and develop appropriate interventions to promote coping (Berman & Rose, 1998).

e. Encourage personal spirituality with the nurturing of friends, community, and family (Walton, Craig, Derwinski-Robinson, & Weinert, 2004).

f. Educate the family about the impact of chronic illness on the roles and responsibilities of those with chronic illness (Walton et al., 2004).

5. Research study findings

a. Polio survivors have been known for positive coping, resulting in achievements in family, social, and professional lives. Postpolio syndrome presents new challenges to independence and functional abilities. Life satisfaction scores of polio survivors are high, but postpolio syndrome is associated with declining scores. People with postpolio syndrome have new challenges such as muscle weakness, scoliosis, elimination problems, fatigue, and pain (Stuifbergen, 2005).

b. A survey of 230 people with SCI indicated that there was a significantly positive correlation between life satisfaction and spirituality. This study supported prior research demonstrating that levels of life satisfaction correlated with levels of spirituality. Spirituality included the concepts of faith, submission, and peace of mind (Brillhart, 2005).

c. In a descriptive study that examined the role of coping strategies as predictors of physical function and social adjustment in people with SCI, a sample of 128 community-residing people with SCI completed a structured questionnaire that included demographic characteristics and the Ways of Coping Questionnaire, Modified Barthel Index, and Social Adjustment Scale. Coping, physical function, and social adjustment, respectively, were measured. Among the eight factors of the Ways of Coping Questionnaire, planful problem solving was used most often by the participants (Song & Nam, 2010).

d. Parents of school-aged children with disabilities indicated by survey that parental coping was enhanced most often by spiritual support, passive appraisal, reframing, and mobilizing the family to accept help. The least common mechanisms for coping included maintaining family integration and understanding the child's health condition (Smith, Jackson, & Sharpe, 2006).

B. Stress

1. Definition: *Stress* has been delineated as a condition or circumstance that disturbs physical or psychological functioning in a person (Sadock, Sadock, & Ruiz, 2014). Exposure to a stressor can initiate a cascade of immune, endocrine, and neurotransmitter responses. The outcome of stress can be manifested in physical, social, cognitive, and/or psychological symptoms. A consortium definition by researchers (Koolhaas et al., 2011, p. 1,291) supports that "*stress* should be restricted to conditions in which an environmental demand exceeds the natural regulatory capacity of an organism; in particular, situations that include unpredictability and uncontrollability. Physiologically, stress seems to be characterized by either the absence of an anticipatory response (unpredictable) or a reduced recovery (uncontrollable) of the neuroendocrine reaction."

2. Middle-range theory

a. Testing a portion of the stress, appraisal, and coping model, Strom and Kosciulek (2007) developed a theoretical model that indicated that higher levels of perceived stress predicted higher levels of self-reported depression, higher levels of depression predicted lower levels of dispositional hope, and dispositional hope predicted increased life satisfaction and work productivity.

3. Assessment

a. Observe for physiological manifestations of stress (e.g., gastrointestinal distress, cardiac palpitations, anxious facial expressions, tremors).

b. Observe for emotional manifestations of stress (e.g., anxiety, emotional lability, restlessness, fright).

c. Observe for intellectual manifestations of stress (e.g., difficulty in concentration and memory, poor coping strategies).

d. Observe for spiritual manifestations of stress (e.g., value conflicts).

e. Observe for social manifestations of stress (e.g., role conflict, status incongruity, withdrawal, antagonism, role rigidity).

4. Nursing interventions
   a. Examine the source of stress (e.g., fears of failure, lack of resources, lack of support system, role loss, and ambiguity).
   b. Examine and reinforce prior successful coping measures.
   c. Provide crisis management.
   d. Consult with the client's case managers and social workers.
   e. Encourage the client to appraise stressors and his or her responses to stress and approaches to problem solving.
   f. Encourage the client and family to be flexible with roles and problem solving.
   g. Promote psychological hardiness by fostering control, commitment, and challenge for growth and development.
   h. Encourage the client to seek spiritual counseling and support.
   i. Encourage use of guided imagery as a relaxation technique to decrease stress (Nathenson, 2006, October).
5. Research study findings
   a. Rintala, Robinson-Whelen, and Matamoros (2005) reported that stressors among men with SCI were focused on problems with physical abilities, health, and finances. Stress was positively related to depression and anxiety and negatively related to life satisfaction. Finally, those with low levels of social support were more vulnerable to negative effects of stress.
   b. Ostwald, Swank, and Khan (2008) identified predictors of functional independence and perceived stress for stroke survivors discharged home from inpatient rehabilitation with a spousal caregiver. Stroke survivors perceived a 50% recovery in their function upon discharge from inpatient rehabilitation. Variables that predict the stroke survivors' recovery are complex, because the severity of the stroke combines with demographic and economic variables and depression to predict functional independence and perceived stress.

V. Psychosocial Disorders

This section provides an overview of relevant psychosocial disorders that can be experienced by patients who require rehabilitation nursing care. Mental health disorders are common in the United States and abroad and are experienced across the life span. It is believed that almost half of all lifetime cases of mental illness begin to emerge by the age of 14 years (National Institute of Mental Health [NIMH], 2009). In addition, individuals with one psychosocial disorder may be at increased risk for additional psychosocial comorbidities.

Nursing care can be especially challenging when working with patients with serious mental illness (SMI). It is estimated that almost 10,000,000 adults, or 4% of Americans, experience SMI (Substance Abuse and Mental Health Services Administration, 2012). SMI includes behavioral, emotional, or mental disorders that result in marked functional impairment and can impede the rehabilitation process. It has been determined that significant functional impairment, with concerns such as lower levels of physical activity and poor dietary habits, are commonly experienced by those with SMI and can contribute to poor overall health and early mortality (Happell, Stanton, Hoey, & Scott, 2014). Also, clients with SMI may make poor individual lifestyle choices such as smoking, have psychiatric symptoms that impair their ability to participate in treatment regimens for rehabilitation or recovery from physical disorders, and experience disparities when trying to access health care (De Hert, Cohen, et al., 2011; De Hert, Correll, et al., 2011). In addition, medications for those with SMI contribute to higher rates of obesity, metabolic syndrome, diabetes mellitus, and cardiovascular disease that can markedly affect recovery from both acute and chronic physical illness.

In this section, exemplars of SMI are reviewed, and relevant assessment and nursing interventions based on evidence-based practice are identified. Criteria listed in this section are based on disorders and diagnostic criteria classified in the *Diagnostic and Statistical Manual of Mental Disorders*, 5th edition (American Psychiatric Association [APA], 2013), the standard reference for clinical practice in the mental health field.

A. Anxiety Disorders/Generalized Anxiety Disorder (GAD)
   1. Description: Anxiety is a common human experience; often an adaptive and normal response that can serve as a warning of both external and internal threats. Anxiety can be experienced in a number of physical, often autonomic, symptoms such as headache, profuse sweating, and chest tightness. Anxiety becomes maladaptive and pathological when symptoms cause great distress and impairment in function. Often, comprehensive medical workups are completed to establish this diagnosis to rule out other causal entities such as medication side effects, medical conditions, or substance abuse (Parese, 2012). Medical conditions that can cause anxiety include hypoglycemia, irritable bowel syndrome, neurological disorders, cardiovascular disease such as congestive heart

failure and myocardial infarction, endocrine disorders such as thyroid disease, and inflammatory disorders such as lupus erythematosus.

a. Anxiety disorders include generalized anxiety disorder, phobic disorders, panic disorder, agoraphobia, specific phobia, substance/medication-induced anxiety disorder, separation anxiety disorder, and selective mutism (APA, 2013).
   1) Differ from each other by the type of objects or situations that induce avoidance behavior, fear, and/or anxiety plus related cognitive ideation
   2) Anxiety experienced within these disorders is beyond what would be considered a normative or developmentally appropriate anxiety or fear.
   3) Are typically long lasting—usually 6 months or longer.
   4) Individuals who experience anxiety disorders usually overestimate the danger in situations or conditions they fear or avoid.
   5) Women experience anxiety disorders twice as often as men do. Older adults are more likely to underreport or minimize anxiety symptoms, which could predict cognitive decline by as much as four times (Martin-Plank, 2014).
b. Anxiety disorders can have a profound influence on clients who are undergoing rehabilitative nursing care.
   1) Heightened psychological stress and anxiety impairs the physiological pathways of wound healing because of increased glucocorticoid and catecholamine production with diminished local proinflammatory cytokine production (Gouin & Kiecolt-Glaser, 2012).
   2) High levels of stress and anxiety can also increase susceptibility to infection and enhance wound hypoxia.
   3) Factors associated with high levels of stress and anxiety can hinder recovery from both surgery and illness and prolong the healing process.
c. Elevated anxiety symptoms as manifested in anxiety disorders can cause chronic disease processes to exacerbate and can place one at increased risk for morbidity and mortality.
   1) Watkins and colleagues (2013) found that heightened generalized anxiety was associated with a twofold increase in risk for mortality in clients with coronary heart disease.
   2) In a recent meta-analysis, elevated anxiety symptoms were associated with increased complications in diabetes, worsened blood glucose levels, greater symptom burden, and increased disability (Smith et al., 2013).
   3) Elevated anxiety symptoms were cited in another recent meta-analysis as being predictive of negative outcomes of chronic obstructive pulmonary disease, including chronic lung disease exacerbation and/or mortality (Atlantis, Fahey, Cochrane, & Smith, 2013).
d. The etiology of generalized anxiety disorder is unknown (Saddock, Saddock, & Ruiz, 2014)
   1) Possible biological causal factors: Dysfunction in regions such as the amygdala, hippocampus, locus ceruleus, and cortico-striato-thalamo-cortical circuits; changes in sleep architecture substance; subsensitivity of adrenergic receptors; alterations in basal ganglia; and white matter metabolic rates.
   2) Possible psychological causal factors: incorrect and inaccurate perception of danger, negative view of one's own ability to cope, and distortion in information processing.
e. Criteria for GAD (APA, 2013)
   1) Must have excessive worry and anxiety about several events or activities that occur more days than not for at least 6 months
   2) Client must find it difficult to control worry.
   3) Three or more of these symptoms must be present if an adult, or only one if a child:
      a) Feeling "keyed up" or restless
      b) Easily fatigued
      c) Feeling as if the mind is going blank or having difficulty with concentration
      d) Irritability
      e) Muscle tension
      f) Sleep disturbance
   4) The symptoms must cause clinically significant impairment or distress that is not attributable to or better explained by another mental disorder.

2. Assessment
   a. Scales and instruments
      1) Beck Anxiety Inventory
      2) Hamilton Anxiety Rating Scale-A
      3) Zung Self-Rated Anxiety Scale
      4) Self-Report for Childhood Anxiety Related Emotional Disorders

b. Related nursing diagnoses (NANDA International [NANDA-I]): anxiety, ineffective coping, readiness for enhanced coping, and fear (Stuart, 2013)
c. Symptoms of generalized anxiety can include heightened awareness of physical symptoms and sensations such as palpitations, syncope, feeling shaky, exaggerated startle response, upset stomach, and sweating, as well as awareness of feeling nervous or frightened.

3. Nursing interventions
a. Maintain and reassure safety in the environment, especially as it relates to the client's medical condition.
b. Encourage verbalization of fears with discussion of reality of the situation.
c. Assist client to face underlying feelings and developmental roots of worries that could be contributing to their irrational fears.
d. Assist client to rehearse and demonstrate adaptive ways of coping with stressors.
e. Support client to enhance self-efficacy in place of worry.
f. Teach stress management skills to interrupt escalating anxiety and promote the physical recovery process (e.g., progressive relation, deep breathing exercises/ breathing retraining, meditation, music therapy, body movement/exercise, grounding techniques, and yoga).
g. Medication administration and related patient teaching: Primarily selective serotonin reuptake inhibitors (SSRIs), serotonin and norepinephrine reuptake inhibitors (SNRIs), noradrenergic agents, benzodiazepines, buspirone, pregabalin, and gabapentin (Stahl, 2013)
h. Support services: Individual psychotherapy such as cognitive behavioral therapy that focuses on the impact of behaviors and emotions in the development and maintenance of anxiety (Behar, DiMarco, Hekler, Mohlman, & Staples, 2009).

B. Depressive Disorders/Major Depressive Disorder

1. Description: Mood disorders are one of the most common psychiatric problems encountered in both primary care and hospital settings. The World Health Organization ranks depression as the number-one cause of disability across the world (World Health Organization, 2012). Symptoms of depressive disorders can be affective and include depressed mood, irritability, anhedonia, and low motivation. They can also be vegetative in nature and can include lack of interest in usual activities, loss of appetite and weight, insomnia, psychomotor agitation or retardation, fatigue, and low energy. Cognitive symptoms of depression include feelings of worthlessness, excessive guilt, impaired concentration, and difficulty making decisions. Mood symptoms also can include thoughts of death with suicidal ideation. Up to 15% of those with depression have thoughts of suicide.
a. Groups at higher risk for depression include women and minorities (i.e., ethnic, racial, sexual), military personnel, and older adults.
1) Women, when in states of high hormonal fluctuation related to changing estrogen levels during puberty, intermittently during the menstrual cycle, and the postpartum and perimenopausal phases, are up to 70% more likely to experience depressive symptoms in comparison with men (Stahl, 2013).
2) Data from military samples yield significant findings (between 23% through 31% endorsement of depressive symptoms) on self-report (Ramsawh et al., 2014).
3) The Substance Abuse and Mental Health Services Administration (2008) reports that 9.3 % of veterans 21 to 39 years of age (312,000 persons) experienced at least one major depressive episode during the past year.
4) Up to 20% of those older than 65 years have experienced depressive symptoms in the United States (Centers for Disease Control and Prevention, 2014).
b. Only half of those identified with mood symptoms receive treatment, and only one fourth of those who enter treatment receive interventions that are evidence based (Mitchell, Vaze, & Rao, 2009).
c. Comorbidity with physical disease processes is documented.
1) Higher levels of depressive symptoms in clients have been linked to suboptimal glycemic control (Kendzor et al., 2014).
2) Associations have been identified between the presence of depressive disorders and subsequent development of micro- and macrovascular complications in those with type 2 diabetes (Pouwer, Nefs, & Nouwen, 2013.
3) Vascular complications can lead to an increased risk for blindness, amputations, myocardial infarction, stroke, end-stage renal disease, and death.

4) Indirectly, poor appetite, sleep impairment, and self-neglect experienced by some clients with depressive disorders can interfere with the immune system by disrupting the endocrine environment and macrophage and lymphocyte functioning in immune responses (Cole-King & Harding, 2001).
5) If the sleep-wake cycle is interrupted, the secretion of proinflammatory cytokines can be altered and cause disruption to the normal healing process.
6) Nurse-led proactive interventions that integrate the management of psychological and medical disease and illness have improved outcomes and rehabilitation for clients who experience depression and coronary heart disease, and/or diabetes (Katon et al., 2010).

d. The etiology of depression is thought to be multicausal (Stahl, 2013):
   1) Biological factors
      a) Monoamine transmitter system dysfunction (i.e., serotonin, dopamine, and norepinephrine) at receptor and cascade system beyond the point of regulation of gene expression
      b) Hypothalamic-pituitary-adrenal axis abnormalities
      c) Neurotropic model
      d) Cholinergic-adrenergic balance: Depression develops when norepinephrine and dopamine are low relative to acetylcholine.
      e) Role of chronic inflammation/infection on cortisol and immune system functioning: Cortisol receptors become desensitized, leading to increased activity of the proinflammatory immune mediators and neurotransmitter disturbances.
   2) Genetics
      a) Vulnerability genes and many environmental stressors that affect information processing in brain circuits and produce depressive symptoms
      b) Variability in genetic coding for serotonin transporter
   3) Psychological theories
      a) Cognitive theory: Cognitive distortions make people susceptible to depression, with a negative view of self, negative interpretation of experience, and negative view of the future.
      b) Learned helplessness: Depression can result from situations in which a person has lost (real or perceived) control over negative life events.
      c) Behavioral: Depressive symptoms result from either inadequate or insufficient positive reinforcement or the client's inability to take advantage of the reinforcement.
      d) Psychodynamic: Early loss causes vulnerability to depression and is associated with loss of relationships or other attachments.
      e) Object relations: Depression results when people's relationships leave them feeling unsafe and insecure.

e. Criteria for major depressive disorder (APA, 2013)
   1) Must have either depressed mood (irritable mood can be a symptom in a depressed child or teen) or anhedonia (i.e., a loss of interest or pleasure for most of the day) almost every day for 2 weeks, according to subjective report/observation by others.
   2) In addition, four or more of the following symptoms must be present:
      a) Weight changes: either loss or gain
      b) Sleep changes: hypersomnia or insomnia almost every day
      c) Psychomotor agitation or vegetation nearly every day
      d) Worthlessness or excessive/inappropriate guilt nearly every day
      e) Indecisiveness or decreased ability to concentrate nearly every day
      f) Recurrent suicidal ideation, suicide attempt or plan, or recurrent thoughts of death
   3) There has been no episode of mania or hypomania.
   4) The symptoms must cause clinically significant impairment or distress that is not attributable to or better explained by another mental disorder.

2. Assessment
   a. Scales and instruments
      1) Beck Depression Inventory
      2) Center for Epidemiological Studies Depression Scale
      3) Edinburg (postpartum)
      4) Geriatric Depression Scale
      5) Hamilton Depression Rating Scale
      6) Patient Health Questionnaire
      7) Zung Depression Scale
      8) PRIME-MD 2 Question Screen

b. Related nursing diagnoses (based on NANDA-I) involving maladaptive emotional responses include low self-esteem, hopelessness, powerlessness, risk for suicide, spiritual distress, and increased risk for self-directed violence (Stuart, 2013)

c. Symptoms of major depressive disorder (mild to severe) could include apathy, guilt, helplessness, hopelessness, low self-esteem, somatic complaints such as gastrointestinal distress and anergy ambivalence, pessimism, uncertainty, agitation, irritability, tearfulness, psychosis, and social withdrawal.

3. Nursing interventions
   a. Educate the client about depression, its causes, and the various treatments.
   b. Identify the interpersonal context of depression as it relates to symptom development and overall impact on the rehabilitation process.
   c. Inquire about suicidal ideation.
   d. Maintain and reassure safety related to risk of self-harm, and create a safety plan if appropriate.
   e. If vegetative symptoms are prominent, support the client to meet his or her basic self-care needs.
   f. Give the client more time to respond if he or she has decreased psychomotor energy. Allow for more time when performing self-care tasks, and break activities down into more manageable tasks.
   g. Augment patient teaching with written materials for later reference.
   h. Intervene to assist patient with weight gain or loss and related nutritional support.
   i. Discuss interaction between lifestyle, environment, and sleep, and create a sleep hygiene plan with client that includes the following: optimal sleep environment, sleep routines, over-the-counter sleep aids, and use of progressive relaxation.
   j. Use of cognitive strategies to include assisting the client to increase his or her sense of control over behavior and goals, increase self-esteem, and modify dysfunctional thinking patterns.
   k. Help client to focus on present activities versus past or future orientation.
   l. Provide reinforcement of positive aspects of client's behavior and self-control.
   m. Develop and encourage use of healthy support systems.
   n. Instruct and model more effective social skills.
   o. Assist the client to establish realistic goals for recovery.
   p. Medication administration and related patient teaching: SSRIs, SNRIs, serotonin partial agonist/reuptake inhibitors (SPARIs), bupropion, mirtazapine, trazodone, monoamine oxidase inhibitor inhibitors, and tricyclic antidepressants (Stahl, 2013).
   q. Can assist client and prepare for additional treatments such as electroconvulsant therapy in some settings.
   r. Support services
      1) Individual psychotherapy
         a) Cognitive behavioral therapy (CBT): Identify and categorize distorted automatic thoughts; identify underlying maladaptive assumptions and negative schema; use of a wide variety of techniques to challenge client thoughts, assumptions, and schemas; and use behavioral interventions to target characteristic deficits and excesses of behavior.
         b) Interpersonal therapy: focuses on the connection between interactions between people and the development of a person's psychiatric symptoms
         c) Problem-solving therapy
      2) Group/peer support
      3) Computer-based delivery of CBT and other treatment modalities
      4) Psychoeducation and bibliotherapy

C. Bipolar and Related Disorders: Bipolar Disorder I

1. Description: Bipolar disorder is less common than depressive disorders and is thought to affect about 1% of all adults (Stuart, 2013). Bipolar disorder is also associated with high comorbidity rates of substance abuse or dependence (60%–70%) and high rates of mortality. In comparison with the general population, rates of suicide attempt are higher in clients experiencing any of the bipolar disorders (Parese, 2012). The majority of individuals who experience manic episodes also have periods of major depressive episodes throughout their lives. Between 22% and 81% of clients with bipolar disorders have had an associated comorbid medical condition or conditions such as cardiovascular disease, diabetes, hypertension, obesity, migraine headaches, hepatitis, and multiple sclerosis (Parese, 2012). Hypertension and cardiovascular disease can occur more than a decade earlier in those with bipolar disorder than in those without this disorder. Clients who experience bipolar disorder will miss twice as many workdays

as those who experience only depressive episodes. This makes it imperative for nurses to inquire about medical comorbidity and lifestyle practices.

a. Etiology
    1) Biological factors (similar to depressive disorders) (Parese, 2012; Stahl, 2013)
        a) Monoamine transmitter system dysfunction (serotonin, dopamine, gamma-aminobutyric acid [GABA], and norepinephrine) at receptor and cascade system beyond the point of regulation of gene expression regulation of gene expression
        b) Hypothalamic-pituitary-adrenal axis and kindling: Over time, environmental stress that is early/prolonged lowers the stress threshold at which mood changes occur until episodes of mania and hypomania occur spontaneously.
        c) Neurotropic model
        d) Voltage-gated ion channel abnormalities
        e) Cholinergic-adrenergic balance: Mania develops when norepinephrine and dopamine are high relative to acetylcholine.
        f) Brain structure abnormalities: decreased pituitary volumes, enlargement of the thalamus, smaller prefrontal lobe volumes, decreased hippocampal volume, larger caudate nuclei, and enlargement of the cortical sulci
    2) Genetics (Saddock, Saddock, & Ruiz, 2014)
        a) If one parent has bipolar disorder, the child has a 28% chance of developing a unipolar or bipolar mood disorder.
        b) Concordance rates for bipolar disorder are 33%–90% in monozygotic twins and 5%–25% in dizygotic twins.
    3) Psychosocial theories
        a) Psychodynamic: Mania could be an individual's attempt to compensate for feelings of loss and depression.
        b) Other associated factors: experiencing adverse life events, poor social support, and a dysfunctional cognitive style

b. Criteria for Bipolar I Disorder (APA, 2013)
    1) One or more manic episodes, which may have been preceded or followed by a major depressive episode or hypomanic episode
    2) The occurrence of the manic and major depressive episodes are not better explained by other disorders such as schizophrenia, delusional disorder, unspecified schizophrenia spectrum disorder, psychotic disorder, schizoaffective disorder, or schizophreniform disorder.
    3) A *manic episode* is a period of persistently elevated and abnormally expansive or irritable mood that lasts for at least a week and presents almost every day, nearly all day, or any duration of time if hospitalization has become necessary. Can include three or more of the following symptoms (or four if mood is only irritable): grandiosity or inflated self-esteem, decreased need for sleep, talk activity, flight of ideas, distractibility, increased goal-directed activity, and excessive involvement in high-risk activities.
    4) A hypomanic episode differs from manic episode only in temporal quality. It lasts at least for days and presents almost every day, nearly all day, and the episode is not severe enough to cause major impairment in social or occupational functioning and does not involve hospitalization.
    5) The symptoms must cause clinically significant impairment or distress that is not attributable to or better explained by another mental disorder.

2. Assessment
    a. Scales and instruments
        1) Mood Disorder Questionnaire
        2) Hypomania Checklist
        3) Young Mania Rating Scale
    b. Related nursing diagnoses (based on NANDA-I): self-care deficit, chronic low self-esteem, disturbed energy field, risk-prone health behavior, ineffective activity planning, social isolation, and risk for suicide (Stuart, 2013)
    c. Symptoms of bipolar I disorder could include elation or euphoria; inflated self-esteem; distractibility; grandiosity; delusions; verbosity; loose associations; poor judgment; expansiveness; little need for sleep; inadequate nutrition; irritability; argumentativeness; emotional liability; excesses in behaviors (such as hypersexuality, aggressiveness, and increased motor activity); and psychosis. In addition, depressive symptoms can be present during a manic episode.

3. Nursing interventions
    a. Some interventions are similar to those used for depressive disorders.
        1) Educate the client about bipolar disorder, its causes, and the various treatments.

2) Inquire about suicidal ideation.
3) Maintain and reassure safety related to risk for self-harm, and create a safety plan if appropriate.
4) Augment patient teaching with written materials for later reference.
5) Discuss interaction between lifestyle, environment, and sleep, and create a sleep hygiene plan with client that includes the following: optimal sleep environment, sleep routines, over-the-counter sleep aids, and use of progressive relaxation.
6) Use of cognitive strategies that include assisting the client to increase his or her sense of control over behavior and goals, increase self-esteem, and modify dysfunctional thinking patterns.
7) Help client to focus on present activities versus past or future orientation.
8) Provide reinforcement of positive aspects of client's behavior and self-control.
9) Develop and encourage use of healthy support systems.
10) Instruct and model more effective social skills.
11) Assist the client to establish realistic goals for recovery.

b. Medication administration and related patient teaching: Antimania (lithium), anticonvulsants (valproic acid, lamotrigine, carbamazepine, oxcarbazepine, topiramate), and atypical antipsychotic drugs (risperidone, olanzapine, quetiapine, and aripiprazole)
c. Psychosocial treatment includes cognitive behavioral therapies (to help evaluate thought problems such as grandiosity, overestimation of self, and the pursuit of unrealistic goals and activities); group therapies; and behavioral therapies.

D. Substance-Related and Addictive Disorders/Alcohol Use Disorder

1. Description: The United States has one of the highest levels of drug addiction and abuse in the world (Stuart, 2013). Common substances of abuse include alcohol, cocaine, heroin, lysergic acid diethylamide (LSD), marijuana, methamphetamine, methylenedioxymethamphetamine, gamma-hydroxybutyrate, flunitrazepam, phencyclidine, ketamine, anabolic steroids, ephedra, and inhalants (e.g., glue). Approximately 18 million people (or roughly 8% of the American population) are alcohol dependent or abusing alcohol. Most experimentation with drugs occurs during adolescence. Underage drinking increases the risk for motor vehicle accidents, high-risk sexual behaviors, and suicide.

a. Alcohol is a central nervous system depressant that acts on opioid synapses.
1) Is thought to cause the release of dopamine in the nucleus accumbens (Stahl, 2013)
2) Alcohol also acts to increase the activity of GABA, an inhibitory neurotransmitter, and decreases glutamate, an excitatory neurotransmitter.
3) Effects: GABA neurotransmitters are what produce the hyperexcitable state that is observed when a client withdraws from alcohol.
4) If an individual has an onset of alcohol withdrawal syndrome, medical intervention is necessary to prevent severe symptoms such as hallucinations, grand mal seizures, delusions, respiratory depression, and, potentially, death.
5) GABAergic medications such as the benzodiazepines are the primary drugs used to treat a client with alcohol withdrawal syndrome.

b. The client who experiences a prolonged alcohol related disorder can have up to a 10-year reduction in life expectancy (Rehm, 2011).
1) Chronic alcohol abuse and dependence are associated with cerebral degeneration; peripheral neuropathy; recurrent pancreatitis; increased incidence of cancers (i.e., of the mouth, esophagus, stomach, liver, pancreas); depression of pulmonary functioning; elevated blood pressure; increased pulse; myocardial infarction; congestive heart failure; unintentional injuries such as motor vehicle accidents; aggression; and suicide risk.
2) Korsakoff's psychosis (anterograde amnesia) can occur and is characterized by impaired memory and confabulation and has a poor prognosis for recovery.
3) There is a high comorbidity with alcohol abuse and other psychiatric disorders as well as other substance abuse disorders.
4) Few clients who experience alcohol-use disorders will seek treatment.

c. Etiology is thought to be multifactorial (Enoch, 2014).
1) Biological factors
a) Alcohol causes differential alteration of $GABA_A$ receptors.

b) Early life stress can create change in neural plasticity.
c) Gender differences in metabolism
2) Genetics
a) Some subtypes can be heritable; that is, likely to involve numerous functional genetic variants.
b) Genetic polymorphism in metabolizing alcohol and amount of dopamine released varies among races.
c) Twin studies: heritability at ~ 50%
3) Psychological theories
a) Behavioral: Operant reinforcement, overlearned maladaptive habit
b) Cognitive: Distorted ways of thinking about alcohol use

d. Criteria for alcohol use disorder (APA, 2013)
1) A 12-month period of a problematic pattern of alcohol use that causes distress or clinically significant impairment
2) Two or more of the following occur:
a) Alcohol is consumed in large amounts or over a longer period than was intended
b) Unable to cut down or control alcohol use
c) Craving or strong urge to use alcohol
d) Spends much time obtaining and using alcohol or recovering from effects
e) Unable to fulfill major roles at work, school, or home because of use
f) Continues to use alcohol even though it causes major problems, both social and interpersonal
g) Giving up important activities because of alcohol use
h) Using alcohol even if physically hazardous
i) Tolerance: need for larger amounts, diminished effect with continued use
j) Withdrawal
k) Continuing to use alcohol even if physical problems or psychological problems have worsened

2. Assessment
a. Scales and instruments
1) CAGE questionnaire
2) Alcohol Use Disorders Identification Test
3) CRAFFT Screen (drugs and alcohol use in teens)
4) Michigan Alcoholism Screening Test
5) Clinical Institute Withdrawal Assessment of Alcohol Scale, revised

b. Related nursing diagnoses (based on NANDA-I): disturbed sensory perception, acute confusion, low self-esteem, ineffective coping, risk for self-directed violence, risk for other-directed violence, and dysfunctional family processes: alcoholism (Stuart, 2013)

c. Laboratory studies
1) Baseline could include urinalysis, toxicology screen, electrolytes, blood urea nitrogen, glucose, creatinine clearance
2) Blood alcohol concentrations may be drawn; 0.08 g/dL is the legal limit for operating a motor vehicle in most states.

d. Symptoms
1) Look for physical signs of alcohol abuse such as telangiectasia, Dupuytren's contracture, and palmar erythema.
2) Behavioral: labile mood, euphoria, outbursts, loss of sexual inhibition, impaired judgment, and decreased ability to concentrate
3) Later signs of alcoholism can include delirium tremens, peripheral neuropathy, ataxia, and a wide stance.

3. Nursing interventions
a. Women and the elderly are often underscreened, so be sure to ask every client about substance use.
b. Often questions about smoking and less threatening subjects are first utilized.
c. Use open-ended questions such as "How much alcohol do you drink?"
d. Follow up with quantity and frequency inquiry.
e. Get collateral information to enhance accuracy from family members and significant others.
f. Check for common laboratory findings suggestive of ethanol abuse, including elevated liver enzymes with aspartate aminotransferase greater than alanine aminotransferase, elevated gamma glutamyl transferase, and mild macrocytosis (Fischbach, 2012).
g. Discuss contraceptive options for alcohol-dependent women of childbearing age to avoid childbirth and potential fetal alcohol syndrome.
h. Address issues of malnutrition, a common consequence of alcohol dependence. Common vitamin deficiencies include vitamins B, A, C, D, and E. Serum magnesium and albumin levels can be low as well.
i. Restore physiologic homeostasis. Thiamine is administered before glucose administration

in suspected Wernicke's encephalopathy (i.e., ataxia, delirium, opthalmoplegia triad).

j. Patient teaching and administration of benzodiazepines, barbiturates, or antiseizure medicines—carbamazepine/valproate for treatment of alcohol withdrawal syndrome.

k. Patient teaching and administration of medications such as naltrexone (oral or extended-release injectable), acamprosate, and disulfiram for treatment of alcohol dependence after detoxification has occurred.

l. Psychosocial treatment includes cognitive behavioral therapies, motivational interviewing (i.e., exploring ambivalence), group therapies, 12-step programs, and behavioral therapies.

E. Trauma- and Stressor-Related Disorders: Posttraumatic Stress Disorder

1. Description: From very early times, it has been well observed that a link exists between exposure to traumatic events and psychopathology. Much of our current knowledge about posttraumatic stress disorder (PTSD) and theories of trauma have arisen from past work with combat soldiers. Examples of contemporary traumatic events could include military combat, severe motor vehicle accidents, diagnosis with a life-threatening illness, capture and torture, or violent personal assault. Although most of us will have experienced some type of traumatic event in our lifetime, only 10% of us will go on to develop a trauma-related disorder (Parese, 2012). The development of PTSD is influenced by the intensity of the closeness of exposure to the trauma, degree of physical injury, loss of significant others or loved ones, and the type of traumatic event. Individual resilience or protective factors also influence the potential development of stress- or trauma-related response. Risk factors can include genetic vulnerability, early separation from parents or adverse childhood events, negative self-appraisal or catastrophic thinking, prior exposure to trauma or polytrauma experiences, lower economic status, or limited social support. Nurses could be the first healthcare provider to assist a client after exposure to trauma.

a. Nurses will encounter clients who have long-standing trauma-related disorders such as PTSD and are entering outpatient or hospital-based care for medical conditions or illness.

1) It has been established that greater fear or distress before surgery can lead to postoperative complications, longer hospital stays, and poorer prognosis (Gouin & Kiecolt-Glaser, 2012).

2) Higher rates of comorbidity with physical diseases and medical conditions such as hyperlipidemia, hypertension, joint disorders, sleep disturbance, and allergies have also been associated with the diagnosis of PTSD (Frayne et al., 2011; Pacella, Hruska, & Delahanty, 2013).

3) Hypercatecholaminergic and hypocortisolemic states have been identified in individuals experiencing PTSD; these can lead to a chronic proinflammatory state.

b. Etiology

1) Exposure to traumatic event or stressor

2) Biological factors (Parese, 2012; Stahl, 2013)

a) Increased autonomic nervous system arousal with resultant dysregulation

(i) Amygdala signals to hypothalamus

(ii) Amygdala activates fight-or-flight response

(iii) Pituitary release adrenocorticotropic hormone

(iv) Adrenal gland: release of cortisol

b) Functional and structural changes from trauma response (in the neurotransmitters norepinephrine, serotonin, GABA, and in the thalamus, prefrontal cortex, amygdala, hippocampus, and other areas of the brain)

3) Self-regulatory system impairment with resultant problems with emotional regulation, dissociation, impulse control, and impaired attention

4) Psychological theories

a) Behavioral: Based on learning theory. Fear associated with the stimuli elicits the response of anxiety and related change in mood behavior and physical functioning.

b) Cognitive behavioral: Trauma changes assumptions about safety, one's ability to evaluate situations, response patterns, and self-efficacy.

c. Criteria for PTSD (APA, 2013)

1) Exposure to serious injury, sexual violation, or actual death/threatened death

2) Presence of one or more intrusive symptoms such as distressing memories, dreams, or dissociative reactions

3) Avoidance of stimuli associated with the traumatic event

4) Negative alterations in cognitions and/or mood associated with the traumatic event, with two or more symptoms such as dissociative amnesia, feelings of detachment, or exaggerated negative beliefs
5) Hypervigilance or heightened arousal with two or more symptoms such as exaggerated startle response, problems with concentration, or irritable behavior
6) The symptoms must cause clinically significant impairment or distress that is not attributable to or better explained by another mental disorder.

2. Assessment
   a. Scales and instruments
      1) PTSD checklists (PCL): (PCL-M [military], PCL-C [civilian], and PCL-S [linked to a specific trauma/event])
      2) Clinician-Administered PTSD Scale
      3) Trauma Symptom Inventory, second edition
      4) Life Events Checklist
      5) Minnesota Multiphasic Personality Inventory-2® posttraumatic stress disorder scales (Keane PTSD Scale and PTSD Scale)
      6) Mississippi Combat Scale for PTSD
      7) Trauma Symptoms Checklist for Children
   b. Related nursing diagnoses (based on NANDA-I): anxiety, fear, ineffective coping, defensive coping, readiness for enhanced coping, and risk for suicide (Stuart, 2013)
   c. Symptoms (Saddock, Saddock, & Ruiz, 2014)
      1) Can be months to years before symptoms manifest after a traumatic event is experienced
      2) Common symptoms can be hyperarousal, painful reexperiencing of an event, emotional numbness, and avoidance behaviors related to the experienced event, as well as impaired memory and attention.
      3) Feelings of guilt, humiliation, and rejection can be endorsed.
      4) Additional associated symptoms can include aggression, irritability, impaired impulse control, depression, and substance abuse.
      5) Children could have nightmares, flashbacks, distressing dreams, regressive behaviors, repetitive acting out of the trauma, withdrawal, decreased play, or replaying traumatic memories during their play. Older children can become more aggressive, act out sexually, or engage in substance abuse.

3. Nursing interventions (Gerardi et al., 2010; Jeffreys, 2014; Parese, 2012; Stahl, 2014)
   a. Be empathetic when you first elicit a history of traumatic exposure and be careful not to retraumatize through disclosure.
   b. Help the client to understand the biopsychosocial mechanisms for his or her symptoms to reduce stigmatization and improve the potential continued care for PTSD.
   c. Have resources and specific follow-up instructions ready to include sources for care and community referral.
   d. Nurses as first responders can use techniques such as Trauma First Aid/Psychological First Aid to reestablish safety and provide separation from the trauma.
   e. Patient teaching and administration of medications to provide symptom reduction such as SSRIs (sertraline and paroxetine). In addition, SNRIs (fluoxetine and venlafaxine) have been used, although they have not yet been approved for PTSD treatment by the U. S. Food and Drug Administration. Alpha-1 antagonists (e.g., prazosin) have also been used to prevent nightmares and improve sleep. Off-label use of beta blockers for hyperarousal symptoms has been effective in some cases.
   f. Psychosocial treatment including cognitive behavioral therapies such as prolonged exposure therapy and cognitive processing therapy are thought to have greater treatment efficacy than medication. Other therapies include eye movement desensitization and reprocessing, stress inoculation training, structured writing therapy, Internet and Web-based treatments, virtual reality exposure, nonexposure psychotherapies, and group or peer counseling.
   g. Teach stress-management skills to interrupt escalating anxiety and to promote the physical recovery process (e.g., progressive relation, deep breathing exercises/breathing retraining, meditation, music therapy, body movement/exercise, grounding techniques, and yoga). Exercise and body-based relaxation techniques have been associated with a reduction in symptomatology.

References

Abjornsson, G., Orbaek, P., & Hagstadius, S. (1998). Chronic toxic encephalopathy: Social consequences and experiences from a rehabilitation program. *Rehabilitation Nursing, 23*(1), 38–43.

American Psychiatric Association. (2013). *Diagnostic and statistical manual of mental disorders* (5th ed.). Washington, DC: Author.

Anderson, H. (2010). Common grief, complex grieving. *Pastoral Psychology, 59*(2), 127–136. doi: 10.1007/s11089-009-0243-5

Association of Rehabilitation Nurses (ARN). (2014). ARN competency model for professional rehabilitation nursing. Retrieved from http://www.rehabnurse.org/uploads/files/education/ARN_Rehabilitation_Nursing_Competency _Model_FINAL_-_May_2014.pdf

Aujoulat, I., Luminet, O., & Deccache, A. (2007). The perspective of patients on their experience of powerlessness. *Qualitative Health Research, 17*(6), 772–785.

Bamm, E. L., & Rosenbaum, P. (2008). Family-centered theory: Origins, development, barriers, and supports to implementation in rehabilitation medicine. *Archives of Physical Medicine & Rehabilitation, 89*(8), 1618–1624.

Bandura, A. (1977). Self-efficacy: Toward a unifying theory of behavioral change. *Psychological Review, 84*, 191–215.

Barry, M., Clarke, A., Jenkins, R., & Patel, V. (2013). A systematic review of the effectiveness of mental health promotion interventions for young people in low and middle income countries. *BMC Public Health, 13*(1), 835.

Behar, E., DiMarco, I. D., Hekler, E. B., Mohlman, J., & Staples, A. M. (2009). Current theoretical models of generalized anxiety disorder (GAD): Conceptual review and treatment implications. *Journal of Anxiety Disorders, 23*(8), 1011–1023. doi: http://dx.doi.org/10.1016/j.janxdis.2009.07.006

Bennett, I. J., & Madden, D. J. (2014). Disconnected aging: Cerebral white matter integrity and age-related differences in cognition. *Neuroscience, 276*(0), 187–205. doi: http://dx.doi.org/10.1016/j.neuroscience.2013.11.026

Bennett, I. J., Motes, M. A., Rao, N. K., & Rypma, B. (2012). White matter tract integrity predicts visual search performance in young and older adults. *Neurobiology of Aging, 33*(2), e421–433. doi: http://dx.doi.org/10.1016/j.neurobiolaging.2011.02.001

Berglund, M., Westin, L., Svanström, R., & Sundler, A. J. (2012). Suffering caused by care—Patients' experiences from hospital settings. *International Journal of Qualitative Studies on Health and Well-being, 7*, 10.3402/qhw.v3407i3400.18688. doi: 10.3402/qhw.v7i0.18688

Berman, C., & Rose, L. (1998). Examination of a patient's adaptation to quadriplegia. *Physical Therapy Case Reports, 1*(3), 148–156.

Bethoux, F., Calmels, P., Gautheron, V., & Minaire, P. (1996). Quality of life of spouses of stroke patients: A preliminary study. *International Journal of Rehabilitation and Health, 2*(3), 189–198.

Bhat, A. A., DeWalt, D. A., Zimmer, C. R., Fried, B. J., & Callahan, L. F. (2010). The role of helplessness, outcome expectation for exercise and literacy in predicting disability and symptoms in older adults with arthritis. *Patient Education, 81*(1), 73–78.

Boraz, M., & Heinemann, A. (1996). The relationship between social support and alcohol abuse in people with spinal cord injuries. *International Journal of Rehabilitation and Health, 2*(3), 189–199.

Brillhart, B. (2005). A study of spirituality and life satisfaction among persons with spinal cord injury. *Rehabilitation Nursing, 30*(1), 31–34.

Brillhart, B., & Johnson, K. (1997). Motivation and the coping process of adults with disabilities: A qualitative study. *Rehabilitation Nursing, 22*(5), 249–256.

Brzuzy, S., & Speziale, B. (1997). Persons with traumatic brain injuries and their families: Living arrangements and well-being post injury. *Social Work in Health Care, 26*(1), 77–88.

Butcher, L. A. (1994). A family-focused perspective on chronic illness. *Rehabilitation Nursing, 19*(2), 70–74.

Captain, C. (1995). The effects of communication skills training on interaction and psychosocial adjustment among couples living with spinal cord injury. *Rehabilitation Nursing Research, 4*(4), 111–118.

Cardol, M., Elvers, J., Oostendorp, R., Brandsma, J., & deGroot, I. (1996). Quality of life in patients with amyotrophic lateral sclerosis. *Journal of Rehabilitation Sciences, 9*(4), 99–103.

Carpenito-Moyet, L. J. (2010). *Handbook of nursing diagnosis.* Philadelphia: Lippincott Williams, & Wilkins.

Centers for Disease Control and Prevention. (2014). Depression is not a normal part of growing older. Retrieved from http://www.cdc.gov/aging/mentalhealth/depression.htm

Cole-King, A., & Harding, K. G. (2001). Psychological factors and delayed healing in chronic wounds. *Psychosomatic Medicine, 63*(2), 216–220.

Cormier-Daigle, M., & Stewart, M. (1997). Support and coping of male hemodialysis-dependent patients. *International Journal of Nursing Studies, 34*(6), 420–430.

Coutu, M. F., Baril, R., Durand, M. J., Côté, D., & Rouleau, A. (2007). Representations: An important key to understanding workers' coping behaviors during rehabilitation and the return-to-work process. *Journal of Occupational Rehabilitation, 17*(3), 522–544.

Craven, R., & Hirnle, C. (2009). *Fundamentals of nursing: Human health and function* (6th ed.). Philadelphia: Lippincott, Williams & Wilkins.

Dausch, B. M., & Saliman, S. (2009). Use of family focused therapy in rehabilitation for veterans with traumatic brain injury. *Rehabilitation Psychology, 54*(3), 279–287.

Davidhizar, R. (1997). Disability does not have to be the grief that never ends: Helping patients adjust. *Rehabilitation Nursing, 22*(1), 32–35.

De Bruin, A. F., Diederiks, J. P. M., De Witte, L. P., Stevens, F. C. J., & Philipsen, H. (1994). The development of a short generic version of the Sickness Impact Profile. *Journal of Clinical Epidemiology, 47*, 407–418.

De Hert, M., Cohen, D., Bobes, J., Cetkovich-Bakmas, M., Leucht, S., Ndetei, D. M., . . . Correll, C. U. (2011). Physical illness in patients with severe mental disorders. II. Barriers to care, monitoring and treatment guidelines, plus recommendations at the system and individual level. *World Psychiatry, 10*(2), 138–151.

Delmar, C., Bøje, T., Dylmer, D., Forup, L., Jakobsen, C., Møller, M., . . . Pedersen, B. D. (2006). Independence/dependence: A contradictory relationship? Life with a chronic illness. *Scandinavian Journal of Caring Sciences, 20*(3), 261–268.

Deutsch, P. M., Allison, L., & Cimino-Ferguson, S. (2005). Life care planning assessments and their impact on life in spinal cord injury. *Topics in Spinal Cord Rehabilitation, 10*(4), 135–145.

Diener, E. (1984). Subjective well-being. *Psychological Bulletin, 95*(3), 542–575.

Donovan, N. J., Heaton, S. C., Kimberg, C. I., Wen, P. S., Waid-Ebbs, J. K., Coster, W., …Velozo, C. A. (2011). Conceptualizing functional cognition in traumatic brain injury rehabilitation. *Brain Injury, 25*(4), 348–364. doi: 10.3109/02699052.2011.556105

Elfstrom, M. L., Ryden, A., Kreuter, M., Taft, C., & Sullivan, M. (2005). Relations between coping strategies and health-related quality of life in patients with spinal cord lesion. *Journal of Rehabilitation Medicine, 31*(1), 9–16.

Enoch, M. A. (2014). Genetic influences on response to alcohol and response to pharmacotherapies for alcoholism. *Pharmacology Biochemistry and Behavior, 123*(0), 17–24. doi: http://dx.doi.org/10.1016/j.pbb.2013.11.001

Faulkner, M. (2001). The onset and alleviation of learned helplessness in older hospitalized people. *Aging & Mental Health, 5*(4), 379–386.

Ferguson, A. D., Richie, B. S., & Gomez, M. J. (2004). Psychological factors after traumatic amputation in landmine survivors: The bridge between physical healing and full recovery. *Disability and Rehabilitation, 26*(14/15), 931–938.

Ferrans, C. E. (1996). Development of a conceptual model of quality of life. *Scholarly Inquiry for Nursing Practice: An International Journal, 10*(3), 293–304.

Ferrin, J. M. (2002). Acceptance of loss after an adult-onset disability: Development and psychometric validation of the Multidimensional Acceptance of Loss Scale. Doctoral dissertation, University of Wisconsin–Madison.

Fischbach, F. (2012). *A manual of laboratory and diagnostic tests* (7th ed.). Philadelphia: Lippincott Williams & Wilkins

Flannery, J. (1998). Using the Levels of Cognitive Functioning Assessment Scale with patients with traumatic brain injury in an acute care setting. *Rehabilitation Nursing, 23*(3), 88–94.

Folstein, M. F., Folstein, S. E., & McHugh, P. R. (1975). "Mini-mental state." A practical method for grading the cognitive state of patients for the clinician. *Journal of Psychiatric Research, 12*(3), 189–198.

Forhan, M., & Backman, C. (2010). Exploring occupational balance in adults with rheumatoid arthritis. *OTJR: Occupation, Participation and Health, 30*(3), 133.

Freysteinson, W. M. (2009). Therapeutic mirror interventions: An integrated review of the literature. *Journal of Holistic Nursing, 27*(4), 241–255.

Gazzaniga, M., Ivry, R., & Mangun, G. (2013). *Cognitive neuroscience: The biology of the mind* (4th ed.). New York: W.W. Norton & Company.

Gerardi, M. B., Wright, S. E., Nicolas-Wedige, R., Berkowitz, A. C., West, A. J., Morel, R. J., & Saucedo, D. K. (2010). Trauma first aide in primary care: Treating physiological symptoms induced by trauma. *American Journal for Nurse Practitioners, 14* (9/10), 44–53.

Geue, K., Goetze, H., Buttstaedt, M., Kleinert, E., Richter, D., & Singer, S. (2010). An overview of art therapy interventions for cancer patients and the results of research. *Complementary Therapies in Medicine, 18*(3–4), 160–170. doi: http://dx.doi.org/10.1016/j.ctim.2010.04.001

Goffman, E. (1974). *Stigma*. New York: Jason Aronson.

Goodman, J. (2014). The horror of stigma: Psychosis and mental health environments in twenty-first- century horror film (Part 1). *Perspectives in Psychiatric Care, 50*(3), 201–209.

Gouin, J.-P., & Kiecolt-Glaser, J. K. (2012). The impact of psychological stress on wound healing: methods and mechanisms. *Critical Care Nursing Clinics of North America, 24*(2), 201.

Gray, C. (2013). Assessment of the suicidal patient in the emergency department. In L. Zun (Ed.), Behavioral emergencies for the emergency physician (pp. 60–68). New York: Cambridge University Press.

Grant, S., St. John, W., & Patterson, E. (2009). Recovery from total hip replacement surgery: "It's not just physical." *Qualitative Health Research, 19*(11), 1612–1620.

Happell, B., Stanton, R., Hoey, W., & Scott, D. (2014). Knowing is not doing: The relationship between health behaviour knowledge and actual health behaviours in people with serious mental illness. *Mental Health and Physical Activity, 7*(3), 198–204. doi: http://dx.doi.org/10.1016/j.mhpa.2014.03.001

Hartley, S. M., Vance, D. E., Elliott, T. R., Cuckler, J. M., & Berry, J. W. (2008). Hope, self-efficacy, and functional recovery after knee and hip replacement surgery. *Rehabilitation Psychology, 53*(4), 521–529.

Hill, W., Schillo, L., & Weinert, C. (2004). Effect of a computer-based intervention on social support for chronically ill rural women. *Rehabilitation Nursing, 29*(5), 169–173.

Holland, J. M., & Neimeyer, R. A. (2010). An examination of stage theory of grief among individuals bereaved by natural and violent causes: A meaning-oriented contribution. *Omega: Journal of Death & Dying, 61*(2), 103–120.

Howell, D. (1998). Reaching to the depths of the soul: Understanding and exploring meaning in illness. *Canadian Oncology Nursing Journal, 8*(1), 22–23.

Isaksson, G., Skar, L., & Lexell, J. (2005). Women's perceptions of changes in the social network after a spinal cord injury. *Disability and Rehabilitation, 27*(17), 1013–1021.

Jahiel, R. I., & Scherer, M. J. (2010). Initial steps towards a theory and praxis of person-environment interaction in disability. *Disability & Rehabilitation, 32*(17), 1467–1474.

Janssen, D. J. A, Franssen, F, M. E, & Wouters, E. F. M. (2011). Impaired health status and care dependency in patients with advanced COPD or chronic heart failure. *Quality of Life Research, 20*(10), 1679–1688. doi: 10.1007/s11136-011-9892-9

Jeffreys, M. (2014). Clinician's guide to medications for PTSD. Retrieved from http://www.ptsd.va.gov/professional/treatment/overview/clinicians-guide-to-medications-for-ptsd.asp

Kales, H. C., Gitlin, L. N., Lyketsos, C. G., & Detroit Expert Panel on Assessment and Management of the Neuropsychiatric Symptoms of Dementia (2014). Management of neuropsychiatric symptoms of dementia in clinical settings: Recommendations from a multidisciplinary expert panel. *Journal of the American Geriatrics Society, 62*(4), 762–769. doi:10.1111/jgs.12730

Katon, W. J., Lin, E. H. B., Von Korff, M., Ciechanowski, P., Ludman, E. J., Young, B., . . . McCulloch, D. (2010). Collaborative care for patients with depression and chronic illnesses. *New England Journal of Medicine, 363*(27), 2611–2620. doi: doi:10.1056/NEJMoa1003955

Kautz, D. D. (2006, October). Inspiring hope in our patients, their families, and ourselves. Paper presented at the conference of the Association of Rehabilitation Nurses, Chicago, IL.

Kautz, D. D., & Van Horn, E. (2009). Promoting family integrity to inspire hope in rehabilitation patients: Strategies to provide evidence-based care. *Rehabilitation Nursing, 34*(4), 168–173.

Kendzor, D. E., Chen, M., Reininger, B. M., Businelle, M. S., Stewart, D. W., Fisher-Hoch, S. P., . . . McCormick, J. B. (2014). The association of depression and anxiety with glycemic control among Mexican Americans with diabetes living near the U.S.-

Mexico border. *BMC Public Health, 14*(1). doi: 10.1186/1471-2458-14-176

Kent, E. E., Smith, A. W., Keegan, T. H. M., Lynch, C. F., Wu, X.-C., Hamilton, A. S., . . . Harlan, L. C. (2013). Talking about cancer and meeting peer survivors: Social information needs of adolescents and young adults diagnosed with cancer. *Journal of Adolescent and Young Adult Oncology, 2*(2), 44–52. doi: 10.1089/jayao.2012.0029

Kiera, S., Stachow, R., Petermann, F., & Tiedjen, U. (2010). Medical inpatient rehabilitation influences on self-esteem and self-efficacy of chronically ill adolescents. *Rehabilitation, 49*(4), 248–255.

Kinavey, C. (2007). Adolescents born with spina bifida: Experiential worlds and biopsychosocial developmental challenges. *Issues in Comprehensive Pediatric Nursing, 30*(4), 147–164.

Koolhaas, J. M., Bartolomucci, A., Buwalda, B., de Boer, S. F., Flügge, G., Korte, S. M., . . . Fuchs, E. (2011). Stress revisited: A critical evaluation of the stress concept. *Neuroscience & Biobehavioral Reviews, 35*(5), 1291–1301. doi: http://dx.doi.org/10.1016/j.neubiorev.2011.02.003

Knopman, D., & Petersen, R. (2014). Mild cognitive impairment and mild dementia: A clinical perspective. *Mayo Clinic Proceedings, 89*(10), 1452–1459.

Lawson, S., Delamere, F. M., & Hutchinson, S. L. (2008). A personal narrative of involvement in post-traumatic brain injury rehabilitation: What can we learn for therapeutic recreation practice? *Therapeutic Recreation Journal, 42*(4), 236–250.

Lobb, E. A., Kristjanson, L. J., Aoun, S. M., Monterosso, L., Halkett, G. K. B., & Davies, A. (2010). Predictors of complicated grief: A systematic review of empirical studies. *Death Studies, 34*(8), 673–698.

Lohne, V. (2008). The battle between hoping and suffering: A conceptual model of hope within a context of spinal cord injury. *Advances in Nursing Science, 31*(3), 237–248.

Lohne, V., & Severinsson, E. (2006). The power of hope: Patients' experiences of hope a year after acute spinal cord injury. *Journal of Clinical Nursing, 15*(3), 315–523.

Lund, M. L., Nordlund, A., Nygard, L., Lexell, J., & Bernspang, B. (2005). Perceptions of participation and predictors of perceived problems with participation in persons with spinal cord injury. *Journal of Rehabilitation Medicine, 37*(1), 3–8.

Lutterman, D. (1984). *Counseling with the communicatively disordered and their families*. Boston: Little, Brown.

Lutterman, D. (2001). *Counseling persons with communication disorders and their families* (4th ed.). Austin, TX: Pro-Ed.

Maciejewski, P. K., Zhang, B., Block, S. D., & Prigerson, H. G. (2007). An empirical examination of the stage theory of grief. *Journal of the American Medical Association, 297*(7), 716–723.

Millen, J. A., & Bray, S. R. (2009). Promoting self-efficacy and outcome expectations to enable adherence to resistance training after cardiac rehabilitation. *Journal of Cardiovascular Nursing, 24*(4), 316–327.

Missiuna, C., DeMatteo, C., Hanna, S., Mandich, A., Law, M., Mahoney, W., & Scott, L. (2010). Exploring the use of cognitive intervention for children with acquired brain injury. *Physical & Occupational Therapy in Pediatrics, 30*(3), 205–219.

Mitchell, A. J., Vaze, A., & Rao, S. (2009). Clinical diagnosis of depression in primary care: a meta-analysis. *The Lancet, 374*(9690), 609–619. doi: http://dx.doi.org/10.1016/S0140-6736(09)60879-5

Moi, A. L., & Gjengedal, E. (2008). Life after burn injury: Striving for regained freedom. *Qualitative Health Research, 18*(12), 1621–1630.

Moses, K. (1989). *Fundamentals of grieving: Relating to parents of the disabled*. Evanston, IL: Resource Networks.

Nathenson, N. (2006, October). A new model in outpatient cardiac rehabilitation. Paper presented at the conference of the Association of Rehabilitation Nurses, Chicago, IL.

Nir, Z., Wallhagen, M., Doolittle, N., & Galinsky, D. (1997). A study of the psychosocial characteristics of patients in a geriatric rehabilitation unit in Israel. *Rehabilitation Nursing, 22*(3), 143–151.

Nypaver, J., Titus, M., & Brugler, C. (1996). Patient transfer to rehabilitation: Just another move? *Rehabilitation Nursing, 21*(2), 94–97.

Olson, M., & Dossey, B. (2013). Dying in peace. In B. Dossey & L. Keegan (Eds.), *Holistic nursing: A handbook for practice* (6th ed., pp. 463–489). Burlington, MA: Jones & Bartlett Learning.

Ostwald, S. K., Swank, P. R., & Khan, M. M. (2008). Predictors of functional independence and stress level of stroke survivors at discharge from inpatient rehabilitation. *Journal of Cardiovascular Nursing, 23*(4), 371–377.

O'Sullivan, D., & Strauser, D. R. (2009). Operationalizing self-efficacy, related social cognitive variables, and moderating effects: Implications for rehabilitation research and practice. *Rehabilitation Counseling Bulletin, 52*(4), 251–258.

Parese, E. (2012). *Psychiatric advanced practice nursing: A biopsychosocial foundation for practice*. Philadelphia: F. A. Davis Company

Paterson, J., & Stewart, J. (2002). Adults with acquired brain injury: Perceptions of their social world. *Rehabilitation Nursing, 27*(1), 13–18.

Pedersen, P. M., Jorgensen, H. S., Nakayama, H., Raaschou, H. O., & Olsen, T. S. (1996). Orientation in the acute and chronic stroke patient: Impact on ADL and social activities. The Copenhagen Stroke Study. *Archives of Physical Medicine & Rehabilitation, 77*(4), 336–339.

Pescosolido, B. A., Martin, J. K., Lang, A., & Olafsdottir, S. (2008). Rethinking theoretical approaches to stigma: A Framework Integrating Normative Influences on Stigma (FINIS). *Social Science & Medicine, 67*(3), 431–440.

Ponsford, J., Bayley, M., Wiseman-Hakes, C., Togher, L., Velikonja, D., McIntyre, A., . . . Tate, R. (2014). INCOG recommendations for management of cognition following traumatic brain injury, part II: Attention and information processing speed.. *The Journal of Head Trauma Rehabilitation, 29*(4), 321–337. doi: 10.1097/HTR.0000000000000072

Pouwer, F., Nefs, G., & Nouwen, A. (2013). Adverse effects of depression on glycemic control and health outcomes in people with diabetes. A Review. *Endocrinology and Metabolism Clinics of North America, 42*(3), 529–544. doi: 10.1016/j.ecl.2013.05.002

Ramsawh, H. J., Fullerton, C. S., Mash, H. B. H., Ng, T. H. H., Kessler, R. C., Stein, M. B., & Ursano, R. J. (2014). Risk for suicidal behaviors associated with PTSD, depression, and their comorbidity in the U.S. Army. *Journal of Affective Disorders, 161*(0), 116–122. doi: http://dx.doi.org/10.1016/j.jad.2014.03.016

Rehm, J. (2011). The risks associated with alcohol use and alcoholism. *Alcohol Research & Health, 34*(2), 135–143. doi: fea-ar&h-65

Resnick, B., Zimmerman, S., Magaziner, J., & Adelman, A. (1998). Use of the Apathy Evaluation Scale as a measure of motivation in elderly people. *Rehabilitation Nursing, 23*(3), 141–147.

Rintala, D. H., Robinson-Whelen, S., & Matamoros, R. (2005). Subjective stress in male veterans with spinal cord injury. *Journal of Rehabilitation Research and Development, 42*(3), 291–304.

Rintala, D., Young, M., Spencer, J., & Bates, P. (1996). Family relationships and adaptation to spinal cord injury: A qualitative study. *Rehabilitation Nursing, 21*(2), 67–74.

Sadock, B., Sadock, V., & Ruiz, P. (2014). *Kaplan & Sadock's synopsis of psychiatry: Behavioral sciences/clinical psychiatry* (11th ed.). Philadelphia: Wolters Kluwer.

Saltapidas, H., & Ponsford, J. (2007). The influence of cultural background on motivation for and participation in rehabilitation and outcome following traumatic brain injury. *The Journal of Head Trauma Rehabilitation, 22*(2), 132–139.

Satir, V. (1988). *The new peoplemaker.* Mountain View, CA: Science and Behavior Books.

Schrank, B., Hayward, M., Stanghellini, G., & Davidson, L. (2011). Hope in psychiatry. *Advances in Psychiatric Treatment, 17*(3), 227–235. doi: 10.1192/apt.bp.109.007286

Schreuer, N., Rimmerman, A., & Sachs, D. (2006). Adjustment to severe disability: Constructing and examining a cognitive and occupational performance model. *International Journal of Rehabilitation Research 29*(3), 201–207.

Secrest, J. A. (2006). The relationship of continuity, functional ability, depression, quality of life over time in stroke survivors. Paper presented at the conference of the Association of Rehabilitation Nurses, Chicago, IL.

Sheridan, N. F., Kenealy, T. W., Kidd, J. D., Schmidt-Busby, J. I. G., Hand, J. E., Raphael, D. L., . . . Rea, H. H. (2012). Patients' engagement in primary care: powerlessness and compounding jeopardy. A qualitative study. *Health Expectations, 18*(1), 32–43.. doi: 10.1111/hex.12006

Sherman, J. E., Sperling, K. B., & DeVinney, D. J. (2004). Social support and adjustment after spinal cord injury: Influence of past peer-mentoring experiences and current live-in partner. *Rehabilitation Psychology, 49*(2), 140–149.

Smith, A., & Schwirian, P. (1998). The relationship between caregiver burden and the TBI survivor's cognition and functional ability after discharge. *Rehabilitation Nursing, 23*(5), 252–257.

Smith, C. R., Jackson, L., & Sharpe, L. (2006). Coping behaviors of parents with school age/latency age children with disabilities. *Pediatric Physical Therapy, 18*(1), 106.

Smith, K. J., Béland, M., Clyde, M., Gariépy, G., Pagé, V., Badawi, G., . . . Schmitz, N. (2013). Association of diabetes with anxiety: A systematic review and meta-analysis. *Journal of Psychosomatic Research, 74*(2), 89–99. doi: http://dx.doi.org/10.1016/j.jpsychores.2012.11.013

Song, H. (2005). Modeling social reintegration in persons with spinal cord injury. *Disability and Rehabilitation, 27*(3), 131–141.

Song, H., & Nam, K. A. (2010). Coping strategies, physical function, and social adjustment in people with spinal cord injury. *Rehabilitation Nursing, 35*(1), 8–15.

Soyupek, F., Aktepe, E., Savas, S., & Askin, A. (2010). Do the self-concept and quality of life decrease in CP patients? Focusing on the predictors of self-concept and quality of life. *Disability & Rehabilitation, 32*(13), 1109–1115.

Spillers, C. S. (2007). An existential framework for understanding the counseling needs of clients. *American Journal of Speech-Language Pathology, 16*(3), 191–197.

Stahl, S. (2013). *Stahl's Essential Psychopharmacology: Neuroscientific Basis and Practical Applications.* New York: Cambridge University Press.

Stahl, S. (2014). *Prescriber's Guide: Stahl's Essential Psychopharmacology.* New York: Cambridge University Press.

Staniute, M., Brozaitiene, J., & Bunevicius, R. (2013). Effects of social support and stressful life events on health-related quality of life in coronary artery disease patients. *Journal of Cardiovascular Nursing, 28*(1), 83–89.

Stanley, B., & Brown, G. K. (2012). Safety planning intervention: A brief intervention to mitigate suicide risk. *Cognitive and Behavioral Practice, 19*(2), 256–264. doi: http://dx.doi.org/10.1016/j.cbpra.2011.01.001

Stephens, M., & Yoshida, K. K. (1999). Independence and autonomy among people with rheumatoid arthritis. *Canadian Journal of Rehabilitation, 12*(4), 229–243.

Strom, T. Q., & Kosciulek, J. (2007). Stress, appraisal and coping following mild traumatic brain injury. *Journal of Brain Injury, 21*(11), 1137–1145.

Struchen, M. A., Clark, A. N., Sander, A. M., Mills, M. R., Evans, G., & Kurtz, D. (2008). Relation of executive functioning and social communication measures to functional outcomes following traumatic brain injury. *NeuroRehabilitation, 23*(2), 185–198.

Stuart, G. (2013). *Principles and practice of psychiatric nursing.* St. Louis: Mosby.

Stuifbergen, A. (2005). Secondary conditions and life satisfaction among polio survivors. *Rehabilitation Nursing, 30*(5), 173–178.

Substance Abuse and Mental Health Services Administration (2013). *Results from the 2012 National Survey on Drug Use and Health: Mental Health Findings*, NSDUH Series H-47, HHS Publication No. (SMA) 13-4805. Rockville, MD: Author.

Tew, J. (2006). Understanding power and powerlessness: Towards a framework for emancipatory practice in social work. *Journal of Social Work, 6*(1), 33–51.

Tollen, A., & Ahlstrom, G. (1998). Assessment instrument for problem-focused coping: Reliability of APC, Part I. *Scandinavian Journal of Caring Sciences, 12*(1), 18–24.

Tyrrell, E. F., Levack, W. M., Ritchie, L. H., & Keeling, S. M. (2012). Nursing contribution to the rehabilitation of older patients: Patient and family perspectives. *Journal of Advanced Nursing, 68*(11), 2466–2476. doi: 10.1111/j.1365-2648.2012.05944.x

U.S. Department of Health and Human Services, National Institutes of Health, National Institute of Mental Health (NIMH). (2009). Treatment of Children with Mental Illness (NIH Publication No. 09-4702). Retrieved from http://www.nimh.nih.gov/health/publications/treatment-of-children-with-mental-illness-fact-sheet/NIMH-Treatment-Children-Mental-Illness-FAQ_34669.pdf

Van Orden, K. A., Witte, T. K., Cukrowicz, K. C., Braithwaite, S. R., Selby, E. A., & Joiner, T. E., Jr. (2010). The interpersonal theory of suicide. *Psychological Review, 117*(2), 575–600. doi: 10.1037/a0018697

Vespa, A., Jacobsen, P. B., Spazzafumo, L., & Balducci, L. (2011). Evaluation of intrapsychic factors, coping styles, and spirituality of patients affected by tumors. *Psycho-Oncology, 20*(1), 5–11. doi: 10.1002/pon.1719

Vickery, C. D., Evans, C. C., Sepehri, A., Jabeen, L. N., & Gayden, M. (2009). Self-esteem stability and depressive symptoms in acute stroke rehabilitation: Methodological and conceptual expansion. *Rehabilitation Psychology, 54*(3), 332–342.

Walton, J., Craig, C., Derwinski-Robinson, B., & Weinert, C. (2004). I am not alone: Spirituality of chronically ill rural dwellers. *Rehabilitation Nursing, 29*(5), 164–168.

Watkins, L. L., Koch, G. G., Sherwood, A., Blumenthal, J. A., Davidson, J. R., O'Connor, C., & Sketch, M. H. (2013). Association of anxiety and depression with all-cause mortality in individuals with coronary heart disease. *Journal of the American Heart Association, 2*(2), e000068.doi: 10.1161/JAHA.112.000068

Weeks, S., & O'Connor, P. (1997). The FAMTOOL family assessment tool. *Rehabilitation Nursing, 22*(4), 188–191.

Willer, B., Ottenbacher, K. J., & Coad, M. L. (1994). The community integration questionnaire: A comparative examination. *American Journal of Physical Medicine & Rehabilitation, 73*(2), 103–111.

Williams, A. M., & Dahl, C. W. (2002). Patient and caregiver perceptions of stroke survivor behavior: A comparison. *Rehabilitation Nursing, 27*(1), 19–24.

Willmott, C., Ponsford, J., Hocking, C., & Schönberger, M. (2009). Factors contributing to attentional impairments after traumatic brain injury. *Neuropsychology, 23*(4), 424–432. doi: 10.1037/a0015058

Wilson, B. (2013). Memory deficits. In M. Barnes & D. Good (Eds.) *Neurological rehabilitation: Handbook of clinical neurology* (pp. 357– 363). New York: Elsevier.

World Health Organization (WHO). (2012). *Depression* (Fact sheet No. 369). Retrieved from http://www.who.int/mediacentre/factsheets/fs369/en/#

Wu, L.-F. (2011). Group integrative reminiscence therapy on self-esteem, life satisfaction and depressive symptoms in institutionalised older veterans. *Journal of Clinical Nursing, 20*(15-16), 2195–2203. doi: 10.1111/j.1365-2702.2011.03699.x

Wyman-Chick, K. A. (2012). Combining cognitive-behavioral therapy and interpersonal therapy for geriatric depression with complicated grief. Clinical Case Studies. doi: 10.1177/1534650112436679

Yalom, I. (1980). *Existensial psychotherapy*. New York: Basic Books.

Yalom, I. (1986). *Love's executioner*. New York: Basic Books.

Yoshida, K. K., Self, H., Renwick, R. M., Forma, L. L., King, A. J., & Fell, L. A. (2009). Consumer values as a basis for future SCI practice models: Application to women with SCI and body issues. *Topics in Spinal Cord Injury Rehabilitation, 15*(1), 1–14.

Zhang, T., Shi, C., Hu, A., Xu, H., Zheng, M., & Liang, M. (2014). Correlation between acceptance of disability and social relational quality in patients with colostomy. *International Journal of Nursing Sciences, 1*(1), 102–106. doi: http://dx.doi.org/10.1016/j.ijnss.2014.02.019

Online Resources

American Association of Suicidology:
http://www.suicidology.org/home

Mental Help Net:
http://www.mentalhelp.net

National Alliance on Mental Illness:
http://www.nami.org

National Association of Pediatric Nurse Practitioners: Mental Health Resources:
http://www.napnap.org/ProgramsAndInitiatives/MentalHealth/MentalHealthResources.aspx

National Center for PTSD:
http://www.ptsd.va.gov/public/web-resources/web-families.asp

National Institute of Mental Health:
http://www.nimh.nih.gov/index.shtm

Nonprofit resource for mental health:
http://www.helpguide.org

Substance Abuse and Mental Health Services Administration:
http://www.samhsa.gov

Section V

Nursing Management of Patients with Common REHABILITATION DISORDERS

Chapter 21

Patients with Acute and Chronic Neurological Diseases

Joan P. Alverzo, PhD CRRN
Kathryn Doeschot, MSN RN CRRN
Meghan Leah Leibas, BSN RN CRRN

LEARNING OUTCOMES

- Differentiate the epidemiology, etiology, pathophysiology, diagnosis and treatment for key chronic neurological conditions.
- Outline rehabilitation nursing interventions to prevent complications and modify the effects of key chronic neurological conditions.

KEY CHAPTER TOPICS

- Multiple sclerosis
- Parkinson's disease
- Amyotrophic lateral sclerosis
- Guillain-Barré syndrome
- Myasthenia gravis
- Postpolio syndrome

PROFESSIONAL REHABILITATION NURSING DOMAINS AND COMPETENCIES

- Domain 1: Competencies 1.1, 1.2, 1.3, 1.4
- Domain 2: Competencies 2.1, 2.2 (Association of Rehabilitation Nurses [ARN], 2014)

Introduction

Life with a chronic illness is still life. Rehabilitation nurses play an important role in caring for people with a wide variety of chronic illnesses and disabilities. Understanding these conditions and the treatment options form the basis for establishing an effective nursing plan of care. Coping with a chronic condition is very stressful. Rehabilitation nurses are the ideal practitioners to provide and coordinate patient and family education and interventions to help patients integrate the effects of their illness into daily life and remain as independent as possible. It is important for rehabilitation nurses to have current knowledge and the requisite skills to prevent complications and modify the effects of chronic conditions regardless of the practice setting.

I. Multiple Sclerosis (MS)

A. Overview

1. A chronic autoimmune demyelinating disease that affects the white matter of the central nervous system (CNS)
2. Affects primarily adults in the prime years of life, with an increasing incidence in children and adolescents
3. Characterized by numerous etiologic possibilities, an uncertain prognosis, and a course that consists of episodes of remission and relapse
4. An unpredictable disease that can result in diverse neurological impairments and necessitates a collaborative approach to care
5. A degenerative, progressive disease characterized by inflammation, *demyelination* (loss of the myelin sheath that surrounds the nerve fiber tracts), plaques in the white matter of the CNS, and scarring of the myelin sheath in the CNS
6. Involves partial or complete destruction of the myelin sheath followed by sclerotic plaques or scar tissue formation
7. Associated with various signs and symptoms caused by the loss of myelin sheath integrity that interferes with the efficiency of nerve impulse conduction in the CNS
8. The term *multiple sclerosis (MS)* signifies that myelin is lost in multiple areas, leaving scar tissue.

B. Epidemiology

1. Incidence
   a. Currently, approximately 350,000–500,000 people are affected with MS in the United States, and 2.5 million people are affected worldwide (Multiple Sclerosis Foundation, 2009b)

b. Approximately 200 MS cases are diagnosed every week.
c. Average age at diagnosis is between 20 and 50 years (Multiple Sclerosis Foundation, 2009b)
d. A major cause of disability and economic hardship in young adults between the ages of 20 and 40 years
e. Occurs more often in women than men, in people who live in colder northern latitudes, in whites, and in people who have first-degree relatives with MS (Multiple Sclerosis Association of America, 2014; Multiple Sclerosis Foundation, 2013; National Multiple Sclerosis Society, n.d.a)
f. Strong association between ultraviolet radiation and MS distribution, with a higher rate in areas with a low ultraviolet index (Beretich & Beretich, 2009)
g. The number of children with MS is increasing, and statistics suggest there may be 20,000 undiagnosed pediatric MS cases in the United States. Healthcare providers do not typically associate MS with children (Steefel, 2006).
h. Unique diagnostic challenges exist with pediatric MS due to the frequency of other childhood disorders. Children would benefit from specialized comprehensive mutltidisciplinary care that includes pediatric and adult MS experts (National Multiple Sclerosis Society, n.d.b). Three percent to 5% of all pediatric patients with MS experience their first attack during childhood; they have a higher relapse rate than those with adult-onset MS, and cognitive impairment can occur early in the disease's course (Bigi & Banwell, 2012).
i. Recent early evidence suggests an increased risk of MS with vitamin D deficiency, but further research is needed. This could have implications for sunscreen use for those who live in northern climates (Smolders, 2010).
j. The overall pattern of lower paid employment among people with MS compared with other chronic diseases is related to delayed symptom management, with men likely to leave the workplace earlier than women (Simmons, Tribe, & McDonald, 2010).

2. Disease patterns
   a. Relapsing-remitting MS (RRMS) is the most typical pattern of the disease.
      1) Defined by episodes with clear relapses (also known as exacerbations or acute attacks) followed by complete or partial recovery periods (remission) free of disease progression
      2) Involves no disease progression between relapses
      3) Approximately 85% of people are initially diagnosed with this disease pattern (Kalb, 2012).
   b. Secondary progressive MS (SPMS)
      1) Can begin as a relapsing-remitting course followed by progression that is unpredictable
      2) Involves acute attacks that can result in a progressive worsening level of disability
      3) Of the 85% who have an initial diagnosis of RRMS, more than 50% will develop SPMS within 10 years, and 90% within 25 years (Kalb, 2012).
   c. Primary progressive MS (PPMS) is identified by a slow but continuous worsening of the patient's disability but with no actual relapses or remissions. There is less than 5% progression from onset (Ferri, 2013).
   d. Progressive relapsing MS (PRMS)
      1) Marked by disease progression from the onset with definite acute relapses
      2) Involves disease progression that continues to escalate between relapses
      3) At diagnosis, approximately 10%–15% of people have this disease pattern (Ferri, 2013).
   e. Benign MS
      1) Neurological systems can be fully functional 15 years after onset of disease (Thompson & Mauk, 2012).
      2) Involves complete recovery and normal functioning after a symptomatic period
   f. Malignant MS (Thompson & Mauk, 2012)
      1) Shortly after onset, disease has rapid progression (Thompson & Mauk, 2012).
      2) Can cause significant disability or death within 5 years (Thompson & Mauk, 2012)
      3) Considered to be extremely rare (Thompson & Mauk, 2012)

C. Etiology
   1. The specific cause remains unknown.
   2. Causes of MS are multifactorial. Autoreactive T cells and B cells, along with an interaction between multiple genes that influence the immune system under the influence of various environmental factors, are thought to be key in the process.

a. A latent viral infection can lead to inflammation of white matter or trigger an autoimmune reaction that precipitates demyelination.
   1) Viruses identified have included Epstein-Barr and human herpes virus 6.
b. Studies have shown that people born in an area with a high risk of MS who move, before the age of 15 years, to a geographic location with a lower incidence of MS acquire the lower risk associated with their new location (Kalb, 2012; Multiple Sclerosis Foundation, 2009a; National Multiple Sclerosis Society, n.d.a)
c. Although there is no specific genetic pattern of transmission for MS, researchers support a multigenic predisposition that makes certain people susceptible to the disease (National Multiple Sclerosis Society, 2010).
d. Even though MS is not believed to be hereditary, having a first-degree relative significantly increases a person's risk of developing the disease (Multiple Sclerosis Foundation, 2009b)
e. Various stressors including emotional stress, fatigue, pregnancy, viral infection, extreme physical exertion, trauma, and secondary illness have been suggested as triggers for MS.
f. Other factors that increase risk for MS include a low level of vitamin D, smoking, and lack of sun exposure.

D. Pathophysiology

1. Overview
   a. Normally, an intact blood-brain barrier protects the brain from immune-cell activity. In MS, the primary neuropathic condition is an autoimmune process orchestrated by activated T cells. The protective barrier is breached as activated T cells migrate into the CNS, triggering an antibody-antigen reaction (inflammatory response) that leads to demyelination of axons (Lewis, Dirksen, Heitkemper, & Bucher, 2014).
   b. Activation of T cells by environmental factors or virus in genetically susceptible individuals with resultant T-cell migration to CNS is likely the initial event in the development of MS (Lewis et al., 2014).
   c. Demyelination appears as diffuse, discrete lesions (plaques) throughout the brain and spinal cord.
      1) Although *remyelination* (natural healing) by oligodendrocytes can restore some myelin function, the characteristic plaque formation or sclerosis interferes with normal nerve conduction. With ongoing inflammation, myelin loses the ability to regenerate. Damage eventually occurs to the underlying axon.
      2) Nerve impulses slow down initially; eventually, with permanently damaged nerve fibers, the impulses become completely blocked.
      3) Sites of demyelination can occur anywhere within the CNS and produce a wide range of signs and symptoms; however, progressive scarring leads to progressive deterioration in neurological function (Lewis et al., 2014).
2. Clinical manifestations (**Table 21-1**)
   a. Primary symptoms
      1) Occur as the result of the nerve-conduction deficits caused by demyelination and plaque formation
      2) Reflect a specific area of dysfunction in the CNS

Table 21-1. Symptomatic Manifestations of Multiple Sclerosis

Primary Symptoms	Secondary Symptoms	Tertiary Symptoms
Muscle weakness, paralysis, spasticity, and hyperreflexia	Falls, fractures, skin breakdown, contractures, and other injuries	Loss of job
Mild to disabling fatigue	Marked reduction in carrying out all aspects of self-care	Complete change in roles
Visual impairments (e.g., diplopia, scotoma, decreased acuity)	Decreased safety caused by decreased visual input	Social isolation
Numbness, tingling, pain, and tremors	Interruption in rest and disrupted sleep	Divorce
Bowel, bladder, and sexual dysfunction	Urinary tract infections, bowel and bladder incontinence or retention, and marked decline in libido and orgasmic ability	Ineffective coping with anxiety, denial, anger, reactive depression, and suicide
Ataxia, nystagmus, dysarthria (scanning speech), and dysphagia	Problems affecting a safe gait pattern, communication ability, and swallowing function	Loss of financial stability, self-esteem, and self-worth
Cognitive changes (e.g., memory loss, impaired judgment), emotional lability, and depression	Marked decline in healthy and effective coping strategies	

3) Symptoms can range from mild to severe; symptoms are unpredictable and vary from person to person and from time to time in the same person.

b. Secondary symptoms
   1) Occur as a consequence of primary symptoms
   2) Include problematic complications resulting from decreased neurological function

c. Tertiary symptoms
   1) Evolve as the cumulative and detrimental effects of the disease affect all aspects of the person's life
   2) Include psychosocial, vocational, financial, and emotional problems

d. Research has begun to show that MS symptoms can present as clusters of symptoms
   1) Heat intolerance, fatigue, and cognitive and vision loss have been shown to be interrelated (Newland, Thomas, Riley, Flick, & Fearing, 2012).
   2) Women with RRMS have been shown to have symptom clusters of pain, fatigue, depression, sleep disturbance, and impaired cognitive function (Newland, Fearing, Riley & Neith, 2012).

3. Diagnosis

a. There is no specific laboratory or radiological test to definitively diagnose MS.

b. Because MS can mimic other diseases, and the initial symptomatic presentation varies and fluctuates so greatly in severity, diagnosing MS is challenging, and a process of eliminating all other possibilities is required.

c. Diagnostic tests that can support a suspected MS diagnosis include the following:
   1) Magnetic resonance imaging (MRI)
      a) Extremely sensitive to white-matter lesions and useful in identifying demyelinated plaques in the CNS
      b) Is used to distinguish between old and new lesions and to monitor disease progression
      c) MRI of head with gadolinium, MRI of cervical spine also helpful. More than 95% of patients with clinically definite MS have an abnormal brain MRI, and the presence of high-signal, bright lesions is so characteristic of MS that a normal brain MRI might suggest an alternate diagnosis (Goldman & Schafer, 2012). However, a normal MRI of the brain does not conclusively exclude MS (Ferri, 2013).
   2) Cerebrospinal fluid (CSF) analysis reveals elevated immunoglobulin G and the presence of oligoclonal (immunoglobulin G) bands and increased protein.
   3) Evoked potential studies (i.e., somatosensory, auditory, and visual) demonstrate a slow, absent, or abnormal response in electrical impulse conduction.
   4) The Schumacher criteria and the revised McDonald criteria are commonly used criteria for diagnosis of MS.
      a) Schumacher criteria include an abnormal neurological exam; white matter involvement; two or more sites of the CNS; pattern of relapsing, remitting, and progressing; age 10 to 50 years; and no other explanation of symptoms (Mattson, 2002).
      b) McDonald criteria include the number of clinical attacks and number of objective lesions on MRI. In some categories, other additional data including demonstration of dissemination in space and/or dissemination in time; in other categories, CSF findings and criteria for diagnosing PPMS (Mattson, 2002; Polman et al., 2011).

4. Prognosis (Kalb, 2012)

a. A more favorable course is seen with the following factors:
   1) Female gender
   2) Onset before age 35 years
   3) Single area of CNS involvement
   4) Complete recovery after an exacerbation

b. A more unfavorable course is seen with the following factors:
   1) Male gender
   2) Onset after age 35 years
   3) Symptoms indicating brain-stem involvement
   4) Multiple areas of CNS involvement
   5) Poor recovery following exacerbations
   6) Frequent attacks

E. Management Options

1. Goal: To decrease the number and frequency of relapses, enhance recovery from exacerbations, alleviate symptoms, maintain independence, and ensure the best quality of life (Lewis et al., 2014; Monahan, Sands, Neighbors, Marek, & Green, 2007)

2. Pharmacotherapy (**Figure 21-1**)

Figure 21-1. Medications Used to Treat MS*	
Disease-Modifying Agents	Teriflunomide (Aubagio®)
	Interferon beta-1a (Avonex®)
	Interferon beta-1b (Betaseron®)
	Glatiramer acetate (Copaxone®)
	Interferon beta-1b (Extavia®)
	Fingolimod (Gilenya®)
	Mitoxantrone (Novantrone®)
	Peginterferon beta-1a (Plegridy®)
	Interferon beta-1a (Rebif®)
	Dimethyl fumarate (Tecfidera®)
	Natalizumab (Tysabri®)
Managing Relapses	High-dose intravenous Solu-Medrol
	High-dose oral prednisone (Deltasone®)
	Adrenocorticotropic hormone (H.P. Acthar® Gel)

*Refer to appropriate pharmacological references to learn more about dosing, side effects, and precautions.

From "Treating MS: Medications," by National Multiple Sclerosis Society, n.d.c, retrieved from http://www.nationalmssociety.org/Treating-MS/Medications. Copyright by National Multiple Sclerosis Society. Reprinted with permission.

a. The necessity of early treatment for MS has been established; providing early intervention can potentially mitigate the progression of the disease.
b. Treatments can change the course of the disease by decreasing the number and severity of relapses, slowing the progression of the disease, and reducing the accumulation of new lesions (Multiple Sclerosis Foundation, 2014)
   1) Interferon-beta products seal off the blood–brain barrier and inhibit T-cell activation, thereby preventing the T cells from entering the CNS and destroying myelin, and ultimately, nerve axons. These drugs are given by subcutaneous injection or intramuscular injection. They are considered to be first-line therapies. These drugs include interferon beta-1a (Avonex®, Rebif®) and interferon beta-1b (Betaseron®, Extavia®).
   2) Glatiramer acetate (Copaxone®) suppresses the immune system's attack on myelin by decreasing the T cells that damage the myelin and is administered by subcutaneous injection (Courtney, 2014).
   3) Natalizumab (Tysabri®) is a humanized monoclonal antibody and works by blocking the white blood cell receptors that allow them to enter the brain and spinal cord, leading to decreased inflammation, and is administered by intravenous (IV) infusion (Multiple Sclerosis Foundation, 2014). It may also enhance remyelination and stabilize damage to the myelin sheath. Patients who have taken Natalizumab have an increased risk of developing progressive multifocal leukoencephalopathy. Natalizumab is generally recommended for patients who have not responded adequately to, or who cannot tolerate, another treatment for MS (Courtney, 2014; Miller, Karpinski & Jezewski, 2012).
   4) Fingolimod (Gilenya®) is a sphingosine 1-phosphate receptor modulator, a member of the immunomodulatory class of drugs, which inhibits potentially damaging T cells from leaving the lymph nodes, thereby decreasing their numbers in the blood and tissues. It has the potential to reduce damage to the CNS and augment the repair of damaged nerves within the CNS (Courtney, 2014). Studies have shown that it significantly reduces moderate renal inflammatory activity (Miller & Umhauer, 2011). Fingolimod is administered orally.
   5) Teriflunomide (Aubagio®) is an immunomodulator that affects the production of T cells and B cells. It is thought to leave intact the immune system's response to infection, so that the ability to fight infection is maintained while taking this medication. In addition, by reducing production of free radicals, it may inhibit nerve degeneration (Courtney, 2014). Studies have shown that its use promotes a reduction in the

number of combined unique active lesions on MRI, fewer T1 enhancing lesions, fewer new or enlarging T2 lesions per scan, and decreased relapse rate (Miller & Umhauer, 2011). This medication is administered orally.

6) Dimethyl fumarate (Tecfidera®) does not have a known mechanism of action and is still under investigation; however, it may have a distinct dual mechanism of action. First, it is an immunomodulator with anti-inflammatory properties that generate anti-inflammatory cytokines and appear to suppress damaging macrophage cell activity. Second, it may have neuroprotective effects due to its activation of a substance that is critical for resistance to cellular damage as well as for normal immune function. This medication is administered orally (Courtney, 2014).

7) Mitoxantrone (Novantrone®) is a type II topoisomerase inhibitor that disrupts DNA synthesis in cells (Turkoski, 2013). It has been correlated with a high incidence of leukemia and a higher than expected rate of cardiac dysfunction (potentially fatal congestive heart failure can occur during treatments or months to years after use [Epocrates, 2014]) and is therefore rarely used. However, it is indicated for worsening and progressive forms of MS (National Multiple Sclerosis Society, n.d.c). It is administered once every 3 months for a maximum of 2 to 3 years. The total dose is limited to avoid the risk of damage to the heart (Courtney, 2014).

8) Steroid treatment is used to shorten the duration of acute attacks but does not reduce the frequency of exacerbations.

9) Dalfampridine (Ampyra®) is used to improve walking speed for MS patients with gait problems (Turkoski, 2013).

c. Treatment to manage symptoms can be extensive (**Table 21-2**).

d. Baclofen is most often used to treat spasticity and tremor.

e. Injections of glatiramer acetate or interferon can produce local reactions, including itching, pain, swelling, or redness, and reduce adherence to the regimen (Pardo, Boutwell, Conner, Denney, & Loeen-Burkey, 2010).

3. MS has become increasingly expensive to manage because of the cost of the medications, but this has been counterbalanced by a decrease in exacerbation and hospitalizations, influencing many national insurance companies to cover the medications (Lad et al., 2010).

4. Alternative approaches (e.g., bee venom therapy, massage, herbal treatment, dietary modifications) (National Multiple Sclerosis Society, n.d.c)
   a. Approximately 75% of people with MS use some form of complementary and alternative medicine.
   b. Patients using alternative therapies should inform their physicians because of the potential for interactions with other medications.
   c. Alternative medicine should not be substituted for conventional therapies.
   d. Research on the impact of these alternative approaches is difficult, because the course of the disease is so variable.

5. Use of a collaborative team of professionals, including, but not limited to physicians, nurses, physical and occupational therapists, spiritual advisers, social workers, psychologists, vocational rehabilitation specialists, and legal advisors

6. Psychological support (Kalb, 2012)
   a. Disease-related education
   b. Diagnosis and treatment of emotional and cognitive problems
      1) Cognitive-behavioral programs have improved outcomes for many patients, particularly women (Sinclair & Scroggie, 2005).
   c. Family interventions and family support
      1) Ensure that relatives and caregivers have an understanding of the diagnosis (Bowen, MacLehose, & Beaumont, 2011).
      2) Facilitate adjustment to new roles within the family (Bowen et al., 2011).
      3) Facilitate decisions related to care options, especially related to care facilities (Bowen et al., 2011).
   d. Support to remain productively employed and/or support to transition out of the workforce
   e. Provide assistance to access available resources

7. Exercise
   a. Aquatic or water therapy gives buoyancy to the body, allowing performance of activities that otherwise would not be possible.
   b. Yoga and tai chi can be beneficial.
   c. Exercises that are fatiguing should be avoided.

8. Nutritional therapy
   a. A high-protein, low-fat, low-cholesterol diet with supplemental vitamins is recommended (Lewis, Heitkemper, & Dirkesen, 2004; Multiple Sclerosis Foundation, 2009b).

Table 21-2. Medications Commonly Used to Treat Symptoms of Multiple Sclerosis*

Symptom	Drug
Weakness	Dalfampridine (Ampyra)
Bladder: Failure to store urine, urgency, frequency, incontinence, nocturia	Onabotulinum toxin A (Botox®)
	Oxybutynin (Ditropan)
	Tolterodine tartrate (Detrol)
Fatigue	Amantadine
	Modanifil (Provigil)
	Methylphenidate (Ritalin)
Depression, anxiety	SNRI medications
	SSRI medications
Pseudobulbar effect	Dextromethorphan + Quinidine (Nuedexta)
	SSRI medications
	Tricyclic antidepressants
Central neuropathic pain-continuous (dysesthesias)	Tricyclic antidepressants
	Antiepileptic medications (pregabalin, gabapentin)
Central neuropathic pain—intermittent (trigeminal neuralgia)	Carbemazepine
	Oxcarbazepine
	Lamotrigine
	Baclofen
Retro-orbital pain	High-dose IV steroids
Sexual dysfunction—male	Sildenafil
	Vardenafil
	Tadalafil
	Injectable:Alprostadil
Spasticity	Baclofen
	Tizanidine
	Dantrolene
	Clonazepam
	Gabapentin
	Levatiracetam
	Clonidine
	Diazepam
	Botox®
Tremor	Propranalol
	Clonazepam
	Hydroxizine
	Primidone
	Isoniazid
	Topiramate
	Buspirone
	Ondansetron
	Gabapentin
Vertigo	Meclizine
	Benzodiazepines
	High-dose corticosteroids
Visual disturbances	High-dose corticosteroids

*Refer to appropriate pharmacological references to learn more about dosing, side effects and precautions of these medications.

Abbreviations: IV, intravenous; SNRI, serotonin norepinephrine reuptake inhibitor; SSRI, selective serotonin reuptake inhibitor.

Adapted from "Symptom Management," by National Multiple Sclerosis Society, n. d., retrieved from http://www.nationalmssociety.org/For-Professionals/Clinical-Care/Managing-MS/Symptom-Management/. Copyright by National Multiple Sclerosis Society. Adapted with permission; "Management of MS-Related Fatigue," by National Clinical Advisory Board of the Multiple Sclerosis Society, 2006, retrieved from http://www.nationalmssociety.org/NationalMSSociety/media/MSNationalFiles/Brochures/ExpOp_Fatigue.pdf. Copyright 2006 by National Multiple Sclerosis Society. Adapted with permission.

b. Natural fiber is encouraged to promote bowel regularity.
c. Research has shown that, at times, vitamin deficiency and malnutrition are overlooked, and more research is needed related to nutritional intake, inflammatory biomarkers, and the MS disease course over time (Plow & Finlayson, 2012)

9. Neuropathic pain, including central neuropathic pain, occurs in more than 40% of people with MS and is described as a constant, often spontaneous burning feeling, most often in the lower limbs (Solaro & Messmer Uccelli, 2010).
   a. Treatment includes tricyclic antidepressants and antiepileptic medication. Cannabinoids can be useful for some people.
   b. Antispasticity medications such as baclofen and benzodiazepines are often used to manage spasticity-related pain.
10. Spasticity and incontinence symptoms may be treated with botulinum toxin injections, but studies to confirm its efficacy are still pending (Habek, Kami, Balash, & Gurevich, 2010).

F. Nursing Process

1. Assessment
   a. Obtain a complete health history and information about current symptoms, time of onset, and history of relapses, including recent or past viral infections or vaccinations, physical or emotional stress, pregnancy, or exposure to extremes of heat and cold based on their potential to trigger an exacerbation (Hickey, 2009).
   b. Pay particular attention to mental state and overt coping abilities.

c. Determine how the disease has affected the patient's lifestyle and family.
d. Observe the patient's overall appearance.
e. Investigate physical mobility, urinary elimination, self-care activities, and safety concerns.
f. Assess for spasticity, weakness, incontinence, and visual and hearing impairments.
g. Investigate use of and compliance in taking prescription medications and alternative approaches.

2. Plan of care
   a. Nursing diagnoses
      1) Impaired physical mobility related to neuromuscular impairment (e.g., weakness, spasticity, and tremor)
      2) Fatigue related to the MS disease process
      3) Self-care deficits (e.g., bathing, dressing, feeding, toileting) related to weakness, spasticity, and tremor
      4) Altered urinary elimination (e.g., retention, frequency, urgency) related to spinal cord involvement and decreased functional ability
      5) Knowledge deficit related to the variable nature of symptoms and multifaceted treatment options
      6) Ineffective individual coping related to the variability of the disease course, cognitive impairments, decreased independence, and changes in family and vocational roles
      7) Sensory perception alterations: visual, related to optic nerve involvement (e.g., diplopia, nystagmus, blurred vision)
      8) Chronic pain related to neuropathy
      9) Impaired communication related to impaired speech muscles
      10) High risk for aspiration related to impaired muscles for swallowing
      11) Ineffective breathing patterns related to impaired respiratory muscles
      12) Altered nutrition, less than required, related to inability to swallow (Hickey, 2009)
   b. Goals
      1) Maintain maximal level of mobility.
      2) Demonstrate safety in mobility and recognize the need for appropriate assistive devices.
      3) Conserve energy and verbalize understanding of ways to integrate energy-conservation principles into daily activities.
      4) Attain maximal level of function in activities of daily living (ADLs).
      5) Maintain continence and identify symptoms of urinary tract infection.
      6) Verbalize understanding of the disease process, significant implications, and prescribed regimens.
      7) Verbalize appropriate plans for coping with stress.
      8) Attain maximal visual functioning, and demonstrate satisfactory use of compensatory measures when needed.
      9) Verbalize satisfactory pain relief.
      10) Maintain maximal level of cognitive function (Thompson & Mauk, 2012)
3. Nursing interventions
   a. Improve mobility and neuromuscular function.
      1) Encourage progressive, resistive exercises according to the prescribed physical therapy program to maintain function of the uninvolved nerves.
      2) Gradually build up tolerance through a daily exercise program.
      3) Use assistive devices (e.g., walker, cane, wheelchair, motorized scooter).
      4) Avoid physical and emotional stressors.
      5) Avoid exposure to extreme heat, and schedule activities to occur during the cooler part of the day; ensure that air conditioning is available in warm weather.
   b. Conserve energy (Burnett, 2013)
      1) Counseling to identify factors contributing to fatigue
      2) Identification of symptom patterns
      3) Use of energy-conservation techniques (e.g., setting priorities, delegating tasks to others, consolidating tasks through planning, using labor-saving devices, pacing activities, establishing periods for short naps)
      4) Avoid vigorous exercise.
   c. Maintain independence in ADLs.
      1) Encourage a balance between assisted and independent activities.
      2) Encourage the use of assistive devices to promote independence.
      3) Avoid extremes in body temperature and use air conditioning when needed.
   d. Improve bladder function and prevent complications.
      1) Avoid caffeinated beverages and encourage high daily fluid intake (approximately 3,000 mL per day).
      2) Administer medications to improve muscle tone of bladder and facilitate emptying,

and instruct patient on effective use of medication.

3) Teach intermittent self-catheterization or external catheter procedures.
4) Use Credé's maneuver or manual reflex stimulation for emptying reflexic bladder (unless contraindicated by complications such as detrusor sphincter dyssynergia).
5) Instruct the patient to identify and prevent urinary tract infections.

e. Improve bowel function and prevent complications.
 1) Teach importance of consistent schedule, limiting irritants, increasing fluid intake, and increasing dietary fiber if tolerable.
 2) Teach scheduling of bowel program 40–45 minutes after a meal (or hot beverage) to stimulate the gastrocolic and duodenocolic reflexes.
 3) Administer medications as necessary to maintain a regular bowel regimen (Thompson & Mauk, 2012).

f. Improve knowledge.
 1) Provide information to help manage the disease on a continuous basis.
 2) Encourage the patient to ask questions.
 3) Review educational information with the patient and family.

g. Develop effective coping strategies to adjust to the illness.
 1) Encourage the patient and family to verbalize feelings and concerns.
 2) Refer the patient and family to support groups (e.g., Multiple Sclerosis Association of America, National Multiple Sclerosis Society).
 3) Make referrals for psychological counseling as necessary.

h. Maintain visual functioning.
 1) Administer treatment as needed (eye patch or occluder, medications).
 2) Instruct patients to rest their eyes when fatigue is noticed.
 3) Advise patients of availability of large-type material and talking books.

i. Promote comfort.
 1) Provide medication as ordered for pain control and instruct on effective use of medications and precautions.
 2) Manage spasticity, including a medication regimen and positioning or movement to reduce the incidence of spasticity.
 3) Encourage use of alternative pain relief measures (e.g., distraction, relaxation, imagery, music, massage).
 4) Assess effectiveness of pain relief measures.

j. Maintain nutritional status.
 1) Assess for swallowing difficulties.
 2) Develop an appropriate dysphagia management plan with patient, care partner, and interdisciplinary team.
 3) Monitor weight at each visit.
 4) Reinforce education with patient and care partner on safe swallowing strategies (Thompson & Mauk, 2012).

k. Maintain cognitive functioning.
 1) Screen for elements that could increase cognitive difficulties, such as medications, sleep disturbance, inadequately controlled pain, and any other untreated symptoms.
 2) Provide instruction both verbally and in handouts, recognize the need to decrease distractions, and implement a safety plan (Thompson & Mauk, 2012).

II. Parkinson's Disease

A. Overview

1. *Parkinson's disease* (PD) is a slowly progressive neurodegenerative disease of the brain.
2. PD involves manifestations that occur when there is significant damage to or destruction of dopamine-producing neurons in the substantia nigra within the basal ganglia of the brain. Approximately 60% of these neurons will have degenerated before clinical symptoms present (Goldman & Schafer, 2012, p. 2327).
3. PD begins insidiously and is characterized by a prolonged course of illness.
4. Loss of dopamine causes neurons to fire out of control, leading to marked disability with the initiation and execution of smooth, coordinated voluntary movements and balance.
5. There is no known way to stop or cure the disease.
6. PD is one of the most common chronic diseases of the nervous system, second only to Alzheimer's disease (Goldman & Schafer, 2012, p. 2326).
7. Types
 a. Primary PD
  1) A chronic debilitating disease caused by an idiopathic dopamine deficiency in the basal ganglia of the brain
  2) Characterized by tremor at rest, rigidity, bradykinesia, and postural instability.
 b. Secondary parkinsonism or parkinsonism syndrome: A group of symptoms (e.g., tremors, stiffness, slow movements) in which there is a

known cause of injury to the dopamine-producing cells.

B. Epidemiology and Incidence

1. Approximately 1 million Americans have PD, with the greatest incidence in whites, and the lowest in Asians and African Americans (Ferri, 2013). Worldwide, 7–10 million people are living with PD (Parkinson's Disease Foundation, 2012).
2. Approximately 60,000 new cases are diagnosed annually in the United States (Parkinson's Disease Foundation, 2012).
3. PD occurs slightly more often in men than in women.
4. PD is diagnosed at an average age of 60 years and incidence increases with age (Parkinson's Disease Foundation, 2012).
5. Approximately 4% of people with PD are younger than age 50 years (young onset PD) (Parkinson's Disease Foundation, 2012).

C. Etiology

1. Primary PD is idiopathic.
2. A number of theories of causation for PD are being tested and include viral, vascular, metabolic, environmental, and genetic; however, PD currently is believed to be associated with a combination of genetic and environmental factors (e.g., viruses, toxins, free radical exposure) (Monahan et al., 2007).
3. There is some suggestion that the use of nonsteroidal antiinflammatory drugs could provide some protection from development of the disease (Gagne & Power, 2010).
4. Secondary parkinsonism could be linked to a variety of causes: Response to antipsychotic, antihypertensive, and neuroleptic agents; metoclopramide (Reglan®); or illicit drug use (e.g., amphetamine, methamphetamine); response to brain trauma, hydrocephalus, tumors, ischemia, encephalitis infections, and arteriosclerosis; response to neurotoxins such as cyanide, manganese, carbon monoxide, and pesticides (Lewis et al., 2014)

D. Pathophysiology

1. Overview
   a. The Braak hypothesis proposes that the earliest evidence of PD is found in the medulla and olfactory bulb and that the disease progresses to the substantia nigra and cortex (Hayes, Fung, Kimber, & O'Sullivan, 2010).
   b. Degenerative changes in several areas in the basal ganglia deplete the inhibitory neurotransmitter dopamine, normally provided to the basal ganglia by the neurons in the substantia nigra.
      1) Dopamine is a neurotransmitter essential for the functioning of the extrapyramidal system, which includes control of upright posture, support, and voluntary motion.
      2) Normally, there is a balance between the neurotransmitters dopamine and acetylcholine (ACh), which are responsible for controlling and refining motor movements and have opposing effects.
   c. An increase in the excitatory effects of ACh caused by depletion of dopamine causes the manifestations of PD and prevents affected brain cells from performing their normal inhibitory function in the CNS.
   d. A shift in the balance of neurotransmitter activity is responsible for the patient's difficulty in controlling and initiating voluntary movements; manifestations occur with 80% destruction of neurons in the substantia nigra (Lewis et al., 2014).
   e. As the disease progresses, dopamine receptors in the basal ganglia are reduced.
2. Clinical features: Classic manifestations (Lewis et al., 2014)
   a. Tremor is often the first sign.
      1) Occurs in the tongue, lips, jaw, chin, head, diaphragm, and limbs
      2) May involve a pill-rolling movement of the thumb and finger
      3) Is present at rest and diminishes with active movement
   b. Rigidity or cogwheeling: Resistance to movement caused by constant contraction of opposing muscle groups, caused by abnormal muscle stiffness and jerky movements with passive motion
   c. Bradykinesia or akinesia: Inability to initiate movement or change movement, which results in abnormal slowness
   d. Postural instability, which causes a stooped-over, flexed posture and a shuffling propulsive gait with no arm swing. Diminished postural reflexes lead to frequent falls that are associated with balance and coordination problems.
   e. Other symptoms: Masklike facial appearance; difficulty chewing and swallowing; voice changes; autonomic disturbances (e.g., orthostatic hypotension, constipation, excessive perspiration, oily skin); and numerous cognitive losses (e.g., memory, problem solving, depression)

3. Diagnosis (Lewis et al., 2014)
   a. Diagnosis is made clinically from the patient's history and presenting symptoms of at least two of three signs of classic triad (i.e., tremor, rigidity, bradykinesia).
   b. No specific laboratory or radiologic studies are available to support a positive diagnosis.
   c. Definitive diagnosis can be confirmed after assessment of the patient's response to antiparkinson medications.

E. Management Options
1. General notes
   a. Currently, there is no known treatment that halts or reverses neuronal degeneration (Hayes et al., 2010).
   b. Current options provide symptomatic relief and improve quality of life.
   c. Nonmotor symptoms (e.g., sleep dysfunction, sensory symptoms, autonomic dysfunction, depression, mood disorders, anxiety disorders, apathy, fatigue, and cognitive dysfunction and dementia, add to the morbidity and may not have effective treatment options) (Fox et al., 2011).
   d. Recent studies have demonstrated increased risk of osteoporosis and osteopenia for patients with PD. Patients with PD have lower bone mineral density and have a greater risk of fractures (Torsney et al., 2014).
2. Types of treatment: motor symptoms
   a. Pharmacotherapy involves the use of drugs from various classes (e.g., monoamine oxidase B inhibitor, levodopa, dopamine agonist, anticholinergic, and catechol-O-methyltransferase inhibitor (Fox et al., 2011) (**Table 21-3**).
      1) Multiple drugs have been developed (e.g., dopamine agonists). Medications include transdermal routes of administration. Newer dopamine agonists can be used as monotherapy and as symptomatic adjuncts to levodopa (Fox et al., 2011).
      2) Levodopa with carbidopa traditionally was the first drug used. Has multiple side effects and drug interactions. Although it is the most widely used drug, patients with PD require frequent changes to their regimen related to changes in symptoms and side effects of the drugs.
   b. Prolonged use of levodopa can result in dyskinesia and an unpredictable period of drug effectiveness (i.e., "off/on" periods) (Lewis et al., 2014).

Table 21-3. Parkinson's Disease Drug Therapy

Drug	Mechanism of Action
Dopaminergics ***Dopamine Precursors*** Levodopa (L-dopa) Levodopa/carbidopa (Sinemet, Parcopa [orally dissolving tablet])	Converted to dopamine in basal ganglia
Dopamine Receptor Agonists Bromocriptine (Parlodeil) Pergolide (Permax) Pramipexole (Mirapex) Ropinirole (Requip, Requip XL) Rotigotine (Neupro [skin patch])	Stimulate dopamine receptors
Dopamine Agonists Amantadine (Symmetrel) Apomorphine (Apokyn)	Blocks reuptake of dopamine into presynaptic neurons Stimulates postsynaptic dopamine receptors
Anticholinergics Trihexyphenidyl (Artane) Benztropine (Cogentin) Biperiden (Akineton)	Block cholinergic receptors, thus helping to balance cholinergic and dopaminergic activity
Antihistamine Diphenhydramine (Benadryl®)	Has anticholinergic effect
Monoamine Oxidase Inhibitors Selegiline (Eldepryl, Carbex) Rasagiline (Azilect)	Block breakdown of dopamine
Catechol O-Methyltransferase (COMT) Inhibitors Entacapone (Comtan) Toicapone (Tasmar)	Block COMT and slow the breakdown of levodopa, thus prolonging the action of levodopa

From *Medical-surgical nursing: Assessment and mangement of clinical problems* (9th ed.). by S. K. Lewis, S. R. Dirksen, M. M. Heitkemper, & L. Bucher, 2014, St. Louis: Elsevier. Copyright 2014 by Elsevier. Reprinted with permission.

   c. Duodenal infusion of levodopa is under investigation; for long-term clinical use, a permanent tube fitted via a gastrostomy tube would be required.
3. Monoamine oxidase-B (MAO-B) inhibitors are often used for initial treatment in early PD. A recent Cochrane review noted improved outcomes in quality of life indicators. MAO-Bs provide mild symptomatic benefit with few side effects.
4. Dopamine agonists such as ropirinol and pramipexole are used for moderate symptomatic benefit, and compared with leveodopa, delay the development of dyskinesia.
   a. Frequent adverse events include somnolence, sudden-onset sleep, hallucinations, edema, and impulse control disorders (Hauser, 2014

5. Additional device-aided therapy for treatment of motor problems in advanced PD: continuous subcutaneous apomorphine infusion (Volkmann et al., 2013).
6. Antiparkinson medications used to manage symptoms are effective for 4–6 years.
   a. After this, disability tends to progress despite medical management.
7. Neuroprotective medications are used to try to slow, block, or reverse disease progression.
   a. To slow the loss of dopamine neurons
   b. Agents under investigation include MAO-B inhibitors, creatine, and isradipine (Hauser, 2014).
8. Nonmotor symptom management
   a. Sildenafil citrate (Viagra®) for erectile dysfunction
   b. Polyethylene glycol for constipation
   c. Modafinil for excessive daytime somnolence
   d. Methylphenidate for fatigue
   e. Little evidence for specific pharmacological treatments for orthostatic hypotension, urinary incontinence, anxiety, and rhythmic movement disorder (Hauser, 2014)
   f. Surgical interventions offer some people relief from some symptoms, treat motor complications or serve as symptomatic adjunct to levodopa (Fox et al, 2011; Lewis et al., 2014).
      1) Pallidotomy and thalamotomy destroy groups of brain cells of the thalamus or basal ganglia to prevent involuntary movements, which are among the most distressing symptoms.
         a) Not reversible
      2) Thalamic or deep-brain stimulators have been approved by the U.S. Food and Drug Administration to treat tremor. This procedure can be reversed or adjusted depending on patient outcomes.
         a) Electrodes are surgically implanted into the thalamus, globus pallidus, or subthalamic nuclei and connected to a neurostimulator (i.e., pulse generator) implanted under the skin of the chest (like a pacemaker).
         b) After the system is in place, the device is programmed to deliver electrical stimulation from the neurostimulator through the extension wire and the lead and into the brain to targeted areas that control movement, thereby blocking the abnormal nerve signals that cause tremor and PD symptoms.
         c) The patient can self-activate the device.
         d) Currently, the procedure is used only for people whose symptoms cannot be adequately controlled with medications.
         e) Many people experience reduction of their PD symptoms after undergoing deep-brain stimulation and are able to greatly reduce their medications (Fox et al., 2011).
   g. Transplantation: Still in experimental stages, transplantation of fetal neural tissue into the brain is designed to provide dopamine-producing cells in the brain, allowing these cells to grow and process dopamine with a goal of either halting or reversing the disease process (Brundin, Barker, & Parmar, 2010).
   h. Nonpharmacological therapies (Fox et al., 2011)
      1) Physical therapy is likely efficacious for treatment of motor symptoms as an adjunct to levodopa.
      2) Occupational and speech therapies: Few studies have investigated effectiveness, but both possibly useful as symptomatic therapy adjunct to levodopa
   i. Nutritional intervention
      1) Diet should contain adequate roughage and fruit to prevent constipation.
      2) Low-protein diet with less fat and more carbohydrates; foods high in protein can decrease absorption of levodopa (Lewis et al., 2014)
      3) Food should be cut into bite-sized pieces, and ample time should be planned for eating.
   j. Expiratory muscle strength training (EMST) used effectively for patients with PD (Burnett, 2013)
   k. Treatment of nonmotor symptoms in PD: evidence-based medicine reviews (Seppi et al., 2011)
      1) Pramipexole is efficacious for treatment of depressive symptoms.
      2) Clozapine is efficacious for treatment of psychosis (close monitoring is needed).
      3) Rivastigmine is efficacious for treatment of dementia.
      4) Botulinum toxins A and B are efficacious in treatment of sialorrhea (i.e., hypersalivation). Glycopyrrolate could be effective as a short-term treatment.
      5) Methylphenidate and modafinil for treating fatigue is in an investigational stage.

6) Nonpharmacological measures to treat orthostatic hypotension include sleeping in a head-up position; increasing frequency or decreasing size of meals; performing physical counter-maneuvers (e.g., squatting, bending forward at waist) at onset of presyncopal symptoms; increasing water and salt intake; and wearing support stockings. Midrodrine and fludocortisone are in use on an investigational basis.
7) Investigational use of sildenafil for treatment of erectile dysfunction (contraindicated in patients on nitrate medications for coronary heart disease)
8) L-dopa/carbidopa controlled release, eszopiclone, and melatonin are under investigation for the treatment of insomnia in PD.
9) Investigational use of modafinil for treatment of excessive daytime sleepiness.

F. Nursing Process

1. Assessment
   a. Obtain a complete health history and information about current symptoms, time of onset, and progression, including CNS trauma, exposure to metals and carbon dioxide, encephalitis, and use of tranquilizers or antipsychotic medications.
   b. Pay particular attention to mental status, ability to answer questions, and overt coping abilities.
   c. Determine how the disease has affected the patient and family, and ask which aspects of the disease are most troublesome.
   d. Observe overall appearance, posture, and gait pattern.
   e. Determine level of extremity stiffness, tremors, and ability to move.
   f. Investigate safe mobility, self-care activities, nutritional intake, and verbal communication.
2. Plan of care
   a. Nursing diagnoses (Monahan et al., 2007)
      1) Ineffective individual coping related to depression and increasingly severe physical limitations
      2) Knowledge deficit related to disease progression, treatment, ongoing adaptations, and availability of support systems
      3) Impaired physical mobility related to tremor, rigidity, bradykinesia, and postural instability
      4) Self-care deficits (e.g., bathing, dressing, feeding, toileting) related to tremor, rigidity, bradykinesia, and postural instability
      5) Inadequate nutrition related to difficulty with chewing, swallowing, and drooling
      6) Impaired verbal communication related to low voice, slow speech, and difficulty moving facial muscles
      7) Risk of injury (i.e., falling) related to tremors, bradykinesia, and altered gait (Kerr et al., 2010)
   b. Goals
      1) Verbalize appropriate plans for coping with stress.
      2) Verbalize understanding of the disease process, significant implications, and prescribed regimen.
      3) Maintain maximal level of mobility.
      4) Attain maximal level of function in ADLs.
      5) Verbalize understanding of diet management and achieve adequate hydration and nutritional balance.
      6) Communicate effectively.
      7) Demonstrate safety in mobility, and recognize the need for appropriate assistive devices.
      8) Uses assistive devices appropriately for ambulation and mobility (Lewis et al., 2014).
3. Interventions
   a. Develop positive coping mechanisms.
      1) Allow the patient to freely verbalize feelings and concerns.
      2) Encourage participation in support groups (e.g., Parkinson's Disease Foundation, Parkinson's Support Groups of America, National Parkinson Foundation).
      3) Encourage the patient to establish realistic, attainable goals.
      4) Support the use of prescribed psychotherapy and medication to combat depression.
   b. Develop a sound knowledge base about the disease and treatments.
      1) Teach the patient about the common signs, symptoms, and progression of PD.
      2) Discuss aspects and related terminology of the disease that are unique to PD and the use of antiparkinson drugs (e.g., "on-off," "wearing off," and "freezing" phenomena).
      3) Educate the patient and family about the desired effects and side effects of prescribed medications and surgical treatments.
      4) Offer suggestions to make living with PD easier, including energy conservation, home modifications, and assistive devices for walking or transfers from one surface to another.

5) Inform the patient and family of local and national support groups for assistance and education.

c. Improve mobility and maximize neuromuscular function.

1) Encourage active and passive range of motion (ROM) exercises according to the prescribed physical therapy program.
2) Allow time for rest after activity, and avoid rushing.
3) Administer medications as prescribed to avoid exacerbation of symptoms.
4) Use warm baths and massage to help relax muscles.
5) Teach to concentrate on walking erect by consciously using a wide-based gait and deliberately swinging the arms; teach the patient to pretend to cross over an imaginary line or rock side to side to initiate leg movement to help deal with "freezing" while walking.
6) Provide muscle stretching and massage to reduce rigidity.

d. Maintain independence in ADLs.

1) Encourage the use of devices to make self-care easier (e.g., raised toilet seats, trapeze bars, grab bars, long-handled shoehorns, elastic shoelaces).
2) Allow adequate time to accomplish self-care.
3) Make environmental modifications to increase safety and independence.

e. Achieve satisfactory hydration and nutritional status.

1) Offer oral care before and after meals (improves intake) (Burnett, 2013).
2) Encourage patients to sit upright for all meals.
3) Offer semisolid foods and thickened liquids if choking occurs.
4) Use stabilized plates, plate guards, nonspill cups, and large-handled utensils.
5) Augment caloric intake with supplementary feedings/nutrient-rich snacks. Consider six small meals daily to meet caloric needs (Burnett, 2013).
6) Monitor weight weekly.
7) Consult with speech therapy for a swallowing evaluation if any question about safe swallowing arises (Burnett, 2013).
8) Regular and meticulous oral care with toothbrush is recommended for patients with dysphagia. Evidence indicates foam brushes are not as effective as toothbrushes in removing plaque and preventing gum disease (Burnett, 2013).

f. Use alternative communication methods as needed to interact with others (Lewis et al., 2014).

1) Reinforce oral exercises prescribed by the speech and language therapist.
2) Listen attentively and wait for the patient to answer questions. Encourage patients to repeat words.
3) Use a picture board if muscle involvement has impaired writing and speaking ability.
4) Use simple words and short sentences.
5) Give one simple direction at a time.

g. Maintain safety.

1) Modify the environment to remove hazards and improve lighting.
2) Install devices for safety (e.g., grab bars, raised toilet seats).
3) Change position slowly with orthostatic hypotension.

III. Amyotrophic Lateral Sclerosis

A. Overview

1. Amyotrophic lateral sclerosis (ALS) is a rapidly progressive neurodegenerative disease involving the destruction of motor neurons in the brain stem and the anterior gray horns of the spinal cord and degeneration of pyramidal tracts
2. Variations in disease progression exist. Functional loss can begin with upper-motor neurons, lower-motor neurons, bulbar symptoms only, or a combination.
3. Characterized by muscle weakness, wasting, and atrophy, followed by spasticity and hyperreflexia
4. Onset is often subtle, and first symptoms may be disregarded. Diagnosis consists of a combination of tests. No single test exists to diagnose ALS.
5. There is no known prevention and no known cure for ALS, but treatments exist to assist in slowing deterioration.
6. Rehabilitation focuses on adaptation to increasing losses of function. Caregiver training will become necessary as the disease progresses and the patient loses self-care abilities.
7. This disease was historically called Lou Gehrig's disease because of the national and international attention the baseball star brought to ALS after his 1939 diagnosis, but a new study has cast doubt on whether Gehrig had ALS or another neurological condition (Schwarz, 2010).

B. Epidemiology

1. Approximately 30,000 people in the United States have ALS at any given time. The incidence ranges from 1.5 to 2.5 per 100,000 people (ALS Association, 2014).
2. Estimated 5,600 new cases of ALS are diagnosed in the United States each year (ALS Association, 2014)
3. ALS more common in males than females by ratio of 2:1 (Lewis et al., 2014)
4. ALS incidence rates increase with age, peaking between 70 and 80 years of age. Rate may be lower in some ethnic populations (e.g., American Indians) and significantly higher in locations such as Guam, Japan's Kii Peninsula, and western New Guinea (Gordon, 2013).
5. Life expectancy ranges from months to decades; median survival is 19 months from diagnosis and 30 months from onset on average (Gordon, 2013).

C. Etiology
1. Sporadic, unknown cause (90%–95% of cases); contributing factors could involve genetics, age, tobacco use, and athleticism
2. Genetic (5%–10% of cases): Mutations responsible for ALS have been identified in approximately 60% of cases (Gordon, 2013).

D. Pathophysiology
1. Overview
   a. ALS is characterized by destruction of motor neurons, primarily in the motor nuclei of the brain stem, anterior horn cells of the spinal cord, corticospinal tracts, and Betz's and precentral cells of the frontal cortex.
   b. Asymmetric muscle weakness and wasting occurs most often, leading to paresis, and progression of functional loss varies.
      1) Upper-motor neuron involvement causes reduced strength and spasticity, often beginning with the intrinsic muscles of the hands.
      2) Lower-motor neuron involvement causes fasciculation, cramps, marked weakness, and muscular atrophy (Gordon, 2013).
   c. Cognitive impairment initially was considered uncommon; recent studies have shown a 15% incidence of frontotemporal dementia, and up to 50% of patients have impaired cognitive skills, as measured by neuropsychological tests (Gordon, 2013). Multiple studies have found that a significant proportion of patient with ALS demonstrate cognitive impairment, some with dementia (National Guideline Clearinghouse, 2012).
2. Differentiation of ALS from motor neuron disease with variants (Polak, Richman, Lorimer, Bonton DeSpulveda, & Del Bene, 2004)
   a. Motor neuron disease with variants
      1) Primary lateral sclerosis, with limited upper motor neuron component, with the longest survival (in the decades) and a progressive decline
      2) Progressive bulbar palsy, with bulbar symptoms and upper or lower motor neuron involvement, with a poor prognosis
      3) Progressive muscular atrophy, with lower motor neuron changes and a prognosis similar to that of ALS
   b. ALS
      1) Asymmetric distal weakness greater than proximal weakness
      2) Upper and lower motor neuron symptoms and bulbar and thoracic symptoms
3. Pathophysiological processes (Gordon, 2013)
   a. Mitochondrial dysfunction
   b. Excitotoxicity: Glutamate defect possible in metabolism, transport, or storage
   c. Oxidative stress caused by excessive free radicals
   d. Aggregation of misfolded protein
   e. Inflammation
   f. Apoptosis (programmed cell death)
4. Clinical manifestations
   a. Asymmetric weakness in all extremities occurs progressively with no remission. Ability to perform ADLs and instrumental ADLs is lost as function decreases.
   b. Intrinsic muscles of hands lose function, resulting in inability to perform fine motor movement (e.g., buttoning pants, tying shoes, writing).
   c. Weakening and loss of gross motor muscles result in inability to walk or stand.
   d. Bulbar symptoms affect swallowing ability. Not every person experiences this symptom.
   e. Brain-stem involvement can account for cranial nerve function loss. Fasciculation, flaccidity, or spasticity can occur in the tongue, hands, and upper extremities.
   f. Frontal lobe involvement can result in emotional lability, regardless of intact intellect.
      1) Pseudobulbar affect could improve with amitriptyline, sertraline, or dextromethorphan/quinine (Ferri, 2013)
   g. Loss of bowel and bladder function and eye movement often occurs late in disease progression.

h. Complete paresis often occurs as the disease progresses.
i. Respiratory muscle involvement inhibits proper breathing, necessitating mechanical support at the patient's discretion.
j. Dysarthria in ALS is related to quality of life, and maintaining effective communication is a priority of treatment (Tomik & Gulloff, 2010).
k. Pain is a common symptom in the later stages. There is little research about how to manage pain in ALS, so conventional pain management strategies should be used (Brettschneider, Kurent, Ludolph, & Mitchell, 2008).

5. Diagnosis
   a. "Diagnosis of progressive UMN and LMN findings by history and examination, is accurate 95% of time when made by an experienced clinician" (Gordon, 2013, p. 297). A combination of laboratory testing, electrophysiology studies, neuroimaging studies, and muscle biopsy are combined with history and physical to determine a diagnosis of ALS. There is no single test to diagnose ALS (**Table 21-4**).
   b. Diagnosis is typically made late in the disease. Individual muscle group involvement early on may be mistaken for other health problems.

E. Management Options
1. A multidisciplinary approach is needed to meet the host of patient problems that occur as the disease progresses (Miller et al., 2009). High-risk issues include the following:
   a. Aspiration pneumonia
   b. Malnutrition
   c. Loss of ability to speak
   d. Muscle spasticity and wasting
   e. Respiratory insufficiency
   f. Depression
2. The focus should be on palliative care and comfort.
3. Key decisions related to management must be discussed in advance of a crisis (Rowland & Shineider, 2001).
4. A teaching plan is developed and individualized to the patient and family.
5. The patient is helped to be as independent as possible for as long as possible with the use of assistive techniques and devices.
6. Education about symptom management is prepared and implemented.
7. The patient and family are assisted to reduce the development of complications.
8. Referrals to support groups, medical professionals, and community resources are provided.

Table 21-4. Diagnostics for Amyotrophic Lateral Sclerosis

- History
- Physical, including thorough neurological exam
- Electromyography to measure fasciculation potentials
- Nerve conduction velocity study
- Blood and urine studies
  - High resolution serum protein electrophoresis
  - Thyroid and parathyroid hormone levels
  - 24-hour urine collection for heavy metals
- Spinal tap
- X rays and magnetic resonance imaging
- Myelogram of cervical spine
- Muscle and/or nerve biopsy
- Transcranial magnetic stimulation can be used to measure the connection between the primary motor cortex and the muscle

From "Neuromuscular disorders" (p. 435), by L. Neal Boylan, 2008. In S. P. Hoeman (Ed.), *Rehabilitation nursing: Prevention, intervention, & outcomes* (4th ed.), St. Louis, Mosby. Copyright 2008 by Mosby. Reprinted with permission.

9. The patient and family are assisted to prepare for decisions including gastrostomy tube placement and the use of mechanical ventilation.
   a. Modified barium swallow is performed to assess for aspiration.
10. The patient and family are assisted to prepare for end-of-life decisions such as advance directives and hospice care and to resolve personal affairs.
11. Only one medication, riluzole (approved in 1996), has proven modestly effective as a neuroprotective agent (Gordon, 2013). Recommended treatment with riluzole is 50 mg twice daily (National Guideline Clearing House, 2012).
12. A combination drug consisting of dextromethorphan and quinidine (Nuedexta®) is commercially available to treat symptoms of pseudobulbar affect (Gordon, 2013).

F. Nursing Process
1. Assessment
   a. Obtain a complete health history, including family incidence of ALS and onset of symptoms.
   b. Assess current level of function and ability to perform ADLs and instrumental ADLs.
   c. Ask for a timeline of changes in function to understand progression of the patient's disease.
   d. Evaluate functional status.
   e. Observe gait and evaluate strength and stability.
   f. Assess flaccidity, spasticity, and reported fasciculation in each muscle group.
   g. Evaluate swallowing and chewing ability.
   h. Evaluate respiratory status.

i. Evaluate bowel and bladder function and the patient's ability to use the bathroom, commode, or bedpan.
j. Perform a skin assessment for wounds caused by decreased mobility.
k. Observe patient and family interactions. Consider how they discuss the disease process, their coping strategies, and their preparedness.

2. Plan of care: Nursing diagnoses
   a. Impaired physical mobility related to muscle wasting, weakness, and spasticity
   b. Self-care deficit related to weakness, loss of function
   c. Impaired communication related to impairment of muscles for speech
   d. Ineffective breathing pattern related to impairment of diaphragm and accessory muscles
   e. Altered nutrition: Less than body requirements, related to impaired bulbar muscles
   f. High risk for aspiration related to impaired bulbar muscles
   g. Potential for anxiety related to prognosis
   h. Risk for ineffective coping related to situation and prognosis
   i. Interrupted family processes related to change in health status in family member, modification of family roles, and foreseen loss of family member
   j. Risk for caregiver role strain related to severity of impairment from disease process
3. Goals
   a. Maintain a maximum level of independence with ADLs.
   b. Demonstrate safety in activity and use of appropriate assistive devices.
   c. Limit complications from loss of function.
   d. Maintain nutrition intake.
   e. Maintain skin integrity.
   f. Verbalize an understanding of the disease process.
   g. Ensure comfort.
4. Interventions
   a. Maintain independence with ADLs.
      1) Seek consultation with occupational therapist.
      2) Educate the patient and family on available adaptive devices.
      3) Assess safety with use of mobility aids (e.g., cane, walker).
      4) Encourage expression of feelings about loss of independence to understand what is most important to the patient, and possibly seek consultation with a psychologist.
   b. Limit complications from progressive loss of function.
      1) Ineffective breathing
         a) Consult with a respiratory therapist.
         b) Review energy-conservation techniques.
         c) Assess breathing pattern and presence of cyanosis or other signs of hypoxia.
         d) Provide suction as needed for management of secretions caused by immobility.
         e) Supportive medications typically used: theophylline, antibiotics, mucolytics, expectorants. Pneumonia and influenza vaccinations are recommended (Gordon, 2013).
         f) Teach use of equipment (e.g., assisted cough device, bilevel positive airway pressure, continuous positive airway pressure, oxygen) as it is prescribed for the patient (Gordon, 2013).
         g) Invasive ventilation chosen by fewer than 5% of patients (Gordon, 2013)
      2) Impaired swallowing and decrease in nutritional intake
         a) Consult with a speech pathologist.
         b) Consult with a dietitian.
         c) Auscultate lungs for abnormal sounds.
         d) Evaluate weakness of facial and oral muscles.
         e) Implement dietary modifications as necessary based on the ability to swallow different consistencies of food.
         f) Teach the patient to eat only one type of food consistency at a time.
         g) Avoid milk products and sticky foods (e.g., peanut butter, white bread).
         h) Consider six small meals daily to meet caloric needs (Burnett, 2013).
         i) Regular and meticulous oral care with toothbrush is recommended for patients with dysphagia. Evidence indicates foam brushes are not as effective as a toothbrush in removing plaque and preventing gum disease (Burnett, 2013).
         j) Provide information to assist the patient in decision making about placement of gastrostomy tube as the disease progresses.
      3) Impaired communication
         a) Provide communication tools such as language boards, paper and pen if the patient can still write, or a computer if the patient can type.

b) Crucial to consult with speech therapist (or other knowledgeable technician) to ensure appropriate choice and use of augmentative and alternative communication system (Burnett, 2013)

c) Augmentative and alternative communication systems range from language/picture boards (low technology) to computerized speech synthesizer devices (high technology). Access can be activated through a headmouse system or through switches (e.g., hand, foot, cheek, eyebrow, eye blink, elbow, knee).

d) Encourage patience from family members to ensure that the patient is allowed to fully communicate needs.

e) Research using brain-computer interfaces for communication and moving virtual limbs is under way (Gordon, 2013).

c. Maintain skin integrity.

1) Assess skin for signs of pressure and breakdown.
2) Assess nutritional and fluid intake.
3) Educate the patient and family about identifying the beginning of skin breakdown.
4) Educate the patient and family about weight shifting and turning in bed to avoid pressure ulcers as mobility decreases.
5) When the patient is no longer independent with bed mobility, turn him or her every 2 hours and weight shift every 20 minutes if the patient is in a wheelchair.
6) Educate on keeping skin clean and dry, and suggest use of proper lotions.

d. Conserve energy (Burnett, 2013).

1) Counseling to identify factors contributing to fatigue
2) Identification of symptom patterns
3) Use energy-conservation techniques (e.g., setting priorities, delegating tasks to others, consolidating tasks through planning, using labor-saving devices, pacing activities, establishing periods for short naps)
4) Avoid vigorous exercise.

e. Discuss the disease process with the patient and family.

1) Provide an open and trusting relationship with the patient and family.
2) Encourage expression of feelings.
3) Educate the patient and family about changes in function that will occur with disease progression, and discuss their plan for adjustment at each stage.
4) Provide information to assist the family and patient in decision making about advance directives, gastrostomy tube placement, and mechanical ventilation.
5) Provide referrals to support groups and medical professionals as needed.
6) Assess coping skills and seek consultation as appropriate.
7) Refer to hospice, palliative, or end-of-life care resources as appropriate.
8) Ensure that the patient is comfortable.
9) Assess for pain resulting from immobility or contractures.
10) Provide medication as ordered for pain control, and instruct the patient on effective use of medications and precautions.
11) Encourage the use of alternative pain-relief measures (e.g., distraction, relaxation, imagery, music, massage).
12) Assess effectiveness of pain-relief measures.

IV. Guillain-Barré Syndrome

A. Overview

1. Guillain-Barré syndrome (GBS) is classified as acute inflammatory polyneuropathy with predominantly motor involvement
2. An acute inflammatory disease affecting the myelin of the nerves in the peripheral nervous system primarily. In some cases axonal degeneration can occur (Polak et al., 2004).
3. Autoimmune response that is triggered by a viral or bacterial infection, systemic illness, or immunizations
4. Onset can be a course of hours to about 3 weeks, and this phase ends when no additional deterioration is occurring.
5. The duration can span 3 years.
6. GBS can cause near-complete paralysis, and rehabilitation should be a comprehensive program to assist and support the regaining of function in all body systems.
7. Residual weakness including pain and fatigue that can persist for months or years occurs in approximately 15%–25% of patients (Polak et al., 2004; van Doorn, Ruts, & Jacobs, 2008).
8. Very few patients remain totally paralyzed.
9. The disease can be life threatening and is considered a medical emergency, with mortality of 3%–10% due to complications of the disease rather than the disease itself (van Doorn et al., 2008).

10. Twenty percent of patients are unable to walk at 6 months after development of GBS (van Doorn, 2009).
11. Cognitive function and level of consciousness are not affected by GBS.

B. Epidemiology
1. Incidence
a. The annual incidence of GBS is between 1.1 and 1.8 per 100,000 people (McGrogan, Madle, Seaman, & de Vries, 2009), with GBS in children (15 years and younger) between 0.34 and 1.34 per 100,000.
b. Both genders, all ages, and all ethnicities are equally affected.
c. The incidence increases in those 50 years and older (McGrogan et al., 2009).
d. Hospitalization for GBS has decreased during the past several years, probably because of the widespread availability of intravenous immunoglobulin (van Doorn, 2009).
2. Subtypes exist that vary in symptoms and pattern and in geographic distribution.
a. Acute inflammatory demyelination polyneuropathy (AIDP): Classic GBS, accounting for 90% of all cases in Western world (Vucic, Kiernan, & Cornblath, 2009)
b. Acute motor axonal neuropathy (AMAN): More prevalent in Asia and South and Central America (Vucic et al., 2009)
c. Acute motor sensory axonal neuropathy (AMSAN): More prevalent in Asia and South and Central America (Vucic et al., 2009)
1) More severe sensory involvement and poorer prognosis

C. Etiology
1. The cause of GBS is unknown, but several triggers exist that seem to relate to the autoimmune attack on the body.
a. Most often the patient may have had a respiratory or gastrointestinal virus in the days to weeks before onset. The viruses typically considered to be frequent antecedents include the following:
1) *Campylobacter jejuni*
2) Cytomegalovirus
3) Epstein-Barr virus
4) *Mycoplasma pneumoniae*
5) Hepatitis A, B, or C
6) Human immunodeficiency virus infections
b. Less often, surgery or a vaccination is believed to cause onset. The vaccines considered to be most frequently associated with GBS are as follows:
1) Rabies
2) Swine flu
3) Poliovirus
4) Tetanus
c. There is only minimal evidence of an association between influenza vaccine and GBS (Jefferson et al., 2010).
2. There is no clear understanding of why a person does or does not develop GBS.
3. No specific disease-causing agent has been identified; therefore, GBS is called a *syndrome*.

D. Pathophysiology
1. Overview
a. Immune-mediated cellular and humoral response that triggers antibody production
b. An antimyelin antibody has been identified that causes antimyelination.
c. Normal myelin is attacked by macrophages; inflammatory lesions occur throughout the peripheral nervous system.
1) Schwann cells and myelin sheath, located on segmental peripheral nerves and the anterior and posterior spinal nerve roots, are affected.
2) Severe lesions can cause axonal degeneration.
d. Remyelination occurs slowly.
2. Variations
a. AIDP
1) Most common
2) Numbness and weakness begin in legs and progress upward, ending at cranial nerves.
3) Loss of motor function is symmetric.
4) Sensory loss occurs, typically as mild numbness, and is typically most severe in the toes.
5) Approximately 50% of patients will need respiratory support.
b. AMAN
1) Progression is the same as that of GBS, but no sensory loss occurs.
2) Children and young adults are affected most often.
3) Muscle pain does not generally occur.
4) AMAN is often considered a milder form of GBS.
c. AMSAN
1) Adults are most typically affected.
2) Downward progression begins with motor weakness in brain-stem cranial nerves.
3) Respiratory involvement occurs quickly.

4) Sensory loss and numbness occur distally and are more prominent in hands than in feet.

d. Miller-Fisher syndrome

1) Very rare, occurring in approximately 5% of GBS cases (adults and children)

2) Triad of ophthalmoplegia, ataxia, and areflexia occurs.

3) Sensory loss does not typically occur.

3. Clinical manifestations (vary in severity depending on the individual case)

a. Ascending symmetric motor weakness occurs.

b. Ascending flaccid paralysis is typical.

c. Loss of neurologic function and deep-tendon reflexes occurs.

d. Respiratory insufficiency and failure may result from weakness in the diaphragm and intercostal muscles and mechanical failure.

e. In approximately 50% of cases, damage to the facial nerve (CN VII) causes facial diplegia (Polak et al., 2004).

f. If involved, damage to glossopharyngeal (CN IX) and vagus (CN X) nerves causes dysphagia and laryngeal paralysis.

g. Autonomic dysfunction is very likely to occur because of changes in sympathetic and parasympathetic nervous systems, and is certain to occur if vagus (CN X) nerves are involved.

1) Paroxysmal hypertension

2) Orthostatic hypotension

3) Cardiac arrhythmias

4) Paralytic ileus

5) Urinary retention

6) Syndrome of inappropriate antidiuretic hormone secretion

h. Great sensitivity to touch; paresthesia typically occurs and can include numbness, most often in the hands and feet

i. Pain management can be challenging because of the adverse effects of drugs. Pain management can include opioids, nonsteroidal anti-inflammatory drugs, antidepressants, anticonvulsants, muscle relaxants, benzodiazepines, intravenous magnesium, and local anesthetics.

j. Pain is sometimes reported as cramping in lower extremities followed by acute pain in the trunk and upper extremities (Haroutinunian, Lecht, Zur, Hoffman, & Davidson, 2009).

4. Diagnosis

a. Criteria based on clinical presentation

1) Progressive weakness in two or more limbs due to neuropathy

2) Areflexia

3) Disease course of less than 4 weeks

4) Exclusion of other causes of symptoms

b. History of recent viral infection

c. Electrophysiological study shows slowing of conduction or a block in motor or sensory nerves (this test can help distinguish between variations of disease).

d. Lumbar puncture shows an increase in protein, but that could be delayed until 7–10 days after onset (Ferri, 2013)

E. Management Options

1. Medical management

a. Studies have shown therapeutic plasma exchange or plasmapheresis (TPE) to be effective in GBS that is severe enough to impair independent ambulation or require mechanical ventilation (Cortese et al., 2011). Optimal plasma exchange protocol (i.e., number of exchanges and volumes exchanged) has not been established by research (Cortese et al., 2011). Can be performed every other day for 10 to 15 days to decrease the severity and duration of the disease. Lewis and colleagues (2014) noted that TPE has little value beyond 3 weeks after disease onset.

b. Studies have shown that intravenous immunoglobulin (IVIG) is as effective as plasmapheresis in treating GBS. Research has not established optimal IVIG infusion frequency and total dosage (Patwa, Chaudhry, Katzberg, Rae-Grant, & So, 2012). Intravenous immunoglobulin administration (divided dose of 1–2 mg/kg over 3–5 days) helps to lessen the attack on the nervous system. Lewis et al. (2014) noted that TPE has little value beyond 3 weeks after disease onset.

c. Medication is often needed to assist with complications such as cardiac arrhythmias, blood pressure changes, constipation, urinary retention, and depression.

d. Corticosteroids do not appear to hasten the course of the illness, and oral corticosteroids could delay recovery (Hughes, Swan, & van Doorn, 2010).

2. The disease most often has spontaneous recovery, so the goal is to manage complications that involve numerous body systems and rehabilitative therapies.

a. Respiratory management and support, due to loss of function and loss of mobility, causing the need for secretion management

b. Management of autonomic dysfunction

1) Management of cardiac arrhythmias

2) Blood pressure management
3) Bowel and bladder management
4) Management of electrolyte imbalances

c. Nutrition management
d. Management of complications that arise from immobility
1) Deep vein thrombosis (DVT) and embolism monitoring and prevention
2) Muscle atrophy
3) Skin integrity

e. Psychological intervention for management of depression

F. Nursing Process

1. Assessment
a. Obtain a full health history, with emphasis on any recent illnesses or symptoms, vaccinations, and surgeries.
b. Obtain a list of current symptoms and onset, as well as an approximate timeline of deterioration of function, to assess speed of progression.
c. Assess respiratory function.
d. Assess for pain, paresthesia, numbness, or paralysis.
e. Assess bowel and bladder function.
f. Evaluate cranial nerve involvement with neurological testing.
g. Evaluate swallowing.
h. Assess nutrition and weight.
i. Observe patient and family interaction to assess for psychological and rehabilitative support.

2. Plan of care: Nursing diagnoses
a. Impaired physical mobility related to disease process
b. Ineffective breathing pattern related to neuromuscular weakness of respiratory muscles
c. Altered nutrition: Less than body requirements related to inability to swallow
d. High risk for aspiration related to dysphagia secondary to cranial nerve involvement
e. Impaired communication related to impairment of speech muscles secondary to cranial nerve involvement
f. Risk for impaired skin integrity related to immobility
g. Risk for DVT related to immobility
h. Risk for constipation related to paralytic ileus
i. Risk for urinary retention related to autonomic dysfunction
j. Acute pain related to disease process
k. Self-care deficit related to loss of function
l. Altered sensory perception resulting from disease process
m. Potential for anxiety related to lack of control within environment
n. Risk for depression related to loss of function and independence

3. Goals
a. Limit pain and discomfort.
b. Maintain function in unaffected limbs, and limit extent of atrophy to affected limbs.
c. Maintain oxygenation and an effective breathing pattern.
d. Manage autonomic dysfunction.
e. Provide nutritional support.
f. Provide means for effective communication.
g. Prevent skin breakdown.
h. Prevent DVT formation.
i. Maintain bowel and bladder elimination.
j. Provide means of environmental control to lessen anxiety.
k. Provide psychological and emotional support to the patient and family.

4. Interventions
a. Provide pain management.
1) Assess pain and changes throughout the disease course and consult with the medical team.
2) Administer medications as ordered for pain relief.
3) Help the patient to be positioned comfortably.
4) Educate assistive personnel and family on managing the patient's pain (e.g., placing socks on the patient can cause a high level of pain, so caregivers should adjust their care appropriately).

b. Maintain function in unaffected limbs, and limit the extent of atrophy to affected limbs.
1) Teach active ROM to patients and passive ROM to caretakers.
2) Consult with a physical therapy team.

c. Maintain oxygenation and effective breathing patterns.
1) Consult with a respiratory therapist and pulmonologist.
2) Monitor pulse oximetry.
3) Maintain a ventilator if needed.
4) Provide tracheostomy care.
5) Provide airway management.
6) Administer oxygen as prescribed.
7) Teach effective coughing to clear secretions.
8) Teach and assist with respiratory adjuncts (e.g., incentive spirometer).
9) Educate on energy-conservation techniques.

d. Manage autonomic dysfunction.
   1) Monitor blood pressure in lying and sitting positions.
   2) Provide supportive measures for orthostatic hypotension (e.g., abdominal binders, compression stockings).
   3) Monitor for cardiac arrhythmias.
   4) Monitor electrolyte balance.

e. Provide nutritional support.
   1) Consult with a dietitian.
   2) Monitor patient's weight.
   3) Provide safe gastrostomy or nasogastric tube feedings if needed.

f. Provide a means for effective communication.
   1) Consult with a speech pathologist.
   2) Provide communication boards, and establish an alternative method that the patient can use to respond (e.g., blinking).
   3) Educate the healthcare team and family members on established communication techniques.

g. Prevent skin breakdown.
   1) Assess skin regularly for signs of breakdown.
   2) Apply proper aids such as moisture barrier creams.
   3) Monitor serum protein levels.
   4) Assess fluid intake and monitor for skin turgor changes.
   5) Turn the patient every 2 hours in bed, and weight shift every 20 minutes when patient is in a wheelchair.
   6) Educate the patient and family on identifying signs of skin breakdown and preventive techniques.
   7) Educate the family on turning and weight shifting.

h. Prevent DVT formation.
   1) Provide compression devices as ordered.
   2) Educate the patient and family about signs and symptoms of DVT.

i. Maintain bowel and bladder function.
   1) Insert a Foley catheter if needed and perform proper catheter care.
   2) Closely monitor intake and output, and encourage increased fluid intake to assist with constipation management.
   3) If the patient is voiding independently, monitor postvoid residuals.
   4) Monitor bowel movements.
   5) Assess activity of bowel sounds and distention and firmness of the abdomen.
   6) Administer bowel program as ordered, including medications and suppository administration.

j. Conserve energy (Burnett, 2013).
   1) Provide counseling to identify factors contributing to fatigue.
   2) Identify symptom patterns.
   3) Use energy-conservation techniques (e.g., setting priorities, delegating tasks to others, consolidating tasks through planning, using labor-saving devices, pacing activities, establishing periods for short naps)
   4) Avoid vigorous exercise.

k. Provide control and a comfortable environment for the patient.
   1) Allow patients to make decisions about their environment, including lighting, sounds, open doors, and room temperature.
   2) Because changes occur in pain and paresthesia throughout the disease course, be sure to consistently ask patients what is comfortable for them while providing care.
   3) Provide an accessible nurse call bell (e.g., tent for head activation, sip and puff in case of complete paralysis).

l. Provide psychological and emotional support to the patient and family.
   1) Consult with a psychologist on the healthcare team. Report changes in mood, attitude, affect, and family dynamics to the psychologist.
   2) Educate the patient and family on the disease course.
   3) Offer community support group information and resources.

V. Myasthenia Gravis

A. Overview

1. *Mysathenia gravis* (*MG*) is a chronic autoimmune disease involving the destruction of ACh receptors that results in fluctuating weakness of the voluntary muscle groups.
2. Most common symptoms include muscle fatigue, drooping eyelids, difficulty with speech and swallowing, weakness in extremities, and respiratory difficulty.
3. Weakness increases with activity and improves with rest.
4. MG was first documented by Sir Thomas Willis, an English clinician, in 1672.
5. Variations of the disease exist, including ocular, generalized, and bulbar.

6. Onset can be subtle or fast, and a myasthenia crisis necessitates emergent respiratory support for survival.
7. Numerous treatments exist, and the goals are to keep the patient symptom free and improve quality of life. No cure exists for MG.
8. Typical patients are able to live in the community, where they require acute care and rehabilitation only while in myasthenic or cholinergic crisis.
9. Stages of MG and the Oosterhuis Global Clinical Classification of Myasthenic Severity help to classify the individual case.

B. Epidemiology
1. Affects approximately 1 per 5,000 people in the United States (Myasthenia Gravis Foundation of America, 2010)
2. It is the most common disorder of the neuromuscular junction, affecting 25 to 142 per million (Sivestri & Wolfe, 2012).
3. Can affect all ages and races and both sexes, but the clinical course can vary by age and sex (Grob, Brunner, Namba, & Pagala, 2008)
   a. Greatest incidence in women younger than 40 years of age and men older than 60 years of age
   b. Female-to-male ratio of 3:2 affected before age 50 years. Sex distribution is closer to equal after age 50 years, with more men affected
   c. *Late-onset MG* is defined as first symptoms appearing at or after 65 years of age.
   d. Congenital myasthenic syndromes represent a wide variety of inherited disorders; the majority presents with symptoms during the first 2 years of life. Symptoms include problems with feeding, breathing, droopy eyelids, reduced eye movement, poor muscle tone, muscle weakness, and fatigue (Muppidi, Wolfe, & Barohn, 2012).
   e. Neonatal myasthenia is seen in 12%–20% of babies born to mothers with MG, because some of the mother's antibodies are passed to the child. The child does not produce his or her own antibodies. This is a transient condition, and the general weakness the baby experiences typically subsides within 3–5 weeks.
   f. Ocular myasthenia is the only onset in about 50% of people with MG, with 50–60% developing generalized disease, most within 2 years (Benatar & Kaminski, 2012).
4. Mortality rates and quality of life have improved as a result of thymectomy procedures, use of steroids and immunoglobulins, and plasma exchange for MG crisis (Diaz-Manera, Rojas-Garcia, & Illa, 2009).
5. The most severe weakness and highest mortality rates occur within the first and second year, with some improvement thereafter (Grob et al., 2008).

C. Etiology
1. The cause of MG is unknown, although it is known to be an autoimmune disease.
2. Presence of a thymoma or an abnormal thymus gland is seen in approximately 75% of people with MG. The relationship is not fully understood, but it is believed that a malfunction in the thymus could cause an error in the production of immune cells, resulting in the production of ACh receptor antibodies.
3. MG is not believed to be directly hereditary, although a predisposition for autoimmune disease can be inherited.
4. Disease can go into remission for long periods, during which no treatment is needed.

D. Pathophysiology
1. Overview
   a. For unknown reasons, the body does not recognize the ACh receptors as being part of itself and so produces autoantibodies against these receptors.
   b. Autoimmune attack occurs on the ACh receptors by binding the autoantibodies to the receptors, although the role of the autoantibodies is not fully understood.
   c. ACh can no longer be used in neurotransmission because of mechanical blockage of the receptor, resulting in muscle weakness and fatigue.
   d. Cholinergic receptors of cardiac and smooth muscle have different antigenicity than skeletal muscle and so are not affected.
   e. Weakness increases with activity throughout the day and improves with rest. As the disease progresses, fatigue occurs with less activity.
   f. Two types of crisis can occur.
      1) Myasthenic crisis
         a) Involvement of respiratory and accessory muscles escalates, necessitating mechanical ventilation
         b) Infection, fever, adverse reaction to medication, and insufficient medication are causes for crisis for patients who have respiratory involvement.
      2) Cholinergic crisis
         a) Results from excessive doses of cholinergic treatment medications
         b) Symptoms can mimic organophosphate poisoning (e.g., salivation, lacrimation,

urinary incontinence, gastrointestinal upset, emesis, miosis).
            c) In some cases, symptoms can include flaccid paralysis and respiratory failure, which are clinically indistinguishable from those of MG itself.

2. Clinical manifestations
   a. Onset variable
      1) Most often gradual
      2) Reports of rapid onset when associated with emotional upset or respiratory infection
   b. For all muscles involved, activity throughout the day increases symptoms, and rest can help to relieve symptoms. As the disease progresses, the patient fatigues more easily.
      1) Although weakness is the presenting sign, reflexes, sensation, and coordination are normal.
   c. Exacerbation can result from infection, illness, surgery, pregnancy, menses, changes in thyroid function, heat, or electrolyte imbalances (i.e., hypokalemia). Patients who take other medications must be aware of side effects involving neurotransmission.
   d. Variations of disease
      1) Ocular: Eye and lid muscles are affected.
      2) Bulbar: Muscles of speech, swallowing, and breathing are affected.
      3) Generalized: Proximal muscles of both upper and lower extremities are involved, with ocular or bulbar involvement.
      4) Neonatal transient: Passes to baby from a mother with MG
   e. Muscle groups tend to be affected in patterns.
   f. Early findings include ptosis and diplopia.
      1) Ptosis can be unilateral or bilateral.
      2) Ptosis intensifies with upward gaze.
   g. Secondary muscle groups involve face, speech, neck, and masticator.
      1) Facial expressions become altered by weakness and fatigue of facial muscles.
      2) Chewing becomes tiresome quickly, and rest periods are needed.
      3) The voice becomes weak and fades after conversation and often sounds nasal.
   h. Generalized weakness involves larger muscle groups.
      1) Limb muscle and proximal muscle involvement
         a) Patients may have difficulty lifting their arms over their head and performing ADLs that require this motion (i.e., grooming hair).
         b) Difficulty in reaching for objects
      2) Neck extensor muscle involvement causes the head to fall forward.
      3) Diaphragm and intercostal involvement constitute myasthenic crisis and necessitate respiratory support, intubation, or mechanical ventilation.
      4) Nonmotor symptoms can occur in some patients, and can include (beyond the typical fatigue and weakness) red-cell aplasia, alopecia, limbic encephalitis, and myocarditis (S. Suzuki, Utsugisawa, & Suzuki, 2013).
3. Myasthenia Gravis Foundation of America, Inc., Classification System (**Table 21-5**)
4. Diagnosis
   a. Tensilon testing: This anticholinesterase is administered to test for immediate improvement in muscle strength. If strength improves, the test is positive. Resuscitation resources must be available when the test is done.
   b. Blood test for elevation of ACh receptors (80%–90% of people with MG show antibody titer elevation)
   c. Electrophysiology: Rapid reduction in nerve conduction studies is a positive result.
   d. Single-fiber electromyography: Tests neuromuscular transmission from a single nerve fiber to pairs of muscles. Detection of failure to transmit or delay indicates a positive test, and for MG, a confirmation test proves to be approximately 99% sensitive.
   e. Mediastinal MRI or computed tomography scan: Many people with MG have an enlarged thymus, and this test shows thymoma if present.

E. Management Options
   1. Treatment must be individualized for each patient after the specific type of MG is diagnosed.
   2. In approximately 10% of cases, MG is associated with a thymoma, and surgical removal is often indicated (Gold & Schneider-Gold, 2008).
   3. The goal of treatment is to remain as symptom free as possible to maintain a good quality of life.
   4. Myasthenic crisis is a life-threatening emergency necessitating early diagnosis and respiratory assistance and is typically treated with some combination of high-dose corticosteroids, plasma exchange, immunoglobulins, and respiratory support (Chaudhuri & Behan, 2009).
   5. The use of bilevel positive airway pressure and other external respiratory support systems can prevent the need for intubation or reduce the duration of crises (Argov, 2009).

6. Some medications such as beta blockers, aminoglycoside and quinolong antibiotics, and some antiarrhythmics can aggravate MG and are contraindicated (Ferri, 2013)
7. Pharmacological management including cyclosporin (with or without corticosteroids) has been found to significantly improve MG (Hart, Sharshar, & Sathasivam, 2009).
   a. Acetylcholinesterase inhibitors and immunomodulating therapies are the mainstays of treatment (Shah, 2014).
      1) Symptom management does not treat the underlying cause.
      2) Most commonly used is pyridostigmine (Mestinon®) and occasionally neostigmine (Prostigmin®) (Maggi & Mantegazza, 2011)
         a) First-line therapy for MG
         b) Suitable for long-term treatment
   b. Muscarinic side effects on smooth muscle and glands can occur.
      1) Bradycardia
      2) Bronchial constriction and spasms, increase in secretions, and wheezing
      3) Blurred vision and constricted pupils
      4) Involuntary micturition
      5) Gastrointestinal upset (e.g., abdominal cramping, diarrhea, vomiting)
      6) Diaphoresis
   c. Nicotinic side effects on skeletal muscle can occur, including facial twitching and spasms.
   d. Long-term corticosteroid therapy
      1) Prednisone is the most common choice.
      2) Seventy percent to 80% remission or improvement (Hickey, 2009)
   e. Immunosuppressant agents: Azathioprine (Imuran®) is often chosen if prednisone is contraindicated for a patient.
   f. Intravenous immunoglobulin
      1) Short-term treatment
      2) Known to improve autoimmune conditions
   g. Antibody treatment: Rituximab. Manufactured antibody administered by infusion over several months can provide several years of positive treatment response in some patients with muscle-specific tyrosine kinase myasthenia gravis (MuSK MG) (Diaz-Manera et al., 2012)
8. Plasmapheresis
   a. Short-term treatment to stabilize patients who may be in crisis
   b. Removes ACh receptor antibodies from blood
9. Surgical thymectomy has been a successful treatment strategy since 1940 for long-term improvement of disease.
10. Nursing management

Table 21-5. Myasthenia Gravis Foundation of America, Inc., Classification System

Class I	Any ocular muscle weakness May have weakness of eye closure All other muscle strength is normal
Class II	Mild weakness affecting other than ocular muscles May also have ocular muscle weakness of any severity
Class IIa	Predominantly affecting limb or axial muscles May also have lesser involvement of oropharyngeal muscle
Class IIb	Predominantly affecting oropharyngeal or respiratory muscles May also have lesser or equal involvement of limb or axial muscles
Class III	Moderate weakness affecting other than ocular muscles May also have ocular muscle weakness of any severity
Class IIIa	Predominantly affecting limb or axial muscles May also have lesser involvement of oropharyngeal muscles
Class IIIb	Predominantly affecting oropharyngeal or respiratory muscles May also have lesser or equal involvement of limb or axial muscles
Class IV	Severe weakness affecting other than ocular muscles May also have ocular muscle weakness of any severity
Class IVa	Predominantly affecting limb or axial muscles May also have lesser involvement of oropharyngeal muscles
Class IVb	Predominantly affecting oropharyngeal or respiratory muscles May also have lesser or equal involvement of limb or axial muscles
Class V	Defined by intubation, with or without mechanical ventilation, except when used during routine postoperative management; the use of a feeding tube without intubation places a client in class IVb

From "Myasthenia gravis: Recommendations for clinical research standards. Task force of the medical scientific advisory board of the Myasthenia Gravis Foundation of America," by A. Jaretzski III, R. J. Barohn, R. M. Ernstoff, H. J. Kaminski, J. C. Keesey, A. S. Penn, and D. B. Sanders, 2000. *Neurology, 55*(1), 1–23. Copyright 2000 by Myasthenia Gravis Foundation of America. Reprinted with permission.

a. Monitoring for crisis events
b. Monitoring for side effects of treatments
c. Monitoring for individual tolerance and weakness
d. Communicating with medical team for treatment changes based on patient response
e. Assisting the patient to remain as independent as possible with ADLs

F. Nursing Process

1. Assessment
   a. Obtain a full health history and focus on the patient's daily symptoms, including his or her weakest time of day.
   b. Assess and record baseline for the patient to safely monitor for crisis (preferably during the patient's strongest time of day).
      1) Respiratory function
      2) Cardiac function
      3) Bowel and bladder function
      4) Baseline gastrointestinal symptoms
      5) Visual acuity
      6) Strength and mobility
      7) Swallowing
      8) Speech
2. Plan of care
   a. Nursing diagnoses
      1) Knowledge deficit relating to disease process and side effects of treatment
      2) Activity intolerance related to fatigue
      3) Risk for aspiration related to muscle weakness and increased secretions
      4) Risk for falls related to muscle weakness
      5) Risk for medical crisis (myasthenic or cholinergic)
   b. Goals
      1) The patient and family will be able to identify signs and symptoms of disease and side effects of medical treatment.
      2) The patient and family will be able to distinguish signs and symptoms of myasthenic and cholinergic crises and know to seek medical attention immediately.
      3) The patient will learn and use energy-conservation techniques.
      4) Respiratory support will be provided.
      5) Nutritional support will be provided.
      6) Medication side effects will be managed.
      7) A safe environment and assistance to prevent falls will be provided.
      8) The patient will be assisted to manage energy output and provided an appropriate schedule for therapy and activities based on fluctuations in strength throughout the day.
3. Interventions
   a. Education for the patient, family, caretaker
      1) Disease process
      2) Side effects of medications and treatments
      3) Myasthenic crisis
         a) Often precipitated by infection but can occur spontaneously
         b) Signs and symptoms
            (i) Sudden relapse of symptoms
            (ii) Difficulty swallowing
            (iii) Rapid decrease in respiratory function
         c) Seek immediate medical attention for lifesaving treatment.
      4) Cholinergic crisis
         a) Caused by toxicity, overmedication with acetylcholinesterase inhibitors
         b) Signs and symptoms can present more slowly than they do in myasthenic crisis.
            (i) Generalized profound weakness
            (ii) Bradycardia
            (iii) Bronchial constriction and spasms
            (iv) Increase in secretions
            (v) Wheezing cough
            (vi) Blurred vision and constricted pupils
            (vii) Involuntary micturition
            (viii) Gastrointestinal upset (e.g., abdominal cramping, diarrhea, vomiting)
            (ix) Diaphoresis
            (x) Facial twitching
         c) Seek immediate medical attention for lifesaving treatment.
      5) Importance of medic alert bracelet
      6) Conserve energy (Burnett, 2013).
         a) Counseling to identify factors contributing to fatigue
         b) Identification of symptom patterns
         c) Use of energy-conservation techniques (e.g., setting priorities, delegating tasks to others, consolidating tasks through planning, using labor-saving devices, pacing activities, establishing periods for short naps)
         d) Avoid vigorous exercise.
      7) Do not take any over-the-counter medications without consulting the doctor.
      8) Diet choices that require less work to chew and swallow
      9) Causes of relapses (e.g., menstruation, infection, stress, extreme temperatures)
   b. Provide respiratory support if needed.

1) Monitor oxygenation.
2) Provide tracheostomy care if needed.
3) Teach effective coughing to clear secretions.

c. Provide nutritional support.
1) Consult with a speech therapist for safe food choices and techniques for swallowing.
2) Consult with a dietitian to ensure that caloric intake is adequate.
3) Encourage a soft-food diet because it requires less energy to chew and swallow.

d. Manage side effects of medications.
1) Provide a private room and limited exposure for patients on immunosuppressive medications.
2) Monitor for effects of medications on all body systems, report untoward symptoms to the provider (e.g., physician, nurse practitioner, physician assistant), and provide nursing interventions to mitigate any negative side effects.

e. Provide a safe environment to prevent falls.
1) Teach the patient to request assistance when weak.
2) Provide essentials within reaching distance of bed.
3) Consult with a physical therapist to provide proper aids for ambulation.
4) Educate the patient on wearing safe, comfortable footwear.

f. Provide an appropriate schedule for the patient.
1) Consult with a medical team and a therapy team.
a) Individualize the patient's medication schedule.
b) Individualize the patient's therapy schedule to allow for rest periods throughout day.
2) Monitor the patient daily, record how he or she is managing with medications and activities, and adjust accordingly.

VI. Postpolio Syndrome

A. Overview
1. Postpolio syndrome (PPS) affects survivors of polio decades after the acute illness.
2. Major symptoms are pain, fatigue, and weakness, with new weakness being the hallmark of PPS.
3. Patients may have sleeping, breathing, and swallowing problems (Post-Polio Health International, 2010).
4. Patients may experience muscle atrophy or wasting (Post-Polio Health International, 2010).
5. PPS is rarely life threatening.
6. The severity of the initial acute polio illness predicts the severity of the PPS (National Institute of Neurological Disorders and Stroke [NINDS], 2012).

B. Epidemiology
1. Experienced by 25%–40% of polio survivors (Post-Polio Health International, 2010)
2. There are more than 440,000 polio survivors in the United States (NINDS, 2012).
3. More common in women than in men

C. Etiology
1. NINDS (2012) diagnosis criteria.
a. Prior paralytic poliomyelitis with lower motor neuron loss that is confirmed
b. Period of partial or complete recovery for 15 years or more
c. Gradual onset of progressive or persistent new muscle weakness or fatigue, often after surgery or a period of inactivity
d. Symptoms that persist for 1 year
e. Exclusion of other problems as a cause of the symptoms
2. There are no diagnostic tests for PPS, but MRI, CT, neuroimaging, and electrophysiological studies can be useful for investigating the course of decline in muscle strength.
3. Postpolio is diagnosed based on the presence of the following criteria:
a. Prior paralyzing poliomyelitis with evidence of motor neuron loss
b. A period of partial or complete functional recovery
c. Slowly progressive and persistent new muscle weakness, decreased endurance, generalized fatigue, muscle atrophy, and/or muscle/joint pain
d. Symptoms that persist 1 year or more
e. Exclusion of other neuromuscular, medical, or skeletal abnormalities as causes of symptoms (NINDS, 2012).
4. People with PPS are at high risk for fracture (Mohammad, Khan, Galvin, Hardiman, & O'Connell, 2009).

D. Pathophysiology (Boyer et al., 2010)
1. Wechler theory
a. New "sprouts" of nerve cells reconnect the nerve cell to the muscles during recovery from acute polio.
b. New nerve cell sprouts trigger contraction of the muscles and supply more muscle fibers with innervation.
c. New nerve cell sprouts are not stable and degenerate over time through "overexertion"

and no longer contract muscle fibers, leading to the perception of new weakness or loss of function.

2. Associated with an inflammatory process in the CSF and overall inflammation (Boyer et al., 2010)

E. Management Options

1. The primary focus of treatment is energy conservation and lifestyle changes to reduce stress, avoiding both inactivity and overuse (Gonzalez, Olsson, & Borg, 2010).
2. Rehabilitation that is comprehensive and interdisciplinary can have a positive effect on the patient's ability to perform ADLs, his or her view of the illness, and long-term outcomes (Larsson Lund & Lexell, 2010).
3. Bracing to support weak muscles
4. Canes or crutches to enhance safety and relieve weight on weak limbs
5. Orthotics to correct leg length discrepancy and gait disturbances
6. Weight loss
7. Select exercises to avoid disuse or overuse weakness
8. Use of a biphasic positive pressure ventilator at night to treat underventilation
9. Depression
   a. Depression in PPS is common.
   b. Highly correlated among those 65 years and older with the resilience factor of spiritual growth (Pierini & Stuifbergen, 2010)
10. Training programs that include warm water are helpful (Farbu, 2010).
11. Training programs that include low-impact aerobics and low-level muscle strengthening are most effective (Tiffreau et al., 2010).
12. Pharmacology
    a. Steroids, amantadine, pyridostigmine, and coenzyme Q10 are of no benefit.
    b. Intravenous immunoglobulin has demonstrated some positive effect on the disease, including reduced pain and increased quality of life (Farbu, 2010).
13. Pain is a persistent and common problem in PPS (Stoelb et al., 2008).
    a. Nociceptive pain is more common than neuropathic pain (Werhagen & Borg, 2010).
    b. Pain is worse in younger people.
    c. Pain is worse in females.
    d. Pain is worse with a younger age of onset of the initial acute polio.
14. Adjustment and education
    a. Experience with initial polio as a child can influence adjustment to PPS.
    b. Late-onset deterioration is feared by many patients.
    c. Must consider individual experiences and the underlying components of fatigue and pain (Yelnik & Laffont, 2010)
15. Prevent pathological fracture and reduce the risk of falls.

F. Nursing Process

1. Assessment
   a. Obtain a full health history, with emphasis on the initial acute polio illness, recovery, functional level, work history, and the onset of PPS symptoms.
   b. Obtain a list of current symptoms and onset and approximate timeline of deterioration of function.
   c. Obtain a history of the exacerbations of symptoms and associated factors, including things that improve symptoms and things that make symptoms worse.
   d. Assess for pain, paresthesia, numbness, and paralysis.
   e. Assess bowel and bladder function.
   f. Observe patient and family interaction to assess for psychological and rehabilitative support.
2. Plan of care: Nursing diagnosis
   a. Impaired physical mobility related to disease process
   b. Decreased activity tolerance related to muscle weakness, pain, and overuse syndrome
   c. Ineffective breathing pattern related to neuromuscular weakness of respiratory muscles
   d. Altered nutrition: Less than body requirements
   e. Risk for DVT related to change in gait and mobility
   f. Risk for constipation related to change in activity and medication effect
   g. Acute pain related to disease process
   h. Self-care deficit related to loss of function
   i. Altered sensory perception due to disease process
   j. Potential for anxiety related to lack of control within environment and change in lifestyle
   k. Risk for depression related to loss of function and independence
3. Goals
   a. Implement energy-conservation strategies.
   b. Maintain function in unaffected limbs and limit extent of atrophy of affected limbs.
   c. Maintain breathing patterns and oxygenation.
   d. Provide nutritional support.
   e. Prevent DVT formation.

f. Maintain bowel and bladder elimination.
g. Provide psychological and emotional support to the patient and family.

4. Interventions
   a. Conserve energy (Burnett, 2013).
      1) Provide counseling to identify factors contributing to fatigue.
      2) Identify symptom patterns.
      3) Use energy-conservation techniques (e.g., setting priorities, delegating tasks to others, consolidating tasks through planning, using labor-saving devices, pacing activities, establishing periods for short naps)
      4) Avoid vigorous exercise.
   b. Maintain function in unaffected limbs, and limit the extent of atrophy of affected limbs.
      1) Teach active ROM to patients and passive ROM to caregivers.
      2) Consult with a physical therapy team.
   c. Maintain oxygenation and effective breathing patterns.
      1) Consult with a respiratory therapist and pulmonologist.
      2) Monitor pulse oximetry and teach the patient how to monitor at home.
      3) Based on respiratory needs, teach the use of ventilator devices for home use.
      4) Teach effective coughing to clear secretions.
      5) Teach and assist with respiratory adjuncts (e.g., incentive spirometer).
   d. Provide nutritional support.
      1) Consult with a dietitian.
      2) Monitor the patient's weight.
      3) Instruct the patient in maximizing nutritional intake.
   e. Prevent DVT formation.
      1) Provide compression devices as ordered.
      2) Educate the patient and family on signs and symptoms of DVT.
   f. Maintain bowel and bladder elimination.
      1) Assess any urinary functional changes and develop a plan to address urinary dysfunction, including the use of assistive devices and equipment.
      2) Teach the patient management strategies to use at home to achieve continence or manage incontinence.
      3) Assess for any signs of constipation or diarrhea.
      4) Develop a plan with the patient that involves dietary intake, fluid intake, and the use of medications to achieve regular bowel movements.
   g. Provide control and a comfortable environment for the patient.
      1) Allow patients to make decisions about their environment including lighting, sounds, open doors, and room temperature.
      2) With respect to the changes in pain and paresthesia that occur throughout the disease course, consistently ask the patient what is comfortable for him or her while providing care, and strategize with the patient on ways to maintain a comfortable home environment.
   h. Provide psychological and emotional support to the patient and family.
      1) Consult with a psychologist on the healthcare team. Report changes in mood, attitude, affect, and family dynamics to the psychologist.
      2) Educate the patient and family on the disease course.
      3) Offer community support group information and resources.

References

ALS Association. (2004). FYI...Epidemiology of ALS and suspected clusters. Retrieved from http://www.alsa.org/assets/pdfs/fyi/fyi_epidemiology.pdf

ALS Association (2014). Facts you Should Know. Retrieved from www.alsa.org/about-als/facts-you-should-know.html

Argov, Z. (2009). Management of myasthenia conditions: Nonimmune issues. *Current Opinions in Neurology, 22*(5), 493–497.

Association of Rehabilitation Nurses (ARN). (2014). ARN competency model for professional rehabilitation nursing. Retrieved from http://www.rehabnurse.org/uploads/files/education/ARN_Rehabilitation_Nursing_Competency _Model_FINAL_-_May_2014.pdf

Benatar, M. & Kaminski, H. (2012). Medical and surgical treatment for ocular myasthenia. *Cochrane Database of Systematic Reviews,* December 12;12:CD005081. doi:10.1002/14651858.CD005081

Beretich, B. D., & Beretich, T. M. (2009). Explaining multiple sclerosis prevalence by ultraviolet exposure: A geospatial analysis. *Multiple Sclerosis, 15*(8), 891–898.

Bigi, S., & Banwell, B. (2012). Pediatric multiple sclerosis. *Journal of Child Neurology, 27*(11), 1378–1383.

Bowen, C., MacLehose, A., & Beaumont J. G. (2011). Advanced multiple sclerosis and the psychosocial impact on families. *Psychology and Health, 26*(1), 113–127.

Boyer, F. C., Tiffeau, V., Rapin, A., Laffont, I., Percebois-Macadre, L., Supper, C.,...Yelnik, A. P. (2010). Post-polio syndrome: Pathophysiological hypotheses, diagnosis criteria, drug therapy. *Annals of Physical Rehabilitation Medicine, 53*(1), 34–41.

Brettschneider, J., Kurent, J., Ludolph, A., & Mitchell, J. D. (2008). Drug therapy for pain in amyotrophic lateral sclerosis or motor neuron disease. *Cochrane Database of Systematic Reviews, 16*(3), CD005226.

Brundin, P., Barker, R. A., & Parmar, M. (2010). Neural grafting in Parkinson's disease: Problems and possibilities. *Progress Brain Research, 184,* 265–294.

Burnett, S. D. (Ed.). (2013). *Evidence-based rehabilitation nursing: Common challenges and interventions* Chicago: Association of Rehabilitation Nurses.

Chaudhuri, A., & Behan, P. O. (2009). Myasthenic crisis. *QJM, 102*(2), 97–107.

Cortese, I., Chaudhry, V., So, Y. T., Cantor, F., Cornblath, D. R., Rae-Grant, A. (2011). Evidence-based guideline update: Plasmapheresis in neurological disorders. *Neurology, 76*(3): 294–300. doi:10.1212/WNL.0b013e318207b1f6

Courtney, S. W. (Ed.). (2014). *MS Research Update.* Cherry Hill, NJ: Multiple Sclerosis Association of America.

Cronin, S., Hardiman, O., & Trayor, B. J. (2007). Ethnic variation in the incidence of ALS: A systematic review. *Neurology, 68*(13), 1002–1007.

Diaz-Manera, J., Martinez-Hernandez, E., Querol, L., Klooster, R., Rojas-Garcia, R., Suárez-Calvet, X.,...Vershcuuren, J. J. (2012). Long-lasting treatment of rituximab in MuSK myasthenia. *Neurology, 78,* 189 –193.

Diaz-Manera, J., Rojas-Garcia, R., & Illa, I. (2009). Treatment strategies for myasthenia gravis. *Expert Opinion on Pharmacotherapy, 10*(8), 1329–1342.

Epocrates. (2014). [Medical App]. San Francisco: Epocrates, Inc.

Farbu, E. (2010). Update on current and emergency treatment options for post-polio syndrome. *Therapeutic Clinical Risk Management, 6,* 307–313.

Ferri, F. F. (2013). *Ferri's clinical advisor 2014.* Philadelphia: Elsevier.

Fox, S. H., Katzenschlager, R., Lim, S-Y, Ravina, B., Seppi, K., Coelho, M.,...Sampaio, C. (2011). The Movement Disorder Society evidence-based medicine review update: Treatments for the motor symptoms of Parkinson's disease. *Movement Disorders, 26*(S3), S2–S40.

Gagne, J. J., & Power, M. C. (2010). Anti-inflammatory drugs and risk of Parkinson disease: A meta-analysis. *Neurology, 74*(12), 995–1002.

Gold, R., & Schneider-Gold, C. (2008). Current and future standards in treatment of myasthenia gravis. *Neurotherapeutics, 5*(4), 535–541.

Goldman, L., & Schafer, A. I. (2012). *Goldman's Cecil medicine* (24th ed.. pp. 2326, 2327). Philadelphia: Saunders Elsevier.

Gonzalez, H., Olsson, T., & Borg, K. (2010). Management of postpolio syndrome. *Lancet Neurology, 9*(6), 634–642.

Gordon, P. H. (2013) Amyotrophic lateral sclerosis: An update for 2013. Clinical features, pathophysiology, management and therapeutic trials. *Aging and Disease, 4*(5), 295–310.

Grob, D., Brunner, N., Namba, T., & Pagala, M. (2008). Lifetime course of myasthenia gravis. *Muscle and Nerve, 37*(2), 141–149.

Habek, M., Kami, A., Balash, Y., & Gurevich, T. (2010). The place of the botulinum toxin in the management of multiple sclerosis. *Clinical Neurology and Neurosurgery, 112*(7), 592–596.

Hauser, R. A., & Lyons, K. E. (2014). Parkinson Disease Treatment & Management. Retrieved from http://emedicine.medscape.com/article/1831191-overview

Haroutinunian, S., Lecht, S., Zur, A. A., Hoffman, A., & Davidson, E. (2009). The challenge of pain management in patients with myasthenia gravis. *Journal of Pain, Palliative Care, and Pharmacotherapy, 23*(3), 242–260.

Hart, I. K., Sharshar, T., & Sathasivam, S. (2009). Immunosuppressant drugs for myasthenia gravis. *Journal of Neurology, Neurosurgery, and Psychiatry, 80*(1), 5–6.

Hayes, M. W., Fung, V .S., Kimber, T. E., & O'Sullivan, J. D. (2010). Current concepts in the management of Parkinson disease. *Medical Journal of Australia, 192*(3), 144–149.

Hickey, J. V. (2009). Neurodegenerative diseases. In J. Hickey (Ed.), *The practice of neurological and neurosurgical nursing* (6th ed.). New York: Lippincott Williams & Wilkins.

Hughes, R. A., Swan, A. V., & van Doorn, P. A. (2010). Corticosteroids for Guillain-Barré syndrome. *Cochrane Database of Systematic Reviews, 2.* CD001446.

Jefferson, T., DiPietrantonj, C., Rivetti, A., Bawazeer, G. A., Al-Ansary, L. A., & Ferroni, E. (2010). Vaccine for preventing influenza in healthy adults. *Cochrane Database of Systematic Reviews, 7,* CD001269.

Jaretzki, A. III, Barohn, R. J., Ernstoff, R. M., Kaminski, H. J., Keesey, J. C., Penn, A. S. , and Sanders, D. B. (2000). Myasthenia gravis: recommendations for clinical research standards. Task Force of the Medical Scientific Advisory Board of the Myasthenia Gravis Foundation of America. *Neurology, 55*(1),16–23.

Kalb, R. (Ed.). (2012). *Multiple sclerosis: A focus on rehabilitation.* Waltham, MA: National Multiple Sclerosis Society.

Kerr, G. K., Worringham, C. J., Cole, M. H., Lacherez, P. F., Wood, J. M., & Silburn, P. A. (2010). Predictors of future falls in Parkinson disease. *Neurology, 72*(2), 116–124.

Lad, S. P., Chapman, C. H., Vaninetti, M., Steinman, L., Green, A., & Boakye, M. (2010). Socioeconomic trends in hospitalizations for multiple sclerosis. *Neuroepidemiology, 35*(2), 93–99.

Larsson Lund, M., & Lexell, J. (2010). A positive turning point in life: How persons with late effects of polio experience the influence of an interdisciplinary rehabilitation programme. *Journal of Rehabilitation Medicine, 42*(6), 559–565.

Lewis, S. K., Dirksen, S. R., Heitkemper, M. M., & Bucher, L. (2014). *Medical-Surgical Nursing: Assessment and Mangement of Clinical Problems* (9th ed). St. Louis: Elsevier.

Lewis, S. M., Heitkemper, M. M., & Dirksen, S. R. (2004). *Medical-surgical nursing: Assessment and management of clinical problems* (6th ed.). St Louis: Mosby.

Maggi, L., & Mantegazza, R. (2011). Treatment of myasthenia gravis: Focus on pyridostigmine. *Clinical Drug Investigations, October 1:31*(10), 691 –701. doi:10.2165/11593300-000000000-00000

Mattson, D. H. (2002). Update on the diagnosis of multiple sclerosis. *Expert Review in Neuro-Therapy, 2*(3), 319–328.

McGrogan, A., Madle, G. C., Seaman, H. E., & de Vries, C. S. (2009). The epidemiology of Guillain-Barré syndrome worldwide: A systematic literature review. *Neuroepidemiology, 32*(2), 150–163.

Miller, C. E., Karpinski, M., & Jezewski, M. A. (2012). Relapsing-Remitting Multiple Sclerosis Patients' Experience with Natalizumab A Phenomenological Investigation. *International Journal of MS Care, 14,* 39–44.

Miller, C. E., & Umhauer, M. A. (2011). Emerging oral therapies for multiple sclerosis. *Journal of Neuroscience Nursing, 43*(1), 3–14.

Miller, R. G., Jackson, C. E., Kasarskis, E. J., England, J. D., Forshew, D., Johnston, W.,…Quality Standards Subcommittee of the American Academy of Neurology (2009). Practice parameter update: The care of the patient with amyotrophic lateral sclerosis: Multidisciplinary care, symptom management, and cognitive/behavioral impairment (an evidence-based review). Report to the Quality Standards Subcommittee of the American Academy of Neurology. *Neurology, 73*(15), 1227–1233.

Mohammad, A. F., Khan, K. A., Galvin, L., Hardiman, O., & O'Connell, P. G. (2009). High incidence of osteoporosis and fractures in an aging post polio population. *Europe Neurology, 62*(6), 369–374.

Monahan, F. D., Sands, J. K., Neighbors, M., Marek, J. F., & Green, C. J. (2007). *Phipps' medical-surgical nursing: Health and illness perspectives* (8th ed.). St. Louis: Mosby Elsevier.

Multiple Sclerosis Association of America. (2014). About MS: MS overview. Retrieved from http://www.mymsaa.org/about-ms/overview/

Multiple Sclerosis Foundation. (2009a). Who gets Multiple Sclerosis? Retrieved from http://www.msfocus.org/who-gets-multiple-sclerosis.aspx

Multiple Sclerosis Foundation. (2009b). What causes Multiple Sclerosis? Retrieved from http://www.msfocus.org/causes-multiple-sclerosis.aspx

Multiple Sclerosis Foundation (2013). Facts about MS. Retrieved from http://www.msfocus.org/Facts-About-MS.aspx.

Multiple Sclerosis Foundation (2014). Treatments for Multiple Sclerosis. Retrieved from http://www.msfocus.org/Treatments-for-multiple-sclerosis.aspx

Muppidi, S., Wolfe, G. I., & Barohn, R. J. (2012). Diseases of the neuromuscular junction. In K. F. Swaiman S. Ashwal, D. M. Ferriero, & N. F. Schor (Eds.), *Pediatric neurology: Principles and practice* (5th ed., pp. 1549–1569). Philadelphia, PA: Elsevier Saunders.

Myasthenia Gravis Foundation of America (2010). What is Myasthenia Gravis? Retrieved from http://myasthenia.org/WhatisMG.aspx

National Guideline Clearinghouse. (2012). EFNS Guidelines on the Clinical Management of Amyotrophic Lateral Sclerosis (MALS): Revised Report of an EFNS Task Force. Retrieved from http://www.guideline.gov/content.aspx?id=38469

National Institute of Neurological Disorders and Stroke (NINDS). (2012). Post-Polio Syndrome Fact Sheet. Retrieved from http://www.ninds.nih.gov/disorders/post_polio/detail_post_polio.htm#261623172

National Multiple Sclerosis Society. (n.d.a). Who Gets MS? (Epidemiology). Retrieved from http://www.nationalmssociety.org/What-is-MS/Who-Gets-MS

National Multiple Sclerosis Society (n.d.b). Pediatric MS. Retrieved from http://www.nationalmssociety.org/What-is-MS/Who-Gets-MS/Pediatric-MS

National Multiple Sclerosis Society (n.d.c). Treating MS: Medications. Retrieved from http://www.nationalmssociety.org/Treating-MS/Medications

National Multiple Sclerosis Society (n.d.d). What Causes MS? Retrieved from http://www.nationalmssociety.org/What-is-MS/What-Causes-MS

National Multiple Sclerosis Society (n.d.e). Rehabilitation. Retrieved from http://www.nationalmssociety.org/For-Professionals/Clinical-Care/Managing-MS/Rehabilitation

Newland, P. K., Fearing, A., Riley, M., & Neith, A. (2012). Symptom clusters in woman with relapsing-remitting multiple sclerosis. *Journal of Neuroscience Nursing, 44*(2), 66–71.

Newland, P. K., Thomas, F. P., Riley, M., Flick, L. H., & Fearing, A. (2012). The use of focus groups to characterize symptoms in persons with multiple sclerosis. *Journal of Neuroscience Nursing, 44*(6), 352–357.

Pardo, G., Boutwell, C., Conner, J., Denney, D., & Loeen-Burkey, M. (2010). Effect of oral antihistamine on local injection site reactions with self-administered glatiramer acetate. *Journal of Neuroscience Nursing, 42*(1), 40–46.

Parkinson's Disease Foundation (2012). Parkinson's Disease Q & A (6th ed.) Retrieved from http://www.pdf.org/pdf/pubs_parkinson_qa_12.pdf

Patwa, H. S., Chaudhry, V., Katzberg, H., Rae-Grant, A. D., & So, Y. T. (2012). Evidence-based guideline: Intravenous immunoglobulin in the treatment of neuromuscular disorders. *Neurology, 78*(13), 1009–1015. doi:10.1212/WNL.0b013e31824de29

Pierini, D., & Stuifbergen, A. K. (2010). Psychological resilience and depressive symptoms in older adults diagnosed with post-polio syndrome. *Rehabilitation Nursing, 35*(4), 167–175.

Plow, M., & Finlayson, M. (2012). A qualitative study of nutritional behaviors in adults with multiple sclerosis. *Journal of Neuroscience Nursing, 44*(6), 337–350.

Polak, M., Richman, J., Lorimer, M., Boynton-DeSepulveda, L., & Del Bene, M. (2004). Neuromuscular disorders of the nervous system. In M. K. Bader & L. R. Littlejohn (Eds.), *AANN core curriculum for neuroscience nursing* (4th ed.). Glenview, IL: American Association of Neuroscience Nursing.

Polman, C. H., Reingold, S. C., Banwell, B., Clanet, M., Cohen, J. A., Filippi, M.,...Wolinsky, J. S. (2011). Diagnostic criteria for multiple sclerosis: 2010 revisions to the McDonald criteria. *Annals of Neurology, 69*(2), 292–302.

Post-Polio Health International. (2010). Post-Polio Syndrome: A New Challenge for the Survivors of Polio. Retrieved from www.post-polio.org/edu/pps.html

Rowland, L. P., & Shineider, N. L. (2001). Amyotrophic lateral sclerosis. *New England Journal of Medicine, 344*(22), 1688–1700.

Schwarz, A. (2010, August 17). Study says brain trauma can mimic ALS. *The New York Times*, A1.

Seppi, K., Weintraub, D., Coelho, M., Perez-Lloret, S., Fox, S. H., Katzenschlager, R.,...Sampaio, C. (2011). The Movement Disorder Society evidence-based medicine review update: Treatments for the motor symptoms of Parkinson's disease. *Movement Disorders, 26*(S3), S42–S80.

Shah, A. K. (2014). Myasthenia gravis differential diagnoses. Retrieved from http://emedicine.medscape.com/article/1171206-treatment

Simmons, R. D., Tribe, K. L., & McDonald, E. A. (2010). Living with multiple sclerosis: Longitudinal changes in employment and the importance of symptom management. *Journal of Neurology, 257*(6), 926–936.

Sinclair, V. G., & Scroggie, J. (2005). Effects of a cognitive-behavioral program for women with multiple sclerosis. *Journal of Neuroscience Nursing, 37*(5), 249–257, 276.

Sivestri, N. J., & Wolfe, G. I. (2012). Myasthenia gravis. *Seminars in Neurology, 32*(3), 215–226.

Smolders, J. (2010). Vitamin D and multiple sclerosis: Correlations, causality, and controversy. *Autoimmune Diseases*, October 5, 2011:629538. doi:10.4061/2011/629538

Solaro, C., & Messmer Uccelli, M. (2010). Pharmacological management of pain in patients with multiple sclerosis. *Drugs, 70*(10), 1245–1254.

Steefel, L. (2006, May 22). Not just for grown-ups: The number of children with multiple sclerosis is climbing at an alarming rate. *Nursing Spectrum*, 16–17.

Stoelb, B. L., Carter, G. T., Abresch, R. T., Purekal, S., McDonald, C. M., & Jensen, M. P. (2008). Pain in persons with postpolio syndrome: Frequency, intensity and impact. *Archives of Physical Medicine and Rehabilitation, 89*(10), 1933–1940.

Suzuki, S., Utsugisawa, K., & Suzuki, N. (2013). Overlooked non-motor symptoms in myasthenia gravis. *Journal of Neurology, Neurosurgery and Psychiatry, 84*(9), 989–994.

Thompson, H. J., & Mauk, K. L. (Eds.). (2012). *Nursing management of the patient with multiple sclerosis*. Chicago, IL: American Association of Neuroscience Nurses.

Tiffreau, V., Rapin, A., Serafi, R., Percebolis-Macadre, L., Supper, C., Jolly, D., & Boyer, F. C. (2010). Post-polio syndrome and rehabilitation. *Annals of Physical and Rehabilitation Medicine, 53*(1), 42–50.

Tomik, B., & Gulloff, R. J. (2010). Dysarthria in amyotrophic lateral sclerosis: A review. *Amyotrophic Lateral Sclerosis, 11*(1–2), 4–15.

Torsney, K. M., Noyce, A. J., Doherty, K. M., Bestwick, J. P. Dobson, R., & Lees, A. J. (2014). Bone health in Parkinson's disease: A systematic review and meta-analysis. *Journal of Neurology, Neurosurgery & Psychiatry, 85*(10). doi:10.1136/jnnp-2013-307307

Turkoski, B. (2013).Your patient has multiple sclerosis: Understanding the challenge. *Orthopaedic Nursing, 32*(1), 45–50.

van Doorn, P. A. (2009). What's new in Guillain-Barré syndrome in 2007–2008? *Journal of Peripheral Nervous System, 14*(2), 72–74.

van Doorn, P. A., Ruts, L., & Jacobs, B. C. (2008). Clinical features, pathogenesis, and treatment of Guillain-Barre syndrome. *Lancet Neurology, 10*, 939–950.

Volkmann, J., Albanese, A., Angelo, A., Chadhuri, K. R., Clarke, C. E., deBie, R. M. A.,...Oertel, W. (2013). Selecting deep brain stimulation or infusion therapies in advanced Parkinson's disease: An evidence-based review. *Journal of Neurology, 260*(11), 2701–2714. doi:10.1007/s00415-012-6798-6

Vucic, S., Kiernan, M. C., & Cornblath, D. R. (2009). Guillain-Barré syndrome: An update. *Journal of Clinical Neuroscience, 16*(6), 733–741.

Werhagen, L., & Borg, K. (2010). Analysis of long-standing nociceptive and neuropathic pain in patients with post-polio syndrome. *Journal of Neurology, 257*(6), 1027–1031.

Yelnik, A., & Laffont, I. (2010). The psychological aspects of polio survivors through their life experience. *Annals of Physical and Rehabilitation Medicine, 53*(1), 60–67.

Chapter 22

Stroke

Linda L. Pierce, PhD RN CNS CRRN FAHA FAAN
Debbie Summers, MSN RN ACNS-BC CNRN SCRN FAHA

LEARNING OUTCOMES

- Identify the stroke process and describe primary prevention measures of stroke.
- Discuss treatment measures for stroke.
- Recognize the nursing process: assess, nursing diagnoses, plan, intervene, evaluate.
- Examine family and caregiver support mechanisms.
- Review the role of advanced practice nursing in stroke care.

KEY CHAPTER TOPICS

- Stroke process
- Primary prevention measures
- Treatment measures
- The nursing process
- Family and caregiver support mechanisms
- Role of advanced practice nursing

PROFESSIONAL REHABILITATION NURSING DOMAINS AND COMPETENCIES

- Domain 1: Competencies 1.1, 1.2, 1.3, 1.4
- Domain 2: Competencies 2.1, 2.2, 2.3
- Domain 3: Competencies 3.3, 3.4
- Domain 4: Competencies 4.2, 4.3 (Association of Rehabilitation Nurses [ARN], 2014a)

Introduction

Alice had a stroke that left her unable to use her left arm and leg; she completed a rehabilitation program 2 years ago. She is unable to climb stairs and uses a wheelchair for mobility. Her health has declined. She has lost weight and inappropriately cries one minute and laughs the next. Her living room was converted to a bedroom in her two-story home. Brownie, her husband, placed a toilet commode near her wheelchair and bed, but he has difficulty transferring her from bed to chair to toilet. He is worried about her safety and is concerned that she could fall and injure herself. If Alice falls, he is concerned that he could not assist her because he has a "bad back." Brownie says that he feels alone, hopeless, and helpless, in caring for his wife because his friends are dying and family members live out of town. He is upset as he begins to think that he can no longer care for his wife at home because of her increasing weakness and his health problems. However, he promised Alice that he would never place her in a nursing home, stating that "family takes care of family." Brownie remembers Alice's rehabilitation nurse and contacts him for guidance.

Alice and Brownie's story is typical in that stroke or "brain attack" (also called cerebrovascular accident [CVA]) affects hundreds of thousands of people each year. The effects of stroke may be slight or severe, temporary or permanent, and can be devastating to the client and family. (Note: The terms client and patient are used interchangeably to denote the person with stroke in this chapter.) Clients who have had a stroke must cope with numerous sensorimotor, visual, perceptual, and language deficits. Rehabilitation should begin when the person is admitted to care. Initially rehabilitation is focused on minimizing complications of the stroke. As the client stabilizes, he or she may be transferred to a rehabilitation unit as soon as 2 days after the stroke has occurred, and rehabilitation should be continued as necessary after the client leaves the facility and returns to the home setting.

Rehabilitation provides an interprofessional team effort (e.g., nurse, physician, social work, therapy) that focuses on helping the person who had a stroke regain as much functional independence as possible. Rehabilitation also plays a major role in helping to prevent secondary complications and minimize long-term disability after stroke. To intervene effectively as a member of the rehabilitation team, the professional nurse, no matter what educational level (associate, bachelor's, master's, or doctoral degree), proficiency level (beginner, intermediate, or advanced), or setting (inpatient or outpatient acute and rehabilitation hospital, skilled/extended care or assisted/transitional living, home and community), must have a good understanding of the physiological, perceptual, and psychological changes that occur after stroke. Nursing goals must focus on maintaining effective tissue perfusion, preventing complications, and enhancing stroke survivors' and caregivers' adjustment and quality of life.

I. Overview of Stroke

Stroke occurs when blood flow to the brain is disrupted (e.g., when a clot or piece of plaque blocks one of the vital blood vessels in the brain or when a blood vessel bursts, spilling blood into surrounding brain tissues). Stroke is a medical emergency, and prompt treatment is vital. Although stroke is a major cause of death, many people survive. Stroke may leave survivors with long-term physical and cognitive difficulties; family members may become informal, unpaid caregivers without any preparation for that role. Rehabilitation after stroke is an important goal for survivors and their caregivers.

A. Description

1. A stroke or CVA is a sudden onset of focal neurological deficit (cerebro) caused by a regional disruption of blood supply (vascular) and oxygen in the brain. Brain cells begin to die, and brain damage occurs (National Stroke Association [NSA], 2014g; Sacco et al., 2013).
2. A stroke, or brain attack, should be treated as a medical emergency; delay of treatment can affect the amount and permanence of the brain damage.
3. Types of stroke include ischemic and hemorrhagic.
    a. An ischemic stroke occurs when a blood clot or piece of plaque blocks a blood vessel or artery and obstructs the blood flow to the brain.
    b. A hemorrhagic stroke occurs when a weakened blood vessel breaks or bursts, interrupting blood flow to an area of the brain and causing bleeding in the brain.
4. When a stroke occurs, blood flow to that part of the brain is disrupted, resulting in tissue anoxia and death of brain cells (infarction). As many as 2 million brain cells die every minute while blood flow is interrupted (NSA, 2014g).
    a. Neurons and other brain cells need oxygen and glucose delivered via the circulatory system to function.
    b. A few minutes of oxygen deprivation (ischemia) is enough to cause permanent damage.
    c. Cell death triggers a cascade of inflammation, edema, and energy depletion that can continue to cause damage for hours to days after the initial insult (National Institute of Neurological Disorders and Stroke [NINDS], 2014b).
5. A transient ischemic attack (TIA) is caused by a temporary clot within a blood vessel that supplies the brain with blood (American Stroke Association [ASA], 2012c; Sacco et al., 2013).
    a. A TIA is a "warning stroke" or "mini-stroke" that produces stroke-like symptoms but no lasting damage. Recognizing and treating TIAs can reduce the risk of a major stroke.
    b. TIA symptoms are the same as those of stroke but typically last 1–2 hours and resolve within 24 hours, leaving no residual deficits (ASA, 2012b; Miller & Summers, 2014).

B. Epidemiology

1. Incidence
    a. Forecasts suggest that by the year 2050 the number of stroke events will expand to a total of 1,334,000 per year in the United States. The majority of this increase will be in older adults and minority (particularly Hispanic) populations (Howard & Goff, 2012). On average, every 40 seconds someone in the United States has a stroke (Go et al., 2013).
    b. Each year, 795,000 Americans have a stroke (Go et al., 2013; NSA, 2014d).
        1) About 600,000 of these are first attacks and 185,000 are recurrent attacks.
        2) Approximately 55,000 more women than men have a stroke each year.
        3) Men's stroke rates are higher than women's at younger ages but not at older ages.
        4) Each year women have more strokes than men, and stroke kills more women than men, possibly because women are older on average when the stroke occurs (ASA, 2012c; The Internet Stroke Center, 2014b; NINDS, 2014b; NSA, 2014e).
    c. More than 140,000 people per year die as a result of a stroke. Between 1995 and 2005, the stroke death rate fell 30% and the actual number of stroke deaths declined 14% (The Internet Stroke Center, 2014b).
    d. About 25% of people who recover from a first stroke will have another stroke within 5 years (NINDS, 2014b).
        1) Second strokes are twice as common in men as women, with 24% of women and 42% of men having a second stroke within 5 years.
        2) Second strokes often have a higher rate of disability and death because parts of the brain that are already damaged by the

original stroke may not be as able to withstand another insult (NSA, 2014g).

e. TIA precedes approximately 40% of strokes and carries a 90-day stroke risk of 10%–15%. An estimated 500,000 TIAs occur in the United States each year (MNT Knowledge Center, 2013; NSA, 2014g).

2. Severity: Stroke is the fourth-leading cause of death in the United States after heart disease, cancer, and lower respiratory disease (Towfighi & Saver, 2011).
3. Risk for stroke: Both modifiable and unmodifiable risk factors contribute to a person's risk of having a stroke.
   a. The incidence of stroke occurring in children is low, about six cases per 100,000 children per year. Strokes are slightly more common in children younger than 2 years old. In all children, 55% of strokes are ischemic, and the remainder are hemorrhagic (NSA, 2014a; Roach et al., 2008). Sixty percent of strokes occur in boys (Lloyd-Jones et al., 2010). Boys have a higher risk of stroke than girls, and African-American children are at a higher risk than Caucasian and Asian children (Lloyd-Jones et al., 2010).
   b. Stroke occurs more often in people with risk factors that cannot be changed, such as being older than 55 years, being male or African American, having a family history of stroke, or having a history of diabetes. Others at risk include those who are of Hispanic or Asian/Pacific Islander origin.
   c. The age-adjusted incidence of stroke is about twice as high in African Americans and Hispanic Americans as in Caucasians. The rate of first strokes in African Americans is almost twice the rate in Caucasians, and African Americans are twice as likely to die from strokes as Caucasians and Hispanics. On average, African and Hispanic Americans tend to experience stroke at younger ages than Caucasians (Go et al., 2013; NINDS, 2014b; NSA, 2009a).
   d. Stroke mortality is unusually high in people living in a cluster of southeastern states—Alabama, Arkansas, Georgia, Louisiana, Mississippi, North Carolina, South Carolina, and Tennessee—known as the "Stroke Belt." A recent study funded by the National Institutes of Health National Institute on Aging suggests that the "belt" is worn from childhood. Higher rates of diabetes and hypertension and possibly poorer socioeconomic conditions for those living in the Stroke Belt, particularly African Americans, contribute to this mortality (NINDS, 2009b).
   e. Risk factors for stroke are controllable or modifiable (preventable) and uncontrollable or unmodifiable. Controllable risk factors fall into two categories: lifestyle and medical. Uncontrollable risk factors include things people cannot change (NINDS, 2009b).
      1) Nonmodifiable or uncontrollable
         a) Age: Risk of stroke doubles for each decade between the ages of 65 and 85 years. In the Framingham Heart Study, among participants younger than age 65 years, the risk of stroke or TIA was 4.2 times higher in subjects with symptoms of depression (Salaycik et al., 2007).
         b) Gender: Stroke is most prevalent in men; however, women are at risk during pregnancy (e.g., risk increases threefold) and menopause (e.g., hormone replacement therapy increases the risk by about 30% in women with an intact uterus and by almost 40% for women who have undergone a hysterectomy and treatment with estrogen) (NINDS, 2009b).
         c) Race and ethnicity: Stroke risk is about twice as high in African Americans and Hispanic Americans as in Caucasians (NINDS, 2009b; NSA, 2009a).
         d) Family history of stroke
         e) Previous stroke, or TIA, or heart attack
         f) Fibromuscular dysplasia
         g) Hole in heart
      2) Modifiable, controllable, or treatable
         a) Hypertension
         b) Heart disease (e.g., atrial fibrillation [AF], heart failure, valvular heart disease)
         c) Diabetes
         d) Dyslipidemia: Elevated low-density lipoprotein cholesterol (LDL-C) and elevated serum triglyceride
         e) Carotid artery disease
         f) TIA or previous stroke
         g) Tobacco use or smoking
         h) Physical inactivity or obesity
         i) Alcohol abuse
         j) Illegal or street drug use (e.g., cocaine, amphetamines)
         k) Blood disorders (e.g., sickle cell anemia, polycythemia)

l) Sleep apnea
m) Hypercoagulation

4. Recovery: Stroke is the leading cause of serious, long-term adult disability (Centers for Disease Control and Prevention [CDC], 2013). A wide range of morbidity is associated with stroke (NSA, 2009c, 2014b, 2014c).
   a. 10% recover almost totally.
   b. 25% are left with minor disabilities.
   c. 40% have moderate to severe problems that necessitate care.
   d. 10% need long-term facility care.
   e. 15% die soon after having a stroke.
5. Annually stroke costs an estimated $36.5 billion, including the cost of healthcare services, medications to treat stroke, and missed days of work (Go et al., 2013).

C. Etiology of Stroke (ASA, 2012b; Markus, Pereira, & Cloud, 2010; NINDS, 2014b; NSA, 2014e).

1. Stroke is the result of an interruption in the blood supply to some part of the brain.
   a. The arterial blood supply to the brain comes from the internal carotid arteries and the vertebral arteries (**Figure 22-1**).
      1) The internal carotid arteries supply the anterior portion of the brain with a greater amount of blood flow and originate from the common carotid arteries. They enter the cranium through the base of the skull, passing through the cavernous sinus and then branching off into the anterior and middle cerebral arteries.
      2) The vertebral arteries are posterior and originate as branches off the subclavian arteries. They pass through the foramen magnum and join at the junction of the pons and medulla oblongata to form the basilar artery. The basilar artery divides at the level of the midbrain to form the two posterior cerebral arteries.
      3) The arterial circle (circle of Willis) is the structure in the brain with the ability to compensate for reduced blood flow from any of the major contributors (collateral blood flow). This circle is formed by the posterior cerebral arteries, posterior communicating arteries, internal carotid arteries, anterior cerebral arteries, and anterior communicating artery.
   b. Ischemic stroke accounts for about 80% of all strokes. It is occlusive in nature as the result of a cerebral embolism or cerebral thrombosis, and it is categorized by vascular distribution or location.
   c. Hemorrhagic stroke has a lower incidence (approximately 20%) than ischemic stroke but is associated with a higher mortality rate. A subarachnoid stroke is a rupture of a large vessel in the protective lining of the brain, and an intracerebral stroke is the rupture of a vessel in the brain itself.

Figure 22-1. Cerebral Arteries and the Areas of the Brain They Supply

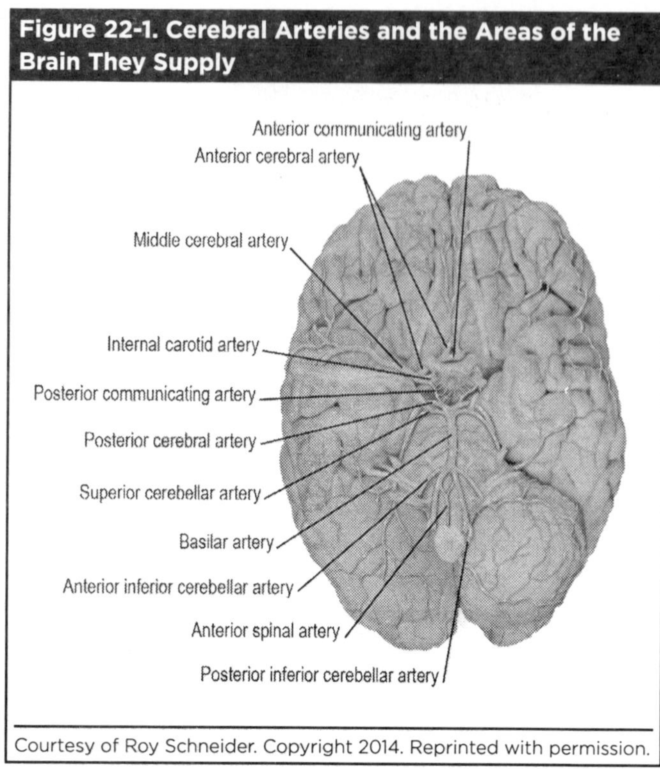

Courtesy of Roy Schneider. Copyright 2014. Reprinted with permission.

2. Metabolic needs of the brain
   a. The brain needs constant circulation of approximately 20% of the body's blood supply to maintain adequate oxygen and nutrients.
   b. Blood flow is autoregulated by the brain itself (Klabunde, 2009).
   c. The physiological demands served by the blood supply of the brain are particularly significant because neurons are more sensitive to oxygen deprivation than other kinds of cells with lower rates of metabolism. In addition, the brain is at risk from circulating toxins and is specifically protected in this respect by the blood–brain barrier.

D. Signs and Symptoms of Stroke (NINDS, 2013)

1. Sudden numbness or weakness of face, arm, or leg, especially unilaterally
2. Sudden confusion, trouble speaking or understanding
3. Sudden trouble seeing in one or both eyes
4. Sudden ataxia, dizziness, or loss of balance or coordination

5. Sudden severe headache with no known cause
6. Act F.A.S.T.:
   a. Face: Has the face fallen on one side; can the person smile?
   b. Arms: Can the person raise both arms and keep them there?
   c. Speech: Is the person's speech slurred?
   d. Time: Call 911 if you see any one of these signs or symptoms of stroke.

E. Pathophysiology
1. TIA (ASA, 2012c; Becker, Wira, & Arnold, 2010; Easton et al., 2009)
   a. Persists for several minutes or hours and then resolves.
   b. Usually lasts 5–15 minutes, followed by full recovery of neurological function within 24 hours; the majority last less than 1 hour.
   c. It has also been defined as "a brief episode of neurological dysfunction caused by focal brain or retinal ischemia, with clinical symptoms typically lasting less than one hour, and without evidence of acute infarction" (Easton et al., 2009, pp. 2276–2277).
   d. Roughly 80% resolve within 60 minutes. Tissue-based definitions are being proposed with magnetic resonance imaging (MRI).
   e. Resolution results in a negative neurological examination, and diagnosis may be based on history.
   f. People who experience TIA may have nine times the risk of a stroke, and often stroke occurs within 30 days of the TIA. (A valid estimate of the incidence of TIA is not available because many TIAs go unreported because of the subtle nature of the symptoms.) After a stroke many clients and families report episodes that were probably TIAs preceding the stroke.
   g. Vertebrobasilar TIA is the result of inadequate blood flow from the vertebral arteries, usually secondary to a partially obstructed subclavian artery, which supplies this area.
   h. Carotid TIA is the result of inadequate blood flow from the carotid artery, usually because of carotid stenosis.
2. Ischemic stroke: Approximately 80% of all strokes (NINDS, 2014b)
   a. Process (Becker et al., 2010; Jauch et al., 2013; Markus et al., 2010; NINDS, 2014b)
      1) Acute ischemic stroke is stroke caused by thrombosis or embolism and is more common than hemorrhagic stroke. On the macroscopic level, ischemic stroke most often is caused by extracranial embolism or intracranial thrombosis, but it may also be caused by decreased cerebral blood flow. On the cellular level, any process that disrupts blood flow to a portion of the brain unleashes an ischemic cascade, leading to the death of neurons and cerebral infarction.
      2) Acute ischemic stroke often begins as a result of atherosclerotic disease and progresses slowly as the affected artery becomes narrowed and eventually occluded. It may also occur as a result of a rupture of an atherosclerotic plaque that travels as an embolus to the brain and blocks blood flow.
      3) Atherosclerotic plaques (stenotic lesions) form at branches and curves in the cerebral circulation. The stenotic area degenerates, which forms an ulcerated vessel wall. Platelets and fibrin adhere to the damaged wall and form clots, which eventually occlude the artery.
      4) The thrombus may enlarge in the vessel distally and proximally, or a portion of the clot may break off and travel up the vessel to a distant site, forming an embolus.
      5) Focal areas of the brain and adjoining brain tissue are deprived of oxygen and glucose. When the deprivation is severe enough and lasts long enough, permanent damage occurs. The timing of the restoration of cerebral blood flow appears to be a critical factor. Time also may prove to be a key factor in neuronal protection.
      6) Neurons near the ischemic or infarcted areas undergo changes that disrupt plasma membranes, causing cellular edema and further compression of capillaries. On the cellular level, the ischemic neuron becomes depolarized as adenosine triphosphate (ATP) is depleted and membrane ion transport systems fail. The resulting influx of calcium leads to the release of a number of neurotransmitters, including large quantities of glutamate, which activates N-methyl-d-aspartate (NMDA) and other excitatory receptors on other neurons. These neurons then become depolarized, causing further calcium influx, further glutamate release, and local amplification of the initial ischemic insult. This massive calcium influx also activates various degradative enzymes, leading to destruction of the

cell membrane and other essential neuronal structures.

7) It is thought that some cortical reorganization and neuroplasticity occurs after a stroke. This process has been described as a "rewiring" of brain cells in response to the environment and experience, including therapy. This change results in a different pattern of movement for the client.

8) Most people survive an initial hemispheric ischemic stroke unless there is massive cerebral edema.

9) Massive brainstem infarcts from basilar thrombosis or embolism almost always are fatal.

b. Types of ischemic strokes (ASA, 2012c; Becker et al., 2010; Easton et al., 2009; Ionita & Levine, 2013; Merck Sharp & Dohme Corporation, 2009–2010; NINDS, 2014b)

1) Embolic stroke

a) A traveling clot, which typically originates from thrombi in the heart or from plaque in the aortic arch or carotid or vertebral arteries that becomes lodged and obstructs cerebral blood flow

b) Commonly associated with a history of cardiac disease, especially atrial fibrillation in older people

c) The sources of cardiogenic emboli include valvular thrombi (e.g., in mitral stenosis, endocarditis, prosthetic valve, mural thrombi, myocardial infarction [MI], AF, dilated cardiomyopathy, severe congestive heart failure, atrial myxoma, and patent foramen ovale). MI is associated with a 2%–3% incidence of embolic stroke, of which 85% occur in the first month after MI.

2) Thrombotic stroke

a) Most common cause of stroke

b) A stationary clot in a large blood vessel, usually caused by atherosclerotic plaque

(i) Plaque forms when calcium and lipids collect and attach to the vessel wall, especially in bifurcations of a large artery. This produces narrowing that impedes or obstructs blood flow.

(ii) Atherosclerosis can produce degeneration of blood vessel walls. This can involve tearing or degeneration of a weakened vessel wall or plaque, which can trigger the normal clotting process, and this congestion further reduces circulation to the area.

(iii) Large-vessel thrombosis: Thrombotic strokes occur most often in large arteries and usually are caused by a combination of long-term atherosclerosis followed by rapid blood clot formation. Clients with thrombotic stroke are likely to have coronary artery disease, and heart attack is a common cause of death in people who have had this type of stroke (NSA, 2014f).

3) Lacunar infarcts (small vessel disease)

a) Thrombotic strokes that affect the small arteries deep within the subcortical white matter of the brain.

b) Are microinfarcts smaller than 1 cm in diameter (usually 2–20 mm) and involve the small perforating arteries, predominantly in the basal ganglia, internal capsules, and pons.

c) Are caused by atherosclerosis.

d) Often result in pure motor, pure sensory, or ataxic hemiparetic deficits.

e) Are closely linked to small-vessel disease found in hypertension or diabetes.

4) Stroke caused by systemic hypoperfusion

a) Caused by inadequate cardiac output with system hypoperfusion.

b) Usually caused by MI, cardiac arrest, and life-threatening ventricular arrhythmias; less commonly caused by pulmonary emboli, acute gastrointestinal bleeding, and shock.

c) Symptoms include pallor, sweating, and hypotension. Neurological deficits are sudden and associated with systemic symptoms related to the underlying problem.

d) Prominent signs include decreased level of consciousness and symmetric depression of hemispheric function.

e) Also called a watershed stroke.

c. Risk factors for ischemic stroke (Becker et al., 2010; The Internet Stroke Center, 2014a; Kernan et al., 2014; NINDS, 2014b)

1) Arterial hypertension; elevated systolic and diastolic blood pressures (BP) are independent risk factors.

2) Smoking increases the risk by 50%.

3) Diabetes increases the risk by 2.5–3.5 times.
4) Insulin resistance is an independent risk factor.
5) Thrombocythemia and polycythemia increase the risk.
6) Impaired cardiac function (coronary artery disease, left ventricular hypertrophy, chronic AF).
7) Chronic atherosclerosis; elevated lipoprotein(a) is an independent risk factor.
8) Hyperhomocystinemia is a strong and independent risk factor.
9) Estrogen deficiency in postmenopausal women increases the risk.
10) Advanced age (the risk doubles every decade).
11) Use of oral contraceptives places a person at a higher risk for an ischemic stroke.
12) Previous cerebrovascular disease can place a person at a higher risk for an ischemic stroke.

3. Hemorrhagic stroke: Intracerebral hemorrhage (ICH) accounts for 10%–15% of all strokes and is associated with higher mortality rates than cerebral infarctions (ASA, 2012a; Esse, Fossati-Bellani, Traylor, & Martin-Schild, 2011; Kuramatsu, Huttner, & Schwab, 2013; Nassisi, 2010; NINDS, 2014b; NSA, 2014f; Sen, Webb, & Selph, 2010; Zebian & Kazzi, 2010)
   a. Process
      1) Spontaneous rupture of a cerebral vessel occurs; blood enters the brain tissue or subarachnoid space.
      2) The most common causes of hemorrhagic stroke are hypertension (up to 60%), ruptured aneurysms, vascular malformations, vasculitis, bleeding into a tumor, hemorrhage from bleeding disorders or anticoagulation, head trauma, and illicit drug use.
      3) The area around the injury dies within a few minutes from lack of oxygen and the failure of the oxygen-dependent ATP metabolic pathway. The broader area of injury is called the penumbra, and this damage is more dynamic, taking 12–24 hours to occur. The release of intracellular calcium initiates the programmed cell death or apoptosis.
      4) With hemorrhagic strokes, focal neurological deficits are found in 80% of people, and altered consciousness occurs in 50% of people.
      5) People with hemorrhagic stroke present with similar focal neurologic deficits but tend to be more ill than people with ischemic stroke. Only 20% of clients regain functional independence.
   b. Types of hemorrhagic stroke
      1) Subarachnoid hemorrhage (SAH)
         a) This is the rupture of a blood vessel located in the subarachnoid space, a fluid-filled space between layers of connective tissue (meninges) that surround the brain. It is caused by some pathologic process, usually rupture of a berry aneurysm or arteriovenous malformation (AVM).
         b) Annual incidence of nontraumatic aneurysmal SAH is six to 25 cases per 100,000. An estimated 10%–15% of people die before reaching the hospital. The mortality rate is as high as 40% within the first week. About half die in the first 6 months.
         c) Presents clinically as a sudden onset of a severe headache ("the worst headache of my life"), nausea and vomiting, signs of meningeal irritation (neck stiffness, low back pain, bilateral leg pain), photophobia and visual disturbances, and varying degrees of neurological dysfunction.
         d) Can result in elevated intracranial pressure, vasospasms, and ischemia, which further reduces cerebral blood flow.
         e) Can also present as prodromal (warning) headaches from minor blood leakage; this is referred to as sentinel headache, with a reported median of 2 weeks before the SAH may occur (30%–50% of aneurysmal SAHs).
         f) More than 25% of people experience seizures close to the acute onset; the location of a seizure focus has no relationship to the location of the aneurysm.
      2) Intracerebral (intraparenchymal) hemorrhage
         a) Often caused by hypertension (blood pressure [BP] is elevated in almost all cases).
         b) Involves small, deep-penetrating blood vessels that rupture and release blood directly into the brain tissue (parenchyma).
         c) An ICH usually invades deep white matter first. ICH has a predilection for

certain sites in the brain, including the thalamus, putamen, cerebellum, and brainstem.

d) Neurological signs and symptoms vary with the site and size of the extravasation of blood (released blood puts pressure on surrounding tissue, which can cause small arterioles and capillaries to tear).

e) It may present clinically as an almost immediate lapse into stupor and coma, with hemiplegia and steady deterioration to death over several hours after initial presentation. More often it presents with a headache, followed within a few minutes by unilateral neurological deficits involving face and limbs.

f) In addition to the area of the brain injured by the hemorrhage, the surrounding brain can be damaged by pressure produced by the mass effect of the hematoma. A general increase in intracranial pressure may occur. This resulting hematoma acts as a space-occupying lesion that, if large enough, will cause brain shifting or herniation.

c. Risk factors for hemorrhagic stroke
   1) High BP is responsible for approximately 60% of ICH and is a controllable stroke risk factor.
   2) Excessive alcohol and illicit drug (cocaine and amphetamines) use is associated with higher incidences of ICH and SAH. For people under the age of 35 years, drug use may be the most predisposing condition for stroke.
   3) Anticoagulant medication may prevent ischemic stroke but may increase the risk of intracerebral hemorrhage if the amount taken exceeds the therapeutic range.
   4) Blood clotting disorders such as hemophilia and sickle cell anemia can increase risk.
   5) Advanced age
   6) History of prior stroke

F. Clinical Manifestations of Stroke: The symptoms of stroke depend on the part of the brain that is damaged by a disruption in arterial blood flow. In some cases, a person may not even be aware that he or she has had a stroke (Patel, Jain, & Wagner, 2008; Markus et al., 2010) (Figure 22-1). See www.strokecenter.org/professionals/brain-anatomy/blood-vessels-of-the-brain/.

1. Each internal carotid artery (Figure 22-1) ascends along one side of the neck and supplies the cerebral hemispheres and diencephalon. These arteries have many twists and turns where plaque can build up, causing a blockage. Such blockages can be identified by sonogram (noninvasive) or by angiogram (invasive). Also, a sound called a bruit can sometimes be heard via stethoscope when a blockage exists. Signs and symptoms of occlusion may include
   a. Headaches
   b. Altered level of responsiveness
   c. Bruits over the carotid artery
   d. Profound aphasia
   e. Ptosis
   f. Unilateral blindness or retinal emboli
   g. Weakness, paralysis, numbness, sensory changes, and visual deficits on the affected side
2. The anterior cerebral artery (one of two main branches of the carotid artery) supplies medial surfaces and upper areas of the frontal and parietal lobes, including the medial aspect of the motor and sensory strip of the hemisphere. Signs and symptoms of occlusion may include
   a. Confusion
   b. Labile emotions, personality changes
   c. Weakness or numbness on affected side
   d. Paralysis of contralateral foot and leg
   e. Impaired mobility, sensation greater in lower extremities than upper extremities, impaired sensory function
   f. Urinary incontinence
   g. Loss of coordination
3. The middle cerebral artery (the most commonly occluded vessel in stroke and the largest branch in the internal carotid artery) supplies part of the frontal lobe and lateral surface of the temporal and parietal lobes, including primary motor and sensory areas for the face, throat, hand, and arm and, in the dominant hemisphere, the areas for speech. Signs and symptoms of occlusion include
   a. Altered level of responsiveness
   b. Alterations in communication, including aphasia, dysphasia, reading difficulty (dyslexia), inability to write (dysgraphia)
   c. Visual field deficits
   d. Alterations in cognition, mobility, and sensation, including contralateral sensory deficit and hemiparesis (more severe in the upper than lower)
4. The anterior communicating artery joins the anterior cerebral arteries of both hemispheres together. Signs and symptoms of occlusion may include:

a. Memory impairments, amnesia
b. Decreased executive functioning

5. The posterior cerebral artery joins the middle cerebral arteries to the posterior cerebral arteries, which are part of the basilar artery system. It supplies the medial and inferior temporal lobes, medial occipital lobe, thalamus, posterior hypothalamus, and visual receptive area. Signs and symptoms of occlusion may include
   a. Hemiplegia
   b. Receptive aphasia
   c. Sensory impairment
   d. Dyslexia
   e. Visual field deficits (cortical blindness from ischemia)
   f. Coma
6. Vertebral or basilar arteries supply the brainstem and cerebellum.
   a. Signs and symptoms of incomplete occlusion
      1) TIA
      2) Unilateral or bilateral weakness of extremities
      3) Visual deficits on affected side such as lack of depth perception, diplopia, or color blindness
      4) Nausea, vertigo, tinnitus
      5) Headache
      6) Dysarthria
      7) Numbness
      8) Dysphagia
      9) "Locked-in" syndrome: No movement except eyelids; sensation and consciousness preserved
   b. Signs and symptoms of complete occlusion
      1) Coma
      2) Decerebrate rigidity
      3) Respiratory and circulatory abnormalities
7. The posterior communicating artery connects the posterior cerebral artery with the internal carotid artery. It also forms part of the circle of Willis. It is more common to develop an aneurysm within the artery than an occlusion.
8. Circle of Willis (circulus arteriosus cerebri) is an anastomotic system of arteries that sits at the base of the brain and is formed by the anterior communicating artery, the two anterior cerebral, the two internal carotid, the two posterior communicating, and the two posterior cerebral arteries. Most aneurysms occur singly, with the most common sites being the circle of Willis and the bifurcation of the middle cerebral artery.

G. Residual Deficits of Stroke (**Table 22-1**) (NSA, 2009c; University of Miami Health System, 2014)

1. Significant alterations in many psychosocial areas
   a. Diminished affect
   b. Increased dependence in activities of daily living (ADLs)
   c. Decreased self-esteem
   d. Altered role performance
   e. Sexual dysfunction
   f. Change in leisure or social activity
   g. Decreased financial earning or vocational capability
2. General sequelae (all of which can influence safety)
   a. Hemiplegia: Weakness or paralysis on one side of the body contralateral to the lesion
   b. Abnormal tone, including flaccidity initially and then hypertonicity or spasticity on the affected side
   c. Sensorimotor problems, ataxia, imbalance
   d. Language deficits if lesion is in the dominant hemisphere
   e. Visuospatial perception impairments
   f. Cognitive deficits
   g. Memory changes
   h. Emotional lability: Inability to control emotions, especially crying and laughter (these may be expressed at inappropriate times)
   i. Fatigue
   j. Depression (may persist for months after the stroke)
   k. Seizure activity
3. Left hemispheric stroke: Common impairments and deficits
   a. Right hemiparesis (weakness) or hemiplegia (paralysis)
   b. Impaired ability to think analytically, shortened retention span, difficulty in learning new information, and problems in conceptualizing and generalizing
   c. Inability to do mathematical computations or interpret symbols
   d. Visual problems, including the inability to see the right visual field of each eye (right homonymous hemianopsia)
   e. Behavioral changes (e.g., slow and cautious, hesitant)
   f. Language difficulty, which includes not only the motor aspect of speech but also the ability to express and understand thoughts, ideas, and symbols in sequence
      1) Expressive (Broca's dysphasia or nonfluent) (ASA, 2013)
         a) Occurs with lesions in the posterior part of the dominant frontal lobe

Table 22-1. Residual Deficits of Stroke and Interventions

Manifestations	Left Hemispheric Damage	Interventions
Paresis or paralysis	Right side	Involve affected side during therapy or activities of daily living (ADLs).
Major deficits	Right homonymous hemianopsia; language deficits (e.g., aphasia, expression, comprehension, word finding); confuses left and right; has trouble gesturing, reading, writing	Incorporate techniques used by the speech therapist when communicating with the client; use a communication board and tools; incorporate the affected side into ADLs and activities; use demonstration and positive feedback.
Thought processes	Has difficulty listening and understanding; cannot process incoming language normally	Be patient; work with clients in short time frames to reduce frustration; offer encouragement; have the same staff work with a client when possible; speak slowly.
Emotional style	Is easily frustrated or depressed; is aware of deficits	Be patient; offer encouragement; exhibit acceptance; educate family on realistic expectations for communication; have a rehabilitation psychologist work with the client.
Attention span	Usually normal	Limit sessions, care, or treatments based on individual need.
Behavioral style	Is slow and cautious; needs encouragement	Allow plenty of time to work with a client; don't appear rushed; don't fragment care.
Manifestations	**Right Hemispheric Damage**	**Interventions**
Paresis or paralysis	Left side	Involve the affected side during therapy or ADLs.
Major deficits	Left homonymous hemianopsia; displays visual, spatial, perceptual deficits (e.g., gets lost, cannot dress self correctly, misjudges distance and position in space, spills things, gets stuck in doorways); has distorted body image; may have agnosia	Use repetition and one-step commands; approach on the left side and place objects in view past midline (e.g., affected arm on table while eating); orient the client in the room so all people enter the room on the left side of the client.
Thought processes	Has poor judgment; may have unrealistic thoughts; has memory deficits; has difficulty with concrete thinking	Always be aware of safety for this client (the client will take risks and act impulsively); establish a routine and stick with it; use a memory book; mark the client's room so it can be easily found with cueing.
Emotional style	Is often cheerful or euphoric; will deny illness or deficits; is unaware of problems; neglects left side; exhibits socially inappropriate behavior	Cue to deficits; constant reminders to call for help; don't leave unattended in bathroom or shower; monitor for inappropriate behavior; educate the family on expectations and deficits (the client will try to convince the family that he or she is fine).
Attention span	Short; is highly distractible	Work with the client one to one in a quiet setting; minimize outside noise and distractions; keep sessions and treatments short.
Behavioral style	Is quick and impulsive; needs supervision to prevent injury	Do not leave clients unattended; may need to use bed and chair alarms or an enclosure bed to prevent injury (clients will not call for help)

(precentral gyrus) and usually is on the left hemisphere

b) Is responsible for the motor aspects of speech

c) Damage in this area results in the inability to form or difficulty forming or finding words; difficulty writing (translating thoughts into symbols, not the physical act of writing); and impaired ability to read letters, numbers, or written material.

d) May have speech that is slow, effortful to produce, and punctuated by long pauses between words; verbal comprehension is largely intact.

e) Altered comprehension of language

f) May have intact automatic speech (e.g., may express a word, phrase, profanity, or song unexpectedly in a clear manner)

g) May have anomia (difficulty finding words and naming objects), perseveration (unintentional repetition of a word or phrase), conductive aphasia (repeating words or phrases on command), and difficulty with sentence construction

2) Receptive (Wernicke's dysphasia or fluent) (ASA 2013)

a) Occurs with lesions in the posterior, superior temporal dominant lobe (superior temporal gyrus)
b) This area is responsible for reception and interpretation of speech.
c) Able to produce verbal language, but language content is meaningless; able to speak fluently, but words may be incorrect or inappropriate in context; unable to detect his or her own errors
d) Besides being impaired with verbal comprehension, is also impaired in naming, reading, and writing

3) Global dysphasia (ASA, 2013)
a) Occurs with lesions in the frontotemporal dominant lobes; anterior and posterior speech areas are extensively impaired.
b) Exhibits comprehension and speaking problems (produces very little speech, a few words or phrases)
c) Impaired reading, naming, and writing skills
d) May have intact automatic speech only for routines such as counting, singing a song, or stating the days of the week

4) Transcortical dysphasias (transcortical sensory dysphasia, mixed transcortical dysphasia, isolated speech center) (Atlanta Aphasia Association, 2006)
a) Occurs with lesions in anterior and posterior presylvian fissures, typically lesion of the inferior left temporal lobe
b) Have the ability to repeat (echolalia) and recite
c) Speech can be fluent but uses paraphrases
d) Inability to read and write
e) Comprehension is impaired

5) Apraxia of speech (National Institute on Deafness and Other Communication Disorders, 2010)
a) Occurs when there is damage to the motor centers in the cortex that control speech
b) Inability to program the position of the speech muscles and the sequence of the muscle movements that is necessary to produce understandable speech
c) Understanding of speech remains intact.
d) Speech may be clear at times and indecipherable the next.
e) Common for perseveration and inconsistency

6) Dysarthria (American Speech–Language–Hearing Association, 2014)
a) Occurs with damage to a central or peripheral motor nerve, brainstem, or cranial nerve
b) Exhibits poorly articulated speech, resulting from interference in the control and execution of the muscles of speech; muscle control of the palate and tongue may be abnormal.
c) May have abnormal voice quality (too soft or loud); speech is slow, may be slurred and hard to understand.

7) Anarthria (Vega, 2008)
a) Total loss of articulation as a result of loss of control of the muscles of speech; inability to articulate words
b) Occurs with damage to a central or peripheral motor nerve or brainstem

4. Right hemispheric stroke: Common impairments and deficits
a. Left hemiparesis (weakness) or hemiplegia (paralysis)
b. Problems with depth perception and spatial relationships
c. Visual disturbances, including an inability to see the left visual field of each eye (homonymous hemianopsia)
d. Inability to distinguish directional concepts such as up–down, front–back, in–out
e. Difficulty distinguishing foreground from background information (figure–ground, spatial–temporal perception)
f. Decreased ability to distinguish between similar shapes and forms (form constancy, spatial–temporal perception)
g. Anosognosia: Lack of awareness or denial of a neurological deficit, especially paralysis, on one side of the body; reduced insight into the ramifications of the impairment
h. Lack of awareness of others' nonverbal communication (e.g., facial expressions, tone of voice, territorial space, gestures); display a flat affect
i. Unilateral neglect: Inability to integrate sensory and perceptual stimuli from one side of the body or environment
j. Behavioral changes (e.g., impulsivity, egocentricity, quickness to try things, risk taking)
k. Social inappropriateness: Sexual disinhibition and inappropriate self-disclosure

l. Difficulty in finding locations, such as one's room, and understanding maps and objects (geographic–topographic memory)

5. Brainstem strokes
   a. Result from ischemic or hemorrhagic process in the midbrain, pons, or medulla
   b. Potential deficits: Many vital centers and nuclei of cranial nerves exist, so deficits can vary greatly, including dysarthria, dysphagia (chewing or swallowing difficulty), ataxia, tetraparesis or tetraplegia, poor balance or coordination, double or blurred vision, pinpoint pupils, horizontal gaze palsy (e.g., eye moves to the side, away from the cerebral lesion), vertigo with nausea, abnormal respiratory patterns, hyperthermia, coma or persistent vegetative state, locked-in syndrome (tetraplegia and facial paralysis, except for eye or eyelid movement; intact cognition; stroke is in the pons).

H. Children and Stroke (AHA, 2014b; International Alliance for Pediatric Stroke, 2014; NINDS, 2011; NSA, 2014a)

1. Etiology
   a. Childhood stroke may occur before birth but most often between 1 month and 18 years of age.
   b. The incidence of stroke in children younger than 15 years old is about 6 cases in every 100,000 children per year. Stroke and other cerebrovascular disorders are among the top 10 causes of death in children in the United States, with rates highest in the first year of life.
   c. Stroke in children is evenly divided between hemorrhagic and ischemic.
   d. A perinatal stroke encompasses a cerebrovascular event that occurs between the last 18 weeks of gestation through 1 month after birth. This may lead to a greater propensity to develop childhood epilepsy.
   e. A stroke that occurs before birth may be called an in-utero stroke, fetal stroke, or prenatal stroke. Stroke occurs more frequently in the perinatal and prenatal age group than in older children.
   f. Babies who have strokes in the womb or within the first month of life are at risk of cerebral palsy.
   g. Premature babies are at risk for stroke during or shortly after delivery if hypoxia occurs.
   h. On average it takes 48–72 hours for children to get to a hospital after their caregivers recognize the first symptom of stroke (this is related to the widespread belief that strokes do not happen to children).
   i. Children have a greater ability to heal because of the greater plasticity or flexibility of their nervous system and brain. The brain is still developing, so it may be more likely to repair itself (children usually recover function with the help of physical and speech therapy).
2. Causes of childhood stroke
   a. Congenital or acquired heart disease
   b. Birth defects
   c. Infections such as meningitis or encephalitis
   d. Trauma
   e. Blood disorders such as sickle cell disease
3. Childhood stroke symptoms
   a. Severe headache (often the first complaint) and seizures (especially in newborns)
   b. Speech difficulties
   c. Problems with eye movement
   d. Numbness, weakness on one side of the body (loss of balance or trouble walking)
4. Stroke-related disabilities
   a. Speech and communication from brain cell damage
   b. Paralysis or weakness unilaterally from brain cell damage (60%)
   c. Cerebral palsy (unique to children; applies to perinatal stroke)
   d. Mental retardation (unique to children)
   e. Epilepsy (unique to children)
5. Stroke education for children
   a. The National Stroke Association (NSA) developed the Hip Hop Stroke Program in 2004, which is being repackaged for easier delivery to children in grades K–12 (see www.stroke.org/site/PageServer?pagename=hiphopstroke).
      1) The program uses children to educate families about stroke, primarily in urban elementary schools.
      2) The program teaches children to develop lifelong healthy habits to prevent stroke and to recognize symptoms of stroke.
      3) The program teaches children to identify stroke as an emergency and to call 911.
   b. NSA Brainiac Kids is a program that is used to teach friends, family, and community about stroke awareness and prevention (see http://support.stroke.org/site/PageServer?pagename=BrainiacKids).
      1) Activities at schools (e.g., act F.A.S.T. skits and games)

2) Activities in the community (e.g., walk-a-thons [encourage physical movements], bake sales [encourage good nutrition])

II. Primary Prevention of Stroke

Evidence is accumulating for more effective prevention strategies and better recognition of people at highest risk for stroke. Risk factors are classified according to potential for modification (nonmodifiable or uncontrolled [e.g., age, gender, race or ethnicity, family history] and modifiable or controllable[e.g., hypertension, diabetes, tobacco use, alcohol consumption]). Certainly some factors are generally not modifiable but identify people who are at increased risk of stroke and who may benefit from rigorous prevention or treatment of other modifiable risk factors (Kernan et al., 2014).

A. Nonmodifiable or Uncontrollable Risk Factors (ASA, 2014; NINDS, 2009b; NSA, 2009a, 2014e)

1. Age: A stroke can happen at any age, but risk doubles every decade after age 55 years.
2. Gender: A stroke is more common in men, but more women than men die from a stroke.
3. Race and ethnicity: A stroke is more common in African Americans (twice the risk) and Hispanics, Asians, and Pacific Islanders.
4. Family history (hereditary factors)
5. Previous stroke, TIA, or heart attack
6. Fibromuscular dysplasia
7. Hole in the heart: Patent foramen ovale

B. Modifiable, Controllable, or Treatable Medical Risk Factors (ASA, 2014; NINDS, 2009b)

1. Hypertension: BP 140 mmHg systolic/90 mmHg diastolic or higher for an extended period of time; however, BP numbers of 120–139 mmHg systolic or 80–89 mmHg diastolic indicate prehypertension.
2. Heart disease: Includes MI, AF, heart failure, and valvular heart disease
3. Diabetes mellitus: Two to four times more likely to have a stroke with increased blood sugar; should have hemoglobin A1c lower than 6
4. Dyslipidemia: Elevated low-density lipoprotein cholesterol (LDL-C) and elevated serum triglyceride have been associated with ischemic stroke and large-artery atherosclerotic stroke. Statin therapy is recommended to reduce risk of stroke in patients with risk of atherosclerosis and an LDL-C of 100 mg/dL or higher (Mora et al., 2012).
5. Carotid or other artery disease: Carotid artery narrowed by 70% or more by atherosclerotic plaque doubles risk of stroke.
6. TIA: Produces stroke-like symptoms but no lasting damage

C. Lifestyle Modifiable, Controllable Risk Factors (ASA, 2014)

1. May be independent of or contribute to medical risk factors that could cause stroke
2. Tobacco use, smoking, or second- and third-hand smoke: Toxic compounds contribute to atherosclerosis, increasing clustering of platelets and increasing clotting time and viscosity.
3. Physical inactivity and obesity: Increased weight puts strain on the circulatory system and increases the risk of stroke. Stress reduction through lifestyle changes decreases release of stress hormones, which contribute to obesity. Get up and move; 30 minutes per day of moderate to vigorous exercise controls obesity and diabetes, lowers BP, and increases high-density lipoproteins, which also lowers risk of stroke, heart attack, and heart disease.
4. Alcohol abuse: An average of more than one alcoholic drink a day for women or more than two drinks a day for men raises BP and can lead to a stroke.
5. Illegal or street drug use: High risk of stroke is linked to intravenous drug use, as is the use of cocaine.
6. Sleep apnea is present in approximately one half to three quarters of patients with stroke or TIA. Sleep apnea is associated with worse functional outcomes. Despite high prevalence, as many as 70% are not diagnosed or treated. A sleep study should be considered in patients with stroke or TIA symptoms, and emerging evidence advices treatment, which has shown to improve outcomes (Bravata et al., 2011; Kernan et al., 2014; Ryan, Bayley, Green, Murray, & Bradley, 2011).
7. The Stroke Risk Scorecard can be used to rate or score personal risk (www.stroke.org/).
8. Ask a healthcare professional about various treatment options to reduce personal stroke medical or lifestyle modifiable or controllable risk factors.

III. Treatment of Stroke

The goal for the acute management of patients with stroke is to stabilize the patient and to perform a complete initial evaluation and neurological assessment. First the interprofessional team must rapidly determine the patient's type of stroke by obtaining brain imaging. If the patient is an ischemic stroke, the team must determine whether the patient is a candidate for acute treatment with intravenous (IV) thrombolytics and the determination of risks and benefits for this intervention. Depending on the patient's presentation, critical decisions may have to focus on the need for intubation, BP control (which differs with ischemic and hemorrhagic strokes), management of increasing brain edema, and determining the best plan of care for the patient and family. This interprofessional team includes all members, starting from the emergency medical services through the inpatient acute area and including rehabilitation to home. The interprofessional team plays a major role in the coordination of acute care and prevention and complications and the recovery process after the stroke.

A. Early Recognition of Stroke
   1. A stroke is a "brain attack."
   2. Time is brain (i.e., early intervention is critical for preventing the loss of cerebral perfusion).
   3. Community education of emergency medical personnel and the general public is key.
   4. Any person experiencing signs and symptoms of a stroke should seek help immediately in a hospital setting. He or she should activate the emergency medical system (call 911) and preferably be transported to the closest appropriate stroke center.
   5. Consultation with a neurosurgeon or neurologist is preferred.
   6. Participation in stroke performance measures that improve client outcomes and save lives is essential.

B. Diagnostic Tests
   1. Brain noncontrast computed tomography (CT) scan (to rule out hemorrhagic stroke in order to be able to administer anticoagulants and recombinant tissue plasminogen activator [rt-PA]) is considered the first choice of imaging.
   2. Magnetic resonance imaging (MRI) may also be ordered with diffusion-weighted imaging. This is especially useful for detecting small infarcts and is superior to CT for diagnosing ischemic stroke.
   3. Advanced imaging to evaluate whether salvageable brain tissue (also referred to as penumbra) is present. These diagnostic tests include CT perfusion or MR perfusion-weighted imaging. Advanced imaging helps determine whether patient is a candidate for additional endovascular stroke intervention.
   4. Blood tests: Complete blood cell count, electrolytes, liver and renal profiles, clotting studies, lipid panel, and markers of cardiac ischemia.
   5. Imaging to evaluate the large extracranial and intracranial arteries of the head and neck. Noninvasive tests include MR angiogram (MRA) and CT angiogram (CTA). An invasive test called digital subtraction angiography (DSA) is also used to evaluate for vessel occlusions in ischemic stroke or to identify an aneurysm in a patient with SAH or rule out an AVM)
   6. Other tests that may be ordered are electrocardiogram, chest radiograph, echocardiogram, electroencephalogram, lumbar puncture, or carotid studies.

C. Medications: Drug therapy is one of the newest ways to combat the damaging effects of a stroke and lessen a person's chance of a recurrent stroke if other lifestyle factors are maintained.
   1. Thrombolytic therapy for ischemic stroke (Jauch et al., 2013; NINDS, 2009b; The Brain Attack Coalition [BAC], 2002)
      a. rt-PA
         1) Only systemic thrombolytic drug approved by the U.S. Food and Drug Administration (in 1996) for ischemic stroke
         2) Enzyme that targets a thrombus within a blood vessel (Lutsep & Berman, 2013)
         3) Must meet the inclusion criteria (arrival in the emergency department [ED] within 4.5 hours of symptom onset, CT rules out hemorrhage, exam consistent with symptoms of stroke)
         4) In the 3-hour window:
            a) Exclusion criteria include significant head trauma or prior stroke in previous 3 months, platelet count less than 100,000, current use of anticoagulants with international normalized ratio (INR) greater than 1.7 or prothrombin time (PT) more than 15 seconds, use of heparin in past 48 hours, and prolonged partial thromboplastin time, elevated BP (systolic greater than 185 mmHg or diastolic greater than 110 mmHg), blood glucose lower than 50 mg/dL, history of previous intracranial or intraspinal surgery, and active internal bleeding (Jauch et al., 2013).
            b) Relative exclusion criteria include minor or rapidly improving stroke symptoms, pregnancy, major surgery or serious trauma within previous 14 days, recent gastrointestinal or urinary tract hemorrhage (within previous 21 days), and recent acute myocardial infarction (within previous 3 months) (Jauch et al., 2013).
         5) In the 3- to 4.5-hour window additional exclusion criteria include aged greater than 80 years, National Institutes of Health Stroke Scale score higher than 25, taking an oral anticoagulant regardless of INR, and history of both diabetes and prior ischemic stroke (Del Zoppo, Saver, Jauch, & Adams, 2009; Jauch et al., 2013)

6) The client is assessed using the National Institutes of Health Stroke Scale, the most widely accepted tool for neurological assessment of stroke; see **Figure 22-2** and www.strokecenter.org/trials/scales/nihss.html for more information (NINDS, 2009a).
7) The Cincinnati Stroke Scale often is used for initial screening of stroke by emergency medical service staff and bedside clinicians; see www.strokecenter.org/professionals/stroke-diagnosis/stroke-assessment-scales/ for more information (The Internet Stroke Center, 2014c).
8) Intravenous rt-PA, 0.9 mg/kg (maximum of 90 mg) is given as a bolus (10% of dose given over 1 minute) and followed by the remaining 90% of the dose as an infusion over 60 minutes.
9) The client is monitored closely for bleeding complications during and after infusion, which includes neurological assessments and control of BP.

b. Antiplatelet and anticoagulation (Furie et al., 2011)
   1) Antiplatelet and anticoagulant drugs are the most common medications used to reduce risk of a secondary stroke.
   2) Aspirin is currently viewed as the gold standard antiplatelet drug because of its effectiveness and low cost. Other antiplatelet drugs used to treat heart disease and ischemic-type stroke include clopidogrel bisulfate (Plavix) and aspirin/extended release dipyridamole (Aggrenox).
   3) Antithrombotic treatment using unfractionated heparin or low-molecular-weight heparin should be initiated within 48 hours for prevention of deep vein thrombosis (DVT). Early mobilization and the use of intermittent compression devices are strategies to decrease risk of DVTs. The use of an antiplatelet such as aspirin (acetylsalicylic acid) should be used only if the patient has a contraindication to antithrombotic (Jauch et al., 2013).
   4) Patients in whom AF is considered the etiology of their stroke should be started on an anticoagulant. Anticoagulation therapy has proven to prevent first and recurrent strokes. The use of antiplatelet therapy or in combination with anticoagulant has a limited role and has not proven to be effective. Warfarin (Coumadin) is the only drug approved for preventing clots in patients with atrial fibrillation. Low-molecular-weight heparin can be used to bridge patients until they are within their therapeutic range during initiation or interruption of warfarin (Jauch et al., 2013).
   5) Recently two new classes of oral anticoagulants have been approved: direct thrombin inhibitors and factor Xa inhibitors for patients in AF. These medications include dabigatran (Pradaxa), the first direct thrombin inhibitor, and two factor Xa inhibitors, rivaroxaban (Xarelto) and apixiban (Eliquis) (Kernan et al., 2014).
   6) Nonpharmacological treatment can be an alternative approach to preventing stroke in AF. A percutaneous device to occlude the left atrial appendage can be implanted. This approach can be used for AF patients who are at high risk of stroke but who are poor candidates for oral anticoagulation (Kernan et al., 2014).

2. Anticonvulsants are controversial. Incidence of seizure after a stroke is estimated at 10% or greater in ischemic stroke (reported higher in hemorrhagic stroke). Currently no studies have shown a benefit from administering anticonvulsants prophylactically. If a patient has a seizure after the stroke, then the patient would be treated with anticonvulsants based on type of seizure (e.g., may use lorazepam [Ativan] initially and phenytoin [Dilantin] in the longer term) (Jauch et al., 2013).
3. Vasopressors may benefit ischemic stroke patients. Although no clear criteria have been validated on using vasopressors, ischemic stroke patients with a large perfusion deficit who demonstrate neurological deterioration when systemic BP decreases may benefit from vasopressors to maintain cerebral perfusion pressure. Nimodipine (Nimotop), a calcium channel blocker, should be used to reduce the deficit produced by delayed cerebral ischemia related to vasospasm that occurs with an aneurysmal subarachnoid hemorrhage (Connolly et al., 2012; Jauch et al., 2013).
4. Support and comfort may be needed, and analgesics, antipyretics, sedation, and pain medication (for central pain syndrome) may be used (ASA, 2014).
5. Statin drugs may be prescribed to treat and prevent hypercholesterolemia and hyperlipidemia (LDL 100 mg/dL or lower with heart disease).
6. Nutripharmaceuticals such as an omega 3–6–9 fatty acid supplement along with a low-fat diet

Figure 22-2. National Institutes of Health (NIH) Stroke Scale

Category	Description	Score
1a. Level of Consciousness (LOC) Obtain verbal or electronic report from a nurse in the facility or on the unit that sent the client.	Alert Drowsy Stuporous Coma	0 1 2 3
1b. LOC questions Ask the client the month and his or her age. The answer must be exactly right.	Answers both correctly Answers one correctly Both incorrect	0 1 2
1c. LOC Commands Ask the client to open/close eyes and then grip/release nonparetic hand.	Obeys both correctly Obeys one correctly Both incorrect	0 1 2
2. Best Gaze Only horizontal movement tested. Oculocephalic reflex is OK, but no calorics. Eyes open—clilent follows finger or face.	Normal Partial gaze palsy Forced deviation	0 1 2
3. Visual Test by confrontation; introduce visual stimulus to the client's upper- and lower-field quadrants.	No visual loss Partial hemianopsia Complete hemianopsia Bilateral hemianopia	0 1 2 3
4. Facial Palsy Ask the client to show teeth/smile, raise eyebrows, and squeeze eye shut.	Normal Minor Partial Complete	0 1 2 3
5a. Motor Arm Left Extend the left arm, palm down, to 90 degrees if sitting or 45 degrees if supine.	No drift Drift Can't resist gravity No effort against gravity No movement Amputation, joint fusion	0 1 2 3 4 UN
5b. Motor Arm Right Extend the right arm, palm down, to 90 degrees if sitting or 45 degrees if supine.	No drift Drift Can't resist gravity No effort against gravity No movement Amputation, joint fusion	0 1 2 3 4 UN
6a. Motor Leg Left Elevate the left leg to 30 degrees and flex at hip, always supine.	No drift Drift Can't resist gravity No effort against gravity No movement Amputation, joint fusion	0 1 2 3 4 UN
6b. Motor Leg Right Elevate the right leg to 30 degrees and flex at hip, always supine.	No drift Drift Can't resist gravity No effort against gravity No movement Amputation, joint fusion	0 1 2 3 4 UN
7. Limb Ataxia Finger-nose, heel-shin tests done on both sides.	Absent Present in one limb Present in two limbs	0 1 2
8. Sensory Use a pinprick to face, arm, trunk, and leg; compare side to side. Assess the client's awareness of being touched.	Normal Partial loss Severe loss	0 1 2

continued

Figure 22-2. National Institutes of Health (NIH) Stroke Scale (continued)

Category	Description	Score
9. Best Language Ask clients to name items, describe a picture, read a sentence; intubated clients should write responses.	No aphasia Mild-to-moderate aphasia Severe aphasia Mute	0 1 2 3
10. Dysarthria Evaluate speech clarity by asking the client to repeat listed words.	Normal articulation Mild to moderate dysarthria Near to unintelligible Intubated or other barrier	0 1 2 UN
11. Extinction and Inattention Use information from prior testing to identify neglect or double simultaneous stimuli testing.	No neglect Partial neglect Complete neglect	0 1 2

Adapted from NIH Stroke Scale, by National Institute of Neurological Disorders and Stroke (NINDS), 2009a. Retrieved from www.strokecenter.org/trials/scales/nihss.html.

may be prescribed to treat and prevent hypercholesterolemia and hyperlipidemia.

7. Neurostimulant agents may be useful in the pharmacological management of neurobehavioral disorders after a stroke.
8. Neuroprotective agents may be useful in making the brain less susceptible to the damaging effects of a stroke. These agents attempt to save ischemic neurons in the brain from irreversible injury. It was thought the treatment would prevent early ischemic injury or prevent reperfusion injury. Clinical trials are looking at the benefits of such agents (Lutsep & Berman, 2013).
   a. Agents that may help prevent early ischemic injury by preventing excitatory neurotransmitter release and reducing the deleterious effects of ischemia on cells in recent clinical study included NMDA antagonists, magnesium, nalmefene, lubeluzole, clomethiazole, and calcium channel blockers. To date, none of the agents have been shown to be beneficial, and no further trials are planned on these agents (Lutsep & Berman, 2013).
   b. Agents to help prevent reperfusion injury by preventing white blood cells from adhering to vessel walls, limiting formation of free radicals, or promoting neuronal repair and possibly protecting the brain from additional injury were also studied, including enlimomab, Hu23F2G, tetracycline antibiotics, and citicoline. None of these agents were shown to be beneficial in preventing reperfusion injury (Lutsep & Berman, 2013).
   c. Recently the focus has been on regulating neuronal healing after ischemia and promoting brain repair. Fiblast, a basic growth factor, was administered in a phase II safety trial that was terminated because of poor risk:benefit ratios. Clinical trials include use of autologous mesenchymal stem cells and GSK249320, a monoclonal antibody that blocks myelin-associated glycoprotein, a molecule inhibiting axonal growth (Lutsep & Berman, 2013).
9. Endovascular treatment for ischemic stroke has become an option during the past decade. The treatment options include intraarterial fibrinolysis and mechanical clot embolectomy with retrieval catheters. The goal is to achieve reperfusion by vascular recanalization of the large intracranial vessels. These procedures are performed within 6–8 hours of stroke onset by an interventional neuroradiologist on patients who are either ineligible for or refractory to IV rt-PA. In addition, angioplasty and stenting may be performed to increase perfusion to the ischemic tissue (Jauch et al., 2013).

D. Surgery

1. Ruptured aneurysms are repaired using a clip, or the aneurysm is treated from inside the vessel by embolization (a metal coil through the artery in the brain that fills the aneurysm and allows a clot to form and prevent more bleeding) (Connolly et al., 2012).
2. AVMs can be treated the same way using interventional neuroradiologic procedures and a coil to clot off the AVM or instillation of glue during an angiogram (keeps blood from flowing through the AVM).
3. An AVM may still warrant surgical excision.
4. Surgical removal of an intracerebral hematoma is controversial. Early surgery can limit injury from the hematoma compression, but surgery increases risk of ongoing bleeding and involves cutting through uninjured brain tissue. Patients with cerebellar hemorrhage should have surgical removal as soon as possible because of the risk of brainstem compression. Also, patients with lobar clots larger than 30 mL and within 1 cm of the surface

may be considered for a craniotomy (Morgenstern et al., 2010).

E. Intensive Care Management (AHA, 2005)

1. Onset to treatment time is critically associated with improved functional outcomes. The ability to identify and treat such events as hypotension, hypertension, and hypoxia is crucial in the first hours after a stroke. Elevated intracranial pressure (ICP) is managed through monitors and ICP catheters or external ventricular drains.
2. Respiratory support is used to maintain oxygen saturation greater than 94% with the least invasive method to achieve normoxia. Endotracheal intubation with mechanical ventilation should be performed if the airway is threatened or if target oxygenation cannot be maintained. Airway protection is important to decrease the risk of aspiration to reduce the incidence of pneumonia. Hyperventilation for treatment of elevated ICP is no longer recommended (Jauch et al., 2013).
3. Cardiovascular support and management of BP: Labetalol (Trandate) or nicardipine (Cardene) is recommended if BP exceeds recommended target levels. BP management after an acute ischemic stroke that has been treated with IV rt-PA must be maintained below 180/105 mmHg during the first 24 hours. This requires close monitoring:BP should be checked and neurological assessment performed every 15 minutes for the first 2 hours, then every 30 minutes for 6 hours, followed by hourly until 24 hours after IV rt-PA bolus. Elevated BP during the first 24 hours after IV rt-PA treatment increases the risk of hemorrhagic transformation of the ischemic tissue. If a patient has not had thrombolytic treatment, the BP medication should be held until BP is greater than 220/120 mmHg. Elevated BP during the acute phase of an ischemic stroke improves cerebral perfusion. BP management in hemorrhagic strokes has a much lower target systolic BP of less than 160 mmHg because of the risk of increased hemorrhage with elevated BP (Connolly et al., 2012; Jauch et al., 2013; Morgenstern et al., 2010).
4. Nutritional support (enteral or parenteral feeding) is provided, and serum glucose is managed (hyperglycemia may increase neuronal damage, and hypoglycemia may extend infarct).
5. Body temperature (hypothermia may be neuroprotective after ischemia) and fluids are managed (avoid aspiration, sustain cerebral perfusion, avoid cerebral edema or fluid overload). Fever reduction with appropriate cooling measures is an essential component of care of the critically ill client. The goal for stroke patients is to maintain normothermia. Isotonic intravenous fluids such as normal saline or Ringer's lactate are often the intravenous fluids of choice when dehydration and hypotension are present because these may exacerbate an infarction.
6. Early rehabilitation and discharge planning should begin at the time of admission. Early identification of rehabilitation needs and an early start to rehabilitation can decrease healthcare costs by reducing dependence, nursing care, and length of stay, and preventing disability (Miller et al., 2010). Physical, occupational, and speech and language therapy; rehabilitation psychology; therapeutic recreation; and consultation with a physical medicine and rehabilitation physician or advanced practice nurse (APN) have been shown to be beneficial.
7. Many hospitals have designated stroke units or are primary or comprehensive stroke centers that provide clients with the complex interventions they need, including medical, nursing, and therapy professionals working as a team from the beginning toward stroke recovery. Early rehabilitation is the emphasis, and active participation by the client and family is encouraged.

F. Stroke Centers

1. Primary stroke centers (AHA, 2014c; Bader & Palmer, 2006; The Joint Commission, 2008, 2014)
   a. In 2000 a multidisciplinary group (BAC) conducted a literature search with the objectives of improving the level of care and standardization of rapid diagnosis, treatment, and care for stroke survivors.
   b. The BAC focused hospitals on prioritizing care with six connecting elements: identification of stroke and rapid transport to a stroke-receiving hospital by emergency medical personnel; ED prioritization of stroke care with rapid triage, protocols for management, and procedures for rt-PA administration; an organized acute stroke team for rapid response to the ED; written care protocols for the multidisciplinary team to follow using evidence-based literature; a designated stroke unit with highly skilled staff; and neurosurgeons available within 2 hours if neurosurgery is needed.
   c. The BAC-recommended support services include a stroke center medical director; 24-hour, 7-days-a-week neuroimaging and laboratory services; outcome and quality improvement tracking for client outcomes; and educational programs for staff and the community.

d. The goal of a primary stroke center is to provide the personnel and infrastructure to stabilize and treat the majority of clients.
e. Development of primary stroke centers led to further recommendations by the BAC and the American Stroke Association (ASA) to work with the Joint Commission on establishing criteria for certification of primary stroke center programs (Joint Commission, 2014).
f. The ASA and the Joint Commission provide tools and resources to help hospitals become ready for certification (e.g., Acute Stroke Treatment Program toolkit, Get with the Guidelines/Stroke Quality Improvement program) and numerous professional education opportunities (online continuing medical education, International Stroke Conference) (AHA, 2014c; Joint Commission, 2008, 2014).
g. For more information on the JC Primary Stroke Center certification or accreditation programs, visit www.jointcommission.org (AHA, 2014; Joint Commission, 2014).
h. A state-by-state list of stroke centers is available from the NSA website at www.strokecenter.org/trials/centers?utf8=%E2%9C%93&search=64081.

2. Comprehensive stroke centers (AHA, 2014a; Bader & Palmer, 2006; Joint Commission, 2008, 2014)
   a. The BAC met in late 2004 and 2005 and used an evidence-based approach to establish criteria for the development of comprehensive stroke center (CSC) models. Thirteen quality measures were identified.
   b. A CSC has the personnel and infrastructure to care for clients needing high-intensity care with specialized tests or neurointerventional therapies.
   c. A CSC must have neurologists and neurosurgeons capable of taking care of clients with strokes involving larger areas of the brain (acute ischemic strokes and complex hemorrhagic strokes). A CSC must have a medical director, surgeons with expertise performing carotid endarterectomy (CEA), diagnostic radiologists, physicians with expertise in interventional endovascular neuroradiology procedures and techniques, ED personnel and links to emergency medical services (EMS), radiology technologists, nursing staff who are trained in the care of stroke patients, APNs, physicians with expertise in critical care or neurointensive care, echocardiography, carotid ultrasound (U/S), and transcranial Doppler (TCD), physicians and therapists with training in rehabilitation, and case managers and social workers.
   d. A CSC provides more advanced care and serves as a resource for a primary stroke center. The ASA and the Joint Commission developed criteria for certification of CSC programs.
   e. Defined core measure elements are required to be tracked and submitted to maintain primary and comprehensive stroke certification. Several regulatory agencies are certifying stroke centers; these include the Joint Commission, DNV Healthcare, and Healthcare Facilities Accreditation Program (HFAP).
3. The Commission on Accreditation of Rehabilitation Facilities (CARF) offers an additional certification for a stroke specialty program. Standards need to be met that address serving the person with a stroke with services that focus on prevention, minimizing impairment, reducing activity limitations, and maximizing the quality of life of people who have had a stroke (CARF, 2014).

G. Future Treatment for Strokes
1. To date, IV rt-PA is the only pharmacological agent approved by the U.S. Food and Drug Administration for the treatment of acute ischemic stroke. All prior clinical trials using neuroprotective and plasminogen activator agents have not shown efficacy and improved outcomes in the treatment of acute ischemic stroke. Early reperfusion has shown to be a favorable predictor of good outcomes in acute stroke treatment. Therefore, the focus of most current clinical trials is early recanalization through the use of mechanical thrombectomy of the clot. Multimodal treatment with IV rt-PA and endovascular treatment with intraarterial thrombolytic and mechanical endovascular treatment is increasingly being used. Current strategies include imaging-guided selection of patients; looking at the diffusion and perfusion difference to determine whether the patient inside and outside the time window is appropriate for endovascular treatment is under investigation.
2. Therapeutic hypothermia is being used in combination with IV rt-PA for its presumed neuroprotective effect, and ultrasound-enhanced thrombolysis is being tested to attempt faster clot lysis (Hennerici, Kern, & Szabo, 2013).
3. Other strategies, including determining the patient's collateral flow through imaging, determining whether the brain tissue is salvageable, and

using different techniques to augment cerebral collateral perfusion, are under research.
4. Research continues to focus on reperfusion or protecting the dying cerebral tissue to halt or reduce the impact of the stroke on patient disability.

IV. Family and Caregiver Support

Informal, unpaid caregivers—family and friends—play a critical role in recovery for the person with stroke, particularly as time spent in hospitals and rehabilitation facilities continues to decrease and home care commitments increase. Providing long-term care and support for a stroke survivor during rehabilitation and recovery can be an extremely rewarding experience. However, caregivers need to care for themselves, because being thrust into the caregiver role with little or no warning can disrupt work and life, in general, causing high levels of emotional, mental, and physical stress.

A. General Facts

1. A stroke changes life not only for the client but also for the entire family (blood relatives and friends), more than any other type of disability.
2. Strokes are the most common cause of adult disability, costing more than $36 billion, including the cost of healthcare services, medications to treat stroke, and missed days of work (CDC, 2014).
3. Stroke survivors are often left with major disabilities and loss of functional independence.
4. Home-based care can be financially cost effective and preserve the gains already made in rehabilitation.
5. Many stroke survivors are able to remain in the home or community when they have the support of a family member.
6. The reliance on family members as care providers (informal, unpaid caregivers) creates multiple stressors for the family because of their own life circumstances, which may include competing demands of work, child care responsibilities, and their own chronic diseases and decline.
7. Caregivers must meet an enormous challenge in caring for the physical and emotional needs of the stroke survivor without neglecting their own needs.
8. Caregivers must suspend their own feelings of grief, fear, and frustration to take care of the stroke survivor. The caregiver may be grieving the loss of companionship and may feel a lack of support and be at risk for depression (Family Caregiver Alliance [FCA], 2013; NSA, 2009b).

B. Education

1. Informal caregivers need information about stroke, its impact, the expected prognosis, and the rehabilitation process.
2. Caregivers need to understand the physical and psychological needs of the stroke survivor. Psychosocial factors include grief at the loss of function, independence, and employment. Social isolation, decreased self-esteem, relationship or sexual difficulties, and difficulties in managing finances should also be considered as psychosocial factors that a caregiver may need to deal with (Pfeil, Gray, & Lindsay, 2009).
3. Caregivers need assistance improving their own caring and coping skills. Caring for a family member after a stroke is demanding and overwhelming. Caregivers of stroke survivors have a role in providing extensive and comprehensive care, along with their previous role as a family member. The pressure from these new roles might cause the caregiver to experience physical and emotional strain (Lockwood-Koehn, 2014; Visser-Meily et al., 2006).
4. Caregivers need to understand their own role changes that evolve when they become caregivers. They may need to take on roles they are not familiar with, such as shopping, cooking, finances, or home maintenance and repair.
5. Caregivers need to understand the changes that occur in the person with stroke, such as fatigue, frustration, egocentricity, or depression. Poststroke depression is a comorbidity that has a negative effect on overall stroke outcomes (National Institute of Mental Health [NIMH], 2011). Reports on poststroke depression duration of symptoms are contradictory and range from weeks to years (Qamar, 2011).
6. Caregivers need support groups to share ideas, information, and coping, including peer counseling in which they can share methods with others in the same situation. Caring for a family member who survived a stroke has been shown to be strongly associated with depression in the caregiver (FCA, 2012). Physical disability of the stroke survivor (e.g., poor motor function, impaired memory, and behavior changes) increases the burden on the caregiver. As this burden increases, caregivers are more likely to have depression (Deno et al., 2013).
7. Caregivers need to be aware of community services and resources available to them. Informal caregivers rely on the Internet more now than in the past; however, not all caregivers have Internet access, and not all Internet resources are reliable.

C. Considerations by the Interprofessional Team
   1. The age and health of the informal, unpaid caregiver and stroke survivor must be considered. As the average lifespan lengthens and medical care improves, there are more people living beyond the age of 80 years who have a high quality of life. Increases in life expectancy and advances in treatment and management of stroke have contributed to greater number of people surviving stroke or providing care for a family member (Sanossian & Ovbiagele, 2009).
   2. Risk factor profiles differ between the sexes. Recent studies show that men more often have a history of MI or diabetes and are more likely to have a history of hypertension and prestroke dementia (Gall et al., 2010).
   3. The culture of the stroke survivor and caregiver (e.g., role of the "sick" person, role of the informal caregiver) and sharing of information may have an effect on the survivor's stroke recovery and on the survivor's and caregiver's coping mechanisms.
   4. The survivor and caregiver may have limited resources because of job losses.
   5. Safety concerns for caregivers (e.g., handling emergencies such as falls or safety in the bathroom; aspiration related to dysphagia) must be addressed.
   6. Caregiver stress can lead to neglect or abuse of the survivor.
   7. Each year more women than men have a stroke. The average life expectancy for women is greater than for men (AHA, 2013c). Therefore, a spouse may not be available to act as caregiver.

D. Problems Identified by Caregivers (Pierce, Steiner, Govoni, Thompson, & Friedemann, 2007; Pierce, Steiner, Hicks, & Holzaepfel, 2006; Pierce, Thompson, Govoni, & Steiner, 2012)
   1. Losing self or independence (not enough personal time or ability to maintain own role in society); feeling of being controlled by another
   2. Struggling with emotions (anger, frustration, fear, isolation); being bothered by physical tasks and household chores, as well as behavioral problems; worrying about own health and who would care for survivor if they were not able
   3. Balancing duties (e.g., caregiver role versus potentially new roles); taking care of a house and finances
   4. Having a partner with physical or emotional limitations (change in relationship between the stroke survivor and caregiver; role reversal); looking for a normal or usual routine
   5. Running on empty or changes in sleep and rest (increase in duties, worry, and physical exhaustion)
   6. Lacking support (spiritual or emotional support present initially and decline after the acute phase of the stroke); feeling overwhelmed and inadequate

E. Resources for Informal Caregivers and Families
   1. American Stroke Association (888.4.STROKE; http://www.strokeassociation.org) provides information on signs and symptoms of stroke, provides information in English and Spanish about stroke, distributes Stroke Connection magazine, lists stroke-certified hospitals, and is a division of the American Heart Association.
   2. The National Family Caregivers Association (http://www.thefamilycaregiver.org) is a grassroots organization created to educate, support, empower, and advocate for the millions of Americans who care for their ill, aged, or disabled loved ones.
   3. The National Alliance for Caregiving (http://www.caregiving.org) is a nonprofit coalition of national organizations focusing on advancing family caregiving through research, innovation, and advocacy. Alliance members help family caregivers learn about videos, pamphlets, and other information sources that have been reviewed and approved as providing solid information.
   4. The Friends' Health Connection (http://www.friendshealthconnection.org/) connects people with illness or disability and their family caregivers with others experiencing the same challenges, offering a personalized support network and educational and motivational programs.
   5. The Well Spouse Association (http://www.wellspouse.org/) is a national membership organization that gives support to husbands, wives, and partners of the chronically ill and disabled. Well Spouse has a network of support groups and a newsletter.
   6. Disability.gov (https://www.disability.gov/) is a U.S. government website that provides easy access to disability-related information and resources with links to relevant programs and services offered by numerous federal government agencies.
   7. The Centers for Medicare & Medicaid Services (http://www.medicare.gov/campaigns/caregiver/caregiver.html) for caregiving provides resources, stories, and newsletters about taking care of someone on Medicare.
   8. Lotsa Helping Hands (http://www.lotsahelpinghands.com/) is a volunteer coordination service

using a Web calendar that organizes a community of family and friends to help with tasks, meals, rides, and other needs.

V. Nursing Process

Evidence has shown a decrease in stroke death when organized inpatient and postacute stroke care is delivered in the first 4 weeks by an interprofessional healthcare team (Briggs, Felberg, Malkoff, Bratina, & Grotta, 2001; Evans, Harraf, Donaldson, & Kalra, 2002). Despite the positive achievements in stroke treatment during the past 2 decades, there remains an estimated 50 million stroke survivors worldwide. Not only is the stroke survivor affected for the rest of his or her life, but so is the family and other caregivers. This team has a very important but limited time to educate the survivor and family. The team must approach this care transition holistically and provide interactive learning. Information shared with the patient must be comprehensive, providing pathophysiological processes related to stroke and the functional and societal impact of the stroke. The nurse often plays the central role in coordinating care through the continuum of recovery.

A. Assessment by Nurses and the Interprofessional Rehabilitation Team

1. Assessment of a new patient admitted from any facility or unit is the first step (**Figure 22-3**). The Modified Rankin Scale is a commonly used scale for measuring the degree of disability or dependence in activities for stroke patients (**Figure 22-4**). Also used is the National Institutes of Health stroke scale to measure a patient's neurological deficits by asking the patient to answer questions and to perform several physical and mental tests. Administer the items in the order listed on this stroke scale (Figure 22-2). The performance in each category is recorded after each subscale exam. Do not go back and change scores. Follow directions provided for each exam technique. Scores should reflect what the client does, not what the clinician thinks he or she can do. The clinician should record answers while administering the exam and work quickly. Except where indicated, the client should not be coached (e.g., helping with verbal or nonverbal cues, repeating requests to the client to make a special effort). The aphasic patient can be encouraged with urgency in the voice and pantomime but not noxious stimulation.
2. Medical management: Assessed by the registered nurse (RN), physicians (e.g., rehabilitation physiatrist, primary physician, and consulting physicians), and licensed independent practitioner (e.g., advance practice nurses, nurse practitioners, and clinical nurse specialists).

Figure 22-3. Assessment of a New Client with Stroke

- Obtain verbal or electronic report from a nurse in the facility or on the unit that sent the client.
- Make an appropriate room assignment based on deficits (e.g., turn affected side toward the door for stimulation, place close to the nursing station if at high risk for falls).
- When the client arrives, assist with his or her transfer to bed. The nursing assessment begins now as the nurse observes how much the client can do during the transfer.
- Determine whether the client can answer questions and is cognitively aware. This can be determined in a short time with conversation while welcoming him or her to the unit. If the client is unable to provide his or her own history, ask a family member to attend the assessment.
- Assess general data (e.g., allergies, medications, identification band on).
- Obtain a complete medical history and complete a head-to-toe assessment, including neurological checks (e.g., for strength, orientation). During this time, also assess communication and cognition skills.
- Assess bowel and bladder function using information obtained from the report of other nurses, combined with information from the client and family. This assessment may not be complete until the nurse actually toilets the client during the first 24 hours.
- Obtain histories for sleep, nutrition, safety, and sex.
- Assess psychosocial history and educational wants, needs, and preferences for learning style.
- Assess leisure interests, community reentry needs, and discharge planning needs.
- Provide the client and family with verbal and written orientation information about the unit and the staff.
- Communicate pertinent information to team members as soon as possible.
- Provide the client with necessary safety equipment (e.g., bed alarm, wheelchair alarm) as soon as the assessment is complete.
- Follow the assessment pattern of the unit but keep in mind that the client may get tired or frustrated if several team members assess the same things at different times.

Figure 22-4. Modified Rankin Scale

Grade	Description
0	No symptoms at all.
1	No significant disability despite symptoms. Able to carry out all usual duties and activities.
2	Slight disability: Unable to carry out all previous activities but able to look after own affairs without assistance.
3	Moderate disability: Needs some help but able to walk without assistance.
4	Moderately severe disability: Unable to walk without assistance and unable to attend to own bodily needs without assistance.
5	Severe disability: Bedridden, incontinent, and needing constant nursing care and attention.

From "Interobserver agreement for the assessment of handicap in stroke patients.," by J. C. van Swieten, P. J. Koudstaal, M. C. Visser, H. J. Schouten, and J. van Gijn, 1988, *Stroke, 19*(5), 604–607. Copyright 1988 by the American Heart Association. Reprinted with permission. Available at http://en.wikipedia.org/wiki/Modified_Rankin_Scale

a. Client's medical stability is the primary focus in rehabilitation. The client should be medically stable before admission to an inpatient rehabilitation facility (Miller et al., 2010).
b. Assessment of medical needs that can impede rehabilitation progress if left unmanaged (e.g., comorbidities such as hypotension, hypertension, hyperglycemia, oxygen saturation, cardiac irregularities, or other chronic illnesses affecting medical stability)

3. Overall function and progress: Assessed by the RN, MD, registered occupational therapist (OTR), physical therapist (PT), speech–language pathologist (SLP), psychologist (if available)
   a. The Functional Independence Measure™ (FIM™), the primary measure of patient progress and outcomes, which is required by Medicare for the Prospective Payment System (PPS), is highlighted in Chapter 7.
   b. The FIM™ system enables providers and programs to document the severity of patient disability and the results of medical rehabilitation and establishes a common measure for the comparison of rehabilitation outcomes.
   c. More information is available at http://www.udsmr.org/WebModules/FIM/Fim_About.aspx.
4. Communication: Assessment by SLP, RN, and OTR (Lubkin & Larsen, 2013; Mauk, 2014; Miller et al., 2010)
   a. Request a consult with the SLP; do not ignore or dismiss language and speech errors.
   b. Evaluation should include assessment of language, cognition, pragmatics, and speech.
   c. Presence of aphasia; expressive or receptive communication
   d. Other methods of communication (e.g., nodding, pointing, gesturing, using symbols)
   e. Premorbid communication pattern: History from family or significant other and developmental level of client
   f. Vocalization problems from motor inability; tracheostomy
   g. Agnosia, apraxia, dysarthria
   h. Hearing aid or glasses
5. Memory: Assessed by SLP, OTR, RN, and PT (Mauk, 2014; Miller et al., 2010)
   a. Premorbid ability
   b. Short-term memory
   c. Long-term memory
   d. Memory problems involving auditory or visual information
6. Problem-solving ability: Assessed by RN, SLP, OTR, PT (Lubkin & Larsen, 2013; Mauk, 2014; Miller et al., 2010)
   a. Premorbid ability
   b. Ability to make appropriate choices
   c. Ability to find solutions
   d. Presence of planning or organizational skills
7. Sensory and visual perception: Assessed by RN, OTR, PT (Mauk, 2014; Miller et al., 2010)
   a. Premorbid use of hearing aid or glasses
   b. Perceptual responses; acuity of senses (e.g., vision, hearing, touch, taste, smell)
   c. Medications that may change sensation or perception
8. ADLs and self-care: Assessed by RN, OTR (Lubkin & Larsen, 2013; Mauk, 2014; Miller et al., 2010)
   a. Ability to bathe, dress, or toilet self
   b. Premorbid abilities
   c. How much help is needed?
   d. Ability to gather needed equipment, supplies, clothing
   e. Mobility to carry out activities
   f. Adaptive equipment needed (e.g., bath sponge, reacher, shoe horn)
9. Dysphagia and swallowing: Assessed by RN, SLP, OTR (Donovan et al., 2013; Hinchey, Shepherd, Furie, Smith, Wang, & Tonn, 2005; Mauk, 2014; Miller et al., 2010)
   a. Must be assessed before any oral medication or food is given
   b. Ability to feed self; amount of assistance needed
   c. Ability to chew, drink, and swallow without difficulty
   d. Correct diet and consistency ordered
   e. Adequate caloric and fluid intake
   f. Use of correct position for eating, alertness
   g. Presence of drooling and pocketing, not swallowing
   h. Presence of cough and gag reflex
   i. Voice quality (e.g., wet, gurgling, nasal while eating)
   j. Use and fit of dentures
   k. Use of upper extremities (e.g., grip, able to lift utensils, able to cut and prepare food)
   l. Ability to see food (e.g., hemianopsia)
   m. Dysphagia screening: Pass/fail procedure to identify a person who may or may not need a complete dysphagia assessment. RN can do a dysphagia screen, if trained.
   n. Swallowing assessment: Performed by SLP; an evaluation of swallowing function that consists

of an extensive cranial nerve direct examination of swallowing and the effects of compensatory strategies (e.g., chin tuck, thickened liquids)

10. Bowel management: Assessed by RN (Consortium for Spinal Cord Medicine, 1998; Mauk, 2014; Miller et al., 2010)
    a. Neurogenic bowel (uninhibited or reflexive type; sudden, involuntary defecation)
    b. Continence history before stroke; bowel history (e.g., when, how often)
    c. Current pattern of elimination
    d. Assess diet and hydration.
    e. Review current medications.
    f. If necessary, assess sphincter tone.
    g. Cognitive ability: Awareness of need to defecate
    h. Medication use
    i. Bowel sounds, abdominal tenderness or distention, rigidity
    j. Transfer skills, sitting tolerance
    k. Ability to get to bathroom, ability to don and doff clothing
    l. Hygiene needs, assistance needed
    m. Positioning, privacy
11. Bladder management: Assessed by RN (Consortium for Spinal Cord Medicine, 2006; Mauk, 2014; Miller et al., 2010)
    a. Neurogenic bladder: Decreased capacity and involuntary voiding as soon as urge is perceived; usually uninhibited type. Also noted some urinary retention in a small percentage of clients.
    b. Continence history before stroke
    c. Current pattern of elimination
    d. Review of current medications
    e. Premorbid history (e.g., nocturia, stress incontinence)
    f. Recent history (e.g., urgency, frequency, urinary tract infection)
    g. Cognitive ability: Awareness of need to urinate, cognition
    h. Transfer skills, sitting tolerance
    i. Ability to perform toileting and to ambulate or call for assistance or get to the bathroom
    j. Hygiene needs, assistance, privacy
    k. Catheter (e.g., intermittent, indwelling): Indwelling should be avoided if at all possible, and if necessary it should be removed as soon as possible.
    l. Fluid intake
    m. Medication use
    n. Consistent implementation interventions that are evidence based by an interprofessional rehabilitation team can influence bladder management skills in stroke survivors (Cournan, 2012).
12. Mobility: Assessed by RN, PT, OTR (Mauk, 2014; Miller et al., 2010)
    a. Bed mobility: Moving up, down, side to side; bridging; sitting up; amount of assistance needed
    b. Transfers: Bed to chair, wheelchair to toilet, to bath bench or shower chair, to car; amount of assistance and type of lift equipment needed
    c. Wheelchair mobility: Type of wheelchair, ability to self-propel, amount of assistance needed
    d. Gait, sitting, standing; need for devices (e.g., walker, cane, crutches)
    e. Endurance, strength, balance, tone, and proprioception
    f. Environment (e.g., lighting, open space)
13. Sexual functioning: Assessed by RN, physician, licensed independent practitioner, psychologist (Lubkin & Larsen, 2013; Mauk, 2014; Miller et al., 2010)
    a. Premorbid sexual history (e.g., preferences, frequency, initiation [partner or self])
    b. Sensory deficits
    c. Mobility
    d. Ability to communicate; visual or perceptual deficits
    e. Emotional status, fear
    f. Fatigue
    g. Knowledge
    h. Positioning
    i. Libido
    j. Need for birth control
    k. Bowel and bladder management before sex
14. Skin integrity: Assessed by RN, PT, OTR, skin care nursing consultant (if available) (Mauk, 2014; Miller et al., 2010)
    a. Immobility
    b. Loss of sensation
    c. Incontinence and hygiene
    d. Presence of pressure, friction, shearing
    e. Presence of any pressure ulcers or skin breakdown
    f. Poor circulation
    g. Risk of skin breakdown: Use of skin assessment scales such as Norton, Braden, or Risk Assessment Pressure Sore
    h. Hydration and nutrition: Nutrition consults

15. Equipment: Assessed by OTR, PT, RN, social worker (SW), discharge planner, case manager (Miller et al., 2010)
    a. Need for assistance with mobility
    b. Need for assistance with ADLs
    c. Financial resources available
16. Psychosocial needs: Assessed by RN, SW, psychologist (Lubkin & Larsen, 2013; Mauk, 2014)
    a. Role changes
    b. Relationships with family members
    c. Family and community support
    d. Coping skills and stressors
    e. Problems with self-image
    f. Depression
17. Leisure: Assessed by RN and certified therapeutic recreation specialist (Mauk, 2014)
    a. Premorbid leisure history
    b. Current physical ability and endurance related to leisure interest
    c. Cognitive status
18. Education: Assessed by each rehabilitation team member (Lubkin & Larsen, 2013; Mauk, 2014)
    a. Cognitive status, intellectual capacity
    b. Attention span
    c. Premorbid learning needs (e.g., visual, auditory, kinesthetic, combination)
    d. Level of formal education
    e. Ability to read or write
    f. Language and cultural barriers
    g. Motivation and readiness to learn
    h. Environmental barriers
    i. Knowledge of disability and self-care needs
    j. Support and presence of caregivers
19. Safety: Assessed by each rehabilitation team member (Lubkin & Larsen, 2013; Mauk, 2014)
    a. Cognition and awareness
    b. Risk for and history of falls
    c. Environment (e.g., hospital, home)
    d. Medication that changes level of consciousness
    e. Sensory impairments
20. Comfort and pain level: Assessed by RN (Lubkin & Larsen, 2013; Mauk, 2014; Miller et al., 2010)
    a. Subluxation and shoulder pain: Subluxation (loss of normal muscle tone in supraspinatus and deltoid muscles) is painless; however, manipulation and improper positioning of a subluxed shoulder cause pain. Prevent through support of affected shoulder, proper positioning, and range of motion exercise.
    b. Shoulder–hand syndrome
    c. Pain and its location and frequency; use a different pain scale for nonverbal aphasic clients (e.g., Wong–Baker FACES Pain-Rating scale available at www.partnersagainstpain.com/printouts/A7012AS6.pdf).
    d. Pain related to activity or randomly occurring location and description of pain
    e. What relieves pain or makes it worse
    f. Effectiveness of pain medicine
    g. Alternatives to medication: Repositioning, visual imagery, music
    h. Changes in sleep pattern; may have reversal of sleep–wake cycle
    i. Sleep history (e.g., normal bedtime, need for white noise, lights)
    j. Sleep problems: Onset, frequent awakenings, nocturia
    k. Environmental (e.g., hot, cold, comfortable bed)
21. Spiritual: Assessed by RN, SW, and chaplain (Lubkin & Larsen, 2013; Mauk, 2014)
    a. Sources of hope and strength
    b. Religious practices
    c. Scheduled time for privacy
22. Discharge planning: Assessed by discharge planner, SW, and case manager in conjunction with rehabilitation team (Lubkin & Larsen, 2013; Mauk, 2014; Miller et al., 2010)
    a. Physical deficits and need for adaptive equipment
    b. Caregiver knowledge and support
    c. Financial resources available
    d. Need for community resources
    e. Adaptations needed for home environment with rehabilitation team input
23. Nutrition: assessed by dietitian in conjunction with SLP (Paquereau et al., 2014; Miller et al., 2010)
    a. Risk of malnutrition and weight loss affects 35%–50% and is an indicator of poor outcome
    b. At risk for not eating because of changes in level of consciousness, dysphagia, depression, sensory or perceptual deficits
    c. Diet modifications must be individualized according to the type and extent of these impairments.

B. Nursing Diagnoses (**Table 22-2**)
1. Impaired physical mobility
2. Self-care deficits (specify level)
3. Sensory–perceptual alteration
4. Impaired verbal communication or communication barrier
5. Altered elimination (bowel and bladder)
6. High risk of aspiration or impaired swallowing
7. Potential for injury or risk for falls

Table 22-2. Nursing Diagnoses, Desired Outcomes, and Interventions in the Care of the Client with Stroke

Nursing Diagnosis	Nursing Outcomes Classification (NOC)	Nursing Interventions Classification (NIC)
Transfer ability, impaired	0202 Balance; body positioning, self-initiated; 0208 Mobility	0200 Exercise promotion; 6490 Fall prevention; 0840 Positioning
Self-care deficit	0300 Self-care (ADL)	1801 Self-care assistance (SCA): bathing/hygiene; 1802 SCA: Dressing/grooming; 1803 SCA: Feeding; 1804 SCA: Toileting; 1806 SCA: Transfers
Communication, impaired	0902 Communication	4976 Communication enhancement, speech deficit
Knowledge deficit	1803 Knowledge of disease process	5602 Teaching: Disease process
Swallowing, impaired	1010 Swallowing status	1056 Enteral tube feeding; 1860 Swallowing therapy; 1710 Oral health maintenance
Urinary incontinence Urinary retention	0502 Urinary incontinence	0560 Pelvic muscle exercise; 0640 Prompted voiding; 0610 Urinary incontinence care; 0620 Urinary retention care
Caregiver role strain	2202 Caregiver homecare readiness; 2205 Caregiver performance: direct care; 2203 Caregiver lifestyle disruption	7040 Caregiver support; 5430 Support group

8. Impaired home maintenance management and discharge planning
9. Impaired thought processes
10. Disturbance in body image
11. Altered sexuality pattern
12. Caregiver distress
13. Ineffective coping
14. Ineffective family coping
15. Spiritual distress
16. Alteration in skin integrity
17. Knowledge deficit
18. Alteration in comfort with or without pain
19. Altered sleep patterns
20. Risk for impaired nutrition
21. Activity intolerance, fatigue

C. Planning and Client Goals: Nursing Outcomes Classification (NOC) (University of Iowa, n.d.b) (Table 22-2)
1. Demonstrate maximal independence in mobility.
2. Perform ADLs at the optimal level of independence with or without the use of assistive devices.
3. Be free from falls or injury.
4. Identify diversional therapy and recreational activities to decrease stress (by caregivers).
5. Verbalize level of satisfaction with sexuality.
6. Identify negative feelings related to self-image.
7. Verbalize understanding of the diagnosis and treatment of stroke or CVA.

D. Interventions: Nursing Interventions Classification (NIC) (University of Iowa, n.d.a) (Table 22-2)
1. Medical management
   a. Monitor vital signs and baseline and ongoing neurological assessment (more frequently during early rehabilitation); medication for hypertension as needed; intravenous fluids for hypotension (if the patient is hypotensive, hemoconcentration can occur and cerebral perfusion decreases, potentially worsening the infarct and manifesting as change in client's neurological status).
   b. Monitor blood glucose and regulate with insulin as needed.
   c. Use intravenous solutions of normal saline.
   d. Provide oxygen as ordered and titrate to 94% or more.
   e. Use telemetry monitoring or electrocardiogram for cardiac abnormalities.
   f. Check lung sounds and risk of aspiration; perform dysphagia screening on all newly admitted patients; reevaluate if patient has change in neurological status or has signs of aspiration.
   g. Check for fever (e.g., for possible urinary tract infection, pneumonia).
   h. Check lab values (e.g., activated partial thromboplastin time, hemoglobin and hematocrit, electrolytes).
   i. Measure legs daily for swelling; assess for DVT, implement DVT prophylaxis measures.
2. Communication: "Language is the most human of mental skills" (Mace & Rabins, 1981, p. 29). Without language, the person with a stroke is lonely, depends on others, and loses self-confidence.
   a. Determine communication method: All disciplines should use consistent methods.
   b. Ensure that hearing aids and glasses are available if needed.
   c. Use symbols and communication boards.
   d. Provide a supportive environment; be patient and calm.
   e. Include the family when possible.
   f. Use music therapy: The person may be unable to speak but able to sing.

g. Use pet therapy; it provides mental stimulation, outward focus, and psychological well-being and helps with physical mobility.
h. Speak slowly and distinctly; use short, simple sentences; maintain eye contact.
i. Establish yes/no reliability.
j. Try cueing; prompt if the direction of verbalization is understood.
k. Provide opportunities for success; offer praise.

3. Memory
   a. Use memory books.
   b. Use cueing and repetition.
   c. Use memory games and allow the patient to reminisce.
   d. Work from simple to complex concepts and promote success.
   e. Present material in different ways (e.g., written, verbal, pictures, demonstration).
4. Problem-solving ability
   a. Allow the client to make choices, beginning with safe and simple options.
   b. Help with planning.
   c. Organize and prioritize information.
   d. Break problems into steps and cue the client through the steps.
5. Sensory and visual perception
   a. Provide adaptive equipment (e.g., glasses, hearing aids).
   b. Ensure appropriate lighting and color contrast.
   c. Make large-print books and materials available.
   d. Place items to allow for visual cuts (homonymous hemianopsia) and teach the client to visually scan the environment.
   e. Reduce environmental noise (e.g., radio, television).
   f. Adapt the environment to accommodate hearing loss (e.g., flashing light for phone).
   g. Use aromatherapy.
   h. Provide various textures and temperatures.
   i. Ensure safety (e.g., hot or cold, especially with decreased sensation).
   j. Serve foods of various colors, tastes, and smells.
   k. Review medications (e.g., sedatives).
   l. Set up the room to stimulate the neglected side.
   m. Eliminate spatial difficulties (e.g., place colored food on a white plate).
6. ADLs and self-care
   a. Ensure privacy and a safe environment (e.g., grab bars, tub bench).
   b. Establish a bathing and toileting routine and provide adaptive equipment for bathing, dressing, and toileting.
   c. Involve caregivers in ADL training.
   d. Incorporate crossover neurodevelopmental techniques (NDTs; e.g., the client's uninvolved side helps the involved side during activity).
   e. Provide an ongoing comprehensive history and assessment for ADL training and for determining the client's home care assistance needs (documentation of this may be required by the client's insurance company).
   f. Adapt the home environment for a wheelchair, equipment, and accessibility.
   g. Allow the client to choose his or her clothing; encourage use of clothing that is loose or easy to put on.
   h. Allow time for activity and rest between self-care activities and promote energy-saving techniques, beginning in bed and progressing throughout the day.
   i. Dress the client's affected side first.
7. Dysphagia and swallowing
   a. Evaluate swallowing (via bedside or radiology) as identified by a video fluoroscopic swallow study.
   b. Position the client upright for feeding and administering medication.
   c. Ensure the correct level of dysphagia diet and consistency (e.g., thicken if needed); ensure that dentures fit properly; obtain a dental consult.
   d. Observe during meals for pocketing, drooling, and swallowing.
   e. Provide adaptive equipment (e.g., divided plate, cutout cup).
   f. Crush medications into applesauce; turn the client's head to the affected side if he or she has difficulty swallowing medications.
   g. Monitor weight changes and lab values.
   h. Consult with a dietitian about the client's food preferences.
   i. Monitor hydration: Clients on oral dysphagia diets need adequate fluids to avoid dehydration.
   j. Use supplemental tube feedings: Check for residual and placement of the tube and position the client upright for feedings.
   k. Use supplemental parental nutrition: Maintain the tube site and monitor labs. Evidence-based literature suggests that the Frazier water protocol helps prevent dehydration.
8. Bowel management

a. Verify the client's premorbid bowel evacuation routine and adapt a bowel program to accommodate the previous routine.
b. Increase fluid intake, bulk, and fiber; monitor intake and output.
c. Monitor bowel sounds and abdominal distention; avoid gas-forming foods.
d. Position the client upright; use a toilet or commode rather than a bedpan; allow time for complete evacuation.
e. Provide appropriate medications (e.g., stool softeners, enemas, and suppositories; laxatives and enemas should be used sparingly).
f. Encourage the client to wear loose clothing and use good hygiene after each stool.

9. Bladder management
   a. Determine continence history and provide adequate lighting if the client has a history of nocturia.
   b. Set up a bladder program to decrease or prevent incontinence.
   c. Assess medications that contribute to incontinence (e.g., diuretics, sedatives, anticholinergics, antihypertensives).
   d. Provide adequate hydration (i.e., fluid intake of 2,000–3,000 mL per day if tolerated or if not contraindicated because of comorbidity) and monitor intake and output.
   e. Use a bladder scan and catheterize for postvoid residuals greater than 150 mL generally or greater than 300 mL if the client is unable to void.
   f. Provide time, privacy, and adaptive equipment for hygiene.
   g. Provide medication to facilitate bladder tone and emptying.
10. Mobility
   a. Work with the client on bed mobility, bridging, bracing lower extremities, sitting up, moving up and down, and increasing endurance.
   b. Use general concepts of neurodevelopmental treatment (e.g., normalizing muscle tone, integration versus compensation, meaningful activities versus simulated activities) to help with proprioception.
   c. Consider use of NDTs for transfers.
   d. Use general concepts of neurointegrative functional rehabilitation and habilitation (Neuro-IFRAH Organization, 2005).
   e. Provide a safe environment for mobility practice (space and lighting).
   f. Encourage the client to wear sturdy shoes to prevent foot drop.
   g. Ensure safety when the client attempts to sit or stand. According to clinical experience, more than one third of falls in clients who have had a stroke occur during rising or sitting down.
   h. Use adaptive equipment as necessary, including lifts if needed.
   i. Moving safely is very important; 40% of all stroke survivors suffer serious falls after their stroke. Stroke survivors are prone to spasticity, which can interfere with walking. Treatment of spasticity may include learning to stretch, medications, injections, or surgery. A home safety check should be done by a member of the rehabilitation team to make modifications to help the client regain independence but avoid falling and injuring self (NSA, 2011).
11. Sexual functioning
   a. Encourage the use of times of day when the client is most rested.
   b. Provide education and support to the client's significant other.
   c. Teach positioning (e.g., supine or on affected side, use pillows for support).
   d. Discuss fear of another stroke.
   e. Instruct the client's partner on the emotional lability of the client.
   f. Encourage tactile stimulation to enhance communication, especially if the client is aphasic.
   g. Discuss birth control methods.
   h. Encourage the client to evacuate the bowel and bladder before sex.
12. Skin integrity
   a. Inspect skin regularly for friction, shearing, and pressure.
   b. Teach weight-shifting techniques.
   c. Use pressure-relieving devices.
   d. Keep the client clean and dry.
   e. Consult with a dietitian for nutritional needs to promote healing.
   f. If the client has sensory loss, guard against contact with extreme hot and cold temperatures (e.g., bath water).
   g. Assess for medications that may alter level of consciousness, sensation, or awareness.
13. Equipment
   a. Provide adaptive equipment as needed; attempt to increase the client's functional ability without equipment if possible.
   b. Verify insurance payment for durable medical equipment (usually done by the SW or case manager).
   c. Reinforce the use of equipment that therapists have obtained.

14. Psychosocial needs
    a. Provide time for verbalization and counseling for the client and family with a psychologist.
    b. Facilitate team and family conferences as needed.
    c. Provide socialization opportunities (e.g., eating meals in the dining room, group therapy, stroke support groups).
    d. Role changes occur and should be discussed with the client and family.
    e. Allow the client and family to grieve their losses (e.g., function, role, relationships).
    f. Reduce stress when possible and allow the client and family to have as much control over care as possible.
15. Leisure
    a. Incorporate the client's leisure interests into therapy (e.g., card games).
    b. Promote community reentry using adaptive equipment (e.g., outing to a wheelchair-accessible fishing dock using a mounted fishing rod holder).
    c. Use memory games to work on cognition in group therapy.
    d. Use NDTs during games (e.g., incorporate the hemiplegic side using the strong side hand over hand to hit a balloon or reach for cards).
    e. Try to adapt the client's leisure interests that use equipment (e.g., fasten an embroidery hoop to a wheelchair).
    f. Encourage pet therapy.
16. Education
    a. Determine readiness and motivation to learn.
    b. Provide information at the client's ability and intellectual level.
    c. Use a variety of teaching methods.
    d. Use an interpreter if language barriers exist.
    e. Plan family teaching sessions.
    f. Reduce distraction and noise when teaching.
    g. Make use of the time when the client is most alert, attentive, and rested.
    h. Test cognition and use return demonstration or verbalization.
    i. Check awareness of current status and build the knowledge base.
17. Safety
    a. Ensure the environment is free of hazards.
    b. Use bed alarms, electronic wristband monitors, and vest restraints as necessary. Use alternative measures whenever possible to decrease use of restraints (e.g., locate the client close to the nursing station, have a family member stay overnight, do hourly rounds, establish a timed voiding program).
    c. Assess medications that may alter awareness.
    d. Evaluate the client's home (e.g., handrails, throw rugs, wheelchair ramp) with assistance from an OTR, case manager, or SW and family or caregivers.
    e. Ensure kitchen and bathroom safety for clients with sensory impairments (e.g., stove, hot and cold water) with assistance from an OTR, case manager, or SW and family or caregivers.
    f. Teach postmorbid impulse control and fall-prevention techniques.
18. Comfort and pain level
    a. Position the client comfortably, be aware of shoulder pain (subluxation possible), and position in bed so the client's shoulder is protracted (**Figure 22-5**).
    b. Do not use the client's arms or shoulders to move the client up in bed. This can cause shoulder injury (torn rotator cuff).
    c. Assess the intensity and location of pain and medicate as appropriate.
    d. Watch for shoulder–hand syndrome: Reduce edema; maintain range of motion of metacarpal phalangeal, proximal interphalangeal, and distal interphalangeal joints; maintain wrist in slight extension; encourage movement of the involved shoulder; and maintain correct bed positioning.
    e. Allow rest periods throughout the day, but decrease frequency if the client cannot sleep at night.
    f. Provide night lighting and white noise if needed.
    g. Monitor the room with cameras if the client is impulsive at night.
19. Spiritual
    a. Notify the chaplain if requested.
    b. Make spiritual readings available (e.g., scriptures, daily devotions).
    c. Arrange for the client to attend chapel services if requested.
    d. Schedule time for meditation and prayer.
20. Discharge planning (in conjunction with case manager or SW)
    a. Discharge planning starts at the time of admission.
    b. Discuss discharge goals and education with the client and family or caregiver at conferences.
    c. Set up follow-up appointments.
    d. Arrange home healthcare, outpatient therapy, or long-term care placement.

Figure 22-5. Bed Positioning

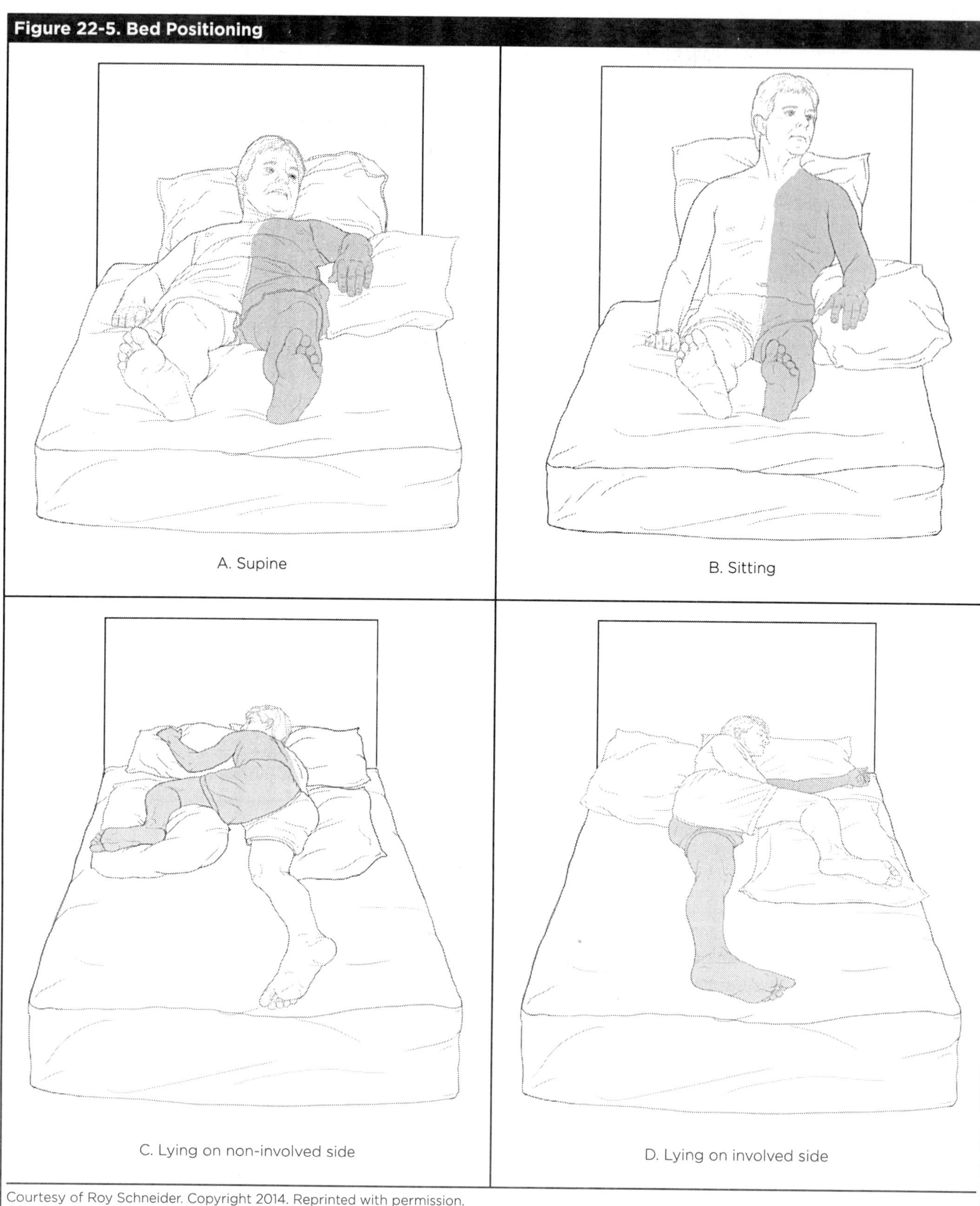

e. Obtain durable medical equipment.
f. Arrange for prescriptions.
g. Provide discharge instructions and explain medications (e.g., side effects, administration).
h. Assist with financial and community resource information.

21. Nutrition
    a. Assess nutrition and hydration, including monitoring intake, urinary and fecal outputs, caloric counts, level of serum protein, electrolytes, blood counts, and body mass index.
    b. Obtain diet history before stroke and work with family to educate client and caregiver on menu choices (e.g., work with them to bring in food patient likes).
    c. Plan nutrition needs based on functional and safety issues, hydration, and nutritional status.
    d. Provide dietary advice if client has elevated lipids, diabetes, or other needs to reduce risk of secondary strokes.
    e. Individual strategies and devices may be needed to improve ability to eat. (e.g., divide feedings into small amounts and give frequently, promote pleasant and relaxing environment; including socialization during meals).

E. Evaluation and Expected Outcomes
   1. Evaluate the client's optimal level of functioning.
   2. Individualize each client's outcomes based on goals related to nursing diagnoses.

F. Posthospitalization Follow-Up
   1. Education about stroke prevention is essential because stroke can be a recurring disorder.
   2. Stroke survivors may go through a predictable recovery process. If so, nursing interventions may be targeted to the client's unique needs throughout the rehabilitation process and after discharge to the home setting (Mauk, 2006; NINDS, 2014a).
   3. Stroke recovery may be facilitated by several controllable and uncontrollable factors such as age, life experience, knowledge of the cause of stroke, expectations, social support, and faith (Mauk, 2006, 2014) **(Figure 22-6)**.
   4. Rehabilitation nurses can gain insight into the concerns and challenges facing stroke survivors who have returned to the community by assessing their learning needs and making referrals for follow-up care.
   5. Many people who have had a stroke experience depression, lack of concentration, anxiety, fatigue that continues even years after stroke, and memory loss (Easton, 2001). Depression can be caused by brain biochemical changes or a normal psychological reaction to the losses related to the stroke. Depression may cause the client to not progress in rehabilitation and may affect thinking skills or concentration. Client and family must be informed of increased risk of depression and seek help from physician (consult a psychologist or psychiatrist, seek out a stroke support group; medication may be needed) (AHA, 2013a). Several depression scales can be used to screen for depression. For an example, see http://www.strokecenter.org/professionals/stroke-diagnosis/stroke-assessment-scales-overview/.

Figure 22-6. The Mauk Model for Poststroke Recovery

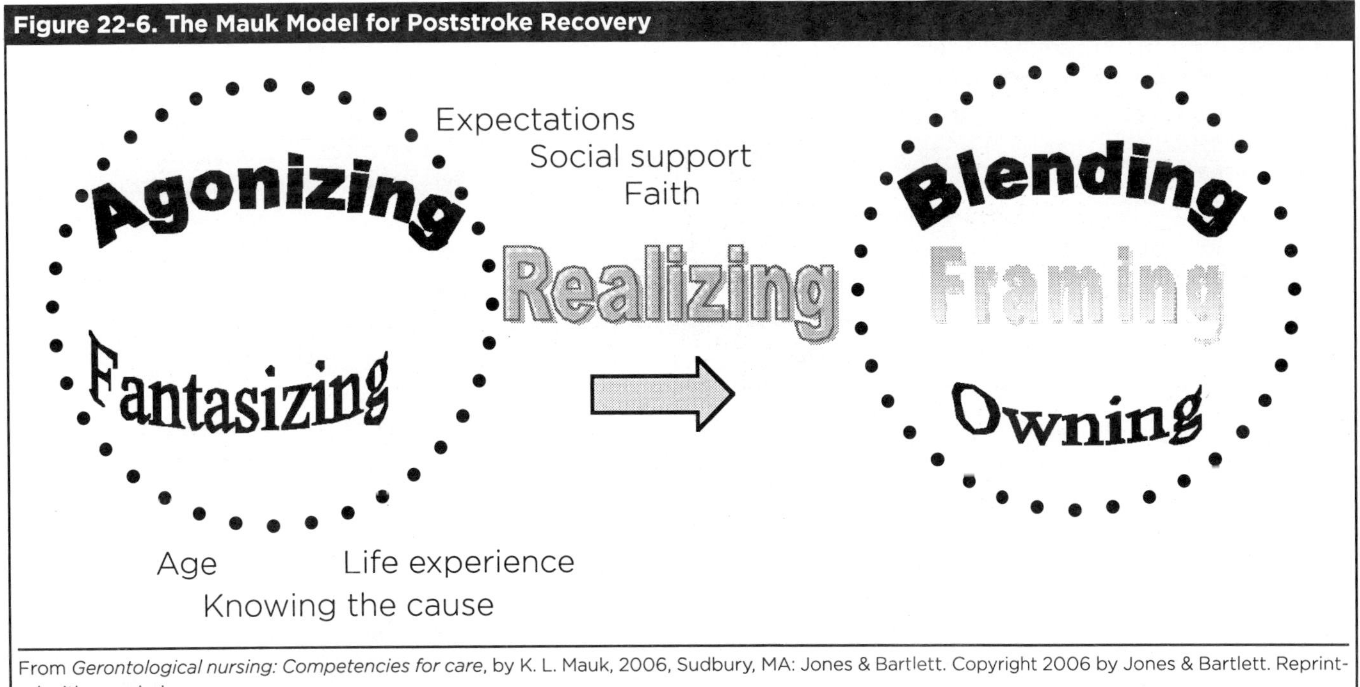

From *Gerontological nursing: Competencies for care*, by K. L. Mauk, 2006, Sudbury, MA: Jones & Bartlett. Copyright 2006 by Jones & Bartlett. Reprinted with permission.

6. Quality of life is also affected by stroke (Secrest, 2002).
7. It is important to refer the client and family for counseling if needed.

G. Managing Stroke Care Transitions (Canadian Stroke Network, 2010)
1. Management of transitions between care environments
2. Assessment of patient, family, and caregiver needs
3. Support for patients, families, and caregivers (written discharge instructions, access to contact person, access to social services, referrals to community agencies)
4. Patient and caregiver education about stroke at all stages across the continuum of stroke care (prevention, acute care, rehabilitation, community reintegration)
5. Interprofessional communication during transitions
6. Discharge planning
7. Early supported discharge
8. Community reintegration

H. Palliative Care (Holloway et al., 2014)
1. Stroke is serious and can be life-threatening, forcing the family to make complex decisions.
2. The family is faced with deciding what treatments should be initiated during this time.
3. A primary palliative care team should be available to patients and family after the stroke and throughout the continuum of care.
4. The interprofessional team must practice patient- and family-centered care, provide the family with estimated prognosis as effectively as possible, assist in determining appropriate care decisions, assist with care coordination and consult a palliative care specialist or the hospice team, and allow the family time and provide bereavement resources.

I. Future Reimbursement
1. In this time of chronic disease management, rehabilitation plays an important role in the clinical management of stroke.
2. According to the AHA (2009), the estimated direct and indirect cost of stroke for 2009 was nearly $73.1 billion. The total projected cost of stroke using 2012 dollars is $95 billion in 2015 and $185 billion in 2030 (AHA, 2013b).
3. Reimbursement changes affect the length of stay in rehabilitation units.
4. Rehabilitation nurses will be challenged to meet clients' needs more rapidly and with fewer resources available.

VI. Advanced Practice (ARN, 2004, 2014b)

Advanced practice registered nurses (APRNs) are often primary care providers and play a pivotal role in the future of healthcare. They are professional registered nurses educated at the master's or post-master's level and in a specific role and patient population. Some APRNs hold a doctor of nursing practice degree. APRNs are prepared by education and certification to assess, diagnose, and manage patient problems, order tests, and prescribe medications. Rehabilitation APRNs may function in a variety of roles, including nurse practitioners, clinical nurse specialists, case managers, administrators, educators, researchers, staff nurses, and consultants, and can play a significant role in the care of stroke survivors and their families. Whether as direct care providers, educators, consultants, researchers, theorists, or leaders, APRNs should be at the forefront in improving the quality of life for stroke survivors and their informal or unpaid caregivers.

A. Clinician: The APRN possesses advanced assessment skills. APRNs should be knowledgeable about current best practices for the care of stroke survivors. Specifically, the APRN specializing in stroke could reasonably be expected to have mastered knowledge related to the content of this chapter but with greater depth and expertise.
1. Practice settings may include:
   a. Emergency department (ED)
   b. Acute care hospital
   c. Acute rehabilitation
   d. Transitional care
   e. Skilled care
   f. Long-term care facility
      1) Intermediate or skilled care
      2) Independent living
      3) Assisted living
   g. Home care
   h. Community (living in a home or residential setting after stroke)
   i. Private practice
2. Additional skills as a direct care provider (clinical nurse specialist or nurse practitioner) may include:
   a. Comprehensive physical exam
   b. Thorough history
   c. Screening for dysphagia, risk for skin breakdown, DVT risk
   d. Identification of risk factors for stroke
   e. Assessment of stroke severity using standardized scales
   f. Assessment of cranial nerve function
   g. Clinical management of acute stroke
   h. Knowledge of stroke rehabilitation principles and concepts

i. Appropriate referrals to stroke service and initiation of rehabilitation
j. Outpatient follow-up visits with survivor and family
k. Coordination of stroke support groups
l. Staff, client, and family education about treatment plan and discharge plans, including ordering of appropriate adaptive equipment
m. Care management or coordination
n. Home care supervision
o. Management of potential common complications
  1) Skin breakdown
  2) Dysphagia
  3) DVT
  4) Aphasia
  5) Ongoing functional limitations including gait disorders, hemiplegia
  6) Depression and anxiety
  7) Sleep disorders
  8) Shoulder subluxation
  9) Altered nutrition or dehydration
p. Prescribing and managing medications

B. Educator: The APRN as educator focuses on identifying areas of need; providing essential knowledge of stroke prevention, treatment, and rehabilitation to the target audience; and fostering a positive learning environment.
  1. Educates various populations in all levels of stroke prevention
    a. Nursing staff
    b. Clients and families
    c. Interdisciplinary team members
    d. Communities
    e. Students
  2. Educates in various settings
    a. Hospitals
    b. Acute rehabilitation units
    c. Transitional care
    d. Long-term care facilities
    e. Academia: Universities and colleges of nursing
    f. Communities
  3. Uses evidence-based practice to develop teaching strategies in areas of need to improve the quality of care
    a. Promotes use of evidence-based practice in the clinical setting
    b. Reviews literature for current evidence-based practice
    c. Develops interventions
    d. Educates staff regarding best practice
    e. Implements best practice
    f. Nursing follow-up after patient discharge shows positive results.

C. Leader: The APRN as leader may also be active in organizations at the local, regional, state, national, and international levels. The APRN may also demonstrate leadership through civic and professional involvement, presentations at conferences, publications, consulting work, and research programs.
  1. Tasks as leader
    a. Advocate for social reform.
    b. Act as a change agent by holding office in professional organizations.
    c. Assist with the development of clinical practice and policy guidelines.
    d. Participate on committees in professional organizations and interdisciplinary national organizations of interest.
    e. Hold positions of influence or lobby in appropriate political arenas to support the rights of those with disabilities.
    f. Write grants for funding of stroke research.
    g. Become a fellow in a national organization such as the American Heart Association (AHA) or American Stroke Association (ASA).
  2. Organizations for involvement
    a. AHA and ASA
    b. National Stroke Association (NSA)
    c. Association of Rehabilitation Nurses (ARN)
    d. American Geriatrics Society (AGS)
    e. American Association of Neuroscience Nurses (AANN)

D. Consultant: As a consultant, the APRN may engage in a variety of activities. The role of consultant is continually redefined as professional nurses increase their expertise in areas related to rehabilitation. These areas may include the following:
  1. Legal consulting
    a. Expert opinion
    b. Expert testimony, written and in court
    c. Clinical expert in law practice
    d. For attorneys, insurance companies, private clients, companies
  2. Educational consulting
    a. For academic institutions, on site
    b. For private clients needing one-on-one teaching
    c. For rehabilitation units providing educational seminars related to stroke
    d. For rehabilitation facilities or private companies that provide outreach in different parts of the country
  3. Clinical consulting
    a. Expert clinician on research team

b. Expert consultant for grant applications and funding
c. Expert on complex cases (in a variety of settings)
d. Share expertise with other team members
e. Author or reviewer of publications (books, articles, case studies) or grants

4. Guardianship: Generally court appointed; often complex cases that do not have appropriate family involvement or that require involvement of a healthcare expert
5. Advocacy: Care planning and mediation for those in care settings; interacting with the interdisciplinary team to ensure quality of care and continuity
6. Life care planning (Mauk, 2012)
   a. "A Life Care Plan is a dynamic document based upon published standards of practice, comprehensive assessment, data analysis and research, which provides an organized, concise plan for current and future needs with associated costs, for individuals who have experienced catastrophic injury or have chronic health care needs" (Weed & Berens, 2010, p. 3).
   b. Advanced practice status is not needed, but APRNs generally have more credibility when involved in legal matters where credentialing and advanced education are important; a background in case management is helpful.
   c. Life care planning for stroke survivors could involve:
      1) Estimating the lifetime cost of care and other needs related to medical malpractice in a lawsuit (e.g., in which the injured party had a stroke)
      2) Predicting lifetime care costs in relation to care coordination or management over time

E. Researcher: The APRN as researcher will study and facilitate the use of evidence-based practice for stroke survivors. Some APRNs may hold positions with a major emphasis on research related to stroke.

1. Examples of APRN involvement in stroke research
   a. Stroke program coordinator
      1) In acute care hospital (including those with primary or comprehensive stroke centers)
      2) In acute rehabilitation
      3) In freestanding rehabilitation facilities
   b. Researcher in research institutions or academic settings
   c. Research scientist in large rehabilitation institutes
   d. Writer or reviewer of grants to seek funding for stroke research
2. Examples of current areas of stroke research by rehabilitation APRNs
   a. Gonzalez and Bakas (2013) explored demographic and theory-based factors associated with survivors' bothersome behaviors as identified by family caregivers.
   b. King and colleagues (2012) study assessed the efficacy of a caregiver problem-solving intervention on stroke caregiver physical and psychosocial adaptation compared with a waitlist control treatment and assessed the mediating effects of coping on outcomes.
   c. Mauk model for poststroke recovery (Mauk, 2006, 2012), a grounded theory that suggests targeting of nursing interventions to each phase of stroke recovery was investigated.
   d. Pierce, Steiner, Khuder, Govoni, and Horn (2009) examined the experiences of stroke caregivers' well-being and care recipients' use of healthcare services in a randomized controlled trial (RCT). Pierce and Steiner (2013) evaluated the Web-based supportive intervention for the stroke caregivers used in that RCT.
   e. Efficacy of evidence-based urinary guidelines in the management of poststroke incontinence was the focus of Vaughn's (2009) study.
3. Evidence-based practice example (Department of Veterans Affairs and The Department of Defense, 2010)
   a. Background on evidence-based practice related to sensory impairment or vision/seeing (hemianopsia) for stroke survivors
      1) People are visual beings.
      2) The ability to take in and perceive visual information accurately is key to being successful in activities of daily living.
      3) After a person has a stroke, many of these visual processes may be compromised.
      4) Visual impairments (e.g., field cuts and motility impairments or diplopia) are associated with increased disability from stroke.
   b. The clinical question: How to improve these vision problems for stroke survivors?
   c. Appraisal of evidence: Visual impairments after stroke are common; however, there is little evidence on how to improve these problems. Sources of evidence for hemianopsia are flawed by weakness in methods used to measure visual field changes and a lack of generalizability to everyday function. Studies are small and often nonrandomized, with mixed

outcomes. The majority of this research is with people with traumatic brain injury. There are few studies centered on ocular motility interventions in stroke.

d. This review is limited to intervention studies for visual field cuts or hemianopsia. Three sources were found and evaluated with the following results: Level of evidence (LOE) = I; overall quality rating (QR) = Fair; strength of recommendation (SR) rating = I.
   1) Level of evidence (LOE):
      a) I: At least one properly done randomized controlled trial (Khan, Leung, & Jay, 2008; Pelak, Dubin, & Whitney, 2007; Poggel, Kasten, & Sabel, 2004)
      b) II-1: Well-designed controlled trial without randomization
      c) II-2: Well-designed cohort or case-controlled analytic study
      d) II-3: Multiple time series evidence with or without intervention, dramatic results of uncontrolled experiments
      e) III: Opinion of experts, descriptive studies, case reports, respected committees
   2) Quality rating (QR): Consistent findings from a number of higher-quality studies across a broad range of populations; supports a high degree of certainty that the results of these studies are true, and therefore the entire body of evidence would be considered "good" quality. "Fair" quality is assigned to the body of evidence indicating that the results could be due to true effects or to biases present across some or all of the studies. For a "poor" quality body of evidence, any conclusion is uncertain because of serious methodological shortcomings, sparse data, or inconsistent results.
   3) Strength of recommendation rating (SR):
      a) A: Good evidence was found; strong recommendation to provide the intervention to eligible patients; concludes benefits substantially outweigh the harm.
      b) B: Fair evidence was found; recommendation to provide the service to eligible patients; concludes benefits outweigh the harm.
      c) C: No recommendation for or against the routine provision of the intervention; concludes the balance of benefits and harms is too close to justify a general recommendation.
      d) D: Recommendation against routinely providing the intervention to asymptomatic patients; concludes at least fair evidence that the intervention is ineffective or that harm outweighs benefits.
      e) I: Evidence is insufficient to recommend for or against routinely providing intervention; evidence is lacking, of poor quality, or conflicting that the intervention is effective, and the balance of benefits and harms cannot be determined.

e. Recommendations for best rehabilitation practice
   1) Recommendations include: Patients who have visual field cuts, hemianopsia, or eye motility impairments after stroke should be provided with an intervention program for that visual impairment or compensatory strategies (SR = I). Consider scanning training, visual field stimulation, prisms, and eye exercises as restorative interventions strategies. Consider prisms and patching as compensatory intervention strategies.
   2) The evidence cited here is insufficient and of fair quality about the recommendation for best practice; other considerations are suggested.
   3) More LOE I from higher-quality studies is needed to determine other evidence-based practice recommendations for sensory impairment in stroke survivors.

ACKNOWLEDGMENTS

We would like to recognize Paddy Garvin-Higgins, MN RN CNS CRRN; Delilah Hall-Towarnicke, MSN RN CNS CRRN; and Carla J. Howard, ACNP-BC CRRN, for their work on this chapter in the previous edition of this book. We thank Director Bobbi Vaughan, MS BS, for her support and Manager Roy Schneider, MS, for his illustrations at the Center for Creative Instruction at the University of Toledo.

References

American Heart Association (AHA). (2005). Critical care and emergency medicine neurology in stroke. *Stroke, 36,* 205.

American Heart Association (AHA). (2009). Primary stroke center certification program. Retrieved from www.heart.org/idc/groups/heart0public/@wcm/@mwa/documents/downloadable/ucm_315542.pdf

American Heart Association (AHA). (2013a). Depression trumps recovery. Retrieved from http://www.strokeassociation.org/STROKEORG/LifeAfterStroke/RegainingIndependence/EmotionalBehavioralChallenges/Depression-Trumps-Recovery_UCM_309731_Article.jsp

American Heart Association (AHA). (2013b). Projected total costs of cardiovascular disease, 2015–2030 (2012 $ in billions) in the United States. Retrieved from https://www.heart.org/idc/groups/heart-public/.../ucm_449849.pdf

American Heart Association (AHA). (2013c). Statistical fact sheet 2013 update: Women & cardiovascular diseases. Retrieved from https://www.heart.org/idc/groups/heart-public/.../ucm_319576.pdf

American Heart Association (AHA). (2014a). Comprehensive stroke certification program. Retrieved from www.heart.org/HEARTORG/HealthcareResearch/MissionLifelineHomePage/Comprehensive-Stroke-Center-Certification_UCM_455446_SubHomePage.jsp

American Heart Association (AHA). (2014b). Facts knowing no bounds: Stroke in infants, children, and youth. Retrieved from www.strokeassociation.org/idc/groups/stroke.../ucm_311389.pdf

American Heart Association (AHA). (2014c). Primary stroke certification program. Retrieved from https://www.heart.org/HEARTORG/HealthcareResearch/MissionLifelineHomePage/Primary-Stroke-Center-Certification_UCM_439155_SubHomePage.jsp

American Speech–Language–Hearing Association. (2014). Dysarthria. Retrieved from http://www.asha.org/public/speech/disorders/dysarthria/

American Stroke Association (ASA). (2012a). Let's talk about hemorrhagic stroke. Retrieved from www.strokeassociation.org/idc/groups/stroke.../ucm_309710.pdf

American Stroke Association (ASA). (2012b). Stroke risk factors. Retrieved from http://www.strokeassociation.org/STROKEORG/AboutStroke/UnderstandingRisk/Understanding-Stroke-Risk_UCM_308539_SubHomePage.jsp

American Stroke Association (ASA). (2012c). Types of stroke. Retrieved from http://www.strokeassociation.org/STROKEORG/AboutStroke/TypesofStroke/Types-of-Stroke_UCM_308531_SubHomePage.jsp

American Stroke Association (ASA). (2013). Types of aphasia. Retrieved from www.strokeassociation.org/STROKEORG/LifeAfterStroke/RegainingIndependence/CommunicationChallenges/Types-of-Aphasia_UCM_310096_Article.jsp

American Stroke Association (ASA). (2014). Central pain syndrome. Retrieved from www.strokeassociation.org/STROKEORG/LifeAfterStroke/RegainingIndependence/PhysicalChallenges/Central-Pain-Syndrome-Treatment_UCM_309892_Article.jsp

Association of Rehabilitation Nurses (ARN). (2004). Role descriptions: The advanced practice rehabilitation nurse. Retrieved from http://www.rehabnurse.org

Association of Rehabilitation Nurses (ARN). (2014a). *ARN competency model for professional rehabilitation nursing.* Retrieved from http://www.rehabnurse.org/uploads/files/education/ARN_Rehabilitation_Nursing_Competency _Model_FINAL_-_May_2014.pdf

Association of Rehabilitation Nurses (ARN). (2014b). Position statement: Advanced practice in rehabilitation nursing. Retrieved from http://www.rehabnurse.org

Atlanta Aphasia Association. (2006). Types of aphasia. Retrieved from http://www.atlantaaphasia.org/WhatIsAphasia02.html

Bader, M., & Palmer, S. (2006). What's the "hyper" in hyperacute stroke? *AACN Advanced Critical Care, 17*(2), 194–214.

Becker, J., Wira, C., & Arnold, J. (2010). Ischemic stroke. Medscape. Retrieved from http://emedicine.medscape.com/article/793904-overview

The Brain Attack Coalition (BAC). (2002). TPA Stroke Study Group guidelines. Retrieved from www.stroke-site.org/guidelines/tpa_guidelines.html

Bravata, D., Concato, J., Fried, T., Ranjbar, N., Sadarangani, T., McClain, V., . . . Yaggi, H. (2011). Continuous positive airway pressure: Evaluation of a novel therapy for patients with acute ischemic stroke. *Sleep, 34,* 1271–1277.

Briggs, D. E., Felberg, R., Malkoff, M., Bratina, P., & Grotta, J. C. (2001). Should mild or moderate stroke patients be admitted to an intensive care unit? *Stroke, 32,* 871–876.

Canadian Stroke Network. (2010). Managing stroke care transitions. In M. Lindsay, G. Gubitz, M. Bayley, M. Hill, C. Davies-Schinkel, S. Singh, & S. Phillips (Canadian Stroke Strategy Best Practices and Standards Writing Group), *Canadian best practice recommendations for stroke care* (pp. 129–150). Ottawa, ON, Canada: Author.

Centers for Disease Control and Prevention (CDC). (2013). Stroke fact sheet. Retrieved from www.cdc.gov/dhdsp/data_statistics/fact_sheets/fs_stroke.htm

Centers for Disease Control and Prevention (CDC). (2014). Stroke facts. Retrieved from www.cdc.gov/stroke/facts.htm

Commission on Accreditation of Rehabilitation Facilities (CARF). (2014). *Quality across the lifespan® accreditation programs.* Retrieved from www.carf.org/Programs/

Connolly, E., Rabinstein, A., Carhuapoma, J., Derdeyn, C., Dion, J., Higashida, R., . . . Vespa, P. (2012). Guidelines for the management of aneurysmal subarachnoid hemorrhage: A guideline for healthcare professionals from the American Heart Association/American Stroke Association. *Stroke, 43*(6), 1711–1737.

Consortium for Spinal Cord Medicine. (1998). *Clinical practice guidelines: Neurogenic bowel management in adults with spinal cord injury.* Washington, DC: Paralyzed Veterans of America.

Consortium for Spinal Cord Medicine. (2006). *Clinical practice guidelines: Bladder management for adults with spinal cord injury.* Washington, DC: Paralyzed Veterans of America.

Cournan, M. (2012). Bladder management in female stroke survivors: Translating research into practice. *Rehabilitation Nursing, 37*(5), 220–230.

Del Zoppo, G., Saver, J., Jauch, E., & Adams, H. (2009). Expansion of the time window for treatment of acute ischemic stroke with intravenous tissue plasminogen activator: A science advisory from the American Heart Association/American Stroke Association. *Stroke, 40,* 2945–2948.

Deno, M., Gillard, P., Graham, G., DiBonaventura, M., Goren, A., Varon, S., & Zorowitz, R. (2013). Anxiety and depression associated with caregiver burden in caregivers of stroke survivors with spasticity. *Archives of Physical Medicine and Rehabilitation, 94*(9), 1731–1736.

Department of Veterans Affairs (VA) and The Department of Defense (DoD). (2010). *VA/DoD Clinical practice guideline: The management of stroke rehabilitation.* Washington, DC: Author.

Donovan, N., Daniels, S., Edmiaston, J., Weinhardt, J., Summers, D., & Mitchell, P. (2013). American Heart Association Council on Cardiovascular Nursing and Stroke Council. Dysphagia screening: State of the art: Invitational conference proceeding from the State-of-the-Art Nursing Symposium, International Stroke Conference 2012. *Stroke, 44*(4), e24–31.

Easton, J. D., Saver, J., Albers, G., Alberts, M., Chaturvedi, E., Feldmann, E., . . . Sacco, R. (2009). Definition and evaluation of transient ischemic attack: A scientific statement for healthcare professionals from the American Heart Association/American Stroke Association Stroke Council; Council on Cardiovascular Surgery and Anesthesia; Council on Cardiovascular Radiology and Intervention; Council on Cardiovascular Nursing; and the Interdisciplinary Council on Peripheral Vascular Disease. *Stroke, 40*(6), 2276–2293.

Easton, K. L. (2001). *The post-stroke journey: From agonizing to owning.* Doctoral dissertation, Wayne State University, Detroit, MI.

Esse, K., Fossati-Bellani, M., Traylor, A., & Martin-Schild, S. (2011). Epidemic of illicit drug use, mechanisms of action/addiction and stroke as a health hazard. *Brain and Behavior, 1*(1), 44–54.

Evans, A., Harraf, F., Donaldson, N., & Kalra L. (2002). Randomized controlled study of stroke unit care versus stroke team care in different stroke subtypes. *Stroke, 33,* 449–455.

Family Caregiver Alliance (FCA). (2012). Selected caregiver statistics. Retrieved from http://www.caregiver.org/caregiver/jsp/content_node.jsp?nodeid=439&expandnodeid=384

Family Caregiver Alliance (FCA). (2013). Daily or in-home caregiver. Retrieved from http://caregiver.org/daily-or-home-caregiver

Furie, K., Kasner, S., Adams, R., Albers, G., Bush, R., Fagan, S., . . . Wentworth, D. (2011). Guidelines for the prevention of stroke in patients with stroke or transient ischemic attack: A guideline for healthcare professionals from the American Heart Association/American Stroke Association. *Stroke, 42*(1), 227–276.

Gall, S. L., Donnan, G., Dewey, H. M., Macdonell, R., Sturm, J., Gilligan, A., . . . Thrift, A. (2010). Sex differences in presentation, severity, and management of stroke in a population-based study. *Neurology, 74*(12), 975–981.

Go, A., Mozaffarian, D., Roger, V., Benjamin, E., Berry, J., Borden, W., . . . Turner, M. (2013). Heart disease and stroke statistics—2014 update: A report from the American Heart Association. *Circulation, 129*(1), e28–e292. doi:10.1161/CIR.0b013e31828124ad

Gonzalez, C., & Bakas, T. (2013). Factors associated with stroke survivor behaviors as identified by family caregivers. *Rehabilitation Nursing, 38*(4), 202–211.

Hennerici, M., Kern, R., & Szabo, K. (2013). Non-pharmacological strategies for the treatment of acute ischemic stroke. *Lancet Neurology, 12*(6), 572–584.

Hinchey, J. A., Shepherd, T., Furie, K., Smith, D., Wang, D., & Tonn, S. (2005). Formal dysphagia screening protocols prevent pneumonia. *Stroke, 36,* 1972–1976.

Holloway, R., Arnold, R., Creutzfeldt, C., Lewis, E., Lutz, B., McCann, R., . . . Zorowitz, R. (2014). Palliative and end-of-life care in stroke: A statement for healthcare professionals from the American Heart Association/American Stroke Association. *Stroke.* Retrieved from http://stroke.ahajournals.org/content/early/2014/03/27/STR.0000000000000015

Howard, G., & Goff, D. (2012). Population shifts and the future of stroke: Forecasts of the future burden of stroke. *Annals of the New York Academy of Sciences, 1268,* 14–20. doi:10.1111/j.1749-6632.2012.06665.x

International Alliance for Pediatric Stroke. (2014). About pediatric stroke: Fast facts. Retrieved from http://www.iapediatricstroke.org/about_pediatric_stroke.aspx

The Internet Stroke Center. (2014a). Reducing your risk. Retrieved from www.strokecenter.org/patients/stroke-treatment/reducing-your-risk/

The Internet Stroke Center. (2014b). Stroke statistics. Retrieved from www.strokecenter.org/patients/about-stroke/stroke-statistics/

The Internet Stroke Center. (2014c). Stroke assessment scales. Retrieved from www.strokecenter.org/wp-content/uploads/2011/08/cincinnati.pdf

Ionita, C., & Levine, S. (2013). Lacunar infarction. MedLink Neurology. Retrieved from http://www.medlink.com/medlinkcontent.asp

Jauch, E., Saver, J., Adams, H., Bruno, A., Connors, J., Demaerschalk, B., . . . Yonas, H. (2013). Guidelines for the early management of patients with acute ischemic stroke: A guideline for healthcare professionals from the American Heart Association/American Stroke Association. *Stroke, 44*(3), 870–947.

The Joint Commission (JC). (2008). *Disease-specific care certification program. STROKE Performance measurement implementation guide* (2nd ed., 2a). Retrieved from www.jointcommission.org/assets/1/18/stroke_pm_implementation_guide_ver_2a.pdf

The Joint Commission (JC). (2014). *Advanced certification comprehensive stroke centers.* Retrieved from www.jointcommission.org/certification/primary_stroke_centers.aspx

Kernan, W., Ovbiagele, B., Black, H., Bravata, D., Chimowitz, M., Ezekowitz, M., . . . Wilson, J. (2014). Guidelines for the prevention of stroke in patients with stroke and transient ischemic attack: A guideline for healthcare professionals from the American Heart Association/American Stroke Association. *Stroke.* Retrieved from http://www.ncbi.nlm.nih.gov/pubmed/24788967

Khan, S., Leung, E., & Jay, W. (2008). Stroke and visual rehabilitation. *Topics in Stroke Rehabilitation, 15*(1), 27–36.

King, R., Hartke, R., Houle, T., Lee, J., Herring, G., Alexander-Peterson, B., & Raad, J. (2012). A problem-solving early intervention for stroke caregivers: One year follow-up. *Rehabilitation Nursing, 37*(5), 231–243.

Klabunde, R. (2009). Autoregulation of organ blood flow. *Cardiovascular Physiology Concepts.* Retrieved from http://www.cvphysiology.com/Blood%20Flow/BF004.htm

Kuramatsu, J., Huttner, H., & Schwab, S. (2013). Advances in the management of intracerebral hemorrhage. *Journal of Neural Transmission, 120*(Suppl l), S35–41.

Lloyd-Jones, D., Adams, R., Brown, T., Carnethon, M., Dai, S., De Simone, G., . . . Wylie-Rosett, J. (2010). Heart disease and stroke statistics—2010 update: A report from the American Heart Association. *Circulation, 121*(7), e46–e215. doi:10.1161/CIRCULATIONAHA.109.192667

Lockwood-Koehn, T. (2014). Stroke groups benefit stroke survivors and caregivers. *StrokeSmart Magazine.* Retrieved from http://www.strokesmart.org/new?id=199

Lubkin, I., & Larsen, P. (Eds.). (2013). *Chronic illness: Impact and interventions* (8th ed.). Sudbury, MA: Jones and Bartlett.

Lutsep, H., & Berman, S. (2013). *Neuroprotective agents in stroke: Overview of neuroprotective agents.* Medscape. Retrieved from http://emedicine.medscape.com/article/1161422-overview.

Mace, N. L., & Rabins, P. V. (1981). *The 36-hour day.* Baltimore: Johns Hopkins University Press.

Markus, H., Pereira, A., & Cloud, G. (2010). *Stroke medicine.* New York: Oxford University Press.

Mauk, K. L. (2006). Nursing interventions within the Mauk model of poststroke recovery. *Rehabilitation Nursing, 31*(6), 267–263.

Mauk, K. (2012). *Rehabilitation nursing: Contemporary approach to practice.* Burlington, MA: Jones & Bartlett Learning.

Mauk, K. (Ed.). (2014). *Gerontological nursing competencies for care* (3rd ed.). Sudbury, MA: Jones and Bartlett.

Merck Sharp & Dohme Corporation. (2009–2010). Introduction to cerebrovascular accident. Retrieved from www.merck.com/mmpe/sec16/ch211/ch211a.html

Miller, E., Murray, L., Richard, L., Zorowitz, R. D., Bakas, T., Clark, P., & Billinger, S. (2010). Comprehensive overview of nursing and interdisciplinary rehabilitation care of the stroke patient: A scientific statement from the American Heart Association. *Stroke, 41,* 2402–2448.

Miller, E., & Summers, D. (2014). State-of-the-science nursing review update on transient ischemic attack nursing care. *Stroke, 45*(5), e71–3. doi:10.1161/STROKEAHA.114.005320.

MNT Knowledge Center. (2013). What is a mini-stroke? What is a transient ischemic attack (TIA)? Retrieved from http://www.medicalnewstoday.com/articles/164038.php

Mora, S., Glynn, R. J., Boekholdt, S. M., Nordestgaard, B. G., Kastelein, J. J., & Ridker, P. M. (2012). On-treatment non-high-density lipoprotein cholesterol, apolipoprotein B, triglycerides, and lipid ratios in relation to residual vascular risk after treatment with potent statin therapy: JUPITER (justification for the use of statins in prevention: An intervention trial evaluating rosuvastatin). *Journal of the American College of Cardiology,* 59, 1521-1528.

Morgenstern, L., Hemphill, J., Anderson, C., Becker, K., Broderick, J., Connolly, E., . . . Tamargo, R. (2010). Guidelines for the management of spontaneous intracerebral hemorrhage: A guideline for healthcare professionals from the American Heart Association/American Stroke Association. *Stroke, 41*(9), 2108–2129.

Nassisi, D. (2010). Hemorrhagic stroke. Medscape. Retrieved from http://emedicine.medscape.com/article/1916662-overview

National Institute of Mental Health (NIMH). (2011). Stroke and depression. Retrieved from http://www.nimh.nih.gov/health/publications/depression-and-stroke/index.shtml

National Institute of Neurological Disorders and Stroke (NINDS). (2009a). NIH stroke scale. Retrieved from www.strokecenter.org/trials/scales/nihss.html

National Institute of Neurological Disorders and Stroke (NINDS). (2009b). Stroke challenges, progress, and promise. Retrieved from http://stroke.nih.gov/materials/strokechallenges.htm#Factors

National Institute of Neurological Disorders and Stroke (NINDS). (2011). Recognition and treatment of stroke in children. Retrieved from http://www.ninds.nih.gov/news_and_events/proceedings/stroke_proceedings/childneurology.htm

National Institute of Neurological Disorders and Stroke (NINDS). (2013). *K*now stroke. Know the signs. Act in time. Retrieved from www.ninds.nih.gov/disorders/stroke/knowstroke.htm#symptoms

National Institute of Neurological Disorders and Stroke (NINDS). (2014a). Post-stroke rehabilitation. Retrieved from http://www.ninds.nih.gov/disorders/stroke/poststrokerehab.htm

National Institute of Neurological Disorders and Stroke (NINDS). (2014b). Stroke: Hope through research. Retrieved from http://www.ninds.nih.gov/disorders/stroke/detail_stroke.htm

National Institute on Deafness and Other Communication Disorders. (2010). Apraxia of speech. Retrieved from http://www.nidcd.nih.gov/health/voice/pages/apraxia.aspx

National Stroke Association (NSA). (2009a). African Americans and stroke. Retrieved from www.stroke.org/site/PageServer?pagename=AAMER

National Stroke Association (NSA). (2009b). Caregivers and families. Retrieved from www.stroke.org/site/PageServer?pagename=care

National Stroke Association (NSA). (2009c). Recovery. Retrieved from www.stroke.org/site/PageServer?pagename=recov

National Stroke Association (NSA). (2011). Mobility after stroke. Retrieved from www.stroke.org/site/DocServer/mobility06.pdf?docID=2801

National Stroke Association (NSA). (2014a). Kids and pediatric stroke. Retrieved from http://www.stroke.org/site/PageServer?pagename=kids

National Stroke Association (NSA). (2014b). Recovery after stroke: Recurrent stroke. Retrieved from http://www.stroke.org/site/DocServer/NSAFactSheet_RecurrentStrokerevised.pdf?docID=998

National Stroke Association (NSA). (2014c). Rehabilitation therapy after stroke. Retrieved from http://www.stroke.org/site/PageServer?pagename=REHABT

National Stroke Association (NSA). (2014d). *S*TARS: Steps against recurrent stroke. Retrieved from www.stroke.org/site/PageServer?pagename=STARS

National Stroke Association (NSA). (2014e). Uncontrollable risk factors. Retrieved from http://www.stroke.org/site/PageServer?pagename=uncont

National Stroke Association (NSA). (2014f). What is stroke? Retrieved from http://www.stroke.org/site/PageServer?pagename=stroke

National Stroke Association (NSA). (2014g). What is a TIA? Retrieved from http://www.stroke.org/site/PageServer?pagename=tia

Neuro-IFRAH Organization. (2005). What is Neuro-IFRAH? Retrieved from www.neuro-ifrah.org/faq.aspx

Paquereau, J., Allart, E., Romon, M., & Rousseaux, M. (2014). The long-term nutritional status in stroke patients and its predictive factors. *Journal of Stroke Cerebrovascular Disease, pii,* S1052–3057.

Patel, S., Jain, R., & Wagner, S. (2008). The vasculature of the human brain. In *Neuroscience in medicine* (pp. 147–166). Totowa, NJ: Humana Press.

Pelak, V., Dubin, M., & Whitney, E. (2007). Homonymous hemianopia: A critical analysis of optical devices, compensatory training, and NovaVision. *Current Treatment Options in Neurology, 9*(1), 41–47.

Pfeil, M., Gray, R., & Lindsay, B. (2009). Depression and stroke: A common but often unrecognized combination. *British Journal of Nursing, 18*(6), 365–369.

Pierce, L., & Steiner, V. (2013). Usage and design evaluation by family caregivers of a stroke intervention website. *Journal of Neuroscience Nursing, 45*(5), 254–261.

Pierce, L., Steiner, V., Govoni, A., Thompson, T., & Friedemann, M. (2007). Two sides to the caregiving story. *Topics in Stroke Rehabilitation, 14*(2), 13–20.

Pierce, L. L., Steiner, V., Hicks, B., & Holzaepfel, A. L. (2006). Problems of new caregivers of persons with stroke. *Rehabilitation Nursing, 31*(4), 166–172.

Pierce, L., Steiner, V., Khuder, S., Govoni, A., & Horn, L. (2009). The effect of a web-based stroke intervention on carers' well-being and survivors' use of healthcare services. *Disability and Rehabilitation, 31*(20), 1676–1684.

Pierce, L., Thompson, T., Govoni, A., & Steiner, V. (2012). Caregivers' incongruence: Emotional strain in caring for persons with stroke. *Rehabilitation Nursing, 37*(5), 368–366.

Poggel, D., Kasten, E., & Sabel, B. (2004). Attentional cueing improves vision restoration therapy in patients with visual field defects. *Neurology, 63*(11), 2069–2076.

Qamar, Z. (2011). *Depression among stroke patients and relation with demographic and stroke characteristics.* Umeå, Sweden: Umeå University.

Roach, E. S., Golomb, M., Adams, R., Biller, J., Daniels, S., deVeber, G., . . . Smith, E. (2008). Management of stroke in infants and children: A scientific statement from a special writing group of the American Heart Association Stroke Council and the Council on Cardiovascular Disease in the Young. *Stroke, 39*(9), 2644–2691.

Ryan, C., Bayley, M., Green, R., Murray, B., & Bradley, T. (2011). Influence of continuous positive airway pressure on outcomes of rehabilitation in stroke patients with obstructive sleep apnea. *Stroke, 42,* 1062–1067.

Sacco, R., Kasner, S., Broderick, J., Caplan, L., Connors, J., Culebras, A., . . . Vinters, H. (2013). An updated definition of stroke for the 21st century: A statement for healthcare professionals from the American Heart Association/American Stroke Association. *Stroke, 44*(7), 2064–2089. doi:10.1161/STR.0b013e318296aeca

Salaycik, K., Kelly-Hayes, M., Beiser, A., Nguyen, A. H., Brady, S., Kase, C., & Wolf, P. (2007). Depressive symptoms and risk of stroke: The Framingham Study. *Stroke, 38,* 16–21.

Sanossian, N., & Ovbiagele, B. (2009). Prevention and management of stroke in very elderly patients. *Lancet Neurology, 8,* 1031–1041.

Secrest, J. S. (2002). How stroke survivors and primary support persons experience nurses in rehabilitation. *Rehabilitation Nursing, 24*(6), 240–246.

Sen, S., Webb, S., & Selph, J. (2010). E-medicine neurology. Retrieved from http://emedicine.medscape.com/article/1160167-media

Towfighi, A., & Saver, J. (2011). Stroke declines from third to fourth leading cause of death in the United States. *Stroke, 42,* 2351–2355.

University of Iowa (n.d.a). *Nursing interventions classification (NIC), 5th edition interventions labels & definitions.* Retrieved from www.nursing.uiowa.edu/excellence/nursing_knowledge/clinical_effectiveness/documents/LabelDefinitionsNIC5.pdf

University of Iowa (n.d.b). *Nursing outcomes classification (NOC).* Retrieved from www.nursing.uiowa.edu/excellence/nursing_knowledge/clinical_effectiveness/noc.htm

University of Miami Health System (UMHS). (2014). Effects of stroke. Retrieved from http://uhealthsystem.com/health-library/neuro/disorder/stroke/effects

van Swieten, J. C., Koudstaal, P. J., Visser, M. C., Schouten, H. J., & van Gijn, J. (1988). Interobserver agreement for the assessment of handicap in stroke patients. *Stroke, 19*(5), 604–607.

Vaughn, S. (2009). Efficacy of urinary guidelines in the management of post-stroke incontinence. *International Journal of Urological Nursing, 3*(1), 4–12.

Vega, J. (2008). Anarthria. Retrieved from http://stroke.about.com/od/glossary/g/anarthria.htm

Visser-Meily, A., Post, M., Gorter, J., Berlekom, S. B. V., van den Bos, T., & Lindeman, E. (2006). Rehabilitation of stroke patients needs a family-centered approach. *Disability Rehabilitation, 28*(24), 1557–1561.

Weed, R., & Berens, D. (Eds.). (2010). *Life care planning and case management handbook* (3rd ed.). Boca Raton, FL: CRC Press Taylor and Francis Group.

Zebian, R., & Kazzi, A. (2010). Subarachnoid hemorrhage. Medscape. Retrieved from http://emedicine.medscape.com/article/794076-overview

Suggested Resources

Alexander, S. (2013). Evidence-based nursing care for stroke and neurovascular conditions. Ames, IA: John Wiley & Sons, Inc.

American Stroke Association. (2014a). My American heart for professionals. Retrieved from http://my.americanheart.org/professional/index.jsp

American Stroke Association. (2014b). Statements and guidelines. Retrieved from http://my.americanheart.org/professional/StatementsGuidelines/Statements-Guidelines_UCM_316885_SubHomePage.jsp

Corrigan, M., Escuro, A., & Kirby, D. (2013). Handbook of clinical nutrition and stroke. New York: Humana Press Springer.

Hickey, J. (2013). The clinical practice of neurological & neurosurgical nursing (7th ed.). Philadelphia: Lippincott Williams & Wilkins.

Lindsay, M., Gubitz, G., Bayley, M., Hill, M., Davies-Schinkel, C., Singh, S., & Phillips, S. (2010). Managing stroke care transitions (pp. 129–150). Ottawa, ON: Canadian Stroke Network.

National Stroke Association (NSA). (2014a). Healthcare professionals. Retrieved from http://www.stroke.org/site/PageServer?pagename=medpro

National Stroke Association (NSA). (2014b). Stroke prevention. Retrieved from www.stroke.org/site/DocServer/NSAStrokePreventionBrochure_sm.pdf?docID=3324-23k

Perry, A., Potter, P., & Ostendorf, W. (2013). Clinical nursing skills and techniques (8th ed.). St. Louis: Mosby Elsevier.

Williams, J., Perry, L., & Watkins, C. (2010). Acute stroke nursing. Oxford: Wiley-Blackwell.

Community Resource Index for Stroke and Caregivers

Access to Respite Care and Help (ARCH). (2014). ARCH National Respite Network and Resource Center. Retrieved from http://archrespite.org

American Association of Retired Persons (AARP). (2014). Caregiving Resource Center. Retrieved from www.aarp.org/home-family/caregiving/

American Heart Association (AHA). (2014). Caregiver. Retrieved from www.heart.org/HEARTORG/Caregiver/Caregiver_UCM_001103_SubHomePage.jsp

American Office on Aging (AoA). (2014). National family caregiver support program. Retrieved from http://aoa.gov/aoa_programs/hcltc/caregiver/

American Stroke Association (ASA). (2014a). Stroke community resources and education. Retrieved from www.strokeassociation.org/STROKEORG/Professionals/Stroke-Resources-for-Professionals_UCM_308581_SubHomePage.jsp

American Stroke Association (ASA). (2014b). Stroke resources for professionals. Retrieved from www.strokeassociation.org/STROKEORG/Professionals/Stroke-Resources-for-Professionals_UCM_308581_SubHomePage.jsp

Canadian Stroke Network and McGill University. (2014). Stroke engine: Family support. Retrieved from http://strokengine.ca/family/

CaringBridge. (2014). Stroke patient resource. Retrieved from https://www.caringbridge.org

Center for Disease Control and Prevention (CDC). (2013). Stroke other resources. Retrieved from www.cdc.gov/stroke/other_resources.htm

Family Caregiver Alliance (FCA). (2014). National Center on Caregiving. Retrieved from www.caregiver.org

The Internet Stroke Center. (2014a). Additional resources and general stroke information. Retrieved from www.strokecenter.org

The Internet Stroke Center. (2014b). Stroke resources for health professionals. Retrieved from www.strokecenter.org/professionals/

Johnson & Johnson. (2014). Strength for caring: Providing enhanced resources for caregivers. Retrieved from www.strengthforcaring.com

Lotsa Helping Hands, Inc. (2014). It takes a community to care for the caregiver. Retrieved from www.lotsahelpinghands.com

National Institute on Aging (NIA). (2014). Caregiving. Retrieved from www.niapublications.org/shopdisplayproducts.asp?id=29&cat=Caregiving

National Institutes of Health (NIH) and National Institute of Neurological Disorders and Stroke (NINDS). (2014). Health professional resources. Retrieved from http://stroke.nih.gov/resources/

National Stroke Association (NSA). (2014a). Acute Stroke Resource Center. Retrieved from www.stroke.org/site/PageServer?pagename=acute

National Stroke Association (NSA). (2014b). Brainiac Kids. Retrieved from http://support.stroke.org/site/PageServer?pagename=BrainiacKids

National Stroke Association (NSA). (2014c). Healthcare professionals. Retrieved from www.stroke.org/site/PageServer?pagename=medpro

National Stroke Association (NSA). (2014d). Hip Hop Stroke Program. Retrieved from www.stroke.org/site/PageServer?pagename=hiphopstroke

National Stroke Association (NSA). (2014e). Resources for your community. Retrieved from www.stroke.org/site/PageServer?pagename=medpro3

The Stroke Network. (2014). Online stroke support and information resources. Retrieved from www.strokenetwork.org

University of Toledo Medical Center. (2014). Caring~Web: Education and support for caregivers of stroke survivors. Retrieved from http://utmc.utoledo.edu/clinics/neurology/caringweb/

Chapter 23

Traumatic Injuries: Traumatic Brain Injury and Spinal Cord Injury

Tiffany LeCroy, MSN RN CRRN FNP-C ACNS-BC
Joan McMahon, MSA BSN CRRN

LEARNING OUTCOMES

- Review the epidemiology and etiology of traumatic brain injury (TBI) and spinal cord injury (SCI).
- Differentiate between classifications of types of TBI and SCI.
- Discuss prevention of common complications of TBI and SCI.
- Identify the nurse's role in caring for patients with TBI and SCI.
- Describe assessment instruments and tools used in TBI and SCI.

KEY CHAPTER TOPICS

- TBI statistics, epidemiology, causation, classification, pathophysiology, assessment, treatment, and nursing care
- SCI statistics, epidemiology, causation, classification, pathophysiology, assessment, treatment, and nursing care

PROFESSIONAL REHABILITATION NURSING DOMAINS AND COMPETENCIES

- Domain 1: Competencies 1.2, 1.3, 1.4
- Domain 2: Competencies 2.1, 2.2 (Association of Rehabilitation Nurses [ARN], 2014)

Introduction

Catastrophic injuries of the brain and spinal cord affect millions of people in the United States each year. Falls, motor vehicle accidents, violence, and sporting and recreational mishaps are the major causes of these injuries. Annually, about 12,000 new spinal cord injuries (SCIs) occur (National Spinal Cord Injury Statistical Center [NSCISC], 2013) and an estimated 1.7 million people sustain a traumatic brain injury (TBI) (Centers for Disease Control and Prevention [CDC], 2010a). Both types of injuries affect primarily the younger population and tend to occur more often in males. Both types of injuries have effects that vary according to the specific location and severity of injury. These injuries often need rehabilitation.

Victims of catastrophic injuries need assistance from healthcare professionals to improve health function and learn to adapt to changes in their functional status in the home and community settings. Rehabilitation nurses play a vital role in improving patient outcomes through astute assessment, timely interventions, and thorough evaluation. The rehabilitation process for TBI and SCI is interprofessional and aimed at improving all aspects of the patient's life.

I. TBI

A. Overview

1. Definitions
    a. *TBI* is defined as an alteration in brain function or other evidence of brain pathology, caused by an external force (Brain Injury Association of America [BIAA], 2014).
    b. May produce altered levels of consciousness, changes in cognition and behavior, and physical limitations (BIAA, 2014)
    c. The severity of brain injury may range from mild to moderate or severe (BIAA, 2014).
    d. The result may be long-term or short-term problems with independent function (BIAA, 2014).
2. Impact
    a. Affects roles and relationships for the patient and family (Baggerly & Le, 2001)

b. Often affects employment, finances, and leisure activities (Baggerly & Le, 2001)

c. Brain damage from external injuries can be immediate or secondary to a variety of pathophysiological changes and may lead to long-term or lifelong needs for assistance from others (Lunney, MaGuire, Endozo, & McIntosh-Waddy, 2010).

3. General symptoms (**Table 23-1**)

B. Types of Brain Injuries

1. *Concussion* is also known as *mild traumatic brain injury (mTBI)*.

a. CDC definition: "A case of mild traumatic brain injury is an occurrence of injury to the head resulting from blunt trauma or acceleration or deceleration forces with one or more of the following conditions attributable to the head injury during the surveillance period:

1) Any period of observed or self-reported transient confusion, disorientation, or impaired consciousness

2) Any period of observed or self-reported dysfunction of memory (amnesia) around the time of injury

3) Observed signs of other neurological or neuropsychological dysfunction, such as

a) Seizures acutely following head injury

b) Among infants and very young children: irritability, lethargy, or vomiting following head injury

c) Symptoms among older children and adults such as headache, dizziness, irritability, fatigue, or poor concentration, when identified soon after injury, can be used to support the diagnosis of mild TBI, but cannot be used to make the diagnosis in the absence of loss of consciousness (LOC) or altered consciousness. Further research may provide additional guidance in this area.

4) Any period of observed or self-reported loss of consciousness lasting 30 minutes or less" (CDC, 2003).

b. Symptoms: May or may not report unconsciousness (Evans, 2003), momentary loss of reflexes or memory, headache, confusion, dizziness, irritability, and visual and gait disturbances (Hickey, 2003b)

2. *Contusion*: Bruising to the brain cortex; may be moderate or severe; outcomes vary according to location and severity of injury (Blank-Reid & Barker, 2002).

a. Found most commonly in the frontal and temporal lobes and at the frontotemporal junction; causes changes in attention, memory, affect, emotion, and executive function

b. Less commonly found in occipital and parietal lobes

c. Small contusions can coalesce into a large intracranial hematoma.

d. May be evidenced by immediate LOC, changes in respirations, hypotension, bradycardia, and temporary loss of reflexes. Vital signs can return to normal within a few seconds, reflexes return, and then consciousness is regained (Huether & McCance, 2012).

3. Hemorrhagic injuries

a. Subdural hematoma (SDH)

1) Results from bleeding between the dura mater and arachnoid interface

2) May be acute, subacute, or chronic

a) Acute SDH develops rapidly and is usually located at the top of the skull.

Table 23-1. General Symptoms of Traumatic Brain Injury

Physical	Cognitive and Behavioral
Paresis	Poor initiation
Dysphagia	Disinhibition
Dysarthria	Agitation
Cerebrospinal fluid leaks	Restlessness
Balance and coordination impairments	Impulsivity
Visual impairments	Aphasias
Loss of bowel control	Memory and thinking deficits
Loss of bladder control	Sequencing difficulties
Spasticity and loss of tone	Attention and concentration deficits
Seizures	Problem solving and reasoning deficits
Dysautonomia ("storming")	Anxiety
Sleep-wake disturbance	Depression
Pain	Emotional lability
Metabolic effects (higher nutritional needs)	Loss of social competence

Data from Baggerly & Le, 2001; Hickey, 2003b, 2003c; Model Systems Knowledge Translation Center, n.d.

b) Subacute SDH develops more slowly, from 48 hours to 2 weeks after injury.
c) Chronic SDH is found more often in the older adult and with chronic alcohol abuse, often related to brain atrophy with stretching of bridging veins (Huether & McCance, 2012).

3) Occurs in 10%–20% of people with intracranial injuries and is more common in older adults
4) SDH expands and compresses brain tissue, also compressing blood vessels and compressing the bleeding veins. Thus, the bleeding that causes the SDH can be stopped, but the volume of blood in the subdural space can lead to elevated intracranial pressure and related symptoms and signs. Changes in level of consciousness, headache, agitation, slowed cognition, restlessness and confusion, seizure, and paresis occur (Huether & McCance, 2012).
5) Surgical evacuation may be needed for larger sizes (more than 1 cm in adults); smaller sizes may benefit from medical management (Chanda & Nanda, 2003; Huether & McCance, 2012).

b. Epidural hematoma
1) Develops as a rapid arterial or venous bleed, often associated with skull fracture or a lacerated meningeal artery (most common cause)
2) More common in young adults and adults older than age 60 years
3) Accounts for approximately 2% of traumatic intracranial insults
4) Changes in level of consciousness, elevated intracranial pressure and associated symptoms, seizure, paresis
5) Usually warrants surgical management (Chanda & Nanda, 2003)

c. Intracerebral hemorrhage
1) In 2%–3% of people with TBI
2) Develops from bleeding into the cerebral tissue and is associated with contusions
3) May act as a space-occupying lesion compressing brain tissue; poor prognosis. Increases intracranial pressure, compresses brain tissue, and leads to cerebral edema (Huether & McCance, 2012)
4) Headache, deteriorating consciousness, coma, contralateral paresis, ipsilateral dilated pupil, signs of herniation (Huether & McCance, 2012)

d. Subarachnoid hemorrhage
1) Develops from bleeding into the subarachnoid space
2) Is associated with severe head injury and aneurysmal ruptures
3) Symptoms related to elevated intracranial pressure and meningeal irritation (Hickey, 2003b)

4. Penetrating injuries
a. Missile injuries (high-velocity trauma)
1) Caused by bullets, rocks, shell fragments, knives, and blunt instruments; the location, path of injury, and depth of penetration directly affect the severity of the injury.
2) Bone fragments can worsen the injury.
3) May be associated with infection caused by bone fragments, hair, and skin entering the brain with the missile (Blank-Reid & Barker, 2002; Huether & McCance, 2012)
4) Herniation of brain tissue is possible.

b. Missile injuries (low-velocity trauma): Local parenchymal damage, most commonly caused by a bullet or sharp object, is the most important factor in determining the extent of injury (Blank-Reid & Barker, 2002).
c. Stab wounds
1) Refers to the piercing of the scalp, skull, or brain by a foreign object (e.g., knife, ice pick, pencil, scissors)
2) May cause severe neurologic impairment depending on the location of the insult (Vinas et al., 2013)

C. Epidemiology
1. It is estimated that more than 5.3 million people live with disabilities resulting from TBI (CDC, 2010b).
2. Direct medical costs and indirect costs of TBI, such as loss of work, totaled an estimated $76.5 billion in the United States every year (CDC, 2010b).
3. Brain injury in sports has attracted new attention.
a. Repeated concussions in sports lead to dementia, amyotrophic lateral sclerosis (ALS), and Parkinson's disease.
b. Professional football receives the most media attention, but concern is increasing in any sport with contact, including boxing, soccer, and lacrosse.
4. Based on 2001–2010 data about emergency room (ER) visits, hospitalizations, and deaths, the CDC (2010c) reported:

a. Rates of TBI-related ER visits increased by 70%, hospitalization rates increased by 11%, and death rates decreased by 7%.
b. In 2010, approximately 2.5 million ER visits, hospitalizations, or deaths were associated with TBI.
   1) TBI contributed to more than 50,000 deaths.
   2) TBI was diagnosed in more than 280,000 hospitalizations and 2.2 million ER visits.

5. The CDC (2010b) also reported the following 2006–2010 data:
   a. Men have higher rates of TBI hospitalizations and ER visits and are three times more likely to die than women.
   b. TBI-related hospitalization rates are highest among people 65 years and older.
   c. ER rates are highest among children age 0–4 years.
   d. Falls are the leading cause of TBI-related ER visits for all age groups. Blunt trauma is the second leading cause of TBI-rated ER visits among children 5–14 years old.
   e. Falls are the leading cause of TBI-related hospitalization among children 0–14 years and adults 45 years and older.
   f. Motor vehicle accidents are the leading cause of TBI-related hospitalizations for adolescents and young adults age 15–44 years.

D. Etiology and Causes of TBI (CDC, 2010c; Faul, Waid, & Coronado, 2010)
   1. Falls are the leading cause of TBI (40%). Falls cause approximately half (55%) of the TBIs among children age 0–14 years, compared with 81% among adults age 65 years and older.
   2. 15% of TBIs are unintentional blunt trauma (i.e., being hit by an object). In children less than 15 years of age, 24% of all TBIs are related to blunt trauma.
   3. Motor vehicle accidents are the third leading cause of TBI (14%) and the second leading cause of TBI-related deaths (26%).
   4. 10% of TBIs are related to assaults. The majority (75%) of assaults associated with TBI occur in young adults ages 15–44 years.
   5. 19% of TBIs have other or unknown causes.
   6. Blasts are a leading cause of TBI in deployed military personnel (Defense and Veterans Brain Injury Center [DVBIC], 2014).

E. Pathophysiology
   1. Although some degree of irreversible damage occurs at the moment of impact (the primary injury), TBI is a process in which additional and progressive secondary and tertiary injury evolves over minutes, hours, and days after the injury (Huether & McCance, 2012).
   2. Primary brain injury
      a. Primary injury is damage to the brain that occurs at the moment of impact (Gennarelli & Graham, 2005). Involves neural injury, primary glial injury, and vascular responses (Huether & McCance, 2012)
      b. Acceleration and deceleration injuries are caused by changes in velocity, when the head moves rapidly and then stops abruptly, which causes strain on the brain tissue in the form of compression, tension, or shearing (Hickey, 2003b). They are associated with motor vehicle crashes, falls, and objects striking the head (Blank-Reid & Barker, 2002).
      c. Diffuse axonal injuries (DAIs)
         1) DAIs are caused by microscopic damage to neuronal axons; microscopic lesions are not seen on traditional computed tomography (CT) and conventional magnetic resonance imaging (MRI) scans; they may appear as small areas of hemorrhage (Flanagan, Cantor, & Ashman, 2008; Meythaler, Peduzzi, Eleftheriou, & Novack, 2001; Wasserman & Smirniotopoulos, 2012).
         2) Diffusion tensor imaging, a newer MRI technique, produces in vivo images of white matter tracts, allowing visualization of neural pathways to determine connectivity and assist in establishing the presence of DAI (Xu, Rasmussen, Lagopoulos, & Haberg, 2007).
         3) Destruction occurs in the cerebral hemispheres, corpus callosum, and brainstem; it is often seen in areas where brain densities differ, such as the junctions of gray and white matter.
         4) Severity depends on the magnitude of the acceleration forces involved in the traumatic event and usually is worse than what is noted on imaging studies (Wasserman & Smirniotopoulos, 2012).
         5) Physical consequences can include physical, cognitive, and behavioral problems.
            a) Paralysis, swallowing disorders, visual and hearing deficits
            b) Confusion, short attention span, poor judgment, memory deficits
            c) Agitation, impulsiveness, blunted affect, depression (Huether & McCance, 2012)

6) Classified as mild, moderate, or severe; about 45% of patients fall into the moderate category, with incomplete recovery in those who survive (Hickey, 2003b).

d. Focal injuries are damage resulting from a localized trauma, involving consolidated areas of tissue destruction such as contusions, lacerations, hematomas, and intracranial hemorrhages; symptoms vary according to type, extent, and location of injury (Hickey, 2003b).

3. Secondary brain injury
   a. A cascade of cellular and molecular processes triggered by the primary insult to the brain. Secondary brain injury can be preventable or at least treatable (Baxter & Wilson, 2012).
   b. Most secondary injury occurs in the first 12–24 hours after trauma but may occur up to 10 days after injury in very severe brain injury (Elovic, Baerga, & Cuccurullo, 2004).
   c. Causes (Blank-Reid & Barker, 2002; Huether & McCance, 2012; Povlishock & Katz, 2005)
      1) Cerebral edema
      2) Elevated intracranial pressure
      3) Hypoxia and ischemia
      4) Infection and inflammatory response
      5) Hypotension
      6) Electrolyte imbalance, hypocapnia
      7) Hyperthermia
      8) Vasospasm
      9) Decreased cerebral perfusion pressure
      10) Release of excitatory neurotransmitters such as glutamate and aspartate
   d. Postinjury complications (National Institute of Neurological Disorders and Stroke [NINDS], 2014c)
      1) Pain
      2) Infections
      3) Seizures
      4) Pressure ulcers
      5) Hydrocephalus
      6) Cerebrospinal fluid leaks
      7) Vascular injuries
      8) Cranial nerve injuries
      9) Multiple organ system failure
      10) Polytrauma
      11) Elevated intracranial pressure
      12) Altered hemodynamic states
      13) Herniation
      14) Respiratory complications
      15) Stress ulcers
      16) Deep vein thrombosis
4. Tertiary brain injury causes
   a. Ongoing inflammation
   b. Epigenetic changes
   c. Systemic complications that contribute to brain injury
      1) Infection
      2) Immobility (Huether & McCance, 2012)
      3) Social issues

F. Assessment
1. Classification
   a. Mild brain injury
      1) Description
         a) May result in an LOC for 30 or fewer minutes (National Center for Injury Prevention and Control [NCIPC], 2003)
         b) Glasgow Coma Scale (GCS) scores of 13–15 (BIAA, 2014; NCIPC, 2003) and negative neuroimaging (**Table 23-2**)
         c) Posttraumatic amnesia (PTA) less than 24 hours (DVBIC, 2010)
         d) A complicated mild brain injury has the same GCS score but with positive CT findings (Kennedy et al., 2006).
         e) About 75%–90% of TBIs are classified as mild (CDC, 2014).
      2) Symptoms may include dizziness, headache, insomnia, fatigue, decreased memory, irritability, confusion, vision changes, tinnitus, unpleasant taste, decreased concentration, and attention deficits (CDC, 2014; NINDS, 2014c).
      3) Most people will have a good recovery, but a minority will have ongoing problems.
         a) Tinnitus, visual changes, headache
         b) Balance problems
         c) Memory, judgment, impulsiveness
         d) Irritability, anger, violence
         e) Sleep disorders, posttraumatic stress disorder
   b. Moderate brain injury
      1) Description
         a) LOC more than 30 minutes but less than 24 hours (DVBIC, 2010)
         b) GCS scores ranging from 9 to 12 (BIAA, 2014; Department of Defense [DoD] and Veteran's Head Injury Program & Brain Injury Association of America, 1999; van Baalen et al., 2003)
         c) Posttraumatic amnesia 24 hours to 7 days (DVBIC, 2010)
         d) Abnormal CT findings
      2) May have a good recovery or learn to compensate for neurological deficits with proper treatment (Barker, 2002)
   c. Severe brain injury

Table 23-2. Glasgow Coma Scale Categories

Category	Response	Score
Eye opening	Spontaneous: Eyes open spontaneously without verbal or noxious stimulation.	4
	To speech: Eyes open with verbal stimuli but not necessarily to command.	3
	To pain: Eyes open with various forms of noxious stimuli.	2
	None: No eye opening with any type of stimulation.	1
Verbal response	Oriented: Aware of person, place, time, reason for hospitalization, and personal data.	5
	Confused: Answers not appropriate to question but correct use of language.	4
	Inappropriate words: Disorganized, random speech, no sustained conversation.	3
	Incomprehensible sounds: Moans, groans, and mumbles incomprehensibly.	2
	None: No verbalization, even to noxious stimuli.	1
Best motor response	Obeys commands: Performs simple tasks on command and able to repeat task on command.	6
	Localizes to pain: Organized attempt to localize and remove painful stimuli.	5
	Withdraws from pain: Withdraws extremity from source of painful stimuli.	4
	Abnormal flexion: Decorticate posturing that occurs spontaneously or in response to noxious stimuli.	3
	Extension: Decerebrate posturing that occurs spontaneously or in response to noxious stimuli.	2
	None: No response to noxious stimuli; flaccid.	1

From *Clinical practice of neurological and neurosurgical nursing* (4th ed.), by J. Hickey, 1996, Philadelphia: Lippincott Williams & Wilkins. Copyright 1996 by Lippincott WIlliams & Wilkins. Reprinted with permission.

1) Description
   a) LOC more than 24 hours (DoD and Veteran's Head Injury Program & Brain Injury Association of America, 1999)
   b) GCS scores lower than 8 (BIAA, 2014; van Baalen et al., 2003)
   c) Posttraumatic amnesia lasting longer than 7 days (DVBIC, 2010)
   d) May make significant improvements but often are left with permanent residual neurological deficits (DoD and Veteran's Head Injury Program & Brain Injury Association of America, 1999) (**Table 23-3**)
2) Severe brain injury results in disorders of consciousness (DOC), where there is a lack of awareness of self and the environment (Giacino et al., 2002; Giacino & Whyte, 2005). Twenty percent to 40% of people with DOC do not survive. As people recover from severe brain injury, they usually pass through various phases of recovery. Recovery can stop at any one of these phases. People with less severe injuries may transition through stages more rapidly and are likely to make better recoveries than people who had longer periods of unconsciousness (Sherer, Vaccaro, Whyte, Giacino, & the Consciousness Consortium, 2007).
   a) *Coma*: Complete absence of arousal or responsiveness
      (i) The eyes do not open spontaneously or in response to stimulation.
      (ii) Absent sleep–wake cycle
      (iii) No purposeful motor activity, distinct defensive movements, or localization to noxious stimuli
      (iv) No ability to follow commands, no intelligible verbalization
      (v) No conscious awareness of self or environment
   b) *Vegetative state*: No distinct evidence of conscious awareness of self or environment. About 50% of people who are in a vegetative state 1 month after TBI eventually recover consciousness.
      (i) Eyes open spontaneously.
      (ii) The sleep–wake cycle resumes; arousal is sluggish, poorly sustained.
      (iii) No signs of intentional, purposeful, or reproducible behavioral responses to stimuli
      (iv) No signs of language perception or communication
   c) *Minimally conscious state*: Distinct behavioral signs of conscious awareness as evidenced by at least one of the following:

(i) Basic command following
(ii) Intelligible verbalization
(iii) Yes–no responses, whether verbal or by gesture
(iv) Nonreflexive emotional or motor behavior that occurs in response to related environmental stimuli (e.g., affective responses to emotional content, object manipulation, pursuit eye movements)
(v) People in a minimally conscious state may do these things inconsistently.
(vi) Once a person can communicate, follow commands, or use an object consistently, they are no longer in a minimally conscious state (**Table 23-4**).

d) Locked-in syndrome
(i) Eye opening is present; eye movement is the primary mode of communication.
(ii) Basic cognitive function is evident on exam.
(iii) Clinical evidence of quadriplegia
(iv) Often occurs as a result of a lesion in the pons

e) *Akinetic mutism*: Condition characterized by diminished neurologic drive or inattention; movement and speech are extremely deficient.
(i) Eye opening and spontaneous visual tracking are present.
(ii) Can be considered a subcategory of minimally conscious state because purposeful responses often are inconsistent but can be elicited after application of stimulation

2. Assessment instruments and tools
a. Agitated Behavior Scale
1) Used for ongoing assessment of presence and intensity of agitation during the acute phase of recovery (Bogner, Corrigan, Bode, & Heinemann, 2000)
2) Composed of 14 items that are each rated from 1 (*absent*) to 4 (*present to an extreme degree*)
3) The best overall indicator for agitation is the total score, although subscales for disinhibition, aggression, and lability can be calculated (Corrigan & Bogner, 1994).

b. Coma/Near Coma (Rappaport, 2000, 2005)
1) Designed to expand the upper range of the Disability Rating Scale
2) Measures clinical changes in vegetative and persistent vegetative state
3) Has eight items grouped into five categories, ranging from extreme coma to no coma

Table 23-3. Classification of Brain Injury

Mild	LOC less than 30 minutes	GCS 13–15	PTA less than 24 hours
Complicated mild	LOC less than 30 minutes	GCS 13–15	PTA less than 24 hours Changes seen on CT scan
Moderate	LOC greater than 30 minutes but less than 24 hours	GCS 9–12	PTA 24 hours to 7 days
Severe	LOC greater than 24 hours	GCS 8 or less	PTA more than 7 days

Abbreviations. GCS, Glasgow Coma Scale; LOC, loss of consciousness; PTA, posttraumatic amnesia.

Data from Defense Centers of Excellence and Psychological Health and Traumatic Brain Injury & the Defense and Veterans Brain Injury Center, 2010; Defense and Veterans Brain Injury Center, 2014; National Center for Injury Prevention and Control (NCIPC), 2003.

Table 23-4. Comparison of Coma, Vegetative State, and Minimally Conscious State

	Coma	Vegetative State	Minimally Conscious State
Eye opening	No	Yes	Yes
Sleep-wake cycles	No	Yes	Yes
Visual tracking	No	No	Often
Object recognition	No	No	Inconsistent
Command following	No	No	Inconsistent
Communication	No	No	Inconsistent
Contingent emotion	No	No	Inconsistent

From *Facts About the Vegetative and Minimally Conscious States After Severe Brain Injury*, 2007, by M. Sherer, M. Vaccaro, J. Whyte, J. T. Giacino, and the Consciousness Consortium. Copyright 2007 by Model Systems Knowledge Translation Center (MSKTC). Retrieved from http://www.msktc.org/lib/docs/Factsheets/TBI_Vegetative_States_after_TBI.pdf. Reprinted with permission.

c. Coma Recovery Scale Revised (Giacino, Kalmar, & Whyte, 2004; Kalmar & Giacino, 2005)
   1) Designed to assess subtle changes in cognitive status and predict outcome in patients with severe disorders of consciousness
   2) Differentiates between vegetative and minimally conscious state

d. Disability Rating Scale
   1) Designed to quantitatively assess moderate to severe brain injury along a wide continuum of recovery, from severe vegetative state to no disability (Wright, 2000)
   2) Composed of eight items that are divided into four categories: arousability, cognitive ability for self-care, degree of dependence, and employability (Rappaport, 2005; van Baalen et al., 2003)

e. FIM™ (Grosswasser, Schwab, & Salazar, 1997; van Baalen et al., 2003)
   1) Constructed to provide a uniform measure of function across rehabilitation settings
   2) Measures items of self-care, sphincter control, mobility, locomotion, communication, and social cognition

f. Galveston Orientation and Amnesia Test: Used to measure the duration of posttraumatic amnesia after a brain injury (Levin, O'Donald, & Grossman, 1975; van Baalen et al., 2003)

g. Glasgow Coma Scale (see Table 23-2)
   1) Used to assess the level of consciousness and neurological functioning after a brain injury
   2) Categorized into three main assessment areas: motor, verbal, and eye-opening responses
   3) Is very useful in the acute care setting (Rosebrough, 1998)

h. Glasgow Outcome Scale (**Table 23-5**): Developed to assess general outcome after brain injury; categories include good recovery, moderate disability, severe disability, persistent vegetative state, and death (van Baalen et al., 2003)

i. Mayo Portland Adaptability Inventory (MPAI) (Malec, 2005)
   1) To assist in the clinical evaluation of people during the postacute (posthospital) period after acquired brain injury (ABI)
   2) To assist in the evaluation of rehabilitation programs designed to serve these people

j. Neurobehavioral Functioning Inventory (Kreutzer, Seel, & Marwitz, 1999)
   1) Used to assess the frequency of a variety of behaviors and symptoms that may occur after brain injury
   2) Composed of 76 items divided into six categories: depression, somatic, memory and attention, communication, aggression, and motor

k. Neuropsychological testing
   1) Refers to a variety of tests and test batteries that are used to measure cognitive function
   2) May include measures of attention, memory, concentration, reasoning, processing speed, and executive function (Girard et al., 1996)

l. Rancho Los Amigos Levels of Cognitive Functioning Scale: Used to interpret the cognitive recovery process after a brain injury (Duke Medicine, 2014) (**Table 23-6**)
   1) Levels range from 1 to 10; lower scores indicate a more severe impairment of consciousness.
   2) Hagen (personal communication, October 25, 2006) states that the Rancho Los Amigos Levels of Cognitive Function Scale was created as a team treatment scale.
   3) Patients will progress at different rates from level to level and may plateau (stop recovery) at any level of the scale.
   4) All members of the team help identify the factors that cause the patient to remain at his or her most common level of cognitive functioning, the factors that facilitate movement to higher levels, and the factors that cause regression so that appropriate interventions can be planned to support progression.

m. The Orientation Log (O-Log) (Novack, 2000)
   1) Developed to measure orientation to time, place, and circumstance in a rehabilitation population
   2) A 10-item serial assessment of orientation

n. Sensory Stimulation Assessment Measure: Designed to expand the GCS and used to standardize sensory presentation (Duff & Wells, 1997; O'Dell & Riggs, 1996; Rader, Alston, & Ellis, 1989)

o. Western Neuro Sensory Stimulation Profile
   1) Used to assess auditory and visual comprehension; tracking; object manipulation; and attention, arousal, tactile, and olfactory function
   2) Contains 33 items in six areas (Ansell & Keenan, 1989)

Table 23-5. Glasgow Outcome Scale

The Glasgow Outcome Scale (GOS) is a global scale for functional outcome that rates patient status into one of five categories: Dead, Vegetative State, Severe Disability, Moderate Disability or Good Recovery. The Extended GOS (GOSE) provides more detailed categorization into eight categories by subdividing the categoriesof severe disability, moderate disability and good recovery into a lower and upper cateogry: Table 1: Extended Glasgow Outcome Scale (GOSE)

1	Death	D
2	Vegetative state	VS
3	Lower severe disability	SD -
4	Upper severe disability	SD +
5	Lower moderate disability	MD -
6	Upper moderate disability	MD +
7	Lower good recovery	GR -
8	Upper good recovery	GR +

Use of the structured interview is recommended to facilitate consistency in ratings.

From *Structured interviews for the Glasgow Outcome Scale and the Extended Glasgow Outcome Scale: Guidelines for their use*, by J. T. L. Wilson, L. E. L. Pettigrew, & G. M. Teasdale, 1997. *Journal of Neurotrauma, 15*(8), 573–585. Copyright 1997 by *Journal of Neurotrauma*. Retrieved from www.tbi-impact.org/cde/mod_templates/12_F_01_GOSE.pdf. Reprinted with permission.

Secondary source: *Assessment of outcome after severe brain damage*, by B. Jennett & M. Bond, 1975. *Lancet, 1*(7905), 480–484.

3. Physical assessment
   a. General: Determine location of brain injury and corresponding symptoms (**Tables 23-7** and **23-8**)
   b. Neurologic
      1) Assess cognitive, motor, and sensory status, reflexes, and cranial nerves.
      2) Monitor anticonvulsant levels.
      3) Monitor for signs and symptoms of elevated intracranial pressure.
      4) Monitor changes in behavior (excesses and deficits).
      5) Monitor changes in level of consciousness.
      6) Monitor effects of medications prescribed for cognition and behavior (at present most of these are often used off label).
   c. Respiratory: Assess airway patency, oxygen saturation, nature of sputum, lung fields, and potential for aspiration.
   d. Cardiovascular: Assess blood pressure, pulse, heart rate, rhythm, risk for or existence of deep vein thrombosis, and risk factors for emboli (atrial fibrillation), presence of dysautonomia.
   e. Nutritional: Assess weekly weights, intake and output, daily hydration status, and dietary intake; anticipate the patient will have higher metabolic demands; modify the diet if dysphagia is present (e.g., use of thickener).
   f. Sensory and perceptual: Assess responses to various types of stimuli, sleep–wake cycles, level of consciousness, and presence of neglect.
   g. Elimination
      1) Assess bowel sounds and premorbid bowel patterns.
      2) Assess premorbid elimination history, urinary output, and bowel movements.
      3) Assess bowel and bladder continence and effectiveness of bowel and bladder programs (e.g., scheduled toileting programs, medications).
      4) Monitor for potential alterations in elimination (e.g., constipation, diarrhea, urinary tract infection, and retention).
   h. Musculoskeletal
      1) Assess for heterotopic ossification, orthopedic injuries, premorbid history of joint disease, contractures, tone, spasticity, range of motion (ROM), and need for adaptive equipment.
      2) Observe safety with transfers, gait, and mobility as appropriate.
      3) Assess handedness.
      4) Assess padding and positioning needs to maintain ROM.
   i. Integumentary: Assess skin condition (turgor, color, wounds, and high-risk places under pressure such as areas with orthotic devices).
   j. Communication: Assess for expressive, receptive, and global aphasias, dysarthria, and alternative communication strategies (e.g., augmentative communication devices).
   k. Behavior: Assess for behavior excesses (e.g., agitation, disinhibition, impulsivity, poor judgment, motor restlessness, perseveration, emotional lability) and deficits (e.g., apathy, poor initiation).
   l. Safety
      1) Assess for risk of falls, wandering, impulsivity, balance, strength, judgment, and insight.
      2) Assess need for least restrictive restraint or one-on-one sitter if necessary.
   m. Psychosocial: Assess family support, coping mechanisms, and potential response to fear and anxiety.
   n. Sexual: Assess function issues and related physical, cognitive, and behavioral alterations.
      1) Last menstrual period
      2) Pregnancy at time of admission
      3) Premorbid sexual problems
      4) Developmental stage
   o. Educational needs of patient and caregiver

Table 23-6. Rancho Los Amigos Levels of Cognitive Functioning Scale—Revised	
Cognitive Level	**Expected Behavior**
Level I No Response: Total assistance	Complete absence of observable change in behavior when presented visual, tactile, proprioceptive, vestibular, or painful stimuli.
Level II Generalized response: Total assistance	Demonstrates generalized reflex response to painful stimuli Responds to repeated auditory stimuli with increased or decreased activity Responds to external stimuli with physiological changes generalized, gross body movement and/or not purposeful vocalization Responses noted above may be the same regardless of type and location of stimulation Responses may be significantly delayed
Level III Localized response: Total assistance	Demonstrates withdrawal or vocalization to painful stimuli Turns toward or away from auditory stimuli Blinks when strong light crosses the visual field Follows a moving object passed within visual field Responds to discomfort by pulling tubes or restraints Responds inconsistently to simple commands Responses directly related to type of stimulus May respond to some people (especially family and friends) but not to others
Level IV Confused/agitated: Maximal assistance	Alert and in heightened state of activity Purposeful attempts to remove restraints or tubes or crawl out of bed May perform motor activities such as sitting, reaching and walking, but without any apparent purpose or upon another's request Very brief and usually nonpurposeful moments of sustained alternatives and divided attention Absent short-term memory May cry out or scream out of proportion to stimulus even after its removal May exhibit aggressive or flight behavior Mood may swing from euphoric to hostile with no apparent relationship to environmental events Unable to cooperate with treatment efforts Verbalizations are frequently incoherent and/or inappropriate to activity or environment
Level V Confused, inappro-priate non-agitated: Maximal assistance	Alert, not agitated, but may wander randomly or with a vague intention of going home May become agitated in response to external stimulation and/or lack of environmental structure Not oriented to person, place, or time Frequent, brief periods, nonpurposeful sustained attention Severely impaired recent memory, with confusion of past and present in reaction to ongoing activity Absent goal-directed, problem-solving, self-monitoring behavior Often demonstrates inappropriate use of objects without external direction May be able to perform previously learned tasks when structured and cues provided Unable to learn new information Able to respond appropriately to simple commands fairly consistently with external structures and cues Responses to simple commands without external structure are random and nonpurposeful in relation to the command Able to converse on a social, automatic level for brief periods of time when provided external structure and cues Verbalizations about present events become inappropriate and confabulatory when external structure and cues are not provided

continued

Table 23-6. Rancho Los Amigos Levels of Cognitive Functioning Scale—Revised (continued)	
Cognitive Level	**Expected Behavior**
Level VI Confused, appropriate: Moderate assistance	Inconsistently oriented to person, time, and place Able to attend to highly familiar tasks in nondistracting environment for 30 minutes with moderate redirection Remote memory has more depth and detail than recent memory Vague recognition of some staff Able to use assistive memory aid with maximum assistance Emerging awareness of appropriate response to self, family, and basic needs Moderate assist to problem solve barriers to task completion Supervised for old learning (e.g., self-care) Shows carryover for relearned familiar tasks (e.g., self-care) Maximum assistance for new learning with little or no carryover Unaware of impairments, disabilities, and safety risks Consistently follows simple directions Verbal expressions are appropriate in highly familiar and structured situations
Level VII Automatic, appropriate: Minimal assistance for daily living skills	Consistently oriented to person and place within highly familiar environments; moderate assistance for orientation to time Able to attend to highly familiar tasks in a nondistraction environment for at least 30 minutes with minimal assist to complete tasks Minimal supervision for new learning Demonstrates carryover of new learning Initiates and carries out steps to complete familiar personal and household routine but has shallow recall of what he/she has been doing Able to monitor accuracy and completeness of each step in routine personal and household activities of daily living (ADLs) and modify plan with minimal assistance Superficial awareness of his/her condition but unaware of specific impairments and disabilities and the limits they place on his/her ability to safely, accurately, and completely carry out his/her household, community, work, and leisure ADLs Minimal supervision for safety in routine home and community activities Unrealistic planning for the future Unable to think about consequences of a decision or action Overestimates abilities Unaware of others' needs and feelings Oppositional/uncooperative Unable to recognize inappropriate social interaction behavior

continued

Table 23-6. Rancho Los Amigos Levels of Cognitive Functioning Scale—Revised (continued)	
Cognitive Level	**Expected Behavior**
Level VIII Purposeful, appropriate: Stand-by assistance	Inconsistently oriented to person, time, and place
	Able to attend to highly familiar tasks in nondistracting environment for 30 minutes with moderate redirection
	Remote memory has more depth and detail than recent memory
	Vague recognition of some staff
	Able to use assistive memory aid with maximum assistance
	Emerging awareness of appropriate response to self, family, and basic needs
	Moderate assist to problem solve
	Consistently oriented to person, place, and time
	Independently attends to and completes familiar tasks for 1 hour in distracting environments
	Able to recall and integrate past and recent events
	Uses assistive memory devices to recall daily schedule and "to do" lists and record critical information for later use with stand-by assistance
	Initiates and carries out steps to complete familiar personal, household, community, work, and leisure routines with stand-by assistance and can modify the plan when needed with minimal assistance
	Requires no assistance once new tasks/activities are learned
	Aware of and acknowledges impairments and disabilities when they interfere with task completion, but requires stand-by assistance to take appropriate corrective action
	Thinks about consequences of a decision or action with minimal assistance
	Overestimates or underestimates abilities
	Acknowledges others' needs and feelings and responds appropriately with minimal assistance
	Depressed
	Irritable
	Low frustration tolerance/easily angered
	Argumentative
	Self-centered
	Uncharacteristically dependent/independent
	Able to recognize and acknowledge inappropriate social interaction behavior while it is occurring and takes corrective action with minimal assistance e barriers to task completion
	Supervised for old learning (e.g., self-care)
	Shows carryover for relearned familiar tasks (e.g., self-care)
	Maximum assistance for new learning with little or no carryover
	Unaware of impairments, disabilities, and safety risks
	Consistently follows simple directions
	Verbal expressions are appropriate in highly familiar and structured situations

continued

Table 23-6. Rancho Los Amigos Levels of Cognitive Functioning Scale—Revised (continued)

Cognitive Level	Expected Behavior
Level IX Purposeful, appropriate: Stand-by assistance on request	Independently shifts back and forth between tasks and completes them accurately for at least two consecutive hours Uses assistive memory devices to recall daily schedule and "to do" lists and record critical information for later use with assistance when requested Initiates and carries out steps to complete familiar personal, household, work, and leisure tasks independently and unfamiliar personal, household, work, and leisure tasks with assistance when requested Aware of and acknowledges impairments and disabilities when they interfere with task completion and takes appropriate corrective action, but requires stand-by assist to anticipate a problem before it occurs and take action to avoid it Able to think about consequences of decisions or actions with assistance when requested Accurately estimates abilities but requires stand-by assistance to adjust to task demands Acknowledges others' needs and feelings and responds appropriately with stand-by assistance Depression may continue May be easily irritable May have low frustration tolerance Able to self monitor appropriateness of social interaction with stand-by assistance
Level X Purposeful, appropriate: Modified independent	Able to handle multiple tasks simultaneously in all environments but may require periodic breaks Able to independently procure, create, and maintain own assistive memory devices Independently initiates and carries out steps to complete familiar and unfamiliar personal, household, community, work, and leisure tasks, but may require more than usual amount of time and/or compensatory strategies to complete them Anticipates impact of impairments and disabilities on ability to complete daily living tasks and takes action to avoid problems before they occur, but may require more than usual amount of time and/or compensatory strategies Able to independently think about consequences of decisions or actions but may require more than usual amount of time and/or compensatory strategies to select the appropriate decision or action Accurately estimates abilities and independently adjusts to task demands Able to recognize the needs and feelings of others and automatically respond in appropriate manner Periodic periods of depression may occur Irritability and low frustration tolerance when sick, fatigued, and/or under emotional stress Social interaction behavior is consistently appropriate

Rancho Los Amigos Levels of Cognitive Functioning Scale—Revised. Reprinted with permission. Original scale coauthored by Hagen, C., Malkmus D., Durham P. (2006). Communication Disorders Service, Rancho Los Amigos Hospital, 1972. Revised 1974 by Hagen, C., Malkmus, D., & Stenderup, K. Revised scale 1997 by Hagen, C.

1) Physical, psychosocial, and safety care
2) Preferred learning style
3) Barriers to learning
4) Readiness to learn

p. Vocational: Assess potential for returning to work, school, or other purposeful activity (e.g., volunteering).

G. Planning: Patient- and Family-Driven Goals

1. Set individualized goals upon admission.
   a. Bowel and bladder continence or established elimination schedules depending on cognition and level of consciousness
   b. Improved cognition
   c. Improved mobility
   d. Improved functional independence
   e. Improved safety (**Table 23-9**)
   f. Improved judgment
   g. Manageable behavior
   h. Increased knowledge to care for self or patient
   i. Resolution of medical problems
   j. Adequate nutritional status
   k. Community reintegration skills
2. Meet at regular intervals to evaluate status of goal achievement.
3. Coordinate the plan with a highly structured interdisciplinary team.
   a. Ensure consistency between providers (nurses, therapists, allied health professionals).

Table 23-7. Location of Injury and Associated Symptoms

Region of Brain	Symptoms
Frontal lobe	Impaired judgment, reasoning, concentration, abstraction, executive functions, behavior, and impulse control; expressive aphasia in dominant hemisphere (usually the left hemisphere); impaired voluntary motor function
Temporal lobe	Impaired somatic, auditory, olfactory, and visual association; receptive aphasia in dominant hemisphere (usually the left hemisphere); impaired learning and detailed memories such as past experiences, conversations, art, music, and taste
Parietal lobes	Impaired sensory association; impaired ability to recognize size, shape, texture, presence of touch, pressure, and body position; impaired recognition of own body parts (often called neglect)
Occipital lobe	Impaired visual perception and visual reflexes
Cerebellum	Impaired fine motor movement, balance, coordination
Brainstem	Abnormalities of cranial nerve function depending on location in brainstem; impaired cardiac, respiratory, and vasomotor function; wakefulness

Data from Barker, 2002; Hickey, 2003c.

Table 23-8. Cerebral Hemispheres and Symptoms

Right Hemisphere	Left Hemisphere
Motor impairment on left side of body	Motor impairments on right side of body
Impulsivity	Impaired speech and language; aphasias
Impaired judgment	Impaired comprehension
Impaired insight into condition (may not realize that deficits exist)	Cautious, slow to perform
Left-sided neglect	Aware of deficits, depression, anxiety
Spatial-perceptual deficits	Impaired right-left discrimination

Data from Barker, 2002.

b. Set interdisciplinary goals.
c. Monitor functional progress and performance.
d. Use predicted goal attainment to guide readiness for discharge and maximize performance.
e. Document coordination of team members and comprehensive care plan daily.

H. Nursing Plan of Care and Interventions for Cognitive Rehabilitation (**Table 23-10**)

I. Evaluation

1. Evaluate progress toward patient and family goals listed in Section G.
2. Use instruments described in Section F.2.

J. Discharge Planning and Community Resources

1. Discharge planning should begin before admission to the rehabilitation facility.
2. Discharge planning should incorporate extensive exploration of community resources for a lifetime of disability management.
   a. Financial resources
      1) Private insurance
      2) Auto insurance
      3) Medicare and Medicaid
      4) Social Security Disability Insurance
      5) Litigation awards
      6) Donations
   b. Continuum of care options
      1) Home
      2) Skilled nursing facilities
      3) Long-term care facilities
      4) Residential programs
      5) Day therapy programs
      6) Assisted living facilities
      7) Clubhouse programs
      8) Cognitive-based centers and neurobehavioral units
   c. Healthcare resources
      1) Home health services
      2) Outpatient programs
      3) Local hospital network
      4) Primary care provider
      5) Durable medical equipment (DME) supplier
      6) Telehealth programs
      7) State-level brain and SCI trust funds
   d. Community resources (for information)
      1) BIAA
      2) American Heart Association
      3) National Stroke Association
      4) Epilepsy Foundation of America
      5) Local library
      6) CDC
      7) DVBIC
      8) National Association of State Head Injury Administrators
      9) National Center for Medical Rehabilitation Research, National Institute of Child Health and Human Development, National Institutes of Health
      10) National Institute on Disability and Rehabilitation Research
      11) NINDS
      12) North American Brain Injury Society
      13) Social Security Administration

Table 23-9. Safety Tips

Don't	Do
Leave sharp objects within reach.	Provide the recommended supervision levels at home (as suggested by the rehabilitation team).
Leave poisons, chemicals, and household cleaners within reach.	Communicate with the client as an adult.
Leave car keys or keys to heavy equipment within reach.	Speak to the client in a regular tone of voice.
Leave the client alone near fire or heat sources (stove, barbecue, matches, lighters, cigarettes).	Praise small accomplishments and do so at the time of occurrence.
Assume the client has the same preinjury abilities or can resume his or her previous roles at home, at work, or in society.	Provide brain injury awareness information to the client's neighbors and fire and police departments.
Leave the client alone near bodies of water (ocean, lakes, swimming pools).	Provide structure and consistency of schedules.
Leave the client unattended and at risk for wandering, falls, or other injuries.	Provide a balance of stimulation and quiet time; recognize signs of impending escalation or fatigue.
Leave the client alone with heavy machinery.	Provide information on positive coping strategies regarding changes in family, work, and social roles.
Leave the client alone or in charge of small children until level of supervision or assistance is known.	Maintain a safe physical environment related to cognitive, behavioral, and physical changes.
Provide meal types or diet textures that are outside the prescribed plan of care.	Reintegrate the client into community activities as appropriate for his or her cognitive and behavioral level.
Overstimulate the client with a multitude of schedule changes, activities, or visitors.	Maintain diet type and texture to prevent aspiration.

From Traumatic Injuries: TBI and SCI by L. Dufour, J. Williams, & K. Coleman, in P. A. Edwards (Ed.), *The specialty practice of rehabilitation nursing: A core curriculum* (4th ed., p. 194). 2000, Glenview, IL: Association of Rehabilitation Nurses. Copyright 2000 by the Association of Rehabilitation Nurses.

14) State Department of Rehabilitation Services
15) Technology recycled equipment exchange programs
16) United Disabilities Services
17) Veterans Health Initiative: Traumatic Brain Injury

e. Assistive technology
1) Can come in many different forms, ranging from simple homemade devices such as ramps to complex computer-integrated systems
2) Pill holders with timed alarms
3) Alarmed wrist watches
4) Noise reduction headphones
5) Light switch dimmers
6) Augmentative communication device
7) Speed dial and memory options on communication devices
8) Voice recognition computer software programs
9) Screen readers or special computer screens, keyboards
10) Devices to assist with activities of daily living (ADLs) such as dressing, grooming, cooking
11) Smart phone applications used to provide exercises targeting memory, attention, speed, flexibility and problem solving
12) Virtual reality technology

K. Preventing TBI
1. Follow safety tips.
a. Always wear a seatbelt when driving or riding in a car.
b. Buckle children in an age-appropriate safety seat every time.
c. Wear headgear when indicated and ensure that children do so (e.g., during contact sports, horseback riding, skateboarding, skiing).
2. Avoid injuries in and around the home.
a. Eliminate slips and falls; use precautions and safety aids (e.g., step stools, grab bars, handrails, window guards, safety gates, nonslip mats, or shock-absorbing material).
b. Store firearms and bullets in different locked cabinets or safes (CDC, 2010a; NINDS, 2014c).

L. TBI Research
1. Aims of research efforts
a. From cellular to social systems
b. Prevention of TBI
c. Reducing TBI-related morbidity
d. Improving outcomes
2. Recent studies focus on new treatment approaches designed to address the different physiological, physical, behavioral, emotional, and cognitive needs of TBI populations (Flanagan, Cantor, & Ashman, 2008; Zitnay et al., 2008).
3. Increased national support for TBI research and care as a result of National Football League, high school sports injuries, and military conflicts in Iraq and Afghanistan

Table 23-10. Plan of Care for Cognitive Rehabilitation

Cognitive Level	Description	Nursing Management for Levels I, II, and III
I: No response	Unresponsive to touch, pain, or auditory or verbal stimuli	Orient client. Encourage family to bring in favorite music, pictures, blankets. Begin to talk to the client about family members and friends. Talk in a normal tone of voice and use short, simple phrases, explaining all nursing tasks. Be careful what you say in front of the client. Guide client to follow simple commands (wink, wiggle fingers). Allow extra time for a response. Introduce smells and tactile, auditory, and visual stimulation. Engage in familiar activities. Nursing assessments and physical care Monitor cardiovascular effects of pharmacological management (neurostimulants). Offer emotional support to family members. Talk to the client about familiar topics of interest, family, and close friends. Schedule nursing tasks to promote sleep-wake cycles. Begin family education; provide materials related to injury. Show family how to interact with the client; model behaviors; teach them not to overstimulate. Provide emotional support.
II: Generalized response	Displays inconsistent, nonpurposeful, reflexic responses to stimuli or pain	
III: Localized response	Responds in a more focused manner to certain types of stimuli (e.g., turns to sound, withdraws from pain, tracks); may follow simple commands inconsistently	

continued

4. In 2014 more than 600 active TBI-related clinical trials were being conducted in the United States.
5. Clinicaltrials.gov is a service of the National Institutes of Health and used as a registry and results database of TBI-related of clinical studies.
6. The Model Systems Knowledge Translation Center (MSKTC) has a TBI database that contains citations for studies conducted by the TBI Model Systems (2014), which is available to view at http://www.msktc.org/publications?sys=T.
7. The Acquired Brain Injury Knowledge Uptake Strategy (ABIKUS) Guideline is designed to provide evidence-based recommendations for the rehabilitation of people with moderate and severe ABI in the postacute period. The primary users of the ABIKUS Guideline are healthcare providers, and the target population for these recommendations is people with moderate and severe ABI. In most instances, these will be people with TBI (ABIKUS, 2011).
8. NINDS funds research on TBI. More information can be found at http://www.ninds.nih.gov/funding/funding_announcements/allcurrent.htm.
9. The CDC also funds TBI research (http://www.brainandspinalcord.org/research-traumatic-brain-injury/index.html).

M. Advanced Practice Considerations: Role of the Advanced Practice Nurse in TBI
   1. Educator
      a. Design a patient and family caregiver education curriculum to be used by rehabilitation nurses in inpatient and outpatient settings (e.g., behavior, safety, cognition and memory, seizures, medications, bowel and bladder, community reentry).
      b. Present professional papers and posters at national and international brain injury meetings.
      c. Coordinate or teach certification review material to facility staff to increase the numbers of certified rehabilitation nurses.
      d. Collaborate with academic institutions to place nursing students in brain injury rehabilitation practicums.
      e. Collaborate with community agencies and academic institutions to teach rehabilitation nursing care for the patient with TBI.
   2. Leader
      a. Collaborate with local and national legislators to advocate for people with TBI regarding rehabilitation benefit coverage, accessibility, community resources, and other funding issues.

Table 23-10. Plan of Care for Cognitive Rehabilitation (continued)		
Cognitive Level	**Description**	**Nursing Management for Level IV**
IV: Confused agitated	Alert and in heightened state of activity; possibly aggressive; may display inappropriate behavior in response to internal confusion; short attention span	Limit the number of visitors to two or three. Provide a quiet, calm, environment; eliminate "noise clutter" from the environment. Reorient frequently. Reassure the client that he or she is safe. Monitor sleep-wake cycles. Provide familiar objects or photos from home. Allow as much freedom of movement as is safe. Do nursing care in short blocks; take a break, then start the next task. Have a helper for safety. Low stimulation during care; explain care in simple terms, avoiding "chatter" Consider 1:1 supervision rather than restraints during certain times of day. Use quiet, low-traffic areas for activities that require attention (e.g., eating). Remove items that might be frightening to the client (TV or news). Use closed-circuit cameras for additional monitoring. Consider an enclosure bed. Do not force the client to do things. Instead, listen to what he or she wants to do and follow his or her lead, within safety limits. Give breaks to prevent agitation or restlessness. Look for patterns. Work with team on this. Change activities frequently; redirect as needed. Consider that the client has no short-term memory, so behavior plans with "consequences" typically don't work. Preventing agitation through control of the external environment and therapeutic use of self is key. Monitor pharmacological management, which may include antianxiety agents. Use structure; same staff, same routine, same way of doing things. Prevention is better than intervention.

continued

   b. Participate on local and state committees such as TBI trust funds (check your local area and state).
   c. Participate in your local chapter of ARN.
   d. Participate in national ARN committees; run for office.
3. Consultant
   a. Serve as a resource for clinical staff in inpatient and outpatient settings for complex patient care problems (assist with treating a complex wound, assess a patient's bowel problems, assist with strategies to facilitate cognitive and behavioral function, assist the case manager with discharge planning supplies related to nursing and medical care).
   b. Attend team conferences and offer information; collaborate with the rehabilitation team.
   c. Collaborate with external case managers regarding funding issues for brain injury rehabilitation stays.
   d. Collaborate with community service agencies serving people with TBI (and their caregivers) for the purpose of providing information and additional resources.
   e. Consult with community-based physicians about the care of their patients with TBI (for questions related to behavior, cognition, spasticity, and nutrition).
4. Researcher
   a. Maintain knowledge of current research findings and up-to-date evidence-based practices.
      1) Journal subscription
      2) Literature reviews
      3) Professional specialty organization membership

Table 23-10. Plan of Care for Cognitive Rehabilitation (continued)

Cognitive Level	Description	Nursing Management for Levels V and VI
V: Confused inappropriate (nonagitated)	Alert, easily distracted, responsive to commands; pays gross attention to environment; displays absent carryover from one situation to another	Use repetition. Reorient frequently to person, place, and time. Use short and simple comments and questions. Assist with activity initiation; set up. Show the client pictures and objects that were of interest before the injury. Provide frequent rest periods; collaborate with the therapy team on schedule. Limit the number of visitors. Monitor nutrition with increased activity. Establish bowel and bladder continence; start toileting programs. Provide tasks appropriate to level (e.g. hygiene, simple meal preparation—cold cereal). Identify areas of motivation for self-care tasks. Schedule rest and quiet time; fatigue or stress is common. Introduce memory aids (e.g., calendars, schedules); help with the schedule. Discuss events of the day to help improve memory. Monitor medication regimen; report sleep-wake, lethargy, agitation patterns to a physician. Begin to incorporate the client in the education process with family. Provide education to the client regarding injury and outcomes. Monitor for safety; it is still an important concern. Structure activities; staff should use a lot of cueing; the goal is for the client to "figure it out" with your help. Provide daily structure. Encourage participation in all therapies. Give immediate positive feedback. May start to use behavior plans with simple rewards.
VI: Confused appropriate	Follows commands consistently but is inconsistently oriented to time and place; has short-term memory deficits; begins to participate in self-care	

continued

4) Conference and lecture attendance
b. Collaborate with TBI researchers.
1) Data collection
2) Identifying subjects
3) Planning and conducting meaningful research
c. Formulate and share research questions based on clinical practice.
d. Attend TBI conferences to learn new knowledge that is not yet published.
e. Develop and maintain facility procedures based on current evidence-based clinical knowledge.
f. Critically evaluate current literature on TBI and apply appropriate findings to practice.

II. SCI

A. Definitions

1. *SCI*: Traumatic insult to the spinal cord resulting in alterations or complete disruption of normal motor, sensory, and autonomic function
2. *Tetraplegia* (replaced the term *quadriplegia*)
    a. Injury to one of the eight cervical segments of the spinal cord
    b. Impairment or loss of motor or sensory function in cervical segments, causing loss of function in all four extremities
3. *Paraplegia*
    a. Impairment or loss of motor or sensory function in the thoracic, lumbar, or sacral segments, causing impairment in trunk, legs, and pelvic organs
    b. Usually occurs as a result of injuries at T2 or below
4. Use of the terms *quadriparesis* and *paraparesis* is discouraged because they do not describe incomplete lesions completely.

B. The Vertebral Segments

1. Cervical vertebrae (7)
2. Thoracic vertebrae (12)
3. Lumbar vertebrae (5)
4. Sacral vertebrae (5)

Table 23-10. Plan of Care for Cognitive Rehabilitation (continued)		
Cognitive Level	**Description**	**Nursing Management for Levels VII and VIII**
VII: Automatic-appropriate	May perform tasks in familiar environment but in a robot-like manner; begins to have insight into deficits; continues to have poor judgment and problem-solving skills	The main goal is to promote reintegration into the community. Ask the client to remember more difficult things from day to day. Reduce environmental structure as necessary. Ask the client to solve problems he or she might encounter at home (e.g., "What would you do if you lost your keys to the house?"). Treat the client as an adult. Provide guidance and assistance in decision making. Encourage and allow the client to use his or her judgment, reasoning, and problem-solving skills within the home and safe community settings. Provide community outings to integrate client back into the social environment. Refer the client to community-based programs that support his or her condition. Encourage the use of memory aids such as note taking, calendars and schedules. Encourage independent functioning. Help the client to set reasonable goals for the future regarding education and employment. Discourage the use of alcohol and drugs. Help the client with conversations relating to social interaction and sexuality. Identify situations that make the client frustrated and discuss strategies for handling these situations. Help the client identify new roles within the family. Decrease barriers that contribute to isolation; transportation and esthetics.
VIII: Purposeful-appropriate	Consistently oriented; has correct responses; intact memory; needs supervision; has realistic planning skills	
Cognitive Level	**Description**	**Nursing Management for Levels IX and X**
IX: Purposeful-appropriate (standby assistance)	Client is aware and acknowledges impairments and disabilities when they interfere with tasks; initiates and carries out steps to complete familiar personal, household, work, and leisure tasks independently and unfamiliar personal, household, work, and leisure tasks with assistance when requested.	Provide breaks with multiple tasks. Continue to provide memory aids with "to do" lists for use with assistance on request. Standby assistance is needed to anticipate a problem before it occurs and to take action to avoid it. Stand-by assistance to adjust to task demands Monitor for depression, irritability, and frustration; counsel as needed; may recommend a neuropsychologist. Stand-by assist to monitor for appropriateness of social interaction Discuss consequences of decision making; the client may take more time than usual or use compensatory strategies to select the appropriate decision. Discuss feelings and needs of others and how to respond to them appropriately. Discourage drugs and alcohol. Discuss difficulties of living with brain injury; provide counseling, resources, and information about support organizations.

continued

5. Spinal cord segments correspond to muscles and associated movements.

C. Epidemiology (NSCISC, 2013)

1. Incidence of SCI
   a. Approximately 40 cases per million occur in the United States, or approximately 12,000 new cases per year
   b. No new overall incidence studies have been done in America since the 1990s.
   c. In the 1970s SCI occurred primarily in young adults 16–30 years of age.
   d. Over time, the median age of people with SCI in the United States has increased.
   e. Since 2005 the median age at injury has been 42.6 years (NSCISC, 2013).
   f. 11.5% of injuries are in those older than 60 years.
   g. 80.7% of those with SCI are male.

Table 23-10. Plan of Care for Cognitive Rehabilitation (continued)

Cognitive Level	Description	Nursing Management for Levels IX and X
X: Purposeful-appropriate (modified independent)	Independently initiates and carries out steps to complete familiar and unfamiliar personal, household, community, work, and leisure tasks, but may need more than the usual amount of time or compensatory strategies to complete them	Client is independent Monitor for depression. Monitor for irritability and low frustration tolerance when sick, fatigued, or under emotional stress. Encourage/support client and family. Encourage participation in a support group. Encourage counseling as needed. Follow up with a physician as needed (medications, outpatient therapy).

Data from Brain Injury Association of America, 2006; Braininjury.com, 2014a, 2014b; Dufour, Williams, & Coleman, 2000; Duke Medicine, 2014; Gatens & Hebert, 2001; Rosebrough, 1998.

h. Since 2010, 67% of SCI injuries have been among Caucasians, 24.4% among African Americans, 0.8% among Native Americans, 7.9% among Hispanics, and 2.1% among Asians.

2. Prognosis (NSCISC, 2013)
   a. Life expectancy after SCI is slightly shorter than normal with paraplegia, and for those with tetraplegia, life expectancy is shorter than that of people with paraplegia.
   b. Mortality rates are significantly higher in the first year after injury and among those who are older at the time of injury. For older patients, mortality rates are higher still in more complete injuries. Mortality rates are also higher for those older than 65 years who are ventilator dependent.
   c. 10%–20% of people with SCI do not survive.
   d. The higher the level of injury, the more negative the effect on life expectancy.
   e. Leading causes of death are pneumonia, pulmonary emboli, and septicemia. Pulmonary complications top the causes of morbidity and mortality because most people with SCI have some respiratory insufficiency (DeViVo & Chen, 2011).
   f. Neurological recovery is poor and the in-hospital mortality rate is high in patients older than 60 years with cervical injuries (Daneshvar et al., 2013).
   g. Recovery of ambulation is significantly lower when injury occurs in those who are older than 50 years of age (Burns, Golding, Rolle, Graziani, & Ditunno, 1997).

D. Etiology (NSCISC, 2013)
1. Motor vehicle accidents account for 36.5% of SCI.
2. Falls account for 28.5% of SCI; they are more common in those older than age 45 years.
   a. The rate of SCI from falls continues to increase steadily as the U.S. population ages.
   b. More than 50% of cervical fractures in those older than 65 years are caused by low-impact mechanisms such as a fall from standing (Pickett, Campos-Benitez, Keller, & Duggal, 2006).
3. Violence accounts for 14.3% of SCI since 2010, after peaking in the 1990s.
4. Sports and recreational injuries account for 9.2%; diving is the most common sport associated with SCI.
5. Other
   a. Tumors
   b. Abscess and infection
   c. Injuries after procedures such as spinal injections or epidural catheter placement
   d. Vertebral fractures
   e. Infarct

E. SCI and the Older Adult
1. Risk factors associated with new SCI in the older person include the following:
   a. Bone changes or arthritis
   b. Higher rate of spinal stenosis
   c. Higher risk for falls
   d. Higher risk of car accidents per miles driven
2. The leading cause of SCI in older adults is falls (Selvarajah et al., 2014).
3. Neurological recovery poor and in-hospital mortality rate high in patients aged 60 or older with a cervical spine injury (Daneshvar et al., 2013).

F. Mechanisms of Injury and Associated Common Abnormalities
1. Direct trauma
   a. Flexion
      1) Occurs when head is thrown violently forward
      2) Occurs when head is struck from behind
      3) Occurs commonly in motor vehicle accidents and falls

b. Flexion with rotation: Occurs when the combination of forces causes severe twisting, resulting in ruptured ligaments and dislocation
c. Hyperextension: Occurs in forward falls in which the face or chin is struck
d. Penetration: Injuries that directly pierce the spinal cord (e.g., gunshot wound, knife wound)

2. Compression
   a. Flexion: Axial
      1) Occurs when vertebral bodies are wedged and compressed
      2) Occurs in the thoracic and lumbar region
      3) Caused by a fall onto the buttocks
   b. Vertical
      1) Occurs when vertebral bodies are shattered and burst into the spinal cord
      2) Typically occurs in the cervical region
      3) Caused by a high-velocity blow to the top of the head (e.g., diving)
   c. Ischemia (spinal cord stroke) (Kamin, 2011; NINDS, 2014b)
      1) Rare
      2) Mechanism unknown
      3) Surgery on aorta puts person at risk

G. Pathophysiology
1. Varying degrees of damage associated with SCI
   a. Severity of bony injury does not always correspond to the extent of neurological impairment.
   b. Common sites of injury—the cervical and thoracolumbar junctures—are the most mobile parts of the spine.
   c. The spinal cord itself may sustain contusion without vertebral fractures or dislocations.
   d. The most common levels of injury in the neck are C4 and C5 and T11 and T12 in the back (Young, 2014).
   e. Progressive tissue destruction occurs in the cord within hours and may involve several responses.
      1) Decrease of microperfusion at site of the injury
      2) Hemorrhage in the gray matter
      3) Development of hematoma and edema
      4) Release of biochemicals at site of injury
      5) Ischemia and necrosis in the cord, secondary chemical cascade causing neurological damage
   f. Clinical presentations include
      1) Spinal shock
         a) Temporary state of reflex depression of cord function occurring after injury
         b) Initial increase in blood pressure
         c) Flaccid paralysis, including bowel and bladder
         d) Lasts several hours to days
      2) Neurogenic shock
         a) Characterized by hypotension, bradycardia, hypothermia
         b) More common in injuries above T6
         c) Need to differentiate between spinal and hypovolemic shock

2. Levels of SCI
   a. Upper motor neuron (UMN) injury
      1) Is evident in lesions above T12–L1 vertebrae
      2) Causes loss of cerebral control over all reflex activity below the level of lesion
      3) Causes spastic paralysis
      4) UMNs lie within the spinal cord.
   b. Lower motor neuron (LMN) injury
      1) Is evident in lesions below T12–L1 level (i.e., conus medullaris, cauda equina)
      2) Causes destruction of the reflex arc
      3) Causes flaccid paralysis
      4) LMNs branch off from the spinal cord.

3. Classifications of incomplete SCI or clinical syndromes (Kirshblum, Anderson, Krassiokov, & Donovan, 2011)
   a. Central cord syndrome: 50% of incomplete injuries and 9% of traumatic SCI
      1) Caused by damage to the central part of the cord
      2) Usually is in the cervical region
      3) Produces loss of motor power and sensation that affects upper limbs more than lower limbs
      4) Produces sacral sparing
   b. Brown-Séquard syndrome: 2%–4% of traumatic SCI
      1) Caused by damage to one side (hemisection) of the cord
      2) Produces loss of motor function and position sense on the same side as the damage and a loss of pain, temperature sensation, and light touch on the opposite side
   c. Anterior cord syndrome: 2.7% of traumatic SCI
      1) Caused by damage to the anterior artery, affecting the anterior two thirds of the cord
      2) Produces paralysis and loss of pain and temperature sensation below the lesion with preservation of position sense
   d. Conus medullaris syndrome

1) Caused by damage to the conus and lumbar nerve roots
2) May produce areflexia (flaccidity) in bladder, bowel, and lower limbs

e. Cauda equina syndrome
1) Caused by damage below conus to lumbar-sacral nerve roots
2) May produce areflexia in bladder, bowel, and lower limbs

H. Assessment (Kirshblum, Burns, Biering-Sorensen, Donovan, et al., 2011)

1. Classification: To be motor incomplete, an SCI must be incomplete (sacral sparing) and have either voluntary anal sphincter contraction or motor function preserved more than three levels below the motor level.

a. Skeletal level of injury: The level at which, by radiographic examination, the greatest vertebral damage is found
1) Stable injury: Occurs when the bone or ligaments support the injured cord area, preventing progression of neurological deficit
2) Unstable injury: Occurs when the bone and ligaments are disrupted and unable to support and protect the injured cord area, possibly causing further neurological deficit

b. Neurological level of injury: The most caudal segment of the spinal cord with normal sensory and antigravity motor function on each side of the body
1) Sensory level
a) Refers to the most caudal segment of the spinal cord with normal sensory function on each side of the body
b) Evaluated at a key sensory point within each of 28 dermatomes on the right and 28 dermatomes on the left side of the body
2) Motor level (**Table 23-11**)
a) Best predictor of a person's functional abilities (McKinley & Silver, 2013)
b) Refers to the most caudal segment of the spinal cord with normal motor function on each side of the body
c) Evaluated at a key muscle within each of 10 myotomes on the right and 10 myotomes on the left side of the body

c. Complete injury: An absence of motor and sensory function in the lowest sacral segment

d. Incomplete injury
1) Results in partial preservation of sensory or motor function below the neurological level and includes the lowest sacral segment
2) Includes sacral sensation at the anal mucocutaneous junction and deep anal pressure
3) Includes motor function of voluntary contraction of the external anal sphincter upon digital examination

e. Zone of partial preservation
1) Consists of the dermatomes and myotomes that are caudal to the neurological level and remain partially innervated
2) Term used only with complete injuries (e.g., a person with a complete C5 injury may have patchy sensation at C6 or C7 but not have any anal reflexes, such as sacral sparing, and thus still be classified as a complete C5 injury)

2. Assessment instruments and tools

a. Assessing impairment: International Standards for Neurological Classification of SCI (ISNCSCI) (Kirshblum et al., 2011; www.ASIA-spinalinjury.org)
1) Frequently used scale that reflects severity of impairment
2) Modified version of the ASIA scale that was built on the Frankel Grading System for SCI
3) Levels of ISNCSCI scale
a) A = Complete: No sensory or motor function is preserved in S4–S5.
b) B = Incomplete: Sensory function (but not motor function) is preserved below the neurological level and extends through S4–S5.
c) C = Incomplete: Motor function is preserved below the neurological level; the majority of muscles below the level are grade 3 or lower.
d) D = Incomplete: Motor function is preserved below the neurological level; the majority of muscles below the level are grade 3 or higher.
e) E = Normal: Normal sensory and motor function.

b. Motor grading scale (Kirshblum et al., 2011): The strength of each muscle is graded on a six-point scale.
1) 0 = Total paralysis
2) 1 = Palpable or visible contraction of the muscle
3) 2 = Active movement: Full ROM with gravity eliminated
4) 3 = Active movement: Full ROM against gravity

5) 4 = Active movement: Full ROM against gravity and moderate resistance in a muscle specific position
6) 5 = Normal active movement, less than full ROM against gravity and sufficient resistance to be considered normal if identified inhibiting factors not present

c. Sensory impairment scale scores (Kirshblum et al., 2011)
1) 0 = Absent
2) 1 = Altered (impaired or partial appreciation, including hyperesthesia)
3) 2 = Normal, or intact (similar as on the cheek)
4) NT = Not testable

d. Other: Spinal Cord Independence Measure (SCIM) assesses 16 categories of self-care, mobility, and respiratory and sphincter function; Quadriplegic Index of Function (QIF) detects slight changes in ADLs among those with tetraplegia; Modified Barthel Index is a 15-item measure of self-care and mobility. The International SCI Pain Basic Data Set (version 2.0) is a shortened tool for measuring pain following SCI (Widerstron-Noga et al., 2014). There are multiple other tools to assist in the functional assessment of people with SCI (SCIRE, 2014).

3. Physical assessment
a. Neurologic
1) Assess cognitive, motor, and sensory status, reflexes, and cranial nerves.
2) Monitor for signs and symptoms of increase or decrease in function, pain, and abnormal sensations.

b. Respiratory: Assess breath sounds, airway patency, oxygen saturation, diaphragm

Table 23-11. Neurological Levels and Functional Potential

Level	Abilities	Functional Goals
C1–C3	Limited movement of head and neck	Breathing: Depends on a ventilator or implant to control breathing.
		Communication: Talking is sometimes difficult, very limited or impossible. If ability to talk is limited, communication can be accomplished independently with a mouth stick and assistive technologies like a computer for speech or typing. Effective verbal communication allows the individual with SCI to direct caregivers in the person's daily activities, like bathing, dressing, personal hygiene, transferring as well as bladder and bowel management.
		Daily tasks: Assistive technology allows for independence in tasks such as turning pages, using a telephone and operating lights and appliances.
		Mobility: Can operate an electric wheelchair by using a head control, mouth stick, or chin control. A power tilt wheelchair also for independent pressure relief.
C4	Usually has head and neck control. Individuals at C4 level may shrug their shoulders.	Breathing: May initially require a ventilator for breathing; usually adjust to breathing full time without ventilator assistance.
		Communication: Normal, may have weaker voice projection
		Daily tasks: With specialized equipment, some may have limited independence in feeding and independently operate an adjustable bed with an adapted controller.
C5	Typically has head and neck control, can shrug shoulder and has shoulder control. Can bend his/her elbows and turn palms face up.	Daily tasks: Independence with eating, drinking, face washing, brushing of teeth, face shaving and hair care after assistance in setting up specialized equipment.
		Health care: Can manage their own health care by doing self-assist coughs and pressure reliefs by leaning forward or side -to-side.
		Mobility: May have strength to push a manual wheelchair for short distances over smooth surfaces. A power wheelchair with hand controls is typically used for daily activities. Driving may be possible after being evaluated by a qualified professional to determine special equipment needs.
C6	Has movement in head, neck, shoulders, arms and wrists. Can shrug shoulders, bend elbows, turn palms up and down and extend wrists.	Daily tasks: With help of some specialized equipment, can perform with greater ease and independence, daily tasks of feeding, bathing, grooming, personal hygiene and dressing. May independently perform light housekeeping duties.
		Health care: Can independently do pressure reliefs, skin checks and turn in bed.
		Mobility: Some individuals can independently do transfers but often require a sliding board. Can use a manual wheelchair for daily activities but may use power wheelchair for greater ease of independence.
C7	Has similar movement as an individual with C6, with added ability to straighten his/her elbows.	Daily tasks: Able to perform household duties. Need fewer adaptive aids in independent living.
		Health care: Able to do wheelchair push-ups for pressure reliefs.
		Mobility: Daily use of manual wheelchair. Can transfer with greater ease.

continued

Table 23-11. Neurological Levels and Functional Potential (continued)

Level	Function	Potential
C8–T1	Has added strength and precision of fingers that result in limited or natural hand function.	Daily tasks: Can live independently without assistive devices in feeding, bathing, grooming, oral and facial hygiene, dressing, bladder management and bowel management. Mobility: Uses manual wheelchair. Can transfer independently.
T2–T6	Has normal motor function in head, neck, shoulders, arms, hands and fingers. Has increased use of rib and chest muscles, or trunk control.	Daily tasks: Should be totally independent with all activities. Mobility: A few individuals are capable of limited walking with extensive bracing. This requires extremely high energy and puts stress on the upper body, offering no functional advantage. Can lead to damage of upper joints.
T7–T12	Has added motor function from increased abdominal control.	Daily tasks: Able to perform unsupported seated activities.
L1–L5	Has additional return of motor movement in the hips and knees.	Mobility: Walking can be a viable function, with the help of specialized leg and ankle braces. Lower levels walk with greater ease with the help of assistive devices.
S1–S5	Depending on level of injury, there are various degrees of return of voluntary bladder, bowel and sexual functions.	Mobility: Increased ability to walk with fewer or no support devices.

From *Rehabilitation functional goals*, by Spinal Injury Network. (2014). Retrieved from www.spinal-injury.net/rehabilitation-goals-sci.htm. Copyright by Spinal Injury Network. Reprinted with permission.

movement, nature of sputum and potential for aspiration, and potential for pulmonary emboli.

c. Cardiovascular: Assess blood pressure, pulse, heart rate, rhythm, edema, deep vein thrombosis, and signs and symptoms of orthostatic hypotension.

d. Nutritional
   1) Assess weekly weight, daily hydration status, and dietary intake.
   2) Monitor complete blood cell count, electrolytes, albumin, and prealbumin levels for anemia, electrolyte imbalance, and nutritional status.

e. Elimination
   1) Assess abdomen for tenderness, distention, masses, and bowel sounds, premorbid and current bowel patterns, current bladder program; assess urine for color, odor, clarity, and amount.
   2) Review effectiveness of bowel and bladder programs. Modify programs as patterns become evident.

f. Musculoskeletal: Assess for swelling, spasticity, ROM, tone, contractures, orthopedic injuries, and heterotopic ossification.

g. Integumentary
   1) Assess the entire body, especially bony prominences, for skin breakdown, redness, warmth, and blanching.
   2) Assess and record size, appearance, and location of any skin breakdown. Staging of a wound should be based on National Database of Nursing Quality Indicator Standards (www.ndnqi.org).
   3) Assess knowledge and practices to prevent skin breakdown.
      a) Turns
      b) Weight shifts every 15–30 minutes lasting 30–90 seconds while in chair (MSKTC, 2009)
      c) Adequate protein in diet

h. Psychosocial: Assess family support, coping mechanisms, adjustment to disability, and potential response to fear and anxiety; monitor for suicidal ideation.

i. Sexual
   1) Assess level of injury in relation to physical capabilities, emotional state, and behavior consistent with denial, anger, or depression.
   2) Assess the current home situation including presence of significant other or spouse, children, and history of birth control practices (if applicable).

I. Planning

1. Setting goals (Byrnes et al., 2012)
   a. Goals should be developed with the patient's strengths and limitations in mind, with consideration of access and resources (comprehensive assessment followed by patient focused goal setting).
   b. Rehabilitation goals should be directed toward helping the patient achieve and maintain

maximum independence and safe performance of self-care activities.

c. Patient involvement in goal setting is fundamental.

d. Goal planning is useful in improving physical, social, and psychological functioning of the patient with SCI.

e. Family involvement with goals from the beginning can influence the success of the patient's rehabilitation.

f. Support and instructions from rehabilitation team members can help the family assist the patient in achieving maximum independence throughout life.

2. Functional outcomes of SCI (see Table 23-11) (www.spinal-injury.net/rehabilitation-goals-SCI.htm)

J. Interventions

1. In the acute phase, interventions emphasize spinal stability, preservation of life, and prevention of complications (Consortium for Spinal Cord Medicine, 2001)

   a. Spinal stability

      1) Use log rolling; avoid twisting.

      2) Surgery may be needed to stabilize the spine (i.e., spinal fusion).

      3) Various orthotics may be used depending on the level of the injury; the name of the brace indicates the part of the spine it immobilizes (Kulkarni, 2013).

         a) Halo brace or cervical tongs immobilize the cervical spine; the halo brace is skeletal traction that provides maximal restriction of movement for those with cervical or high thoracic injuries (to T3).

         b) Cervical collars are used commonly during surgical treatments. However, patients must still observe spinal precautions.

         c) A sternal occipital mandibular immobilizer brace is used in minimally unstable fractures; it allows greater movement than the halo brace but must be fitted correctly; it is ideal for bedridden patients.

         d) Thoracic lumbar sacral orthosis

         e) Thoracolumbar orthosis is used to treat T10–L2 fractures.

         f) Lumbar sacral orthosis stabilizes L1–L4.

      4) Immobilizers often are worn for about 3 months to allow the spine to heal. Physician practices vary as to whether they require bracing at all times, only when out of bed, or not at all.

      5) Emphasize the purpose of immobilization to allow time for healing and prevent further injury that could result in more damage to the spinal cord.

   b. Prevention of secondary complications

      1) Chronic complications of SCI (Abrams & Wakasa, 2014)

         a) Autonomic dysreflexia

         b) Coronary artery disease

         c) Pulmonary complications

         d) Bladder dysfunction: Urinary tract infections, urinary and renal calculi, kidney reflux, renal insufficiency

         e) Sexual dysfunction

         f) Gastrointestinal complications: Constipation, hemorrhoids

         g) Osteoporosis, vitamin D deficiency

         h) Heterotrophic ossification

         i) Contractures

         j) Pressure ulcers

         k) Spasticity: Oral meds versus intrathecal Baclofen Botox

         l) Pain: neuropathic, musculoskeletal

         m) Neurologic deterioration: Syringomyelia, progressive posttraumatic myelomalacic myelopathy

         n) Psychiatric: Depression, suicide, drug addiction, divorce

      2) In older adults the following are more likely (Krassioukov, Furlan, & Fehlings, 2003)

         a) Infections

         b) Psychiatric disorders

         c) Pressure sores

         d) Cardiovascular problems

2. Interventions are determined with the patient and family's input to promote maximum health, independence, and safety.

3. Interventions may involve teaching the patient and family about the problem-solving process, providing adaptive devices as necessary, and educating the patient and family about safe and effective performance of skills.

4. Rehabilitation nurses must encourage the patient and family to work toward achieving goals and to continue to perform goals that have already been accomplished.

5. Additional suggestions for patient care (Hickey, 2003a)

   a. Establish a therapeutic nurse–patient relationship.

   b. Cultivate a climate of trust.

c. Allow the patient to verbalize feelings.
d. Accept the patient's behavior without being judgmental.
e. Let the patient know it will take time to adjust to the disability.
f. Answer questions, referring those you are unable to answer to the appropriate source.
g. Document emotional and psychological reactions in the chart.
h. Incorporate steps for meeting the emotional and psychological needs of the patient into the care plan.
i. Promote a good self-concept and body image by encouraging the patient to use good grooming habits.
j. Use team conferences to discuss the patient's emotional and psychological status.
k. Involve the patient in the decision-making process related to his or her care to foster a feeling of self-control.
l. Address the following concerns expressed by people with SCI in an honest but hopeful manner:
   1) Anticipation of functional return to normal
   2) Prognosis for ambulation
   3) Sexual dysfunction
   4) Pain
   5) Impaired bowel and bladder function
   6) Financial difficulties
   7) Loss of independence; role reversal
   8) Anxiety
m. Adapt strategies for older patients with SCI that optimize the length of stay and provide resources after discharge (Scivoletto, Morganti, Ditunno, Ditunno, & Molinari, 2003).
n. Address the needs of the family caregiver, particularly in the following areas (Lindsey, 1998):
   1) Negative attitudes toward the person with SCI
   2) Feelings of guilt
   3) Frustration at lack of appreciation from the patient
   4) Loss of alone time
   5) Feeling overwhelmed
   6) Setting boundaries in the relationship of caregiving

6. Nursing plan of care (**Table 23-12**).

K. Evaluation

1. Use assessment tools
2. Residual deficits and systemic dysfunction that may occur after SCI (Abrams & Wakasa, 2014)
   a. Neurological manifestations
      1) Loss or decrease of voluntary motor function below level of injury
      2) Loss or decrease of sensation
      3) Loss of normal reflex activity
      4) Autonomic dysfunction caused by loss of normal sympathetic nervous system functioning
      5) Autonomic dysreflexia or hyperreflexia (Stephenson, Berliner, & Klein, 2013; Wan & Krassioukov, 2014)
         a) A medical emergency
         b) Occurs in 48%–90% of those with injuries at or above T6, especially cervical injuries; rare occurrences in injuries as low as T10
         c) More common in males than females (4:1)
         d) Caused by stimulation below the level of injury, often in the area of the sacral segments or lower, such as overdistended bladder, fecal impaction, decubitus ulcers, urological procedures, pregnancy and delivery, gynecological procedures, ingrown toenails, fractures, restrictive shoes or clothing, deep vein thrombosis, sexual activity, and kidney stones
         e) Characterized by hypertension, bradycardia, flushing and perspiration above the level of the lesion, gooseflesh above the level of the lesion, nasal congestion, and an impending sense of doom
         f) Blood pressure 20–40 mmHg above the patient's normal baseline may indicate autonomic dysreflexia.
         g) Treatment involves reducing the causing stimulus (e.g., empty the bladder) and lowering blood pressure by raising the head of the bed and administering appropriate medications.
         h) Untreated, can result in stroke, seizures, coma, pulmonary edema, or death
         i) Many episodes can be prevented with good bowel and bladder care and prevention of pressure ulcers.
      6) Hypotension
      7) Loss of thermoregulation
      8) Loss of vasomotor tone or control
   b. Cardiovascular manifestations
      1) Hypotension and vasodilation, causing decreased cardiac output
         a) Orthostatic hypotension: Rapid drop in blood pressure when the erect position

is assumed; patients with cervical or high thoracic injury have poor vasomotor control, so there is difficulty getting blood out of the lower extremities and back to the heart.

b) Vasodilation: Results from loss of sympathetically induced vasoconstriction, which triggers pooling of blood in abdomen and lower extremities

2) Bradycardia is caused by unopposed vagal tone (10th cranial nerve).

3) Impaired temperature regulation (poikilothermia), a condition in which the body assumes the environmental temperature because of the inability to sweat or shiver below the injury

4) Cardiac dysrhythmias, which usually appear in the first few weeks and are more common in severe injuries

5) Blood clots (risk is three times higher than in a person without SCI)

c. Respiratory manifestations

1) Injury above C4: Results in paralysis of respiratory muscles, including the diaphragm; the patient is dependent on a ventilator. Avoid saline installation into ventilated patients without a working diaphragm; evidence shows this is a harmful and outdated intervention.

2) Injury between C4 and T6: Results in paralysis of the intercostal and abdominal muscles; the patient usually is weaned from the ventilator but needs aggressive pulmonary management.

3) Injury between T6 and T12: Results in paralysis of some abdominal muscles; the patient does not need a daily respiratory program unless an upper respiratory infection is present.

4) Pneumonia is a common complication; intubation increases the risk of ventilator-acquired pneumonia (VAP), which accounts for about 25% of deaths (NINDS, 2014b). Oral hygiene minimizes VAP.

d. Metabolic and musculoskeletal manifestations

1) Negative nitrogen balance

2) Decreased basal metabolic rate and expenditure of energy

3) Hypercalcemia or hypercalciuria

4) Altered secretion of pituitary-derived hormones

5) Heterotopic ossification

6) Contractures

7) Muscle spasms

Table 23-12. Summary of the Collaborative Management of Multisystem Problems in the Acute Phase After Spinal Cord Injury

System-Specific Considerations	Patient Problems/Nursing Diagnosis and Collaborative Problems	Assessment and Monitoring Data	Management and Interventions
Neurological system			
The level and pattern of neurological loss depends on the level of injury and need to be assessed and monitored for change; change can result from extension of injury or ascending edema. As a result of spinal shock,many motor, sensory, and reflex functions are lost. Many specific deficits are listed under the body system that they primarily affect. Hypothermia and orthostatic hypotension are commonly seen in the acute phase. The patient who is tetraplegic is completely dependent on the care provider for self-care and mobility. Often a cerebral concussion was also sustained at the time of injury; often memory isi mpaired for the circumstance of injury.	**Patient problems/Nursing diagnoses** • Risk for altered body temperature • Hypothermia • Knowledge deficit • Impaired memory • Pain, acute • Impaired physical mobility • Self-care deficit, complete • Self-care deficit, instrumental • Sensory/perceptual alterations • Sexual dysfunction • Sleep pattern disturbance • Impaired swallowing • Risk for injury **Collaborative problems** • Increased intracranial pressure if also sustained a brain injury	**Clinical data** • Assess baseline and monitor highest sensory level, motor function, and reflexes. • Monitor vital signs. • Assess baseline and monitor routine neurological signs for evidence of a concomitant brain injury. **Laboratory data** • Magnetic resonance imaging (MRI) or computed tomography (CT) scan • Plain X-rays of spine	Provide for total care needs of patient. Make sure that the patient is on the right type of bed based on the stability of the fracture and personal characteristics of the patient, such as weight. Provide information to patient and family as requested; recognize that information will need to be repeated because of inability to comprehend fully the impact of the injury. Be alert for decreased neurological function as a result of edema.

continued

Table 23-12. Summary of the Collaborative Management of Multisystem Problems in the Acute Phase After Spinal Cord Injury (continued)

System-Specific Considerations	Patient Problems/Nursing Diagnosis and Collaborative Problems	Nursing Management	Level of Injury
Respiratory system			
The probability of certain respiratory complications decreases the lower the injury because the diaphragm and intercostals are spared. Patients who cannot cough or manage their own secretions need a special respiratory management program. Cervical surgery (both the procedure itself and the associated anesthesia) increases the risk of postoperative respiratory complications; thus, an optimal time for surgery (when the respiratory system is in the best condition possible) is recommended. Other risk factors contributing to altered respiratory function include immobilization, bed rest, smoking; preexisting pulmonary disease (e.g., chronic obstructive pulmonary disease), concurrent chest trauma (e.g., fractured ribs, contused lungs), anemia, and gastric distention or paralytic ileus. Gastric distention may be associated with vomiting, aspiration, and compromised lung expansion. Alert: Ascending edema can rapidly cause respiratory difficulty that requires immediate intervention; monitor rate and pattern frequently.	**Patient problems/Nursing diagnoses** • Ineffective airway clearance • Risk for aspiration • Ineffective breathing pattern • Impaired gas exchange • Inability to sustain spontaneous ventilation • Risk for respiratory infection • Risk for altered respiratory function **Collaborative problems** • Hypoxemia • Atelectasis, pneumonia • Pneumothorax • Respiratory arrest	**Clinical data** • Determine baseline respiratorystatus. (Auscultate chest; note breathing pattern; assess the patient's ability to cough and deep breathe effectively.) **Laboratory data** • Chest x-ray studies • Blood gas levels • Complete blood count (CBC) • Sputum cultures • Pulmonary function studies (e.g, vital capacity)	Provide chest physical therapy (PI) and deep breathing exercises every 2-4 h; if the patient is unable to cough effectively, assist with coughing by firmly depressing the abdomen when the patient coughs (place hands below the rib cage and above the umbilicus). Provide for intermittent positive-pressure breathing (IPPB) every 4 h. Provide for use of incentive spirometer every 4 h.
Cardiovascular system			
Loss of sympathetic input from the higher brain centers results in bradycardia and vasomotor paralysis (vasodilation of blood vessels below the level of injury), so blood pressure is lowered. Orthostatic hypotension results in pooling of blood below the level of injury because of vasodilation; this causes hypotension and decreased blood return to the heart. Pooling of blood, coupled with immobility, greatly increases the risk of vascularstasis and orthostatic hypotension.	**Patient problems/Nursing diagnoses** • Impaired gas exchange • Decreased cardiac output • Altered tissue perfusion • Risk for peripheral neurovascular dysfunction **Collaborative problems** • Decreased cardiac output • Dysrhythmias • Deep vein thrombosis (DVT) • Hypovolemia	**Clinical data** • Monitor vital signs. • Provide cardiac monitoring. • Monitor response to elevation of head (orthostatic hypotension). • Observe for signs and symptoms of thrombophlebitis, DVT, and pulmonary embolus. **Laboratory data** • Electrocardiogram • Electrolyte, coagulation studies	Cardiology consult may be necessary, especially if a cardiac contusion is suspected. Assess for arrhythmias by observing the cardiac monitor. Monitor the patient's response to elevation of the head (orthostatic hypotension). Observe for signs and symptoms of DVT and pulmonary embolus.

continued

Table 23-12. Summary of the Collaborative Management of Multisystem Problems in the Acute Phase After Spinal Cord Injury (continued)

System-Specific Considerations	Patient Problems/Nursing Diagnosis and Collaborative Problems	Nursing Management	Level of Injury
Integumentary system			
Loss of vasomotor tone, paralysis, and bed rest contribute to the development of pressure areas and skin breakdown. Once developed, broken areas of skin are very difficult to heal; therefore, use of a bed type to relieve continuous pressure while maintaining alignment should be considered.	**Patient problems/Nursing diagnoses** • Risk for peripheral neurovascular dysfunction • Impaired skin integrity • Impaired tissue integrity • Altered peripheral tissue perfusion **Collaborative problems** • Pressure ulcers	**Clinical data** • Monitor for signs and symptoms of redness or breakdown.	Provide skin care turn patient every 2–4 h. When a special bed (e.g., a Rota Rest bed) is in use, adapt care measures appropriately.
Musculoskeletal system			
Prolonged immobility and paralysis have significant effects on bone, joints, and muscles	**Patient problems/Nursing diagnoses** • Disuse syndrome • Impaired physical mobility • Altered protection **Collaborative problems** • Contractures • Ankylosis • Muscle atrophy • Osteoporosis	**Clinical data** • Monitor range of motion of joints for development of deformities, spasticity, or ankylosis.	Consult with physical therapist to develop individualized PT program. Provide range-of-motion exercises once daily. Position the patient's extremities in proper body alignment.
Gastrointestinal system			
Peristalsis is lost with spinal shock, resulting in paralytic ileus. A distended abdomen interferes with adequate respirations. Stress ulcers and gastric hemorrhage can also occur; because sensation is lost, the patient cannot feel the pain of ulceration. Monitor for constipation.	**Patient problems/Nursing diagnoses** • Ineffective breathing pattern • Risk for altered respiratory • Function • Risk for injury • Bowel incontinence • Constipation **Collaborative problems** • Paralytic ileus • GI bleeding • Constipation	**Clinical data** • Perform abdominal auscultation for bowel sounds. • Monitor stools for occult blood. • Monitor gastric pH. **Laboratory data** • CBC • Decreased hemoglobin	Immediately insert a nasogastric tube to intermittent suction (low) for GI decompression. Maintain patient's NPO status until bowel sounds return and the nasogastric tube is removed. Initiate a bowel program as soon as possible. Maintain a pH >5.0 by using Maalox, 30 ml every 3 h. Administer drugs (e.g., cimetidine) for gastric prophylaxis. Administer stool softeners/laxatives to facilitate a bowel program.

continued

Table 23-12. Summary of the Collaborative Management of Multisystem Problems in the Acute Phase After Spinal Cord Injury (continued)			
System-Specific Considerations	**Patient Problems/Nursing Diagnosis and Collaborative Problems**	**Nursing Management**	**Level of Injury**
Genitourinary system			
Bladder reflexes and control of micturition from higher brain centers are lost with cord injury; atonic bladder results. An atonic bladder (loss of bladder tone) is distended and predisposes the patient to urinary tract infections (UTIs).	**Patient problems/Nursing diagnoses** • Reflex incontinence • Altered pattern of urinary elimination • Urinary retention • Risk for infection **Collaborative problems** • Acute urinary retention • Urinary tract infection	**Clinical data** • Palpate suprapubic area for bladder distention. • Review intake and output record. **Laboratory data** • Urine culture and sensitivity, urinalysis, blood urea nitrogen, and creatinine	Insert an indwelling urinary catheter immediately. Remove catheter and initiate intermittent catheterization program every 6–8 h once the patient is stable. Aggressively treat UTI. Maintain an intake and output record. Use aseptic technique when managing the indwelling catheter.
Metabolic (nutritional) system			
The method of providing nutrition will depend on the associated injuries, level of consciousness, and presence or absence of peristalsis. The body needs sufficient fluid, carbohydrates, and protein for energy and tissue repair.	**Patient problems/Nursing diagnoses** • Altered nutrition: less than body requirements • Fluid volume deficit • Fluid volume excess **Collaborative problems** • Negative nitrogen balance • Electrolyte imbalances • Acidosis • Alkalosis • Hypoglycemia, hyperglycemia	**Clinical data** • Assess skin turgor and mucous membranes for adequacy of hydration. • Monitor weight two times a week. • Monitor muscle mass of extremities. **Laboratory data** • Albumin, electrolytes, and other indications of nutritional levels	Maintain NPO status until peristalsis returns. Nutrition consult is necessary as soon as possible. Total parenteral nutrition may need to be considered. Use GI tract, if not contraindicated, as soon as peristalsis returns
Psychological or emotional response			
If the patient is conscious, he or she is usually in a state of shock and denies what has happened and the impact on lifestyle. Allow the patient to ask questions when ready. The family may require the most support as they begin to comprehend what has happened and its impact on personal and family function.	**Patient problems/Nursing diagnoses** • Impaired adjustment • Anxiety • Body image disturbance • Confusion • Decisional conflict • Defensive coping • Ineffective denial • Diversional activity deficit • Grieving • Ineffective individual coping • Personal identity disturbance • Powerlessness • Impaired social interaction **Collaborative problems** • Depression • Anxiety	**Clinical data** • Assess the patient to determine what he or she is ready to hear. • Assess the family unit and its response to the injury and its impact.	Be supportive of the patient and family. Provide comprehensive information. Make appropriate referrals for support.

From *Clinical practice of neurological and neurosurgical nursing* (6th ed., pp. 435–438), by J. Hickey, 2009, Philadelphia: Lippincott Williams & Wilkins. Copyright 2009 by Lippincott Williams & Wilkins. Reprinted with permission.

8) Alterations in skin integrity

e. Gastrointestinal manifestations
   1) Peristaltic slowing, causing paralytic ileus
   2) Increased acidity, causing gastrointestinal bleeding
   3) Increased potential for pancreatitis after injury (Stiens, Fajardo, & Korsten, 2003)
   4) Abnormal liver function caused by trauma
   5) Neurogenic bowel (see Chapter 19)
   6) Constipation and hemorrhoids

f. Genitourinary manifestations
   1) Neurogenic bladder (see Chapter 19)
      a) Reflexic (UMN dysfunction)
      b) Areflexic (LMN dysfunction)
   2) Urinary outlet sphincter dysfunction

g. Sexual manifestations (see Chapter 19)
   1) Males
      a) Reflexogenic erection
      b) Psychogenic erection
      c) Variability in sperm production, penile erection, fertility, or ejaculation, depending on level of injury
   2) Females
      a) Menses cease and then resume within 6 months to a year.
      b) May still conceive and bear children but should be under the care of a physician specializing in women with SCI
      c) Autonomic dysreflexia may be a problem during delivery.
      d) Discuss contraception practices.
      e) Little research has been done on the unique needs of women experiencing SCI. Women have specific needs that should be addressed (Newman, 2006).

h. Pain manifestations (Starkweather, 2007)
   1) Muscular-skeletal pain
   2) Visceral pain
   3) Neuropathic pain (Cardenas & Jensen, 2006)
      a) Radicular
      b) Transitional zone at level of injury
      c) Below level (most common)

i. Psychosocial manifestations
   1) Stressors and losses
      a) Stressors
         (i) Survival
         (ii) Quality of life
         (iii) Lifestyle and occupational changes
         (iv) Changes in relationships and roles
         (v) Participation in recreational activities
         (vi) Neurogenic pain
      b) Losses
         (i) Sensation
         (ii) Mobility
         (iii) Bowel and bladder control
         (iv) Sexual function
         (v) Control and independence
         (vi) Former roles
         (vii) Self-esteem
   2) Emotions and behaviors
      a) Anxiety
      b) Frustration
      c) Anger
      d) Hostility
      e) Fear
      f) Sarcasm
      g) Regression
      h) Denial
      i) Guilt
      j) Depression
      k) Sensory overload
      l) Pain manifestations with neuropathic pain

L. Discharge Planning
   1. Begins before admission to rehabilitation
   2. Is a collaborative effort between the patient, family, and interdisciplinary team
   3. Includes the following considerations:
      a. Identify key family members who will be learning or performing care.
      b. Provide education for patient and family throughout the rehabilitation stay; teach about the prevention of complications, including bladder infections, pressure sores, respiratory problems, fatigue, and constipation.
      c. Identify the location or setting to which the patient is being discharged.
      d. Perform a home evaluation.
      e. Identify and order necessary DME.
      f. Identify funding sources.
      g. Ensure that the patient is discharged to a safe environment.
      h. Make referrals to a life care planner if needed.

M. Aging with SCI (Charlifue, 2007a, 2007b, 2007c; Charlifue & Gerhart, 2004; Charlifue, Lammertse, & Adkins, 2004; McColl, Arnold, Charlifue, & Gerhart, 2001; McMahon & Howland, 2013; Winkler, 2012)
   1. Typically, the greater the number of years since the injury, the better the psychological adaptation to the injury, up to 30 years. Psychological adjustment improves over time in people aging with SCI. Studies indicate that older adults use better

coping strategies and have more realistic expectations (Krause & Broderick, 2005).

2. A longitudinal study in Great Britain tracked more than 800 people with SCI (NSIC, 2012).
   a. Death rates and causes of death
      1) SCI survivors have a higher death rate than the general population.
      2) Causes of death include cardiovascular disease, pneumonia, septicemia, cancer, and suicide.
      3) The rate of cardiovascular disease is more than 200% higher in people with SCI than people the same age without spinal injury (Winkler, 2012).
   b. Morbidity (illnesses and complications)
      1) Urinary tract infections
      2) Pressure ulcers
      3) Chest infections, spasticity, perceived abdominal pain, and general malaise (more likely in people with tetraplegia)
      4) Musculoskeletal problems such as joint pain, stiffness, pressure sores, and diarrhea (especially in people with paraplegia)
      5) Increased fractures, cystitis, and motor and sensory changes (especially in people with incomplete injuries)
      6) Functional decline or decreasing physical independence
      7) Gastrointestinal problems are common and worsen with age, including hemorrhoids and difficulty with bowel evacuation (Winkler, 2012).
   c. General health, life satisfaction, and stress
      1) More than 75% reported feeling generally healthy, and 74% were generally satisfied with their lives.
      2) Stress and depression decreased as years passed since the injury.
      3) Stress was related to adaptation and coping but unrelated to injury severity or physical independence.
   d. Risk factors
      1) Pressure ulcers
         a) More likely in people with paraplegia
         b) More likely in people who have already developed one pressure sore
         c) Higher risk for those with abnormal pulses in feet and lower extremities
         d) Higher risk with unemployment
         e) The number of pressure ulcers increased with time (NSCISC, 2012)
      2) Upper extremity pain (Consortium for Spinal Cord Medicine, 2005)
         a) Increases with the age of the SCI
         b) Decreased psychosocial well-being coincided with increase in upper extremity pain.
         c) Limitations in ROM increased the risk of upper extremity pain.
      3) Life satisfaction
         a) Younger participants who had greater psychosocial well-being and financial resources reported greater life satisfaction.
         b) Participants who reported social involvement had less fatigue and were less likely to be overweight.
         c) Declined over time (Charlifue & Gerhart, 2004)
         d) Less life satisfaction was associated with less community reintegration.
      4) Factors related to decreased physical independence
         a) Advanced age, especially among people with paraplegia
         b) Changes in DME
         c) Changes in bladder management program
         d) Increased fatigue over time: Those with a poor self-perception of health had more fatigue.
      5) Community integration and social support (Charlifue & Gerhart, 2004)
         a) A general decline in community integration over time related to decreased physical independence, decreased mobility, and a lack of social integration.
         b) Life satisfaction was related to community reintegration.
      6) Spirituality and depression (Charlifue, 2007a)
         a) No significant relationship between spiritual well-being and age or length of time since injury
         b) People reporting better spiritual well-being were less depressed and reported better quality of life.

3. Conclusions
   a. Pressure ulcers and respiratory problems appear to be more common with advancing age.
   b. Musculoskeletal problems are associated more with longer durations of injury.
   c. Life satisfaction and quality of life are vital concepts, neither of which is totally dependent on the level or severity of the disability or on the number of medical complications;

however, each seems to be very important as a predictor of future outcomes.
  d. Fatigue, depression, and decreased life satisfaction should not go unaddressed because they may lead to costly and compromising complications.
  e. There is a general decline in community integration based on a variety of factors.

N. Prevention (www.asia-spinalinjury.org/committees/prevention_facts.php)
  1. Always wear a seat belt.
  2. Children under 12 years of age should be properly restrained in the back seat.
  3. Obey speed limits and rules of the road when driving.
  4. Athletes should wear proper safety gear and use spotters as appropriate and never perform head-first moves.
  5. Swimmers should make sure that water is deep enough and clear enough to see objects under the water. They should enter the water feet first.
  6. Firearms should be kept unloaded and secured.
  7. Never drive under the influence of alcohol or drugs.
  8. Homes with children should have safety gates and window guards.
  9. Avoid tripping and falling hazards, especially in homes of older adults. Install grab bars in bathroom, banisters and railings; use nonslip bath mats and avoid throw rugs.

O. Research
  1. Basic science: Current research is focused on advancing our understanding of five key principles of spinal cord repair (NINDS, 2014b)
    a. Neuroprotection: Protecting surviving nerve cells from further damage (e.g., by use of antibiotics, erythropoietin, hypothermia, manipulation of macrophages, use of ALS drug riluzole)
    b. Regeneration: Stimulating the regrowth of axons and targeting their connections appropriately (e.g., by use of antiinflammatory drugs, antibody use, targeting inhibiting proteins, getting past glial scar through use of chondroitinase ABC, development of matrix to bridge lesion)
    c. Cell replacement: Replacing damaged nerve or glial cells (e.g., through research involving human oligodendrocyte progenitor cells, Schwann cells, bone marrow stromal cells, and nasal olfactory ensheathing cells)
    d. Retraining central nervous system circuits and plasticity to restore body functions (looking at the effects of exercise and active rehabilitation to increase function and prevent early cardiovascular disease). The central pattern generator is a group of nerve cells that synchronizes muscle activity during alternating stepping of the legs.
    e. Electrophysiology of the spinal cord: Researchers have identified the appearance of a newly formed reflex, which demonstrates that nerve circuits may be altered and new connections formed after injury in humans.
  2. Epidural stimulation: Use of electrical stimulation and therapy to initiate function. Many scientists are investigating this method for various functions, such as:
    a. University of Louisville (Angeli, Edgerton, Gerasimenko, Harkema, 2014)
    b. Newcastle University movement lab (http://speakingofresearch.com/2014/05/19/spinal-cord-stimulation-restores-monkeys-ability-to-move-paralysed-hand/)
  3. Functional electric stimulation (FES): Computer electrode systems to enable more natural but complex functions to occur (Gater, Dolbowa, Tsuib, & Gorgey, 2011)
    a. Cardiac
    b. Phrenic nerve
    c. Diaphragmatic pacing
    d. Breathing
    e. Coughing
    f. Grasping
    g. Stepping
    h. Truncal stabilization
    i. Bladder and bowel function
    j. Exercise
    k. Experiments in transcranial direct current stimulation
    l. Neural prostheses: Bioengineers are trying to restore functional connections through computers and functional electrical stimulation systems to control the muscles of the arms and legs, especially to stimulate walking, reaching, and gripping.
    m. See also the Cleveland FES center website (http://fescenter.org/index.php?option=com_content&view=section&id=3&Itemid=2)
  4. Robotic-assisted therapy: Research testing restoration of function of people with chronic paralysis (Sale, Franceschini, Waldner, & Hesse, 2012). There are many products on the market
    a. Lokomat
    b. AMES

c. Body-weight-supported treadmill training with robotic gait trainer
   1) The navigator
   2) Zero G
   3) LiteGait
   4) Smart Step
d. Reo Go
e. InMotion robots
f. Exoskeletons
   1) Ekso bionics
   2) Indego
   3) ARGO
g. Biofeedback and monitoring system
   1) Auto Ambulator
   2) Hand Mentor/Bioness
h. Robotic assisted tilt-table therapy (RATTT; Craven, Gollee, Coupaud, Purcell, & Allan, 2013); clear trends in acute exercise responses to RATTT in a small and complex case mix of early-stage SCI

5. Brain–computer interfaces: The goal is to bypass the damaged nerve circuits in the spinal cord and establish a direct link between the brain and an assistive implanted device to restore voluntary muscle movement and coordination of muscles.
   a. Walking simulator (King, Wang, Chui, & Nenadic, 2013)
   b. Brain–computer interface in medicine, Mayo Clinic (Shih, Krusienski, & Wolpaw, 2012)
   c. Scientists at Northwestern University in Chicago, with funding from the National Institutes of Health, successfully bypassed the spinal cord and restored fine motor control to paralyzed limbs using a brain–computer interface.
6. Pain research
   a. Pain research group is evaluating the effect of SCI pain on quality of life.
   b. Pain treatment: Chronic pain syndromes are thought to continually trigger functional changes in neurons.
   c. Drugs that interfere with neurotransmitters related to pain syndromes are being investigated.
7. Spasticity: Drug interventions, surgery, and electrical stimulation below the injury may decrease spasms. Spasticity and fatigue in paralyzed muscle provide essential information for designing exercise programs that optimize function in muscles that have lost some or all of their nerve supply.
8. The Christopher & Dana Reeve Foundation NeuroRecovery Network (CDRF NRN) provides body weight support treadmill training for patients with SCI. This treatment program gathers data about the use of a specialized treadmill. The treadmill training is intended to promote a focus of neurorecovery of signals that are being affected through physical training. It is believed that neuro pathways are affected by physical training. Reeve Foundation NeuroRecovery Network (2014) highlights:
   a. 568 patients have completed or are currently enrolled in NRN therapy protocols.
   b. 80 participants are now walking in the home and community.
   c. 243 patients enrolled in community fitness and wellness activity-based therapy/NRN programs.
9. General notes
   a. No one theory or approach will encompass all the effects of SCI.
   b. Many scientists believe that significant new treatments will be found not in a single approach but rather in a combination of techniques.
   c. Currently 590 SCI research studies in all stages are listed on clinicaltrials.gov.
   d. Many research studies start strong and turn out to be statistically weak.
   e. Technology innovation: Can require significant fiscal resources, but evidence for efficiency outcomes can be challenging

P. Advocacy Organizations
   1. Christopher & Dana Reeve Foundation: www.crpf.org
   2. National Spinal Cord Injury Association: http://www.spinalcord.org
   3. United Spinal Association: http://www.unitedspinal.org
   4. Facing Disability.Com: http://www.facingdisability.com

Q. Professional Organizations
   1. Academy of Spinal Cord Injury Professionals: http://academyscipro.org
   2. Association of Rehabilitation Nurses: http://www.rehabnurse.org
   3. American Spine Injury Association: http://www.asia-spinalinjury.org

R. Advanced Practice Considerations: Role of the Advanced Practice Nurse in SCI Rehabilitation
   1. Educator
      a. Work alongside the rehabilitation team as a clinical nurse specialist to develop education platforms for patients and families in both inpatient and postacute care settings. This would include addressing community reintegration challenges.

b. Present professional papers and posters at national and international symposiums and professional educational events.
c. Coordinate or teach certification review material related to SCI to rehabilitation staff to increase the number of certified rehabilitation nurses.
d. Assist with the placement of nursing students in the spinal cord clinical setting to increase overall understanding of the care of patients with SCI.
e. Advocate by educating the community, related healthcare agencies, and academia to increase the knowledge base of healthcare professionals who care for the patient and family.

2. Advocate and leader
   a. Collaborate with local and national legislators to advocate for people with SCI regarding rehabilitation benefit coverage, accessibility, community resources, and other funding issues.
   b. Participate on local and state committees.
   c. Participate with the local chapter of ARN while providing education and advocacy for people with SCI.
   d. Participate in ARN on a national level.
3. Consultant
   a. Provide direct rehabilitation nursing services to patients with SCI and their families who help care for them, actively addressing the often complicated issues that arise from complex neurological deficits.
   b. Serve as a vital component of the rehabilitation team by providing expert knowledge in the treatment and complex care of the patient with SCI.
   c. Collaborate with all rehabilitation team disciplines to ensure receipt of coordinated care throughout the healthcare continuum and beyond into the community.
   d. Advocate financial assistance by providing guidance and sharing knowledge about assistive organizations to care managers, social workers, family, and the patient with SCI.
4. Researcher and catalyst of change
   a. Remain active in the field of research for SCI as a reviewer, assisting in active research, participating in pilot testing for new strategies.
   b. Address areas of complications, patient challenges, and creative ideas as an opportunity to further support clinical education and services.
   c. Develop and maintain facility procedures based on evidence-based clinical practice.

References

Abrams, G., & Wakasa, M. (2014). *Chronic complications of spinal cord injury.* Retrieved from www.uptodate.com/contents/chronic-complications-of-spinal-cord-injury

Acquired Brain Injury Knowledge Uptake Strategy (ABIKUS). (2010). *ABIKUS guideline.* Retrieved from www.abiebr.com/abikus

American Spinal Injury Association (ASIA) website. (2014). Prevention. Retrieved from www.asia-spinalinjury.org/committees/prevention_facts.php

Angeli, C. A., Edgerton,V. R., Gerasimenko, Y. P., & Harkema, S. J. (2014) Altering spinal cord excitability enables voluntary movements after chronic complete paralysis in humans. *Brain, 137*(5), 1394-1409.

Ansell, B., & Keenan, J. (1989). The Western Neuro Sensory Stimulation Profile: A tool for assessing slow-to-recover head injured patients. *Archives of Physical Medicine and Rehabilitation, 70,* 104–108.

Association of Rehabilitation Nurses (2014). ARN competency model for professional rehabilitation nursing. Retrieved from http://www.rehabnurse.org/uploads/files/education/ARN_Rehabilitation_Nursing_Competency _Model_FINAL_-_May_2014.pdf

Baggerly, J., & Le, N. (2001). Nursing management of the patient with head trauma. In J. B. Derstine & S. D. Hargrove (Eds.), *Comprehensive rehabilitation nursing* (pp. 331–367). Philadelphia: W.B. Saunders.

Barker, E. (2002). Neuroanatomy and physiology of the nervous system. In E. Barker (Ed.), *Neuroscience nursing: A spectrum of care* (pp. 3–50). St. Louis: Mosby.

Baxter, D., & Wilson, M. (2012). The fundamentals of head injury. *Neurosurgery, 30*(3), 116–121.

Blank-Reid, C., & Barker, E. (2002). Neurotrauma: Traumatic brain injury. In E. Barker (Ed.), *Neuroscience nursing: A spectrum of care* (pp. 409–437). St. Louis: Mosby.

Bogner, J. A., Corrigan, J. D., Bode, R. K., & Heinemann, A. W. (2000). Rating scale analysis of the Agitated Behavior Scale. *The Journal of Head Trauma Rehabilitation, 15*(1), 656–669.

Brain Injury Association of America. (2006). Scales and measurements of function. Retrieved from www.biausa.org/Pages/what_is_the_rehab_process.html#ways

Brain Injury Association of America (BIAA). (2014). About brain injury. Retrieved from www.biausa.org/about-brain-injury.htm

Brain injury.com. (2014a). Recovery and rehabilitation. Retrieved from www.braininjury.com/recovery.shtml

Brain injury.com. (2014b). Symptoms of brain injury. Retrieved from www.braininjury.com/symptoms.shtml

Burns, S. P., Golding, D. G., Rolle, W. A., Graziani, V., & Ditunno, J. F. (1997). Recovery of ambulation in motor-incomplete tetraplegia. *Archives of Physical Medicine and Rehabilitation, 78*(11), 1169–1172.

Byrnes, M., Beilby, J., Ray, P., McLennan, R., Ker, J., & Schug, S. (2012) Patient-focused goal planning process and outcome after spinal cord injury rehabilitation: Quantitative and qualitative audit. *Clinical Rehabilitation, 26*(12), 1141–1149.

Cardenas, D. D., & Jensen, M. P. (2006). Treatments for chronic pain in persons with spinal cord injury: A survey study. *Journal of Spinal Cord Medicine, 29*(2), 109–117.

Centers for Disease Control and Prevention (CDC). (2010a). Heads up: Preventing brain injuries. Retrieved from www.cdc.gov/ncipc/pub-res/tbi_toolkit/patients/preventing.htm

Centers for Disease Control and Prevention (CDC). (2010b). Injury prevention and control: Traumatic brain injury. Retrieved from http://cdc.gov/traumaticbraininjury/statistics.html

Centers for Disease Control and Prevention (CDC) (2010c). Brain injury in the United States: Facts sheet. Retrieved May 4, 2014 from http://www.cdc.gov/traumaticbraininjury/get_the_facts

Centers for Disease Control and Prevention (CDC). (2014). Heads up: Brain injury in your practice. Retrieved from www.cdc.gov/concussion/HeadsUp/physicians_tool_kit.html

Chanda, A., & Nanda, A. (2003). Subdural and epidural hematomas. In R. W. Evans (Ed.), *Saunders manual of neurologic practice* (pp. 500–506). Philadelphia: Saunders.

Charlifue, S. (2007a). A collaborative longitudinal study of aging with spinal cord injury: Overview of the background and methodology. *Topics in Spinal Cord Injury Rehabilitation, 12*(3), 1–14.

Charlifue, S. (2007b). Effects of aging on individuals with chronic SCI. *Topics in Spinal Cord Injury Rehabilitation, 12*(3), 1–96.

Charlifue, S. (2007c). Living well: Aging and SCI: Some good news. *PN/Paraplegia News, 61*(1), 12–13.

Charlifue, S., & Gerhart, K. (2004). Community integration in spinal cord injury of long duration. *NeuroRehabilitation, 19*(2), 91–101.

Charlifue, S., Lammertse, D. P., & Adkins, R. J. (2004). Aging with spinal cord injury: Changes in selected health indices and life satisfaction. *Archives of Physical Medicine and Rehabilitation, 85*(11), 1848–1853.

Consortium for Spinal Cord Medicine. (2005). *Preservation of upper limb function following spinal cord injury: A clinical practice guideline for health-care professionals.* Washington, DC: Paralyzed Veterans of America.

Corrigan, J. D., & Bogner, J. A. (1994). Factor structure of the Agitated Behavior Scale. *Journal of Clinical and Experimental Neuropsychology, 16*(3), 386–392.

Craven, C. T., Gollee, H., Coupaud, S., Purcell, M. A., & Allan, D. B. (2013). Investigation of robotic-assisted tilt-table therapy for early-stage spinal cord injury rehabilitation. *Journal of Rehabilitative Research and Development, 50*(3), 367–378.

Daneshvar, P., Roffey, D. M., Brikeet, Y. A., Tsai, E. C., Bailey, C. S., & Wai, E. K. (2013). Spinal cord injuries related to cervical spine fractures in elderly patients: Factors affecting mortality. *The Spine Journal, 13*(8), 862–866.

Defense Centers of Excellence and Psychological Health and Traumatic Brain Injury (DCoE) and the Defense and Veterans Brain Injury Center (DVBIC). (2010). *Mild traumatic brain injury pocket guide (CONUS).* Retrieved from http://dvbic.dcoe.mil/sites/default/files/DCoE_mTBI-Pocket-Guide.pdf

Defense and Veterans Brain Injury Center (DVBIC). (2014). What are the causes? Retrieved from http://dvbic.dcoe.mil/about-traumatic-brain-injury/article/tbi-basics

Department of Defense (DOD) and Veteran's Head Injury Program & Brain Injury Association of America. (1999). *Brain injury and you.* Washington, DC: Author.

DeVivo, M. J., & Chen, Y. (2011). Epidemiology of traumatic spinal cord injury. In S. Kirshblum, & D. I. Campagnolo (Eds.), *Spinal cord medicine* (2nd ed., pp. 72–84). Philadelphia: WoltersKluwer/Lippincott Williams and Wilkins.

Duff, D., & Wells, D. (1997). Postcomatose unawareness/vegetative state following severe brain injury: A content methodology. *Journal of Neuroscience Nursing, 29*(5), 305–317.

Dufour, L., Williams, J., & Coleman, K. (2000). Traumatic injuries: TBI and SCI. In P. A. Edwards (Ed.), *The specialty practice of rehabilitation nursing: A core curriculum* (4th ed., pp. 196–198). Glenview, IL: Association of Rehabilitation Nurses.

Duke Medicine. (2014). Patient and family guide to traumatic brain injury. Retrieved from www.dukehealth.org/repository/dukehealth/2011/02/24/11/32/42/2572/TBI.pdf

Elovic, E., Baerga, E., & Cuccurullo, S. (2004). Mechanism and recovery of head injury. In S. Cuccurullo (Ed.), *Physical medicine and rehabilitation board review*. New York: Demos Medical Publishing.

Evans, R. W. (2003). Mild head injury and postconcussion syndrome. In R. W. Evans (Ed.), *Saunders manual of neurologic practice* (pp. 488–493). Philadelphia: Saunders.

Faul, M. X. L., Waid, M. M., & Coronado, V. G. (2010). *Traumatic brain injury in the United States: Emergency department visits, hospitalizations and deaths 2002–2006*. Atlanta: Centers for Disease Control and Prevention, National Center for Injury Prevention and Control.

Flanagan, S. R., Cantor, J. B., & Ashman, T. A. (2008). Traumatic brain injury: Future assessment tools and treatment prospects. *Neuropsychiatric Disease and Treatment, 4*(5), 877–892.

Gater, D., Dolbow, D., Tsui, B., & Gorgey, A. (2011). Functional electrical stimulation therapies after spinal cord injury. *NeuroRehabilitation, 28*(3), 231–248.

Gatens, C., & Hebert, A. R. (2001). Cognition and behavior. In S. Hoeman (Ed.), *Rehabilitation nursing: Process, application and outcomes* (pp. 599–630). St. Louis: Mosby.

Gennarelli, T. A., & Graham, D. I. (2005). Neuropathology. In J. M. Silver, T. W. McAllister, & S. C. Yudofsky (Eds.), *Textbook of traumatic brain injury* (pp. 27–50). Washington, DC: American Psychiatric Publishing.

Giacino, J. T., Ashwal, S., Childs, N., Cranford, R., Jennett, B., Katz, D. I., . . . Zasler, N. D. (2002). The minimally conscious state: Definition and diagnostic criteria. *Neurology, 58*(3), 1–11.

Giacino, J., Kalmar, K., & Whyte, J. (2004). The JFK Coma Recovery Scale–Revised: Measurement characteristics and diagnostic utility. *Archives of Physical Medicine and Rehabilitation, 85*(12), 2020–2029.

Giacino, J., & Whyte, J. (2005). The vegetative and minimally conscious states. *Journal of Head Trauma Rehabilitation, 20*(1), 30–50.

Girard, D., Brown, J., Burnett-Stolnack, M., Hashimoto, N., Hier-Wellmer, S., Perlman, O. Z., & Siegerman, C. (1996). The relationship of neuropsychological status and productive outcomes following traumatic brain injury. *Brain Injury, 10*, 663–676.

Grosswasser, Z., Schwab, K., & Salazar, A. (1997). Assessment of outcome following traumatic brain injury in adults. In R. Herndon (Ed.), *Handbook of neurologic rating scales* (pp. 187–208). New York: Demos Vermande.

Hickey, J. (1997). *Clinical practice of neurological and neurosurgical nursing* (4th ed.). Philadelphia: Lippincott Williams & Wilkins.

Hickey, J. (2003a). *Clinical practice of neurological and neurosurgical nursing* (5th ed.). Philadelphia: Lippincott Williams & Wilkins.

Hickey, J. (2003b). Craniocerebral trauma. In J. Hickey (Ed.), *Clinical practice of neurological and neurosurgical nursing* (5th ed., pp. 373–406). Philadelphia: Lippincott Williams & Wilkins.

Hickey, J. (2003c). Overview of neuroanatomy and neurophysiology. In J. Hickey (Ed.), *Clinical practice of neurological and neurosurgical nursing* (5th ed., pp. 45–92). Philadelphia: Lippincott Williams & Wilkins.

Huether, S. E., & McCance, K. L. (2012). *Understanding pathophysiology* (5th ed.). St. Louis: Elsevier.

Jennett, B., & Bond, M. (1975). Assessment of outcome after severe brain damage. *Lancet, 1*(7905), 480–484.

Kalmar, K., & Giacino, J. T. (2005). The JFK Coma Recovery Scale—Revised. *Neuropsychological Rehabilitation, 15*(3–4), 454–460.

Kamin, S. (2011). Vascular, nutritional and other nontraumatic conditions of the spinal cord. In S. Kirshblum & D. Campagnolo (Eds.), *Spinal cord medicine* (2nd ed., pp. 600–601). Philadelphia: Lippincott Williams & Wilkins.

Kennedy, R. E., Livingston, L., Marwitz, J. H., Gueck, S., Kreutzer, J. S., & Sander, A. M. (2006). Complicated mild traumatic brain injury on the inpatient rehabilitation unit: A multicenter analysis. *Journal of Head Trauma Rehabilitation, 21*(3), 260–271.

King, C. E., Wang, P. T., Chui, L. A., Do, A. H., & Nenadic. Z. (2013). Operation of a brain-computer interface walking simulator for individuals with spinal cord injury. *Journal of Neuroengineering and Rehabilitation 10*(1), 77, 2013.

Kirshblum, S., Anderson, K., Krassioukov, A., & Donovan, W. (2011). Assessment and classification of traumatic spinal cord injury. In S. Kirshblum & D. Campagnolo (Eds.), *Spinal cord medicine* (2nd ed., pp. 85–105). Philadelphia: Lippincott Williams & Wilkins.

Kirshblum, S. C., Burns, S. P. , Biering-Sorensen, F., Donovan, W., Graves, D. E., Jha, A., …Waring, M..(2011). International standards for neurological classification of spinal cord injury. *Journal of Spinal Cord Medicine, 34*(6), 535–546.

Krassioukov, A. V., Furlan, J. C., & Fehlings, M. G. (2003). Medical co-morbidities, secondary complications, and mortality in elderly with acute spinal cord injury. *Journal of Neurotrauma, 29*(4), 391–399.

Krause, J. S., & Broderick, L. (2005). 25 year longitudinal study of the natural course of aging after spinal cord injury. *Spinal Cord, 43*(6), 349–356.

Kreutzer, J. S., Seel, R. T., & Marwitz, J. H. (1999). *Neurobehavioral Functioning Inventory (NFI)*. San Antonio, TX: The Psychological Corporation, Harcourt Brace & Company.

Kulkarni, S. (2013). Spinal orthotics. Retrieved from www.emedicine.medscape.com/article/314921-overview

Levin, H., O'Donald, V., & Grossman, R. (1975). The Galveston orientation and amnesia test: A practical scale to assess cognition after head injury. *Journal of Nervous and Mental Disease, 167*, 675–686.

Lindsey, L. (1998). *Caring for caregivers*. SCI InfoSheet #17. Spinal Cord Injury Information Network. Retrieved from www.spinalcord.uab.edu/show.asp?durki=22479

Lunney, M., MaGuire, M., Endozo, N., & McIntosh-Waddy, D. (2010). Consensus-validation study identifies relevant nursing diagnoses, nursing interventions, and health outcomes for people with traumatic brain injuries. *Rehabilitation Nursing, 35*(4), 161–165.

Malec, J. (2005). *The Mayo Portland Adaptability Inventory*. The Center for Outcome Measurement in Brain Injury. Retrieved from www.tbims.org/combi/mpai

McColl, M. A., Arnold, R., Charlifue, S., & Gerhart, K. (2001). Social support and aging with a spinal cord injury: Canadian and British experiences. *Topics in Spinal Cord Injury Rehabilitation, 6*(3), 83–101.

McKinley, W., & Silver, T. M. (2013). Functional outcomes per level of spinal cord injury. Retrieved from http://emedicine.medscape.com/article/322604-overview

McMahon, J. K., & Howland, W. A. (2013). Spinal cord injury. In D. Apuna-Grummer & W. A. Howland (Eds.), *A core curriculum for nurse life care planning* (pp. 83–153). Bloomington, IN: iUniverse, LLC.

Meythaler, J. M., Peduzzi, J. D., Eleftheriou, E., & Novack, T. A. (2001) Current concepts: Diffuse axonal injury associated traumatic brain injury. *Archives of Physical Medicine and Rehabilitation, 82*(10), 1461–1471.

Model Systems Knowledge Translation Center (MSKTC). (2009). Skin care & pressure sores: Preventing pressure sores. Retrieved from www.msktc.org/sci/factsheets/skincare/Preventing-Pressure-Sores

Model Systems Knowledge Translation Center (MSKTC). (2014). TBI. Retrieved from www.msktc.org/publications?sys=T

Model Systems Knowledge Translation Center (MSKTC). (n.d.). Traumatic brain injury factsheets. Retrieved from www.msktc.org/tbi/factsheets

National Center for Injury Prevention and Control (NCIPC). (2003). *Report to Congress on mild traumatic brain injury in the United States: Steps to prevent a serious health problem.* Atlanta: Centers for Disease Control and Prevention.

National Institute of Neurological Disorders and Stroke (NINDS). (2014a). Spinal cord infarction. Retrieved from www.ninds.nih.gov/disorders/spinal_infarction/spinal_infarction.htm#What_is

National Institute of Neurological Disorders and Stroke (NINDS). (2014b). Spinal cord injury: Hope through research. Retrieved from www.ninds.nih.gov/disorders/sci/detail_sci.htm

National Institute of Neurological Disorders and Stroke (NINDS). (2014c). Traumatic brain injury: Hope through research. Retrieved from www.ninds.nih.gov/disorders/tbi/detail_tbi.htm

National Spinal Cord Injury Statistical Center (NSCISC). (2012). Annual report for the spinal cord injury model systems. Retrieved from www.nscisc.uab.edu/

National Spinal Cord Injury Statistical Center (NSCISC). (2013). Facts and figures at a glance. Retrieved from www.nscisc.uab.edu/

National Spinal Injuries Center (NSIC). (2012). Research activity. Retrieved from www.buckinghamshirehealthcare.nhs.uk/spinal

The NeuroRecovery Network. (2014). Retrieved from www.christopherreeve.org/site/c.ddJFKRNoFiG/b.6241709/k.498C/NeuroRecovery_Network_Mission.htm

Newman, S. D. (2006). *Community integration of women with spinal cord injury: A case for participatory research.* SCI Nursing. Retrieved from www.unitedspinal.org/publications/nursing/2006/08/27/community-integration-of-women-with-spinal-cord-injury-a-case-for-participatory-research/

Novack, T. (2000). *The orientation log.* The Center for Outcome Measurement in Brain Injury. Retrieved from www.tbims.org/combi/olog

O'Dell, M., & Riggs, R. (1996). Management of the minimally responsive patient. In L. Horn & N. Zasler (Eds.), *Medical rehabilitation of traumatic brain injury* (pp. 103–132). Philadelphia: Hanley & Belfus.

Pickett, G. E., Campos-Benitez, M., Keller, J. L., & Duggal, N. (2006). Epidemiology of traumatic spinal cord injury in Canada. *Spine, 31*(7), 799–805.

Povlishock, J. T., & Katz, D. J. (2005). Update on neuropathology and neuronal recovery after traumatic brain injury. *Journal of Head Trauma Rehabilitation, 20*(1), 76–94.

Rader, M., Alston, J., & Ellis, D. (1989). Sensory stimulation of severely brain injured patients. *Brain Injury, 3,* 141–147.

Rappaport, M. (2000). The Coma/Near Coma Scale. The Center for Outcome Measurement in Brain Injury. Retrieved from www.tbims.org/combi/cnc

Rappaport, M. (2005). The Disability Rating and Coma/Near-Coma scales in evaluating severe head injury. *Neuropsychological Rehabilitation, 15*(3–4), 442–453.

Rosebrough, A. (1998). Traumatic brain injury. In P. A. Chin, D. Finocchiaro, & A. Rosebrough (Eds.), *Rehabilitation nursing practice, major neurological deficits and common rehabilitation disorders* (pp. 223–244). New York: McGraw-Hill.

Sale P., Franceschini M., Waldner A., & Hesse S. (2012) Use of the robot assisted gait therapy in rehabilitation of patients with stroke and spinal cord injury. *European Journal of Physical and Rehabilitation Medicine, 48*(1), 111–121.

SCIRE. Spinal Cord Injury Rehabilitation Evidence website. (2014). Retrieved from http://www.scireproject.com/rehabilitation-evidence

Scivoletto, G., Morganti, B., Ditunno, P., Ditunno, J. F., & Molinari, M. (2003). Effects on age on spinal cord lesion patients' rehabilitation. *Spinal Cord, 41*(8), 457–464.

Selvarajah, S., Hammond, E. R., Haider, A. H., Abularrage, C. J., Becker, D., Dhiman, N., . . . Schneider, E. B. (2014). The burden of acute traumatic spinal cord injury among adults in the United States: An update. *Journal of Neurotrauma, 31*(3), 228.

Sherer, M., Vaccaro, M., Whyte, J., Giacino, J., & the Consciousness Consortium. (2007). *Facts about the vegetative and minimally conscious states after severe brain injury.* Vienna, VA: Brain Injury Association of America.

Shih,J. J., Krusienski, D.J., & Wolpaw, ,J. R. (2012). Brain-computer interfaces in medicine. *Mayo Clinic Proceedings, 87*(3), 268–279.

Starkweather, A. R. (2007). Chronic pain after spinal cord injury: An overview of treatment options. *Spinal Cord Injury Nursing, 24*(3), 18–25.

Stephenson, R., Berliner, J., & Klein, M. (2013). Autonomic dysreflexia in spinal cord injury. Medscape reference. Retrieved from http://emedicine.medscape.com/article/322809

Stiens, S. A., Fajardo, N. R., & Korsten, M. A. (2003). The pancreas: Increased risk for pancreatitis. In V. W. Lin, D. D. Cardenas, N. C. Cutter, et al. (Eds.), *Spinal cord medicine: Principles and practice.* New York: Demos Medical Publishing.

van Baalen, B., Odding, E., Maas, A. I. R., Ribbers, G. M., Bergen, M. P., & Stam, H. J. (2003). Traumatic brain injury: Classification of initial severity and determination of functional outcome. *Disability and Rehabilitation, 25*(1), 9–18.

Vinas, F. C., Nosko, M. G., Talavera, F., Pluta, R. M., Zamboni, P., Koppell, B. H., & Pilitsis, J. (2013). Penetrating head trauma. Retrieved from http://emedicine.medscape.com/article/247664-overview

Wan, D., & Krassioukov, A. V. (2014). Life-threatening outcomes associated with autonomic dysreflexia: A clinical review. *The Journal of Spinal Cord Medicine, 37*(1), 2–10.

Wasserman, J. R., & Smirniotopoulos, J. G. (Eds.). (2012). Diffuse axonal injury imaging. Retrieved from http://emedicine.medscape.com/article/339912-overview

Widerstrom-Noga, E., Biering-Sorensen, F., Bryce, T. N., Finnerup, N. P., Jensen, M. P., Richards, J. S., & Siddall, P. J. (2014). The International Spinal Cord Injury Pain Basic Data Set (version 2.0). *Spinal Cord, 52,* 282–286.

Wilson, J. T. L., Pettigrew, L. E. L., & Teasdale, G. M. (1997). Structured interviews for the Glasgow Outcome Scale and the Extended Glasgow Outcome Scale: Guidelines for their use. *Journal of Neurotrauma, 15*(8), 573–585.

Winkler, T. (2012). Spinal cord injury and aging. Retrieved from http://emedicine.medscape.com/article/322713-overview

Wright, J. (2000). Introduction to the Disability Rating Scale. The Center for Outcome Measurement in Brain Injury. Retrieved from www.tbims.org/combi/drs

Xu, J., Rasmussen, I. A., Lagopoulos, J., & Haberg, A. (2007). Diffuse axonal injury in severe traumatic brain injury visualized using high-resolution diffusion tensor imaging. *Journal of Neurotrauma, 24,* 753–765.

Young, W. (2014). Spinal cord injury levels & classification. Travis Roy Foundation Website. Retrieved from http://www.travisroyfoundation.org/sci/resources/spinal-cord-injury-levels-classification/

Zitnay, G. A., Zitnay, K. M., Povlishock, J. T., Hall, E. D., Marion, D. W., Trudel, T., …Barth, J. T. (2008). Traumatic brain injury research priorities: The Conemaugh International Brain Injury Symposium. *Journal of Neuortrauma, 25*(10) 35–52.

Suggested Reading

Apuna-Grummer, D., & Howland, W. A. (Eds.). *A core curriculum for nurse life care planning.* Bloomington, IN: iUniverse, LLC.

Azouvi, P., Jokic, C., Attals, N., Denys, P., Markabi, S., & Bussel, B. (1999). Carbamazepine in agitation and aggressive behavior following severe closed-head injury: Results of an open trial. *Brain Injury, 13*(10), 797–804.

Baguley, I. J., Cameron, I. D., Gree, A. M., Slewayounan, S., Marosszeky, J. E., & Gurka, J. A. (2004). Pharmacological management of dysautonomia following traumatic brain injury. *Brain Injury, 18*(5), 409–417.

Bell, K. R., & Williams, F. (2003). Use of botulinum toxin type A and type B for spasticity in upper and lower limbs. *Physical Medicine and Rehabilitation Clinics of North America, 14,* 821–835.

Brain Injury.com. (2014a). Recovery and rehabilitation. Retrieved from www.braininjury.com/recovery.shtml

Brain Injury.com. (2014b). Symptoms of a brain injury. Retrieved from www.braininjury.com/symptoms.shtml

Brooke, M. M., Patterson, D. R., Questad, K. A., Cardenas, D., & Farrel-Roberts, L. (1992). The treatment of agitation during initial hospitalization after traumatic brain injury. *Archives of Physical Medicine and Rehabilitation, 73,* 917–921.

Brooke, M. M., Questad, K. A., Patterson, D. R., & Bashak, K. J. (1992). Agitation and restlessness after closed head injury: A prospective study of 100 consecutive admissions. *Archives of Physical Medicine and Rehabilitation, 73,* 320–323.

Burnett, M. D., Kennedy, R. E., Cifu, D. X., & Levenson, J. (2003). Using atypical neuroleptic drugs to treat agitation in patients with a brain injury: A review. *Neurorehabilitation, 13,* 165–172.

Centers for Disease Control and Prevention (CDC). (2003). *Report to Congress on mild traumatic brain injury in the United States: Steps to prevent a serious health problem.* National Center for Injury Prevention and Control. Retrieved from www.cdc.gov/ncipc/pub-res/mtbi/mtbireport.pdf

Cicerone, K. D., Dahlberg, C., Malec, J. F., Langenbahn, D. M., Felicetti, T., Kneipp, S. S., . . . Catanese, J. (2005). Evidence-based cognitive rehabilitation: Updated review of the literature from 1998 through 2002. *Archives of Physical Medicine and Rehabilitation, 86,* 1681–1692.

Consortium for Spinal Cord Medicine. (1997). *Prevention of thromboembolism in spinal cord injury.* Washington, DC: Paralyzed Veterans of America.

Consortium for Spinal Cord Medicine. (1998a). *Depression following spinal cord injury: A clinical practice guideline for primary care physicians.* Washington, DC: Paralyzed Veterans of America.

Consortium for Spinal Cord Medicine. (1998b). *Neurogenic bowel management in adults with spinal cord injury.* Washington, DC: Paralyzed Veterans of America.

Consortium for Spinal Cord Medicine. (1999a). *Depression: What you should know: A guide for people with spinal cord injury.* Washington, DC: Paralyzed Veterans of America.

Consortium for Spinal Cord Medicine. (1999b). *Neurogenic bowel: What you should know: A guide for people with spinal cord injury.* Washington, DC: Paralyzed Veterans of America.

Consortium for Spinal Cord Medicine. (1999c). *Outcomes following traumatic spinal cord injury.* Washington, DC: Paralyzed Veterans of America.

Consortium for Spinal Cord Medicine. (2001). *Acute management of autonomic dysreflexia in individuals with spinal cord injury presenting to health care facilities. A guide for people with spinal cord injury* (2nd ed.). Washington, DC: Paralyzed Veterans of America.

Consortium for Spinal Cord Medicine. (2003). *Pressure ulcer prevention and treatment following spinal cord injury: A clinical practice guideline for health-care professionals.* Washington, DC: Paralyzed Veterans of America.

Consortium for Spinal Cord Medicine. (2005a). *Preservation of upper limb function following spinal cord injury: A clinical practice guideline.* Washington, DC: Paralyzed Veterans of America.

Consortium for Spinal Cord Medicine. (2005b). *Respiratory management following spinal cord injury.* Washington, DC: Paralyzed Veterans of America..

Consortium for Spinal Cord Medicine. (2006). *Bladder management for adults with spinal cord injury: A clinical practice guideline for health-care providers.* Washington, DC: Paralyzed Veterans of America.

Consortium for Spinal Cord Medicine. (2008a). *Early acute management in adults with spinal cord injury. A clinical practice guideline.* Washington, DC: Paralyzed Veterans of America.

Consortium for Spinal Cord Medicine. (2008b). *Preservation of upper limb function: What you should know: A guide for people with spinal cord injury.* Washington, DC: Paralyzed Veterans of America.

Consortium for Spinal Cord Medicine. (2010a). *Bladder management following spinal cord injury: What you should know. A guide for people with spinal cord injury.* Washington, DC: Paralyzed Veterans of America.

Consortium for Spinal Cord Medicine. (2010b). *Sexuality and reproductive health in adults with spinal cord injury. A clinical practice guideline*. Washington, DC: Paralyzed Veterans of America.

Demark, J., & Gemeinhardt, M. (2002). Anger and its management for survivors of acquired brain injury. *Brain Injury, 16*(2), 91–108.

Francisco, G. E., Hu, M. M., Boake, C., & Ivanhoe, C. B. (2005). Efficacy of early use of intrathecal baclofen therapy for treating spastic hypertonia due to acquired brain injury. *Brain Injury, 19*(5), 359–364.

Giacino, J. T., Ashwal, S., Childs, N., Cranford, R., Jennett, B., Katz, D. I., . . . Zasler, N. D. (2002). The minimally conscious state: Definition and diagnostic criteria. *Neurology, 58*(3), 1–11.

Giacino, J., & Whyte, J. (2005). The vegetative and minimally conscious states: Current knowledge and remaining questions. *Journal of Head Trauma Rehabilitation, 20*, 30–50.

Glen, M. B. (1998). Methylphenidate for cognitive and behavioral dysfunction after traumatic brain injury. *Journal of Head Trauma Rehabilitation, 13*(5), 87–90.

Harvey, C. V. (2005). Spinal surgery patient care. *Orthopaedic Nursing, 24*(6), 426–440.

Hughes, S., Colantonio, A., Santaguida, P. L., & Paton, T. (2005). Amantadine to enhance readiness for rehabilitation following severe traumatic brain injury. *Brain Injury, 19*(14), 1197–1206.

Kajs-Wyllie, M. (2002). Ritalin revisited: Does it really help in neurological injury? *Journal of Neuroscience Nursing, 43*(6), 303–313.

Kirshblum, S., & Campagnolo, D. (Eds.). (2011). *Spinal cord medicine* (2nd ed.). Philadelphia: Lippincott Williams & Wilkins.

Kraus, M. F., Smith, G. S., Butters, M., Donnell, A. J., Dixon, E., Yilong, C., Marion, D. (2005). Effects of dopaminergic agent and NMDA receptor antagonist amantadine on cognitive function, cerebral glucose metabolism and D2 receptor availability in chronic traumatic brain injury: A study using positron emission tomography. *Brain Injury, 19*(7), 471–479.

Leone, H., & Polsonetti, B. W. (2005). Amantadine for traumatic brain injury: Does it improve cognition and reduce agitation? *Journal of Clinical Pharmacy and Therapeutics, 30*, 101–104.

Levy, M., Berson, A., Cook, T., Bollegala, N., Seto, E., Turanski, S., et al. (2005). Treatment of agitation following traumatic brain injury: A review of the literature. *Neurorehabilitation, 20*, 279–306.

Llemke, D. M. (2004). Riding out the storm: Sympathetic storming after traumatic brain injury. *Journal of Neuroscience Nursing, 36*(1), 4–7.

Martinkewiz, P., Furr, B. J., Farnan, C., & Martinez, P. G. (2011). Traumatic injuries: Traumatic brain injury and spinal cord injury. In C. D. Jacelon (Ed.), *The specialty practice of rehabilitation nursing: A core curriculum* (6th ed., pp. 251–287). Glenview, IL: Association of Rehabilitation Nurses.

Maryniak, O., Manchanda, R., & Velani, A. (2001). Methotrimeprazine in the treatment of agitation in acquired brain injury patients. *Brain Injury, 15*(2), 167–174.

Meythaler, J., Brunner, R., Johnson, A., & Novack, T. (2002). Amantadine to improve neurorecovery in traumatic brain injury–associated diffuse axonal injury: A pilot double-blind randomized trial. *Journal of Head Trauma Rehabilitation, 17*(4), 300–313.

Meythaler, J. M., Clayton, W., Davis, L. K., Guin-Renfroe, S., & Brunner, R. C. (2004). Orally delivered baclofen to control spastic hypertonia in acquired brain injury. *Journal of Head Trauma Rehabilitation, 19*(2), 101–108.

Meythaler, J. M., Depalma, L., Devivo, M. J., Guin-Renfroe, S., & Novack, T. A. (2001). Sertraline to improve arousal and alertness in severe traumatic brain injury secondary to motor vehicle crashes. *Brain Injury, 15*(4), 321–331.

Mooney, G. F., & Haas, L. J. (1993). Effect of methylphenidate on brain injury–related anger. *Archives of Physical Medicine and Rehabilitation, 74*, 153–160.

Pachet, A., Friesen, S., Winkelaar, D., & Gray, S. (2003). Beneficial behavioral effects of lamotrigine in traumatic brain injury. *Brain Injury, 17*(8), 715–722.

Pena, C. G. (2003). Seizure emergency. *American Journal of Nursing, 103*, 73–81.

Port, A., Willmott, C., & Charlton, J. (2002). Self-awareness following traumatic brain injury and implications for rehabilitation. *Brain Injury, 16*(4), 277–289.

Povlishock, J. T., & Katz, D. J. (2005). Update on neuropathology and neuronal recovery after traumatic brain injury. *Journal of Head Trauma Rehabilitation, 20*(1), 76–94.

Rao, V., & Lyketsos, C. G. (2002). Psychiatric aspects of traumatic brain injury. *Psychiatric Clinics of North America, 25*(1), 1–24.

Rhijn, J. V., Molenaers, G., & Ceulemans, B. (2005). Botulinum toxin type A in the treatment of children and adolescents with an acquired brain injury. *Brain Injury, 19*(5), 331–335.

Schiff, N. D., Rodriguez-Moreno, D., Kamal, A., Kim, K. H. S., Giacino, J. T., Plum, F., . . . Hirsch, J. (2005). fMRI reveals large-scale network activation in minimally conscious patients. *Neurology, 64*, 514–523.

Schneider, W. N., Drew-Cates, J., Wong, T. M., & Dombovy, M. L. (1999). Cognitive and behavioral efficacy of amantadine in acute traumatic brain injury: An initial double-blind placebo-controlled study. *Brain Injury, 13*(11), 863–872.

Shoumitro, D., & Crownshaw, T. (2004). The role of pharmacotherapy in the management of behavior disorders in traumatic brain injury patients. *Brain Injury, 18*(1), 1–31.

Silver, J. M., Kourmara, B., Chen, M., Mirski, D., Potkin, S. G., Reyes, P., . . . Gunay, I. (2006). Effects of rivastigmine on cognitive function in patients with traumatic brain injury. *Neurology, 67*, 748–755.

Stanislav, S. W., & Childs, A. (2000). Evaluating the usage of droperidol in acutely agitated persons with brain injury. *Brain Injury, 14*(3), 261–265.

Sugden, S. G., Kile, S. J., Farrimond, D. D., Hilty, D. M., & Bourgeois, J. A. (2006). Pharmacological intervention for cognitive deficits and aggression in frontal lobe injury. *Neurorehabilitation, 21*, 3–7.

Thorley, R. R., Wertsch, J. J., & Klingbeil, G. E. (2001). Acute hypothalamic instability in traumatic brain injury: A case report. *Archives of Physical Medicine and Rehabilitation, 82*, 246–249.

Walker, W. C., Ketchum, J. M., Marwitz, J. H., Chen, T., Hammond, F., Sherer, M., & Meythaler, J. A. (2010). Multicentre study on the clinical utility of post-traumatic amnesia duration in predicting global outcome after moderate–severe traumatic brain injury. *Journal of Neurology, Neurosurgery, and Psychiatry, 81*, 87–89.

Whiteneck, G. (Ed.). (1993). *Aging with spinal cord injury*. New York: Demos.

Wiercisiewski, D. R. (2001). Pharmacologic management of behavior in traumatic brain injury. *Physical Medicine and Rehabilitation: State of the Art Review, 15*(2), 267–281.

Wroblewski, B. A., Joseph, A. B., Kupfer, J., & Kalliel, K. (1997). Effectiveness of valproic acid on destructive and aggressive behaviors in patients with acquired brain injury. *Brain Injury, 11*(1), 37–47.

Zafonte, R. D., Lexell, J., & Cullen, N. (2001a). Possible applications for dopaminergic agents following traumatic brain injury: Part 1. *Journal of Head Trauma Rehabilitation, 16*(1), 1179–1182.

Zafonte, R. D., Lexell, J., & Cullen, N. (2001b). Possible applications for dopaminergic agents following traumatic brain injury: Part 2. *Journal of Head Trauma Rehabilitation, 16*(1), 112–116.

Chapter 24

Rehabilitation for the Patient with a Musculoskeletal Condition

Paula Stangeland, PhD RN CRRN NE-BC
Cheryl Lehman, PhD RN CNS-BC RN-BC CRRN

LEARNING OUTCOMES

- Review select skeletal conditions, including osteoporosis, arthritis, and fractures.
- Examine a variety of soft tissue injuries, including sprains, strains, and dislocations.
- Distinguish between surgical interventions for musculoskeletal conditions.
- Identify key aspects of physical assessment and rehabilitation nursing interventions for complications related to musculoskeletal conditions that are encountered in the rehabilitation setting.
- Apply rehabilitation nursing principles to the care of patients with a musculoskeletal condition.

KEY CHAPTER TOPICS

- Skeletal conditions
- Soft tissue injuries
- Surgical interventions
- Other complications

PROFESSIONAL REHABILITATION NURSING DOMAINS AND COMPETENCIES

- Domain 1: Competencies 1.2, 1.3
- Domain 2: Competency 2.2
- Domain 4: Competency 4.2 (Association of Rehabilitation Nurses [ARN], 2014)

Introduction

Knowledge of musculoskeletal conditions, potential complications, and musculoskeletal rehabilitation is important for rehabilitation nurses across settings and patient populations and throughout the continuum of care. Musculoskeletal rehabilitation is evolving in the United States, primarily due to the evolution of the Centers for Medicare and Medicaid (CMS) regulations. For example, in the past, the majority of orthopedic rehabilitation for patients with joint replacement, major fractures, and multiple traumas took place in acute inpatient rehabilitation facilities. With the CMS regulations changes, orthopedic rehabilitation increasingly is taking place in skilled nursing facilities and nursing homes. Nurses in many settings are likely to encounter patients with musculoskeletal conditions as a primary or secondary diagnosis.

Although this chapter focuses on the rehabilitation patient with a primary diagnosis of musculoskeletal condition, it is important to remember that a musculoskeletal condition can be a secondary diagnosis, rather than the primary reason for admission. For instance, a patient with traumatic brain injury (TBI) might exhibit severe muscle spasticity related to the brain injury, or a non–weight-bearing patient might be at high risk for osteoporosis and bone fractures.

The function of bones, muscles, and joints is a key factor in mobility and independence and requires the rehabilitation nurse to remain alert to potential complications in the musculoskeletal system that can affect patient independence and quality of life. The rehabilitation nurse must also remain aware of preventive activities that can help rehabilitation patients maintain the health and function of the musculoskeletal system. Education on muscle and bone health is important for all patients, regardless of their primary diagnosis.

This chapter offers the learner the opportunity to review rehabilitation nursing care for patients with soft tissue injury or a skeletal condition. Key rehabilitation-related aspects of surgical interventions are reviewed, as are complications related to musculoskeletal conditions.

I. Skeletal Conditions

A. Osteoporosis

1. A common metabolic bone disease evidenced by decreased bone mass and poor bone quality
   a. Progressive, chronic disease
   b. Microarchitectural deterioration of bone tissue
   c. Reflects inadequate bone accumulation during growth and maturation, or excessive losses after that
   d. Increases risk of hip, spine, and wrist fracture
   e. Preventable
2. Can be primary or secondary in nature
   a. Primary osteoporosis most common form, more common in women
      1) Postmenopausal osteoporosis, age-associated osteoporosis, idiopathic form in premenopausal women and middle-aged men
   b. Secondary osteoporosis, more common in men
      1) Associated with inflammatory disorders, disorders of bone marrow, endocrine disorders of bone remodeling, medications
3. Ten million people in the United States have osteoporosis, and 18 million more are at risk.
   a. Another 34 million Americans are at risk for osteopenia (i.e., low bone mass) (American Academy of Orthopaedic Surgeons [AAOS], 2009; Jacobs-Kosmin, 2013)
   b. Occurs in both sexes, all races, and all age groups
   c. One in two women and one in eight men older than age 50 years will sustain an osteoporosis-related fracture during their lifetime.
   d. More than one third of men who develop a hip fracture related to osteoporosis will die within 1 year (U. S. Preventive Services Task Force, 2011)
4. World Health Organization (WHO) definition of osteoporosis (WHO, 2004)
   a. Key diagnostic test is X ray for bone mineral density, expressed as T-score
      1) Normal: T-score > -1
      2) Osteopenia: T-score between -1 and -2.5
      3) Osteoporosis: T-score < -2.5
      4) Severe osteoporosis: T-score < -2.5 with fragility fractures
   b. Alternative scoring for the bone mineral density is the Z-score, which is used for premenopausal women and for men and children. Z-scores can also be adjusted for ethnicity and race.
   c. The 10-year risk for osteoporotic fractures can be calculated for individuals with the use of the WHO fracture risk assessment (FRAX® tool: http://www.shef.ac.uk/FRAX/index.aspx?lang=En).
5. Not all causes are clear, but genetics, endocrine system, and lifestyle factors can contribute.
   a. Nonmodifiable risk factors for osteoporosis
      1) Age > 50 years, female, and postmenopausal
      2) Family history of osteoporosis; being thin and underweight
      3) A history of fractures; white or Asian background
   b. Modifiable risk factors for osteoporosis
      1) A diet low in vitamin D and calcium
      2) A diet low in fruits and vegetables
      3) A diet high in protein, caffeine, and sodium
      4) An inactive lifestyle
      5) Smoking, alcohol abuse, or weight loss
      6) Certain medications
         a) Aluminum-containing antacids, heparin, Dilantin®, phenobarbital, cancer chemotherapy, lithium, Depo-Provera®
         b) Methotrexate, proton pump inhibitors, selective serotonin reuptake inhibitors and other antidepressants, or steroids
         c) Thiazolidinediones, excess thyroid hormone, Tamoxifen®, Tacrolimus® (National Osteoporosis Foundation [NOF], n.d.)
   c. Diseases that can cause osteoporosis
      1) Autoimmune disorders: rheumatoid arthritis, multiple sclerosis, lupus erythematosus, and ankylosing spondylitis
      2) Digestive and gastrointestinal disorders: celiac disease, inflammatory bowel disease, weight loss surgery, gastrectomy, and gastrointestinal bypass procedures (NOF, n.d.)
      3) Endocrine, hormonal disorders: diabetes, hyperparathyroidism, hyperthyroidism, Cushing's syndrome, thyrotoxicosis, amenorrhea, premature menopause, and low testosterone levels in men
      4) Hematologic, blood disorders: leukemia, lymphoma, multiple myeloma, sickle cell

disease, blood and bone marrow disorders, thalassemia
    5) Chronic kidney disease
    6) Neurological disorders: TBI, SCI, stroke, Parkinson's disease, multiple sclerosis
    7) Mental illness: depression, eating disorders
    8) Cancer: breast, prostate
    9) Other: HIV/AIDS, chronic obstructive pulmonary disease, female superathletes, chronic kidney disease, liver disease, organ transplant, polio and postpolio syndrome, weight loss (NOF, n.d.)
6. There are usually no symptoms of osteoporosis until a fracture occurs.
    a. Screening measures are key components of prevention and early detection.
    b. Could see a loss of height or curvature of spine (NOF, n.d.)
7. Laboratory tests are used to rule out other diseases that could be causing bone loss and to establish baseline condition. These tests include
    a. Complete blood count, serum calcium, phosphate, alkaline phosphatase, vitamin D, creatinine, parathyroid hormone, magnesium, iron, ferritin, liver function tests, and thyroid stimulating hormone.
8. Treatment goals
    a. Prevention
    b. Screening to discover disease early
        1) Evidence is lacking about optimal intervals for performing bone density screening and whether repeated screening is needed in a woman whose initial test was negative.
        2) Evidence is lacking regarding the efficacy of bone density screening for males.
    c. Preserve existing bone tissue.
    d. Depending upon the cause, medications such as estrogens, parathyroid hormone, bisphosphonates, raloxifene, and calcitonin can be used, along with vitamin D and calcium supplementation and weight-bearing exercise.
9. Implications for the rehabilitation team
    a. Most, if not all, patients in the rehabilitation setting are at high risk for bone loss, osteopenia, and osteoporosis resulting from a medical condition, immobility, nonweight bearing, dietary deficiencies, medications, and other individual risk factors such as age, smoking, and family history.
    b. Osteoporosis can develop over time, with effects appearing after discharge.
        1) Emphasize importance of risk factor assessment and patient teaching in the rehabilitation setting.
    c. Rehabilitation team should consider recommending bone density testing before or after discharge, depending on patient's condition and risk factors.
    d. Dietary consultation and education are also important during the rehabilitation stay.
    e. The team should remain aware that osteoporosis-related fractures could occur in the rehabilitation setting.
    f. As the population ages, more rehabilitation patients could be at risk for osteoporosis.
10. Rehabilitation nursing implications
    a. Risk factor assessment for all patients, including medications
    b. Ongoing monitoring for fracture potential
        1) Diet, activity, weight bearing, diagnosis, age, balance, and mobility
    c. Safety interventions for transfers and ambulation
    d. Patient education on personal risk factors and interventions
        1) Diet, weight-bearing exercise
        2) Current evidence indicates caution when recommending routine calcium supplementation for persons whose laboratory levels of this substance is unknown, due to risk of other side effects.
            a) Too much calcium supplementation can impair iron absorption and can also cause kidney stones, cardiac arrhythmias, constipation, and possibly even heart disease.
            b) Blood levels should be known before supplementation is recommended.
        3) Don't forget sunshine! Exposure to sun is important for vitamin D production in the body. Twenty minutes of sun exposure per day, without sunscreen, is currently recommended. Vitamin D supplementation might be needed if sun exposure is not possible.

B. Arthritis
1. Osteoarthritis (OA)
    a. Not a normal consequence of aging
        1) Twenty-seven million people in the United States have OA (Arthritis Foundation, 2014)
    b. Characterized by degeneration of cartilage and the underlying bone within a joint, as well as bony overgrowth

1) Biochemical breakdown of articular cartilage in synovial joints (Lozada, 2014)
2) Leads to pain and joint stiffness
3) Most commonly affects the knees, hips, hands, spine
4) Gradual onset
5) Does not always progress into severe disease
6) Noninflammatory

c. Two types—idiopathic and secondary
1) Idiopathic OA can be localized or generalized.
a) Localized OA most commonly affects hands, feet, knee, hip, or spine.
b) Generalized or can involve three or more joint sites
2) Secondary due to other conditions that cause or enhance of the risk of OA
a) Trauma, congenital or developmental disorders, osteonecrosis, rheumatoid arthritis, gouty arthritis, septic arthritis, or Paget's disease of the bone
b) Diabetes mellitus, acromegaly, hypothyroidism, or frostbite (Kalunian, 2013)
c) Menopause, some occupations that require frequent kneeling and stooping

d. Primary symptom is joint pain
1) Begins with soreness or stiffness
2) Develops into joints that are sore or stiff after inactivity or overuse
3) Pain then becomes worse after activity or toward the end of the day.
4) Pain can be moderate and come and go, not affecting ability to do ADLs (Arthritis Foundation, 2014).
5) Can also have reduced range of motion and crepitus
6) Morning stiffness usually lasts less than 30 minutes.
7) Systemic symptoms are not present with OA, distinguishing it from inflammatory joint disorders such as rheumatoid arthritis.

e. Diagnostic studies done after the patient presents with symptoms consist of physical examination, X ray, and laboratory work to rule out other conditions.
1) Laboratory work includes erythrocyte sedimentation rate, rheumatoid titer factors, and evaluation of synovial fluid (Kalunian, 2013).

f. Common risk factors for OA include increasing age, obesity, previous or repeated joint injury, overuse of the joint, weak thigh muscles, and genetics (Arthritis Foundation, 2014).

g. There is no cure for OA.

h. Goals of treatment include reduction of pain and improvement of functional status.
1) Combination of nonpharmacological and pharmacological interventions
2) Medications are used to reduce or relieve pain (American College of Rheumatology recommendations).
a) Hand
(i) Topical capsaicin
(ii) Topical nonsteroidal antiinflammatory drugs (NSAIDs)
(iii) Oral NSAIDs
(iv) Tramadol
b) Knee
(i) Acetaminophen
(ii) Oral NSAIDs
(iii) Topical NSAIDs
(iv) Tramadol
(v) Intra-articular injections of corticosteroids
c) Hip
(i) Acetaminophen
(ii) Oral NSAIDs
(iii) Tramadol
(iv) Intra-articular injections of corticosteroids (Lozada, 2014)
3) Physical therapy (PT) and occupational therapy (OT) address joint function and muscle strength.
4) Complementary interventions can be used.
a) Acupuncture, yoga, massage, guided imagery, therapeutic touch
b) Glucosamine and chondroitin medications could be prescribed by some practitioners.
5) Surgery is considered with the presence of severe pain or severely impaired mobility or function.
a) Arthroscopy
(i) For removal of meniscal tears and loose bodies, debridement of articular cartilage (Lozada, 2014)
b) Osteotomy
(i) For patients < 60 years with malaligned knee or hip joint
(ii) Can lessen pain and help defer knee replacement until later
(iii) Helps to shift weight from damaged cartilage on medial aspect

of knee to healthy lateral aspect (Lozada, 2014)

c) Arthroplasty (knee, hip)
   (i) Surgical removal of joint surface and insertion of metal and plastic prosthesis
   (ii) Performed only after all other interventions have failed or if patient cannot perform ADLs despite maximal therapy (Lozada, 2014)

d) Fusion
   (i) Union of the bones on either side of a joint
   (ii) Relieves pain but prevents motion and puts stress on surrounding joints

6) Weight reduction is an important aspect in symptom relief, especially in knees and hips.

7) Other treatment interventions include application of heat and cold

i. Implications for rehabilitation team
   1) OA could be a secondary condition for the rehabilitation patient—not the reason for admission, but present regardless
      a) Or it could have been the primary cause of joint replacement or other surgery that resulted in a rehabilitation admission.
   2) OA as a secondary condition could interfere with rehabilitation for the primary condition.
      a) Pain, limited joint range of motion, lessened ability to do ADLs
   3) Other patient conditions/diagnoses can exacerbate symptoms of OA and need to be addressed in rehabilitation.
      a) Obesity
   4) The patient with chronic OA could require medication to address pain and inflammation, even if the OA was not the reason for admission.

j. Rehabilitation nursing implications
   1) Functional and pain assessments
   2) Pain management
      a) Around the clock
      b) Special dosing pretherapy
   3) Patient education
      a) Weight loss
      b) Diet
      c) Pain management
      d) Joint protection
      e) Home safety
   4) Implement adaptive equipment for ADLs as prescribed by PT and OT to address limitations caused by OA.
   5) Safety precautions for limited joint mobility and pain that interferes with transfers and ambulation
   6) Home evaluation with OT and PT

2. Rheumatoid arthritis (RA)
   a. Chronic systemic inflammatory disease of unknown cause
      1) External trigger (e.g., infection, trauma) initiates an autoimmune reaction
         a) Genetic, environmental, hormonal, immunologic, and infectious factors can play roles, as can socioeconomic, psychological, and lifestyle factors (Temprano, 2014).
         b) Leads to synovial hypertrophy, chronic joint inflammation
         c) Extra-articular (systemic) manifestations possible
         d) Parental history of substance abuse can increase risk (Temprano, 2014).
   b. Affects all populations; incidence three cases per 10,000 population worldwide
      1) 1.5 million people in the United States have been diagnosed with RA.
      2) Women affected three times as often as men
      3) Sex differences decrease with increased age.
      4) Most commonly begins between ages 30 and 60 years
      5) Higher risk with complications of pregnancy such as hyperemesis, preeclampsia, and gestational hypertension
      6) Juvenile RA is the most common type of arthritis in children.
   c. Clinical picture includes exacerbations and remissions
      1) Forty percent of people with RA are disabled within 10 years.
      2) Clinical course can be worsening and progressive, but some people have self-limiting disease.
      3) Early diagnosis and treatment can help limit exacerbations and achieve remission.
      4) Unfavorable diagnosis with
         a) Extra-articular manifestations, large number of joints involved, age younger than 30 years, female sex, systemic symptoms, insidious onset, HLA-DRB*04/04 genotype, high serum titer of autoantibodies (Temprano, 2014)

5) Diagnosis made on consideration of symptoms, X rays, laboratory results
    a) Laboratory tests include erythrocyte sedimentation rate, C-reactive protein level, CBC, rheumatoid factor assay, antinuclear antibody assay, anticyclic citrullinated peptide, and antimutated citrullinated vimentin assays.

d. Signs and symptoms
    1) Symmetrical polyarthritis
        a) On both sides of body, especially hands and feet
        b) Joint inflammation and swelling
        c) Pain
    2) Extra-articular (systemic) involvement
        a) Rheumatoid nodules, subcutaneous
            (i) Olecranon processes, proximal ulna, back of heel, occiput, and ischial tuberosities are the most common sites (Temprano, 2014)
        b) Other body systems: cardiac, pulmonary, renal, gastrointestinal, vascular, hematological, neurological, and ophthalmological

e. Complications
    1) Infection, anemia, osteoporosis, heart disease, Sjögren's syndrome, leukopenia, or splenomegaly
    2) Progressive deterioration of joints with deformity
    3) Progressive difficulty with ADLs
    4) "Constitutional" symptoms
        a) Fatigue, malaise, morning stiffness, weight loss, and low-grade fever

f. Treatment
    1) Goals include reducing inflammation, managing pain, maintaining joint function, and preventing joint deformity.
    2) Pharmacological and nonpharmacological
        a) NSAIDs, disease-modifying antirheumatic drugs, immunosuppressants, corticosteroids
        b) Surgical interventions include synovectomy, tenosynovectomy, tendon realignment, reconstructive surgery, arthrodesis
        c) Massage, exercise, diet, stress reduction
        d) Physical and occupational therapy for joint protection, heat and cold application, exercise, and patient education

g. Implications for rehabilitation team
    1) Can be admitted to inpatient rehabilitation for initial assessment and prescription of adaptive equipment, pain management, mobility and safety training, splinting
    2) Can also be managed in outpatient rehabilitation clinic
    3) RA could be the secondary diagnosis in a patient admitted to rehabilitation for a primary condition such as stroke or traumatic injury.
        a) Can affect rehabilitation for primary condition
    4) Home evaluation and modifications could be necessary.

h. Patient education
    1) Pain management
    2) Reducing disability
    3) Joint protection
        a) Maintain joint position in neutral position.
        b) Use strongest joint available for any activity.
        c) Distribute weight over several joints instead of a single joint.
        d) Change positions frequently.
        e) Avoid repetitive movements.
        f) Modify chores to minimize stress on joints (Lewis, Dirksen, Heitkemper, Bucher, & Camera, 2011)
    4) Range of motion (ROM) exercises

3. Gout and gouty arthritis
    a. A form of inflammatory arthritis with a sudden, acute onset of pain, swelling, and tenderness, often in the big toe
        1) Also called crystal-induced arthropathy because of the role of uric acid crystals (i.e., monosodium urate monohydrate crystals)
        2) One of the oldest diseases in the medical literature, known since the time of the ancient Greeks
        3) If untreated, joint destruction and renal damage can occur.
    b. Can be a primary or secondary condition
        1) Primary related to underexcretion or overproduction of uric acid
            a) Dietary excesses or alcohol overuse and metabolic syndrome
        2) Secondary related to medications or conditions that cause hyperuricemia
            a) Myeloproliferative diseases
            b) Renal failure
            c) Renal tubular disorders
            d) Lead poisoning
            e) Starvation or dehydration
            f) Hyperproliferative skin disorders

g) Enzymatic defects (Rothschild, 2014)

3) Diseases that increase the risk of developing gout

a) Hypertension, diabetes mellitus, renal insufficiency, hypertriglyceridemia, and hypercholesterolemia

b) Obesity, anemia, psoriasis, and psoriatric arthritis

c) Consumption of fructose-rich foods and beverages also increase the risk of gout in men and women

c. Diagnosis is based on finding urate crystals in aspirated synovial fluid.

1) Signs and symptoms

a) Podagra (pain in the great toe related to gout)

b) Arthritis in other sites: instep, ankle, wrist, finger joints, knee

c) Monoarticular (i.e., single joint) involvement

d) Abrupt painful attacks that reach maximum intensity within 8–12 hours

e) Becomes polyarticular (i.e., multiple joints) over time without treatment

f) Can resemble RA if untreated over time

g) Swelling, warmth, tenderness, erythema over joint, fever, tophi in soft tissues

h) Eye involvement can occur if untreated over time (Rothschild, 2014)

2) Complications

a) Severe degenerative arthritis

b) Secondary infections

c) Renal damage, renal stones

d) Fractures in joints with tophaceous gout (Rothschild, 2014)

d. Diagnosis includes laboratory testing, X rays, and ultrasound

1) Laboratory tests can include synovial fluid analysis, serum uric acid level, 24-hour uric acid evaluation, white blood cells, triglycerides, high-density lipoprotein (HDL), glucose, and renal and liver function tests (Rothschild, 2014).

e. Treatment goals include treating acute attacks of gout, providing prophylaxis to prevent flare-ups, and lowering excess stores of urate.

1) Other goals are pain management, preventing disease progression, and preventing deposition of uric acid crystals in the renal system.

2) Treatment can include

a) Acute stage medications: NSAIDs, corticosteroids (oral or intra-articular injections), adrenocorticotropic hormone (ACTH), colchicine

b) Long-term medications are used to lower uric acid levels.

(i) allopurinol, febuxostat, and probenecid

c) Nonpharmacological interventions include dietary restrictions of high-purine foods, avoiding alcohol (especially beer), avoiding high fructose corn syrup, limiting use of naturally sweet fruit juices as well as table sugar and table salt, maintaining high level of water intake, low-cholesterol/low-fat diet, and weight reduction if obese.

d) Surgery could be indicated with joint infection, joint deformity, spinal cord impingement, intractable pain, and ulcers related to tophi.

f. Implications for the rehabilitation team

1) An attack of gouty arthritis could occur in the rehabilitation setting as a secondary condition in a patient admitted for another diagnosis.

2) Any rehabilitation patient can be on chronic medications and dietary restrictions for gout, even if admitted for another condition. It is important that these medications and dietary restrictions continue throughout the rehabilitation stay.

3) Gouty arthritis can also occur for the first time in a patient in the rehabilitation setting who has been admitted for another condition, meaning that initial workup, treatment, and patient education must be accomplished before discharge.

g. Implications for the rehabilitation nurse

1) For acute attacks

a) Assessment, pain management, medication administration

2) For chronic gout

a) Medication administration, functional and pain assessment, dietary restrictions

3) Patient education on medications, dietary restrictions, adaptive equipment, safety

4. Avascular necrosis (AVN)

a. Also called osteonecrosis, bone infarction, aseptic necrosis, ischemic bone necrosis

b. Cellular death of bone components due to interruption of blood supply

1) Bone cells begin to die within 12–48 hours of loss of blood supply.

2) Bone marrow fat cells die within 5 days.
3) Bone structures then collapse, with destruction of bone, loss of function, and pain.
4) Usually involves epiphysis of long bones
   a) Femoral and humoral heads
   b) Most common in hip
   c) Can occur in smaller bones (Tofferi, 2012)
5) Use of bisphosphonate medications has recently been associated with AVN of the jaw.
6) Progressive process, with bone destruction within 5 years if not treated

c. New cases: 15,000 in United States each year
   1) Results in 10% of all total hip replacement surgeries performed in the United States
   2) 380 cases of osteonecrosis of jaw reported with bisphosphonate use
   3) Not associated with race or ethnicity, except for cases of AVN in African Americans with sickle cell disease
   4) Mostly found in males, but in females, more cases associated with systemic lupus erythematosus
   5) Disease of middle age, occurring most often in ages 40–50 (Tofferi, 2012)

d. Risk factors
   1) Organ transplant or corticosteroid use
   2) Alcohol abuse, radiation therapy, hypertension, vasculitis, sickle cell anemia, traumatic injury, vascular compression, arterial embolism and thrombosis, chemotherapy, decompression sickness, Gaucher's disease, RA, or lupus

e. Signs and symptoms
   1) Often found by accident on routine X rays ordered for other purposes
   2) May be asymptomatic
   3) Symptoms depend on joint affected
      a) Hands, feet often symptomatic
   4) Primary symptom is pain in the affected joint
      a) With femoral head AVN, pain is felt in groin and worsens with weight bearing.
      b) Pain worsens over time.
      c) Large infarcts associated with severe pain (Tofferi, 2012)

f. Diagnosis is based on symptoms and radiologic findings.
   1) MRI most sensitive test
   2) Bone biopsy can be performed but is not routinely ordered because of high sensitivity and specificity of MRI (Tofferi, 2012).

g. Treatment depends upon severity, location, and patient's age.
   1) There is no known way to prevent or stop this disease process.
   2) Conservative treatment includes limiting weight bearing and pain management.
   3) Immobilization is sometimes used.
   4) Bisphosphonates can be used but sufficient evidence not available to support this practice
   5) Statin therapy can prevent corticosteroid-induced AVN.
   6) Surgery is required for advanced cases.
      a) Core decompression to decrease intermedullary pressure on blood vessels
         (i) Holes are drilled into the bone to relieve pressure on blood vessels and create channels for new blood vessel growth.
         (ii) Prevents progression to severe arthritis in 25%–85% of cases (American Academy of Orthopaedic Surgeons [AAOS], 2014)
      b) Bone graft with core decompression
      c) Osteotomy to transfer weight-bearing forces and prevent fracture
      d) Total hip arthroplasty (Tofferi, 2012)

h. Implications for the rehabilitation team
   1) A patient with AVN can be admitted for mobility and gait training and equipment prescription or can be admitted postoperatively.
   2) Rehabilitation interventions depend on the reason for admission.
   3) Safety training is important, as is pain management.
   4) Home safety evaluation by PT, OT, and nurses is necessary.

i. Implications for the rehabilitation nurse
   1) Pain assessment and management
   2) Evaluation of function and safety
   3) Assist with mobility, gait, and ADLs.
   4) Ensure safety.
   5) Patient education on pain management, safety
   6) Caregiver training

5. Legg-Calve-Perthes (LCP) disease
   a. Also called ischemic necrosis of the hip, coxa plana, osteochondritis, and AVN of the femoral head
      1) AVN of the proximal femoral head resulting from poor blood supply (Harris, 2013)
      2) Rare condition

3) Found only in children

b. Affects 4 in 100,000 children
   1) Age at diagnosis usually between 2 and 12 years; average age is 7 years.
   2) Males comprise 75% of cases (Harris, 2013).

c. Cause unknown
   1) Usually unilateral
   2) Bilateral in < 10% of cases, but not simultaneously (Harris, 2013)
   3) Rapid growth occurs in relation to blood supply available.
      a) Stages of LCP: interruption of blood supply, necrosis of bone, removal of necrotic tissue by body, natural replacement with newer bone
      b) Bone replacement can be normal (Harris, 2013).

d. Risk factors
   1) Active children who are small for their age
   2) Asians, Eskimos, whites
      a) Lower incidence in Australian Aboriginals, Native Americans, Polynesians, Blacks
   3) Exposure to secondhand smoke (National Osteonecrosis Foundation [NONF], 2000)

e. Symptoms
   1) Intermittent limp (abductor lurch), especially after exertion
   2) Mild or intermittent pain in anterior thigh
   3) Pain in hip, groin, or knee (Harris, 2013; NONF, 2000)

f. Diagnosis
   1) X ray (NONF, 2000)

g. Treatment
   1) Goals
      a) Eliminate hip irritability.
      b) Restore and maintain good ROM in hip.
      c) Prevent femoral epiphyseal collapse.
      d) Attain spherical femoral head when hip heals (Harris, 2013).
   2) Initial treatment
      a) Minimal weight bearing
         (i) Crutches if able
      b) Positioning and protection of joint with abducted, internally rotated femur
         (i) Using bracing (nonsurgical treatment) or osteotomy (surgery) (Harris, 2013)

h. Implications for the rehabilitation team
   1) The patient with LCP can be seen in the inpatient or outpatient setting
      a) Mobility training
      b) Equipment prescription and training
      c) Education on safety
      d) Caregiver training

i. Implications for rehabilitation nurse
   1) Pain assessment and management
   2) Education on safety, skin care
   3) Reinforce PT/OT education on equipment and mobility training.
   4) Train caregiver.

C. Fractures

1. Bone fractures can be the primary reason for admission to the rehabilitation setting, or fractures can occur within the rehabilitation setting secondary to falls or other trauma. Several types of fractures are discussed in this section.
2. A *fracture* is the disruption of the integrity of a living bone, involving injury to bone marrow, periosteum, and nearby tissues.
3. Examples of fracture types include pathological, stress, and greenstick.
4. Caused when force applied to the bone exceeds the strength of the bone
   a. Direct or indirect trauma (Buckley, 2014)
5. Fractures can be classified or described on the basis of
   a. Anatomy
      1) Specific bone and location within the bone
         a) Diaphysis, metaphysis, physis, or epiphysis (Buckley, 2014)
      2) Articular surface involvement
         a) Intra-articular (Buckley, 2014)
      3) Displacement
         a) Degree or percentage to which distal fragment is displaced compared with proximal fragment (Buckley, 2014)
      4) Rotation
      5) Shortening
      6) Fragmentation
         a) Multifragmentary
      7) Soft tissue involvement
   b. Simple fractures are spiral, oblique, or transverse.
   c. Multifragmentary fracture has more than two fragments as the result of multiple breaks in the bone.
   d. Wedge fractures allow the proximal and distal fragments to remain in contact with each other.
   e. Complex multifragmentary fracture has no contact between distal and proximal fragments without bone shortening.
   f. Open fracture has soft tissue injury (Buckley, 2014).

6. There are 5.6 million fractures annually in the U.S.
   a. In males, higher incidence in young men and men > 60 years of age (bimodal distribution)
   b. In women, unimodal pattern with highest incidence around time of menopause (Buckley, 2014)
7. Can heal in two ways
   a. Primary healing
      1) Anatomic reduction with compression is achieved, no callus is formed, internal modeling
   b. Secondary/indirect healing
      1) Anatomic reduction not achieved or compression not possible, bony callus forms with external remodeling to bridge the gap (Buckley, 2014)
   c. Phases of bone healing
      1) Fracture and inflammatory phase
      2) Granulation tissue/soft callus formation
      3) Hard callus formation
      4) Remodeling and lamellar bone creation (Buckley, 2014)
   d. Factors with worse bone healing
      1) Advanced age, multiple comorbidities, smoking, poor nutrition, open fracture with poor blood supply, multiple traumatic injuries, local infection (Buckley, 2014)
   e. Initial treatment includes realignment and immobility, with close assessment of neurological and vascular status
      1) Hemostasis and prevention of infection important in open fractures
      2) Pain management important
      3) Operative and nonoperative fracture management possible
         a) Nonoperative
            (i) Closed reduction
         b) Operative
            (i) Failed closed management, unstable fractures, displaced intra-articular fractures, multiple trauma, open wounds, nonunion, injury to growth plate
            (ii) Surgery is not performed with active soft tissue or bone infection, excessive soft tissue injury or swelling, complicated comorbidities such as myocardial infarction (MI), when amputation is the better choice.
8. Pathological fracture
   a. A bone fracture at a site where bone has already been weakened by another disease, such as cancer, osteoporosis, or infection
      1) Occurs during normal activities
      2) Fragility fracture is one type of pathological fracture.
   b. Fracture and underlying disease process both need to be addressed.
   c. Diagnosis includes studies to consider or rule out another disease.
      1) Bone scan
      2) Biopsy of bone
      3) Laboratory work including CBC, sedimentation rate, serum calcium
   d. Implications for rehabilitation team
      1) Several patient populations in the rehabilitation setting are at high risk for pathological fracture.
         a) Older adults
         b) Patients with cancer
         c) Patients with inherited bone disease
      2) Even if admitting diagnosis is not bone related, rehabilitation team members must remain aware of fracture risk in these patients.
         a) Ensure safety education and safe transfers and ambulation.
         b) Appropriate equipment prescription and use
         c) Use of gait belts
            (i) Caution with bony metastasis of the spine
      3) Include evaluation of bone health with any falls in high-risk populations.
         a) Hip fracture
9. Stress fractures
   a. Two types
      1) Insufficiency fractures: due to normal stress on osteoporotic bones
      2) Stress fractures: when normal bone is subjected to abnormal stress (Kishner, 2014)
   b. Most common in lower extremities, but location depends of amount of force and direction of force
      1) Running, jumping, sports
   c. Causes
      1) Disrupted bone homeostasis and inadequate bone repair with repetitive overload
   d. Incidence 5%–30% among athletes and military
      1) Among the five most common injuries reported by runners
   e. Risk factors

1) Genetics, white, female, very active people
2) Low bone-mineral density, lower limb malalignment
3) Tall stature, poor athletic conditioning, strength imbalance, weakness
4) Pathological bone condition, endocrine abnormalities
5) Intense athletic training, continued activity even with pain, worn-out athletic shoes or equipment, poor nutrition, medications such as steroids

f. Symptoms
1) Insidious onset of activity-related pain
a) Occurs toward the end of a particular activity in early stages
b) As worsens, occurs earlier during same activity
c) Rest can relieve symptoms in early stages
2) Pain can also be felt in other areas as weight is shifted and movements are changed to relieve pain, placing stress on other parts of the musculoskeletal system.
3) Pain on palpation or percussion of affected area
4) Localized swelling and possible erythema

g. Diagnosis
1) Computed tomography, magnetic resonance imaging (MRI)

h. Treatment
1) Fracture care as indicated
2) Activity modification
3) Pain management—NSAIDs
4) Medications—bisphosphonates
5) PT

i. Rehabilitation team implications
1) Education on risk factors and prevention
2) Pain management
3) Fracture care
4) Athletic equipment: must fit, must be functional for the activity, and must not be worn out (e.g., shoes)

10. Greenstick fractures
a. Occurs when a bone bends and cracks, instead of breaking into pieces
1) Incomplete fracture of long bones
2) More common in children
b. Normally causes pain
1) Difficult to diagnose in babies or young children who cannot verbalize pain
c. Symptoms include
1) Swelling, redness, and bruising
d. Classified as a stable fracture
e. Treatment is splinting in most cases.

11. Rehabilitation team implications with fractures
a. When fracture and repair are the admitting diagnoses for rehabilitation care, interventions depend on severity, location, and type of fracture and repair mechanisms.
1) Key interventions involve functional assessment, equipment prescription and training, mobility, and safety.
2) Must also be alert for complications of fracture and fracture care
a) Pain, infection, malalignment, fat embolism, and venous thromboembolism

12. Rehabilitation nursing implications
a. Functional assessment
b. Pain assessment and management
c. Patient education, including safety
d. Reinforce PT and OT interventions.
e. Monitor for signs of healing, nonhealing, and other complications.

II. Soft Tissue Injuries

A. Sprains and Strains
1. A *sprain* is a stretching or tearing of ligaments (Mayo Clinic, 2014d).
a. *Ligaments* are the bands of fibrous tissue that connect one bone to another in the joints.
2. A *strain* is a stretching or tearing of muscle or tendon.
a. *Tendons* are fibrous threads of tissue that connect muscles to bones.
3. Incidence and prevalence
a. According to the U.S. Department of Labor, Bureau of Labor Statistics (2013), sprains, strains, and tears are the leading causes of injury and account for 38% of the total injury and illness cases requiring days away from work.
b. The ankle is the most common location for a sprain.
c. It has been reported that approximately 23,000 ankle sprains occur each day in the United States (Young, 2014).
d. Strains often occur in the lower back and hamstring muscle.
4. Risk factors
a. Poor conditioning leaves muscles weak and more likely to sustain injury.
b. Fatigued muscles are unable to provide good support for joints.
c. Improper warmup before physical activity leaves muscles tight.
1) Warming up properly before vigorous physical activity loosens the muscles and increases joint range of motion, making the

muscles less tight and less prone to trauma and tears.

5. Causes and precipitating features
   a. Sprains
      1) Ankle: Walking or exercising on uneven surfaces
      2) Knee: Pivoting during athletic activities (e.g., basketball)
      3) Wrist: Landing on hand during a fall
   b. Strains: Acute or chronic
      1) Acute strain occurs when muscles are pulled and can tear when overstretched (Mayo Clinic, 2014d).
         a) Slipping or falling on a wet surface
         b) Running, jumping, or throwing objects
         c) Lifting heavy objects, especially while in an awkward position
      2) Chronic strains result from repetitive movements of muscles in activities such as the following:
         a) Gymnastics
         b) Rowing
         c) Tennis
6. Acute signs and symptoms
   a. Symptoms vary depending on severity of injury.
      1) Sprains
         a) Pain
         b) Edema
            (i) Decreased sensation with severe edema
         c) Ecchymosis/bruising
            (i) Excessive bruising can indicate a broken bone.
         d) Limited ability to move affected joint
         e) Might hear or feel a "pop" in affected joint
      2) Strains
         a) Pain
         b) Swelling
         c) Muscle spasms
         d) Inability or limited ability to move affected muscle
7. Acute treatment modalities of sprains and strains
   a. Depends on the location and severity of injury
      1) Assess neurovascular status of involved area.
      2) Elevate involved area.
      3) Apply ice.
      4) Immobilize.
      5) Use medications.
         a) Over-the-counter pain reliever such as ibuprofen or acetaminophen
      6) Surgery could be required if ligament or tendon is torn or ruptured.
8. Chronic treatment
   a. Heat treatments to help relax and loosen tissues, and stimulate blood flow to the area
9. Acute care relevant to rehabilitation care and therapy
   a. Increase/maintain movement
   b. Nursing care and interventions
      1) Assessment of affected area
      2) Ice to reduce pain and swelling
10. Potential complications in rehabilitation setting
    a. Pain
    b. Instability of joint/reinjury
11. Goals of rehabilitation
    a. The main goal of rehabilitation is to restore normal joint function.
    b. Recover a pain-free range of motion.
    c. Increase strength.
12. Rehabilitation nursing implications
    a. Protect the injured joint or muscle.
    b. Patient education: Teach proper strengthening to prevent reinjury.
    c. Reinforce necessity of performing exercises to increase flexibility.
13. Age-related issues
    a. Older adults at risk of falls are more likely to sprain the knee or ankle joints.
    b. Early onset of arthritis in joints is associated with history of sprains and strains.

B. Dislocation and Subluxation
1. *Dislocation*
   a. Severe injury of the ligaments that surround a joint
2. *Subluxation*
   a. Partial or incomplete dislocation of joint surface
3. Incidence and prevalence
   a. Occurs most frequently in fingers and shoulders
   b. The overall incidence rate is 1.69 dislocations per 1,000 person-years.
4. Risk factors, causes, and precipitating features
   a. Significant demographic risk factors
      1) Falls
         a) Increase the possibility of a dislocated joint, especially if one uses the arm or hand to brace or reduce the impact of the fall
   b. Heredity

1) Some people are born with ligaments that are looser and more prone to injury than those of most people.

c. Participation in sports
   1) Increases risk for dislocation, especially in high-impact or contact sports
   2) Contact sports: football, hockey, and other sports that coud involve falls
   3) Basketball players and football players also commonly dislocate joints in their fingers and hands by accidentally striking the ball, the ground, or another player.

d. Motor vehicle accidents are the most common cause of hip dislocations.
   1) Can greatly reduce the risk of injury by wearing a seat belt

5. Acute signs and symptoms
   a. Visibly out of place or deformity
   b. Edema or discoloration
   c. Extremely painful
   d. Loss of function
   e. Could experience numbness or tingling near or below the injury
   f. Major complication is avascular necrosis (bone cell death related to inadequate blood supply to area)
6. Acute treatment modalities
   a. Treat as a fracture when first aid is administered.
      1) Check for pulse distal to the location.
      2) Keep the patient as still as possible.
      3) Move person as a whole unit.
   b. Dislocation must be reduced by a surgeon as soon as possible.
      1) Closed reduction
      2) Open reduction
7. Key points of acute care relevant to rehabilitation care and therapy: assessment, healing, and nursing care and interventions
   a. Nursing care and interventions
      1) Pain relief
      2) Support and protection of joint
      3) Immobilization (brace, splint, or sling to allow time to heal)
8. Potential complications in rehabilitation setting
   a. Increased risk for recurring dislocation secondary to loose ligaments
9. Goals of rehabilitation
   a. Pain management
   b. Return to normal function
10. Rehabilitation nursing implications
    a. Assess risk factors.
    b. Monitor safety.
    c. Educate patient, family, and significant other.
       1) Signs and symptoms of subluxation or dislocation
       2) Prevention of reinjury
       3) Don/doff immobilization device (e.g., brace, splint, or sling)
       4) Reinforce exercise routine.
11. Age-related issues
    a. Increased time to heal
    b. Poor healing

C. Repetitive Strain Injuries (RSI)
1. Occur from trauma caused by repeated physical movements, prolonged force, and poor posture, which damages tendons, nerves, muscles, and other soft body tissues (Lewis et al., 2011)
2. According to the Bureau of Labor Statistics (BLS; BLS, 2014), repetitive strain injuries are the nation's most common and costly occupational health problem.
3. Approximately 5 million American workers suffer from RSI (OSHA, 2013).
4. Risk factors
   a. Advancing age
   b. Poor posture
   c. Stress
      1) Muscles that are tight are more susceptible to strains.
   d. Poorly trained athletes
5. Causes and precipitating features
   a. People at high risk for injury include dancers; musicians; people who frequently use computers with mouse and keyboard; people who work with vibrating tools (e.g., jackhammers); and competitive and poorly trained persons who play sports on a regular basis (e.g., football, swimming, soccer, horseback riding) (Lewis et al., 2011).
   b. Assembly line worker
   c. Lifting too much weight or lifting improperly
   d. Climbing
   e. Painting
   f. Typing
   g. Tool operations
6. Acute signs and symptoms
   a. Numbness and tingling in affected area
   b. Pain
7. Acute treatment modalities
   a. Immobilization with splint (especially at night, rest affected area)
   b. Ice to reduce inflammation
8. Key points of acute care relevant to rehabilitation care and therapy: assessment, healing, nursing care and interventions

9. Potential complications in rehabilitation setting
    a. Reinjury
    b. Pain
10. Goals of rehabilitation
    a. Increased function
    b. Decreased pain
    c. Alternatives to completing task and maintaining any restrictions
11. Rehabilitation nursing implications
    a. Patient education
        1) Using proper ergonomics in the workplace
        2) Taking breaks and participating in injury-specific stretch and exercise programs that focus on strengthening weak, injured tendons and muscles.
        3) Stretching overly tight, restricted muscles to maintain or increase circulation, which in turn brings oxygenated blood to the
    b. Pain control
12. Age-related issues
    a. Aging adults have a higher incidence of poor healing.
    b. Older adults could require a longer healing period.

D. Carpal Tunnel Syndrome (CTS)

1. Compression of the median nerve located within the confines of the carpal tunnel
    a. Commonly associated with hobbies or occupations that require continuous movement
    b. Ligaments and bones within the wrist for the carpal tunnel
    c. Some consider CTS an inflammatory disorder caused by repetitive stress, physical injury, or a medical condition.
2. Incidence and prevalence
    a. CTS can affect anyone who uses their wrists repetitively at work or play.
    b. Persons at greater risk for CTS are those with diabetes mellitus and hypothyroidism.
    c. Women are more likely than men to develop CTS due to their smaller carpal tunnel.
3. According to the Mayo Clinic (2014b), risk factors associated with CTS include the following
    a. Previous dislocations or fractures of the wrist
    b. Rheumatoid arthritis
    c. Osteoarthritis of the wrist and carpus
    d. Obesity
    e. Medication use
        1) Insulin
        2) Sulphonylureas
        3) Metformin
        4) Thyroxine
    f. Female (smaller carpal tunnel)
    g. Medical conditions such as diabetes mellitus, menopause, obesity, thyroid disorders, and kidney failure can increase the chances of carpal tunnel syndrome development (Mayo Clinic, 2014a).
    h. Workplace conditions that require prolonged repetitive conditions such as assembly line work and working with vibrating equipment
4. Causes and precipitating features
    a. The biological mechanisms leading to carpal tunnel syndrome are unclear except with certain underlying diseases.
    b. Research suggests that no single cause can be identified (Peters, Page, Coppieters, Ross, & Johnston, 2013). However, causes can be a combination of risk factors that contribute to the development of CTS.
5. Acute signs and symptoms
    a. Carpal tunnel syndrome is characterized by pain, numbness, tingling, weakness, and problems performing fine hand movements due to pressure on the median nerve in the wrist.
    b. Physical assessment findings include a positive Tinel's sign (percussion over medial nerve in wrist elicits tingling) and Phalen's maneuver (allow wrist to flex naturally and freely for 60 seconds; if positive, a tingling sensation occurs in hand).
6. Acute treatment modalities
    a. Initially, mild symptoms can be treated at home. The sooner treatment is started, the less likely that permanent nerve damage will occur.
        1) Stop activities that cause numbness and pain.
        2) Rest wrist for longer periods between activities.
        3) Apply ice to wrist for 10 to 15 minutes one or two times per hour.
        4) NSAIDs are recommended to relieve pain and reduce swelling.
        5) Wear a wrist splint at night (takes pressure off the median nerve).
        6) Injections of corticosteroids can provide short-term relief of symptoms.
    b. Carpal tunnel release (a surgical intervention) could be necessary if symptoms last beyond 6 months.
        1) Open-release surgery (incision into wrist)
        2) Endoscopic carpal tunnel release (two to three small punctures)
7. Key points of acute care relevant to rehabilitation care and therapy: assessment, healing, nursing care and interventions

a. Nursing care and interventions
   1) Begin mobilization immediately postoperatively.
   2) Decrease edema with elevation.
   3) Pain reduction
      a) NSAIDs
      b) Ice therapy (three to four times a day)
   4) Education for patient and family
      a) Education on CTS, basic anatomy, and causes of compression
      b) Provide verbal and written instructions related to home exercise program.
      c) Provide information related to ergonomics, body mechanics, adaptive equipment, and adaptations as needed during activities of daily living.
      d) Teach with return demonstration of splint don/doff, wearing schedule, and hygiene.
      e) Patients should be educated on the importance of maintaining the wrist in an elevated position during the initial rehabilitation phase.

8. Goals of rehabilitation
   a. Reduce edema.
   b. Decrease pain.
   c. Increase strength.
   d. Increase mobilization.
9. Rehabilitation nursing implications
   a. Assess for risk factors, including medication.
   b. Maintain safety.
   c. Educate about prevention and maintenance.
10. Age-related issues
   a. Everyone is susceptible to CTS; however, it is unusual for persons to develop CTS before age 20, and the incidence increases with age.
   b. Older persons could take longer to heal.

E. Rotator Cuff (RTC) Injury

1. The rotator cuff is a group of muscles (i.e., supraspinatus, infraspinatus, teres minor, and subscapularis) and tendons that surround the shoulder joint, and keep the head of the humerus (upper arm bone) firmly seated within the glenoid fossa (the shallow socket of the shoulder). A rotator cuff injury or tear can be caused by a gradual degenerative process or occur with acute injury (Mayo Clinic, 2014c).
2. Incidence and prevalence
   a. A recent study by Schmidt, Claudius, and Brown (2015) reported approximately 18 million Americans present with shoulder pain yearly. In addition, these researchers state a large percentage are a result of rotator cuff disease. The AAOS reports that 5%–40% of people without shoulder pain could have a torn rotator cuff (AAOS, 2014).
   b. According to a recent study with a sample population of 683 people (1,366 shoulders) ranging in age from 22–87 years when examined, 20.7% of the population had full-thickness rotator cuff tears. In addition, 16.7% of the study population without symptoms also had rotator cuff tears (Yamamoto et al., 2010).
3. Risk factors
   a. Age
      1) Risk of a rotator cuff injury increases with age.
      2) Rotator cuff tears are most common in people older than 40 years.
   b. Sports
      1) Baseball pitchers, archers, and tennis players are at greater risk of having a rotator cuff injury because of the repetitive arm movements.
   c. Occupations such as carpentry or house painting require repetitive arm motions, often occurring overhead, that can damage the rotator cuff over time.
4. Acute signs and symptoms
   a. Pain
      1) Outside of the shoulder and in the upper arm
      2) Worsens when performing overhead activities (with the arm above head height)
   b. Severe injury and pain can awaken individuals anytime during sleep.
   c. Decreased strength
   d. Inability to perform normal tasks
5. Rehabilitation nursing implications
   a. Assess for risk factors.
   b. Education on related causes, prevention, and maintenance
   c. Maintain pain goals and pain control.
   d. Mobility
6. Age-related issues
   a. Recent research found that persons older than 60 years of age were two times more likely to experience a large RTC tear and three times more likely to experience a massive RTC tear compared with younger persons (Gumina et al., 2013).
   b. Time to heal after surgery increases with age.

F. Meniscus injury

1. *Menisci* are crescent-shaped fibrocartilage located in the knee and other joints.

a. There are two menisci in the knee; each is located between the femur and tibia.
   1) One meniscus is located on the medial (inner side) of the knee, and one is located on the lateral (outer side) of the knee.

2. Injuries to the menisci commonly occur in athletes engaging in sports such as basketball, soccer, football, and hockey (Lewis et al., 2011).
   a. The two most common causes of a meniscus tear are the result of traumatic injury (often seen in athletes) and degenerative processes (seen in older patients who have more brittle cartilage).
   b. It is common for injury to the meniscus to occur in conjunction with other injuries within the knee.
   c. Other injuries can occur to structures including the anterior cruciate ligament (ACL) and the medial collateral ligament.
3. Acute signs and symptoms
   a. Usually experience pain and swelling as the primary symptoms
   b. A common complaint is *joint locking*, which is the inability to completely straighten the knee joint.
      1) Joint locking is the result of torn cartilage preventing the normal movement of the knee.
   c. The most common symptoms of a meniscus tear
      1) Knee pain
      2) Swelling of the knee
      3) Tenderness when the meniscus is pressed
      4) Popping or clicking in the knee joint
      5) Limited motion
4. Acute treatment modalities
   a. Diagnosis is made with X ray or MRI.
      1) X ray helps determine whether arthritis exists in the joints.
      2) MRIs are completed to determine whether the meniscus is torn.
   b. Treatment
      1) A tear does not always mean that surgery is required.
      2) Treatment depends on several factors: the type of tear, the activity level of the patient, and the patient's response to initial treatment measures.
      3) Initial treatment includes
         a) Ice
         b) Rest
         c) Antiinflammatory medications (cortisone injections can be helpful in reducing inflammation)
         d) Physical therapy
5. Key points of acute care relevant to rehabilitation care and therapy: assessment, healing, and nursing care and interventions
   a. Nursing care and interventions
      1) Assess for risk factors.
      2) Provide education on related causes, prevention, and maintenance.
      3) Maintain pain goals and pain control.
      4) Decrease risk of reinjury.
         a) Teach patients to perform warm-up activities before participating in sports.
         b) Teach to bear weight as tolerated especially while on crutches.
         c) Use immobilizer or brace as ordered.
      5) Increase mobility.
         a) Encourage patient to participate in physical therapy to increase knee flexion and muscle strength.
6. Potential complications in rehabilitation setting
   a. Infections
   b. Pain
   c. Decrease in flexion and muscle strength related to pain and poor participation
   d. Reinjury with possible nerve injury
7. Goals of rehabilitation
   a. Increase mobility.
   b. Decrease pain.
   c. Protect the postsurgical knee
   d. Restore normal knee extension.
   e. Eliminate effusion (swelling).
   f. Restore leg control.
8. Age-related issues
   a. It is recommended that young athletes and young adults have follow-up studies, as they are at high risk for osteoarthritis after meniscus or ACL injury (Maffulli, Longo, Gougoulias, Loppini, & Denaro, 2010).
   b. Research found that a meniscal tear in middle-aged and elderly persons without previous knee surgery commonly increases the risk of osteoarthritis (Englund et al., 2009).

G. Anterior Cruciate Ligament Injury
1. Background
   a. More than 50% of sports injuries involve the knee.
      1) The ACL is the most commonly injured ligament.

2) ACL injuries occur most often during non-contact, such as when an athlete pivots, jumps, or slows down when running.

2. Acute signs and symptoms
   a. Common reports of landing on the ground or surface, twisting the knee, and hearing a popping sound
      1) The sound is usually associated with pain that occurs immediately after the popping sound.
   b. Persons with an ACL injury complain of the knee feeling unstable and are unable to continue playing.
   c. Positive Lachman's test: the best test for determining ACL injury.
      1) The Lachman's test involves positioning the patient in a prone position with the knee flexed at approximately 20–30 degrees. The examiner places one hand behind the tibia and the other hand on the thigh of the patient. The examiner slowly pulls on the tibia, noting the performance of the ligament. If the ligament is intact and working properly, the ligament will limit the ROM to a normal amount. If the ligament is torn, excessive movement will occur, and there will be an end point that is soft to the touch.
      2) X ray and MRI are used to diagnose the condition.
3. Acute treatment modalities
   a. For an injured intact ACL, conservative treatment includes ice, rest, NSAIDs, elevation of the limb, and ambulation as tolerated with crutches.
   b. Knee immobilizer to support knee during healing
   c. Physical therapy to maintain ROM and strength
   d. Reconstructive surgery is often recommended for active patients.
4. Key points of acute care relevant to rehabilitation care and therapy: assessment, healing, and nursing care and interventions
   a. Nursing care and interventions
      1) Assess and reassess for pain control.
      2) Educate on treatment modalities.
      3) Maintain immobilization of knee before surgery.
      4) Encourage ROM soon after surgical repair.
5. Goals of rehabilitation
   a. Return to optimal level of functioning as before the injury.
6. Rehabilitation nursing implications
   a. Assess risk factors for recurrence.
   b. Educate related to causes, prevention, maintenance, and recovery.
      1) Inform patient it could take up to 8 months or more for optimal functioning to return.
   c. Encourage physical therapy participation.
   d. Encourage progressive weight bearing.
7. Age-related issues
   a. Persons with a history of ACL injuries are at a greater risk for osteoarthritis as they age.

H. Bursitis

1. Background
   a. *Bursitis* is a painful condition that affects the bursae (small fluid-filled sacs lined with synovial membranes).
      1) Bursae act as cushions to prevent friction between bones, tendons, and muscles near joints.
      2) Bursitis occurs when bursae become inflamed (Mayo Clinic, 2014a).
   b. Bursitis is most commonly found in the shoulder, elbow, and hip.
      1) It can also be found in areas such as knees, heels, and big toe.
      2) Bursitis often occurs near joints used for repetitive motions.
2. Risk factors
   a. Age: Bursitis is more common in the elderly population.
   b. Occupations or hobbies requiring repetitive motion or pressure on particular bursae
   c. Other medical conditions such as rheumatoid arthritis, gout, and diabetes increase the risk of developing bursitis.
3. Causes and precipitating features
   a. Repetitive joint movements
      1) Throwing a baseball
      2) Lifting something overhead repeatedly
      3) Leaning on elbows for long periods
      4) Extensive kneeling (e.g., while laying carpeting or scrubbing floors)
      5) Prolonged sitting on hard surfaces
4. Acute signs and symptoms
   a. Pain
   b. Edema in area
   c. Warmth at and around site
   d. Limited ROM
5. Symptoms requiring physician intervention
   a. Joint pain that interferes with activities of daily living or is disabling
   b. Prolonged pain for more than 1–2 weeks
   c. Affected joint area has excessive edema with redness, bruising, or a rash.

d. Sharp or shooting pain, especially when exercising or during other types of exertion
e. Fever

6. Acute treatment modalities
   a. Diagnosed with ultrasound or MRI
   b. Rest the affected joint and protect joint from additional trauma: This is often the only treatment needed to heal.
   c. Ice to decrease pain and localized inflammation.
   d. NSAIDs
   e. Find and remove the cause.
   f. In most cases, bursitis pain goes away within a few weeks with proper treatment, but recurrent flare-ups of bursitis are common.
7. Goals of rehabilitation
   a. Increase and maintain optimal function.
   b. Decrease pain.
8. Rehabilitation nursing implications
   a. Assess risk factors for recurrence.
   b. Educate patient and family about causes, prevention, maintenance, and recovery.
   c. Inform patient and family that recovery can take up to 8 months or more to achieve optimal functioning.
   d. Encourage physical therapy participation.
9. Age-related issues
   a. Aging population is at increased risk of bursitis
   b. Prolonged healing secondary to age-related changes

III. Surgical Interventions

A. Joint Replacement

1. Background
   a. *Joint replacement surgery* is the replacement of a joint with an artificial prosthesis
   b. The joints most commonly replaced are the hips and knees.
2. Incidence and prevalence
   a. In older adults, joint replacement surgery is the type of orthopedic surgery most commonly performed.
3. Risk factors
   a. Older age
   b. Disease processes such as OA
   c. Lack of exercise
4. Acute treatment modalities
   a. The goals of surgical intervention for an orthopedic problem are to relieve the pain in the joint caused by the damage done to the cartilage and to increase mobility.
5. Key points of acute care relevant to rehabilitation care and therapy: assessment, healing, and nursing care and interventions
   a. Nursing care and interventions
      1) Educate pre- and postoperatively and ensure that the patient understands limitations.
         a) Teach deep breathing and coughing prior to surgery.
         b) Positioning and use of bedpan and bedside commode
         c) Assess neurovascular system.
         d) Monitor intake and output.
         e) Administer antibiotics.
         f) Monitor pain level; can have a patient-controlled analgesia pump
         g) Educate about signs and symptoms of complications such as increased pain, fever, drainage, and dislocation.
         h) Set realistic goals.
6. Potential complications in rehabilitation setting
   a. Infection
   b. Blood clots
   c. Dislocation
   d. Prosthetic breakage
   e. Nerve injury
   f. Wear and loosening
7. Goals of rehabilitation
   a. Decrease pain.
   b. Increase mobility.
   c. Provide education related to causes; prevention; and mobility, including restrictions.
8. Rehabilitation nursing implications
   a. Most joint replacement recovery modalities are applicable to all joint replacements. However, some differences exist depending on the joint involved.
      1) Knee replacements
         a) Do not place pillows under the operated knee.
            (i) Pillows contribute to a decrease in ROM, can cause contractures, and impair recovery and mobility.
         b) Placing a pillow under the calf is OK, as long as the pillow does not affect ROM of the knee.
         c) The patient must get into bed on his or her unaffected side, and get out of bed on the affected, or surgical, side of his or her body.
      2) Hip replacements
         a) Do not cross legs.
         b) Do not bend at hips past 90 degrees.
         c) Do not lie on the side of the body that was not operated on.

d) Keep toes pointed forward when lying, standing, and walking.
e) Prevent adduction or abduction of affected hip.
f) Get into bed on the unaffected side and get out of bed on the affected side.
g) Weight bearing on the operative leg will be restricted for up to 6 to 8 weeks.

3) Shoulder replacements
a) Avoid lifting heavy objects until physician directs it is safe to do so.
b) Continue active range of motion within pain limit.
c) Inform patient and family that optimal benefits from surgery could take up to a year to achieve.

9. Age-related issues
a. Coexisting morbidities can contribute to poor or prolonged healing.
b. Aging adults are at increased risk for OA after joint replacement.
c. Older adults are at increased risk for fractures near the replacement hardware.

B. Amputation
1. Background
a. *Amputation* is the removal of a limb or part of the body that is usually the result of a surgical procedure but can also be a result of trauma. Amputation is a permanent condition that leaves the person with self-care, psychosocial, and body image deficits.

2. Incidence and prevalence
a. According to the Amputee Coalition (2014), approximately two million persons in America have experienced amputations or were born with limb anomalies. Another 28 million people in America are at risk for amputation.
b. The most common reason for amputation is a lack of blood supply to the limb. Peripheral vascular disease (PVD) and peripheral arterial disease (PAD) are reported to be the most common disease processes associated with amputation (Centers for Disease Control [CDC], 2013b).
c. In 2009, the hospital discharge rate for toe amputation was 2.5 per 1,000 diabetic populations for males and 1.1 per 1,000 diabetic populations for females (CDC, 2013a).

3. Risk factors
a. Age
1) Risk for amputation increases with age.
b. Sex
1) Strong evidence exists that men are more likely to experience an amputation than women (Peek, 2011).
c. Race
1) African Americans, especially women, have a greater incidence of amputation (Nguyen et al., 2009).
d. Smoking
e. Consumption of caffeine and alcohol
f. Lack of weight-bearing exercise
g. Lack of osteoporotic medication
h. Diabetes
1) PVD/PAD: diseases in which circulation is compromised

4. Causes and precipitating features
a. The causes for amputation depend on underlying disease process and trauma.
b. *Congenital*: occurring at birth
1) A congenital limb deficiency can involve either the upper or lower limb. However, in rare instances, multiple limbs are affected. Congenital deficiencies can involve the complete absence of a limb, but more commonly a portion of the affected limb is missing.
c. Acquired (trauma, disease, or surgical)
1) Malignant tumor: Bone tumors can be primary (i.e., originating in the bone) or metastatic (spreading to the bone from another point of origin). Primary bone cancer is less common than metastatic bone cancer (National Cancer Institute at the National Institutes of Health, 2013).
2) Diabetes/PVD/PAD
3) Osteomyelitis: Loss of epithelial tissue predisposes the bone to infection. Persons with diabetes and diabetic foot ulcers are more prone to developing osteomyelitis. Infection of the bone is treated with more conservative treatment, such as antibiotics, before amputation is considered.

5. Acute signs and symptoms
a. Acquired
1) Absence of peripheral pulses
2) Necrotizing tissue
3) Pale skin
4) Cool-to-cold skin to the touch
5) Decreased-to-absent sensation
6) Arteriography/venography: no visible circulation
7) Doppler ultrasound without pulsations
8) Increased white blood cell count

6. Acute treatment modalities

a. Antibiotics
b. Surgical intervention to remove necrotic tissue

7. Key points of acute care relevant to rehabilitation care and therapy: assessment, healing, nursing care, and interventions
   a. Nursing care and interventions
      1) Preoperative care
         a) Reinforce education about the reasons for amputation.
         b) Teach the importance of performing upper body exercise to maintain strength for crutch walking.
         c) Provide education about postoperative positioning to prevent complications.
         d) Inform about the possibility of phantom pain.
         e) Provide general postoperative teaching (e.g., cough, deep breathing, and incentive spirometry).
      2) Postoperative care
         a) Depends on the type of amputation, the patient's age, and state of health
         b) Monitor vital signs and dressing for signs and symptoms of hemorrhage.
         c) Have a tourniquet available for emergency use.
         d) Maintain sterile technique when changing dressing to prevent infection.
         e) Assess affected limb for signs of irritation, excoriation, or odor.
         f) Frequently assess areas particularly prone to pressure.
         g) Maintain proper compression bandage and/or limb shrinker.
            (i) Remove compression bandage and/or shrinker to provide care, and reapply snugly but ensure it is not too tight.
            (ii) Assess circulation.
         h) Prevent contractures.
            (i) Limit sitting in a chair to 1 hour or less.
            (ii) Do not place pillows under surgical extremity.
            (iii) Have patient lie prone (unless contraindicated) for 30 minutes three or four times per day.
         i) Mobility is started as soon as possible.
            (i) Ensure understanding of mobility orders to prevent injury.
            (ii) Before discharge, reinforce instructions related to weight bearing, crutch walking, signs and symptoms of infections, prevention of contractures, and the importance of follow-up care.

8. Potential complications in rehabilitation setting
   a. Chronic pain
   b. Phantom limb pain
   c. Contractures
   d. Abduction
   e. Scar formation
   f. Wounds
   g. Fatigue
   h. Feelings of helplessness, especially after upper-extremity amputations, brought on by difficulty completing tasks with one hand

9. Goals of rehabilitation
   a. Prepare residual limb for prosthesis.
   b. Fit prosthetic and train in its use.
   c. Improve strength and control.
   d. Restore ability to perform ADLs and promote independence.
   e. Provide education related to assistive devise and artificial limbs.
   f. Provide emotional support and/or counseling to deal with grief related to loss of limb and changes in body image.

10. Rehabilitation nursing implications
   a. Assessment
      1) Complete a through history, physical examination, and functional assessment.
      2) Provide positive support to encourage independent performance of activities of daily living.
      3) Provide comprehensive education for the patient, family, and significant others related to
         a) Diagnosis
         b) Disease processes
         c) Pain management
         d) Weight management
         e) Medications
         f) Psychosocial issues
         g) Sexuality
         h) Complications associated with condition
         i) Community resources.

11. Age-related issues
   a. Increasing age and coexisting morbidities can contribute to poor healing.
   b. Aging is associated with increased risk for diabetes and OA associated with amputation.
   c. Children and adolescents
      1) Can be more sensitive to changes in body image

2) Decreased self-esteem is commonly seen secondary to perceived nonacceptance by peers and changes in appearance and functional abilities.
3) Delayed growth and development
4) Persons older than age 65 years might require a longer rehabilitation.
5) Multiple comorbidities and age-related changes in older adults commonly cause problems during rehabilitation.

C. Fracture Fixation

1. Background
   a. A fracture can be a complete or incomplete break in the continuity of the structure of a bone.
   b. Fractures are also classified according to the direction of the fracture line (i.e., transverse, oblique, greenstick, comminuted, spiral, stress, and pathological).
   c. Fractures can also be classified as nondisplaced or displaced.
2. Incidence and prevalence
   a. According to the AAOS (2012), more than 7 million bones are broken each year in the United States. The majority of these fractures occur in men 45 years of age and younger and women older than 45 years. These incidents account for more than 14 million visits to medical facilities, resulting in about $21 billion a year in medical expenses (AAOS, 2012).
3. Types of fractures
   a. Colles' fracture: fracture of the distal radius. Most common fracture in adults.
   b. Fracture of humerus: common in young and middle-aged adults
   c. Pelvic fracture: ranges from benign to life threatening and is associated with the highest mortality rate
   d. Hip fracture: most common in older adults, and more than 90% of incidents are associated with a fall
4. Risk factors
   a. Sports activities
      1) Basketball
      2) Football
      3) Rugby
      4) Wrestling
      5) Hockey
      6) Skiing
      7) Snowboarding
      8) In-line skating
   b. Health conditions
      1) Osteoporosis
      2) Bone disease
      3) Calcium deficiency
5. Causes and precipitating features
   a. Falls
   b. Sports injuries
   c. Motor vehicle accidents
6. Acute signs and symptoms
   a. Immediate pain
   b. Decreased function
   c. Edema
   d. Muscle spasms
   e. Ecchymosis immediately after injury and distal to fracture
   f. Inability to bear weight/inability to use affected body part
   g. Guarding affected area
   h. Obvious bone deformity might or might not be present.
7. Acute treatment modalities
   a. Immobilize the body part in the position in which it was found to prevent further tissue and possible nerve damage.
   b. Manage pain.
   c. Use X ray, computed tomography, or MRI to diagnose classification and extent of damage.
   d. Anatomic realignment
8. Key points of acute care relevant to rehabilitation care and therapy: assessment, healing, and nursing care and interventions
   a. Nursing care and interventions
      1) Complete assessment and history, including physical examination
      2) Fracture reduction
         a) *Closed reduction* is a nonsurgical realignment that uses traction and countertraction to realign affected area.
            (i) Usually completed under general anesthesia
            (ii) Can involve external fixation, splints, braces, or orthoses to maintain immobilization
         b) *Traction* is the application of a device to create a pulling force with counterforce in the opposite direction.
            (i) The purposes of traction
               (1) Reduce pain.
               (2) Decrease possibility of muscle spasms.
               (3) Immobilize a joint.
               (4) Expand joint space.
            (ii) Types of traction
               (1) Skeletal

(2) Skin: usually temporary until skeletal traction or surgery is possible
c) *Open reduction* is a surgical procedure that realigns the bone and usually involves internal fixation such as plates and screws to maintain immobility.
d) Open reduction with internal fixation involving a joint normally requires early ROM.
3) *Casting* is a temporary immobilization of the affected body part and is a common treatment after closed reduction.
a) Types of cast
(i) Sugar-tong splint: commonly used in wrist injuries or when acute injury results in swelling of the injured part
(ii) Short-arm cast: commonly used for wrist or metacarpal injuries. Normally extends from the distal palmer crease to the proximal forearm.
(iii) Long-arm cast: used for stable forearm or elbow fractures. It is similar to the short-arm cast but extends to the humerus.
(iv) Short-leg cast: usually extends from the base of the toes to the inferior of the knee
(v) Long-leg cast: usually extends from the base of the toes to the gluteal crease or groin
(vi) Body-jacket cast: used to support stable spinal injuries of the thoracic and lumbar spine
(vii) Single-hip spica: commonly used in stable femoral fractures and to immobilize the affected limb and trunk
(viii) Double-hip spica: applied to both of the lower extremities and the trunk
b) Nursing care related to fracture and cast
(i) Casts are usually not strong enough to bear weight for approximately 24 to 72 hours.
(ii) Cast needs to be open to air to dry properly. Never cover a fresh cast.
(iii) Avoid direct pressure to cast during drying time.
(iv) Use an open palm to handle cast to prevent denting the cast.
(v) Once the cast is dry, small pieces of tape (petals) might need to be applied to the edges to prevent skin irritation.
(vi) When using a sling, ensure that axilla are well padded to prevent skin excoriation and pressure on the neck.
(vii) Encourage active ROM to unaffected limb to prevent stiffness.
(viii) In the presence of a body jacket
(1) Assess abdomen for bowel sounds (cast could compress the mesenteric artery and duodenum). Common complaints include complaints of feeling fullness, pain, or pressure in abdomen; nausea; and vomiting.
(2) Assess respiratory status, bowel and bladder function, and bony prominences (especially iliac crest).
(ix) Perform frequent neurovascular checks.
(x) In the presence of a double spica, never use the separation bar to assist with turning or moving the patient.
(xi) Use a fracture bedpan to promote comfort and ease of movement on and off the bedpan.
(xii) Asses pain before and after medication.
(xiii) Provide safety measures, as many drugs can alter the level of consciousness and cause weakness, dizziness, respiratory depression, and hypotension.
(xiv) Provide nutritional support (a dietary consultation might be needed). Ample protein, vitamins, and calcium are needed to support healing.

9. Potential complications in rehabilitation setting
a. Pain
b. Muscle spasms
c. Muscle atrophy
d. Contracture
e. Foot drop
f. Compartment syndrome
g. Venous thromboembolism (VTE)
10. Goals of rehabilitation

a. Increase strength and mobility.
b. Provide education related to risk factors, prevention, and treatment.
c. Provide education related to nutritional needs (e.g., increase calcium and vitamin D supplements).
d. Provide an environment of safety in hospital and at home.

11. Rehabilitation nursing implications
    a. Manage pain.
    b. Assess risk factors and educational needs, and prevent future fractures.
12. Age-related issues
    a. Gait and balance problems are common in older adults, increasing the risk for falls.
    b. Inadequate tissue to absorb shock from falls
    c. Polypharmacy: Many older adults take multiple medications that affect balance.
    d. Osteoporotic hip fracture leading to falls

D. Spinal Cord Injury and Spinal Surgery

1. Background
    a. Spinal cord injury is classified as paraplegia or tetraplegia. SCI is further classified according to the mechanism of injury, level of injury, and completeness of injury.
    b. Syndromes associated with incomplete SCI lesions
        1) Central cord syndrome
        2) Anterior cord syndrome
        3) Brown-Séquard syndrome
        4) Posterior cord syndrome
        5) Conus medullaris and cauda equine syndrome
    c. The most common cause for death in SCI is respiratory complications.
    d. Spinal surgery is usually considered a last option. In most cases, nonsurgical treatments and procedures are considered before surgical intervention.
    e. Many types of spinal surgery exist. However, the most common surgical intervention is laminectomy and decompression.
2. Incidence and prevalence
    a. Approximately 200,000 people in the United States currently live with SCI.
    b. Annually, there are 15–40 new cases per million people.
    c. Alcohol has been found to play a major factor in spinal cord injuries (Forchheimer, Cunningham, Gater, Jr., & Maio, 2005).
3. Risk factors
    a. Evidence of cord compression
    b. Progressive neurological impairment
    c. Compound vertebral fractures
    d. Presence of bony fragments
    e. Penetrating wounds
4. Causes and precipitating features
    a. SCIs are caused by trauma such as motor vehicle collisions, falls, acts of violence, sports injuries, and other miscellaneous causes.
    b. Tumors of the spinal cord account for approximately 1% of all neoplasms. These tumors are classified as primary or secondary and further classified as extradural or intradural.
5. Key points of acute care relevant to rehabilitation care and therapy: assessment, healing, nursing care and interventions
    a. Nursing care and interventions
        1) Thorough assessment of all systems
        2) Maintain spine stability
        3) Education and intervention related to complications associated with SCI
            a) Nutritional support
            b) Autonomic dysreflexia
            c) Bowel and bladder management
            d) Respiratory management
            e) Temperature control
            f) Altered sensory perception care plan
            g) Prevention of pressure ulcers
            h) Altered sexuality/sexual function counseling plan
            i) Grief and depression
        4) Provide emotional support to patient, family, and significant others.
        5) Maintain optimal level of mobility and neurological functioning.
6. Potential complications in rehabilitation setting
    a. Pressure ulcers
    b. Autonomic dysreflexia
    c. Bowel and bladder retention or incontinence
    d. Hydronephrosis
    e. Heterotrophic ossification
    f. Depression
7. Goals of rehabilitation
    a. Help the person understand his or her injuries and the details regarding required care.
    b. Become as independent as possible in everyday activities such as bathing, eating, dressing, grooming, and wheelchair use.
    c. Help the person learn to accept a new lifestyle, especially pertaining to sexual, recreational, and housing options.
    d. Educate the person on how to instruct caregivers in assisting with care.
    e. Prepare for vocational rehabilitation.
8. Rehabilitation nursing implications

a. Establish a therapeutic relationship.
b. Allow time for the patient to verbalize feelings, fears, and concerns.
c. Answer and address all questions honestly.
d. Perform physical assessment of all systems.
e. Maintain safety by log rolling and avoiding twisting during the acute phase.
f. Maintain spinal precautions using halo, cervical collars, and orthoses.
g. Educate patient, family, and significant others about immobilizers.
h. Prevent secondary complications.
i. Help to identify and set goals.
j. Assess and monitor psychosocial adjustment.

9. Age-related issues
   a. Older adults with SCI tend to have more complications compared with younger persons with SCI.
   b. Bowel and bladder dysfunction can increase with age.
   c. Rehabilitation in older adults typically takes longer secondary to previous chronic health conditions and poor health at the time of injury.
   d. Cardiovascular disease is prevalent in persons with SCI.
   e. Lack of sensation in persons with high-level injures can mask symptoms of acute myocardial infarction, increasing the mortality rate.

IV. Other Complications

A. Heterotrophic Ossification (HO) (McLean, 2013; Speed, 2015)

1. Background
   a. *Heterotrophic ossification* is the formation of mature lamellar bone in nonbone tissue.
   b. Also called ectopic ossification or myositis ossificans progressiva
   c. Can affect bones or joints
   d. Causes inflammation, pain, restricted joint movement
2. Incidence and prevalence
   a. Incidence is 2%–63% following total hip arthroplasty and acetabular fracture surgery.
   b. Incidence as high as 32% following total knee arthroplasty, and as high as 56% if knee arthroplasty requires surgical revision
   c. High incidence following traumatic injury
      1) Military blast injuries and amputations
   d. Men can be affected more frequently, but women tend to have more severe symptoms.
   e. Peak incidence is from 4 to 12 weeks postinjury and up to 5 months after trauma.
3. Risk factors
   a. Spinal cord injury
   b. Brain injury
   c. Infections of central nervous system
      1) Tetanus
      2) Polio
   d. Central nervous system tumors
   e. Multiple sclerosis
   f. Cardiovascular accident
   g. Joint surgery
   h. Amputation and traumatic amputation
   i. Burns
   j. Previous HO
   k. Hip and pelvic surgery
   l. Genetic predisposition
   m. Anoxic encephalopathy
   n. Intensive rehabilitation, transfer activities, and repeated minor trauma during ADLs
   o. Muscle trauma
   p. Prolonged coma
   q. Spasticity
4. Causes and precipitating features
   a. Osteogenic cells are stimulated to form osteoid, which develops into mature HO.
   b. Inflammation could be the trigger.
      1) Secondary to trauma, infection, or unknown
   c. HO bone contains more osteoblasts than ordinary bone.
   d. Exact etiology not well defined or understood
5. Acute signs and symptoms
   a. Varies in time of onset after injury or surgery
      1) Pain and stiffness
      2) Limits in range of motion
      3) Redness, swelling
      4) Increased limb spasticity
      5) Fever
      6) Joint effusion
6. Acute treatment modalities
   a. Acute stage
      1) Rest the involved joint in functional position.
      2) Gentle, passive ROM
   b. Surgery if extreme pain, nerve entrapment, or stiffness are present
   c. Radiation
   d. Antiinflammatory drugs
   e. Etidronate
7. Key points of acute care relevant to rehabilitation care and therapy: assessment, healing, and nursing care and interventions
   a. Nursing care and interventions
      1) Recognize at-risk patients.

2) Minimize activities and movements that could injure tissue.
    a) Overwork, fatigue, malpositioning
3) Assess all complaints of pain.
    a) Location, intensity, inflammation, swelling, redness, heat, joint range of motion
    b) Report as indicated to physician.
4) Pain management
5) Be alert for interference of HO with fit of prosthetics.
    a) HO can occur on bottom surface of residual limb, causing pressure ulcers when in contact with prosthetic.
    b) HO can change the fit of prosthetics, causing ulceration.

8. Potential complications in rehabilitation setting
    a. Loss of joint range of motion
    b. Pressure ulcers
        1) Infection
    c. Pain
    d. Interference with ADLs
9. Goals of rehabilitation
    a. Manage pain.
    b. Restore and maintain joint function and ROM.
    c. Prevent pressure ulcers and infection.
10. Age-related issues
    a. Incidence of HO can be greater in older patients who have had joint replacement surgery.
    b. HO can be confused with deep vein thrombosis, as signs and symptoms can be similar.
    c. Healing could be prolonged in older patients.

B. Compartment Syndrome

1. Background
    a. *Compartment syndrome* is a serious condition in which elevated intra-compartmental pressure within a confined myofascial compartment interferes with neurovascular function of tissues within the affected area (Lewis et al., 2011).
    b. Compartment syndrome decreases capillary blood flow necessary to maintain viable tissue.
    c. Usually occurs subsequent to a traumatic event, most commonly a fracture of long bones
2. Incidence and prevalence
    a. According to the National Institutes of Health Office of Rare Diseases (National Institutes of Health Office of Rare Disease, 2014), compartment syndrome is listed as a rare disease.
    b. The NIH ORD considers a rare disease to be one that affects fewer than 200,000 people in the United States.
3. Risk factors
    a. Condition that can lead to bleeding in cases of trauma and fractures
        1) Taking anticoagulants
        2) Having a bleeding disorder such as hemophilia
    b. Participation in certain collision or contact sports such as football
    c. Bandages or casts that are worn too tightly or worn for too long
    d. Recent injury to the area
    e. Burns
    f. Swelling of tissues under the skin
4. Causes and precipitating features
    a. Vein obstructions in the extremities secondary to edema
    b. Hemorrhage
    c. Complication of surgery
5. Acute signs and symptoms
    a. According to Lewis et al. (2011), there are six Ps that characterize compartment syndrome.
        1) Paresthesia: numbness or tingling
        2) Pain: severe and distal the injury and not relieved by medication (early sign)
        3) Pressure: feeling of tightness or fullness of muscles
        4) Pallor: pale, shiny skin over affected area
        5) Paralysis: loss of function
        6) Pulselessness: affected area has decreased or absent pulse (usually a later sign)
6. Acute treatment modalities
    a. Rapid diagnosis and treatment are critical to prevent long-term damage to muscles and nerves.
    b. Do not elevate extremity above heart level, as it can impede arterial blood flow.
    c. Do not use cold compresses, because they cause vasoconstriction and can exacerbate condition.
    d. If compartment syndrome is caused by a tight bandage or tight cast, these might need to be removed or loosened.
    e. *Fasciotomy*, a surgical procedure in which a linear incision is made in the tissue to relieve pressure, must be completed as soon as possible to prevent permanent damage.
7. Key points of acute care relevant to rehabilitation care and therapy: assessment, healing
    a. Because the incision is left open for optimal draining and decompression, particular care must be taken to help prevent infection of the wound.
    b. In severe cases of compartment syndrome, amputation could be necessary

c. Compartment syndrome damages muscles and increases myoglobin release, which can result in renal tubular necrosis or acute kidney injury. Therefore it is imperative to monitor urine output.

8. Potential complications in rehabilitation setting
   a. Contractures
   b. Infection
   c. High risk for venous thromboembolism
   d. Acute kidney injury
9. Goals of rehabilitation
   a. Increase function to optimal level.
   b. Decrease complications.
10. Rehabilitation nursing implications
   a. Establish therapeutic relationship.
   b. Allow time for patient to verbalize feelings, fears, and concerns.
   c. Answer and address all questions honestly.
   d. Perform physical assessment of all systems.
   e. Educate patient, family, and significant others about condition and prevention of complications.
   f. Help patient to identify and set goals.
11. Age-related issues
   a. Although compartment syndrome can occur at any age, athletes younger than 40 years of age are at increased risk for chronic compartment syndrome.
   b. Aging adults tend to be more at risk for falls and have a greater incidence of osteoarthritis, which increases their risk for fractures. Consequently, the risk of developing compartment syndrome also increases.
   c. Delayed healing can occur in older adults.
   d. Older persons typically have less strength and endurance than younger people, which can result in increased difficulty in compensating for limitations of injury (Roberts, 2011).

C. Fat Embolism Syndrome

1. Background
   a. *Fat embolism syndrome* (FES) is a disorder in which a particle or several particles of fat globules are released into the bloodstream and become lodged in the pulmonary capillary vessels.
   b. Fat emboli are usually a result of a traumatic injury, particularly a traumatic fracture.
   c. Fat emboli tend to be small and numerous, causing many signs and symptoms.
2. Incidence and prevalence
   a. Recent research detected fat globules in the blood of 67% of orthopedic trauma patients. In addition, when blood was sampled in close proximity of the fracture, the percentage of patients with fat globules in their blood increased to 95% (Kwiatt & Seamon, 2013).
   b. The mortality rate with FES ranges from 5% to 15% (Shaikh, 2009).
3. Risk factors
   a. Young age
   b. Closed fractures
   c. Multiple fractures
   d. Conservative therapy for long-bone fractures
   e. Excessive nailing of the medullary cavity
4. Causes and precipitating features
   a. Fractures
   b. Liposuction
   c. Soft-tissue injuries
   d. Diabetes mellitus
   e. High-dose steroids
5. Acute signs and symptoms
   a. Symptoms usually occur within 1 to 3 days after traumatic injury and most often involve the brain, lungs, and skin. In addition, progression of FES is rapid.
   b. Shortness of breath
   c. Pallor
   d. Tachycardia
   e. Tachypnea
   f. Hypoxemia
   g. Thrombocytopenia
   h. Petichial rash
   i. Agitation
   j. Confusion
   k. Coma
   l. Severe cases can lead to multiorgan dysfunction.
   m. Most patients (approximately 90%) recover completely within 1 year. According to recent studies, residual deficits range from subtle personality changes and memory loss to long-term focal deficits (Shaikh, 2009).
6. Acute treatment modalities
   a. Treatment of FES is aimed at prevention and symptom management.
   b. Early immobilization of fracture is an important aspect in prevention of developing FES.
   c. The treatment is usually supportive, providing adequate oxygenation including oxygen via mask. In severe cases, the patient could require mechanical ventilation.
   d. Fluid resuscitation for the prevention of hypovolemic shock and correction of acidosis
   e. Monitor intake and output.

7. Key points of acute care relevant to rehabilitation care and therapy: assessment, healing, nursing care and interventions
8. Potential complications in rehabilitation setting
   a. Pulmonary edema
   b. Acute respiratory distress syndrome
   c. Death
9. Goals of rehabilitation
   a. Reverse the changes related to FES.
   b. Optimize functional and respiratory status.
10. Rehabilitation nursing implications
   a. Encourage exercise to increase strength.
   b. Educate about self-management, medications, and nutrition
   c. Assess psychosocial status.
   d. Help patient identify and set goals, and revise as necessary.
   e. Provide encouragement.
   f. Acknowledge fears and anxiety.
   g. Assist with coping mechanisms.
   h. Evaluate patient's understanding of goals.
   i. Stress the importance of follow-up care.
11. Age-related issues
   a. Young people are at increased risk for FES.
   b. Poor outcomes of FES are commonly associated with aging persons who have multiple underlying medical diagnoses and decreased physiological reserves.

D. Infection
1. Background
   a. Multiple microorganisms are linked to infections.
   b. The most common microorganisms include
      1) Bacteria
      2) Viruses
      3) Fungi
      4) Protozoa.
   c. Bacteria cause disease either by entering the body or growing inside cells and secreting toxins. Bacteria are also classified by their shape.
   d. *Viruses* are simple infectious microorganisms that do not have a cellular structure. Viruses contain a small amount of ribonucleic acid and deoxyribonucleic acid.
   e. *Fungi* are microorganisms similar to plants but do not contain chlorophyll. Diseases caused by fungi are called mycoses.
   f. *Protozoa* are small, single-celled microorgan isms that usually live in soil or water.
2. Incidence and prevalence
   a. A recent study isolated 35 various bacterial strains and found that of 73% of patients (n = 2,061) who had orthopedic surgeries, 65.72% had gram positive bacteria and 34.28% had gram negative bacteria (Li, Guo, Ou, Dong, & Zhou, 2013).
   b. According to the CDC, 1 in 25 hospitalized patients has experienced at least one hospital-acquired infection (CDC, 2015.
   c. Surgical-site infections and device-associated infections accounted for approximately 48% of all hospital-acquired infections.
3. Risk factors
   a. Smoking
   b. Lack of preoperative antibiotics
   c. Length of surgery (> 3 hours)
   d. Diabetes mellitus
   e. Previous surgeries
   f. Compromised immune system
4. Causes and precipitating features
   a. Failure to wash hands between patients
5. Acute signs and symptoms
   a. Increased pain, swelling, redness, or warmth around the affected area
   b. Red streaks extending from the affected area
   c. Drainage from the affected area
   d. Fever
   e. Fatigue
   f. Increased white blood cell count
6. Key points of acute care relevant to rehabilitation care and therapy: assessment, healing, and nursing care and interventions
   a. Nursing care and interventions
      1) Wash hands before and after seeing patients.
      2) Review signs and symptoms of infection.
      3) Keep dressing clean and intact.
      4) Monitor lab values complete blood count for infection.
7. Potential complications in rehabilitation setting
   a. Illness in the patient
   b. Longer stay
   c. Longer recovery time
   d. Costs associated with a longer stay in hospital and longer recovery time
8. Goals of rehabilitation
   a. The patient is free of infection.
   b. Function is increased to optimal ability.
9. Rehabilitation nursing implications
   a. Provide increased safety measures, as infections can cause increased weakness and increased risk for falls.
   b. Provide education related to signs and symptoms of infection.
   c. Monitor vital signs and labs for signs of infection.

d. Monitor glucose levels, as these tend to be elevated in the presence of infection.

10. Age-related issues
    a. Infection rates in older adults are 2–3 times higher than in younger patients.
    b. Age-related changes such as decreased immune system, physical disabilities, and multiple comorbidities increase risk of infection in older adults.

E. Pain

1. Background
   a. Pain is associated with many musculoskeletal conditions as well as treatments for musculoskeletal conditions.
   b. Pain can limit activity and affect joint motion, strength, mobility, and independence.
2. Risk factors
   a. Overuse of a joint or muscle
   b. Inflammation and infection
   c. Disease
      1) RA, OA, rheumatic pain
      2) Fibromyalgia
      3) Spinal disc disease
   d. Trauma
      1) Fracture
      2) Strain, sprain
   e. Tumor
      1) Invasion into bone
      2) Pressure on nerves
   f. Poor posture, positioning
   g. Surgery
3. Causes and precipitating features
   a. Nerve impingement
   b. Poor vascular supply
   c. Poor positioning
   d. Inflammation, infection
4. Acute signs and symptoms
   a. Complaints of pain
   b. Impaired tissue function
   c. Decreased ROM in joints
5. Acute treatment modalities
   a. Antiinflammatories
   b. Pain medications
   c. Heat, cold
   d. Braces and supports
6. Key points of acute care relevant to rehabilitation care and therapy: assessment, healing, and nursing care and interventions
   a. Nursing care and interventions
      1) Assessment
         a) Pain
         b) Joint function
         c) Progress or regression
         d) Pain management
7. Potential complications in rehabilitation setting
   a. Impaired ADLs
   b. Loss of mobility
   c. Longer length of stay
   d. Discharge to location other than home
      1) Skilled nursing facilities, nursing home
8. Goals of rehabilitation
   a. Prevent pain.
   b. Manage pain.
   c. Assess pain complaints thoroughly.
9. Age-related issues
   a. Care must be taken to consider pain complaints seriously.
      1) Do not assume that "all old people have pain" or that pain in elderly people is due to arthritis and rheumatism.

F. Venous Thromboembolism (VTE)

1. Background
   a. VTE is a disease that encompasses both deep vein thrombi and pulmonary embolus. According to the CDC (2012a), DVTs (blood clots) are underdiagnosed and represent a serious, potentially preventable medical condition. Pulmonary emboli occur when part of a clot or an entire clot breaks off and travels through the bloodstream to the lungs. Pulmonary embolisms can be fatal.
   b. Virchow's triad includes three broad categories that contribute to the etiology of venous thrombosis. The categories are venous stasis, damage to the endothelium, and blood hypercoagulability.
2. Incidence and prevalence
   a. The exact incidence of VTE is unknown; however, the CDC (2012b) reported that estimates in the United States range from 300,000 to 900,000 annually.
   b. Almost half of all VTEs occur during or soon after discharge from a hospital stay or surgery.
   c. The number of Americans who die from VTEs each year is estimated to be 60,000–100,000.
3. Risk factors
   a. According to Goldhaber (2010), risk factors can be divided into the following categories:
      1) Hospitalized patients
      2) Recurrent VTE
      3) Genetics
      4) Long-haul air trips
      5) Community acquired
      6) Women's health
   b. All categories have precipitating factors.
4. Causes and precipitating factors

a. Hospitalized patients
    1) Major surgery
    2) Cancer
    3) Congestive heart failure
    4) Chronic obstructive pulmonary disease
    5) Chronic kidney disease
b. Recurrent VTE risk factors while taking anticoagulant therapy
    1) Immobilization
    2) Cancer
    3) Chronic obstructive pulmonary disease
    4) Discontinuation of anticoagulant therapy
    5) Overweight/obesity
    6) Low levels of high-density lipoprotein cholesterol
    7) Male
    8) Presenting with symptoms of pulmonary embolus instead of DVT
    9) Lack of recanalization of DVT on ultrasound examination
c. Genetics
    1) V leiden factor
    2) Prothrombin gene mutation
d. Long-haul air trips
    1) Immobility
    2) Constrictive clothing
    3) Community acquired
    4) A history of prior VTE
    5) Venous insufficiency
    6) Pregnancy
    7) Trauma
    8) Frailty
    9) Immobility
e. Women's health
    1) Pregnancy
    2) Oral contraceptives
    3) Postmenopausal hormone therapy

5. Acute signs and symptoms
    a. A patient can have a DVT with unilateral leg edema, pain in an extremity, paresthesias, warm skin, erythema, and temperature of 100.4 or higher.
        1) Note: Homan's sign has been shown to be an unreliable and invalid assessment for DVT. It should not be performed, because it has no value in determining the presence or absence of a DVT.
6. Potential complications in rehabilitation setting
    a. VTE is sometimes fatal and its victims face long-term risk of postthrombotic leg swelling and ulceration.
7. Goals of rehabilitation
    a. Assist individuals to achieve the highest level of independence and quality of life possible.
    b. Decrease risk of complications.
8. Rehabilitation nursing implications
    a. Assess for risk factors and complications.
    b. Educate about risk factors, causes, treatment, and prevention.
    c. Provide support for patient, family, and significant others.
9. Age-related issues
    a. Advanced age is associated with a higher risk of mortality.

References

American Academy of Orthopaedic Surgeons (2009). Position Statement: Osteoporosis/Bone Health as a National Public Health Priority. Retrieved from http://www.aaos.org/about/papers/position/1113.asp

American Academy of Orthopaedic Surgeons (2013). Fact Sheet: The Role of Orthopaedics. Retrieved from http://anationinmotion.org/wp-content/uploads/2013/05/Ortho-Consumer.pdf

American Academy of Orthopaedic Surgeons (2014). Total Joint Replacement. Retrieved from http://orthoinfo.aaos.org/topic.cfm?topic=A00233

Amputee Coalition (2014). About Us. Retrieved from http://www.amputee-coalition.org/about-us/

Arthritis Foundation (2014). Osteoarthritis. Retrieved from http://www.arthritis.org/arthritis-facts/disease-center/osteoarthritis.php

Association of Rehabilitation Nurses (ARN). (2014). ARN competency model for professional rehabilitation nursing. Retrieved from http://www.rehabnurse.org/uploads/files/education/ARN_Rehabilitation_Nursing_Competency _Model_FINAL_-_May_2014.pdf

Buckley. R. (2014). General principles of fracture care treatment and management. Retrieved from http://emedicine.medscape.com/article/1270717-treatment

Bureau of Labor Statistics (2014). News release: Nonfatal; Occupational injuries and illnesses requiring days away from work, 2013. Retrieved from http://stats.bls.gov/news.release/archives/osh2_12162014.pdf

Centers for Disease Control and Prevention (2012a) Venous thromboembolism (VTE). Retrieved from http://www.cdc.gov/ncbddd/aboutus/annualreport2012/documents/ar2012-vte-printversion.pdf

Centers for Disease Control and Prevention (2012b). Venous thromboembolism in adult hospitalizations—United States, 2007–2009. *Morbidity and Mortality Weekly Report, 61*(22), 401–4.

Centers for Disease Control and Prevention (2013a). Age-Adjusted Hospital Discharge Rates for Nontraumatic Lower Extremity Amputation (LEA) per 1,000 Diabetic Population, Toe Amputation By Sex, United States, 1993–2009. Retrieved from http://www.cdc.gov/diabetes/statistics/lealevel/table10_toe.htm

Centers for Disease Control and Prevention (2013b). Number (in Thousands) of Hospital Discharges for Nontraumatic Lower Extremity Amputation With Diabetes as a Listed Diagnosis, United States, 1988–2009. Retrieved from http://www.cdc.gov/diabetes/statistics/lea/fig1.htm

Centers for Disease Control (2015). Data and Statistics. Antimicrobial use prevancle survey. Retrieved from http://www.cdc.gov/HAI/surveillance/

Englund, M., Guermazi, A., Roemer, F. W., Aliabadi, P., Yang, M., Lewis, C. E.,… Felson, D. T. (2009). Meniscal tear in knees without surgery and the development of radiographic osteoarthritis among middle-aged and elderly persons: The Multicenter Osteoarthritis Study. *Arthritis & Rheumatology, 60*(3), 831–839. doi:10.1002/art.24383

Forchheimer, M., Cunningham, R., Gater, Jr., D., & Maio, R. (2005). The relationship of blood alcohol concentration to impairment severity in spinal cord injury. *Journal of Spinal Cord Medicine, 28*(4). 303–7.

Goldhaber, S. Z. (2010). Risk factors for venous thromboembolism. *Journal of the American College of Cardiology, 56*(1), 1–7. doi:10.1016/j.jacc.2010.01.057

Gumina, S., Carbone, S., Campagna, V., Candela, V., Sacchetti, F. M., & Giannicola, G. (2013). The impact of aging on rotator cuff tear size. *Musculoskeletal Surgery, 97*(Suppl. 1), 69–72.

Harris, G. D. (2013). Legg-Calve-Perthes disease. Retrieved from http://emedicine.medscape.com/article/1248267-overview

Jacobs-Kosmin, D. (2013). Osteoporosis. Retrieved from http://emedicine.medscape.com/article/330598-overview#a0101

Kalunian, K. C. (2013). Diagnosis and classification of osteoarthritis. Retrieved from http://www.uptodate.com/contents/diagnosis-and-classification-of-osteoarthritis?source=preview&language=en-US&anchor=H1#H1

Kishner, S. (2014). Physical medicine and rehabilitation for stress fractures. Retrieved from http://emedicine.medscape.com/article/309106-overview

Kwiatt, M. E., & Seamon, M. J. (2013). Fat embolism syndrome. *International Journal of Critical Illness and Injury. 3*(1), 64–8.

Lewis, S., Dirksen, S., Heitkemper, M., Bucher, L., & Camera, I. (2011). *Medical surgical nursing: assessment and management of clinical problems.* St. Louis: Elsevier Mosby.

Li, G. Q., Guo, F. F., Ou, Y., Dong, G. W., & Zhou, W (2013). Epidemiology and outcomes of surgical site infections following orthopedic surgery. *American Journal of Infection Control. 41*(12), 1268–1271. doi: 10.1016/j.ajic.2013.03.305

Lozada, C. J. (2014). Osteoarthritis. Retrieved from http://emedicine.medscape.com/article/330487-overview

Maffulli, N., Longo, U. G., Gougoulias, N., Loppini, M., & Denaro, V. (2010). Long-term health outcomes of youth sports injuries. *British Journal of Sports Medicine, 44*, 21–5. doi:10.1136/bjsm.2009.069526

Mayo Clinic (2014a). Bursitis: Diseases and conditions. Retrieved from http://www.mayoclinic.org/diseases-conditions/bursitis/basics/definition/con-20015102

Mayo Clinic (2014 b). Carpal tunnel syndrome: risk factors. Retrieved from http://www.mayoclinic.org/diseases-conditions/carpal-tunnel-syndrome/basics/risk-factors/con-20030332

Mayo Clinic (2014c). Rotator cuff injury. Retrieved from http://www.mayoclinic.org/diseases-conditions/rotator-cuff-injury/basics/causes/con-20031421

Mayo Clinic (2014d). Sprain and Strains. Retrieved from http://www.mayoclinic.org/diseases-conditions/sprains-and-strains/basics/definition/CON-20020958

McLean, C. (2013). Traumatic heterotopic ossification. Retrieved from http://emedicine.medscape.com/article/1254416-overview#a5

National Cancer Institute at the National Institutes of Health (2013). Fact sheet: bone cancer. Retrieved from http://www.cancer.gov/cancertopics/factsheet/Sites-Types/bone

National Institutes of Health Office of Rare Disease (2014). Compartment syndrome. Retrieved from http://rarediseases.info.nih.gov/gard/6141/compartment-syndrome/resources/1

National Osteonecrosis Foundation (NONF). (2000). Legg-Calve-Perthes disease. Retrieved from http://nonf.org/perthesbrochure/perthes-brochure.htm

National Osteoporosis Foundation (NOF). (n.d.). Medications that may cause bone loss. Retrieved from http://nof.org/articles/2

Nguyen, L. L., Hevelone, N., Rogers, S. O., Bandyk, D. F., Clowes, A. W., Moneta, G. L.,...Conte, M. S. (2009). Disparity in outcomes of surgical revascularization for limb salvage. Race and gender are synergistic determinants of vein graft failure and limb loss. *Vascular Medicine, 14*(4), 397–9. doi:10.1177/1358863X09107006

Peek, M. E. (2011). Gender differences in diabetes related lower extremity amputations. *Clinical Orthopaedics and Related Research, 469*(7), 1951–5. doi:10.1007/s11999-010-1735-4

Peters, S., Page, M., Coppieters, M., Ross, M., & Johnston, V. (2013). Rehabilitation following carpal tunnel release. *Cochrane Database System Review, 5*(6). doi:10.1002/14651858.CD004158.pub2

Roberts, D. (2011). Arthritis and connective tissue diseases. In S. L. Lewis, S. R. Dirksen, M. M. Heitkemper, L. Bucher, & I. M. Camera (Eds.). *Medical-surgical nursing: Assessment and management of clinical problems* (8th ed., p. 1658). St. Louis: Elsevier.

Rothschild, B. M. (2014). Gout and Pseudogout. Retrieved from http://emedicine.medscape.com/article/329958-overview#a0101

Schmidt, C., Claudius, J., and Brown, B. (2015). Management of rotator cuff tears. *The Journal of Hand Surgery. 40*(2), 399–408.

Shaikh, N., (2009). Emergency management of fat embolism. *Journal of Emergency trauma Shock. 3*(1), 29–33.

Speed, J. (2015). Heterotopic ossification. Retrieved from http://emedicine.medscape.com/article/327648-overview

Temprano, K. K. (2014). Rheumatoid arthritis. Retrieved from http://emedicine.medscape.com/article/331715-overview

Tofferi, J. K. (2012). Avascular Necrosis. Retrieved from http://emedicine.medscape.com/article/333364-overview

U. S. Department of Labor, Bureau of Labor Statistics (2013). Nonfatal occupational injuries and illnesses requiring days away from work, 2012. Retrieved from http://www.bls.gov/news.release/pdf/osh2.pdf

U.S. Preventive Services Task Force (2011). Osteoporosis: Screening. Retrieved from http://www.uspreventiveservicestaskforce.org/uspstf10/osteoporosis/osteors.htm

World Health Organization (2004). WHO scientific group on the assessment of osteoporosis at the Primary Health Care Level. Retrieved from http://www.who.int/chp/topics/Osteoporosis.pdf

Yamamoto, A., Takagishi, K., Osawa, T., Yanagawa, T., Nakajima, D., Shitara, H., & Kobayashi, T. (2010). Prevalence and risk factors of a rotator cuff tear in the general population. *Journal of Shoulder Elbow Surgery, 19*(1), 116–20. doi:10.1016/j.jse.2009.04.006

Young, C.C. (2014). Ankle Sprain. Retrieved from: http://emedicine.medscape.com/article/1907229-overview#a0156

Chapter 25

Cardiac and Pulmonary Rehabilitation

Cheryl Lehman, PhD RN CNS-BC RN-BC CRRN

LEARNING OUTCOMES

- Discuss select cardiac and pulmonary conditions requiring rehabilitation.
- Review indications and contraindications for cardiac and pulmonary rehabilitation.
- Identify the goals of cardiac and pulmonary rehabilitation.
- Identify key aspects of physical assessment and rehabilitation nursing interventions for complications related to the cardiac and pulmonary conditions that can be seen in the rehabilitation setting.
- Apply rehabilitation nursing principles to care of the patient with a cardiac or pulmonary condition.

KEY CHAPTER TOPICS

- Cardiac rehabilitation
- Cardiovascular diseases requiring rehabilitation
- Pulmonary rehabilitation
- Pulmonary disease requiring rehabilitation

PROFESSIONAL REHABILITATION NURSING DOMAINS AND COMPETENCIES

- Domain 1: Competencies 1.2, 1.3
- Domain 2: Competency 2.2
- Domain 4: Competency 4.2 (Association of Rehabilitation Nurses [ARN], 2014)

Introduction

Cardiac and pulmonary rehabilitation are specialty-specific forms of rehabilitation that have the following similar goals:

- Identify, modify, and manage risk factors to reduce disability, morbidity, and mortality.
- Improve functional capacity.
- Alleviate/lessen symptoms.
- Educate patients about the management of disease.
- Improve quality of life (American Association of Cardiovascular and Pulmonary Rehabilitation [AACVPR], 2014).
- Cardiac and pulmonary rehabilitation can also stop or slow the progression of disease.

Cardiac and pulmonary rehabilitation can take place in the inpatient rehabilitation setting, but it can also be provided in medical specialty units, on an outpatient basis, or in the home. Newer modalities are under investigation, including Internet-based training and monitoring and telerehabilitation.

I. Cardiac Rehabilitation

A. History

1. 1930s—patients with heart attacks were prescribed 6 weeks of bed rest
2. 1940s—patients with heart attacks were allowed to sit up in a chair
3. 1950s—3–5 minutes per day of walking was allowed, beginning 4 weeks after the heart attack
4. 1950s—Dr. Herman Hellerstein (1916–1993) introduced the concept of cardiac rehabilitation (Singh, 2013)

B. Background

1. Statistics on cardiac disease in the U.S. population continue to be alarming.
   a. The most recent data show that more than 2,150 Americans die every day from cardiovascular disease.
      1) One death every 40 seconds (American Heart Association

[AHA]/American Stroke Association [ASA], 2015)

b. 787,000 people in the United States died from heart disease, stroke and other cardiovascular diseases in 2011 (AHA/ASA, 2015)

c. Cardiovascular diseases kill more people than all forms of cancer combined (AHA/ASA, 2015)

d. Nearly half of all African-American adults have some form of cardiovascular disease (48% of women, 46% of men) (AHA/ASA, 2015).

e. In 2011, 326,200 people had an out-of-hospital cardiac arrest in the United States. Of those treated by emergency medical services, 10.6% survived. 31.4% of the bystander-witnessed out-of-hospital cardiac arrests survived (AHA/ASA, 2015).

f. Every year, 209,000 people have a cardiac arrest in the hospital setting (AHA/ASA, 2015).

g. The total number of cardiovascular operations and procedures in the United States increased 28% between 2000 and 2010.

h. The total and indirect costs of cardiovascular disease (CVD) and stroke in the United States in 2010 are estimated to be $315.4 billion. CVD care costs are more than that for any other diagnostic group, including cancer (Go et al., 2014).

2. Heart disease is the leading cause of death for both males and females.
   a. More than half of heart disease deaths in 2009 were in men.
3. Statistics on the percentage of deaths caused by heart disease by ethnicity and race in 2008:
   a. Whites 25.1%
   b. African Americans 24.5%
   c. Asians or Pacific Islanders 23.2%
   d. Hispanics 20.8%
   e. American Indians or Alaska Natives 18% (Centers for Disease Control and Prevention [CDC], 2014a)
4. Between 2007 and 2009, the number of deaths from heart disease was highest in the South and lowest in the western United States (CDC, 2014a).
5. Only 10%–30% of eligible patients in the United States are receiving cardiac rehabilitation (AACVPR, 2014).

C. Cardiac Rehabilitation

1. According to the AHA, cardiac rehabilitation is "a professionally supervised program to help people recover from heart attacks, heart surgery and percutaneous coronary intervention (PCI) procedures such as stenting and angioplasty. Cardiac rehab programs usually provide education and counseling services to help heart patients increase physical fitness, reduce cardiac symptoms, improve health, and reduce the risk of future heart problems, including heart attack" (AHA, 2015a).
2. Benefits of cardiac rehabilitation have been shown to include
   a. Reduced risk of fatal MI (≥ 25%)
   b. Decreased severity of angina and need for antiangina medications
   c. Decreased hospitalizations
   d. Decreased cost of physician office visits and hospitalizations (≤ 35%)
   e. Fewer emergency department visits
   f. Decreased cardiac event rates
   g. Decreased all-cause mortality (AACVPR, 2014)
3. Patient-specific benefits include
   a. Improved functional capacity
   b. Increased knowledge of heart disease
   c. Improved adherence to positive lifestyle changes
   d. Enhanced compliance with medical regimen
   e. Increased self-esteem and confidence
   f. Reduced subsequent morbidity and mortality (AACVPR, 2014)
4. Eligible patients include those who have or have had
   a. Heart attack
   b. Coronary artery disease (CAD)
   c. Heart failure
   d. Heart procedure or surgery
      1) Stenting, coronary artery bypass graft
      2) Valve replacement, pacemaker insertion
      3) Implantable defibrillator
      4) Transplant
   e. Cardiomyopathy
   f. Congenital defects
5. Cardiac rehabilitation is contraindicated in patients with
   a. Unstable angina
   b. Uncompensated heart failure
   c. Uncontrolled arrhythmias
   d. Severe ischemia, left ventricular dysfunction, or arrhythmia during exercise testing
   e. Poorly controlled hypertension
   f. Hypertension or hypotension induced with exercise
   g. Unstable concomitant medical problems
      1) Diabetes
      2) Fever
      3) Transplant rejection
      4) Other (Singh, 2013)

6. Medicare covers cardiac rehabilitation for
   a. Stable angina
   b. Post myocardial infarction
   c. Post percutaneous coronary intervention (PCI)
   d. Post coronary artery bypass graft
   e. Post valve repair or replacement
   f. Post heart transplant (AACVPR, 2014)
7. Private insurers may also cover rehabilitation for
   a. Peripheral arterial disease
   b. Heart failure
   c. Cardiomyopathy (AACVPR, 2014)
8. Short-term goals
   a. Reconditioning
   b. Limiting the effects of heart disease, both physiological and psychological
   c. Decreasing the risk of sudden cardiac arrest or reinfarction
   d. Controlling the symptoms of heart disease
9. Long-term goals
   a. Identification and treatment of risk factors
   b. Stabilizing or reversing the atherosclerotic process
   c. Enhancing the psychological status of the patient
10. The program includes
    a. Staff
       1) Doctor of medicine (MD); registered nurse (RN) with cardiac experience; exercise specialist, physical therapist, or exercise physiologist
       2) As needed: dietitian, psychologist or behavioral therapist, vocational counselor, social worker
    b. Counseling so patient can understand and manage the disease process
    c. An exercise program
       1) In cardiac rehabilitation, the modification of risk factors is achieved through a supervised exercise program and education.
       2) The exercise component consists of aerobic exercise, strength training, and flexibility exercises.
       3) Aerobic exercises contribute to cardiovascular health by increasing the strength of the heart, reducing risk factors, and increase feelings of well-being.
       4) Strength training promotes the ability to manage activities of daily living (ADLs) and bone health.
       5) Flexibility training protects patients from injury.
    d. Counseling on nutrition
    e. Assistance with modifying risk factors such as hypertension, smoking, high cholesterol, physical inactivity, obesity, and diabetes
    f. Vocational guidance for returning to work
    g. Information on physical limitations
    h. Emotional support
    i. Counseling on medications
11. Phase 1: initiated while the patient is in the hospital
    a. Visit by member of cardiac rehabilitation team
    b. Education about the disease and recovery process
    c. Personal encouragement
    d. Inclusion of family
    e. Assisted range of motion within 24–48 hours of MI
    f. In cardiac care unit: low-risk patients getting up to a chair and performing ADLs
       1) Grooming, sponge bath
       2) Shaving
    g. In step-down unit: sit, stand, walk in room or hallway two times daily with monitoring (Singh, 2013)
12. Phase 1.5: after the patient returns home, for 2–6 weeks
    a. More education on heart health
    b. Medical status supervised
    c. Low-level exercise and physical activity
    d. Instruction on changes needed for resumption of active lifestyle (Singh, 2013)
13. Phase 2: a supervised ambulatory outpatient program spanning 3–6 weeks
    a. Has completed hospitalization and 2–6 weeks of recovery at home
    b. Team formulates level of exercise necessary to meet patient's needs
    c. Exercise treatments three times per week at rehabilitation facility
    d. Constant medical supervision by nurse and exercise specialist, and use of exercise electrocardiograms (Singh, 2013)
14. Phase 3: a lifetime maintenance phase in which physical fitness and additional risk factor reduction are emphasized
    a. Sessions scheduled three times per week
    b. Exercises that the patient prefers such as walking, bicycling, or jogging
    c. RN supervises classes
    d. Electrocardiogram monitoring usually not necessary
15. Chest pain management
    a. Medications as needed
    b. Oxygen

c. Monitor vital signs and oxygenation.
d. Assess and intervene as necessary.

D. Education Content
1. Disease process and anticipated outcomes
2. Medications
3. Energy conservation
4. Dietary restrictions
5. Prevention of infection
6. Counseling for school, sports, sexual activity, genetics, employment, cardiopulmonary resuscitation
7. Guidance on when to call the provider

E. Cardiovascular Diseases Requiring Rehabilitation
1. Types
a. Coronary artery disease
b. Heart failure
c. Cardiomyopathy
d. Congenital defects
e. Valvular defects
2. Risk factors
a. Modifiable and nonmodifiable
1) Heredity, race, gender, age
2) Smoking, hypertension, cholesterol, diabetes
3) Sedentary lifestyle, stress, birth control pills, alcohol, obesity
3. Disease processes
a. Coronary heart disease (CHD) or coronary artery disease: A disorder of the coronary arteries that leads to disruption of the blood flow that supplies oxygen and nutrients to the myocardium (**Figure 25-1**) (Boudi, 2014)
1) Epidemiology: An atherosclerotic disease of the coronary arteries that results in a narrowing of the vessel lumen
a) Single largest killer of men and women in the United States (Boudi, 2014)
2) Etiology: A disorder with periods of activity and periods of quiescence (Boudi, 2014)
a) Vascular damage caused by aging, diabetes, dyslipidemia, hypertension, nicotine exposure, or infection initiates a chain of events that leads to atherosclerosis (Boudi, 2014)
3) Pathophysiology: Arteriosclerosis (thickening, reduced elasticity, and calcification of the coronary arteries) and atherosclerosis (plaque buildup) in the coronary arteries
a) Endothelial damage allows infiltration of lipids and inflammatory cells into the endothelial and subendothelial spaces
b) Secretion of cytokines and growth factors promotes formation of atheroma, which can eventually rupture, leading to acute coronary syndrome or MI (Boudi, 2014).
4) Risk factors for CHD (**Figure 25-2**): Some of these factors, such as age and family history, cannot be changed. However, other factors can be changed; these are called modifiable risk factors. Making changes that reduce risk can help stop the progression of heart disease.

Figure 25-1. Atherosclerosis

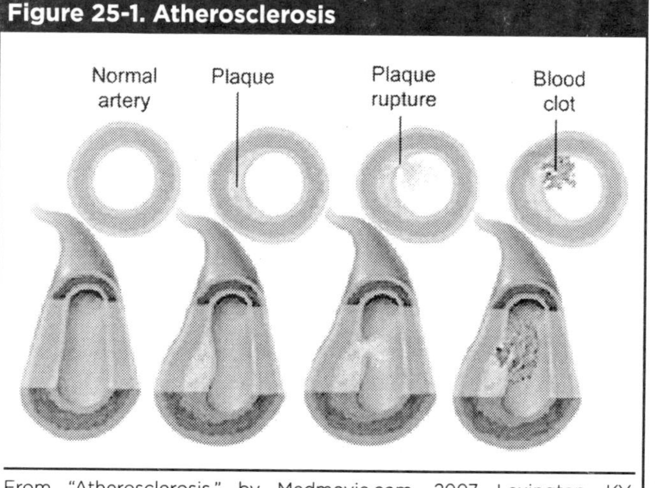

From "Atherosclerosis," by Medmovie.com, 2007, Lexington, KY: Medmovie.com. Copyright 2007 by Medmovie.com. Reprinted with permission.

Figure 25-2. Cardiovascular Risk Factors

The American Heart Association offers a downloadable CV Risk Calculator and other cardiac-related prevention guideline tools for Apple and Android products, available at the Apple App Store and on Google Play.

For more information, visit http://my.americanheart.org/professional/StatementsGuidelines/PreventionGuidelines/Prevention-Guidelines_UCM_457698_SubHomePage.jsp.

a) Tobacco smoke
b) Air pollution
c) Hyperlipidemia and dyslipidemia
d) Hypertension
e) Physical inactivity
f) Overweight and obesity
g) Diabetes mellitus
h) Stress
i) Alcohol consumption
(i) More than two drinks a day for men
(ii) More than one drink a day for women
j) Diet and nutrition

k) Advanced age (AHA, 2015c; Boudi, 2014)

5) Complications
   a) Angina: 10.2 million people per year experience angina, or transient chest pain, due to myocardial ischemia.
      (i) Stable: Triggered by a predictable degree of exertion, its duration, and frequency
      (ii) Unstable: Transitory syndrome in which a thrombus forms but is lysed, and there are no residual deficits
      (iii) Variant, Prinzmetal's, or vasospastic angina, caused by vasospasms
   b) Myocardial infarction (MI): 8.5 million people per year experience an MI, or death of myocardial tissue from inadequate coronary perfusion, when blood supply to a portion of the heart is severely reduced or stopped. MI can occur at rest or with exertion. Pain can last longer than 30 minutes, is continuous, and is unrelieved by rest, position change, or nitroglycerin tablets.
      (i) Symptoms
         (1) Chest pain characterized as crushing, squeezing, stabbing, or heavy pressure
         (2) Can radiate down the left arm and to neck, jaws, teeth, epigastric area, and back
         (3) Extreme fatigue
         (4) Diaphoresis
         (5) Syncope
         (6) Dyspnea, orthopnea
         (7) Nausea, vomiting
         (8) Dysrhythmias: Include premature atrial and ventricular contractions, conduction abnormalities, and tachycardia and bradycardia

6) Treatment
   a) Invasive interventions (Zafari, 2014)
      (i) Percutaneous transluminal coronary angioplasty is an invasive nonsurgical procedure performed via a catheter introduced into the coronary artery. Patency is restored to the coronary artery by inflating and deflating a balloon at the distal end of the catheter to compress plaques in the arteries.
      (ii) Stent placement: After angioplasty, a small metal stent is inserted to maintain patency of the arterial lumen.
      (iii) Ablation: This is a laser procedure that focuses on an area of the heart that is causing a dysrhythmia; the area is lysed to stop the cycle.
   b) Surgical procedures
      (i) Coronary artery bypass graft: Conduits for blood are created from arteries or veins, bypassing areas of stenosis.
      (ii) Pacemaker or automatic implantable cardioversion-defibrillator placement (for dysrhythmias)
      (iii) Medications, which can be used alone or in combination, depending on the CHD and the severity of symptoms
   c) Management measures (AHA, 2015c): Risk factor modification for CHD
      (i) Stop smoking.
      (ii) Control blood pressure.
      (iii) Control cholesterol: AHA-recommended cholesterol levels
         (1) Lower LDLs to < 100 mg/dL.
         (2) Raise HDLs to > 50 mg/dL (women) or > 40 mg/dL (men).
         (3) Maintain total cholesterol level of < 200 mg/dL.
            (a) Lower fasting triglyceride level to < 150 mg/dL.
         (4) Ways to lower elevated cholesterol levels
            (a) Diet
            (b) Exercise
            (c) Weight control
            (d) Medications
            (e) Smoking cessation
            (f) Diabetes management
            (g) Physical activity
            (h) Consultation with a physician before beginning an exercise program
         (i) Manage stress.
         (j) Note: This year, there is less focus by the AHA on treating "numbers" and more focus on calculating and addressing

overall risk and managing a healthy lifestyle.

b. Congestive heart failure or heart failure: A complex condition in which the heart fails to pump at a rate necessary to supply the blood needed by the tissues of the body, or is able to supply bodily requirements only when diastolic filling pressures are elevated (Dumitru, 2014).
   1) Epidemiology: Affects 5.7 million Americans of all ages and is responsible for more hospital admissions than all cancers combined (Dumitru, 2014)
      a) Expected to increase in incidence as the population ages (Dumitru, 2014)
   2) Etiology: Structural abnormalities, abnormal biochemical and physiologic conditions, precipitating events, and genetics can lead to heart failure (Dumitru, 2014)
      a) The above mentioned conditions can include
         (i) Diabetes
         (ii) Hypertension
         (iii) CAD
         (iv) Arrhythmias
         (v) Valvular disease
         (vi) Medications
         (vii) Infections
         (viii) Inflammation
         (ix) Alcohol abuse
         (x) Cardiomyopathy (Dumitru, 2014)
   3) Pathophysiology: Loss or dysfunction of the cardiac muscle or an inability of the ventricle to fill or pump blood (Linton, 2015) due to
      a) Cardiac hypertrophy
      b) Arrhythmias
      c) Cardiac wall stiffness
      d) Action of atrial natriuretic peptides and brain natriuretic peptides
      e) Action of neurohormonal systems (Dumitru, 2014)
   4) New York Heart Association Functional Classification of Heart Failure:
      a) Class I: without limitation of physical activity
      b) Class II: with slight limitation of physical activity, in which ordinary physical activity leads to fatigue, palpitation, dyspnea, or anginal pain; patients are comfortable at rest
      c) Class III: with marked limitation of physical activity, in which less than ordinary activity results in fatigue, palpitation, dyspnea, or anginal pain; patients are comfortable at rest
      d) Class IV: not only unable to perform any physical activity without discomfort but also has symptoms of heart failure or the anginal syndrome even at rest; patients' discomfort increases if any physical activity is undertaken (Dumitru, 2014).
   5) Treatment
      a) Nonpharmacological
         (i) Exercise
            (1) "A 2012 meta-analysis showed that aerobic exercise training, particularly long-term, can reverse left ventricular remodeling in clinically stable heart failure patients, while strength training had no effect on remodeling" (Dumitru, 2014).
         (ii) Diet and nutrition
            (1) Weight monitoring
            (2) Restricted sodium and fluids as ordered
               (a) 2–5 g sodium/day
               (b) 2 L fluid restriction with sodium N 130 mEq/dL or in those whose status is difficult to control with diuretics
            (3) Calorie supplementation for those with cardiac cachexia (Dumitru, 2014).
      b) Device therapy: Pacemakers (including cardiac resynchronization therapy), implantable cardiac defibrillators, and mechanical assist devices
      c) Cardiac transplantation
      d) Medications
         (i) Angiotensin-converting enzyme inhibitors
         (ii) Angiotensin II receptor blockers
         (iii) Beta-adrenergic blockers
         (iv) Diuretics
         (v) Digoxin
         (vi) Aldosterone antagonists
         (vii) Anticoagulant and antiplatelet agents
         (viii) Hydralazine and nitrates
         (ix) Inotropes

(x) Avoid or use with extreme caution calcium channel blockers, nonsteroidal antiinflammatory drugs (NSAIDs), and antiarrhythmics, as they can exacerbate heart failure (Dumitru, 2014).

c. Cardiomyopathy: Diseases that affect the myocardium, resulting in enlargement or restriction, leading to cardiac dysfunction. Types include dilated (accounts for 87% of all cardiomyopathies), nonobstructive, obstructive, and restrictive cardiomyopathies. This section describes dilated cardiomyopathy. With dilated cardiomyopathy, the myocardium is dilated and there is impaired contraction of the ventricles.
   1) Epidemiology: Found in all ages, but symptoms usually become apparent during the third and fourth decades of life (Goswami, 2013).
      a) True incidence in unknown but appears to be increasing (Goswami, 2013).
   2) Etiology: CHD is the most common cause of dilated cardiomyopathy, accounting for more than half of the cases.
      a) Genetics, infections, and toxins can also play a role (Goswami, 2013).
      b) Multiple other potential causes include thiamine deficiency, collagen vascular disease, and transplant rejection (Goswami, 2013).
   3) Pathophysiology: Ventricular chamber enlargement, increase in ventricular filling capacity, little or no wall hypertrophy (Goswami, 2013).
      a) Can lead to mitral and tricuspid valve regurgitation, further dilation, and myocardial dysfunction (Goswami, 2013).
   4) Complications: CHF and dysrhythmias
   5) Treatment
      a) Medications: Treat symptoms (e.g., heart failure)
      b) Surgical
         (i) Heart transplantation
         (ii) Left ventricular assist device
         (iii) Implanted cardioverter-defibrillator
         (iv) Ventricular restoration surgery
         (v) Biventricular pacing (Goswami, 2013).
      c) Management measures are the same as those for CHF.

d. Congenital heart defects: Structural or functional abnormalities of the heart or great vessels existing from birth that obstruct blood flow in and to the heart and cause the blood to flow abnormally through the heart. The severity ranges from life threatening to undetected (CDC, 2014b)
   1) Ventricular septal defect is the most common type (CDC, 2014b).
   2) Epidemiology: Congenital heart defects (CHD) occur in approximately 0.9% of live births in the United States (CDC, 2014b).
      a) Estimated that 2 million children and adults in the United States are living with CHDs (CDC, 2014b).
   3) Etiology: Congenital heart defects occur during heart development, which occurs soon after conception. In most cases the cause is not known, although sometimes medications, maternal infections, maternal health condition, maternal exposures, and genetics can be responsible. Smoking, diabetes, and maternal obesity have been linked to CHD development (CDC, 2014b).
   4) Pathophysiology: This depends on the particular defect: atrial, ventricular, or valvular. Venous and arterial defects are all possible.
   5) Complications (CDC, 2014b): These defects can result in a number of medical conditions:
      a) Congestive heart failure (CHF)
      b) Pulmonary hypertension
      c) Dysrhythmias
   6) Treatment (CDC, 2014b)
      a) Medication: Treats symptoms
      b) Surgery: Used for repair of defects
      c) Management measures are the same as for CHF.

e. Cardiac valve disease: Classified according to the valve involved and the functional alterations (Linton, 2015)
   1) Epidemiology, etiology, and pathophysiology depend on the valve involved. For example, the most common cause of mitral regurgitation is rheumatic heart disease.
   2) Complications can include CHF and dysrhythmias.
   3) Treatment (Linton, 2015)
      a) Invasive treatments: Surgery
      b) Annuloplasty: Corrects regurgitation by repairing the enlarged annulus
      c) Valvuloplasty: Repair of the valve leaflet

d) Prosthetic heart valves: Replacement of valves with a mechanical or biological valve
e) Management measures (Linton, 2015)
  (i) Monitor vital signs.
  (ii) Auscultate for heart murmurs
  (iii) Assess activity tolerance
  (iv) Monitor coagulation.
  (v) Check for bleeding.
  (vi) Educate patient on medications, diet, and activity

F. Effects of CVD

1. Arrhythmias
2. Ischemia and MI
3. Poor tissue perfusion
4. Exercise intolerance
5. Deconditioning
6. Pain
7. Dyspnea
8. Edema
9. Malnutrition
10. Hypoxic encephalopathy
11. Hypoxemia

G. Nursing Process

1. Assessment (Linton, 2015)
  a. Subjective elements
    1) Palpitations, dizziness, lightheadedness, syncope, shortness of breath, fatigue, poor appetite, insomnia, restlessness, anxiety and fear, nausea, jaw pain, indigestion
    2) Chest discomfort: Quality, location, precipitating factors, duration, alleviating factors
  b. Objective elements
    1) Skin: Pallor, diaphoresis
    2) Cardiac output: Tachycardia, bradycardia, irregular heart rhythm, heart murmur, hypotension, hypertension, confusion, decreased urine output, peripheral edema, sacral or genital edema, weight gain, abdominal distention, electrocardiogram changes, elevated cardiac serum enzymes (creatine kinase myocardial band) and muscle proteins
    3) Pulmonary status: Crackles; wheezes; dyspnea; labored breathing; frothy, blood-tinged sputum; cyanosis
    4) Nutritional: Anorexia, decreased skin turgor and integrity
  c. History
    1) Health habits
    2) Medical
    3) Surgical
    4) Social support
    5) Previous independence level
    6) Medications
  d. Diagnoses (Doenges, Moorhouse, & Murr, 2010; Linton, 2015)
    1) Activity intolerance
    2) Anxiety
    3) Cardiac output, decreased
    4) Shock, risk for
    5) Coping, ineffective
    6) Electrolyte imbalance, risk for
    7) Fatigue
    8) Fear
    9) Fluid volume, imbalanced, risk for
    10) Health maintenance, ineffective
    11) Health-seeking behavior
    12) Knowledge deficit
    13) Mobility, impaired
    14) Self-care deficits (e.g., feeding, bathing, grooming, dressing, toileting)
    15) Nutrition, readiness for enhanced
    16) Pain
    17) Perfusion, risk for decreased
    18) Powerlessness, risk for
    19) Skin integrity, risk for impaired
    20) Sleep pattern, disturbed
    21) Spiritual distress, risk for
    22) Therapeutic regimen management, ineffective
    23) Tissue integrity, impaired
    24) Tissue perfusion, ineffective
    25) Gas exchange, impaired
  e. Plan: Goals for patient and family (Linton, 2015)
    1) Demonstrate understanding of exercise plan, and verbalize understanding of activity intolerance by modifying activity and resting to prevent fatigue, palpitations, shortness of breath, and diaphoresis.
    2) Verbalize that pain will be relieved after measures are taken, and reduce symptoms of angina, dyspnea, and fatigue.
    3) Demonstrate understanding of and participation in self-management, including ADLs, exercise programs, dietary management, and lifestyle changes.
    4) Maintain adequate nutritional status to lower risk of progression of cardiac disease and promote healing.
    5) Maintain adequate mentation, heart rate, rhythm, and urine output.
    6) Demonstrate decreased anxiety and verbalize understanding of disease, procedures, and expected outcomes.

7) Identify stressors and develop strategies to decrease stress.
8) Verbalize an understanding of the importance of taking medications as prescribed, actions of medications, how to administer medications, and potential side effects.
9) Maintain skin integrity.
10) Verbalize and demonstrate an understanding of the importance of following therapeutic and medical treatment recommendations.
11) Verbalize improved health-related quality of life.
12) Reduce hospitalizations and use of medical resources (AACVPR, 2014).

f. Implementation (Linton, 2015)
1) Activity intolerance; mobility impairment; self-care deficits, fatigue
a) Monitor activities that aggravate the condition (e.g., type of activity, intensity, frequency of symptoms).
b) Monitor blood pressure, heart rate, and respiratory rate before, during, and after exercise, staying within target heart rate parameters.
c) Increase activities gradually.
2) Cardiac pain management
a) Administer medications for chest pain and symptoms.
b) Administer oxygen therapy as ordered to increase oxygen to myocardium.
c) Monitor vital signs.
d) Assess effectiveness of interventions.
3) Nutrition; readiness for enhanced
a) Consult with a dietitian for special dietary instructions and meal planning.
b) Monitor weight daily.
c) Offer caloric supplements (if needed).
d) Offer measures to improve appetite (e.g., appropriate environment, good oral care, and small, frequent meals).
e) Administer antiemetics before meals (if necessary).
f) Administer medications so as not to interfere with meals.
4) Tissue perfusion, impaired or ineffective; cardiac output, decreased; fluid volume, imbalanced, risk for; perfusion, risk for decreased; shock, risk for; skin integrity, risk for
a) Monitor level of consciousness, signs and symptoms of hypoxemia
b) Monitor laboratory values of blood urea nitrogen, creatinine, and electrolytes.
c) Monitor vital signs for changes.
d) Monitor electrocardiogram.
e) Document changes in the patient's condition.
5) Anxiety; coping, ineffective; fear; powerless, risk for; spiritual distress, risk for; sleep pattern, disturbed
a) Explain procedures, disease process, and expected outcomes.
b) Allow the patient to express feelings.
c) Involve the family, significant other, and spiritual counselor.
d) Encourage participation in the decision-making process and lifestyle changes.
e) Provide information about support groups, social services, and vocational counseling.
6) Fluid volume excess; electrolyte imbalance, risk for
a) Administer diuretics as ordered and monitor their effectiveness (e.g., increased urine output, decreased edema, clear lung sounds).
b) Monitor weight daily and report weight gain of 2 pounds in 24 hours.
c) Restrict sodium and fluid intake.
1) Knowledge deficit; health-seeking behaviors; health maintenance, ineffective
a) Instruct about disease process and expected outcomes.
b) Instruct about medications: Purpose, dosage, how to administer, potential side effects, take only as prescribed, and the importance of follow-up with physician.
c) Practice energy-conservation techniques; instruct on signs and symptoms of overexertion.
d) Instruct on dietary restrictions and infection prevention.
e) Offer counseling for employment, genetics, marriage, childbearing, contraceptive use, resuming sexual relations, and learning cardiopulmonary resuscitation.
f) Instruct about oxygen safety.
g) Instruct about proper protection of sternum (and grafts) if the patient has had surgery.
h) Instruct on modification of risk factors.

i) Include significant other and family members in all instructions.

8) Gas exchange
   a) Monitor chest X ray.
   b) Elevate the head of the bed.
   c) Monitor breath sounds and respiratory function.
   d) Encourage coughing and deep breathing.

9) Therapeutic regimen, ineffective
   a) Promote performance of ADLs.
   b) Promote therapeutic regimen.
   c) Teach proper incision care for surgical patients.
   d) Assess the patient's and family members' readiness to learn and follow the therapeutic regimen.
   e) Stress the importance of administering medications as prescribed, reporting untoward reactions or responses to medications and difficulties obtaining recommended medications (e.g., affordability, accessibility).
   f) Assess understanding of the treatment regimen.

10) Evaluation
   a) Assess the efficacy of the treatment regimen.
   b) If goals are not met as originally designed, reassessment should be done and revisions to the plan of care developed.

II. Pulmonary Rehabilitation

Pulmonary rehabilitation is indicated for those with chronic pulmonary disease who are symptomatic despite optimal medical treatment.

A. Benefits of Pulmonary Rehabilitation
   1. Increased strength of peripheral and respiratory muscles
   2. Decreased anxiety and depression
   3. Fewer abnormalities of nutrition
   4. Improvements in overall and exertional dyspnea
   5. Better quality of life
   6. Increases in maximal exercise capacity and endurance

B. Eligibility
   1. Presence of chronic respiratory impairment with reduced exercise tolerance or restricted activities, even with optimal medical management
   2. Persistence of symptoms, disability, and handicap

C. Setting
   1. Inpatient
   2. Outpatient
   3. Home
   4. Telerehabilitation
   5. Other modalities under investigation

D. Interventions
   1. Interprofessional team: MD, RN, physical therapist (PT) or exercise physiologist, occupational therapist, psychologist, respiratory therapist, dietitian, others as needed
   2. Patient and family education
      a. Energy conservation and work simplification
      b. Medications and other therapies
      c. End of life education
   3. Exercise training
      a. Targeted at 60% of maximal workload for 20–30 minutes, two to five times per week.
   4. Psychosocial and behavioral interventions
      a. Coping, managing anxiety and depression
   5. Risk reduction
      a. Smoking cessation
   6. Outcome assessment
      a. Dyspnea
      b. Exercise tolerance
      c. Health status
      d. Activity levels
   7. Medications
   8. Vaccines
      a. Flu, pneumonia
   9. Nutritional assessment
   10. Prevention, recognition, and early treatment of morbidities
   11. Inpatient, outpatient, and extended care of patients with chronic respiratory illness

E. Consequences of Pulmonary Disease
   1. Peripheral muscle dysfunction
   2. Respiratory muscle dysfunction
   3. Nutritional abnormalities
   4. Cardiac impairment
   5. Skeletal disease
   6. Sensory deficits
   7. Psychosocial dysfunction

F. Mechanism of Morbidities
   1. Deconditioning
   2. Malnutrition
   3. Effects of hypoxemia
   4. Steroid myopathy or intensive care unit neuropathy
   5. Hyperinflation of lungs
   6. Diaphragmatic fatigue
   7. Frequent hospitalizations
   8. Effects of medications
   9. Psychosocial dysfunction due to anxiety, depression, guilt, dependency, and sleep disturbance

G. Causes of Disability

1. Muscle dysfunction
2. Poor endurance
3. Combination of impairments
4. Inadequate finances
5. Inadequate family support
6. Public policies

H. Pulmonary Diseases Requiring Rehabilitation

1. Obstructive
    a. Chronic bronchitis
        1) Four percent of the American population has been diagnosed with chronic bronchitis.
            a) Many more cases are suspected due to underreporting.
            b) Affects males more than females
            c) More frequent with low socioeconomic status and urban, industrialized areas
        2) Characterized by inflammation of bronchial tubes
            a) Defined as cough with sputum for at least 3 months of the year during the most recent 2 years
            b) Associated with hypertrophy of mucus-producing glands in the airways
            c) Progressive airflow limitation will occur, and fibrotic emphysematous changes will be seen.
        3) Causes include respiratory viruses, smoking, bacterial infection, air pollution, and workplace exposures.
        4) Treatment is aimed at alleviating symptoms.
            a) Medications
                (i) Mucolytics
                (ii) Cough suppressants
                (iii) Short-acting, long-acting beta-agonists
                (iv) Antiinflammatories and/or antibiotics for acute flare-ups (Fayyaz, 2014).
    b. Emphysema
        1) Rate of emphysema in the population unchanged since 2000
            a) Eighteen cases per 1,000 people in the United States
            b) Worldwide prevalence is 10.1%
            c) Increasing in women (Demerjian, 2012)
        2) Characterized by permanent enlargement of the alveoli, with decline in the surface area available for gas exchange
            a) Loss of elastic recoil of alveoli
            b) Airway narrowing due to loss of alveolar supporting structure (Demerjian, 2012)
        3) Causes
            a) Genetics modified by environmental exposures
                (i) Cigarette smoke
                (ii) Workplace fumes
                (iii) Air pollution (Demerjian, 2012)
            b) Exposures lead to inflammation.
                (i) Inflammation amplified by proinflammatory mediators, oxidative stress, and proteases.
                (ii) Results in destruction of elastin and structural elements (Demerjian, 2012)
        4) Treatment
            a) "...to relieve symptoms, prevent disease progression, improve exercise tolerance and health, prevent and treat complications and exacerbations, reduce mortality" (**Figure 25-3**) (Demerjian, 2012)
            b) Smoking cessation
            c) Education
            d) Medications
                (i) Bronchodilators
                    (1) Short acting
                    (2) Long acting
                (ii) Phosphodiesterase inhibitors
                (iii) Antiinflammatories
                (iv) Mucolytics
                (v) Proton pump inhibitors
                (vi) Oxygen
                (vii) Alpha-1 antitrypsin (AAT) replacement if deficiency (Demerjian, 2012)
    c. Asthma
        1) Most common chronic disease in childhood
            a) Seven million children affected
                (i) Affects 5%–10% of the overall population
                    (1) 23.4 million persons
            b) In the United States, prevalence is greater in African Americans than in whites, as well as in older and younger age groups.
            c) Common in industrialized nations (Morris, 2014)
        2) Characterized by
            a) Airway inflammation
            b) Intermittent airflow obstruction
            c) Bronchial hyperresponsiveness (Morris, 2014)
        3) Causes
            a) Contributing factors include
                (i) Environmental allergens
                (ii) Infections

Figure 25-3. Breathing Techniques

Certain exercises can be used to improve your breathing. They include pursed-lip breathing and abdominal breathing.

Pursed-Lip Breathing

- Pursed-lip breathing decreases how often you take breaths and keeps your airways open longer. This allows more air to flow in and out of your lungs so you can be more physically active.
- To do pursed-lip breathing, you breathe in through your nostrils. Then you slowly breathe out through slightly pursed lips, as if you're blowing out a candle. You exhale two to three times longer than you inhale. Some people find it helpful to count to two while inhaling and to four or six while exhaling.
- Illustrations are available at www.nhlbi.nih.gov/health/dci/Diseases/pulreh/pulreh_during.html
- The illustration shows the pursed-lip breathing technique. The "inhale" illustration shows how to inhale correctly using this technique. The "exhale" illustration shows how to exhale correctly. Click your mouse on the "inhale" and "exhale" tabs at the top of the illustration to view each step of the technique.

Abdominal Breathing

- Abdominal breathing is the process of contracting the diaphragm, the muscle that separates the lungs from the stomach and liver. It enables the lungs to expand more fully and expel carbon dioxide more effectively.
  1. Adjust your posture so that your lungs, chest, and abdomen can expand fully (standing, sitting or lying down).
  2. Place your hand on your abdomen to assess the effectiveness of your breathing.
  3. Breathe in through the nose slowly, feeling your abdomen expand.
  4. Rest for a moment.
  5. Slowly exhale through your mouth.
  6. Repeat the process for several minutes or as tolerated.

From *Pursed-lip breathing*, by the National Heart, Lung, and Blood Institute, National Institutes of Health, 2010. Retrieved from www.nhlbi.nih.gov/health/dci/Diseases/pulreh/pulreh_during.html

(iii) Exercise
(iv) Gastrointestinal (GI) reflux disease
(v) Chronic sinusitis or rhinitis
(vi) Medication sensitivity
(1) Acetylsalicylic acid, NSAIDs, sulfites
(vii) Use of beta blockers
(1) Including eye drops
(viii) Obesity
(ix) Air pollution
(x) Cigarette smoke
(xi) Stress
(xii) Environmental fumes (Morris, 2014)

b) Prematurity, advanced maternal age, prenatal exposure to tobacco smoke (Morris, 2014)

4) Treatment
a) Goals
(i) Prevent symptoms.
(ii) Minimize morbidity in acute episodes.
(iii) Maintain lifestyle.
b) Acute and chronic
c) Control agents
(i) Inhaled corticosteroids
(ii) Inhaled cromolyn or nedocromil
(iii) Long-acting bronchodilators
(iv) Theophylline
(v) Leukotriene modifiers
(vi) Anti-IgE antibodies
d) Relief medications
(i) Short-acting bronchodilators
(ii) Systemic corticosteroids
(iii) Ipratropium (Morris, 2014)

d. Cystic fibrosis (CF)
1) Autosomal recessive inherited disease
a) Most common lethal hereditary disease in the white population
b) Prevalence in the United States
(i) Whites: one case per 3,200–3,500 people
(ii) Hispanics: one case per 9,200–9,500 people
(iii) African Americans: one case per 15,000–17,000 people
(iv) Asian Americans: one case per 31,000 people
c) Females have more severe course and younger mean age at death (Sharma, 2014)
2) Characterized by decreased secretion of chloride and increased reabsorption of sodium and water across epithelial cells
a) Sticky mucus
(i) Promotes infection and inflammation
(ii) Occurs in respiratory tract, pancreas, GI tract, sweat glands, and other exocrine tissues
b) Pancreatic enzyme deficiency
c) Principle cause of death is end-stage lung disease (Sharma, 2014)

- 3) Cause
    - a) Inherited defect in CF gene
- 4) Treatment
    - a) Goals
        - (i) Maintaining normal lung function
        - (ii) Maintaining adequate nutrition and growth
        - (iii) Managing complications
    - b) Chest physiotherapy and postural drainage
        - (i) With forced expiratory technique and positive expiratory pressure mask
        - (ii) Can use ThAIRapy Vest® for CPT
    - c) Nebulizers
    - d) Medications
        - (i) Bronchodilators
        - (ii) Mucolytics
        - (iii) Antibiotics
        - (iv) Pancreatic enzyme supplements
        - (v) Multivitamins
        - (vi) Medications to reverse abnormal chloride transport (e.g., Ivacaftor)
        - (vii) Bisphosphonates to prevent bone loss
    - e) Regular diet with added calories and unrestricted fat intake
        - (i) Additional salt intake in warm climates
        - (ii) Nutritional supplements
    - f) Regular exercise
    - g) Long-term monitoring
        - (i) Growth and development
        - (ii) Lung function
        - (iii) Infection
        - (iv) GI tract health
        - (v) Psychosocial issues (Sharma, 2014)

e. Alpha-1 antitrypsin deficiency

- 1) Related to emphysema
- 2) AAT is a protein whose role is to neutralize neutrophil elastase, an enzyme that breaks down elastin.
- 3) Loss of AAT predisposes to elastolysis and an early onset of panacinar emphysema.
- 4) Deficiency of AAT is inherited as an autosomal codominant condition
- 5) Levels < 11 mmol/L increase risk of emphysema (Demerjian, 2012)

f. Bronchiectasis

- 1) Abnormal and permanent distortion of conducting bronchi or airways, often after and due to an infection
    - a) Chronic wet cough in children that does not respond to antibiotics may be bronchiectasis (Emmons, 2014)
- 2) Characterized by airways that are inflamed and easily collapsible, resulting in obstruction of air flow with resultant dyspnea, impaired clearance of secretions
    - a) Can progress to respiratory failure
    - b) Rare (Emmons, 2014)
- 3) Symptoms include
    - a) Cough
    - b) Daily mucopurulent sputum production
    - c) Hemoptysis
    - d) Dyspnea, wheezing, fever, weight loss, weakness
- 4) Causes include
    - a) Infection
    - b) Aspiration
    - c) Cystic fibrosis
    - d) AAT deficiency
    - e) Autoimmune diseases
    - f) Toxic gas exposure
    - g) Connective tissue disorders
    - h) Immunodeficiency
    - i) Autosomal dominant polycystic kidney disease (Emmons, 2014)
- 5) Treatment
    - a) Goals
        - (i) Improve symptoms
        - (ii) Prevent complications
        - (iii) Reduce exacerbations
    - b) Antibiotics and chest physiotherapy
    - c) Bronchodilators
    - d) Corticosteroid therapy
    - e) Oxygen

2. Restrictive

a. Characterized by reduced lung volumes

- 1) Intrinsic disorders
    - a) Lung volumes reduced due to excessive elastic recoil of the lungs in comparison with forces from the chest wall. Expiratory airflow is reduced.
- 2) Extrinsic disorders
    - a) Lung volumes are reduced from chest wall pressures or muscular disorders.

b. Examples

- 1) Interstitial lung disease
    - a) Disease of lung parenchyma
        - (i) Causes inflammation or scarring of lung tissue
    - b) Causes
        - (i) Idiopathic fibrotic diseases
        - (ii) Connective tissue diseases

(iii) Drug-induced diseases
(iv) Sarcoidosis and other primary lung diseases
(v) Exposures: dust, metals, organic solvents, farming, and agriculture

2) Neuromuscular and neurologic diseases
a) Causes
(i) Myasthenia gravis
(ii) Amyotrophic lateral sclerosis
(iii) Myopathy
(iv) Spinal cord injury
(v) Others

3) Chest wall abnormalities
a) Causes
(i) Kyphoscoliosis
(1) Associated with long-term wheelchair use
(2) Congenital
(ii) Obesity
(iii) Ascites
(iv) Congenital
(v) Trauma

c. Symptoms
1) Progressive exertional dyspnea
2) Dry cough
3) Fatigue
4) Impaired control of secretions
5) Recurrent infections

d. Treatment depends on condition (Caronia, 2014)

3. Other lung conditions
a. Lung cancer
1) Small and non-small cell types
a) Second most common cancer in men and women, not counting skin cancer
b) Estimated 224,210 new cases in the United States in 2014
c) Leading cause of cancer death (American Cancer Society, 2014)
2) Goals of rehabilitation
a) Improve ability to exercise and do ADLs
b) Lessen complications of surgery
c) Improve pulmonary function
d) Improve quality of life
e) Improve coexisting medical conditions such as chronic obstructive pulmonary disease and emphysema
f) Preoperative rehabilitation to improve surgery outcomes

b. Lung transplant
1) First transplant performed in 1963; patient survived 18 days
a) Ongoing issues with rejection and healing
b) Immunosuppressant research in the 1980s improved outlook for transplants.
c) First successful transplant done in 1986 (Moffat-Bruce, 2014)
2) Indications
a) Advanced disease with life expectancy < 2–3 years despite optimal medical management, and class III and IV New York Heart Association symptoms, with stable nutritional status, motivation for rehabilitation, and support systems in place
(i) Chronic obstructive pulmonary disease
(ii) Idiopathic pulmonary fibrosis
(iii) Alpha-1-antitrypsin disease
(iv) Primary pulmonary hypertension (Moffat-Bruce, 2014)
3) Contraindications
a) Cancer during the last 2 years
b) Noncurable chronic infections such as hepatitis B or C, human immunodeficiency virus (HIV)
c) Advanced dysfunction of a major body system that is not treatable
d) Current cigarette smoking
e) Poor nutritional status
f) Poor rehabilitation potential
g) Psychosocial issues, substance abuse, history of noncompliance (Moffat-Bruce, 2014)
4) Outcomes and prognosis
a) 1-year survival rate of 8% and 5-year survival rate of 51%
b) Mortality rate highest during first year
c) Exercise training after surgery is recommended to improve health, function, and blood pressure (Moffat-Bruce, 2014)

c. Obesity
1) Multiple implications for respiratory health
a) Effects on lung and chest wall compliance
b) Loads chest wall and reduces functional residual capacity
c) Increases oxygen consumptions and carbon dioxide secretion
d) Breathlessness, especially during exercise
e) Associated with asthma (Salome, King, & Berend, 2010)

f) Obstructive sleep apnea increased
g) Increased risk of deep vein thrombosis and pulmonary embolism
h) Hypoventilation
i) Increased pulmonary hypertension (Friedman & Andrus, 2012)

d. Sleep apnea
1) Central versus obstructive
a) Obstructive
(i) Recurrent episodes of upper airway collapse during sleep
(ii) Signs/symptoms
(1) Snoring
(2) Witnessed apnea
(3) Gasping and choking sensations
(4) Nocturia
(5) Insomnia, restless sleep (Downey, 2014)
(iii) Causes
(1) Structural abnormalities
(a) Down syndrome
(b) Marfan syndrome
(c) Prader-Willi syndrome
(d) High, arched palate
(e) Brachycephalic head form
(f) Others
(2) Nonstructural
(a) Obesity
(b) Central fat distribution
(c) Male gender
(d) Alcohol or sedatives
(e) Smoking
(f) Supine sleep position
(g) Rapid eye movement sleep
(h) Older age
(i) Postmenopausal women
(3) Others
(a) Hypothyroidism
(b) Stroke
(c) Neurological syndromes
(d) Acromegaly
(e) Environmental exposures (Downey, 2014)
(iv) Treatment
(1) Weight loss
(2) Sleep on side
(3) Avoid alcohol, sedatives
(4) Continuous positive airway pressure, bilevel positive airway pressure (Downey, 2014)
(5) Surgery for structural abnormalities
b) Central
(i) Absence of respiratory effort
(1) Cessation of airflow for 10 seconds or longer without an identifiable respiratory effort (Becker, 2014)
(ii) Causes
(1) Ventilatory instability
(2) Depression of brain-stem respiratory centers or chemoreceptors
(3) Narcotics
(4) Brain-stem lesions
(iii) Treatment
(1) Continuous positive airway pressure
(2) Bilevel positive airway pressure
(3) Inhaled carbon dioxide
(4) Atrial pacing

e. Ventilator dependency
1) Iron lung first used in 1929
a) Vacuum pump created negative pressure, expanding the patient's chest
b) Vacuum would shut off to allow passive exhalation
2) Positive pressure machines began to be used in the 1950s and are still in use
a) Airway pressure pushes the air into the lung through an endotracheal tube or tracheostomy tube (Byrd, 2013).
3) Some indications
a) Bradypnea or apnea with respiratory arrest
b) Acute lung injury
c) Tachypnea
d) Respiratory muscle fatigue
e) Coma
f) Hypotension
g) $PaCO_2 > 50$ mmHg with an arterial pH < 7.25
h) Vital capacity < 15 mL/kg
i) Neuromuscular disease tube (Byrd, 2013)
4) Complications
a) Alveolar damage, rupture from high ventilator pressures or volumes
b) Oxygen toxicity
c) Ventilator-associated pneumonia
d) Stress ulcers
e) Sedation-related ileus

f) Increased intracranial pressure
g) Delirium
h) Sleep deprivation
i) Fluid retention
j) Cardiac effects tube (Byrd, 2013)

5) Rehabilitation
a) Caregiver training
b) Weaning
c) Equipment trial, setup, adjustment
d) Home evaluation
e) PT, occupational therapist
(i) Strengthening, seating, posture, ADLs

I. Rehabilitation Nursing Interventions

1. Assessment (Linton, 2015)
a. Medical and family history
1) Medical history
2) Surgical history
3) Use of supplemental oxygen, medical devices, and knowledge of appropriate use
4) Medications: Including allergies and drug intolerance
5) Triggers in work and home environments
b. Lifestyle
1) Smoking history
2) Work and home activities
c. Recent illnesses
d. Self-care skills
e. Knowledge and use of medications
f. Test results: Pulmonary function, blood tests, electrocardiogram, chest radiography

2. Physical
a. Activity
b. Physical limitations (e.g., strength, functional ability, orthopedic limitations)
c. Exercise tolerance, need for supplemental oxygen, cardiac function
d. Neurological: Cognition changes, lethargy, restlessness
e. Pulmonary: Dyspnea, tachypnea, wheezes, crackles, rhonchi, decreased breath sounds, cough, hoarseness, clubbed fingers, chest retractions, barrel chest, decreased chest wall movement, productive thick sputum that may be odorous, hemoptysis, postnasal drainage
f. Cardiovascular: Tachycardia, dysrhythmia, fatigue, chest pain, edema
g. Gastrointestinal
1) General: Weight loss or gain, appetite, oral sores, constipation, dehydration, reflux
2) Special gastrointestinal considerations for patients with CF: Bulky, foul-smelling, pale, or watery stool; intestinal obstruction; fecal impaction; and tarry stools if bleeding; jaundice; ascites; abnormal liver function laboratory results
h. Skin: Decreased skin turgor with dehydration, diaphoresis
1) Color
2) Temperature
i. Nutritional: Weight loss, lack of appetite, loss of taste, swallowing difficulties, constipation, hydration, serum albumin
j. Psychosocial
1) Support systems
2) Individual and family coping
3) Psychosocial: Fear of suffocation, sleep disturbance, depression, anxiety
4) Willingness to participate in program, health-changing behavior
5) Symptoms of depression
k. Knowledge of disease process, description and interpretation of medical tests

3. Nursing diagnoses (Doenges et al., 2010; Linton, 2015)
a. Airway clearance, ineffective
b. Anxiety
c. Coping, ineffective
d. Activity intolerance
e. Constipation, risk for
f. Electrolyte imbalance, risk for
g. Fatigue
h. Fluid balance, risk for imbalance
i. Gas exchange, impaired
j. Infection, risk for
k. Knowledge deficit
l. Mobility, impaired
m. Nutrition, imbalanced, less or more than body needs
n. Powerlessness, risk for
o. Self-care deficit (e.g., bathing and hygiene, dressing and grooming, feeding, toileting)
p. Sexual dysfunction
q. Skin integrity, risk for impaired
r. Spiritual distress, risk for
s. Stress, overload
t. Therapeutic regimen management, readiness for enhanced
u. Tissue perfusion, ineffective

4. Plan: Goals for patient and family (American Lung Association [ALA], 2010; Linton, 2015)
a. Demonstrate effective breathing patterns without fatigue, and use energy conservation measures.
b. Demonstrate improved airway clearance through use of postural drainage when

appropriate, coughing, deep breathing, and taking medications as directed (**Figure 25-4**).

c. Demonstrate resolution of cognitive changes if they have not become permanent; resolve cyanosis.

d. Demonstrate ability to perform ADLs using compensation measures when necessary to prevent dyspnea or fatigue; for children, demonstrate ability to participate in normal activities using preactivity medications.

e. Demonstrate stable weight for age and size, take adequate caloric intake daily, and have a normal albumin level.

f. Have regular bowel movements without constipation or dehydration, and take in adequate amounts of fluid daily.

g. Remain free of infection and prevent influenza and pneumonia.

h. Demonstrate adequate sleep patterns for rest and rejuvenation.

i. Verbalize decreased spiritual distress, increasing sense of integrity while living with chronic disease.

j. Demonstrate support for the person with the disability, and verbalize resources available for family support.

k. Acknowledge fear and anxiety, and demonstrate ways to decrease anxiety (e.g., hobbies, social activities, relaxation techniques).

l. Verbalize understanding of compensation measures while engaging in sexual activity.

m. Verbalize knowledge of the disease process and precipitating factors of respiratory difficulties and how to avoid or minimize effects, administer medication and oxygen therapy properly, and know when to call the physician.

n. Verbalize and demonstrate understanding of the therapeutic regimen and the importance of self-monitoring and compliance with therapeutic recommendations.

5. Interventions (ALA, 2010; Linton, 2015)

a. Observe respiration depth and rate, dyspnea, nasal flaring.

b. Inspect thorax or symmetry of respiratory movement, chest muscle retractions, changes in skin color and capillary refill, and changes in mentation or behavior.

c. Auscultate lungs for adventitious sounds.

d. Administer oxygen, bronchodilators, antibiotics, corticosteroids, and other medications as directed.

e. Teach breathing techniques and exercises to conserve energy (Figure 25-3).

f. Identify ways to conserve energy in daily activities. Consult occupational therapist for energy conservation techniques with ADLs.

g. Adapt ways to increase endurance and conserve energy.

h. Slowly increase activity as tolerance allows, promoting as much independence as possible.

i. Encourage a regular exercise program with planned rest periods between activities.

j. Teach patients receiving intermittent, continuous, or nocturnal ventilator support to do the following:

1) Strengthen skeletal muscles that have atrophied from illness and bed rest.
2) Strengthen skeletal muscles by beginning exercises during periods in which the patient is receiving ventilator support, adjusting ventilator settings as needed, and including strengthening techniques (e.g., free weights, gravity, manual resistance, elastic bands).
3) Improve nutritional support through supplements, considering the possibility of using a feeding tube to increase muscle strength and endurance. Patients with a tracheotomy have limited speech and are at risk of aspiration.
4) Assist with communication by exploring different modalities.
5) Prevent aspiration by teaching compensatory swallowing techniques.
6) Provide uninterrupted periods of rest.

k. Identify triggers.

1) Air particles (indoor and outdoor)
2) Cold air or sudden temperature change
3) Tobacco or smoke from burning wood or leaves
4) Perfume, paint, hairspray
5) Allergens (e.g., dust mites, pollen, pollution, animal dander)
6) Common cold, influenza, or respiratory illness
7) Vigorous exercise
8) Stress or excitement
9) Certain foods

l. Control measures (ALA, 2010)

1) Do skin testing as ordered to identify allergens.
2) Keep an asthma diary to identify triggers.
3) Use pillow and mattress covers.
4) Remove carpets.
5) Use air-filtering devices or air conditioning.
6) Keep pets out of bedrooms.

Figure 25-4. Airway Clearance Techniques

If a client has a condition that is causing a buildup of mucus in his or her airways such as cystic fibrosis, he or she will be taught how to loosen and expel the mucus. These are called airway clearance techniques (ACTs). The following is a brief overview of ACTs. The ACTs a client uses will be based on his or her needs and his or her disease.

Coughing

Coughing is the most basic and effective of ACTs. Mucus is cleared from the lung by the speed of the airflow. However, coughing a lot can make a client feel short of breath. One type of coughing is called huffing. The technique involves taking a breath in and actively exhaling. To huff, imagine breathing onto a mirror and steam it up. Although huffing is not as forceful as a cough, it can be very effective and is not as tiring.

Chest Physical Therapy (CPT or Chest PT) or Postural Drainage & Percussion (PD&P)

CPT or chest PT or PD&P is an ACT that includes postural drainage and chest percussion. Postural drainage involves the client getting into certain positions (postures) that drain mucus from different parts of the lung. It works by using gravity to it drain from airways where it can be coughed. Chest percussion involves clapping and using vibration to dislodge and move mucus.

Oscillating Positive Expiratory Pressure (Oscillating PEP)

Oscillating PEP is an ACT in which the client exhales many times through a device. Breathing with these devices vibrates the large and small airways and dislodges mucus so it can be expelled. After blowing through the device many times, the client coughs or huffs to expel the mucus. This entire process is repeated many times.

High-Frequency Chest Wall Oscillation

High-frequency chest wall oscillation is done with an inflatable vest attached to a machine that vibrates it at high frequency. The vest vibrates the chest to loosen the mucus so it can be expelled. Every 5 minutes the client turns off the machine and coughs or huffs to expel the mucus.

PEP Therapy

PEP therapy moves air into the lungs and behind the mucus using extra (collateral) airways. PEP keeps the airways open. A PEP system includes a mask or mouthpiece attached to a resistor. During this treatment, the client breathes in normally and breathes out a little harder against the resistance.

Active Cycle of Breathing Technique (ACBT)

ACBT involves breathing techniques. It can be changed to meet each person's needs. It moves mucus through air pressure and decreases airway spasm. ACBT includes the following:

- Breathing control: This is normal, gentle breathing of the lower chest while relaxing the upper chest and shoulders.
- Thoracic expansion exercises: During thoracic expansion exercises, the client inhales deeply. Some people hold their breath for 3 seconds to increase its effectiveness. This may be combined with chest clapping or vibrating, followed by breathing control.
- Forced expiration technique: huffs of varied lengths with breathing control.

Autogenic Drainage (AD)

AD is self-drainage. It uses varied airflows to move mucus from small to large airways. AD has three parts

- Dislodging mucus
- Collecting mucus
- Clearing mucus

The client inhales at different levels and then adjusts exhalation to increase airflow and move mucus. AD takes practice to be successful, and it is most effectively used with people older than 8 years.

From *Airway clearance techniques*, by Cystic Fibrosis Foundation, 2010. Retrieved from www.cff.org/treatments/Therapies/Respiratory/AirwayClearance/#Airway_clearance_techniques. Copyright 2010 by Cystic Fibrosis Foundation. Reprinted with permission.

7) Ensure early detection of respiratory infections.
8) Stop smoking.
9) Monitor the pollution index and adjust outdoor activities accordingly.
10) Avoid exposure to colds and influenza, and encourage vaccinations against influenza and pneumonia.

m. Promote caloric intake to support adequate growth.
1) Provide frequent small meals to lessen fatigue.
2) Provide appropriate food consistency to enhance energy conservation during meals.
3) Maintain good oral care.
4) Monitor for swallowing difficulties and risk for aspiration.
5) Monitor for nutritional risk.
6) Weigh daily and monitor for dehydration (keep records of intake and output and skin turgor).
7) Monitor intake.
8) Monitor albumin levels, and offer protein supplements as needed for healing and weight maintenance.
9) Administer vitamins and pancreatic enzymes for patients with CF as ordered.

n. Monitor stools.
1) Encourage fluids, fiber, stool softeners, or laxatives.
2) Encourage ambulation.

3) Note color, amount, consistency, frequency, and presence of blood.

o. Teach about medications.
   1) Explain usage and symptoms of effectiveness, ineffectiveness, and toxicity.
   2) Monitor theophylline levels (if prescribed).

p. Maintain inhalation equipment.

q. Teach about safe oxygen use in the home.
   1) Explain that oxygen is combustible and must be kept away from open flames and heat, including a running gas stove or gas or kerosene space heater.
   2) Prevent leakage.
      a) Keep the tank upright.
      b) Turn off the system when not in use.
      c) Do not place anything over the tubing.
      d) Keep an all-purpose fire extinguisher available.
      e) In case of fire, turn off the oxygen and leave the home.
      f) Notify the fire department that there is oxygen in the home. Many fire departments offer free safety inspections.
   3) Monitor for symptoms of insufficient or excessive amounts of oxygen.
      a) Difficult, irregular, or slow breathing
      b) Restlessness or anxiousness
      c) Tiredness or drowsiness
      d) Difficulty waking up
      e) Persistent headache
      f) Confusion, difficulty concentrating, or slurred speech
      g) Cyanotic fingertips or lips
   4) Teach the patient to notify the practitioner if any of these symptoms occur, and never change the flow rate without guidance from the physician.

r. Teach about diagnostic tests, disease processes, prognoses, and therapies.

s. Assist the patient and family with coping and stress reduction.
   1) Develop trust with the patient and family, encourage family members to express feelings, assist in problem solving, identify support systems, and offer support network as needed.
   2) Promote normal growth and development.
   3) Encourage personal control.
   4) Teach relaxation and stress-reduction techniques.
   5) Consult with the chaplain or the patient's spiritual guide to offer spiritual support.

t. Offer education on sexual and other physical activity.

5. Evaluation
   a. Patient follow-up is crucial.
   b. Evaluate the patient's understanding of instructions and how the interventions are affecting them, positively or negatively.
   c. Revise goals and interventions with the patient and the physician as needed.

References

American Heart Association (AHA)/American Stroke Association (ASA). (2015). Heart disease and stroke statistics. Retrieved from http://www.heart.org/HEARTORG/General/Heart-and-Stroke-Association-Statistics_UCM_319064_SubHomePage.jsp

American Association of Cardiovascular and Pulmonary Rehabilitation (AACVPR). (2014). Cardiac rehabilitation: Low cost, low technology, great medicine! Retrieved from https://www.aacvpr.org/Portals/0/resources/professionals/CRPresentationforPhysiciansAHA_Jan2013.pdf

American Cancer Society. (2014). What are the key statistics about lung cancer? Retrieved from http://www.cancer.org/cancer/lungcancer-non-smallcell/detailedguide/non-small-cell-lung-cancer-key-statistics?utm_source=msn&utm_medium=cpc&utm_campaign=Lung+Cancer+-+Exact+Term&utm_content=Sitelinks&utm_term=lung%20cancer

American Heart Association (AHA). (2015a). Cardiac rehabilitation. Retrieved from http://www.heart.org/HEARTORG/Conditions/More/CardiacRehab/What-is-Cardiac-Rehabilitation_UCM_307049_Article.jsp

American Heart Association (AHA). (2015b). Heart disease and stroke statistics. Retrieved from http://www.heart.org/idc/groups/ahamah-public/@wcm/@sop/@smd/documents/downloadable/ucm_470704.pdf

American Heart Association (AHA). (2015c). Coronary artery disease http://www.heart.org/HEARTORG/Conditions/More/MyHeartandStrokeNews/Coronary-Artery-Disease---Coronary-Heart-Disease_UCM_436416_Article.jsp

Association of Rehabilitation Nurses (ARN). (2014). ARN competency model for professional rehabilitation nursing. Retrieved from http://www.rehabnurse.org/uploads/files/education/ARN_Rehabilitation_Nursing_Competency _Model_FINAL_-_May_2014.pdf

Becker, K. (2014). Central sleep apnea. Retrieved from http://emedicine.medscape.com/article/304967-overview

Boudi, F. B. (2014). Coronary artery atherosclerosis. Retrieved from http://emedicine.medscape.com/article/153647-overview#aw2aab6b2b2

Byrd, R. P. (2013). Mechanical ventilation. Retrieved from http://emedicine.medscape.com/article/304068-overview

Caronia, J. R. (2014). Restrictive lung disease. Retrieved from http://emedicine.medscape.com/article/301760-overview

Centers for Disease Control and Prevention (CDC). (2014a). Heart disease facts. Retrieved from http://www.cdc.gov/heartdisease/facts.htm

Centers for Disease Control and Prevention (CDC). (2014b). Congenital heart defects. Retrieved from http://www.cdc.gov/ncbddd/heartdefects/data.html

Condon, M. C. (2004). *Women's health: An integrated approach to wellness and illness.* Upper Saddle River, NJ: Prentice Hall.

Cystic Fibrosis Foundation (2010). Airway clearance techniques. Retrieved from www.cff.org/treatments/Therapies/Respiratory/AirwayClearance/#Airway_clearance_techniques

Demirjian, B. G. (2012). Emphysema. Retrieved from http://emedicine.medscape.com/article/298283-overview

Doenges, M. E., Moorhouse, M. F., & Murr, A. C. (2010). *Nursing diagnosis manual: Planning, individualizing & documenting client care.* Philadelphia: F. A. Davis.

Downey, R. (2014). Obstructive sleep apnea. Retrieved from http://emedicine.medscape.com/article/295807-overview

Dumitru, I. (2014). Heart failure treatment & management. Retrieved from http://emedicine.medscape.com/article/163062-treatment#aw2aab6b6b2

Eliopolous, C. (2004). *Integrative health promotion: Conceptual bases for nursing practice.* Thorofare, NJ: Slack.

Emmons, E. E. (2014). Bronchiectasis. Retrieved from http://emedicine.medscape.com/article/296961-overview

Fayyaz, J. (2014). Bronchitis. Retrieved from http://emedicine.medscape.com/article/297108-overview

Friedman, S. E., & Andrus, B. W. (2012). Obesity and pulmonary hypertension: A review of pathophysiologic mechanisms. *Journal of Obesity*, 2012, Article ID 505274. doi:10.1155/2012/505274

Go, A. S., Mozaffarrian, D., Roger, V., Benjamin, E. J., Berry, J. D., Blaha, M. J.,...Ford, E. S. (2014). American Heart Association: Statistical Update: Heart Disease and Stroke Statistics—2014 Update. Retrieved from http://circ.ahajournals.org/content/129/3/399.full

Goswami, V. J. (2013). Dilated cardiomyopathy. Retrieved from http://emedicine.medscape.com/article/152696-overview

Linton, A. D. (Ed.) (2015). Introduction to medical surgical nursing (6th ed.). St. Louis: Elsevier Saunders.

Madison, H. E. (2010). What women want to know: Assessing the value, relevance, efficacy, and self-management intervention for rural women with coronary heart disease. Unpublished manuscript. University of Massachusetts, Amherst, MA.

Medmovie. (2007). Atherosclerosis. Retrieved from http://medmovie.com/topic/cvml_0070a/cvml-0070a-atherosclerosis-1280x720/

Moffatt-Bruce, S. D. (2014). Lung transplantation. Retrieved from http://emedicine.medscape.com/article/429499-overview

Morris, M. J. (2014). Asthma. Retrieved from http://emedicine.medscape.com/article/296301-overview

National Heart and Blood Institute. (2010). Pursed-lip breathing. Retrieved from www.nhlbi.nih.gov/health/dci/Diseases/pulreh/pulreh_during.html

Salome, C. M., King, G. G., & Berend, N. (2010). Physiology of obesity and effects on lung function. *Journal of Applied Physiology, 108*, 206–211. Retrieved from http://jap.physiology.org/content/108/1/206

Sharma, G. D. (2014). Fibrosis. Retrieved from http://emedicine.medscape.com/article/10016

Singh, V. N. (2013). Cardiac rehabilitation. Retrieved from http://emedicine.medscape.com/article/319683-overview#aw2aab6b3

Zafari, A.M. (2014). Myocardial infarction treatment and management. Retrieved from http://emedicine.medscape.com/article/155919-treatment#aw2aab6b6b8

Online Resources

American Association for Cardiovascular and Pulmonary Rehabilitation (AACVPR): www.aacvpr.org

About Cardiac and Pulmonary Rehabilitation: https://www.aacvpr.org/About/AboutCardiacPulmonaryRehab/tabid/560/Default.aspx

Cardiac Rehabilitation Fact Sheet: https://www.aacvpr.org/Portals/0/resources/patients/CRFactSheet112.pdf

Cardiac Rehabilitation Fact Sheet In Spanish: https://www.aacvpr.org/Portals/0/resources/patients/CRFactSheet_Spanishversion04.12.pdf

Pulmonary Rehabilitation Fact Sheet: https://www.aacvpr.org/Portals/0/resources/patients/PR%20Fact%20Sheet%202.12.pdf

Academy of Nutrition and Dietetics Heart Health and Diet: http://www.eatright.org/Public/content.aspx?id=6820

National Sleep Foundation: www.sleepfoundation.org/

Chapter 26

Other Disease Processes Requiring Rehabilitation Interventions

Patricia A. Haldi, MS CRRN CDE
Susan Wirt, MSN RN CRRN CCM CLCP CRP CNLCP

LEARNING OUTCOMES

- Discuss strategies for the rehabilitation nurse and team to use to inspire positive self-care management behaviors for individuals diagnosed with diabetes mellitus.
- Identify the clinical manifestations of human immunodeficiency virus (HIV)/acquired immune deficiency syndrome (AIDs) that the rehabilitation nurse and team can most effectively address in care management.
- Recognize appropriate rehabilitation team strategies in the management of individuals diagnosed with cancer.
- Identify risks and benefits for various weight loss programs for obesity and the impact on the overall rehabilitation plan of care.

KEY CHAPTER TOPICS

- Diabetes mellitus
- HIV/AIDS
- Cancer
- Obesity

PROFESSIONAL REHABILITATION NURSING DOMAINS AND COMPETENCIES

- Domain 1: Competencies 1.1, 1.2, 1.3, 1.4
- Domain 2: Competencies 2.1, 2.2
- Domain 4: Competency 4.2 (Association of Rehabilitation Nurses [ARN], 2014)

Introduction

Rehabilitation nurses play an important role in caring for people with disabilities who are often dealing with a wide variety of underlying chronic diseases. This chapter reviews the diseases that warrant rehabilitation nursing interventions:

- Diabetes mellitus (DM)
- HIV and AIDS
- Cancer
- Obesity

Learning to live with an acute disability is challenging; with the addition of one or more chronic diseases, the challenge is even greater. Many times the chronic disease complicates and extends the rehabilitation and recovery process. In these cases, the rehabilitation nurse, as a key member of the patient's treatment team, is vital in educating the client, family, and fellow team members about ways to prevent complications related to chronic conditions. Rehabilitation nurses in all care settings must be knowledgeable about and skilled in the most current evidenced-based standards of care to maintain credibility in the role of team leader.

I. Diabetes Mellitus

A. Overview

1. Diabetes mellitus (DM) is a group of metabolic diseases characterized by hyperglycemia that results from defects in insulin secretion, insulin action, or both.
2. DM is a comorbidity associated with conditions commonly treated by rehabilitation teams (e.g., stroke, heart disease, amputation, renal failure, orthopedic conditions).

3. DM represents a significant health burden in terms of increased hospital length of stay and costs.
   a. This is often due to disease progression with potential acute complications resulting from prolonged hypoglycemia and hyperglycemia.
4. The daily care and prevention of acute complications of DM in all rehabilitation practice is complex. It entails addressing many issues aside from glycemic control and requires a partnership between the client and the health professional for medical care and self-management.
5. Substantial progress has been made in the treatment and management of diabetes, and many new treatment options are being researched and marketed.
6. Rehabilitation nurses can make a difference in client outcomes by using current standards of care in diabetes management with effective client teaching to empower behavioral changes (e.g., lifestyle changes related to diet, exercise, stress management, and self-administration of medications).

B. Types (Centers for Disease Control and Prevention [CDC], 2014a)
1. Type 1
   a. Affects 5% of the total number of people with diabetes
      1) Results from B-cell destruction in the pancreas and usually leads to absolute insulin deficiency
   b. To survive, people with type 1 diabetes must have insulin delivered by injection, an insulin pump, or inhaled insulin (Doheny, 2014)
2. Type 2
   a. Affects 90%–95% of the total number of people with diabetes
   b. Results from a progressive insulin secretory defect on the background of insulin resistance
   c. People with type 2 diabetes have a variety of treatment options that include diet and exercise, oral agents, insulin delivered by injection or a pump, or inhaled insulin (Doheny, 2014).
3. Gestational diabetes (American Diabetes Association ADA, 2015; CDC, 2014a)
   a. Hyperglycemia that first appears in pregnancy, usually around 24–28 weeks or later, and usually resolves at birth
   b. An estimated 200,000 American women (approximately 5% of total pregnancies) are diagnosed with gestational diabetes annually.
   c. 5%–10% of those with gestational diabetes are found to have diabetes, and 40%–60% could develop diabetes within the next 5–10 years
   d. Treatment for gestational diabetes is diet, exercise, and tight glucose control with insulin delivery by injection or an insulin pump.
4. Other types
   a. Result from specific genetic conditions (e.g., maturity-onset diabetes of youth), surgery, drugs, malnutrition, infections, and other illnesses)
   b. Account for less than 5% of all diagnosed cases (CDC, 2014a)

C. Epidemiology and Incidence (CDC, 2014a)
1. Diabetes is a global epidemic and burden. More than 347 million people worldwide have diabetes.
2. In the United States, 29.1 million people (9.3% of the population) have diabetes—21.0 million with diagnosed diabetes and 8.1 million with undiagnosed diabetes.
3. Ethnic minorities (Hispanics and Latinos, American Indians, some Asian Americans, and Native Hawaiians) and older adults are expected to be disproportionately affected by the increase, with the number of Hispanics with diabetes predicted to increase almost six fold.
4. People 65 years or older account for more than 25% of the U.S. population, and the aging of the overall population is a significant driver of the diabetes epidemic (Kirkman et al., 2012).
5. Diabetes is the seventh most common cause of death in the United States and is the leading cause of adult blindness, chronic renal failure, and nontraumatic lower-extremity amputations.
6. People with diabetes have a risk of death about twice that of people of the same age without diabetes.
7. People with diabetes have two to four times the risk of atherosclerosis and are three to four times more likely to have a heart attack or stroke than people without diabetes.
8. The direct and indirect costs of diabetes are staggering, having totaled more than $174 billion in 2007. However, the full burden of diabetes is hard to measure, because death records often fail to reflect the role of diabetes, and the costs related to undiagnosed diabetes are unknown.
9. Diabetes is the fourth most common comorbid condition among patients discharged from the hospital.
10. Martz et al. (2006) reported a 31% rate of known diabetes in people hospitalized with stroke and an additional 16% of people with unrecognized diabetes and hospital-related hyperglycemia.

D. Etiology (ADA, 2015)

1. *Type 1 diabetes* is an autoimmune disorder that involves B-cell destruction by islet cell antibodies, leading to absolute insulin deficiency.
2. *Type 2 diabetes* is the result of a progressive defect in the secretion of insulin on the background of insulin resistance.
3. *Gestational diabetes* is a form of glucose intolerance diagnosed during pregnancy that, if uncontrolled, places both mother and baby at risk for complications during the pregnancy; the mother has a 20%–50% chance of developing diabetes within the next 5–10 years.
4. Other types of diabetes result from specific genetic defects in B-cell function, genetic defects in insulin action, diseases of the exocrine pancreas (e.g., cystic fibrosis), and drug or chemical-induced diabetes (e.g., in the treatment of AIDS or after organ transplantation).
5. Categories of increased risk (ADA, 2015)
   a. *Prediabetes* is an elevated risk of developing diabetes, as indicated by an impaired fasting glucose (IFG), impaired glucose tolerance (IGT), or higher than normal levels of hemoglobin A1C (HbA1C).
      1) Note: The term *HbA1c* refers to glycated hemoglobin. It develops when hemoglobin, a protein within red blood cells that carries oxygen throughout the body, joins with glucose in the blood, becoming "glycated." HbA1c is a useful indicator of how well the blood glucose level has been controlled over 2 to 3 months. In healthy people, the HbA1c level is less than 6% of total hemoglobin. Studies have demonstrated that the complications of diabetes can be delayed or prevented if the HbA1c level is kept below 7%. It is recommended that treatment of diabetes be directed at keeping an individual's HbA1c level as close to normal as possible (i.e., < 6%) without episodes of hypoglycemia (i.e., low blood glucose levels). HbA1c is also referred to as hemoglobin A1c or simply A1c (Stoppler, 2014).
   b. *IFG* is a condition in which the fasting blood sugar level is elevated (i.e., 100–125 mg/dl or 5.5–6.9 mmol/l) after an overnight fast but is not high enough to be classified as diabetes.
   c. *IGT* is a condition in which the blood sugar level is elevated (i.e., 140–199 mg/dL or 7.7–11.0 mmol/l) after a 2-hour oral glucose tolerance test but is not high enough to be classified as diabetes.
   d. A HbA1C level between 5.7 and 6.4 is at the borderline of diagnosis but not high enough to be classified as diabetes.
   e. Progression to diabetes among those at elevated risk is not inevitable because weight loss and increased physical activity can prevent or delay diabetes and can return blood glucose levels to normal.
   f. People in this category are already at elevated risk for other adverse health outcomes such as heart disease and stroke.
   g. The CDC estimated that at least 86 million American adults age 20 years or older had prediabetes in 2012. (CDC, 2014a)
   h. **Figure 26-1** gives the recommended treatment options for prediabetes, beginning with lifestyle modifications and obesity prevention. Further treatment options follow the progression to full diabetes.

E. Risk Factors for Diabetes
1. Type 1 (Gale, 2014)
   a. Family history of diabetes, genetic
   b. Age: Usually associated with children and young adults, although disease onset can occur at any age
   c. Prenatal environmental factors: Babies with higher birth weight and the children of older mothers have a slightly higher risk of diabetes
   d. Postnatal environmental factors: Exposure to enteroviruses, early diet, levels of vitamin D, and routine vaccinations
   e. Other, more general, factors: Lack of immune stimulation due to an antigen-free environment (the hygiene hypothesis) or childhood over nutrition resulting in increased insulin resistance (the accelerator hypothesis)
2. Type 2 (Lyssenks & Laakso, 2013)
   a. Obesity: Body fat of more than 25% for men and more than 30% for women
   b. Physical inactivity
   c. Environmental factors: smoking; diet, including low amounts of fiber and high amounts of saturated fat; history of non-diabetic elevated blood sugar, fasting or 2-hour glucose; elevated blood pressure; dyslipidemia; and different drug treatments (e.g., diuretics, unselected beta-blockers)
   d. Family history of diabetes or history of gestational diabetes
   e. Race or ethnicity: African Americans, Hispanics and Latinos, American Indians, and some Asian Americans and Native Hawaiians or

Figure 26-1. Prediabetes Algorithm

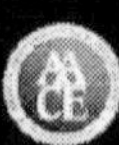

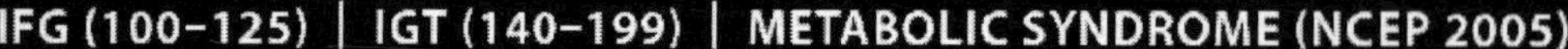

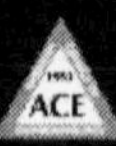

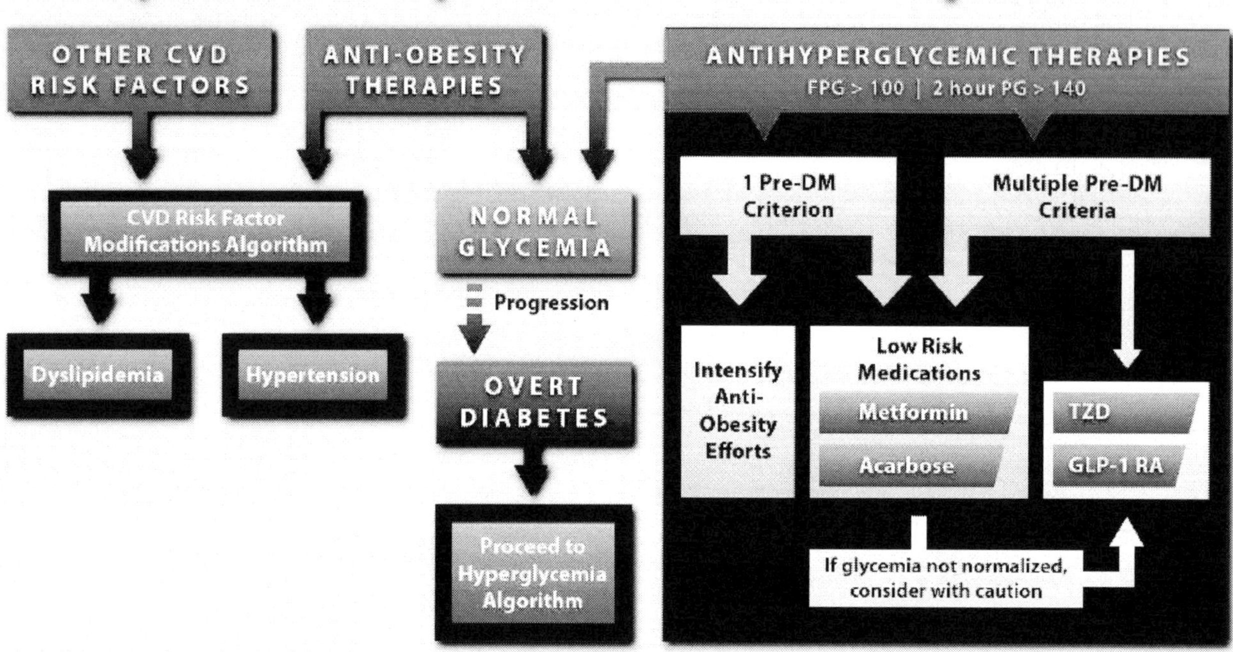

From "American Association of Clinical Endocrinologists comprehensive diabetes management algorithm," by A. J. Garber et al., 2013, *Endocrine Practice, 19*(Suppl. 2), 329. Retrieved from https://www.aace.com/files/aace_algorithm.pdf. Copyright 2013 by the American Association of Clinical Endocrinologists. Reprinted with permission.

other Pacific Islanders are at particularly high risk for type 2 diabetes and its complications.

f. Age: Usually associated with older adults, but type 2 diabetes in children and adolescents is being diagnosed more frequently, particularly in the nonwhite populations listed previously

g. Previous IGT or IFG

h. Polycystic ovary disease (in women)

i. Hypertension (i.e., ≥ 140/90 or on therapy for hypertension)

j. High-density lipoprotein (HDL) cholesterol level < 35 mg/dl (1.9 mmol/l) or triglyceride level > 250

k. History of cardiovascular disease

F. Pathophysiology (ADA, 2015)

1. Impaired release of insulin from the pancreas

   a. Normal

      1) Phase 1: Stored insulin from beta cells is released within the first 5 minutes after glucose ingestion.

      2) Phase 2: More insulin is released and newly synthesized by beta cells.

   b. In diabetes

      1) Type 1: Endogenous insulin release is deficient.

      2) Type 2: Endogenous insulin release can be normal, inefficient, or deficient.

2. *Insulin resistance* (need for the beta cells of the pancreas to make more insulin to accommodate, or secondary hyperinsulinemia)

   a. A condition in which normal amounts of insulin are inadequate to produce a normal insulin response from fat, muscle, and liver cells

   b. Insulin resistance in fat cells results in hydrolysis of stored triglycerides, which elevates free fatty acids in the blood plasma.

Table 26-1. Symptomatic Manifestations of Diabetes Mellitus

Primary Symptoms	Secondary Symptoms	Tertiary Symptoms
Poor wound healing Skin and feet	Infection, chronic ulceration, limb amputation Dryness and cracking, callus formation, ulceration, deformities (e.g., Charcot's foot)	Dysfunctional denial Dysfunctional grief Body image crisis Social isolation
Peripheral neuropathy (e.g., numbness, tingling, pain, decreased sensation in extremities)	Cold intolerance, rest and sleep disturbance, inadequate hand and finger movement (e.g., carpal tunnel syndrome)	Ineffective coping with anxiety, reactive depression, anger
Gastroparesis (e.g., bowel, bladder, sexual dysfunction)	Constipation, urinary retention, urinary tract infections, gastroparesis, vaginal dryness, decreased libido and orgasmic ability	Marital conflict or divorce Loss of job, financial stability, self-esteem, and self-worth Loss of ability to provide adequate self-care, causing loss of independence and control over life, living situation, location (i.e., often needing nursing home placement if unable to do self-insulin management)
Blurred vision, cataracts, blindness, retinopathy	Errors with insulin drawing and mixing, declining ability to visually inspect skin and feet	Falls, accidents End-stage renal disease Microvascular disease Macrovascular disease
Hypoglycemia	Mild symptoms (e.g., sweating, trembling, impaired concentration, dizziness), severe symptoms (e.g., mental confusion, lethargy, unconsciousness)	
Hyperglycemia	Specific symptoms (e.g., polyuria, polydipsia, blurred vision, polyphagia, weight loss), nonspecific symptoms (e.g., weakness, malaise, lethargy, headaches), gastrointestinal symptoms (e.g., nausea, vomiting, abdominal pain), respiratory symptoms (e.g., Kussmaul's, ketonuria, metabolic acidosis, hyperventilation, coma)	
Weight changes (e.g., more or less than ideal body weight)	Obesity (body fat more than 25% in men and 30% in women), central adipose tissue accumulation, inadequate nutrition	
Chronic systemic dysfunction	Orthostatic hypertension, cardiac denervation, hypoglycemia unaware, proteinuria	

Table 26-2. Criteria for the Diagnosis of Diabetes

1. A1C ≥ 6.5%. The test should be performed in a laboratory using a method that is NGSP certified and standardized to the DCCT assay.*

OR

2. FPG ≥ 126 mg/dL (7.0 mmol/L). Fasting is defined as no caloric intake for at least 8 h.*

OR

3. 2-h plasma glucose ≥ 200 mg/dL (11.1 mmol/L) during an OGTT. The test should be performed as described by the World Health Organization, using a glucose load containing the equivalent of 75 g anhydrous glucose dissolved in water.*

OR

4. In a patient with classic symptoms of hyperglycemia or hyperglycemic crisis, a random plasma glucose ≥ 200 mg/dL (11.1 mmol/L).

*In the absence of unequivocal hyperglycemia, results should be confirmed by repeat testing.

From "Standards of Medical Care in Diabetes—2015, by the American Diabetes Association, 2015, *Diabetes Care, 38*(Suppl. 1), S9. Copyright 2015 by the American Diabetes Association. Reprinted with permission.

c. Insulin resistance in muscle reduces glucose uptake, whereas insulin resistance in the liver reduces glucose storage, with both effects elevating blood glucose.
d. High plasma levels of insulin and glucose caused by insulin resistance often lead to metabolic syndrome and type 2 diabetes.
e. Leads to insulin deficiency as the pancreas works harder to meet the increasing need to overcome the resistance

3. Insulin deficiency
   a. Primary problem in type 1 diabetes
   b. Common in thin people with type 2 diabetes
   c. Increases in type 2 diabetes with longevity of the disease
4. Clinical manifestations (**Table 26-1**)

G. Diagnostic Criteria (ADA, 2014a): Diagnosis for type 1 or type 2 is confirmed by one of the methods outlined in **Table 26-2**. Test results should be repeated when feasible.

1. A1C 6.5 or higher. The test should be performed in a laboratory using a method that is National Glycohemoglobin Standardization Program (NGSP) certified and standardized to the Diabetes Control and Complications Trial (DCCT) assay.
2. It is unclear whether the same cut point should be used to diagnose children or adolescents.
3. Fasting plasma glucose (FPG) at or above 126 mg/dl (7.0 mmol/L). Fasting is defined as no caloric intake for at least 8 hours.
4. Two-hour postprandial glucose at or above 200 mg/dl (11.1 mmol/L) during an oral glucose tolerance test (OGTT). The test should be performed as described by the World Health Organization (WHO), using a glucose load containing the equivalent of 75 g anhydrous glucose dissolved in water.

Figure 26-2. Glycemic Control Algorithm

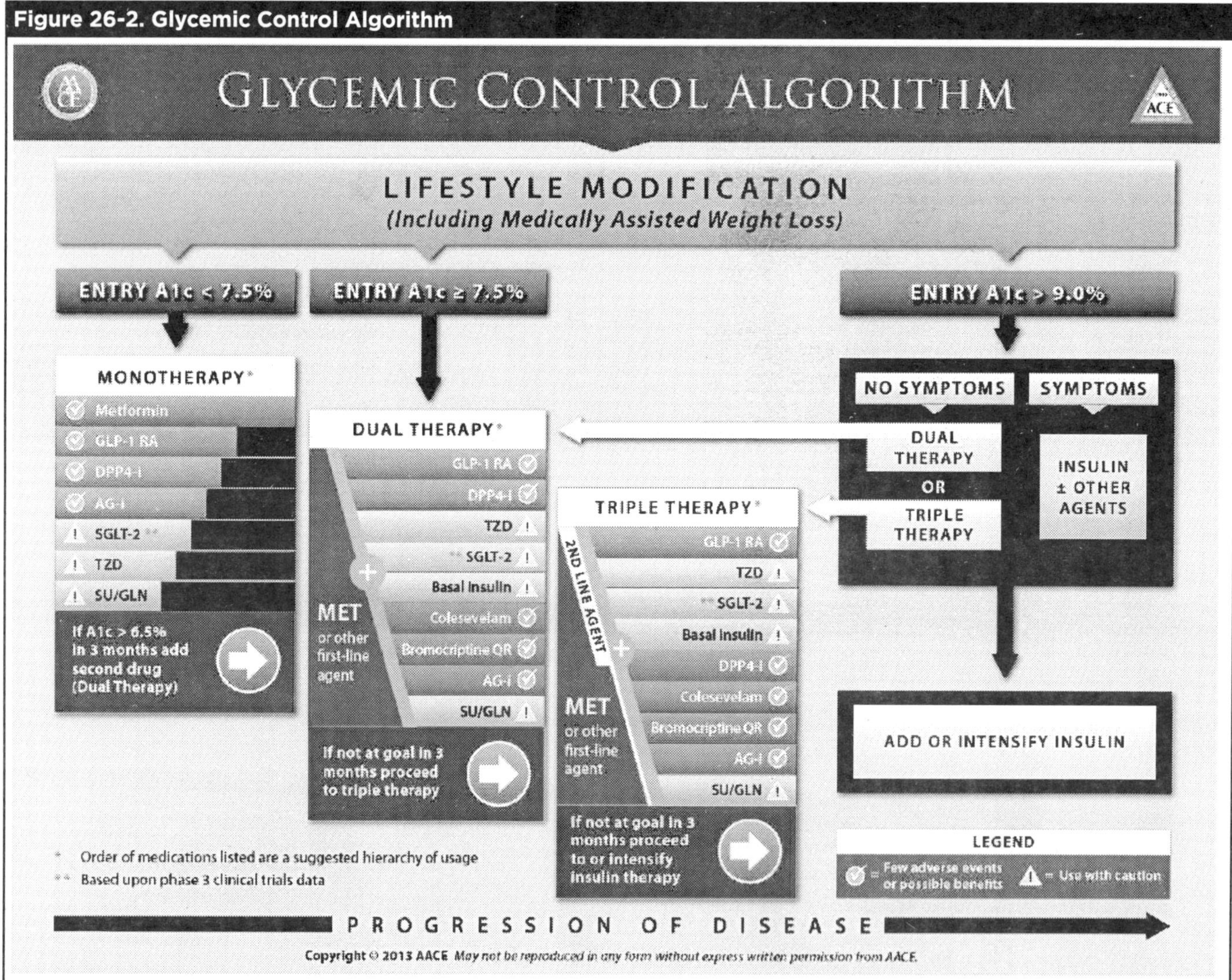

From "American Association of Clinical Endocrinologists comprehensive diabetes management algorithm," by A. J. Garber et al., 2013, *Endocrine Practice, 19*(Suppl. 2), 329. Retrieved from https://www.aace.com/files/aace_algorithm.pdf. Copyright 2013 by the American Association of Clinical Endocrinologists. Reprinted with permission.

5. Random non-fasting plasma glucose testing (any time of day without consideration of last meal) at or greater than 200 mg/dL (11.1 mmo/L).

H. Management Options (ADA, 2015)

1. Glycemic control (**Figure 26-2**)
   a. Optimal target for a pre-meal blood glucose, as recommended by the ADA, is now 80–130 mg/dl instead of 70–130 mg/dl, to reflect new studies comparing blood glucose levels with A1C targets.
   b. Three primary techniques to measure glycemic control
      1) Self-monitoring of blood glucose (SMBG) recommendations
         a) SMBG frequency and timing should be dictated by the patient's specific needs and goals. SMBG is especially important for patients treated with insulin to monitor for and prevent asymptomatic hypoglycemia and hyperglycemia.
         b) Patients on multiple-dose insulin or insulin-pump therapy should do SMBG before meals and snacks, occasionally postprandial, at bedtime, before exercise, when they suspect they might have low blood glucose levels, after treating low blood glucose until they are normoglycemic, and before performing critical tasks such as driving.
         c) SMBG accuracy is instrument and user dependent. It is important to evaluate each patient's monitoring technique.
      2) Interstitial glucose (ADA, 2015)
         a) Real-time continuous glucose monitoring (CGM), done by measuring interstitial glucose (which correlates well with plasma glucose), is possible with the use of CGM devices and sensors. These sensors are particularly useful in patients who have hypoglycemia unawareness and/or frequent hypoglycemic episodes. Uses are primarily associated with insulin pumps and require advanced training for patients as well as practitioners.
      3) A1C (ADA, 2015)
         a) A1C targets are determined by individual patient treatment plans with consideration of risk for significant hypoglycemia or other adverse effects of treatment.
         b) Appropriate patients for tight control might include those with short duration of diabetes, long life expectancy, and no significant cardiovascular disease.
         c) Less stringent A1C goals, such as an A1C > 7, could be appropriate for patients with a history of severe hypoglycemia; limited life expectancy; advanced microvascular or macrovascular complications; and long-standing diabetes, in which the general goal is difficult to attain despite appropriate glucose monitoring and effective doses of multiple glucose-lowering agents including insulin.

I. Medical Nutritional Therapy (ADA, 2014a; Boucher & Evert, 2014)

1. Nutritional therapy is recommended as an effective component of the overall treatment plan for all people with type 1 and type 2 diabetes.
2. Individualized medical nutrition therapy (MNT) as needed to achieve treatment goals should be provided by a registered dietitian familiar with diabetes MNT.
   a. Education and training in intensive flexible insulin therapy using the carbohydrate-counting, meal-planning approach can result in improved glycemic control for individuals with type 1 diabetes.
   b. Using fixed daily insulin doses and consistent carbohydrate intake with respect to time and amount can result in improved glycemic control and reduce the risk for hypoglycemia.
   c. A simple meal-planning approach such as portion control or healthful food choices could be better suited for older adults and patients with type 2 diabetes who have health and numeracy literacy concerns.
3. Energy balance and weight
   a. Individuals with type 2 diabetes who are obese or overweight would benefit from modest weight loss, achieved by reducing calorie intake while maintaining a healthful eating pattern.
   b. For some individuals, especially those early in the disease process, modest weight loss can provide improvement in glycemia, hypertension, and/or lipid levels.
   c. Recommendations for modest weight loss include counseling on nutrition therapy, physical activity, and behavioral change, along with ongoing support.
4. Macronutrients
   a. A registered dietitian should provide individualized meal plans, with specific amounts of

carbohydrates, fats, and protein according to height, weight, eating habits, food preferences, lipid profile, blood protein, and other medical conditions (e.g., end-stage renal disease).
   b. For all patients with diabetes, the percentage of calories from carbohydrates, protein, and fat needs to be individualized.
   c. Combinations of different foods or food groups are acceptable. Personal preference regarding tradition, culture, religion, health beliefs, and economics should be considered when recommending an eating pattern.
5. Carbohydrates
   a. Both the amount (grams) of carbohydrate and the type of carbohydrate in a food influences blood glucose level.
   b. Monitoring carbohydrate intake, whether by counting carbohydrates or estimating based on experience, remains a key strategy in achieving glycemic control.
   c. For good health, carbohydrate intake from vegetables, fruits, whole grains, legumes, and dairy products should be advised over intake from other carbohydrate sources, especially those that contain added fats, sugar, or sodium.
6. A glycemic index food chart can be helpful in substituting low-glycemic-load foods for higher-glycemic-load foods and could modestly improve glycemic control.
7. Protein
   a. Individuals with diabetes and no evidence of diabetic kidney disease should have individualized goals for an ideal amount of protein intake for optimizing glycemic control.
   b. Individuals with diabetic kidney disease need not reduce the amount of protein below usual intake due to evidence that it does not alter glycemic measures, cardiovascular risk measures, or the course of glomerular filtration rate decline.
   c. Individuals with type 2 diabetes should not use carbohydrate sources high in protein to treat or prevent hypoglycemia, because protein increases insulin response without increasing plasma glucose concentrations.
8. Fats
   a. Total amount of fat intake for individuals with diabetes should be individualized, because evidence for an ideal amount is inconclusive.
   b. A Mediterranean-style diet high in monounsaturated fats (i.e., a MUFA-rich diet) eating pattern could benefit glycemic control and cardiovascular disease risk factors.
   c. At least two servings a week of foods containing omega-3 fatty acids, such as fatty fish, are recommended, because of the beneficial effects on lipoproteins and role in the prevention of heart disease.
   d. Recommended amounts of dietary saturated fat, cholesterol, and trans fat is the same for individuals with diabetes as for the general public.
   e. Individuals with diabetes and dyslipidemia might be able to modestly reduce total and LDL cholesterol by including 1.6–3 grams per day of plant sterols found in enriched foods.
9. Fiber
   a. Recommended amount of dietary fiber and whole grains are the same as for the general public.
10. Nonnutritive sweeteners and sugar alcohols are safe when consumed within the acceptable daily intake levels established by the U.S. Food and Drug Administration (FDA).
11. Alcohol
   a. Recommendation for alcohol consumption is moderation (one drink or less per day for adult women and two drinks or less per day for men).
   b. One drink is defined as 12 ounces of beer, 5 ounces of wine, or 1.5 ounces of distilled spirits.
   c. Alcohol consumption can present a risk for delayed hypoglycemia, especially if taking insulin or insulin secretagogues.
   d. Education and awareness regarding the recognition and management of delayed hypoglycemia is necessary for those who choose to consume alcohol.
12. Sodium
   a. Sodium intake is recommended to be less than 2,300 mg/day.
   b. Individuals with diabetes and hypertension should consume even less sodium than the recommended amount, and the intake should be individualized.
13. Supplements
   a. Routine supplementation with antioxidants, such as vitamins E and C and beta-carotene, is not advised because of lack of evidence of efficacy and concern about long-term safety.
   b. The benefit of chromium supplementation in people with diabetes or obesity has not

been conclusively demonstrated and is not recommended.

c. Individualized meal planning should include optimization of food choices to meet recommended dietary allowances for all micronutrients.

14. Physical activity
    a. Initial physical activity recommendations should be modest and based on the client's willingness and ability, gradually increasing the duration and frequency to 30–45 minutes of moderate aerobic activity 3–5 days per week. The goal is at least 150 minutes/week of moderate-intensity aerobic physical activity (50%–70% maximum heart rate).
    b. In the absence of contraindications, people with type 2 diabetes should be encouraged to perform resistance training three times per week.
    c. Activity levels of at least 1 hour a day of moderate activity (e.g., walking) or 30 minutes a day of vigorous (e.g., jogging) activity may be needed to achieve successful long-term weight loss.
    d. Exercise options and strategies for self-directed exercise can be identified by a physical therapist.
    e. Benefits, effects, risks, and precautions vary depending on
        1) Age and type of diabetes
        2) Physical conditioning and presence of other chronic diseases
        3) Presence of ketonuria
    f. Providers should assess clients for comorbidities that might predispose clients to injury (e.g., hypertension, diabetic neuropathy, unstable proliferative retinopathy).
15. Bariatric surgery (ADA, 2014a)
    a. Should be considered for adults with a body mass index (BMI) greater than 35 kg/m^2 and type 2 diabetes, especially if the client is unable to control diabetes with lifestyle and pharmacological therapy. (There is not enough evidence to recommend surgery in clients with a BMI less than 35.)
    b. Bariatric surgery has been shown to lead to near or complete normalization of glycemia in 40%–95% of patients with diabetes who have a BMI that exceeds 35 kg/m^2, depending on the study and surgical procedure.
    c. Research has shown that quality-of-life measures are significantly better in the bariatric therapy groups than in a medical-therapy group (Schauer et.al., 2014).
    d. Studies have shown that among obese patients with uncontrolled type 2 diabetes, 3 years of intensive medical therapy plus bariatric surgery resulted in glycemic control in significantly more patients than did medical therapy alone (Schauer et al., 2014).
    e. Bariatric surgery is costly in the short term and has associated risks.
    f. People who have had bariatric surgery require lifelong lifestyle support and medical monitoring.
16. Medication therapy
    a. Oral agents (ADA, 2015)
        1) Classifications of oral antidiabetic agents include the following:
            a) Sulfonylureas stimulate the pancreas to make more insulin and include glyburide (Micronase®, Glynase®, and DiaBeta®), glipizide (Glucotrol® and Glucotrol XL®), and glimepiride (Amaryl®).
            b) Meglitinides or nonsulfonylurea secretagogues stimulate the pancreas to make more insulin and include repaglinide (Prandin®) and nateglinide (Starlix®).
            c) Biguanide diabetic medication shuts off the liver's excess glucose production and includes metformin (Glucophage®).
            d) Alpha-glucosidase inhibitors slow absorption of carbohydrates in the intestine and include acarbose (Precose®) and miglitol (Glyset®).
            e) Thiazolidinedione increases the body's sensitivity to insulin and includes rosiglitazone (Avandia®), which was subjected to selling restrictions in the U.S. because of its potential to increase the risk of cardiovascular events. The restrictions were reversed in 2013 but few providers prescribe it. Pioglitazone (Actos®) has the potential to increase the risk of bladder cancer.
            f) Dipeptide peptidase-4 inhibitors (DPP-4 inhibitors) include sitagliptin (Januvia®), saxagliptin (Onglyza®), linagliptin (Tradjenta®), and aloglipin (Nesina®). These drugs slow the inactivation of incretin hormones and improve pancreatic beta-cell insulin synthesis and release, lower pancreatic alpha-cell glucagon secretion, and reduce hepatic glucose production.

g) Glucagon-like peptide (GLP-1) receptor agonists include exenatide (Byetta/Bydureon®), liraglutide (Victoza®), and lixisenatide (Lyxumia®). Dulaglutide, a compound taken once weekly, has been under investigation since June 2014 and is awaiting FDA approval. GLP-1 agonists work by enhancing glucose-dependent insulin secretion by the pancreatic beta cell, suppressing inappropriately elevated glucagon secretion, and slowing gastric emptying.

h) SGLT2 inhibitors (a new class of drugs as of 2013) include canagliflozin (Invokana®) and dapagliflozin (Farxiga®). These drugs work in the kidneys to block reabsorption of excess glucose, which is then eliminated in the urine.

i) Bile acid sequestrants lower LDL cholesterol and have been approved for use in type 2 diabetes. Includes Colesevelam (Welchol®).

2) Each class of drugs differs in mode and site of action, advantages, and disadvantages, and the choice of agent for each person should be made with consideration of the person's overall health status.

3) Medication regimens can be simple or complex, with options for monotherapy or polytherapy.

4) Complexity of the regimen is increased by adding insulin therapy to oral therapy (e.g., bedtime insulin and daytime oral insulin) when oral therapy alone is no longer effective.

5) Evidence supports the combination of biguanides with insulin to improve weight management and glycemic control and reduce congestive heart disease risk.

6) The use of insulin and incretin-based therapies together has recently emerged as a new therapeutic option for patients with type 2 diabetes (Meece, Pearson, & Siminerio, 2014).

a) The addition of incretin-based therapies complements the glucose-lowering potential of basal insulin without increasing the risk of hypoglycemia.

b) The addition of DPP-4 inhibitors could allow for lower doses of insulin and less weight gain.

c) The addition of GLP-1 receptor agonists could help with weight loss.

d) Incretin-based therapies offer advantages over prandial insulin when treating postprandial hyperglycemia.

b. Injectable agents

1) Insulin therapy for type 1 diabetes should consist of multiple daily injections (three to four injections per day of basal and prandial insulin) or continuous subcutaneous insulin infusion.

a) Most patients with type 1 diabetes should be educated on how to match prandial insulin dose to carbohydrate intake, premeal blood glucose, and anticipated activity.

b) Most patients with type 1 diabetes should use insulin analogs to reduce hypoglycemia risk.

2) Patients with type 2 diabetes with markedly symptomatic and/or elevated blood glucose levels or A1C should consider insulin therapy, with or without additional agents, from the time of onset.

a) Patients with type 2 diabetes who are treated with noninsulin immunotherapy at the maximum tolerated dose and who do not achieve or maintain the A1C target over 3 months will need a second oral agent or insulin added according to efficacy, cost, potential side effects, effects on weight, comorbidities, hypoglycemia risk, and patient preferences.

b) Because of the progressive nature of type 2 diabetes, insulin therapy is eventually indicated for most patients.

3) Pramlintide (Symlin®), a synthetic analog of the hormone amylin—found to be deficient in type 1 DM—is used as an adjunct therapy with mealtime insulin. It slows gastric emptying, curbs appetite, suppresses postprandial plasma glucagon and hepatic glucose output, and helps mediate satiety centrally, resulting in decreased caloric intake and promoting weight loss. It is approved for people with type 1 DM and type 2 DM who take insulin. It should not be put into the same syringe used for insulin.

4) Sodium glucose cotransporter 2 inhibition blocks 90% of filtered glucose reabsorption in proximal tubules, resulting in increased glucose excretion via urine.

c. Insulin therapy usually addresses basal insulin (e.g., fasting) and bolus (e.g., preprandial

Table 26-3. Types of Insulin for Diabetes Treatment

Type of Insulin	Brand Name/Generic Name	Onset	Peak	Duration
Rapid acting	NovoLog/aspart	15 min	30–90 min	3–5 hr
	Apidra/glulisine	15 min	30–90 min	3–5 hr
	Humalog/lispro	15 min	30–90 min	3–5 hr
Short acting	Humulin/regular	30–60 min	2–4 hr	5–8 hr
	Novolin/regular	30–60 min	2–4 hr	5–8 hr
Intermediate acting	Humulin/NPH	1–3 hr	8 hr	12–16 hr
	Novolin	1–3 hr	8 hr	12–16 hr
Long acting	Levemir/detemir	1 hr	None	20–26 hr
	Lantus/glargine	1 hr	None	20–26 hr
Premixed neutral protamine Hagedorn (NPH)	Humulin 70/30 70% NPH and 30% regular	30–60 min	Varies	10–16 hr
	Novolin 70/30 70% NPH and 30% regular	30–60 min	Varies	10–16 hr
	Humulin 50/50 50% NPH and 50% regular	30–60 min	Varies	10–16 hr
Premixed insulin lispro protamine suspension and rapid-acting lispro	Humalog mix 50/50 50% insulin lispro protamine and 50% insulin lispro	10–15 min	Varies	10–16 hr
Premixed insulin aspart protamine suspension and rapid-acting insulin aspart	Novolog mix 70/30 70% insulin aspart protamine and 30% insulin aspart	5–15 min	Varies	10–16 hr

Note. Before using in clinical practice, the reader is encouraged to always verify and seek updated information.

From "Types of Insulin," by the National Institute of Diabetes and Digestive and Kidney Diseases, retrieved from http://www.niddk.nih.gov/health-information/health-topics/Diabetes/diabetes-medicines/Pages/insert_C.aspx

glucose level and postprandial excursion) (**Table 26-3**).

1) Insulin regimens are numerous, ranging from simple to complex, and can pose a challenge to the rehabilitation nurse. The following regimens are limited to the basic regimens, because ideally, an individualized program—suited to the person's needs, lifestyle, and resources—would be implemented.
2) Combination regimens
   a) Daily routine doses of long-lasting insulin (basal) (e.g., neutral protamine Hagedorn [NPH], glargine, or detemir) can be combined with a secretagogue with or without additional oral sensitizer for people with type 2 diabetes (but not for patients with type 1 diabetes).
   b) Premixtures (e.g., NPH 50/regular 50, NPH 70/regular 30, Humulin® R 70/30 or Novolin® R 70/30, NPH 75/lispro 25, Humalog® mix 75/25, NPH 70/aspart 30, Novolog® mix 70/30) twice daily, with or without oral sensitizers, are normally used for convenience, low cost, patient preference, and insurance coverage and to improve compliance.
3) Intensive conventional therapy
   a) Multiple daily injections of 0.2–0.6 initial units per kilogram with or without oral sensitizers, 50% bolus (rapid-acting insulin) at meals, and 50% basal

insulin (long-lasting insulin) (i.e., NPH, glargine, or detemir) once or twice a day (percentages can vary depending on individualization of regimen to match the patient's needs)

b) Daily routine doses of basal insulin (i.e., NPH, glargine, or detemir) once or twice daily with fast-acting insulin boluses using carbohydrate/insulin ratios calculated according to future carbohydrate consumption

c) Provides flexibility (e.g., a meal can be delayed and less food consumed, because the bolus amount is determined by the amount of food eaten, a clear advantage over trying to consume the correct amount of food at the right time to match the action of a traditional insulin such as NPH)

d) Correction dose (previously called *sliding scale*): Bolus dose of rapid- or fast-acting insulin calculated on actual blood glucose level

4) Injection therapy

a) Absorption rates differ between injection sites and types of insulin. Absorption is fastest in the abdomen, followed by the arms, thighs, and buttocks. Absorption is less variable with analog insulin.

b) Lipohypertrophy usually slows absorption; this is less of a problem with analog insulin.

c) Exercise increases the rate of absorption by providing increased blood flow to the injection site; this is less of a problem with analog insulin.

5) Afrezzainhaled insulin therapy, was approved by the FDA in June 2014 as an alternative to fast-acting insulin. It is administered via an inhaler with premeasured, rapid-acting insulin and is used before meals. Studies show that Afrezza works equally as well as injected insulin. Due to Afrezza's shorter half-life, there is less weight gain and less chance of its causing very low blood glucose levels (Doheny, 2014).

6) Insulin U-500 (regular human insulin) was introduced in the U.S. market in 1952 for use in patients with extreme insulin resistance caused by allergies to animal insulin. Its use is increasing because of the parallel epidemics of obesity and type 2 diabetes (Cochran, Valentine, Samaan, Corey, & Jackson, 2014).

a) Humulin R U-500 is regular insulin that is five times more concentrated than U-100 insulin (500 units in 1 milliliter instead of the typical 100 units in 1 milliliter).

b) Useful when large doses of insulin are needed without taking large volumes

c) Useful when reduced delivery volume is needed. Results in fewer total injections for patients receiving high doses of insulin, which can lead to improved glycemic control and greater patient satisfaction

d) Starts working within the first hours after injection and lasts up to 12–24 hours

e) Given with a U-100 insulin syringe

f) Requires additional training for both nurses and patients to prevent errors in delivery doses, with increased risk for hypoglycemia

d. Insulin-pump therapy (ADA, 2015)

1) Insulin pumps are devices used for administering insulin that consist of controls, a processing module, batteries, an insulin reservoir, and a catheter to carry the insulin into the subcutaneous tissue.

2) Insulin pumps make it possible to deliver continuous small amounts of fast-acting (basal) insulin and a mealtime bolus dose, providing tighter control over blood sugar and reducing the chance of long-term complications (e.g., blindness, amputation, renal disease).

3) Costs can run into the thousands of dollars for initial setup and continued maintenance and include the costs of insulin, batteries, and infusion catheter sets.

4) Insurance and Medicare can pay up to 80% of the costs of pump therapy.

5) Numbers of insulin pump users continue to increase, and pump features continue to advance.

6) People using their pumps often rebel against forced removal.

7) Rehabilitation nurses must be prepared to deal with any client who continues to use the pump during an inpatient stay.

8) Pump use can be helpful in achieving glycemic control by matching the typical insulin pattern of a person without diabetes.

9) Transitioning onto and off a pump can entail a complex series of insulin management plans and orders from the physician, as well as coordination of pharmacy and nursing staff.
10) A comprehensive plan should be in place for the safe use of an insulin pump. Patients using continuous subcutaneous insulin infusion (CSII) pump therapy in the outpatient setting can be candidates for diabetes management in the hospital, provided that they have the mental and physical capacity to do so. Hospital policy and procedures delineating inpatient guidelines for CSII therapy are advisable, and the availability of hospital personnel with expertise in CSII therapy is essential. It is important that nursing personnel document basal rates and bolus doses taken on a daily basis. (ADA, 2015)
11) An insulin pump, developed by Medtronic known as an "artificial pancreas," was approved by the FDA on September 27, 2013. More studies are expected to be undertaken before the system becomes available on the general market. Medtronic considers this "a baby step towards a fully-automated, closed-loop pancreatic system. The device simulates only one aspect of normal pancreatic function." (Leach, 2013).

J. Hospital Inpatient Diabetes and Glycemic Control (ADA, 2014a; Cobaugh et al., 2013; Nirantharakumar, et al, 2013)

1. Poorly controlled blood glucose levels are associated with increased morbidity and mortality, and greater healthcare costs are caused by increased length of hospital stay, complications, and readmissions.
2. Insulin is considered one of the top five "high alert" medications by the Institute for Safe Medication Practices (ISMP). It is one of the medications commonly implicated in medication errors in hospitals. It can potentially cause serious harm, including death. See **Table 26-4** for a summary of some common high-priority insulin errors.
3. Both undertreatment and overtreatment of hyperglycemia are safety issues in hospitalized clients and are considered errors of omission, because hyperglycemia can negatively affect the treatment of illness and diabetes.
4. All people with diabetes admitted to the hospital should be given an order for blood glucose monitoring, with results made available to the healthcare team.
5. The practice of routine administration of correction/sliding-scale insulin doses as a primary strategy to treat hyperglycemia has been eliminated as an acceptable standard of care.
6. Recommendations are that the use of "free text" insulin orders in electronic and paper medical records be replaced with protocol-driven and evidence-based order sets that allow for the prescription of complex insulin regimens.
7. Ensure that insulin use is linked directly to patients' nutrition status, meal delivery, and point-of-care glucose testing. Insulin administration should be well coordinated and standardized.
8. Nurses must adhere to hospital policies and procedures that require that insulin pens be used for individual patients only. In addition, hospitals must establish policies and educational programs to ensure the safe use of insulin pens and disposable needle tips.
9. Patients and family caregivers should be educated to request administration of rapid-acting insulin when the patient begins his or her meal.
10. In patients with variable nutritional intake, prandial insulin administration should be delayed until completion of the meal.

Table 26-4. Expert Panel-Identified High Priority Insulin Errors by Phase of Medication-Use Process

Phase	Error
Prescribing	Incorrect dosage/irrational insulin orders Nomenclature-related errors
Transcribing	Incorrect transcription of verbal or telephone orders Transcription of an incorrect dose
Dispensing and storage	Failure to double-check insulin products (i.e. preadministration) Look-alike containers Unsecure and/or non-segregated storage in patient care areas and/or pharmacy areas
Administering	Administration of incorrect doses Incorrect use of insulin pens Name confusion Relationship of insulin administration to nutrition
Monitoring	Failure to appropriately monitor for insulin effects and adjust dose accordingly

From "Enhancing insulin-use safety in hospitals: Practical recommendations from an ASHP Foundation expert consensus panel," by D. J. Cobaugh, et al., 2013, *American Journal of Health-System Pharmacy, 70*, 1404-1413. doi:10.2146/ajhp130169. Copyright 2013 by *American Journal of Health-System Pharmacy*. Reprinted with permission.

11. Protocol-driven and evidence-based order sets should be developed for insulin use, and blood glucose should be monitored during planned and unplanned interruptions of enteral nutrition or total parenteral nutrition.
12. Glucose targets for critically ill clients
    a. Insulin therapy to treat persistent hyperglycemia should start at a threshold no greater than 180 mg/dL (10 mmol/l).
    b. Once insulin therapy is started, a glucose range of 140–180 mg/dL (7.7–10 mmol/l) should be maintained.
    c. An intravenous insulin protocol has demonstrated efficacy and safety in achieving this range without increasing the risk for hypoglycemia.
13. More stringent therapy goals, such as 110–140 mg/dL (6.1–7.7mmol/l) could be appropriate for selected patients, as long as the patient is free from hypoglycemia unawareness or recurrent significant hypoglycemia.
14. Glucose targets for noncritically ill patients treated with insulin are generally greater than 140 mg/dl (7.7 mmol/l), with random blood glucose under 180 mg/dl (10 mmol/l), provided these targets can be safely achieved.
15. Lower or higher targets can be recommended for certain people who are at lower or higher risk for hypoglycemia, especially clients receiving physical therapy as part of their rehabilitation program.
16. Protocols or algorithms and order sets guide the management of hyperglycemia and hypoglycemia.
17. Scheduled subcutaneous insulin with basal, nutritional, and correctional components is the preferred method for glucose control in noncritically ill patients.
18. Glucose monitoring should be initiated in any patient not known to be diabetic who receives therapy that is associated with high risk for hyperglycemia, including glucocorticoids, enteral or parenteral nutrition, or other medications such as octreotide or immunosuppressives.
19. Treatment should be considered for patients who have hyperglycemia, and the goals are the same as those for patients with known diabetes.

K. Acute Problems Associated with Diabetes
1. Hypoglycemia
    a. Eating too little; too much insulin or oral diabetes medication; excessive exercise; alcohol; certain cancers; critical illnesses such as kidney, liver, or heart failure; hormonal deficiencies
    b. Symptoms
        1) Mild: Sweating, trembling, difficulty concentrating, lightheadedness, and blurred vision
        2) Specific: Inability to self-treat, mental confusion, lethargy, and unconsciousness
        3) Hypoglycemia unawareness can be present due to autonomic neuropathy, with loss of warning neuroglycopenic symptoms resulting from deficient sympathetic neuronal (norepinephrine) and adrenomedullary (epinephrine) responses to falling glucose levels.
        4) Some medications can mask symptoms (e.g., beta-blockers).
    c. Treatment options (ADA, 2014a)
        1) Begin with administration of 15–20 g (5–10 g for children) of fast-acting carbohydrate (e.g., three glucose tablets or one small tube of glucose gel, 2 tablespoons raisins, 8 ounces of low-fat milk, half a can of regular soda).
        2) Retest the blood glucose level after 15 minutes.
        3) Give an additional 15 g carbohydrate if blood glucose is still lower than 70 mg/dL (3.8 mmol/l).
        4) Consider preference, allergies, and food intolerance when making treatment choices (e.g., give glucose gel to clients with dysphagia).
        5) People taking glucosidase inhibitors (i.e., acarbose or nateglinide) must use glucose (dextrose) tablets, or, if those are unavailable, milk or honey.
        6) Be careful not to overtreat and cause rebound hyperglycemia.
        7) Using a food with added fat (e.g., a chocolate bar) is not recommended, because fat can slow down the body's absorption of the carbohydrate.
        8) The use of protein to keep blood glucose up after it has been at a low level is not necessary and can add calories and promote weight gain.
        9) Follow the treatment with a snack or scheduled meal if it is 2 hours before the next meal.
        10) Severe hypoglycemia can be treated with glucagon injection or intravenous glucose.
        11) Prevention of low blood glucose is the best treatment (e.g., not skipping meals, eating six small meals a day instead of three large ones, taking the fast-acting bolus insulin

after a meal instead of before it, reducing the amount of insulin or oral diabetes medications before exercise, frequently monitoring blood glucose before and after exercise, and taking a snack if indicated before exercising. Consider reassessing the insulin regimen if blood glucose levels fall below 100 mg/dl (5.5 mmol/l). Modifying the regimen is required when blood glucose values are below 70 mg/dl (3.8 mmol/l), unless there is a reason for the low level (e.g., example, a missed meal).

2. Hyperglycemia
   a. Causes: Eating too much food; not enough insulin or oral diabetes medication; physical stress such as a cold, infection, or the flu; emotional stress such as family conflict; problems with the insulin; or other medications (e.g., corticosteroids, phenytoin)
   b. Symptoms
      1) Specific: Polyuria, polydipsia, blurred vision, dysphagia, weight loss
      2) Nonspecific: Weakness, malaise, lethargy, and headache
      3) Gastrointestinal: Nausea, vomiting, abdominal pain
      4) Respiratory: Kussmaul's breathing, metabolic acidosis, hyperventilation
   c. Treatment: Insulin and fluids
   d. Prevention of hyperglycemia: Eating the correct number and portion sizes of carbohydrates established per individual needs, taking medications on time, limiting snacking, treating infections and illness, controlling stress, increasing exercise, limiting fats
3. Other complications associated with diabetes
   a. Cardiovascular disease is the major cause of mortality for people with diabetes (ADA, 2015).
   b. Diabetes is an independent risk factor for macrovascular disease and its common coexisting conditions (e.g., hypertension and dyslipidemia).
   c. Other complications include Charcot's foot, amputations, neuropathy, gastroparesis, depression, retinopathy, nephropathy, and autonomic nerve disease, which affects nerves that control heartbeat, digestion, and other automatic functions.
4. Self-blood glucose testing and diabetes medication administration
   a. The American Diabetes Association (ADA) position regarding diabetes self-management in the hospital may be applicable if the patient meets the following criteria after the patient and physician consult with the nursing staff and all agree that patient self-management is appropriate while hospitalized (ADA 2015):
      1) Demonstrate a stable level of consciousness
      2) Exhibit reasonable stable daily insulin requirements
      3) Successfully conducted diabetes self-management at home
      4) Maintain physical skills needed to successfully self-administer insulin and perform self-monitoring of blood glucose.
      5) Have adequate oral intake
      6) Demonstrate proficiency in carbohydrate counting
      7) Use multiple daily insulin injections or insulin pump therapy
      8) Understand sick-day management
   b. The rehabilitation nurse often is responsible for initiating newly diagnosed clients' self-monitoring of blood glucose and self-medication administration (e.g., self-administering of insulin) and ensuring that those with previously existing skills are competent, knowledgeable, and safe.
   c. Referral to a certified diabetes educator on staff or in the community might be helpful for a client learning diabetes self-management skills.
   d. Adding the specialty practice of diabetes education is a possibility for every rehabilitation nurse; information about this specialty can be obtained from the American Association of Diabetes Educators (www.diabeteseducator.org).
   e. Facilities need written policies and procedures and medical staff approval to ensure the safety and legality of self-monitoring and self-medication administration programs.
5. Insulin pumps in the hospital setting
   a. The use of insulin pumps in the hospital is becoming more common. A hospital policy must be in place that guides the assessment process when a patient wearing an insulin pump is admitted. Specific procedures must be initiated to ensure the safe use of the equipment and an admitting physician's order for pump settings (e.g., basal dose[s], insulin type, correction factor[s]), as should a method of documentation of bolus doses, a schedule for taking and documenting glucose levels, documentation of

carbohydrate intake, and directives regarding the patient's responsibilities (ADA, 2015).

b. Patients using an insulin pump need orientation to hospital policy regarding the use of the insulin pump, their responsibilities regarding documentation at the bedside, when to notify the nurse of the need for blood glucose check, how to report carbohydrate intake, and how to make corrections to bolus time and amounts.

c. Hospitals that allow patients to use their physician-ordered insulin pumps should have a policy whereby the patient is evaluated for safe use of the device and their ability to make informed decisions. In addition, the rehabilitation physician and/or a clinical psychiatrist should ensure that patients have good problem-solving skills.

d. Hospitals that allow patients to use their insulin pumps should consider referring patients to an insulin-pump diabetes expert for assistance with patient advocacy. Staff training regarding the current standards of care involving insulin-pump use in the hospital is also recommended.

e. The Joint Commission has a certification program for hospitals wanting to establish advanced programs for diabetes management. It is advantageous for any hospital, including rehabilitation hospitals, to acquire this advanced certification. The specific criteria for this advanced certification is described in the 2015 *Comprehensive Certification Manual for Disease-Specific Care - including Advanced Programs for Disease-Specific Care*. This manual is available through The Joint Commission at http://store.jcrinc.com/JCRStore/SearchProductAction.do.

L. Nursing Process

1. Assessment

a. Gather objective data: Determine the type of diabetes and classification. People with hyperglycemia can be classified into one of three categories: previously diagnosed DM, unrecognized DM, or hyperglycemia related to hospitalization.

b. Gather subjective data: Determine the client's self-perceived compliance with medical and nutritional prescriptions for medication administration, blood glucose monitoring, meal planning, exercise, foot and skin care, sick-day management, and treatment and preventive methods for high and low glucose levels.

c. Determine the client's acceptance of the disease, the effect on his or her lifestyle, and perceived social and economic barriers to compliance.

d. Observe the client's functional ability and physical and psychological barriers (e.g., verbal and nonverbal communication, mobility, vision, cognition).

e. Observe the client's ability in self-glucose testing, self-insulin drawing and administration, and foot and skin care.

f. Identify the family support system.

2. Plan of care

a. Nursing diagnoses

1) Ineffective individual coping related to denial and depression

2) Knowledge deficit related to disease cause, progression, and treatments

3) Self-care deficits related to the following:

a) Physical, social, economic, and psychological barriers and limitations (e.g., medication administration, self-glucose testing)

b) Neuropathy, limited mobility, and poor vision (e.g., foot and skin care)

c) Lack of knowledge of target blood glucose levels

d) Lack of financial and social support systems

e) Lack of knowledge about follow-up needs and prevention of further complications related to the disease process

4) Altered nutritional intake (more or less than the body needs) related to lack of awareness about serving sizes, limited self-discipline, and noncompliance with dietary guidelines

5) Sensory/perceptual alterations related to neuropathy

6) Sexual dysfunction related to microvascular and macrovascular impairment

b. Goals

1) State barriers to and develop methods of effective coping with diabetes.

2) Increase level of independent self-administration of medication and glucose testing.

3) Perform or direct daily foot checks and skin care.

4) Identify adequate nutritional intake according to ADA guidelines.

5) Practice selecting proper serving sizes of favorite foods.

6) Identify ways to compensate for altered sensory/perceptual sensations.

7) Identify individual concerns with and compensate for sexual dysfunction.
8) Learn normal and target blood glucose levels.
9) Identify variances of blood glucose levels, corrective actions, and when to call for help.
10) State sick-day care.
11) Identify and obtain needed adaptive equipment (e.g., talking meters, insulin bottle holders, dose-dialing insulin syringes, premixed syringes, magnifying guides).
12) Identify and obtain insurance and Medicare and Medicaid benefits for diabetes education and equipment (e.g., meters, strips, lancets, therapeutic shoes).
13) Maintain appropriate weight loss as needed.
14) Identify proper use and disposal of needles and syringes.
15) Involve family or a significant other in management of diabetes as needed.
16) Learn preventive measures and identification and treatment of acute and chronic complications.

3. Interventions
   a. Teach coping strategies (e.g., stress management, humor, breathing exercises).
   b. Provide opportunities for assisted practice with a self-medication program (e.g., storing, drawing, mixing, and injecting insulin).
   c. Direct daily self-foot checks and skin care (e.g., using skin cream, protective shoes).
   d. Promote identification and selection of the proper number and size of carbohydrate servings for individualized meal programs (e.g., four carbohydrate servings would total 60 g carbohydrate, or 15 g carbohydrate times four food choices).
   e. Suggest ways to compensate for altered sensory/perceptual sensations (e.g., wear diabetic socks at night to increase warmth, circulation, and comfort).
   f. Teach compensation for sexual dysfunction (e.g., cream for vaginal dryness, enhancer medications and pumps for men).
   g. Teach problem-solving skills to treat and prevent blood glucose variances and to know when and how to get help.
   h. Teach use of adaptive equipment (e.g., talking meters, insulin bottle holders).
   i. Teach survival skills and suggest follow-up education and self-management support as needed after dismissal from the hospital.
   j. Discuss insurance and Medicare and Medicaid benefits for education, equipment, and continued assistance (e.g., nursing home or assisted living placement, support groups).
   k. Discuss follow-up care (e.g., annual eye exam, HbA1C test, kidney function test).
   l. Teach sick-day management (e.g., increase frequency of blood glucose testing, know when to call the doctor).
   m. Encourage the client to perform at least 150 minutes per week of moderate-intensity aerobic activity, and if no contraindications, encourage him or her to perform resistance training three times per week after discharge to home.
   n. Teach proper disposal of needles and syringes.
   o. Involve family or a significant other in management of diabetes.
   p. Discuss acute and chronic complications that can occur with diabetes and management of complications.

4. Additional information
   a. Share resources for social support with patients such as ADA support groups; online social media (e.g., blogs and Internet resources); applications for electronic devices that help with insulin management, nutrition, and exercise; and documentation and management tools.

M. Rehabilitation
1. The need for rehabilitation usually results from the complications of diabetes rather than the disease itself.
2. Stroke, heart disease, peripheral neuropathy, and amputation are the consequences of diabetes that rehabilitation nurses treat.
3. Key rehabilitation nursing strategies
   a. Incorporate all interventions identified in the nursing process assessment into the daily care of the client.
   b. Observe for neuropathy, lack of proprioception, and instability as you treat the client.
4. The rehabilitation team should include the following in addition to the basic team:
   a. Nutritional counselor or dietitian
   b. Diabetic educator, if available
   c. Pain management specialist
   d. Endocrinologist or primary care physician who is managing the diabetes

II. HIV and AIDS

A. Overview (CDC, 2014c; Fan, Conner, & Villarreal, 2011; Lee et al., 2014)

1. AIDS was first recognized in 1981 as a serious life-threatening illness and has since become a worldwide epidemic.
2. In 1985 the causative agent HIV was identified, and AIDS was determined to be the end stage of the HIV infection.
3. Although significant breakthroughs in prevention, treatment, and diagnosis have increased survival times, the long-term prognosis for people with HIV and AIDS remains poor.
4. Drug therapy to treat the infection became available in 1987 and has since expanded, but despite research and new developments, no cure or vaccine is available, and the HIV epidemic is far from over (CDC, 2014c; Lewis, Heitkemper, & Dirksen, 2004, Rote & Huether, 2010).
5. HIV/AIDS is the major cause of morbidity and mortality worldwide, and the sub-Saharan region of Africa is the epicenter. The World Health Organization (WHO) reported that 32% of all newly diagnosed HIV infections, as well as AIDS-related deaths in 2006, occurred in this region (Rote & Huether, 2010)
6. It is estimated that 35 million people worldwide have died of AIDS since the start of the epidemic, including 583,298 Americans (Rote & Huether, 2010).
7. Avoiding behaviors that place a person at risk of infection is the only way to prevent the infection.
8. Nurses play a vital role in caring for people with HIV and AIDS and are challenged to stay up to date on the most current research because information in this area is constantly developing.

B. Types
1. *AIDS* is the most advanced stage of a progressive immune function disorder caused by the retrovirus HIV.
2. HIV
    a. Attacks the immune system and leaves the body defenseless against numerous infections and health problems
    b. Includes two strains that cause AIDS and have different geographic distributions
        1) HIV-1 accounts for the majority of infections worldwide (Avert.org., 2010).
            a) Classified into four groups: The "major" group, M, the "outlier" group, O, and two new groups, N and P. These four groups could represent four separate introductions of simian immunodeficiency virus into humans. Group O appears to be restricted to west-central Africa, and group N, a strain discovered in 1998 in Cameroon, is extremely rare.
            b) More than 90% of HIV-1 infections belong to group M.
        2) HIV-2, (a less virulent strain) appears to be prevalent in West African countries but has only limited distribution in other areas.

C. Epidemiology (CDC, 2013; Lee et al., 2014; World Health Organization [WHO], 2010)
1. In 2010, an estimated 35 million people worldwide were living with HIV/AIDs, including 1.2 million people in the United States, and 50,000 new cases are diagnosed each year in the United States. By comparison, in 2006, 4.9–6.1 million newly infected people were located in South Africa (Lee et al., 2014, Rote & Huether, 2010).
2. Of the 1.1 million people in the United States living with HIV, an estimated 1 in 6 do not know they are infected.
3. Advances in treatment slowed the overall progression of HIV infection to AIDS, leading to dramatic decreases in AIDS deaths in the United States. The number of new AIDS diagnoses has remained relatively stable in the United States.
4. AIDS is a disease that affects primarily homosexual males, but it has infiltrated other population groups as well. In 2006, 50% of newly diagnosed cases in the United States were due to male-to-male sexual activity, 33% to high-risk heterosexual contact, and 13% to injected drug abuse; 26% were diagnosed in females, with approximately 74% of cases related to high-risk heterosexual activity (Rote & Huether, 2010).
5. African Americans accounted for 51% of the HIV/AIDS diagnoses made in 2007 in the United States, whites accounted for 29%, and Hispanics and Latinos accounted for 18%. As with many other diseases, individuals of lower socioeconomic status have poorer outcomes due to increased exposure to risk factors; reduced access to early testing and treatment; and cultural, religious, and social influences such as stigma and discrimination (Lee et al., 2014).

D. Etiology
1. The origin of HIV is unknown.
2. The causative agent of HIV infection is HIV, a retrovirus.
3. A person with HIV can be asymptomatic for many years and not even know that he or she is infected; however, as the immune system weakens, the person becomes ill more often.
4. Differentiating between exposure, infection, and disease: When an HIV-infected person has

intimate contact with an uninfected person (exposure), it does not always result in transmission of HIV to the uninfected person. Likewise, not all people who become infected with the virus (infection) develop physical symptoms.

5. HIV is a continuous disease process that ranges from asymptomatic to AIDS, which is characterized by potentially life-threatening opportunistic infections (OIs) (Rote & Huether, 2010).
6. The time between initial infection and appearance of circulating antibodies is referred to as the "window period" (Rote & Heuther, 2010, p. 322).
   a. Primary infection or early chronic infection: Refers to the period between infection with HIV and the development of HIV-specific antibodies, which results in viremia (large amounts of virus in the blood)
      1) Onset is 0–12 weeks from initial infection.
      2) Virus infects white blood cells called CD4+ T-lymphocytes (i.e., T-helper cells), which are the master coordinators of the immune system.
      3) Immune system clears virus to lymphatic organs.
      4) The CD4+ T-cell count declines and is greater than or equal to 500 cells/mm^3.
      5) Clinical manifestation is similar to symptoms of flu or mononucleosis (e.g., fever, fatigue, headache, arthralgia, myalgia, generalized lymphadenopathy, pharyngitis, anorexia, weight loss, and night sweats). Symptoms usually disappear after a week to a month.
   b. Chronic asymptomatic infection
      1) Onset is 12 weeks–12 years or more from initial infection.
      2) Anti-HIV antibodies will have been produced by about 12 weeks and can be detected by antibody screening.
      3) The virus is present primarily in lymphatic tissue and slowly spreads throughout the body.
      4) Clinical symptoms usually are absent or mild. Vague symptoms include fatigue, headache, lymphadenopathy, and night sweats.
      5) As the viral load increases, the CD4+ T-cell count gradually declines (200–499 cells/mm3).
   c. AIDS
      1) As the immune system fails, symptoms increase, and the illnesses that occur become more severe.
      2) Signs and symptoms progress from mild to moderate (e.g., chills, frequent fever, night sweats, dry productive cough, dyspnea, lethargy, confusion, stiff neck, seizures, headaches, malaise, oral lesions, generalized lymphadenopathy, skin rashes, abdominal discomfort, chronic diarrhea, weight loss, fatigue, short-term memory loss, tuberculosis, oral hairy leukoplakia, shingles, thrombocytopenia, pelvic inflammatory disease in women that does not respond to treatment, developmental delays and failure to thrive in children) to life-threatening OIs.
      3) CD4+ T-cell counts continue to decline to less than 200 cells/mm3.
      4) One or more OIs or diseases (i.e., AIDS indicator conditions) develop (**Figure 26-3**). Children can contract the same OIs or diseases as adults, but they can also have severe forms of common childhood bacterial infections such as conjunctivitis, ear infections, and tonsillitis (Health-Disease.org, 2011).

Figure 26-3. Opportunistic Infections Associated with AIDS

Viral: Cytomegalovirus disease, herpes simplex, pneumonitis or esophagitis
Bacterial: *Mycobacterium tuberculosis*, recurrent pneumonia, recurrent *Salmonella septicemia*
Protozoal: *Pneumocystis carinii* pneumonia (PCP), toxoplasmosis of the brain
Fungal: Candidiasis of bronchi, trachea, lungs, or esophagus
Neurological: Dementia, headaches
Neoplastic processes: Lymphoma, Kaposi's sarcoma (KS), cervical carcinoma
Wasting syndrome: Chronic diarrhea, weakness, weight loss, constant or intermittent fever for at least 30 days

      5) Clinical manifestations involve the loss of lean body mass and wasting syndrome.
      6) Without treatment, death occurs within 3–5 years and usually results from infection, cancer, or wasting syndrome.

E. Pathophysiology
   1. Overview (Fan et al., 2011, Rote & Huether, 2010)
      a. *HIV* is a retrovirus that consists of ribonucleic acid (RNA) virus that contains a special viral enzyme called reverse transcriptase, which allows the virus to replicate backward, going from RNA to deoxyribonucleic acid (DNA), and then integrate and take over a cell's own genetic material.

b. HIV cannot replicate unless it is inside a living cell.

c. HIV interacts with human cells that have CD4 receptors on their surface membrane, which include lymphocytes, monocytes, macrophages, astrocytes, and oligodendrocytes (i.e., white blood cells that fight infections); once attached, HIV virus enters the cell.

d. After the virus enters the cell, viral RNA is transcribed into DNA with the assistance of the enzyme reverse transcriptase, becoming a permanent part of the cell's genetic structure and replicated during normal cell processes.

e. HIV uses the cell to make copies of itself, produces new HIV retroviruses, and kills primarily CD4+ T lymphocytes, because they have more CD4+ receptor-bearing cells.

f. Viral load (i.e., the number of circulating HIV retroviruses in the person's serum) increases.

g. Antibodies are produced and detectable between 6 weeks and 6 months after infection; however, these antibodies are not able to fight the infection.

h. Millions of CD4+ T cells are destroyed every day, but the bone marrow and thymus are able to produce enough CD4+ T cells to replace the destroyed cells for many years.

i. Once the ability of HIV to destroy CD4+ T cells exceeds the body's ability to make them, the cells will not be able to regulate immune responses, resulting in the most serious stage of HIV infection—AIDS, with OIs.

j. Immune problems start to occur when the CD4+ T cell count drops to 200–499 cells/mm3; severe problems develop with fewer than 200 CD4+ T cells/mm^3.

2. Transmission

   a. HIV is transmitted from human to human through exposure to infected body fluid (e.g., blood, semen, vaginal secretions, breast milk).

   b. No evidence has been found that HIV is transmitted through tears, sweat, saliva, vomit, urine, or feces.

   c. Common modes of transmission:

      1) Sexual contact (e.g., oral, vaginal, anal)
      2) Sharing a needle or syringe (e.g., intravenous drug use, tattooing, body piercing)
      3) Blood transfusion (risk is extremely small because of blood screening and heat treatment)
      4) Tissue or organ donation
      5) Prenatal contact from mother to infant before or during birth or during breastfeeding
      6) Occupational exposure (e.g., needle stick)

   d. HIV is not spread through casual contact (e.g., touching; hugging; shaking hands; sharing eating utensils; eating food prepared by a person with HIV; coughing; sneezing; using restrooms; touching animals or insects; or living, working, or attending school with an HIV-infected person).

3. Clinical manifestations

   a. Common signs and symptoms of HIV infection include chills, fever, flulike symptoms, rash, fatigue, malaise, arthralgias, headache, loss of appetite, weight loss, myalgias, nausea, vomiting, pharyngitis, oral ulcers, dry productive cough, sore throat, rash, night sweats, shortness of breath, stiff neck, yeast infection, lymphadenopathy, gastrointestinal distress, diarrhea, pain, dementia, confusion, infected gums, sores on anus and genitals, and photophobia (Zingman, 2010).

   b. People with AIDS are susceptible to OIs, which are life-threatening illnesses caused by organisms that normally do not cause problems in healthy people (Fan et al., 2011).

      1) OIs can affect every organ and body system.
      2) Diagnosis and treatment of OIs are essential to increase longevity.
      3) Pneumocystis pneumonia caused by a fungus microbe is a common OI in adults.
      4) Children are susceptible to OIs, conjunctivitis, ear infections, and tonsillitis.

4. Diagnosis

   a. Early testing and routine voluntary testing for HIV will alert the HIV-infected person to avoid high-risk behavior, reducing HIV transmission; enabling appropriate treatment; and resulting in improved health, extended life, and prevention of OIs (Workowski & Berman, 2010).

   b. Recommendations for HIV testing (Workowski & Berman, 2010)

      1) Routine HIV screening for people 13–64 years of age in all healthcare settings after the client is notified that screening will be performed unless he or she declines (opt-out screening) and for all adolescents who are sexually active and/or use injection drugs
      2) HIV testing at least once per year for people at high risk unless the client declines (opt-out screening)
      3) HIV screening included in a panel of prenatal screening tests for all pregnant women

as soon as pregnancy is detected and repeat screening in the third trimester in certain geographical locations with elevated HIV infection rates, unless the client declines (opt-out screening)

4) All persons seeking treatment for any sexually transmitted disease

c. Written consent is not recommended (it is presumed unless specifically declined), and HIV screening should be incorporated into the general consent for medical care.

d. Prevention and pretest counseling are encouraged but not required for diagnostic testing as part of routine screening programs in healthcare settings.

1) Pretest counseling

a) Review test procedures.

b) Explain the meaning of positive and negative test results.

c) Provide information on HIV and AIDS.

d) Form a plan for risk reduction.

e) Describe the importance of follow-up care.

f) Prepare the client for potential psychological and emotional reactions to a positive test result.

2) Posttest counseling

a) If the test is negative, provide advice on retesting (if the person engages in high-risk behavior) and preventing the spread of HIV.

b) If the test is positive, evaluate the person's potential for suicide; provide crisis intervention if needed and information on symptoms of HIV and AIDS; teach health maintenance; refer for medical follow-up and tuberculosis screening, support groups, clinical trials, or experimental protocols; and discuss potential discrimination.

e. Confidentiality with HIV testing is very important because disclosure could result in discrimination.

f. Diagnostic tests available (CDC, 2012; Fan et al., 2011)

1) Antibody testing (rapid test [20 minutes], enzyme-linked immunosorbent assay, Western blot)

a) Detects the presence of antibodies to HIV

b) Involves a delay (window period) of 3 weeks to 6 months before a detectable antibody is produced

c) A positive test should be repeated and then confirmed by an alternative method, usually the Western blot.

d) Most widely used

2) Antigen testing

a) Detects the virus (HIV RNA) in the blood

b) Virus is detectable 1 week earlier than with antibody testing but is labor intensive and costly

c) Can be performed if an antibody test is negative and the person is highly likely to test positive

3) Viral load: Measures plasma HIV RNA levels in a sample of blood, indicating the amount of virus in the person's serum, how well the immune system is controlling the virus, or whether the medication regimen is working

a) Without antiretroviral medication: Viral load every 3–4 months

b) With antiretroviral medication: Viral load 2–8 weeks after initiation of treatment and then every 3–4 months to make sure the drug is still working

4) CD4 cell count: Used to measure the extent of immune damage that has occurred, to stage HIV infection and determine prognosis, and to determine whether the medication regimen is working

5) Drug resistance testing: Determines whether a person's HIV strain is resistant to any anti-HIV medication

F. Management Options (Panel on Antiretroviral Guidelines for Adults and Adolescents, 2014)

1. Early intervention results in improved health outcomes, delay of clinical progression of the disease, and reduced mortality; thus, early diagnosis is essential. Research has focused on antiretroviral agents to inhibit disease progression, prophylactic therapy to prevent OIs, therapy to restore the damaged immune system, and vaccine development (Monahan, Sands, Neighbors, Marek, & Green, 2007; Workowski & Berman, 2010).

2. The primary goals driving the decision to initiate antiretroviral therapy (ART) include the following:

a. Maximally and durably suppress plasma HIV viral load.

b. Reduce HIV-associated morbidity and prolong survival.

c. Improve quality of life.

d. Restore and preserve immunological function.

e. Prevent HIV transmission.
f. Potential for preventing transmission of HIV to newborns with an HIV-positive mother increases when treatment is initiated at or before the first 12 hours after birth (Workowski & Berman, 2010).

3. HIV suppression with ART could also decrease inflammation and immune activation, which are thought to increase rates of cardiovascular and other comorbidities.
4. The FDA has approved a number of drugs for treating HIV infection (Fan et al., 2011).
   a. Nucleoside analog reverse transcriptase inhibitors (NRTIs)
      1) Target the viral enzyme reverse transcriptase. These drugs specifically block the virus from replicating while having little effect on the host.
      2) Include azidothymidine (AZT), zalcitabine (ddC), didanosine (ddI), stavudine (d4T), lamivudine (3TC), abacavir (Ziagen®), tenofovir (Viread®), and emtricitabine (Emtriva®)
   b. Nonnucleoside reverse transcriptase inhibitors (NNRTIs)
      1) Bind to the reverse transcriptase enzyme and prevent it from functioning
      2) Include delavirdine (Rescriptor®), nevirapine (Viramune®), and efavirenz (Sustiva®)
      3) In 2010 a single dose of nevirapine was found to be effective in substantially reducing HIV transmission from pregnant women to their children.
   c. Protease inhibitors
      1) Prevent the virus from making long protein molecules necessary to create a new virus, thus halting replication
      2) Include ritonavir (Norvir®), saquinavir (Invirase®), indinavir (Crixivan®), nelfinavir (Viracept®), lopinavir (Kaletra®), atazanavir (Reyataz®), amprenavir (Agenerase®), darunavir (Prezista®), lopinavir (Kaletra®), tipranavir (Aptivus®), and fosamprenavir (Lexiva®)
   d. Integrase inhibitors
      1) The most recently developed antiviral drugs that target the viral integrase, which is the enzyme responsible for integration of viral DNA into the host cell
      2) Raltegravir (Isentress®) was approved for use in 2007, and when used with other anti-HIV drugs, is effective in controlling viral loads.
   e. Fusion inhibitors
      1) Interfere with HIV-1's ability to enter cells by blocking the merging of the virus with the cell membrane
      2) Include enfuvirtide (T-20, Fuzeon®)
   f. First- and second-line treatments updated in 2010 (WHO, 2010)
      1) First-line therapy recommendations consist of NNRTI and two NRTIs, one of which should be AZT or tenofovir (TDF).
      2) Second-line therapy recommendations consist of ritonavir (RTV)-boosted protease inhibitor and two NRTIs, one of which should be AZT or TDF, depending on what was used in first-line therapy.
      3) Reduce use of d4T in first-line therapy due to long-term toxicities.
5. The most effective treatment strategy is combination drug therapy, which can attack viral replication in several different ways, attack different stages of the HIV life cycle, produce a more sustained antiviral effect in a person with HIV, and decrease the likelihood of drug resistance.
   a. Current recommendations are to monitor a client with HIV and to initiate ART after the CD4T counts drop below 350 cells/mm^3, with or without clinical symptoms (WHO, 2010)
   b. The current guidelines recommend achieving the maximum suppression of symptoms for as long as possible. This used to be called highly active antiretroviral therapy (HAART) but now is referred to as ART (Fan et al., 2011).
   c. In addition, because quality of life is important, the overall goal of AIDS treatment is to find the strongest possible regimen that is also simple and has the fewest side effects.
      1) With effective ART therapies, HIV-infected people experience a drop in viral loads below the level of detectability for several years, and many survive for decades after diagnosis of AIDS (Workowski & Berman, 2010).
      2) ART is not a cure but reduces the amount of virus circulating in the bloodstream.
      3) Drops in viral loads are accompanied by recoveries of T-cell counts, increases in immune function, and the disappearance of AIDS symptoms.
6. A number of treatments are available for some opportunistic diseases (e.g., radiation and chemotherapy for Kaposi's sarcoma and other forms of cancer, ganciclovir to treat cytomegalovirus eye infections, fluconazole to treat yeast and other

fungal infections, and pentamidine or trimethoprim/sulfamethoxazole to treat *Pneumocystis carinii* pneumonia).

7. The influenza vaccine is recommended; people with advanced AIDS could have a poor response to immunization and should be given antiviral medications if they are likely to be exposed to other people with influenza.
8. Alternative and complementary therapies include therapeutic touch, massage therapy, meditation, imagery, tai chi, and herbal medicine.
9. Health promotion and disease prevention can be effective in preventing the spread of infection.
    a. Promote a lifestyle that prevents or decreases the risk of HIV infection.
        1) Abstain from sexual activity or use a condom for all insertive sexual practices with a partner who has or might have HIV.
        2) Don't use intravenous drugs, don't share needles and equipment, use a clean needle and syringe or disinfect them after each use, decrease the number of injections, and avoid engaging in risky sexual activity.
        3) Early testing and routine screening for all clients 13–64 years of age
        4) Screen all potential blood donors for high-risk behaviors and signs and symptoms of AIDS, and test all human tissue intended for transplantation for HIV antibodies.
        5) Adhere to safety guidelines to prevent occupational exposure.
    b. Promote a healthy lifestyle in people who are already infected.
        1) Decrease high-risk behavior.
        2) Attend regular medical and psychiatric evaluations and follow-ups.
        3) Maintain proper nutrition and diet (e.g., high calorie, high protein to prevent weight loss), which improve immune function.
        4) Maintain food safety by keeping food at the proper temperature, cooking food thoroughly, avoiding foods that might be contaminated or harboring bacteria, and washing fruits and vegetables before eating (because people with HIV infection are vulnerable to foodborne illness).
        5) Remove fresh flowers and plants from the patient's environment.
        6) Avoid cleaning the litter box.
        7) Ask visitors to wear a mask if they have a cold.
        8) Maintain proper hand washing.
        9) Reduce and control stress.
        10) Avoid or limit cigarettes, alcohol, and drugs.
        11) Exercise regularly but avoid overexertion. Get plenty of rest.

G. Nursing Process

1. Assessment
    a. Obtain a complete history of current high-risk behaviors that could put other people at risk and signs and symptoms that could indicate the progression of HIV and the presence of OIs.
    b. Perform a neurological evaluation and a cognitive evaluation for onset of deficits, as 50% of patients who are HIV/AIDS positive will experience cognitive problems as a result of the disease process or ART medications (Vance, 2013).
    c. Perform a psychosocial evaluation (e.g., support systems, financial state, employment status, coping strategies).
    d. Observe the client's overall health and appearance and conduct a complete physical and functional assessment, because any body system can be affected.
    e. Investigate nutritional status, energy level, and preventive strategies to protect others and self from further infectious insult.
    f. Assess for weight loss, fever, skin lesions, short-term memory loss, and cold symptoms.
    g. Assess compliance with treatment, effectiveness of the treatment regimen, and side effects.
2. Plan of care
    a. Nursing diagnoses
        1) Hopelessness related to terminal disease process
        2) Fear related to possible death
        3) Anticipatory grieving related to terminal diagnosis
        4) Ineffective individual coping or compromised family coping related to diagnosis
        5) Inadequate nutrition related to the disease process, wasting syndrome, and side effects of the treatment regimen
        6) Pain related to the disease process
        7) Fatigue and deconditioning related to poor nutrition, the disease process, treatment side effects, and muscle weakness
        8) Activity intolerance related to deconditioning and inadequate nutrition
        9) Risk for infection related to deficient immune system
        10) Knowledge deficit related to diagnosis, prognosis, and long-term care
    b. Goals (Lewis et al., 2004)

1) For the asymptomatic stage
   a) Demonstrate a healthy lifestyle.
   b) Verbalize an understanding of measures to prevent further HIV transmission.
   c) Identify and use effective strategies for coping with stressful situations and adjustment to illness.
   d) Verbalize an understanding of the disease process, significant implications, and treatment options.
2) For the symptomatic stage
   a) Verbalize an understanding of the prevention and treatment of OIs.
   b) Verbalize an understanding of and appropriately manage problems caused by HIV infection.
   c) Maintain a maximal level of function to reduce or prevent impairments.
   d) Verbalize understanding of and adhere to the drug regimen to keep the viral load as low as possible for as long as possible.
3) For the terminal stage
   a) Maintain a desired level of comfort.
   b) Verbalize wishes and declare preferences regarding treatment options.
   c) Experience a dignified and comfortable death.

3. Interventions
   a. Asymptomatic stage
      1) Provide education about the diagnosis of HIV, prevention of the spread of HIV, disease progression, and treatment options.
      2) Use strategies to prevent infection.
      3) Provide education for people who are HIV negative and at risk for contracting HIV, and prevent the HIV-infected person from transmitting the virus to others.
      4) Empower the client to take control of preventive measures.
      5) Encourage the client to maintain social and community activities.
      6) Monitor for signs and symptoms of infection, which may indicate disease progression.
      7) Provide emotional support, include significant others in the plan of care, and help identify additional sources of financial and emotional support.
      8) Assess the psychological response to situations.
   b. Symptomatic stage
      1) Provide education about medications and adverse effects.
      2) Assess effectiveness of the treatment regimen (i.e., viral load, CD4+ T-cell count), adverse reactions, and compliance with medication regimens.
      3) Educate about changing treatment options and encourage continued adherence.
      4) Monitor weight and provide a high-calorie, high-protein diet and nutritional supplements as necessary.
      5) Manage and treat HIV-related symptoms with antibiotics, antifungals, or antiviral medication for infection; antiemetics for nausea; analgesics for pain; and antidiarrheal medication for diarrhea.
      6) Balance energy with rest to maintain a normal or nearly normal activity level, and use assistive devices (e.g., wheelchair, cane) to conserve energy and maintain maximum level of function independence.
      7) Encourage verbalization of fears and concerns.
   c. Terminal stage
      1) Assist with end-of-life comfort measures in a suitable care setting and appropriate services (e.g., hospice).
      2) Administer pain medication to relieve pain and discomfort.
      3) Administer antianxiety medication for anxiety and restlessness.
      4) Promote a calm environment.
      5) Provide emotional and spiritual support to the client and significant others.
      6) Maintain the client's dignity and wishes throughout the dying process.
      7) Instruct significant others about the dying process.
      8) Provide bereavement counseling for significant others.
4. Evaluation: Modify care according to the stage of HIV and the client's response to nursing interventions.

H. Rehabilitation
   1. Rehabilitation needs are determined by the stage of HIV, presence and impact of other OIs, and the client's response to nursing interventions. With improved treatments, individuals are living longer and are likely to experience the impact of their disease as well as the aging process.
   2. HIV and AIDS rehabilitation should include the following:
      a. Client and family education and counseling

b. Functional activities with introduction of assistive devices as needed
c. Nutritional counseling
d. An exercise program to help build strength, endurance, and mobility
3. In addition to the basic rehabilitation team members, the team should include the following:
a. Primary care physician or infectious disease specialist
b. Counselor
c. Representative of hospice or palliative care

III. Cancer

A. Overview

1. *Cancer* encompasses a group of diseases characterized by the growth and spread of abnormal cells that result in death if not controlled.
2. Cancer is the second most common cause of death in the United States, exceeded only by heart disease, and smoking causes one third of all cancer deaths (American Cancer Society [ACS], 2014a).
3. Adult cigarette smoking prevalence in the United States has been slowly declining since 1991. The prevalence among adolescents has declined since the late 1990s, but one in five adults and adolescents is a smoker (ACS, 2014a)
4. Prostate, breast, lung, and colorectal cancers are the most common cancers in the United States (ACS, 2014a; National Cancer Institute [NCI], 2011).
5. The cancer incidence rate has declined since the early 2000s. However, incidence rates for some cancers (e.g., melanoma of the skin; non-Hodgkin's lymphoma; childhood cancers; leukemia; and cancers of the kidney, renal pelvis, thyroid, pancreas, liver, testis, and esophagus) are rising (NCI, 2014e).
6. Categories of cancer (NCI, 2014e)
a. *Carcinoma*: Cancer that begins in the skin or internal and external linings of the body (e.g., skin, lungs, breast, pancreas, and other organs and glands)
b. *Sarcoma*: Cancer that begins in bone, cartilage, fat, or other connective tissue (e.g., bone, skeletal muscle, fibrous tissue, or cartilage)
c. *Myeloma*: Cancer of plasma cells of bone marrow
d. *Lymphoma*: Cancer of cells in the glands or nodes of the lymphatic system
e. *Leukemia*: Cancer that affects the blood-forming elements of the bone marrow
f. *Central nervous system (CNS) cancers*: Cancers that begin in the tissues of the brain and spinal cord
g. *Mixed type*: Cancer of multiple tissue types
7. Not all tumors are cancerous.
a. Benign tumors are not cancerous. They can be removed and in most cases do not return.
b. Malignant tumors are cancerous. Cells in these tumors can invade nearby tissues and spread to other parts of the body (i.e., metastasis).
8. Early detection and treatment improve the chances of a cure.

B. Epidemiology and Incidence (ACS, 2014a)

1. Approximately 1,665,540 new cancer cases will be diagnosed in 2014in the United States.
2. Approximately 585,720 Americans are expected to die of cancer in 2014.
3. One of every two American men and one of every three American women will develop cancer during their lifetime.
4. 78% of all cancers are diagnosed in people 55 years and older.
5. The 5-year survival rate for all cancers diagnosed between 2003 and 2009 was 68%, up from 49% during 1975–1977 (ACS, 2014a; Silver, Baima, & Mayer, 2013).
6. Individuals with lower socioeconomic status have a greater cancer risk and less favorable outcomes due to increased exposure to risk factors and reduced access to prevention, screenings, and treatment after cancer is diagnosed (ACS, 2014a)
7. Cancer occurrence rates are increasing in economically developing countries as a result of the adoption of Western lifestyles that include smoking, poor diet, physical inactivity, and reproductive factors (ACS, 2014a; NCI, 2014e).
8. The worldwide impact of cancer is increasing; it is expected that there will be 21.4 million new cases and 13.2 million cancer deaths by 2030 (ACS, 2014a; Silver et al., 2013).

C. Etiology and Risk Factors

1. The exact cause of cancer remains a mystery.
2. Development of cancer is a multistep process that is influenced by many independent variables that cause damage to DNA, resulting in mutation within the genes of cells.
3. Mutations can be caused by chemicals or physical agents, called *carcinogens*, or they can occur spontaneously and be passed down from one generation to the next.
4. Risk factors (ACS, 2014a; NCI, 2014d)
a. Age: The risk of nearly all cancers increases with age.

b. Genetic factors: Some cancers are inherited and create a significant predisposition to cancer. About 5% of cancers are strongly hereditary (an inherited genetic alteration confers a very high risk of developing one or more specific types of cancer).

c. Hormonal factor: Evidence suggests that hormones could be connected with the development of certain cancers.

d. Exposure to environmental factors: 75%–80% of cancer in the United States is attributed to environmental factors.

1) Tobacco smoke is the most lethal known carcinogen (responsible for 30% of cancer deaths in the United States).

2) Radiation: Ionizing and ultraviolet radiation (sunlight) can cause cancer.

3) Poor nutrition, obesity, and inactivity are responsible for 35% of cancer deaths in the United States. Research shows that approximately one third of all cancer deaths are related to an unhealthy diet and lack of physical activity in adulthood (ACS, 2014a).

a) Some research indicates that grilled meats can cause cancer. Cooking meats at high temperatures produces chemicals (i.e., heterocyclic amines) that can increase cancer risk (ACS, 2013).

b) People who have diets high in saturated fats have a greater cancer risk than those who have lower-fat diets.

c) Inactivity has been linked to a higher risk of colon cancer.

4) Certain viruses: A number of cancers have been linked to viruses (e.g., sexually transmitted disease organisms) that suppress the immune system.

5) Occupational exposure (responsible for 4% of cancer deaths in the United States): Exposure to carcinogens (e.g., drugs, chemicals, and radiation) increases the risk of cancer.

6) Alcohol: Drinking alcohol has been linked with an elevated risk of cancer of the esophagus, oral cavity, pharynx, and larynx (ACS, 2014a).

e. Precancerous lesions: Benign lesions and tumors (polyps of the colon and rectum, certain pigmented moles) tend to progress to cancer.

f. Psychosocial factors: Extreme stress activates the body's endocrine (hormone) system, which in turn can cause changes in the immune system. There is no research that directly links cancer with stress.

D. Pathophysiology

1. Overview: Cancer develops when a number of mechanisms, either alone or in combination, cause abnormalities in cell growth and multiplication.

2. Cancer cells

a. Characteristics

1) Variable size and shape

2) Loss of capacity for specialized function

3) Continued growth after division

a) Normal cells usually die after 50–60 divisions; however, cancer cells continue in an uncontrolled growth pattern.

b) Cancer cells continue to grow despite a diminished concentration of growth hormones.

b. Tumor growth

1) Cancer cells accumulate and form a mass of abnormal cells (or tumors) that can compress, invade, and destroy normal tissues.

2) Most cancers form tumors, but not all tumors are cancerous.

a) Benign: Noncancerous tumors that stop growing and do not spread to other parts of the body

b) Malignant: Cancerous tumors

c. Carcinogenesis

1) The process through which cancer develops and abnormal cells grow and proliferate out of control

2) Change or mutation in the nucleus of a cell: Millions of cells in the human body die and are replaced every second. The body's immune system typically recognizes mutant cells and destroys them before they multiply, but some mutant cells survive and cause cancer.

3) Carcinogenesis can occur after exposure to carcinogens, which are substances that start or promote the process (e.g., various chemicals, gases, and other substances found in the air, water, foods, pesticides, and industrial settings; tobacco smoke; cleaning products; paints; certain viruses such as HIV, HPV, hepatitis B, and Epstein-Barr).

4) Two models of carcinogenesis (NCI, 2014e)

a) Vogelstein and Kinzler (2004) emphasized that cancer is ultimately a disease of damaged DNA, which is composed of a sequence of genetic mutations that can turn normal cells into cancerous cells.

b) Hanahan and Weinberg (2000) focused on the hallmark events at the cellular level that lead to a tumor.

d. Metastasis

1) Abnormal cells multiply out of control.

2) A tumor spreads from the original site to another site via the lymphatic system, blood vessels, or natural tissue planes (Virshup, 2010).

3) This uncontrolled growth and spread of cancer cells can eventually interfere with vital organs or functions, resulting in a variety of other tissue changes in the body such as pain, cachexia, lowered immunity, anemia, leukopenia, and thrombocytopenia, and if not controlled, can result in death. Metastasis is the major cause of death from cancer (Virshup, 2010)

4) Once a cancer has metastasized, the same therapies that were used while the tumor was localized are typically ineffective (Virshup, 2010)

5) The primary sites of cancer metastasis are the bone, lymph nodes, liver, lungs, and brain (Virshup, 2010).

6) Cancer is classified according to the body part where it started.

3. Symptoms that could signal the presence of cancer (ACS, 2012)

a. A change in the size, color, shape, or thickness of a wart, mole, or mouth sore

b. A sore that resists healing

c. Persistent cough, hoarseness, or sore throat

d. Thickening or lumps in the breasts, testicles, or elsewhere

e. A change in bowel or bladder habits

f. Any unusual bleeding or discharge

g. Chronic indigestion or difficulty swallowing

h. Persistent headaches

i. Unexplained loss of weight or appetite

j. Persistent fatigue, nausea, or vomiting

k. Persistent low-grade fever, either constant or intermittent

l. Repeated instances of infection

4. Diagnosis

a. Diagnostic testing: Laboratory testing (e.g., complete blood count, chemistry profile, liver function test, tumor markers [i.e., substances measurable in the blood that are not produced or are produced in a lesser amount in healthy people]).

b. Noninvasive: Radiological studies, computed tomography (CT), magnetic resonance imaging (MRI), ultrasonography, and nuclear medicine studies

c. Invasive procedures: Biopsy (a variety of biopsy types are available that range from needle biopsy to surgical procedure), endoscopy

d. Staging

1) Staging is the process used to describe the extent of the disease or the spread of cancer from the original site.

2) The tumor-node-metastasis staging system is a uniform system, developed by the WHO and used worldwide. This staging system assesses tumors in three ways (T describes tumor spread, *N* describes node involvement and *M* describes metastasis) to determine a stage; stages range from I to IV (Monahan et al., 2007; Virshup, 2010).

a) T: Extent of the primary tumor. TX means the primary tumor cannot be evaluated. T0 means there is no evidence of a primary tumor. *Carcinoma in situ* (CIS) means abnormal cells are present but have not spread to neighboring tissue. Although not cancer, CIS could become cancer and is sometimes called preinvasive cancer. T1 to T4 describe the size or level of invasion into nearby structures (the higher the T number, the larger the tumor).

b) N: Absence or presence of regional lymph node involvement. *NX* means regional lymph nodes cannot be evaluated. *N0* means there is no regional lymph node involvement. *N1* to *N3* describe the size, location, or number of lymph nodes involved. The higher the N number, the more involved the lymph nodes are.

c) *M*: Absence or presence of metastases. *MX* means distant metastases cannot be evaluated. *M0* means there are no known distant metastases, and *M1* means that distant metastases are present.

e. Pap smear: Cells found in body secretions are spread, stained, and examined for tissue classification.

f. Tumor marker blood test: Measures for the presence of tumor markers or proteins associated with specific cancers (e.g., CA27–29 for breast cancer, CA125 for ovarian cancer, prostate-specific antigen for prostate cancer

g. Screening examinations by healthcare professionals can help detect cancer of the breast, colon, rectum, cervix, prostate, testis, oral cavity, and skin.
h. Self-examination for breast and skin cancer can result in early detection of tumors.

E. Management Options
1. Prevention measures (ACS, 2014a)
   a. Do not smoke or chew tobacco. Avoid exposure to smoke. Tobacco is believed to play a role in 90% of all lung cancer deaths (ACS, 2014a).
   b. Limit alcohol intake. Alcohol increases the risk of cancers of the mouth, pharynx, larynx, esophagus, liver, and breast, and probably the colon and rectum (ACS, 2014a).
   c. Eat a well-balanced diet.
      1) Studies suggest that people who eat more fruits and vegetables, which are rich sources of antioxidants, could have a lower risk for some types of cancer (ACS, 2014a).
      2) Reduce the intake of fat.
      3) Limit red meat and animal fat.
      4) Avoid processed, smoked, cured, fried, or barbecued foods.
      5) Balance caloric intake with physical activity.
      6) Maintain a healthy weight, and avoid excessive weight gain throughout life.
   d. Practice sun safety and recognize when skin changes occur.
      1) Stay out of the sun between 10 am and 3 pm.
      2) Use sunscreen with a sun protection factor of 15 or higher outdoors. Wear a hat and shirt when in the sun.
      3) Wear ultraviolet-light–filtering sunglasses.
      4) Avoid tanning booths.
   e. Exercise regularly. Exercise reduces the risk of several types of cancer (e.g., breast, colon, endometrium, prostate) and reduces the risk of other health problems (e.g., heart disease, high blood pressure, diabetes, osteoporosis).
   f. Follow occupational hazard guidelines if exposed to carcinogens.
      1) Limit exposure to carcinogens at home.
      2) Avoid using aerosol cleaning products.
      3) Wear gloves when using carcinogenic chemicals.
      4) Follow safety warnings when using paint, solvents, pesticides, household cleaners, and other carcinogenic chemicals.
   g. Have precancerous adenomatous polyps removed to prevent colon cancer.
   h. Practice safe sex.
      1) Human papilloma virus is a known cause for cervical cancer and a risk factor for other cancers.
      2) HIV and AIDS are associated with some types of cancers.
   i. Get screened for cancer regularly. Screening tests such as colonoscopy, mammogram, and Pap smear can detect abnormal changes before they become cancerous.
2. Cancer treatment modalities are used to cure, control, or provide palliation; options depend on the stage of the tumor and the level of metastasis.
   a. Surgery: The oldest form of treatment offers the greatest chance for cure for many types of cancer.
      1) Biopsy: Obtain specimens of suspected tissue.
      2) Curative resection: Resect lesions.
      3) Palliation: Relieve symptoms to improve quality of life.
   b. Radiation: A stream of high-energy particles or waves is used to destroy or damage cancer cells in a specific area.
      1) Used before surgery to shrink a tumor so it can be removed more easily
      2) Used after surgery to stop the growth of cancer cells that remain
      3) Side effects: Irritation of the overlying skin and mucus membranes, nausea, vomiting, anorexia, bone-marrow depression, anemia, thrombocytopenia, and leukopenia
   c. *Chemotherapy* is the use of drugs to treat cancer by interfering with the stages of the dividing cell cycle and is used to treat cancer cells that have metastasized.
      1) Anticancer drugs are more powerful when used in combination. More than 50 anticancer drugs are currently in use.
         a) Drugs of different actions can work together to kill more cancer cells.
         b) The use of multiple drugs can reduce the chance of developing a resistance to one particular drug.
         c) Drugs can be administered by mouth, intravenously, intramuscularly, or topically.
      2) Side effects vary with the drug and the client. They can include nausea, vomiting, fatigue, temporary hair loss, mouth sores or dryness, difficulty swallowing, diarrhea, and increased vulnerability to infection.

d. *Bone marrow transplantation* (BMT) and *peripheral blood stem cell transplantation* (PBSCT) are procedures that restore stem cells that have been destroyed by high doses of chemotherapy or radiation therapy (NCI, 2011).
   1) Autologous BMT: The client's own bone marrow is used.
   2) Allogeneic BMT: The client receives a donor's bone marrow.
      a) Syngeneic: Donor is an identical twin.
      b) Related: Donor is a relative.
      c) Unrelated: Donor is not a relative.
   3) The stem cells used in BMT come from the liquid center of the bone, called the marrow. The stem cells used in PBSCT come from the bloodstream.

e. Hormone therapy consists of drug treatment that interferes with hormone production or action to kill or slow the growth of cancer cells.

f. Biologic therapies (immunotherapy or biologic response modifier therapy) manipulate the immune system through the use of naturally occurring biologic substances or genetically engineered agents that promote or support the immune system's response to cancer.

g. Gene therapy manipulates genetic material inside cancerous cells to make them easier to destroy or prevent their growth, and in some approaches targets healthy cells to increase their ability to fight cancer (Virshup, 2010).

h. No alternative cancer treatments have been found to cure cancer; however, when used in conjunction with traditional therapies, they can relieve certain symptoms and side effects, and can include vitamins, herbs, dietary supplements, or procedures such as acupuncture (NCI, 2014a)
   1) Body work promotes relaxation and reduces cancer-related fatigue (e.g., massage, reflexology).
   2) Exercise controls fatigue, muscle tension, and anxiety.
   3) Mind-body medicine improves quality of life through behavior modification (e.g., guided imagery, hypnotherapy, biofeedback, art or music therapy).
   4) Acupuncture has been found to be effective in the management of chemotherapy-associated nausea and vomiting and in controlling pain associated with surgery (ACS, 2012; NCI, 2014a).

i. Nutrition and diet can play a role in cancer prevention, but no diet can cure cancer. A proper diet with vitamins, minerals, and other nutrients can inhibit the development of cancer by neutralizing carcinogens, ensuring proper immune function, and preventing tissue and cell damage.

3. Treatment of side effects
   a. Pain: The goal of pain management is to relieve suffering and control pain.
      1) Medication
         a) For mild to moderate pain: Nonopioids, including aspirin, acetaminophen, and nonsteroidal anti-inflammatory drugs such as ibuprofen and naproxen
         b) For moderate to severe pain
            (i) Opioids, including morphine, hydromorphone, oxycodone, hydrocodone, codeine, fentanyl, and methadone. A prescription is needed for these medicines. Nonopioids can be used along with opioids for moderate to severe pain.
            (ii) Adjunct medications
         c) For tingling and burning pain: Antidepressants, including amitriptyline, imipramine, doxepin, and trazodone; antiepileptics, including gabapentin and pregabalin
         d) For pain caused by swelling: Steroids, including prednisone and dexamethasone
      2) Other methods: Relaxation techniques, imagery, distraction, music, humor, biofeedback, and hypnosis
      3) Invasive techniques: Surgery, nerve block, acupuncture
   b. Nausea: Provide small, light meals throughout the day rather than heavy meals.
      1) Avoid gas-forming foods.
      2) Eat small, frequent meals to keep the stomach from feeling too full.
      3) Ginger candy, tea, or capsules
      4) Bland foods such as rice, applesauce, crackers, toast
      5) Cold or room-temperature foods
      6) Relaxation, imagery, and distraction techniques
      7) Antiemetics: Dronabinol (Marino®), ondansetron (Zofran®)
      8) Antiulcer medications: Ranitidine (Zantac®), sucralfate (Carafate®), metoclopramide (Reglan®)

9) Lorazepam (Ativan®) could produce adjunct antiemetic therapy.

c. Increased risk for infection
   1) Arises from underlying disease; side effects of treatment (e.g., neutropenia, immune suppression); disruption of mucous membranes or skin; presence of a long-term venous access device; impaired nutrition; and prolonged hospitalization
   2) Can be managed via prevention; prompt recognition of suspected infection; treatment of skin complications; administration of antibiotics, antifungals, or antiviral agents; fever management; or platelet or blood transfusion for bleeding

d. Fatigue
   1) Minimize symptoms that interfere with sleep.
   2) Avoid stimulants.
   3) Pace activities to save energy.
   4) Exercise.

e. Weight loss
   1) Can be caused by treatment side effects that impair nutritional status, uncontrolled pain that impairs appetite, or fatigue that affects the ability to obtain and eat food
   2) Can be treated according to the cause of the weight loss and the overall goals
   3) Can be treated with oral or parenteral nutritional supplementation and appetite-stimulating products

f. Pruritus
   1) Systemic histamine
   2) Topical corticosteroid cream can reduce localized urticaria; antifungal cream can be used for fungal infections.
   3) Tepid bath with aloe vera or oatmeal
   4) Creams containing aloe vera or lanolin for radiation dermatitis
   5) Stop medications suspected of causing pruritus.

g. Arm care precautions for women after breast or axillary surgery
   1) Perform range-of-motion exercises.
      a) Ensures full use and flexibility of the arm to help alleviate damage to the nerves and muscles that accompanies breast cancer surgery
      b) Reduces the risk and severity of lymphedema (i.e., the accumulation of lymph fluid in the tissues of the upper extremity after breast cancer surgery), which occurs most commonly in women with breast cancer who had axillary node dissection followed by radiation
   2) Avoid sunburn and burns while cooking, baking, or smoking.
   3) Wear protective gloves while gardening.
   4) Wear loose-fitting watches, jewelry, and clothing.
   5) Treat cuts immediately and monitor for signs of infection.
   6) Use the unaffected arm for intravenous access, blood draws, and blood pressure; avoid getting chemotherapy in the affected arm.
   7) Avoid carrying heavy objects with the affected arm.

h. Monitor for oncological emergencies: Hypercalcemia, disseminated intravascular coagulation, alterations in blood-clotting mechanisms, septic shock, pleural effusion, spinal cord compression, neoplastic cardiac tamponade, superior vena cava syndrome, elevated intracranial pressure, airway obstruction, urinary obstruction, massive hemoptysis (Monahan et al., 2007).

F. Clinical Management of Cancers Necessitating Rehabilitation

Cancer survival rates (5 years and greater) have increased in recent years as a result of early diagnosis, treatment options, and supportive services; however, most patients have residual challenges that would benefit from rehabilitation and rehabilitation nursing (Silver et al., 2013). Some specific cancers are more likely to require referral to rehabilitation, including:

1. Brain tumors (NCI, 2014b)
   a. Brain cancer is the second leading cause of cancer death in people younger than 20 years of age and accounts for 2% of all malignancies and 2.5% of all cancer deaths (Vogel, Wilson, & Melvin, 2004).
   b. Each year 35,000 people in the United States are diagnosed with a primary brain tumor.
   c. Metastasis to the brain is more common, with an incidence 10 times that of primary brain cancer (Vogel et al., 2004).
   d. Exposure to chemicals such as pesticides, herbicides, fertilizers, petrochemicals, and viruses; bioelectromagnetic fields and cellular telephones have been studied as potential contributors to brain cancer (Muscat et al., 2000; Vogel et al., 2004).
   e. Anaplastic astrocytoma and glioblastoma account for approximately 38% of primary brain tumors; meningiomas and other mesenchymal

tumors account for approximately 27% of these types of tumors.

f. Brain tumors have better outcomes in children than in adults.

g. Clinical manifestations vary according to the location and size of the tumor but can include headache; seizures; nausea and vomiting; memory deficit; and changes in speech, motor skills, and vision.

h. Diagnosis: Neurologic assessment, CT, MRI, biopsy

i. Treatment: Surgery, radiation therapy, and chemotherapy

   1) Chemotherapy can prolong survival in people with some tumor types and has been reported to lengthen disease-free survival in people with gliomas, medulloblastoma, and some germ-cell tumors.

   2) Complications of CNS surgery include intracranial bleeding, cerebral edema, infection, neuromotor deficits, thrombosis, and hydrocephalus.

2. Spinal cord tumors (Mayo Clinic, 2011)

   a. The spine is the third most common site for metastatic cancer, after the lungs and liver. Most tumors that affect the vertebrae have spread to the spine from another site in the body.

   b. Cancerous tumors that originate in the bones of the spine are far less common and include osteosarcomas (i.e., osteogenic sarcomas), the most common type of bone cancer in children, and Ewing's sarcoma, a particularly aggressive tumor that affects young adults.

   c. Spinal cord lymphomas are more common in people whose immune systems are compromised by medications or disease.

   d. Many cases of spinal cord tumors run in families. Examples of these hereditary tumors are neurofibromatosis 2 and Von Hippel-Lindau disease.

   e. Intradural-extramedullary tumors develop in the spinal cord's arachnoid membrane (meningiomas), in the nerve roots that extend out from the spinal cord (schwannomas and neurofibromas), or at the spinal cord base (filum terminale ependymomas).

   f. Intramedullary tumors begin in the supporting cells in the spinal cord. Most are either astrocytomas, which affect mainly children and adolescents, or ependymomas, the most common type of spinal cord tumor in adults.

   g. Clinical manifestations are related to the site and size of tumor and can include pain; weakness; sensory loss (e.g., numbness, decreased skin sensitivity to temperature); muscle spasms; and loss of bowel and bladder control. If left untreated, symptoms can progress to include muscle wasting and paralysis.

   h. Diagnosis: Neurologic assessment, CT, MRI, biopsy

   i. Treatment: Surgery, radiation therapy, and chemotherapy

3. Bone cancer (ACS, 2014b; Memorial Sloan Kettering Cancer Center, 2014; NCI, 2014c)

   a. Cancer that originates in the bone (primary bone cancer) is rare; cancer that spreads to the bones (metastatic cancer) from other parts of the body is more common.

      1) The three most common types of primary bone cancer are osteosarcoma, chondrosarcoma, and Ewing's sarcoma.

      2) Primary bone cancer can occur at any age but is more common in older children and young adults (ACS, 2014b). The likelihood of a cure for primary bone cancer depends on how early it is detected and how rapidly it spreads.

      4) Primary bone cancers make up a small percentage of all cancers, less than 0.20%.

      5) In 2014 there were an estimated 3,200 new cases of cancer of the bones and joints and 1,460 deaths from cancer in the United States (ACS, 2014a).

   b. Symptoms: A hard lump felt on the surface of the bone, pain (especially at night), swelling in bones and joint, spontaneous bone fracture, fever, weight loss, fatigue, and impaired mobility (Memorial Sloan Kettering Cancer Center, 2014; Monahan et al., 2007)

   c. Diagnosis: X rays, other imaging tests, and biopsy

   d. Treatment

      1) Surgical removal when possible. If the cancer is in the arm or leg, amputation usually is avoided, and the bone is reconstructed with a metal prosthesis.

      2) Radiation and chemotherapy

         a) Can be given before surgery to reduce the size of the tumor

         b) Can be used after surgery to kill remaining cells

         c) Used to treat inoperable bone cancer

      3) *Cryosurgery* is the use of liquid nitrogen to freeze and kill cancer cells. This technique

can sometimes be used instead of conventional surgery to destroy the tumor.

4) Therapy should begin as soon as possible to avoid stiffness and improve mobility, and if amputation was unavoidable, to help the client learn how to use the prosthesis.

e. Common types

1) Osteosarcoma

a) Tends to affect people between 10 and 30 years of age

b) Makes up approximately 35% of all primary bone cancers

c) Has an incidence rate twice as high in men as in women

d) Starts most often in bones of the arms, legs, or pelvis

2) Chondrosarcoma

a) Tends to attack middle-aged adults; not often found in people younger than 20 years of age

b) Originates in the cartilage cells

c) Most common sites: pelvic bone, long bones, and scapula

3) Ewing's family of tumors

a) Tend to occur in children and teenagers; not common in adults older than 30 years of age.

b) Occur most often in the white population and are extremely rare in African-American and Asian populations

c) About 60% of Ewing tumors start in bone, but others are found outside the bone in soft tissue.

d) Pelvis is the most common site.

4) Fibrosarcoma

a) Originates in soft tissue around the bones (i.e., ligaments, tendons, fat, and muscle)

b) Tends to occur in older and middle-aged adults

c) Originates most often in legs, arms, or jaw

G. Prehabilitation and Rehabilitation (Cancer.net, 2012; Monahan et al., 2007; Silver & Baima, 2013; Silver, Baima, Newman, Galantino, & Shockney, 2013)

The majority of cancer survivors report significant short- and long-term impairments related to their diagnosis and treatments. The majority of these impairments are reported to be physical rather than psychological; rehabilitation at any stage of cancer treatment can improve function and psychological distress, thereby reducing disability and maximizing independence and quality of life (Silver et al., 2013).

Rehabilitation of cancer patients should focus on the following:

1. Improve the quality of life and reduce impairments and disability for patients with cancer by
   a. Improving physical and emotional health (Silver & Baima, 2013)
   b. Encouraging independence and reducing reliance on caregivers
   c. Helping the person to adjust to actual, perceived, and potential losses due to the disease and treatment
   d. Reducing sleep problems
   e. Addressing pain issues related to cancer and treatments
   f. Decreasing hospitalization and readmissions (Silver et al., 2013)
   g. Identifying potential work issues and barriers to maintaining gainful employment, as more than 50% of adult cancer survivors are younger than 65 years of age (Silver et al., 2013)
2. Cancer rehabilitation should be patient-centered and include
   a. Client and family education and counseling
   b. Pain management
   c. Nutritional counseling
   d. Exercise programs to help build strength, endurance, and mobility
   e. Education and support related to risk factor reduction and elimination
   f. Education for activities of daily living (ADLs) as well as cooking and basic housekeeping with assistive devices as indicated.
3. The cancer rehabilitation team should include but not be limited to oncologist; physiatrist; rehabilitation nurses; therapists (e.g., physical, occupational, and speech), mental health professionals; and vocational counselors (Silver et al., 2013).

H. Nursing Process

1. Assessment
   a. History
      1) Signs and symptoms of underlying disease and side effects of treatment
      2) Pain quality, location, duration, intensity, and relieving factors
      3) Dietary evaluation with food preferences
      4) Use of complementary therapies
      5) Psychosocial evaluation (e.g., support systems, coping strategies)
   b. Complete physical and functional assessment to determine the degree of loss of function
2. Plan of care
   a. Nursing diagnoses

1) Risk of impaired skin integrity related to skin irritation during radiotherapy
2) Pain related to tumor causing pressure on nerves, metastases, and reaction from cancer therapy
3) Fatigue, balance disturbances, and gait changes, and deconditioning related to inactivity, poor nutrition, disease progression, and reaction to cancer treatment
4) Risk of inadequate nutrition related to side effects of cancer therapy
5) Risk of infection related to effects of therapy on bone marrow production of white blood cells and platelets
6) Anxiety related to diagnosis, prognosis, treatment, pain, and changes in body image and self-esteem
7) Ineffective individual coping related to diagnosis, fear, treatment, and pain
8) Ineffective family coping related to diagnosis, treatment, and fear
9) Fear related to prognosis and possible death
10) Anticipatory grieving related to cancer diagnosis and prognosis
11) Stressors related to finances and employment
12) Spiritual distress related to cancer diagnosis and prognosis

b. Goals, according to phase of illness
   1) Acute phase
      a) Demonstrate healthy lifestyle and remain free of signs and symptoms of infection.
      b) Identify and use effective strategies for coping with stressful situations and adjusting to illness.
      c) Verbalize understanding of the disease process and significant implications.
      d) Verbalize understanding of the treatment regimen and side effects.
      e) Verbalize discomfort.
   2) Intermittent or chronic phase
      a) Verbalize understanding of the prevention and management of side effects of the treatment regimen.
      b) Maintain maximal level of function.
      c) Demonstrate safety in mobility and use assistive devices as needed.
      d) Verbalize understanding of diet management, maintain present weight, and maintain fluid hydration.
      e) Verbalize discomfort.
   3) Palliative phase
      a) Maintain a desired level of comfort.
      b) Verbalize wishes and declare preferences regarding treatment options.
      c) Experience a dignified and comfortable death.

3. Interventions
   a. Acute phase: To attain remission, prevent and control side effects of treatment, promote health, and decrease disability
      1) Educate the client and family about the diagnosis, prognosis, treatment, side effects and symptoms, nutritional needs, risk of injury caused by immunosuppression medication, prevention of infections, and support groups.
      2) Provide emotional support by helping the client and family express grief.
      3) Minimize infection and use strategies to prevent infection.
      4) Provide education on pain-relief measures and complications.
      5) Maximize comfort and provide pain relief with prescribed analgesics; accepting the client's report of pain; using a consistent method or scale to evaluate pain; and providing nonpharmacological, complementary methods of pain control (e.g., imagery, distraction, relaxation, music).
      6) Assess psychological response to situations and provide emotional support by helping the client and family express grief.
      7) Ensure adequate hydration and nutrition with vitamin supplements.
      8) Assess employment and work issues (e.g., time off for treatment, health insurance coverage, and financial status) (Silver et al., 2013).
   b. Intermittent or chronic stage: To address side effects of treatment and complications
      1) Provide assistive devices for use in performing ADLs.
      2) Balance rest with activity to conserve energy and reduce fatigue.
      3) Prevent infection, adhere to strict hand-washing protocols, maintain aseptic technique, and monitor for signs and symptoms of infection, administering antimicrobial therapy as needed.
      4) Assess response to pain management and maintain comfort.
   c. Palliative and end-of-life care: To provide comfort, emotional support, and symptom management; promote a peaceful death

1) Neither hasten nor postpone death.
2) Assist with end-of-life comfort measures in a suitable care setting and with appropriate services (e.g., hospice).
3) Help the client achieve as full a life as possible, with relief from pain and other symptoms; administer pain medication to relieve pain and discomfort, antianxiety medication for anxiety and restlessness, and antiemetics for nausea and vomiting.
4) Offer support systems to help the client live as actively as possible until death.
5) Promote a calm environment.
6) Provide emotional and spiritual support to the client and significant others.
7) Maintain the client's dignity and honor the client's spiritual beliefs and wishes throughout the dying process.
8) Educate the client and significant others about the dying process.
9) Provide bereavement counseling for significant others.

4. Evaluation: Modify care according to the client's response to nursing interventions, focusing on quality of life and comfort. See **Table 26-5** for a comprehensive list of rehabilitation strategies for the cancer patient.

IV. Obesity

A. Overview (CDC, 2014c)

1. Obesity has become a public health crisis in the United States and the rest of the developed world.
2. Because many of the complications from excess weight are treated in postacute rehabilitation facilities (e.g., postcardiac surgery, post hip and knee replacement), rehabilitation nurses frequently care for patients who are overweight or obese (**Figure 26-4**).
3. Recent studies (Padwal, Wang, Sharma, & Dyer, 2012; Peitz, 2014) have shown that increased length of stay and costs are associated with severe obesity. Strategies to mitigate these effects are necessary and often part of a rehabilitation nurse's challenge in working with overweight and obese patients.
4. A recent study (Hammond et al., 2012) revealed that higher body mass index is one of the variables associated with readmission to acute care inpatient rehabilitation after traumatic spinal cord injury (SCI).
5. Another recent study (Arreghini, Manzoni, Castelnuovo, Santovito, & Capodaglio, 2014) showed that obese patients with fibromyalgia who undergo comprehensive rehabilitation could have lower functional capacities and increased self-perceived disability, and ultimately could require additional rehabilitation resources.
6. Rehabilitation nurses need to ensure that special accommodations for an overweight or obese patient can be arranged. The rehabilitation nurse needs to model sensitivity, realizing that a lack of proper hospital accommodations is a factor that can compound a general sense of inferiority among overweight or obese patients, who experience discrimination and feel stigmatized, and are thus less likely to seek health care in the future.

B. Obesity and Overweight Defined

1. Both the American Medical Association (Karns, 2013) and the American Association of Clinical Endocrinologists (2013) officially classify obesity as a disease.
2. *Obesity* is a disease with genetic, environmental, and behavioral determinants that confers increased morbidity and mortality. It requires a treatment that incorporates lifestyle, medical, and surgical options; balances risks and benefits; and emphasizes medical outcomes that address the complications of obesity rather than cosmetic goals (Garber et al., 2013).
3. Obesity represents a state of excess storage of body fat.
   a. Grade 1 overweight (also called overweight) is identified by a body mass index (BMI) of 25–29.9 kg/m^2.
   b. Grade 2 overweight (commonly called obesity) is identified by a BMI of 30–39 kg/m^2.
   c. Grade 3 overweight (commonly called morbid obesity) is identified by a BMI of 40 kg/m^2 or higher.
4. Some authorities advocate a definition of obesity based on percentage of body fat, as follows:
   a. Men: percentage of body fat greater than 25%, with 21%–25% being borderline.
   b. Women: percentage of body fat greater than 33%, with 31%–33% being borderline.
5. Obesity occurs when more calories are taken in than are burned through activity and exercise.
6. A waist circumference greater than 35 inches for women and 40 inches for men indicates obesity.
7. In children, being at the 85th percentile indicates overweight, and being at the 95th percentile indicates obesity for age- and sex-matched control subjects.

C. Prevalence, Incidence, and Trends (Jensen et al., 2013)

1. More than 78 million adults in the United States were obese during 2009–2010.

Table 26-5. Common Interdisciplinary Rehabilitation Team Strategies

Service	Purpose	Examples
Diagnostic imaging	Diagnose etiology of impairment	MRI for diagnosis of adhesive capsulitis or "frozen shoulder" in a patient with breast cancer
Electrodiagnosis	Diagnosis of a neuropathy or myopathy	Diagnose long thoracic nerve palsy or "winging scapula" in a patient with lung cancer
Cardiovascular conditioning	Mitigate fatigue	Treat postchemotherapy fatigue
Therapeutic exercise	Address specific muscle imbalances	Address shoulder dysfunction in a patient with head and neck cancer
Manipulation and soft-tissue mobilization	Improve range of motion	Address sequelae associated with radiation fibrosis syndrome
Thermal and electrical modalities	Control pain	TENS for neuropathic pain
Oral and topical analgesics	Control pain	Lidocaine patch for postthoracotomy pain
Injections and implantable pumps	Control pain	Phenol injection of splanchnic nerve for pancreatic cancer pain
Swallowing evaluation	Identify and improve swallowing impairments and avoid or reduce aspiration	Recommend dietary modifications in a patient with laryngeal cancer
Speech evaluation	Identify and improve speech and language impairments	Improve speech in a patient with brain metastasis in the left hemisphere
Assistive devices	Enhance function	Prescribe a reacher for a patient with loss of lumbar motion from metastasis
Orthotics	Compensate for weakness or limited range of motion to improve ambulation and avoid falls	Prescribe an ankle-foot orthosis for a patient with foot drop from neuropathy
Prosthetics	Replace amputated limb	Prescribe prosthesis for a patient with osteosarcoma
Home evaluation	Assess and improve safety of home environment	Assess functional mobility in the home including stairs, for a patient with fixation after metastasis to femur
Work evaluation	Evaluate and improve ability to perform essential job functions	Facilitate return to work after resection for a brain tumor
Driving evaluation	Assess and improve safe driving	Recommend adaptive equipment such as larger mirrors and sensors for a patient with head and neck cancer with limited cervical range of motion
Mental health counseling	Evaluate and improve psychological well-being	Recommend specific coping strategies for decreasing anxiety around returning to work
Neuropsychological testing	Evaluate cognitive deficits in "chemo brain"	Recommend rehabilitation interventions that focus on adaptive strategies to improve memory and concentration as well as function organization in daily life

Abbreviations. MRI, magnetic resonance imaging; TENS, transcutaneous electrical nerve stimulation.

From "Impairment-Driven Cancer Rehabilitation: An essential component of quality care and survivorship," by J. Silver, J. Baima and S. Mayer, 2013, *Cancer: A Journal for Clinicians, 63,* 300. Copyright 2013 American Cancer Society. Reprinted with permission.

2. Current estimates are that 69% of adults are either overweight or obese, and approximately 35.7% are obese.
3. National Health and Nutrition Examination Surveys report that obesity estimates for adult men and women during 2009–2010 did not differ significantly from the 2003–2008 period and that the increases in the prevalence rates of obesity appear to be slowing or leveling off. However, overweight and obesity continue to be highly prevalent in some racial and ethnic minority groups and in those with lower income and less education.
4. During the past 30 years, the prevalence of childhood obesity has more than doubled among children ages 2–5 years and has almost tripled among

Figure 26-4. Complications-Centric Model for Care of the Overweight/Obese Patient

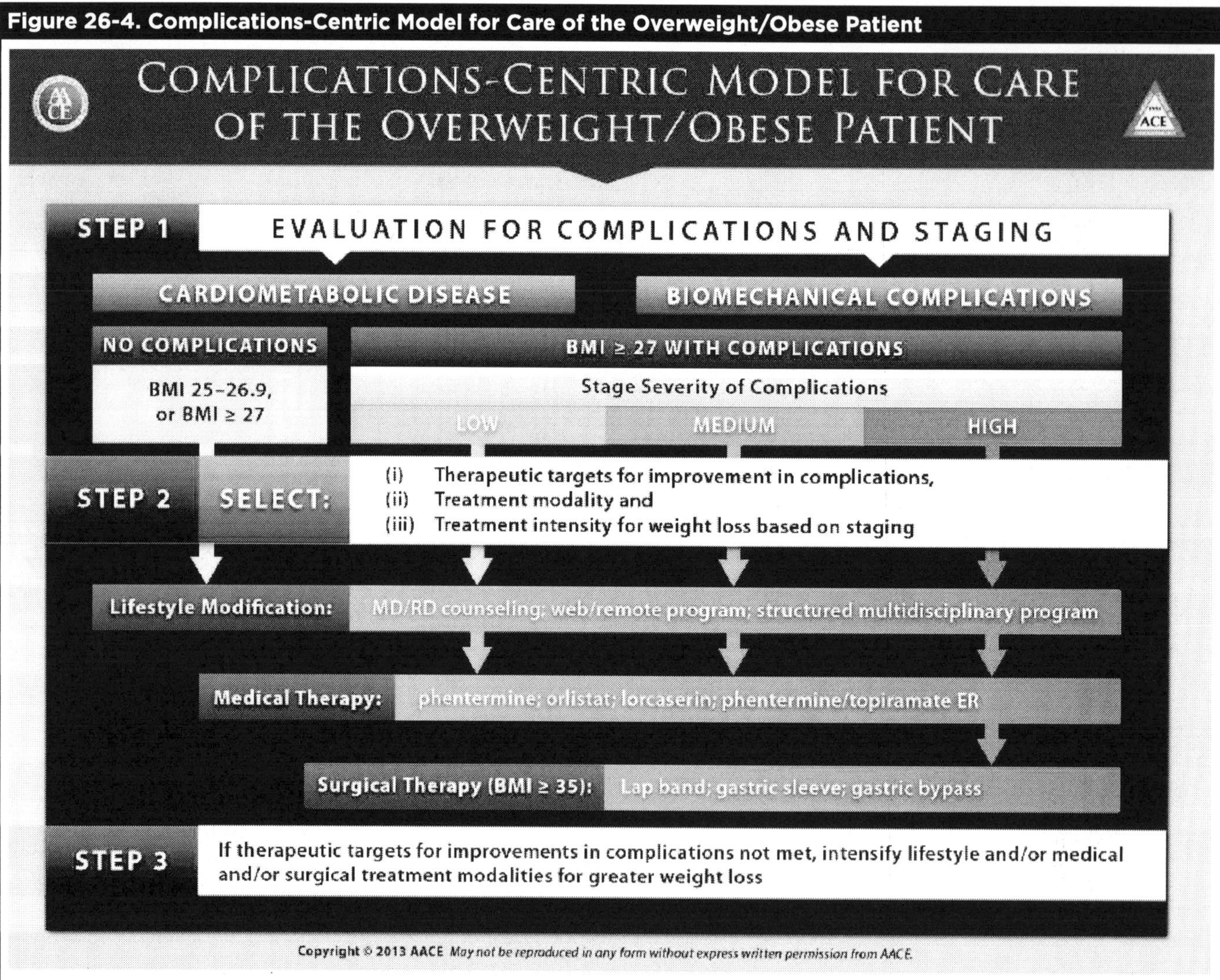

From "American Association of Clinical Endocrinologists comprehensive diabetes management algorithm," by A. J. Garber et al., 2013, *Endocrine Practice, 19*(Suppl. 2), 329. Retrieved from https://www.aace.com/files/aace_algorithm.pdf. Copyright 2013 by American Association of Clinical Endocrinologists. Reprinted with permission.

children ages 6–11 years and adolescents ages 12–19 years.

5. Pima Indians of Arizona and other Native-American populations have a particularly high incidence of obesity.
6. Polynesians, Micronesians, Anurans, Maoris of the West and East Indies, African Americans in North America, and Hispanic populations in North America have high predispositions to obesity.

D. Symptoms Associated with Obesity
   1. Difficulty sleeping
   2. Snoring
   3. Sleep apnea
   4. Joint or back pain
   5. Excessive sweating
   6. Always feeling hot
   7. Rashes or infection in folds of the skin
   8. Feeling out of breath with minor exertion
   9. Daytime sleepiness or fatigue
   10. Depression

E. Comorbidities (Hamdy, Citkowitz, Uwaifo, & Oral, 2014): The following comormidities can manifest with obese conditions:
   1. The American Association of Clinical Endocrinologists states that obesity-related comorbidities can be classified into two general categories:
      a. insulin resistance/cardiometabolic disease
      b. mechanical consequences of excess body weight (Garber et al., 2013)
   2. Respiratory: Obstructive sleep apnea, greater predisposition to respiratory infections, increased incidence of bronchial asthma, and Pickwickian syndrome (i.e., obesity hypoventilation syndrome)

3. Malignant: Association with endometrial, prostate, colon, breast, gall bladder, and possibly lung cancers
4. Psychological: Social stigmatization and depression
5. Cardiovascular: Coronary artery disease, essential hypertension, left ventricular hypertrophy, cor pulmonale, obesity-associated cardiomyopathy, accelerated atherosclerosis, and pulmonary hypertension of obesity
6. CNS: Stroke, idiopathic intracranial hypertension, and meralgia paresthetica
7. Obstetric and perinatal: Pregnancy-related hypertension, fetal macrosomia, and pelvic dystocia
8. Surgical: Increased surgical risk and postoperative complications, including wound infection, postoperative pneumonia, deep venous thrombosis, and pulmonary embolism
9. Pelvic: Stress incontinence
10. Gastrointestinal: Gall bladder disease (cholecystitis, cholelithiasis), nonalcoholic steatohepatitis, fatty liver infiltration, and reflux esophagitis
11. Orthopedic: Osteoarthritis, coxa vera, slipped capital femoral epiphyses, Blount disease and Legg-Calvé-Perthes disease, and chronic lumbago
12. Metabolic: Type 2 diabetes mellitus, prediabetes, metabolic syndrome, and dyslipidemia
13. Reproductive (in women): Anovulation, early puberty, infertility, hyperandrogenism, and polycystic ovaries
14. Reproductive (in men): Hypogonadotropic hypogonadism
15. Cutaneous: Intertrigo (bacterial and/or fungal), acanthosis nigricans, hirsutism, and increased risk for cellulitis and carbuncles
16. Extremity: Venous varicosities, lower-extremity venous and/or lymphatic edema
17. Miscellaneous: Reduced mobility and difficulty maintaining personal hygiene

F. Known causes of and theories about obesity (CDC, 2014b)

1. Energy imbalance: eating too many calories and not getting enough physical activity
2. Body weight is the result of genes, metabolism, behavior, environment, culture, and socioeconomic status.
3. Hormonal imbalance
4. Genetics and gender differences
5. Altered metabolism

G. Secondary Causes of Obesity

1. Hypothyroidism
2. Cushing's syndrome
3. Insulinoma
4. Hypothalamic obesity
5. Polycystic ovarian syndrome
6. Genetic syndromes such as Prader-Willi, Alström's, Bardet-Biedl, Cohen's, Börjeson-Forssman-Lehmann, and Fröhlich's syndromes; and growth hormone deficiency
7. Oral contraceptive use
8. Pregnancy
9. Medications such as phenothiazines, sodium valproate, carbamazepine, tricyclic antidepressants, lithium, glucocorticoids, megestrol acetate, thiazolidinediones, sulfonylureas, insulin, adrenergic antagonists, serotonin antagonists
10. Smoking cessation
11. Eating disorders such as binge eating, bulimia nervosa, night eating disorder
12. Hypogonadism
13. Pseudohypoparathyroidism
14. Tube-feeding–related obesity
15. Traumatic brain injury
16. SCI

H. Assessment

1. Evaluate the following:
   a. Metabolic factors
   b. Genetic factors
   c. Level of activity
   d. Behavior
   e. Endocrine factors
   f. Race, gender, age factors
   g. Ethnic and cultural factors
   h. Socioeconomic status
   i. Dietary habits
   j. Smoking cessation
   k. Pregnancy and menopause
   l. Psychological factors
   m. History of gestational diabetes
   n. Evaluation for the aforementioned secondary causes
2. Consider the following clinical problems that might have similar findings: Dercum's disease, partial lipodystrophies, mesomorphic body states, anasarca (severe edema).
3. Laboratory tests: With no comorbidities, tests will be normal, but comorbid problems should be ruled out.
   a. Full lipid panel: At a minimum, test fasting cholesterol, triglycerides, and HDL cholesterol levels. These levels can be normal, or the typical dyslipidemia associated with metabolic syndrome X could be found. This is characterized by low HDL, elevated LDLs, normal to marginally elevated total cholesterol, and elevated fasting triglyceride concentrations.

b. Hepatic panel: This test is expected to yield normal results, but findings could be abnormal (e.g., elevated transaminase levels in the setting of nonalcoholic steatohepatitis or fatty infiltration of the liver).

c. Thyroid function: The results are typically normal, but checking them to detect primary hypothyroidism (characterized by elevated serum thyrotropin and normal or low levothyroxine or triiodothyronine levels) is worthwhile. Hypothyroidism rarely causes more than mild obesity.

d. Fasting glucose and HbA1c: Obesity and insulin resistance go hand in hand.

I. Treatment

1. The American Association of Clinical Endocrinologists (Garber et al., 2013) advocates its complications-centric model for care of the overweight/obese patient (Figure 26-4).
2. Recommended goals for weight loss (Jensen et al., 2013)
    a. A realistic and meaningful weight loss goal is an important first step.
    b. Sustained weight loss of as little as 3%–5% of body weight can lead to clinically meaningful reductions in some cardiovascular disease (CVD) risk factors. More weight loss produces even greater benefits.
    c. Weight loss requires creating an energy deficit through caloric restriction, physical activity, or both.
    d. Energy deficit of ≥ 500 kcal/day typically can be achieved with dietary intake of 1,200 to 1,500 kcal/day for women and 1,500 to 1,800 kcal/day for men.
    e. The choice of a calorie-restricted diet can be individualized based on the patient's preferences and health status. Very low-calorie diets (< 800 kcal/day) should be used only in limited circumstances in a medical care setting, where medical supervision and a high-intensity lifestyle intervention can be provided.
    f. If a specialized diet for CVD risk reduction, diabetes, or other medical conditions is also prescribed, referral to a nutrition professional is recommended.
    g. Recommendations for management of medical conditions during weight loss: While weight loss treatment is ongoing, manage risk factors such as hypertension, dyslipidemia, and other obesity-related conditions. Monitor the patient's requirements for medication change as weight loss progresses, particularly for antihypertensive medications and diabetes medications that can cause hypoglycemia.
3. Dietary changes: Work with dietitian to decide best dietary changes.
    a. Prescribe a calorie-restricted diet for obese and overweight individuals who would benefit from weight loss, based on the patient's preferences and health status, and preferably, refer patient to a nutrition professional for counseling.
    b. A variety of dietary approaches can produce weight loss in overweight and obese adults (Jensen et al., 2013).
    c. Advise overweight and obese individuals who would benefit from weight loss to participate for ≥ 6 months in a comprehensive lifestyle program that assists participants in comprehensive weight loss interventions provided in individual or group sessions by a trained interventionist.
    d. Electronically delivered weight loss programs (including by telephone) that include personalized feedback from a trained interventionist can be prescribed for weight loss but could result in less weight loss than face-to-face interventions could promote.
    e. Some commercially based programs that provide a comprehensive lifestyle intervention can be prescribed as an option for weight loss, provided they are peer-reviewed, and published evidence exists regarding their safety and efficacy.
    f. Use a very low calorie diet (defined as < 800 kcal/day) only in limited circumstances and only when provided by trained practitioners in a medical care setting where medical monitoring and high-intensity lifestyle intervention can be provided. Medical supervision is required because of the rapid rate of weight loss and potential for health complications.
    g. For weight loss maintenance, prescribe face-to-face or telephone-delivered weight loss maintenance programs that provide regular contact (monthly or more frequently) with a trained interventionist who helps participants engage in high levels of physical activity (i.e., 200–300 minutes/week), monitor body weight regularly (i.e., weekly or more frequently), and consume a reduced-calorie diet (needed to maintain lower body weight).
4. Bariatric surgical treatment for obesity (Schauer et al., 2014a). Adults with a BMI ≥ 40, or those with a BMI ≥ 35 with obesity-related comorbid

conditions who are motivated to lose weight, have not responded to behavioral treatment with or without pharmacotherapy, and have had sufficient weight loss to achieve targeted health outcome goals, can opt for bariatric surgery consideration. This treatment could be an appropriate option to improve health and should be offered along with a referral to an experienced bariatric surgeon for consultation and evaluation.

b. For individuals with a BMI < 35, there is insufficient evidence to recommend for or against undergoing bariatric surgical procedures.

c. Advise patients that choice of a specific bariatric surgical procedure can be affected by patient factors including age, severity of obesity/BMI, obesity-related comorbid conditions, other operative risk factors, risk of short- and long-term complications, behavioral and psychosocial factors, patient tolerance for risk, and provider factors (e.g., surgeon and facility).

d. Quality-of-life measures were significantly better in the bariatric therapy groups than in the medical-therapy group (Schauer et al., 2014).

e. A recent study showed that in obese patients with uncontrolled type 2 diabetes, 3 years of intensive medical therapy plus bariatric surgery resulted in glycemic control in significantly more patients than those that did medical therapy alone (Schauer et al., 2014).

5. Increased physical activity
   a. Exercise is vital to any weight management program, because it helps build muscle mass and increase metabolic activity of the entire body mass.
   b. Exercise helps reduce body fat proportions and decreases the amount of compensatory muscle mass loss.
   c. Consistent moderate exercise is important in maintaining weight and improving overall cardiopulmonary fitness.
   d. Clients should undergo cardiovascular and pulmonary screening before undergoing any exercise program.
6. Behavior changes: The effectiveness depends on both a highly motivated client and a dedicated counselor who is willing to maintain long-term follow-up.
7. Prescription medications (Garber et al., 2013)
   a. Weight-loss medications can be used in combination with lifestyle modification for all patients with a BMI ≥ 27 kg/m^2 and comorbidities. Two drugs, lorcaserin HCL (Belviq®) and phentermine/topiramate (Qsymia®) extended-release (ER), have been approved by the FDA as adjuncts to lifestyle modification in overweight/obese patients.
   b. Both drugs have been shown to improve blood pressure, triglyceride levels, and insulin sensitivity; prevented progression to diabetes during the research period; and improved glycemic control and lipids in patients with type 2 diabetes.
   c. Other medications used to help with weight loss are phentermine and orlistat (Yanovski, 2014).
      1) Orlistat/tetrahydrolipstatin is a prescription drug sold under the trade name Xenical® and over-the-counter as Alli®. Its primary function is preventing the absorption of fats by acting as a lipase inhibitor, thereby reducing caloric intake. It is intended for use in conjunction with a healthcare-provider-supervised, reduced-calorie diet. Alli was recalled from the market in March 2014 due to product tampering, and at the time of this writing has not yet returned to the market.
      2) Phentermine, the name of which is a contraction of phenyl-tertiary-butylamine, is a psychostimulant drug of the phenethylamine class, with pharmacology similar to amphetamine. It is approved as an appetite suppressant to help reduce weight in obese patients when used short term and combined with exercise, diet, and behavioral modification. It is typically prescribed for individuals who are at increased medical risk due to their weight.
8. Population-based strategies that improve social and physical environmental contexts for healthful eating and physical activity are helpful for the entire population (National Institutes of Health [NIH], 2013).
   a. The "EatPlayGrow" curriculum combines the latest science and research from the NIH with the Children's Museum of Manhattan's creative educational approach to teach children ages 2–5 and their parents how to make healthy living choices that are fun and easy to include in daily routines (NIH, 2013).
   b. The "We Can!" and "Let's Move!" programs offer ways to enhance children's activity and nutrition (NIH, 2013).

J. Maintaining Weight Loss (American Heart Association, 2014)

1. To successfully and healthfully achieve weight loss and keep weight off, most people need to continue to learn to use nutritious foods and follow a healthy preparation routine.
2. Use healthy guidelines to make smart choices that benefit the heart and overall health.
3. Get tips on staying heart smart and making healthy food choices at the store.
4. Learn to eat healthfully when dining out.
5. Learn how to read and understand food labels to help make good choices.
6. Regular physical activity that includes 30–60 minutes of moderate-intensity aerobic physical activity, such as brisk walking every day, is highly recommended. Before starting any new physical activity program, the client should first consult with his or her primary physician and/or exercise therapist.
7. Regular muscle-strengthening activities that work all major muscle groups (i.e., legs, hips, back, abdomen, chest shoulders, and arms) will help maintain weight loss, reduce abdominal fat, and preserve muscle mass.

K. Rehabilitation Nursing Key Requirements
1. Provide bariatric furniture and equipment (e.g., commodes, wheelchairs, beds, walkers).
2. Know your facility's safe client handling and moving policy and procedures.
3. Increase the number of staff to assist with procedures, transfers, and moves.
4. Use bariatric lifts and assistive devices for your safety and that of the client.
5. Use blood pressure cuffs that are large enough for your client.
6. Perform frequent skin inspections, turning, and repositioning. Remember to keep skin creases/folds clean and dry.
7. Treat your client with dignity and respect

L. Plan of Care: In addition to the rehabilitation plan of care, the client who is obese has the following needs:
1. Nursing diagnoses
   a. Ineffective individual coping related to denial and depression
   b. Knowledge deficit related to causes of weight gain and treatments for obesity
   c. Self-care deficits related to the following:
      1) Physical, social, economic, and psychological barriers and limitations
      2) Lack of knowledge about complications of obesity
      3) Lack of financial and social support systems
      4) Lack of knowledge about follow-up needs and prevention of further complications related to the disease process
   d. Altered nutritional intake (more than a body needs) related to lack of awareness about serving sizes, limited self-discipline, and noncompliance with dietary guidelines
   e. Activity intolerance related to sedentary lifestyle
2. Goals
   a. State barriers to and develop methods of effective coping to avoid overeating.
   b. Verbalize an understanding of the relationship between weight loss, weight control, and exercise.
   c. Achieve modest weight loss with the help of medical and nutritional consultation to rule out risks.
   d. Identify behavioral modification strategies to avoid overeating.
   e. Practice selecting proper serving sizes of favorite foods.
   f. Identify individual concerns with and compensate for sexual dysfunction.
   g. Identify and obtain needed adaptive equipment.
   h. Exercise as individualized and prescribed by physician and/or exercise therapist.
3. Interventions
   a. Teach coping strategies (e.g., stress management, humor, breathing exercises, support groups).
   b. Discuss current eating habits and strategies to reduce calorie intake.
   c. Promote identification and selection of proper food choices.
   d. Discuss cues that promote eating. Identify strategies to eliminate or reduce these cues.
   e. Teach the strategy of keeping a food diary to monitor dietary pattern changes.
   f. Discuss the role of exercise in weight loss and maintenance.
   g. Instruct the client to keep an exercise record to document time and intensity of exercise.
   h. Teach survival skills, and suggest follow-up education and self-management support as needed after discharge from the hospital.
   i. Discuss follow-up care, lifestyle, and behavior modification strategies to promote successful weight loss.
   j. Discuss fact that the greater the BMI and waist circumference, the greater the risk of CVD,

type 2 diabetes, and all-cause mortality (Jensen et al., 2013).

k. Teach that lifestyle changes that produce even modest, sustained weight loss of 3–5% produce clinically meaningful health benefits such as reductions in triglycerides, blood glucose, and HbAIC, as well as prevention of type 2 diabetes. Greater weight loss reduces blood pressure; improves LDL-C and HDL-C levels; reduces the need for medications to control blood pressure, glucose, and lipids; and further reduces triglycerides and blood glucose levels.

V. Advanced Practice for Specific Disease Processes that Warrant Rehabilitation Interventions

A. Clinician

1. The goal of treatment is to prevent the onset of disease process or injury through education about healthy living, reduction of risk factors, support and treatment of symptoms, and prevention of further complications.
2. Assess history, clinical presentation, and current treatment.
3. Complete a physical examination.
4. Assess effectiveness of treatment and medications.
5. Assess psychosocial and economic factors that could influence the management of the disorder or injury.
6. Assess coping mechanisms and available support systems.
7. Follow up with the client as needed according to the progression of the disease, complications, and effects of current treatment.
8. Role model use of evidence in practice.

B. Educator

1. Educate the client, family, and significant others about the disease process, course, signs and symptoms, and treatment options.
2. Provide education about prescribed medications and adverse effects.
3. Discuss prevention strategies, emphasizing the need to reduce risk factors that can be changed.
4. Educate and encourage participation in local and national support groups.
5. Teach the client, family, and significant others to assist with active and passive exercises to prevent further complications and maintain independence in mobility and ADLs.
6. Teach the importance of eating a nutritious diet according to the disorder and injury.
7. Encourage regular rest periods and daily activity, and teach the client to balance rest with activity to prevent fatigue.

C. Leader

1. Provide in-service education to interdisciplinary staff in acute care about specific disease processes, clinical manifestations, interventions, and treatment options.
2. Provide community education about disease prevention, healthy living, specific disease processes, treatment options, and prevention of further complications.
3. Update protocols and procedures, and implement changes in practice reflecting evidence-based practice.
4. Participate in research and translate research into practice.
5. Keep abreast of current literature and disseminate appropriate articles to clinical staff.
6. Actively participate in specialty nursing organizations that focus on policy and practice.
7. Consider implementing journaling clubs.

D. Consultant

1. Refer to or consult with a specialist (e.g., neurologist, urologist, oncologist, burn specialist, HIV and AIDS specialist, endocrinologist, or obesity surgeon) for an evaluation and complete workup.
2. Function as a liaison with community health professionals.
3. Refer to a national organization or chapters for education and support.
   a. American Diabetes Association: www.diabetes.org
   b. American Association of Diabetes Educators: http://aadenet.org/
   c. National Diabetes Education Program: www.ndep.nih.gov/
   d. CDC National Diabetes Fact Sheets: www.cdc.gov/diabetes/pubs/factsheet.htm
   e. National Association of People with AIDS: www.napwa.org/
   f. CDC HIV/AIDS: www.cdc.gov/hiv/
   g. American Cancer Society: www.cancer.org/
   h. American Association for Cancer Research: www.aacr.org/
   i. National Cancer Institute: www.cancer.gov/
   j. The American Obesity Association: www.obesity.org/
4. Refer to and collaborate with the rehabilitation team for therapy.
5. Refer the client and family for psychological counseling to help them cope with the diagnosis and prognosis.
6. Serve as a client and family advocate.
7. Serve as a resource to staff.

E. Researcher
   1. Review current research on significant diagnostic categories.
   2. Participate in clinical research studies as appropriate and available.
   3. Help staff nurses develop research questions.
   4. Serve as a mentor for staff nurses regarding quality improvement, evidence-based practice, and research.
   5. Locate evidence for staff nurses to assist with bedside research.
   6. Facilitate system change to support use of evidence-based practice.
   7. Support research at the bedside (or clinic).

References

American Association of Clinical Endocrinologists (2013, May/June). Task force on the new comprehensive diabetes algorithm. *Endocrine Practice, 19*(Suppl 2), 1–48.

American Cancer Society (2012). Signs and symptoms of cancer. Retrieved from www.cancer.org/cancer/cancerbasics/signs-and-symptoms-of-cancer

American Cancer Society (2013). A backyard chef's guide to healthier grilling. Retrieved from http://www.cancer.org/cancer/news/features/a-backyard-chefs-guide-to-healthy-grilling

American Cancer Society (2014a). Cancer facts and figures 2014. Retrieved from http://www.cancer.org/acs/groups/content/@research/documents/webcontent/acspc-042151.pdf

American Cancer Society (2014b). What are the most common types of childhood cancer? Retrieved from http://www.cancer.org/cancer/cancerinchildren/detailedguide/cancer-in-children-types-of-childhood-cancers

American Diabetes Association. (2015). Standards of care in diabetes 2015. *Diabetes Care,* 38(S1), S1-S2. Retrieved from http://care.diabetesjournals.org/content/38/Supplement_1/S1.full

American Diabetes Association (2014a). Standards of medical care in diabetes: 2014. *Diabetes Care, 37*(Suppl. 1). S14–S80.

American Diabetes Association (2014b). Insulin pumps. Retrieved from http://www.diabetes.org/living-with-diabetes/treatment-and-care/medication/insulin/insulin-pumps.html

American Diabetes Association (2014c). Oral Medications: What Are My Options? Retrieved from http://www.diabetes.org/living-with-diabetes/treatment-and-care/medication/oral-medications/what-are-my-options.html

American Diabetes Association (2015). *Diabetes Care,* January 2015 38:S1-S2; doi:10.2337/dc15-S001

American Heart Association (2014). Losing Weight. Retrieved from http://www.heart.org/HEARTORG/GettingHealthy/WeightManagement/LosingWeight/Losing-Weight_UCM_307904_Article.jsp

Arreghini, M., Manzoni, G. M., Castelnuovo, G., Santovito, C., & Capodaglio, P. (2014). Impact of fibromyalgia on functioning in obese patients undergoing comprehensive rehabilitation. *PLOS ONE,* March 11, 2014. doi:10.1371/journal.pone.0091392. Retrieved from http://www.plosone.org/article/info%3Adoi%2F10.1371%2Fjournal.pone.0091392

Association of Rehabilitation Nurses (ARN). (2014). *ARN competency model for professional rehabilitation nursing.* Retrieved from http://www.rehabnurse.org/uploads/files/education/ARN_Rehabilitation_Nursing_Competency _Model_FINAL_-_May_2014.pdf

Avert.org (2010). HIV Types, Subtypes Groups and Strains. Retrieved from www.avert.org/hiv-types.htm

Boucher, J. L., & Evert, A. B. (2014). Diabetes nutrition therapy recommendations emphasize importance of individualized approach. *AADE In Practice.* March 2014, 20–28.

Cancer.Net (2012). Rehabilitation. Retrieved from www.cancer.net/patient/Survivorship/Rehabilitation

Centers for Disease Control and Prevention (2012). Draft recommendations: Diagnostic laboratory testing for HIV infections in the United States. Retrieved from http://www..gov/hiv/pdf/policies_Draft_HIV_Testing_Alg_Rec_508.2.pdf

Centers for Disease Control and Prevention (2013). HIV-AIDS in the United States: At a glance. Retrieved from http://www.cdc.gov/hiv/statistics/basics/ataglance.html

Centers for Disease Control and Prevention, (201a). National Diabetes Statistics Report, 2014. Retrieved from http://www.cdc.gov/diabetes/pubs/statsreport14/national-diabetes-report-web.pdf

Centers for Disease Control and Prevention. (2014b). Adult obesity facts. Retreived from http://www.cdc.gov/obesity/data/adult.html

Centers for Disease Control and Prevention (2014c). About HIV/AIDS. Retrieved from http://www.cdc.gov/hiv/basics/whatishiv.html

Cobaugh, D. J., Maynard, G., Cooper, L., Kienle, P. C., Vigersky, R., Childers, D., Cohen, M., et al. (2013). Enhancing insulin-use safety in hospitals: Practical recommendations from an ASHP Foundation expert consensus panel. *American Journal of Health-System Pharmacy, 70,* 1404–1413. doi:10.2146/ajhp130169. Retrieved from http://www.ajhp.org

Cochran, E. K., Valentine, V., Samaan, K. H., Corey, I. B., & Jackson, J. A. (2014). Practice tips and tools for the successful use of U-500 regular human insulin the diabetes educator is key. *The Diabetes Educator, 40*(2), 153–165.

Doheny, K. (2014). Inhaled insulin: What to tell patients. Medscape Multispecialty. Retreived from http://www.medscape.com/viewarticle/827637

Fan, H. Y., Conner, R. F., & Villarreal, L. P. (2011). *AIDS science and society* (6th ed.). Sudbury, MA: Jones & Bartlett.

Gale, E. A. M. (2014). Epidemiology of type 1 diabetes [internet]. (Aug 13); Diapedia 2104085168 rev. no. 39.http://dx.doi.org/10.14496/dia.2104085168.395. Retreived from http://www.diapedia.org/type-1-diabetes-mellitus/epidemiology-of-type-1-diabetes

Garber, A. J., Abrahamson, M. J., Batzilary, J. I., Blonde, L. Bloomgarden, Z. T., Bush, M. A.,…Davidson, M. H. (2013). American Association of Clinical Endocrinologists' comprehensive diabetes management algorithm. *Endocrine Practice, 19*(Suppl. 2), 329. Retrieved from https://www.aace.com/files/aace_algorithm.pdf

Hamdy, O., Citkowitz, E., Uwaifo, G. I., & Oral, E. A. (2014). Obesity: practice essentials. Retreived from http://emedicine.medscape.com/article/123702-overview#showall

Hammond, F. M., Demail, M., Horn, S. D., Smout, R. J., Chen, D., DeJong, G.,…Bloomgarden, J. J., (2012). Acute rehospitalizations during inpatient rehabilitation for spinal cord injury. *Archives of Physical Medicine and Rehabilitation. 94*(4), S98–S105. Retrieved from http://www.scholars.northwestern.edu/pubDetail.asp?id=84875421820&u_id=3719

Hanahan D., & Weinberg R. (2000). The hallmarks of cancer. *Cell, 100* (1), 57–70. doi: http://dx.doi.org/10.1016/S0092-8674(00)81683-9

Health-Disease.org. (2011). Acquired immunodeficiency syndrome: Causes and treatment. Retrieved from www.health-disease.org/immune-disorders/acquired-immunodificiency-syndrome.htm.

Jensen, M. D., Ryan, D. H., Apovian, C. M., Loria, C. M., Ard, J. D., Millen, B. E.,…Yanovski, S. Z. (2013). AHA/ACC/TOS guideline for the management of overweight and obesity in adults. *Journal of the American College of Cardiology.* doi:10.1016/j.jacc.2013.11.004

Karns, B. (2013). The American Medical Association classifies obesity as a disease, overriding committees' recommendations that better measurement metrics and research are needed. Retreived from http://www.healthline.com/health-news/policy-ama-says-obesity-is-not-a-disease-061813

Kirkman, M. S., Briscoe, V. J., Clark, N., Flores, H., Haas, L. B., Halter, J. B.,...Swift, C. S. (2012). Diabetes in older adults. *Diabetes Care, 35*(12), 2650 –2664.

Lee, S., Ko, J., Tan, X., Patel, I., Balkrishnan, R., & Chang, J. (2014). Markov chain modeling analysis of HIV/AIDS progression: A race-based forecast in the United States. *Indian Journal of Pharmaceutical Sciences, 76*(2), 107–115. Retrieved from http://www.ncbi.nlm.nih.gov/pmc/articles/PMC4023279/

Leach, C. (2013). Medtronic's "artificial pancreas" gains FDA approval. *Insulin Nation.* Retreived from http://insulinnation.com/treatment2/artificial-pancreas/medtronics-artificial-pancreas-gains-fda-approval/

Lewis, S. M., Heitkemper, M. M., & Dirksen, S. R. (2004*). Medical-surgical nursing: Assessment and management of clinical problems* (6th ed.). St. Louis: Mosby.

Lyssenks V., & Laakso, M. (2013). Genetic screening for the risk of Type 2 Diabetes. Worthless or valuable? *Diabetes Care, 36*(Supple. 2) S120–S126. Retrieved from http://care.diabetesjournals.org/content/36/Supplement_2/S120.full.pdf+htm

Martz, K., Keresztes, K., Tatschl, C., Nowotny, M., Dachenhausen, A., Brainin, M., & Tuomilehto, J. (2006). Disorders of glucose metabolism in acute stroke patients: An underrecognized problem. *Diabetes Care, 29,* 792–797.

Mayo Clinic (2011). Spinal tumor. Retrieved from www.mayoclinic.com/health/spinal-tumor/DS00594

Meece, J. D., Pearson, T. & L. Siminerio, L. M. (2014). Complementary approaches to improving glucose control-insulin and incretins: Patient case studies in action. *The Diabetes Educator, 40*(Suppl. 1), 4s–26s.

Memorial Sloan Kettering Cancer Center (2014). About primary bone cancer. Retrieved from http://www.mskcc.org/cancer-care/adult/bone/about-primary-bone

Monahan, F. D., Sands, J. K., Neighbors, M., Marek, J. F., & Green, C. J. (2007). *Phipps' medical-surgical nursing: Health and illness perspectives* (8th ed.). St. Louis: Mosby Elsevier.

Muscat, J. E., Malkin, M. G., Thompson, S., Shore, R. E., Stellman, S. D., McRee, D.,...Winder, E. L. (2000). Handheld cellular telephone use and the risk of brain cancer. *Journal of the American Medical Association, 284,* 3001–3007.

National Cancer Institute (2011). Common cancer types. Retrieved from www.cancer.gov/cancertopics/types/commoncancers

National Cancer Institute. (2013). Bone marrow transplantation and peripheral blood stem cell transplantation. Retrieved from www.cancer.gov/cancertopics/factsheet/Therapy/bone-marrow-transplant. National Cancer Institute (2014a). Acupuncture (PDQ®). Retrieved from www.cancer.gov/cancertopics/pdq/cam/acupuncture/HealthProfessional/allpages#Section_1

National Cancer Institute (2014b). Adult brain tumors treatment (PDQ). Retrieved from http://www.cancer.gov/cancertopics/pdq/treatment/adultbrain/HealthProfessional.

National Cancer Institute (2014c). Bone cancer. Retrieved from http://www.cancer.gov/cancertopics/factsheet/Sites-Types/bone

National Cancer Institute (2014d). Cancer prevention overview. Retrieved from www.cancer.gov/cancertopics/pdq/prevention/overview/healthprofessional

National Cancer Institute (2014e). What is cancer? Defining cancer. Retrieved from www.cancer.gov/cancertopics/what-is-cancer

National Institutes of Health (2013). My five senses early childhood health lesson. Retreived from http://www.nhlbi.nih.gov/health/educational/wecan/tools-resources/eatplaygrow-fivesenses.htm

Nirantharakumar, K., Saeed, M., Ian, W., Marshall, T., & Coleman, J. J. (2013). In-hospital mortality and length of stay in patients with diabetes having foot disease. *Journal of Diabetes and Its Complications, 27*(5), 454–458. doi:10.1016/j.jdiacomp.2013.05.003 Retrieved from http://www.jdcjournal.com/article/S1056-8727(13)00111-6/abstract

Padwal, R. S., Wang, X., Sharma, A. M., & Dyer, D. (2012). The impact of severe obesity on post-acute rehabilitation efficiency, length of stay, and hospital costs. *Journal of Obesity, 2012.* Article ID 972365. doi:10.1155/2012/972365

Panel on Antiretroviral Guidelines for Adults and Adolescents (2014). *Guidelines for the use of antiretroviral agents in HIV-1-infected adults and adolescents* (pp. 1–161). Washington, D.C.: Department of Health and Human Services. Retrieved from www.aidsinfo.nih.gov/ContentFiles/AdultandAdolescentGL.pdf

Peitz, G. W. (2014). Obesity may increase costs, hospital stay in patients with chest pain, dyspnea. Circulation: Cardiovascular Quality and Outcomes. doi:10.1161/CIRCOUTCOMES.113.000702. Retrieved from http://www.healio.com/cardiology/chd-prevention/news/print/cardiology-today/%7B4d905982-4a2f-4b15-a9d2-655be5e5e27d%7D/obesity-may-increase-costs-hospital-stay-in-patients-with-chest-pain-

Rote, N., & Huether, S. (2010). Infection. In K. McCance & S. Huether (Eds.), *Pathophysiology: The biological basis for disease in adults and children* (6th ed., pp. 293–326). Maryland Heights, MO: Mosby Elsevier.

Schauer, P. R., Bhatt, D. L., Kirwan, J. P., Wolski, K., Brethauer, S. A., Navaneethan, S. D., ... Kashyap, S. R. (March 31, 2014). Bariatric surgery versus intensive medical therapy for diabetes— 3-year outcomes. *New England Journal of Medicine.* 2002–2013. doi: 10.1056/NEJMoa1401329. Retrieved from http://www.nejm.org/doi/pdf/10.1056/NEJMoa1401329

Silver, J., & Baima, J. (2013). Cancer prehabilitation: An opportunity to decrease treatment-related morbidity, increase cancer treatment options, and improve physical and psychological health outcomes. *American Journal of Physical Medicine and Rehabilitation, 92*(8), 715–727. doi: 10.1097/PHM.0b013e31829b4afe

Silver, J., Baima, J., & Mayer, S. (2013). Impairment driven cancer rehabilitation: An essential component of quality care and survivorship. *Cancer: A Journal for Clinicians* (63), 295–317. doi: 10.3322/caac.21186

Silver, J., Baima, J., Newman, R., Galantino, M., & Shockney, L. (2013). Cancer rehabilitation may improve function in survivors and decrease the economic burden of cancer to individuals and society. *Work, 46,* 455–472. doi:10.3233/WOR-131755

Stoppler, M. C. (2014). What is HbAic? Retrieved from http://www.emedicinehealth.com/hemoglobin_a1c_hba1c/article_em.htm

Vance, D. (2013). Prevention, rehabilitation, and mitigation strategies of cognitive deficits in aging with HIV: Implications for practice and research. *ISRN Nursing,* 1–21. doi:10.1155/2013/297173

Virshup, D. (2010). Biology, clinical manifestations, and treatment of cancer. In K. McCance & S. Huether (Eds.), *Pathophysiology: The biological basis for disease in adults and children* (6th ed., pp. 360–395). Maryland Heights, MO: Mosby Elsevier.

Vogel, W. H., Wilson, M. A., & Melvin, M. S. (2004). *Advanced practice oncology and palliative care guidelines.* Philadelphia: Lippincott Williams & Wilkins.

Vogelstein B. & Kinzler K. (2004). Cancer genes and the pathways they control. *Nature Medicine 10*(8): 789–799. doi:10.1038/nm1087

Workowski, K., & Berman, S. (2010). Sexually transmitted disease treatment guidelines, 2010. *Morbidity and Mortality Weekly Report, 59*(RR12), 1–110. Retrieved from http://www.cdc.gov/mmwr/preview/mmwrhtml/rr5912a1.htm

World Health Organization (2010). Toward Universal Access: Scaling up Priority HIV/AIDS Interventions in the Health Sector: Progress Report 2010. Retrieved from http://whqlibdoc.who.int/publications/2010/9789241500395_eng.pdf

Yanovski. S. Z., & Yanovski, J. A. (2014). Long-term drug treatment for obesity: A systematic and clinical review. *Journal of the American Medical Association, 311*(1), 74 –86. doi:10.1001/jama.2013.281361. Retrieved from http://jama.jamanetwork.com/article.aspx?articleid=1774038

Zingman, B. (2010). Diagnosis and management of acute HIV infection. Retrieved from www.medscape.com/viewarticle/724634

Suggested Reading

Centers for Disease Control and Prevention (2008). *National diabetes fact sheet: General information and national estimates in diabetes in the United States, 2007.* Atlanta: Author.

Suggested Resources

Afrezz–inhaled insulin. For more information refer to the official web page, https://www.afrezza.com

Institute for Safe Medication Practices (2009). Reuse of insulin pen for multiple patients' risks transmission of bloodborne disease. *Acute Care ISMP Medication Safety Alert.* Retrieved from www.ismp.org/newsletters/acutecare/articles/20090212-2.asp

Medical Pharmacies Tablet. (2014). Safe use of insulin and insulin pens. Retrieved from http://www.medicalpharmacies.com/documents/MPGL_Revised November_Tablet_2014.pdf

National Institutes of Health (2014). AIDS info: Offering Information on HIV/AIDS Treatment, Prevention, and Research Website. Retrieved from http://www.aidsinfo.nih.gov/

Oncology Rehab Partners (2104). Advancing survivorship care. Retrieved from http://www.oncologyrehabpartners.com/

Pagoto, S. l., & Appelhans, B. M. (2013). A call for an end to the diet debates. *Journal of the American Medical Association, 310*(7), 687–688.

Scott, C. (2014). FDA Approves Artificial Pancreas You Can Wear. Retrieved from http://singularityhub.com/2013/09/28/fda-approves-artificial-pancreas-you-can-wear/

The Joint Commission. (2015). Comprehensive certification manual for disease-specific care including advanced programs for disease-specific care. The manual can be purchased through Joint Commission Resources. Contact customer service at 877.223.6866 or online at http://store.jcrinc.com/JCRStore/SearchProductAction.do.

Chapter 27

Acute and Chronic Pain

Pamela Masters-Farrell, MSN RN CRRN
Kathleen A. Stevens, PhD RN CRRN NE-BC

LEARNING OUTCOMES

- Define pain.
- Identify common physiological, behavioral, and psychological responses to pain.
- Differentiate pain based on classifications.
- Compare and contrast pain theories.
- Identify key elements in assessment and management of acute and chronic pain.
- Plan evidence-based pain management interventions for at-risk populations.
- Apply concepts of cultural diversity to pain management.

KEY CHAPTER TOPICS

- Pain classifications, pathways, and processes
- Pain theories
- Pain assessment
- Pharmacological and non-pharmacological management of pain symptoms
- Management of adverse effects of pain treatment
- Management of pain in at-risk populations
- Cultural diversity and pain management

PROFESSIONAL REHABILITATION NURSING DOMAINS AND COMPETENCIES

- Domain 1: Competencies 1.2, 1.3, 1.4
- Domain 2: Competencies 2.1, 2.2
- Domain 3: Competency 3.4 (Association of Rehabilitation Nurses [ARN], 2014)

Introduction

Pain is defined as an "unpleasant sensory and emotional experience associated with actual or potential tissue damage, or described in terms of such damage" (International Association for the Study of Pain [IASP], 2011a). In addition, Margo McCaffery's classic definition—"pain is whatever the experiencing person says it is, existing whenever he (or she) says it does" (McCaffery, 1979, p. 11)—should always be kept in mind.

Although these two definitions of pain seem straightforward, effective pain management is one of the most complicated challenges in health care. Successful management relies on continuous holistic care from a multidisciplinary team, not always an easy feat in today's healthcare system. Rehabilitation nurses must evaluate the client's pain in its entirety, including its effects on the client's personal, family, and community roles. It is only through a holistic interdisciplinary team approach that successful pain management outcomes can be achieved.

ARN supports the following definition of the pain management rehabilitation nurse: "The pain management rehabilitation nurse promotes and advances the professional rehabilitation nursing practice of caring for people with pain. Excellence in this specialized practice area is achieved through education, advocacy, research, and networking" (ARN, Role Description," para. 3).

Significance of Pain as a Problem

The societal and economic extent of the pain problem is striking. With 116 million Americans affected by pain, and costs for health care and lost productivity estimated at $560–$635 billion annually, the Institute of Medicine (IOM) (2011) has declared pain to be a major public health problem.

I. Pain Classifications

Pain can be categorized in many ways, including duration, source, mode of transmission, and etiology (Taylor, Lillis, Lemone, & Lynn, 2006).

A. Duration

1. Acute pain stems from tissue damage, is rapid in

onset and protective in nature, and it ranges from mild to severe.

a. When the underlying cause resolves, pain should resolve.
b. If is it not effectively treated, acute pain can progress to a chronic form.
    1) Thus, optimal treatment of chronic pain is prevention through effective acute pain management (Walsh, Santa Maria, & Eckmann, 2010).
c. Burns, fractures, muscle injury, childbirth, and surgery are examples of conditions that cause acute pain.
d. Commonly injured tissues are skin, muscle, bone, ligaments, tendons, and visceral organs (IASP, 2011b).
e. Fewer than 50% of postoperative clients receive adequate pain relief (Apfelbaum, Chen, Mehta, & Gan, 2003).
f. Procedural pain is a form of acute pain that is triggered by a specific procedure in children and adults.

2. Puntillo and colleagues (2001) found that patient-reported procedural pain in the critical care setting was most commonly associated with turning, wound drain removal, and wound care, all procedures commonly performed in the rehabilitation setting.
3. Chronic pain occurs when acute pain persists beyond the expected healing period (longer than 3 months), or it can be present without noticeable past injury. It is a disease process in which pain is a persistent symptom of an autonomous problem (Walsh et al., 2010).
    a. Chronic pain is a multifaceted problem that involves both the peripheral and central nervous systems and is characterized by hyperactive neural circuits. It can lead to debilitation and impaired function of the affective, cognitive, physical, and occupational aspects of life (Brennan, 2014).
    b. Chronic pain is a heterogeneous problem. It is difficult to classify, diagnose, and treat, and it affects one in three primary care patients (Brennan, 2014).
    c. Chronic pain is a subjective experience affected by genetic factors, prior experiences, psychological status, social environment, cultural background, and other health-related states (Brennan, 2014).
    d. Exacerbations of chronic pain can be triggered by the progression of the originating physiological problem, physiological stress, or worsening psychosocial situations (Walsh et al., 2010).
    e. Although anxiety is a characteristic of acute pain, depression, hopelessness, helplessness, and despair are characteristics of chronic pain. Fifty percent to 70% of persons with chronic pain have either primary depression or depression resulting from the ongoing pain cycle (Walsh et al., 2010).
    f. Chronic pain is associated with the following disease conditions: osteoarthritis, rheumatoid arthritis, headache, backache, cancer pain, neuralgias, chronic renal failure, chronic pancreatitis, phantom pain, and complex regional pain syndromes. As acute care management has improved for individuals with spinal cord injury (SCI) resulting in more incomplete injuries, the number of individuals with an SCI has increased. Prevalence rates range from 26% to 93% in individuals who report chronic pain after traumatic SCI (Dijkers, Bryce, & Zanca, 2009).
    g. Clients are often questioned regarding the legitimacy of their pain (Craig, 2006).

B. Source
1. Cutaneous: Involves skin or subcutaneous tissue
2. Somatic: Diffuse and originates in tendons, ligaments, bones, blood vessels, or nerves
3. Visceral: Poorly localized and originates within organs in the thorax, cranium, and abdomen when organs are stretched abnormally. Stretching can create distention, ischemia, or inflammation, which initiates pain (Taylor et al., 2006).

C. Pain Mechanisms
1. *Central pain* is pain initiated or caused by a primary lesion or dysfunction in the central nervous system (IASP, 2011a). Rehabilitation examples include cerebrovascular lesions, multiple sclerosis, and traumatic SCI correlated with sensory abnormalities (primarily related to temperature and pain) and hyperesthesia (Boivie, 2006).
2. *Peripheral neuropathic* pain is pain initiated or caused by a primary lesion or dysfunction in the peripheral nervous system (IASP, 2011a).
    a. Rehabilitation examples include diabetes, polyarteritis, alcoholic nutritional deficiency states, entrapment neuropathies, and amputation stump pain.
    b. Usually localized to affected area
    c. Mechanisms underlying pain in neuropathies remain obscure (Scadding & Koltzenburg, 2006).

3. *Psychogenic pain* is the interpretation and expression of emotional distress in pain language and behavior.
   a. Anxiety, neurosis, hysteria, and depression are most often interpreted in this manner.
   b. This mechanism of pain is often overlooked in persons experiencing chronic pain (Walsh et al., 2010).
4. Operant, or learned, pain-behavior mechanisms are significant factors in chronic pain.
   a. Pain behavior can persist for some time after the initial precipitating event due to environmental reinforcement. Environmental reinforcers can be positive ones such as increased attention, relief provided by medications, avoidance of undesirable activities, or increase in preferred activities. Negative reinforcement can occur if the person is punished by external factors (e.g., overprotectiveness and other social responses) while his or her function is increasing and pain issues are resolving (Walsh et al., 2010).

II. Pain Pathways and Processes: Transduction, Transmission, Modulation, Response (Figure 27-1)

The concept of pain processing and the definitions of terms are the combined work of many scientists. There is no one definitive source on the topic, so summaries from textbooks reflect multiple authors' contributions to the literature.

A. Transduction (Activating Nociceptors)

1. *Nociceptors* are specialized nerve endings found at the ends of small, unmyelinated and myelinated afferent neurons that are preferentially sensitive to a stimulus, such as heat, pressure, or other tissue damage (Meyer, Ringkamp, Campbell, & Raja, 2006). Nociceptors can be polymodal, responding to many different types of stimuli such as heat, chemical, or mechanical, or they can be more specialized and share both afferent and efferent functions (Meyer et al., 2006). The IASP defines a *nociceptor* as a receptor that is preferentially sensitive to a noxious stimulus or to a stimulus that would become noxious if prolonged.
2. Transduction starts with activation of nociceptors by various stimuli.
   a. Chemical or electrical changes (ischemia or substances from injured tissue)
   b. Mechanical (stretching or pressure on organs)
   c. Thermal (temperature changes of heat or cold)
3. Damaged tissue cells release chemicals (e.g., prostaglandins, histamine, bradykinin, serotonin, substance P) that stimulate the pain process (Taylor et al., 2006).

Figure 27-1. Pain Pathways and Processes

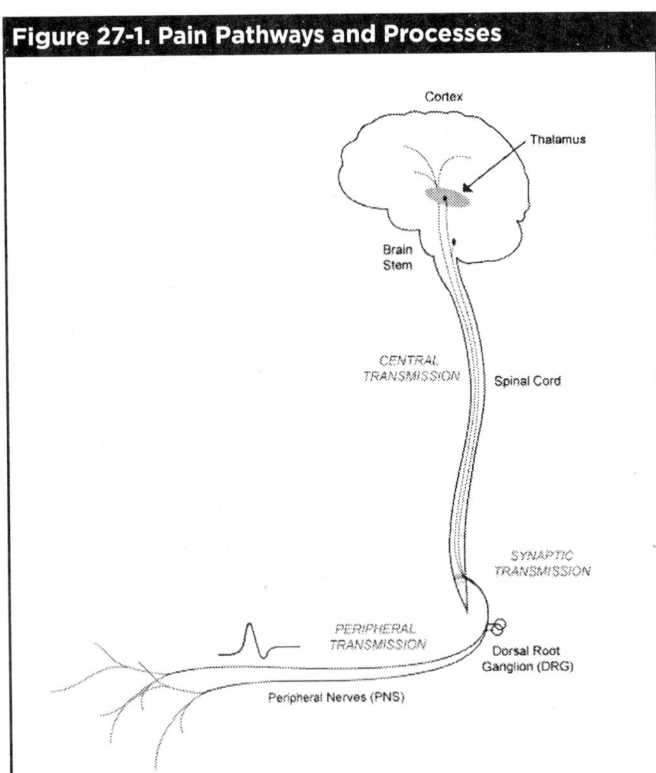

From "Combination drug therapy for chronic pain: A call for more clinical studies," by J. Mao, M. S. Gold, M. Backonja, 2011, *Journal of Pain, 2*(12), 157-166. Copyright 2011 American Pain Society. Reprinted with permission.

B. Transmission

Pain sensations are transmitted to the spinal cord and higher centers.

1. Acute: Localized pain along fast-conducting A-delta fibers
2. Visceral (diffuse): burning, aching pain through slow-conducting C-nerve fibers (Taylor et al., 2006)
3. The transmission of impulses in primary afferent nerves is facilitated by neurotransmitters, particularly glutamate. Other neurotransmitters include aspartate, neuropeptides such as substance P, and calcitonin gene-related peptide (Julius & McKleskey, 2006).
4. Ascending pain impulses are then transmitted contralaterally to pathways in the dorsal horn of the spinal cord (Bradley & McKendree-Smith, 2002).
5. Most afferent impulses ascend via the lateral spinothalamic and spinoreticular tracts (Bradley & McKendree-Smith, 2002).
6. The impulses then ascend to the thalamus and reticular formation in the brain and on to the cortex (Bradley & McKendree-Smith, 2002).
7. Mode of transmission: Referred pain is transmitted to a cutaneous site different from the site of

origin. For example, pain associated with myocardial infarction can be referred to the neck, shoulder, and arm (Taylor et al., 2006).

C. Modulation: *Neuromodulators* (endorphins and enkephalins) are endogenous opioid substances in the brain and spinal cord that alter pain perception.
   1. *Endorphins* are produced at neural synapses in the central nervous system pathway and have powerful analgesic effects and produce euphoria.
   2. *Enkephalins* are less potent than endorphins and hypothesized to reduce pain by inhibiting release of substance P from terminals of afferent neurons (Taylor et al., 2006).

D. Perception of Pain

Perception of pain is formed in the primary and secondary somatosensory cortex, the insular cortex, and other parts of the limbic forebrain (Bradley & McKendree-Smith, 2002). The somatosensory cortex formulates the "affective expression of pain (how . . . pain looks to an observer)" (Huether & DeFriez, 2006, p. 450).
   1. The threat presented by acute and especially chronic pain is based in part on the effect on daily activities, ability to cope with the pain, and potential long-term consequences of the pain or its cause (Bond, 2006).
   2. Personality, environmental factors (e.g., presence or absence of social support), and affective disorders (e.g., depression or anxiety) or other psychiatric conditions also affect the person's expression of pain and behaviors surrounding the pain experience (Brennan, 2014).
   3. Age, gender, and cultural background can also influence pain perception.

E. Neuroplasticity and Pain
   1. The nociceptive system demonstrates significant plasticity that contributes to chronic pain. For example, if a pain-related signal is unchecked, as in a situation in which persistent peripheral inflammation exists, the nervous system can reorganize itself and create a situation in which pain is no longer directly related to tissue damage. This process is called *peripheral sensitization* (Brennan, 2014).
   2. In chronic pain situations, the spinal cord can demonstrate plasticity, resulting in central sensitization; facilitate ascending pain messaging; and reduce the activity of the descending modulatory system that normally inhibits incoming pain-related signals. This allows sensory stimuli that are not typically perceived as painful (e.g., the touch of a feather) to be perceived as painful, and painful stimuli to be perceived as more painful (i.e., hyperalgesia) (Brennan, 2014).

F. Common Responses to Pain (Taylor et al., 2006)
   1. Physiological (involuntary) responses
      a. Sympathetic responses to superficial and moderate pain
         1) Increased blood pressure
         2) Increased pulse and respirations
         3) Pupil dilation
         4) Muscle tension and rigidity
         5) Pallor
         6) Increased adrenalin output
         7) Increased blood glucose
      b. Parasympathetic responses to deep and severe pain
         1) Nausea and vomiting
         2) Fainting
         3) Decreased blood pressure
         4) Decreased pulse rate
         5) Rapid and irregular breathing
   2. Behavioral (voluntary) responses
      a. Moving away from painful stimuli
      b. Grimacing, moaning, or crying
      c. Restlessness
      d. Protecting the area and refusing to move
   3. Psychological responses
      a. Weeping and restlessness
      b. Withdrawal
      c. Stoicism
      d. Anxiety
      e. Depression
      f. Fear
      g. Anger
      h. Anorexia
      i. Fatigue
      j. Hopelessness
      k. Powerlessness

III. Pain Theories

A. Gate Control Theory (Melzack & Wall, 1965): This is the most widely accepted theory of pain, but it remains controversial.
   1. The theory postulates a gating mechanism in the spinal cord.
   2. Nociceptor impulses are transmitted from specific skin sites via large A-delta and small C-nerve fibers to the spinal cord, terminating in the substantia gelatinosa.
   3. The cells of the substantia gelatinosa function as the gate. The large, fast-conducting fibers close the gate, and the small, slower cells open the gate.
   4. The closed gate results in a decrease in the stimulation of trigger cells, a decrease in pain impulses, and a decrease in pain perception. If persistent stimulation of the large fibers occurs, it results in adaptation.

5. The opposite occurs with an open gate. Stimulation of trigger fibers, transmission of impulses, and pain perception increase when the substantia gelatinosa opens the gate.

B. Neuromatrix Theory: This theory proposes an explanation for pain that does not correlate with an actual injury or a specific cause.

1. *Neuromatrix theory* suggests that the central nervous system contains a built-in body-self neuromatrix, which is capable of generating nerve impulses that represent the multidimensional somatosensory experience (Huether & DeFriez, 2006).
2. These nerve impulses, called the *neurosignature patterns*, can be activated by peripheral sensory stimulation or by brain processes to produce persistent pain.
3. *Phantom limb pain* is an example of this activation; there is no actual body part to feel pain, yet the brain perceives that the limb is both present and painful (Huether & DeFriez, 2006; Melzack, 1999).
4. The neuromatrix provides an explanation for chronic pain, which can exist with no discernible cause or stimulus (Huether & DeFriez, 2006; Melzack, 1999).

IV. Middle-Range Nursing Theories Applicable to Pain Management

A. Theory of Symptom Management: Examples applied to pain experiences (Humphreys et al., 2008)

1. Symptom experience. Example: Clients with chronic pain develop distrust because they feel they are not believed and are delegitimized.
2. Symptom management strategies. Example: Clients might keep silent or withhold information from providers. They might not take medications because of misconceptions about or negative implications of taking pain medications.
3. Symptom status outcomes. Example: Pain is not under control, and the client becomes angry and frustrated.

B. Cultural Negotiation Model (Engebretson & Littleton, 2001).

1. The *cultural negotiation model* is an interactive process that enhances the traditional nursing process (**Table 27-1**). The negotiation model holds that the client provides expert knowledge of his or her own condition. McCafferey's (1979) definition of pain is a good fit for the model, because the client who expresses pain has his or her own ideas about what pain is and beliefs about how it should be treated. Often, clients perceive problems with taking pain medication as a result of misinformation or deeply held beliefs.

V. Assessment and Management of Acute Pain

These guidelines have been summarized from the Registered Nurses Association of Ontario's (RNAO) *Assessment and Management of Pain* (2013) with permission.

A. Assessment

1. Screen for the presence or risk of any type of pain.
   a. On admission or visit with a healthcare professional
   b. After a change in medical status
   c. Prior to, during, and after a procedure
2. Perform a comprehensive pain assessment on clients screened having the presence or risk of any type of pain using a systematic approach and appropriate validated tools.
3. Perform a comprehensive pain assessment on clients unable to self-report using a validated tool.
4. Explore the client's beliefs, knowledge, and level of understanding about pain and pain management.
5. Document the client's pain characteristics.

B. Planning

1. Collaborate with the client to identify his or her goals for pain management and suitable strategies to ensure a comprehensive approach to the plan of care.
2. Establish a comprehensive plan of care that incorporates the goals of the client and the interprofessional team that addresses
   a. Assessment findings
   b. The client's beliefs and knowledge and level of understanding
   c. The client's attributes and pain characteristics.

C. Implementation

1. Implement the pain management plan using principles that maximize efficacy and minimize the adverse effects of pharmacological interventions including
   a. Multimodal analgesic approach
   b. Changing of opioids (dose and route) when necessary
   c. Prevention, assessment, and management of adverse effects during the administration of opioid analgesics
   d. Prevention, assessment, and management of opioid risk
2. Evaluate any nonpharmacological (physical and psychological) interventions for the effectiveness and the potential for interactions with pharmacological interventions.
3. Teach the client and his or her family and caregivers about the pain management strategies in the

plan of care and address known concerns and misbeliefs.

D. Evaluation

1. Reassess the client's response to the pain management interventions consistently using the same re-evaluation tool. The frequency of reassessments will be determined by
   a. Presence of pain
   b. Pain intensity
   c. Stability of the patient's medical condition
   d. Type of pain (e.g., acute versus persistent)
   e. Practice setting
2. Communicate and document the patient's responses to the pain management plan.

E. Management

1. Assessing and managing pain in at-risk populations: The RNAO pain management guidelines are used as a starting point, but at-risk populations can have special problems not addressed in the general guidelines. This section provides more detailed information about at-risk populations that rehabilitation nurses could encounter, including older adults and clients who are nonverbal, have dementia, and have had a stroke.
   a. Older adults
      1) Pain assessment is critical to creating a useful treatment plan. Pain assessment in older adults is often more challenging because of comorbidities, sensory and cognitive impairments, and misinformation about pain in aging. Establishing an institutionally appropriate procedure for evaluating pain and response to treatment, followed by regular reassessment using the same methods, is key to effective management (Herr, 2011). The American Geriatrics Society Panel on Persistent Pain in Older Persons (2002) provides the following examples of common pain behaviors in cognitively impaired older adults:
         a) Facial expressions (e.g., frowns, grimaces, closed eyes)
         b) Vocalizations (e.g., sighing, groaning, grunting, calling out, asking for help)
         c) Body movements (e.g., rigid, tense; guarding, fidgeting, pacing, rocking; mobility changes)
         d) Changes in interactions with others (e.g., aggressive, resisting care, disruptive, withdrawn)
         e) Changes in activity patterns (e.g., refusing to eat, changing sleep patterns, suddenly stopping common routines)
         f) Mental status changes (e.g., crying or tears, increased confusion, irritability)
      2) Pain behavior tools useful in cognitively impaired older adults
         a) The City of Hope website includes English-language tools available for assessing pain in nonverbal older adults (http://prc.coh.org/PAIN-NOA.htm).
         b) Pain Assessment in Advanced Dementia and Pain Assessment Checklist for Seniors with Limited Ability to Communicate are tools supported by consensus recommendations from expert groups for use in assessing pain in nonverbal residents in nursing homes

Table 27-1. Nursing Process Expanded with Cultural Negotiation Model

Nursing Process	Cultural Negotiation (Engebretson & Littleton, 2001)
Assess	Exchange of expert knowledge between client and provider
Diagnose • Chronic pain related to neuropathic pain • Anxiety related to potential lifestyle and job changes • Deficient knowledge related to individual pain control needs • Misinformation about use of pain medication	Analysis and interpretation of information about communication of pain symptoms and beliefs about pain medication
Plan (Nursing Outcomes Classification) • Pain control • Quality of life	Joint decision making • Increased family role in housework • Most effective way to inform coworkers about pain • Discussion of beliefs about pain medications
Implement (Nursing Intervention Classification) • Analgesic administration • Pain management • Medication management • Standardized templates often used to create the plan	Mutually derived plans • Desired outcomes for home setting • Desired outcomes for work setting • Desired outcomes for pain control
Evaluate	Outcome appraisal

(Herr, Bursch, Ersek, Miller, & Swafford, 2010).

3) Several factors can impede appropriate pain management in older adults.
   a) Clients fear addiction to or side effects of pain medications.
   b) Clients believe pain is the inevitable consequence of aging or that reporting pain could indicate something more serious is wrong. In addition, if the healthcare provider does not ask about the pain, the older client might perceive that it should not exist.
   c) Clients believe if they admit to pain, family or caregivers will label them "bad patients" (Hanks-Bell, Halvey, & Paice, 2004).
   d) Some healthcare providers might not manage an older adult's pain properly because of the inaccurate perception that older adults experience less pain.
   e) Healthcare providers believe that if the client does not report pain, he or she is not experiencing it.
   f) Older adults' sensitivity to the side effects of pain medications, especially narcotics, could indicate that these medications should be avoided. Older adults experience diminishing renal and liver function, which affects the metabolism of medications commonly used for pain and its sequelae (e.g., opiates, benzodiazepines, and anticholinergics).
   g) Nurses might not be familiar with resources to assess pain in patients who are unable to self-report pain, including older adults with dementia, infants and preverbal toddlers, unconscious patients, persons with intellectual disabilities, or patients at the end of life (Herr, Coyne, McCaffery, Manworren, & Merkel, 2011)

b. Pain assessment in the nonverbal client
1) See Herr et al. (2011) for the American Society for Pain Management Nursing's position statement and clinical practice recommendations.
2) Hierarchy of pain assessment technique
   a) Self-report remains the gold standard of assessment, even in clients with severe cognitive impairment.
   b) Search for potential causes by reviewing acute and chronic conditions and procedures that could affect the client.
   c) Assess pain-related behaviors.
   d) Include surrogate reporting by caregivers, family members, or anyone who knows the client well.
   e) Attempt an analgesic trial to see whether behavior changes.

c. Cancer pain
1) Cancer survival rates have increased, but treatments that allow longer survival can lead to chronic pain syndromes (Paice, 2011).
   a) Chemotherapy-induced painful peripheral neuropathies: Rehabilitation is essential for maintaining and improving function, gait training, muscle strengthening, proper use of assistive devices, and fall-risk assessment and intervention (Stubblefield et al., 2009).
   b) Graft versus host disease: Multiple systems are affected, but treatment has not been well studied (Paice, 2011).
   c) Radiation therapy: Chest pain, cystitis, enteritis, myelopathy, osteoporosis, pelvic fractures, pelvic nerve entrapment, plexopathies, and secondary malignancies can occur (Paice, 2011).
   d) Hormonal therapies and arthralgias
      (i) Aromatase inhibitors are associated with significant joint pain.
      (ii) Treatments have not undergone trials (Paice, 2011).
2) Numerous barriers to cancer pain management remain. Some examples include fear of addiction and developing tolerance to the medication and the ideas that pain is inevitable with cancer, medication will weaken the immune system, and good clients do not complain (Gunnarsdottir, Donovan, Serlin, Voge, & Ward, 2002).
3) The representational approach to client education (e.g., the RIDcancerPain program) is one of the more fully developed educational interventions in cancer pain management (Donovan et al., 2007; Donovan & Ward, 2001). During this counseling intervention, the client is helped to develop an individualized cancer pain management plan.

d. Chronic pain (Brennan, 2014; Walsh et al., 2010)

1) Therapeutic interventions used for acute pain are often contraindicated in chronic pain.
2) Patient self-description of pain is critical to understanding the various aspects of pain and its consequences.
   a) Tools such as the Brief Pain Inventory-Short Form (http://www.partnersagainstpain.com/printouts/A7012AS8.pdf) can be used to evaluate current and recent pain levels, treatment responses, and impacts on function and quality of life.
3) Assessment focuses on factors that cause or exacerbate pain, interventions that have been effective, psychological conditions, life stressors (e.g., employment or personal relationship issues), sleep disturbances, function, and activity levels.
   a) Assessment includes responses to analgesic interventions and personal or familial history of substance abuse.
   b) Chronic pain is typically associated with inactivity that results in compromised cardiovascular function, impaired musculoskeletal strength and flexibility, and impaired joint function, contributing to the loss of overall function.
4) The physical examination focuses on identifying pathophysiological pain mechanisms. A neurological examination is essential.
   a) Imaging and other tests should be reserved for situations in which they will affect the choices for treatments and interventions.
5) Management of chronic pain
   a) A multidisciplinary approach utilizes appropriate team members to effectively address the multidimensional needs of this patient population.
   b) Pharmacological therapy should address the pathophysiological process that is causing pain (e.g. antiinflammatory medications to manage peripheral inflammation or drugs that enhance central inhibitory signals from the brain, such as tricyclic antidepressants to mediate central-pain processing associated with reorganization of nociceptive circuits caused by the neuroplasticity response.)
      (i) Medications should be used cautiously in older patients because of the high risk of adverse drug reactions and increased risk of falls due to potential side effects of the medications.
      (ii) Overall pain relief in chronic pain situations is rare, and education should reinforce the fact that medications are only one component of treatment.
      (iii) Tricyclic medications are the first line of treatment for neuropathic pain. Anticonvulsants, such as gabapentin, valporic acid, and pregabalin, based on off-label use, can also be effective in the treatment of central pain (National Cancer Institute, 2014). Care should be exercised whenever using a medication for off-label use.
6) Physical modalities are often used to increase tolerance to a more active treatment program.
7) Emotional and behavioral intervention is used to teach patients to replace problematic responses with more positive coping behaviors that improve self-management.
   a) Combinations of therapeutic approaches are often needed to overcome emotional burdens and chronic pain behaviors. Psychosocial intervention promotes identification and modification of dysfunctional activities that contribute to disability or prevent appropriate adjustment to the chronic pain condition.
   b) Cognitive behavioral therapy uses a systematic, goal-oriented approach that involves education, coaching, stress management, problem solving, and activity pacing.
   c) Acceptance and commitment therapy promotes a change in expectations from pain elimination to living as well as possible with chronic pain.
   d) Motivational interviewing uses empathy and positive feedback to support self-efficacy, action planning, and goal achievement.
   e) Psychosocial interventions are effective strategies for many clients, as they reduce pain interference, depression, and pain-related anxiety.

VI. Cultural Diversity

A. Strategies for Culturally Appropriate Assessment and Management of Pain (Davidhizar & Giger, 2004, pp. 47–55).

1. Use assessment tools to assist with measuring pain.
2. Appreciate variations in affective response to pain.
3. Be sensitive to variations in communication styles.
4. Recognize that the communication of pain might not be acceptable within a culture.
5. Appreciate that the meaning of pain varies between cultures.
6. Use knowledge of biological variations.
7. Develop personal awareness of values and beliefs that can affect responses to pain.

B. The Clinically Relevant Continuum Model of Cultural Competence (Engebretson, Mahoney, & Carlson, 2008)

1. This model provides a useful framework that links the cultural competency continuum (Cross, Bazron, Dennis, & Isaacs, 1989) and evidence-based practice (**Figure 27-2**). Examples of how the model can be used in client-centered pain care are provided in Figure 27-2.
2. As used in Figure 27-2, "standardization" would equate to clinical practice guidelines, which provide current best practices based on the highest level of evidence available (such as the pain management guidelines).
3. "Outcomes focused" includes measures such as functioning, mood, and depression.
4. The evidence-based practice triangle includes client values and circumstances, provider expertise, and evidence. Provider expertise includes specific knowledge of client populations to help provide anticipatory guidance. For example, clients often do not take their pain medications because they do not want to associate themselves with any negative stereotype of a person who takes pain medication or because of fear of addiction or loss of control. For the provider, this means some clients must be encouraged to take the medication (Monsivais, 2011; Monsivais & McNeill, 2007).
5. Cultural subgroups are created by people who share a chronic illness. Many shared pain-related behaviors exist among people with chronic pain. According to a review of the literature, somatizing, overdramatizing, withholding information from the provider, and leaving the healthcare system when they felt ignored were common pain-related behaviors (Monsivais & Engebretson, 2011). Knowledge of such behaviors forms both research evidence and part of the provider's expertise in recognizing them.

Figure 27-2. Model of Cultural Competency and Evidence-Based Practice

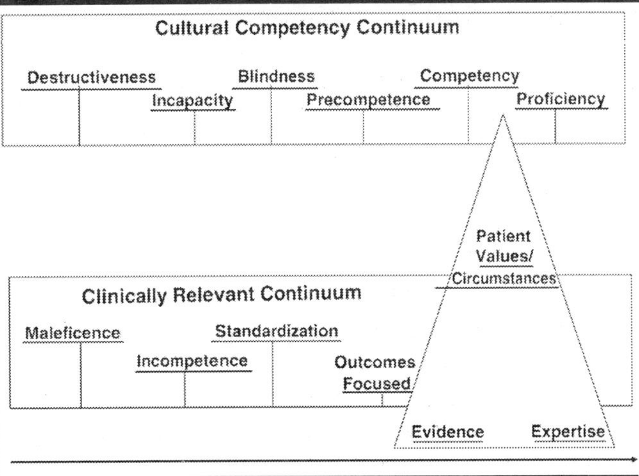

From "Cultural competency in the era of evidence-based practice," by J. Engebretson, J. Mahoney, & E. Carlson, 2008, *Journal of Professional Nursing, 24*(3), pp. 172–178. Copyright 2008 by the American Association of Colleges of Nursing. Reprinted with permission.

Case Study

Mrs. K. is a 45-year-old office worker with a 10-year history of a pain who is the main wage earner in her family. Her husband is disabled and unemployed and she has two teenaged children. Nonsteroidal antiinflammatory drugs alleviated her pain for a brief period when it first started. She works frequently at a computer, and she states that the computer work makes the pain worse, especially at the elbow. She says she takes pain medicines only when she really needs them to get through work or so she can sleep. She admits to being afraid of addiction and the long-term side effects of medication on her body.

When she comes home from work she does some of the housework, although her husband does contribute to cleaning, shopping, and cooking on a regular basis. Mrs. K. says she has been putting in more hours at work and that is when her symptoms worsen. Her coworkers are helpful when she asks for assistance in lifting, but she is worried about asking for too much help, fearing that such requests could jeopardize her job. She tries to work through her breaks because the agency is short-staffed but realizes this habit could be increasing her pain levels.

Discussion Questions

- What assessment tools will you use to create a comprehensive pain assessment for Mrs. K?
- How will you use the results of your assessment to create a client-centered plan that meets best practices? (See Section IV, "Middle-Range Nursing Theories Applicable to Pain Management," for application to the cultural negotiation model.)
- How would you evaluate the outcomes of the pain-management strategies?

References

American Geriatrics Society Beers Criteria Update Expert Panel (2012). American Geriatrics Society updated Beers Criteria for potentially inappropriate medication use in older adults. *Journal of the American Geriatrics Society, 60*(4), 616–631.

American Geriatrics Society Panel on Persistent Pain in Older Persons (2002). The management of persistent pain in older persons. *Journal of the American Geriatrics Society, 50,* S204–S224.

Apfelbaum, J. L., Chen, C., Mehta, S. S., & Gan, T. J. (2003). Postoperative pain experience: Results from a national survey suggest postoperative pain continues to be undermanaged. *Anesthesia and Analgesia, 97,* 534–540.

Association of Rehabilitation Nurses (n.d.). Role Descriptions: The pain management rehabilitation nurse. Retrieved from http://www.rehabnurse.org/pubs/role/Role-Pain-Management-Rehab-Nurse.html

Association of Rehabilitation Nurses (ARN). (2014). *ARN competency model for professional rehabilitation nursing.* Retrieved from http://www.rehabnurse.org/uploads/files/education/ARN_Rehabilitation_Nursing_Competency _Model_FINAL_-_May_2014.pdf

Ballantyne, J. C., Sullivan, M. D., & Kolodny, A. (2012). Opioid dependency or addiction; Is there a difference? *Annals of Internal Medicine, 172*(17), 1342–1343.

Boivie, J. (2006). Central pain. In S. McMahon and M. Koltzenburg (Eds.), *Wall and Melzack's textbook of pain* (5th ed., pp. 1057–1074). Philadelphia: Elsevier.

Bond, M. R. (2006). Psychiatric disorders and pain. In A. B. McMahon & M. Koltzenburg (Eds.), *Wall and Melzack's textbook of pain* (5th ed., pp. 259–266). Philadelphia: Elsevier.

Bradley, L. A., & McKendree-Smith, N. (2002). Central nervous system mechanisms of pain in fibromyalgia and other musculoskeletal disorders: Behavioral and psychologic treatment approaches. *Current Opinion in Rheumatology, 14*(1), 45–51.

Brennan, M. J. (2014). *Best practices in chronic pain management: Multidimensional assessment to multimodal treatment.* Hoboken, NJ: Integritas Communications. Retrieved from http://www.exchangecme.com/ehealthpain

Craig, K. D. (2006). Emotions and psychobiology. In S. McMahon and M. Koltzenburg (Eds.), *Wall and Melzack's textbook of pain* (5th ed., pp. 231–239). Philadelphia: Elsevier.

Cross, T., Bazron, B., Dennis, K., & Issacs, M. (1989). *Towards a culturally competent system of care.* Washington, DC: Georgetown University Child Development Center, Child and Adolescent Service System Program Technical Assistance Center.

Davidhizar, R., & Giger, J. N. (2004). A review of the literature on care of clients in pain who are culturally diverse. *International Nursing Review, 51,* 47–55.

Dijkers, A., Bryce, T., & Zanca, J. (2009). Prevalence of chronic pain after traumatic spinal cord injury: A systematic review. *Journal of Rehabilitation Research & Development, 46*(1), 13–30.

Donovan, H. S., & Ward, S. (2001). A representational approach to patient education. *Journal of Nursing Scholarship, 33*(3), 211–216.

Donovan, H. S., Ward, S. E., Song, M. K., Heidrich, S. M., Gunnarsdottir, S., & Phillips, C. M. (2007). An update on the representational approach to patient education. *Journal of Nursing Scholarship, 39*(3), 259–265.

Engebretson, J., & Littleton, L. (2001). Cultural negotiation: A constructivist-based model for nursing practice. *Nursing Outlook, 49*(5), 223–230.

Engebretson, J., Mahoney, J., & Carlson, E. (2008). Cultural competency in the era of evidence-based practice. *Journal of Professional Nursing, 24*(3), 172–178.

Gunnarsdottir, S., Donovan, H. S., Serlin, R. C., Voge, C., & Ward, S. (2002). Patient-related barriers to pain management: The Barriers Questionnaire II (BQ-II). *Pain, 99*(3), 385–396.

Hanks-Bell, M., Halvey, K., & Paice, J. A. (2004). Pain assessment and management in aging. *Online Journal of Issues in Nursing, 9*(3), 65–82.

Herr, K. (2011). Pain assessment strategies in older adults. *Journal of Pain, 12*(3) (Suppl. 1), 53.

Herr, K., Bursch, H., Ersek, M., Miller, L., & Swafford, K. (2010). Use of pain-behavioral assessment tools in the nursing home: Expert consensus recommendations for practice. *Journal of Gerontological Nursing, 36,* 18–29.

Herr, K., Coyne, P. J., Key, T., Manworren, R., McCaffery, M., Merkel, S.,...American Society for Pain Management Nursing (2006). Pain assessment in the nonverbal patient: Position statement with clinical practice recommendations. *Pain Management Nursing, 7*(2), 44–52.

Herr, K., Coyne, P., McCaffery, M., Manworren, R., & Merkel, S. (2011). Pain assessment In the patient unable to self-report: Position statement with clinical practice recommendations. *Pain Management Nursing, 12*(4), 230–250.

Huether, S. E., & DeFriez, C. B. (2006). Pain, temperature regulation, sleep, and sensory function. In K. L. McCance and S. E. Huether (Eds.), *Pathophysiology: The biologic basis for disease in adults and children* (5th ed., pp. 447–490). Philadelphia,: Elsevier Mosby.

Humphreys, J., Lee, K. A., Carrieri-Kohlman, V., Puntillo, K., Faucett, J., Janson, S., Aouizerat, B., & Doneskly-Cuenco, D. (2008). Theory of symptom management. In M. J. Smith & P. R. Liehr (Eds.), *Middle range theory for nursing* (2nd ed., pp. 145–158). New York, NY: Springer.

Institute of Medicine (2011). *Relieving pain in America: A blueprint for transforming prevention, care, education, and research.* Washington, DC: National Academies Press.

International Association for the Study of Pain (2011a). "Resources" to "IASP Taxonomy" to "Pain Terms." Retrieved from www.iasp-pain.org

International Association for the Study of Pain (2011b). Mechanisms of Acute Pain [Fact sheet]. Retrieved from http://www.iasp-pain.org/files/Content/ContentFolders/GlobalYearAgainstPain2/AcutePainFactSheets/3-Mechanisms.pdf

Julius, D., & McKleskey, E. W. (2006). Cellular and molecular properties of primary afferent neurons. In A. B. McMahon and M. Koltzenburg (Eds.), *Wall and Melzack's textbook of pain* (5th ed., pp. 35–48). Philadelphia: Elsevier.

McCaffery, M. (1979). *Nursing management of the patient with pain* (2nd ed.). Philadelphia: J. B. Lippincott.

Melzack, R. (1999). From the gate to the neuromatrix. *Pain* (Suppl. 6), S121–S126.

Melzack, R., & Wall, P. D. (1965). Pain mechanisms: A new theory. *Science, 150*(699), 971–979.

Meyer, R. A., Ringkamp, M., Campbell, J. N., & Raja, S. N. (2006). Peripheral mechanisms of cutaneous nociception. In A. B. McMahon and M. Koltzenburg (Eds.), *Wall and Melzack's textbook of pain* (5th ed., pp. 3–34). Philadelphia: Elsevier.

Monsivais, D. (2011). Promoting culturally competent chronic pain management using the clinically relevant continuum model. *Nursing Clinics of North America, 46*(2), 163–169.

Monsivais, D., & Engebretson, J. (2011). Cultural cues: Review of qualitative evidence of patient-centered care in patients with non-malignant chronic pain. *Rehabilitation Nursing, 36*(4), 166–171.

Monsivais, D., & McNeill, J. (2007). Multicultural influences on pain medication attitudes and beliefs in patients with nonmalignant chronic pain syndromes. *Pain Management Nursing, 8*(2), 64–71.

National Cancer Institute (2014). Physician Data Query® (PDQ®) Database, Health Professional Version. Retrieved from http://www.cancer.gov/cancertopics/pdq/supportivecare/pain/HealthProfessional

Paice, J. A. (2011). Chronic treatment-related pain in cancer survivors. *Pain, 152*(Suppl.), 84–89.

Puntillo, K. A., White, C., Morris, A., Perdue, S. T., Stank-Hutt, J., Thompson, C. L., & Wild, L. R. (2001). Patients' perceptions and responses to procedural pain: Results from THUNDER II project. *American Journal of Critical Care*, 10, 238–251.

Registered Nurses Association of Ontario (2002). *Assessment and management of pain*. Toronto, ON, Canada: Author.

Registered Nurses Association of Ontario (2007). *Assessment and management of pain: Supplement*. Toronto, ON, Canada: Author.

Scadding, J. W., & Koltzenburg, M. (2006). Painful peripheral neuropathies. In S. McMahon and M. Koltzenburg (Eds.), *Wall and Melzack's textbook of pain* (5th ed., pp. 973–999). Philadelphia: Elsevier.

Stubblefield, M. D., Burstein, H. J., Burton, A. W., Custodio, C. M., Deng, G. E., Ho, M., & Von Roenn, J. H. (2009). NCCN task force report: Management of neuropathy in cancer. *Journal of the National Comprehensive Cancer Network, 7*(Suppl. 5), S1–S26.

Taylor, C. R., Lillis, C., Lemone, P., & Lynn, P. (2006). *Fundamentals of nursing: The art and science of nursing care* (6th ed.). Philadelphia: Lippincott Williams & Wilkins.

Walsh, N. E., Santa Maria, D., & Eckmann, M. (2010). Treatment of the patient with chronic pain. In W. R. Frontera (Ed.), *DeLisa's Physical Medicine & Rehabilitation Principles and Practice* (5th ed., pp. 1273–1318). Philadelphia: Walters Kluwer/Lippincott Williams & Wilkins.

Suggested Resources

The IASP Task Force (see www.iasp-pain.org/AM/Template.cfm?Section=Home&Template=/CM/HTMLDisplay.cfm&ContentID=3011) provides definitions and clear guidelines for desirable characteristics of different types of pain facilities, such as

- Pain treatment facilities
- Multidisciplinary pain centers
- Multidisciplinary pain clinics
- Pain clinics
- Modality-oriented clinics

Additional Sources of Valuable Information

Alliance of State Pain Initiatives: http://trc.wisc.edu/

American Academy of Pain Management: http://www.aapainmanage.org/

American Academy of Pain Medicine: http://www.painmed.org/

American Chronic Pain Association: http://www.theacpa.org/

American Pain Society: http://www.americanpainsociety.org/

American Society for Pain Management Nursing: http://www.aspmn.org/Pages/default.aspx

City of Hope Pain and Palliative Care Resource Center: http://prc.coh.org/

The Coalition Against Pediatric Pain: http://www.tcapp.org/

Consult Geri RN: http://consultgerirn.org/topics/pain/want_to_know_more

Geriatric Pain: http://www.geriatricpain.org/Pages/home.aspx

Partners Against Pain: http://www.partnersagainstpain.com/

Society for Pediatric Pain Medicine: http://www.pedspainmedicine.org/

Chapter 28

Acute and Chronic Complications in the Rehabilitation Patient Population

Gail L. Sims, MSN RN CRRN
Anne Leclaire, MSN RN CRRN
Kathleen Stevens, PhD RN CRRN NE-BC

LEARNING OUTCOMES

- Define complications by system related to rehabilitation diagnoses.
- Describe implications for rehabilitation nurses to prevent complications.
- Promote health and quality of life for people with potential or actual complications associated with primary disability.

KEY CHAPTER TOPICS

- Musculoskeletal complications
- Cardiovascular complications
- Infection
- Neurologic complications
- Dehydration and electrolyte imbalance
- Alteration in body composition
- Genitourinary complications
- Gastrointestinal complications
- Psychiatric complications

PROFESSIONAL REHABILITATION NURSING DOMAINS AND COMPETENCIES

- Domain 1: Competencies 1.2, 1.3
- Domain 2: Competency 2.1 (Association of Rehabilitation Nurses [ARN], 2014)

Introduction and Background

Complications of catastrophic illness or injury can have a negative impact on function and quality of life for people with disabilities. Changing policies and proactive patterns driven by escalating healthcare costs require those with catastrophic events to move through acute hospitalization more quickly than in the past. Higher acuity during inpatient rehabilitation and reduction in length of stay (LOS) in recent years has placed greater pressure on providers across the healthcare continuum to manage all aspects of medical care and rehabilitation in a compressed timeframe.

Return to acute care (RTAC) as it relates to outcomes is a topic that influences every level of care in the continuum. Predictors of RTAC include a longer time from injury to rehabilitation admission. Longer hospitalization LOS influences RTAC, which represents the impact of medical conditions on achievement of rehabilitation milestones and medical stability for discharge readiness. The most serious complications that contribute to rehospitalizations (RTAC) of people with disabilities include respiratory complications, urinary tract infections (UTIs), gastrointestinal disorders, and disorders of skin such as pressure ulcers (Hammond et al., 2013). Long-term morbidities at 1 year after injury or illness include neuropathic musculoskeletal pain, phantom pain syndrome, pneumonia, deep vein thrombosis (DVT), pressure ulcers (PUs), spasticity, shoulder subluxation, joint contracture, dysphagia, urinary incontinence, anxiety, and depression (Kuptniratsaikul, Kovindha, Suethanapornkul, Manimmanakorn, & Archongka, 2013).

The Model Spinal Cord Injury Systems Database identified that rehospitalization occurred in 55% of patients in the first year after spinal cord injury (SCI) and continued at a stable rate of roughly 37% each year during the next 20 years (Cardenas, Hoffman, Kirshblum, & McKinley, 2004). A prior study indicated that secondary medical complications at annual follow-up included pneumonia or atelectasis, pulmonary embolism, pressure ulcers, fractures, and renal calculi (McKinley, Jackson, Cardenas, & Devivo, 1999).

Medical complications after SCI can be minimized or eliminated by provision of early surgical stabilization, resulting in reduced length of stay, fewer secondary complications, early mobilization, and transfer to rehabilitation as soon as the patient is medically stable (Fehing & Singh, 2009). Earthquake survivors who sustained SCI in China were studied to determine the most common medical complications, which included pressure sores, pain, bowel and bladder dysfunction, urinary tract stones, respiratory infections and UTIs, postural hypotension, autonomic hyperreflexia, and deep venous thrombosis (Yongquiang et al., 2012).

Complications after acute stroke include falls, skin breakdown, urinary tract and chest infections, seizures, depression, recurrence of stroke, and painful shoulders (Davenport, Dennis, Wellwood, & Warlow, 1996). Knowing the nature and timing of complications, along with identification of high-risk patients, may help the rehabilitation nurse to plan stroke services. People who have had previous strokes are at greater risk of systemic medical complications during stroke recovery (Kumar, Selim, & Caplan, 2010). Complications may cause a delay in successful rehabilitation, or even death. Problems such as infection, venous thromboembolism, or cardiac disease are considered preventable late effects after stroke. Complications are more common with increasing age, prestroke disability, total anterior circulation strokes, and urinary incontinence. The American Stroke Association states that the decline in stroke mortality is a major public health and clinical medicine success story (Doehner, Schenkel, Anker, Springer, & Audebert, 2013). Strong evidence suggests this decline can be attributed to a combination of interventions and programs based on scientific findings and implemented with the purpose of reducing stroke risks, including improved control of hypertension.

For a number of reasons, rehabilitation patients with all diagnoses in all settings are at risk for medical complications ranging from dehydration to deep venous thrombosis, pulmonary embolus, and infection. The rehabilitation nurse is in a unique position to prevent complications, recognize the signs of complications that do occur, and initiate early intervention to prevent illness, further disability, and even death.

I. Musculoskeletal Complications

A. Bone Mass Loss and Osteoporosis

1. *Osteoporosis* is defined as loss of bone throughout the skeleton, predisposing people to fractures. Osteoporosis of disuse results from a lack of normal functional stress on bones. When immobility occurs as a result of disease or injury, bone density diminishes more rapidly than under normal circumstances. Quantitative computed tomography assesses change in bone mineral to measure loss (Edwards, Schnitzer, & Troy, 2013). The effects of aging and electrical stimulation exercise on bone after SCI must be assessed (Dolbow, Dolbow, Gorgey, Adler, & Gater, 2013). The effects of SCI on bone density and morphology in children were assessed with peripheral quantitative computer tomography (pQCT) (Biggin et al., 2013). Measurement of volumetric bone mineral density (vBMD) provides valuable insight into changes in bone and muscle development in children after SCI.
2. Common rehabilitation populations at risk
   a. Approximately 7% of women over the age of 50 years have osteoporosis. Prevalence is higher among Asian Americans and European Americans than African Americans. Bone loss and the risk of fractures increase with age, immobilization, excess of thyroid hormone, use of corticosteroids and some anticonvulsant drugs; the consumption of alcohol, tobacco, and caffeine; and after menopause. Genetics is a nonmodifiable risk factor that also contributes to osteoporosis (*Taber's 22nd Edition Medical Dictionary*)
   b. SCI: Bone loss after SCI occurs because of pathologic changes in osteoblastic activities caused by mechanical unloading (Sabour et al., 2013). Bone loss and increased risk of fragility fracture around the knees is a complication of SCI (Edwards, Schnitzer, & Troy, 2014).
   c. Stroke: Femoral neck bone mineral density changes are associated with a shift in standing weight in hemiparetic stroke patients (Chang et al., 2014). Patients bearing less weight on the paretic leg have more rapid reduction in femoral neck bone mineral density. It is common for stroke survivors to experience accelerated bone loss and increased fracture risk as a result of impaired mobility (Borschmann et al., 2013). Volumetric bone mineral density within the first year after stroke is related to physical acuity and motor recovery. Increased bone loss and fracture rate is evident in people after stroke (Pang, Yang, & Jones, 2013).
   d. Multiple sclerosis (MS), Guillain–Barré, and other neurological impairments cause disuse-related bone loss from immobilization. Decrease in bone mineral density leads to weakening of the bone and increased risk of fracture (Gisiason et al., 2014).
3. Assessment
   a. Compare any prior bone density assessments.
   b. Note any comments made on radiologic tests since admission for mention of bone loss.
   c. Check lab results for hypercalcemia and hypocalcemia.
   d. Assess for increased risk with certain medications and supplements.
   e. Determine whether there is a history of urinary stones.
   f. Collaborate with dietitian to determine dietary intake of calcium.

g. Assess prior lifestyle activities such as walking, resistance training, and weight lifting to help determine potential for risk of bone mass loss or osteoporosis.
h. Assess risk factors related to bone mass loss or osteoporosis in patients with MS, Parkinsonism, and Guillain–Barré, including loss of function due to pain, fractures, and decreased mobility known as disuse-related bone loss, which affects morbidity, mortality, and cost to the healthcare system (Kazakia et al., 2014).
i. Assess for signs of bone mass loss or osteoporosis, including severe pain, presence of pathological fractures, and decreased functional mobility.
j. Use a risk assessment tool such as the FRAX Tool from the World Health Organization (http://www.shef.ac.uk/FRAX/) to help quantify risk for fracture from osteoporosis

4. Nursing interventions specific to rehabilitation
   a. Standing activities including early mobilization prevents fractures.
   b. Bone loading activities such as physical exercise and functional electrical stimulation (FES) are used to prevent osteoporosis. Electrical stimulation activities administered appropriately are assumed safe, with thousands of documented safe FES cycling sessions (Kazakia et al., 2014).
   c. The results of recent studies may guide rehabilitative programs to improve bone health and promote education on the benefits of both passive and active mobility.
   d. Bisphosphonates and pamidronate have shown evidence in reducing bone loss in acute phase post-SCI, although there may be limited efficacy in preventing long-term bone loss (Charlifue, Jha, & Lammertse, 2010).
   e. Education must be provided on sources of calcium such as milk, cheese, and dietary supplements.
5. Outcomes and long-term considerations
   a. Bone mass loss can be prevented or minimized through mobilization.
   b. Prevention of fractures can minimize complications and promote quality of life for the person with disabilities throughout the lifespan.
   c. Equipment modifications, assessment of and changes to posture, and techniques used in performing functional activities may be necessary, particularly for people with SCI (Charlifue et al., 2010).
   d. A plan should be developed to avoid or minimize risk of falls as mobility and risks change over time.
   e. Periodic bone density evaluations may be warranted, particularly for menopausal and postmenopausal women with SCI.

B. Steroid-Induced Bone Loss
1. Definition: Bone mineral density loss can be caused by prolonged use of corticosteroids for chronic obstructive pulmonary disease (COPD), asthma, rheumatoid arthritis, lupus, and other conditions in which steroids are prescribed.
2. Common rehabilitation populations at risk
   a. Rheumatic disorders such as rheumatoid arthritis and lupus erythematosus
   b. Respiratory disorders such as COPD and asthma
   c. Neurological disorders and injuries such as SCI and MS
   d. Compromised mobility accompanied by long-term steroid use
3. Assessment
   a. Controllable risk factors such as immobility, smoking, and excessive alcohol consumption should be assessed. These risk factors apply to all types of bone loss, not just steroid induced.
   b. Noncontrollable risk factors such as COPD, organ transplant, inflammatory bowel disease, amenorrhea, and hypogonadism in men should also be noted (Picado & Luengo, 1996a).
   c. Complexity of the treatment guidelines for certain conditions and poor patient compliance are attributed to the high rate of occurrence of steroid-induced bone loss.
   d. Dosage and length of steroid use should be determined to assess the degree of potential bone loss.
4. Nursing interventions specific to rehabilitation
   a. Encourage activity, adequate daily calcium intake and supplements, smoking cessation, and avoidance of excessive alcohol intake.
   b. Provide education about the seriousness of steroid-induced bone loss and risk factors, many of which can be controlled by patients.
   c. Encourage minimal use of steroids if other medications are potentially effective.
5. Outcomes and long-term considerations
   a. Steroid-induced bone loss can be caused by prolonged use of steroids.
   b. Rehabilitation nurses can help improve patient outcomes by advocating for minimizing steroid use and suggesting use of other preventive

treatment options such as nonsteroidal anti-inflammatory medications, as well as educating the public on minimizing controllable risk factors.

C. Muscle Atrophy

1. Definition: A decrease of muscle mass caused by disuse, myopathy, or neurogenic causes. Atrophy can lead to decreased strength and contracture formation.
2. Common rehabilitation populations at risk
   a. SCI
   b. Stroke
   c. MS
   d. Guillain–Barré, amyotrophic lateral sclerosis (ALS), neuropathy, muscular dystrophy
   e. Neuropathy
   f. Rheumatoid arthritis
   g. Malnourished
   h. Immobile (e.g., bed rest, casts, splints)
   i. Older adults
3. Assessment
   a. Collaborate with physical and occupational therapists to assess functional mobility and performance of activities of daily living (ADLs) to determine degree of muscle atrophy, tone, movement, and strength.
   b. Therapists and physiatrists should determine the degree of myopathy through manual muscle testing.
   c. Nerve conduction studies performed by a physiatrist or neurologist determine degree of neuropathy. This information provides valuable data that have significant health implications (Singh, Rohilla, Saini, & Kaur, 2014).
   d. Determine presence of pathological fractures, debilitation, and multiple systems' deterioration resulting from bone loss and their contribution to limitations or lack of function.
   e. Assess degree of pain from bone loss that may compromise mobility and patient's perception of contribution of pain to reduction in perceived quality of life.
4. Nursing and team interventions specific to rehabilitation
   a. Promoting active range of motion is valuable in preventing muscle atrophy.
   b. Involving the patient in ADLs to his or her maximum functional ability promotes muscle tone and return of independence.
   c. Application of prescribed splints and repositioning in bed or chair slows or prevents contractures.
   d. Ultrasound and stretching by therapists contribute to improvement and maintenance of functional levels.
   e. Consultation with a nutritionist helps promote adequate protein and fluid intake.
5. Outcomes and long-term considerations
   a. Muscle atrophy from disuse can be reduced by early mobilization.
   b. Physical activity minimizes complications and promotes quality of life for people with disabilities.
   c. For some disorders or conditions, atrophy will continue despite activity.
   d. Atrophy can decrease mobility and increase fall risk, potentially increase pain, and reduce chest wall expansion, thereby increasing risk for pneumonia.
   e. In cases where contractures are interfering with function, surgical intervention may be needed.

D. Dislocation of Hip or Shoulder, Overuse Syndrome, and Shoulder Subluxation

1. Definitions
   a. *Dislocation*: The displacement of any part, especially the temporary displacement of a bone from its normal position in a joint. Shoulder displacement of the head of the humerus extends beyond the boundaries of the glenoid fossa. Inferior dislocation may result from poor muscle tone, as with hemiplegia, and from the weight of the arm pulling the humerus downward. Hip dislocation occurs through the obturator foramen, on the pubis, in the perineum, or through a fractured acetabulum. Stability of shoulder or hip may be compromised, with risk of damage to soft tissue structures.
   b. *Subluxation*: Partial or incomplete dislocation. Subluxation occurs most commonly in the shoulder joint, radial head, or temporomandibular joint, which causes relaxation or stretching of the capsule and ligaments that can result in popping noises during movement or partial dislocation of the joint, such as forward movement of the mandible (*Taber's Medical Dictionary Online, n.d.)*
   c. *Complete dislocation*: A dislocation that separates the joint completely.
   d. *Overuse syndrome*: In the shoulder, overuse occurs as a result of the shoulder's muscular imbalance across the glenohumeral joint, with anterior musculature development significantly greater than posterior. This instability

increases the risk of soft tissue injury (Smith, 2012), including shoulder impingement syndrome and possibly a torn rotator cuff. Severe paralysis increases the likelihood of developing pain and injury. Overuse of the wrist may result in carpal tunnel syndrome, and overuse at the elbow may result in what is known as golfer's or tennis elbow.

2. Common rehabilitation populations at risk
   a. SCI
   b. Stroke
   c. Any person using a cast, manual wheelchair, or crutches
   d. Diabetes
   e. Rheumatoid arthritis
3. Assessment
   a. Shoulder subluxation occurs more frequently in patients with a known presence of fluid in the subhumeral and subdeltoid bursae and in patients with reduced functional capacity, as occurs after a stroke.
   b. Objective assessment of asymmetrical posture and subjective assessment of pain is necessary to determine whether subluxation, dislocation of hip or shoulder, or overuse of shoulder has occurred.
   c. Assess for pattern of pain or numbness at affected site or distally, guarding of site by the patient, muscle atrophy, and palpable or visible gap at shoulder structures.
   d. Common diagnostic tests include radiograph, magnetic resonance imaging, electromyography, ultrasound, and nerve conduction studies.
4. Nursing and therapist interventions specific to rehabilitation
   a. Prevention of damage to shoulder and surrounding tissue is accomplished by entire team approach focusing on positioning and mobilization.
   b. Rehabilitation nurses coordinate care, communicate proper technique, and reinforce education of patient, family, and staff members.
   c. Therapist recommendations and proper application and use of supportive devices such as arm troughs, slings, pillows, and bracing preserve structure, prevents complications, and promotes function.
   d. Promotion of exercise using prescribed technique, body weight management, strength training, and reinforcement of proper techniques for transfers and wheelchair mobility prevent serious complications.
   e. In some cases of extreme pain and unstable joint, less range of motion exercise may promote controlled joint tightening to prevent pain and subluxation and to promote function.
   f. Surgery is performed for impingement or rotator cuff tear when conservative approaches do not resolve the problem. Studies reporting postsurgical outcomes for people with SCI are limited, and they include prolonged and potentially difficult postoperative rehabilitation periods. These procedures can temporarily limit function and must be weighed against long-term benefits and quality of life measures (Charlifue et al., 2010).
   g. Patients at high risk of hemiplegic shoulder pain with severe arm paralysis and supraspinatus tendon pathology need more careful attention to prevent injury during rehabilitation (Kim, Jung, Yang, & Paik, 2014). Modifications such as use of transfer boards, power assist, and power wheelchairs may be necessary, with or without surgery, to promote healing of the affected shoulder.
   h. Robotic protocol consists of linear movement controlled by motorized mechanism to guide the extremity through the range of motion. The robotic protocol for shoulder subluxation in patients with chronic stroke was studied and determined to improve shoulder stability and motor power and resulted in improved functional outcomes 3 months after sessions were completed (Dohle, Rykman, Chang, & Volpe, 2013).
   i. Improvements in functional ADLs were significant in studies using the California tri-pull taping method, involving the application of strips of tape latitudinally over the joint area to provide upper extremity support after stroke was determined to decrease inferior shoulder subluxation (Hayner, 2013).
   j. The orthopedic sling was reported to be used frequently by occupational therapists after stroke despite low evidence for its efficacy (Li, Murai, & Chi, 2011). Caution is advised to not immobilize the upper extremity entirely but to incorporate the limb into functional tasks that do not involve pulling or straining the extremity.
   k. The use of a bed trapeze is discouraged to prevent straining the joint; a bed with elevating head may improve functional mobility and prevent injury.

l. Proper support of the hemiparetic upper extremity with an arm trough promotes correct alignment for wheelchair positioning.
m. In cases of limited arm motor control in the subacute phase after stroke, static stretch positioning combined with the use of electrical stimulation has no statistically significant effect on range of motion (ROM), shoulder pain, basic arm function, or ADLs (de Jong, Dijkstra, Gerritsen, Geurts, & Postema, 2013).

5. Outcomes and long-term implications
   a. Encourage use of adaptive aids and transfer techniques to prevent future loss of function, injury to extremity, and pain.
   b. Consider whether the specific activities done a particular way have the potential to cause injury over time; for example, repetitive opening of a heavy office door can cause trauma to the shoulder joint and may require modification of an electronic mechanism.
   c. Dislocations and subluxations can be prevented through proper extremity positioning and strengthening. Provision of support to weak or paralyzed extremities is critical in the prevention of complications.

II. Cardiovascular Complications

A. Peripheral Edema

1. *Edema* is observable swelling resulting from fluid accumulation in the tissue spaces of lower extremities or dependent arms. Fluid accumulation can be caused by sodium retention, low albumin levels, varicose veins, congestive heart failure, and venous insufficiency as well as trauma, inflammation, and infection. Peripheral edema occurs with congestive heart failure when the heart is too weak to pump blood throughout the body, increasing venous pressure and forcing fluid into the surrounding tissues. Venous insufficiency contributes to edema when the valves of the veins are damaged, resulting in the pooling of blood and escape of fluid into the surrounding tissues (Cunha, 2014). Edema increases the size and changes the shape of the extremity.
2. Common rehabilitation populations at risk
   a. Amputation: Edema often occurs in the residual limb after surgery.
   b. SCI: A loss of vascular tone in lower extremities and the effects of gravity impair venous blood return, leading to blood pooling in legs and feet and moving into the tissue spaces (Krassioukov, Eng, Warburton, & Teasell, 2009).
   c. Stroke: The arm and leg of the affected side lose vascular tone and innervation, leading to an increase in edema from lack of movement.
   d. Orthopedic procedures: Surgical procedures, such as total knee and hip arthroplasties, can lead to increases in lower extremity edema when movement is limited and the extremity is kept in a dependent position.
   e. Cancer treatment: Damage to the lymphatic system from cancer treatments and surgical procedures can cause peripheral edema in that part of the body (lymphedema). The most common cause of lymphedema results from destruction or removal of lymph nodes, which can be a chronic condition.
3. Assessment
   a. Visualize and measure for increase in size or change in shape of involved extremity. Note that newly paralyzed limbs are undergoing muscle atrophy, which may mask edema or swelling.
   b. Note whether the skin appears to be shiny or taut.
   c. Assess for pitting edema, indentation of the skin that remains after pressure is applied to the area.
   d. Note complaints voiced by the patient that the area feels tight, heavy, warm, or painful.
   e. Assess for decreased movement or flexibility in joints surrounding the area.
   f. Pulses must be assessed, but they may be difficult to palpate if edema is present.
4. Nursing interventions specific to rehabilitation
   a. Provide education related to self-management and preventive strategies.
   b. After an amputation, keep the residual limb elevated to prevent fluid from pooling in the dependent extremity and into the surrounding tissue. Edema in the residual limb must be controlled to limit complications, such as wound dehiscence and infection. Once the incision has healed, a compression device such as a shrinker is applied to control and limit edema and to shape the residual limb for future prosthesis (Marshall & Stansby, 2010). (Note: Elevating the postamputation limb must be balanced with preventing contracture at the flexed joint. Thus, periods of residual limb elevation must be alternated with stretching exercises at the nearby joint. Hip flexors are particularly prone to contracture, which can interfere with future ambulation.)

c. Elevate extremities higher than the heart periodically throughout the day to limit edema.
d. Apply compression devices to affected limbs during the day to reduce the effects of gravity on edema and promote vascular return. Compression devices include stockings, elastic wraps, or Coban® (Smith et al., 2012). Use of sequential compression devices while in bed promotes fluid return.
e. Decrease sodium intake.
f. Increase protein in diet to elevate albumin levels if hypoalbuminemia is an issue.
g. Minimize use of constrictive devices and apparel, such as rings, watches, wrinkled stockings or socks, and ill-fitting shoes. Lace shoes will loosen to accommodate edema but can be tightened as edema subsides.
h. Monitor for signs and symptoms of DVT: Redness, warmth, one limb larger than the other. Again, note that newly paralyzed limbs are undergoing muscle atrophy, which may mask swelling.
i. Protect skin from trauma and use padding as needed.
j. Check at-risk skin more frequently in edematous limbs.
k. Administer diuretics as prescribed by physician.

5. Outcomes and long-term considerations
a. Overt bladder distension from urinary retention and prolonged sitting can compress the iliac vessels, which can cause lower extremity edema.
b. Uncontrolled and prolonged residual limb edema impairs the ability to shape a residual limb for prosthetic fitting.
c. Uncontrolled peripheral edema places affected extremities at risk for tissue injury and contributes to slow healing.
d. Lymphedema may become severe and chronic if not properly addressed in the acute phase.

B. Orthostatic Hypotension (OH)

1. *Orthostatic hypotension* is defined as a decrease in systolic blood pressure of at least 20 mmHg or a decrease in diastolic blood pressure of at least 10 mmHg when a person's body is changed from supine to an upright position (Krassioukov et al., 2009). In a third of affected people, this drop in blood pressure is asymptomatic, and in an additional 25% the symptoms have been found to be atypical and misleading to physicians (Arbogast, Alshekhlee, Hussain, McNeeley, & Chelminsky, 2009).

2. Common rehabilitation populations at risk
a. Stroke: Orthostatic hypotension may result from antihypertensive and diuretic medication adjustments after stroke. Lack of muscle tone in paralyzed limbs may also contribute. Fluctuations in blood pressure can result from post-stroke cardiac autonomic dysfunction.
b. SCI: The loss of reflex vasoconstriction, the lack of muscle tone in lower extremities, and the effects of gravity cause excessive blood pooling in the abdominal viscera and lower extremities. Reduced thoracic blood volume leads to decreased end-diastolic volume and decreased left ventricular stroke volume. This decrease in blood pressure can also reduce cerebral blood flow, which can cause cognitive symptoms (Krassioukov et al., 2009). OH is more commonly seen in tetraplegia than paraplegia.
c. Postsurgical (multitrauma, amputation, orthopedic procedures, particularly in cases with significant blood loss): Hypotension can occur from fluid loss during surgery or when restarting antihypertensive medications that were held for surgery.
d. Parkinson's disease
e. Debility: Deconditioning caused by prolonged bed rest changes blood pressure control.
f. Older adults: The prevalence of orthostatic hypotension for adults age 85 years and older is about 50%. In older adults, blood pressure varies directly with vascular resistance, heart rate, and stroke volume, which affects cardiac filling (Gupta & Lipsitz, 2007).
g. Blood pressure lowers in people with orthostasis caused by a change from reclining to upright posture, food ingestion, infection, hyperventilation, hot weather, and lifting of heavy objects (Figueroa, Basford, & Low, 2010).

3. Assessment
a. Monitor for symptoms such as lightheadedness, dizziness, fainting, blurred vision, or muscle weakness with changes in position.
b. Assess patient for evidence of unusual fatigue, backache, or headache.
c. Assess for near or actual syncope (temporary loss of consciousness) with position change.
d. Particularly in older adults, observe for changes in speech, vision, confusion, impaired cognition, and falls (Gupta & Lipsitz, 2007).
e. Measure blood pressure and heart rate at intervals of 1–5 minutes after the person has moved

from supine to standing to identify extent of OH (Gupta & Lipsitz, 2007).
   f. Assess for potential causes of OH when orthostatic blood pressure changes are noted.
4. Nursing interventions specific to rehabilitation
   a. Direct treatment to improve and adjust to symptoms.
   b. Gradual position changes allow the blood pressure to normalize. Slowly work to acclimate the person to 90 degrees. May need to sit patient upright in bed at 90 degrees for a few minutes before transferring to chair to allow blood pressure to acclimate. The use of a tilt table may be necessary to improve out-of-bed tolerance.
   c. Consult pharmacist to review medications that could precipitate hypotension, and work with physician to adjust antihypertensive medications. Older adults may be at greater risk of hypotensive episodes, which may present as frequent falls.
   d. Apply compression stockings to improve venous return. Elastic wraps over stockings or other compression device may also be needed in extreme hypotensive cases.
   e. Apply abdominal binders as indicated to combat thoracic venous pooling. Apply tight enough to exert gentle pressure while lying flat in bed, in the morning and remove when lying supine (Figueroa et al., 2010).
   f. Monitor sodium levels for hyponatremia and increase salt intake as ordered unless contraindicated. Ask physician to consider use of salt tablets or high-salt food items, such as pickles or potato chips, when needed to increase circulating blood volume.
   g. Encourage adequate fluid intake to increase the amount of circulating blood volume.
   h. Promote exercise or passive ROM to stabilize central blood volume.
   i. Consult with therapists about appropriate physical countermaneuvers involving isometrically contracting muscles below waist to reduce venous capacity, increase peripheral resistance, and augment venous return. Specific techniques include toe-raising, intermittent leg-crossing and contraction, thigh muscle co-contraction, bending at waist, slow marching in place, and leg elevation (Bouvette, McPhee, & Opfer-Gehrking, 1994).
   j. FES may be performed as ordered to contract leg muscles, which increases cardiac output and improves stroke volume by redistributing blood volume from lower extremities (Krassioukov et al., 2009).
   k. If nonpharmacologic measures are ineffective, administer prescribed medications that increase vascular tone, which results in increased blood pressure (e.g., midodrine), medications that increase cardiac output and cause vasoconstriction (e.g., ephedrine or pyridostigmine), or increase blood volume (e.g., fludrocortisone) (Krassioukov et al., 2009).
   l. Educate patients and families on the causes of OH and potential treatment options.
   m. Use elevating leg rests and partially reclined chair backs.
   n. Monitor closely during bathing or showering, when compression garments are off and warmth of water dilates blood vessels. Patient may need bed bath, cart shower, or reclining shower chair.
   o. Teach blood pressure measurement and monitoring of safe range to patient and family.
   p. Ensure that family and patient know interventions for OH.
5. Outcomes and long-term considerations
   a. In people with SCI, continued hypotension may contribute to the development of pressure ulcers from reduced tissue perfusion.
   b. Resolving OH improves a person's functional status and reduces the risk of complications.
   c. Orthostatic hypotension in older adults contributes to significant morbidity from falls, fractures, syncope, transient ischemic attacks (TIAs), and myocardial infarction (MI) (Gupta & Lipsitz, 2007).
   d. OH in older adults is predictive of stroke, MI, and increase in overall mortality (Arbogast et al., 2009).
   e. A high percentage of older adults are asymptomatic, so symptom complaints cannot be the only measure used for diagnosis.

C. Myocardial Infarction (MI)
1. Definition: A blocked coronary causes a decrease or interruption in blood flow to the subendocardial areas of the heart, causing myocardial ischemia. Prolonged cardiac ischemia can result in death due to heart muscle being deprived of oxygen and nutrients.
2. Common rehabilitation populations at risk
   a. Amputation: Acute cardiac events are one of the most frequent medical complications for amputees (Meikle, Devlin, & Garfinkel, 2000). People who need amputations due to impaired circulation rather than trauma often have

cardiovascular disease. Posttraumatic lower limb amputees have higher rates of morbidity and mortality from cardiovascular disease. Abnormalities of arterial flow proximal to the amputation site may be the link to cardiovascular risk (Naschitz & Lenger, 2008). Energy expenditure required for either ambulation or wheelchair mobility can exert excessive strain on an already compromised cardiac system (Marshal & Stansby, 2010).

b. Stroke: A common complication of ischemic stroke is cardiac autonomic dysfunction, which causes fluctuation in blood pressure. This dysfunction causes increased risk for ischemic heart damage, hypertension, arrhythmias, and MI (Chen, Lai, Lin, Liou, & Lin, 2011). MIs necessitate transfer to acute care hospitalization in 15.7% of stroke patients (Stineman, Ross, Maislin, Fiedler, & Granger, 2003).

c. Brain tumors may be associated with cardiac arrhythmias and MI due to autonomic cardiac dysfunction.

3. Assessment
   a. Most symptoms occur over several hours
   b. Epigastric pain: May start off feeling like heartburn
   c. Crushing chest pain, like a vise around the chest
   d. Poor facial color, greenish hue
   e. Dizziness
   f. Faintness
   g. Dyspnea
   h. Women may not exhibit typical symptoms
4. Nursing interventions specific to rehabilitation
   a. Contact physician immediately and initiate emergency oxygen.
   b. Administer one baby aspirin (81 mg) as prescribed by MD or advanced cardiac life support protocol.
   c. Obtain stat cardiac enzymes and electrocardiogram.
   d. Monitor vital signs, oxygenation, heart sounds, and cardiac rhythms for changes.
   e. Enforce bed rest until MI ruled in or ruled out.
   f. Educate patient and family on signs and symptoms of MI.
   g. Prepare patient and family for next steps of probable transfer to a cardiac unit for monitoring and further treatment.
5. Outcomes and long-term considerations
   a. In stroke patients, 11.9% of unexpected adverse events were cardiac related, such as hypotension, hypertension, and MI (Ostwald, Godwin, & Fang, 2013).
   b. Cardiopulmonary arrest and chest pain were conditions most associated with increased risk of transfer to acute care during stroke rehabilitation (Stineman et al., 2003).
   c. In new amputees, cardiovascular complications caused death in 23.9% of cases, making it the most common complication causing death (Belmont et al., 2011). Ambulating with a prosthesis expends 25%–40% additional energy for a below-the-knee amputation (BKA) as compared to a normal ambulator. A person with an above-the-knee amputation (AKA) expends 65% to 100% more energy for ambulation. These additional energy needs will severely limit the mobility of patients with existing ischemic disease (Marshal & Stansby, 2010).

D. Arterial Occlusive Disease, Peripheral

1. Definition: Ineffective peripheral tissue perfusion may be related to deficient knowledge of controllable risk factors such as hypertension, smoking, and sedentary lifestyle. Arterial occlusive altered skin characteristics, diminished pulses, claudication, or delayed peripheral wound healing may occur in cases of occlusive vessel disease. Although this is often a chronic disease that occurs slowly over time, acute arterial occlusion, an emergency situation, has also been known to occur in the rehabilitation setting.
2. Common rehabilitation populations at risk
   a. SCI
   b. Stroke
   c. MS
   d. Guillain–Barré
   e. Diabetes
   f. Genetic clotting disorders
3. Assessment
   a. Signs of peripheral arterial occlusion
      1) Intermittent claudication
      2) Pain in the limb at rest
      3) Numbness of the extremity
      4) Muscle atrophy and weakness
      5) Cool extremity
      6) Diminished or absent pulses
      7) Extremity is pale when elevated, dusky red when in dependent position.
      8) Hair loss and thickened toenails in chronic condition
      9) Nonhealing ulcers or other wounds in the affected limb

10) In acute occlusion, sudden pain, pulselessness, pallor (or cyanosis), and coolness are the common symptoms.

b. Assess degree of paralysis or generalized weakness due to deconditioning, which may prevent adequate blood flow.

c. Assess peripheral blood flow using Doppler ultrasound, palpate arteries in the lower extremities, and assess color, temperature, and sensation of pain in the extremities.

4. Nursing interventions specific to rehabilitation

a. Perform passive or active range of motion.

b. Position lower extremities to promote proper blood flow.

c. Educate patients about controllable risk factors such as maintenance of blood pressures in safe range, smoking cessation, and exercise programs.

d. Treat a sudden onset of limb pain with suspicion, and assess for signs of acute arterial occlusion.

5. Outcomes and long-term considerations

a. Promotion of therapeutic environment enables people with disabilities to engage in activities to increase circulation.

b. Collaboration with the interdisciplinary team maximizes function and promotes health and wellness.

c. Healthy lifestyles can be encouraged and promoted through the lifespan, such as weight management, abstaining from smoking, and performing regular exercises.

E. Venous Thromboembolism: Deep Vein Thrombosis and Pulmonary Embolism

1. Definition of *venous thromboembolism* (VTE): A blood clot that forms in a vein and migrates to another location. A deep venous thrombosis that becomes a pulmonary embolism (PE) often results in serious health consequences, such as disability or death. Factors associated with an increased likelihood of VTE, especially in cases of acute ischemic stroke, include history of atrial fibrillation or flutter and receipt of intravenous or intraarterial tissue plasminogen activator (Douds et al., 2014).

2. Common rehabilitation populations at risk

a. SCI: The risk of DVT and PE is significantly higher in SCI patients compared with the general population. The highest risk is seen within the first 3 months after injury (Chung et al., 2014).

b. Stroke: Incidence of DVT after acute stroke within 2 weeks was 12.4% in a large population in China (Chung et al., 2014). One Canadian study indicated that PE was more common (1% with acute ischemic stroke) in patients with severe stroke, history of cancer, previous DVT or PE, or acute DVT. PE is associated with lower short- and long-term survival, greater disability, and longer length of acute hospitalization (Pongmoragot et al., 2013).

c. Traumatic brain injury (TBI): PE or DVT may occur more commonly in people with decreased mobility as a result of severe brain injury.

d. MS: PE or DVT can occur in this population as a result of immobility.

f. Studies suggest PE can present without DVT (Van Gent et al., 2014).

3. Assessment

a. Noninvasive Doppler ultrasound and detection of D-dimer in plasma have been studied for sensitivity and specificity in the detection of DVTs in symptomatic patient (Chappell et al., 2014).

b. Prescreening tools help predict DVT occurrence, such as age over 65 years, sex (female), obesity, active cancer, cerebral hemorrhagic stroke, and extremity muscle weakness.

c. Initial and ongoing assessment for redness, pain, or swelling in any extremity, as well as monitoring for elevation of C-reactive protein and D-dimer, are important in early detection.

d. Assess upon admission if a vena cava filter has been placed before rehabilitation. If DVT is suspected, the presence of the filter can be helpful in determining the actual cause without attempting to place another filter. No specific precautions are needed when an inferior vena cava filter is in place. Filters can be left in place indefinitely, unless there is suspicion that the device is causing infection or that blood flow is impeded.

e. Note: Homan's sign does not have good power for ruling in or ruling out DVT and should no longer be used as an assessment tool.

4. Nursing and team interventions specific to rehabilitation

a. Pharmacologic thromboembolism prophylaxis (Amin, Lin, Thompson, & Weiderkehr, 2013) across the continuum of care can be used to control the number of complications from VTE while avoiding additional intracranial hemorrhage in patients with moderate to severe brain injury (Nickele, Kamps, & Medow, 2013).

b. Physicians may consider interruption of rehabilitation program for implanting inferior vena cava filters (VCFs) in high-risk situations, because PE poses potentially fatal consequences.
c. Prevention of VTE includes early mobilization and prophylactic anticoagulation and may include mechanical methods such as antiembolism stockings, intermittent pneumatic compression, and foot impulse devices that are noninvasive (Robertson & Roche, 2013).
d. Some sources indicate that the efficacy of graduated compression stockings or intermittent pneumatic compression in the population recovering from stroke is not clear (Naccarato, Grandi, Dennis, & Sandercock, 2010).
e. Using a wheelchair knee gatch to elevate lower extremities and avoiding lower extremity trauma during transfers helps to decrease the risk of DVT.
f. Radiation and chemotherapy may increase the risk of DVT and PE. Therefore, prophylaxis may be indicated in these populations. Anticoagulation should be used unless there is ongoing bleeding or severe coagulopathy (Chung, Lee, Kim, & Eho, 2011).
g. Pharmacological prophylaxis significantly decreased the incidence of DVT in subjects with acute SCI (Halim, Chhabra, Arora, & Kumar, 2014).
h. Low-molecular-weight heparin (LMWH) is the preferred method of choice for the prevention of VTE in people who have had ischemic strokes in Polish, European, and American countries (Bembenek & Czlonkowska, 2013)

5. Outcomes and long-term considerations
   a. Results of VTE incidence and patterns of prophylaxis in acute ischemic stroke patients considered appropriate for prophylaxis (nonambulatory) were published in the Get With the Guidelines–Stroke (GWTG-S) Study. There was a high overall rate of prophylaxis used, but the incidence of VTE was 3% and differed between hospitals (Douds et al., 2014).
   b. Patients with TBI were studied in an intensive care setting. Mechanical and pharmacological prophylaxis appears to be the best practice for prevention of DVTs and PEs (Praeger et al., 2012).
   c. It has been shown that patients with DVT or PE receiving anticoagulation with the presence of a vena cava filter prevented recurrence of PE (Young, Tang, & Hughes, 2010).

F. Remote or Extra-Ischemic Intracerebral Hemorrhage or Hemorrhagic Conversion

1. Definition: Intracerebral hemorrhage can occur spontaneously or after intravenous recombinant tissue-type plasminogen activator (tPA) is used to treat patients who have experienced an initial ischemic stroke. This can take place in relation to the infarct or in remote areas from infarcted tissue (Mazya et al., 2014). Intracerebral hemorrhage is an uncommon complication of stroke thrombolysis that increases mortality and decreases functional outcomes.
2. Common rehabilitation populations at risk: Previous stroke and higher age were associated with increased incidence of remote parenchymal hemorrhage.
3. Assessment
   a. Monitor blood pressure readings for variations and trends.
   b. Administer antihypertensives at prescribed intervals.
   c. Communicate with physician regarding elevation of blood pressure above baseline.
4. Nursing and team interventions specific to rehabilitation
   a. Heightened importance must be placed on the assessment of neurological status in people recovering from a stroke, particularly those who have received tPA.
   b. Follow established parameters for administration of additional as-needed antihypertensives to prevent complications.
   c. More research is needed on the effect of preexisting cerebrovascular disease on complications of recanalization therapy in acute ischemic stroke.
5. Outcomes and long-term considerations
   a. Complications of intracerebral hemorrhage can be prevented by close monitoring of blood pressure after an initial ischemic stroke.
   b. When tPA is administered, nurses must be vigilant for signs of a potential hemorrhage, such as cognitive decline, nausea and vomiting, papillary changes, and weakness.
   c. Ensure that patient and family know how to measure blood pressure and frequency required.
   d. Ensure that patient and family know the importance of taking antihypertensives as prescribed.

G. Autonomic Dysreflexia (AD)

1. Definition: AD is a potentially life-threatening medical emergency that affects people with an

SCI at T6 or above. An irritating stimulus below the level of injury sends nerve impulses to the spinal cord, which are blocked at the level of injury. The body does not respond to these impulses as it should and activates unopposed sympathetic activity. Massive vasoconstriction is triggered and elevates the blood pressure. Nerve receptors in the heart and blood vessels sense the rising blood pressure, causing vasodilation above the level of injury. This sequence will continue until the noxious stimulus is removed (Milligen, Lee, McMillan, & Klassen, 2012). Most common causes of AD are

a. Distended bladder (blocked catheter, overfilled bladder, UTI)
b. Distended bowel (constipation, impaction, hemorrhoids)
c. Skin irritation (pressure ulcer, infections, cuts, bruise, abrasions, ingrown toenails, burns, tight or restrictive clothing)
d. Sexual activity
e. Menstrual cramps
f. Bone fractures
g. Abdominal conditions (gastric ulcer, colitis)
h. Labor and delivery.

2. Common rehabilitation populations at risk: People with an SCI at T6 or above
3. Assessment
   a. Hypertension
   b. Bradycardia: less than 60 beats per minute
   c. Pounding headache
   d. Flushed face
   e. Sweating above the level of injury
   f. Goosebumps below the level of injury
   g. Nasal stuffiness
   h. Symptoms may vary by individual
4. Nursing interventions specific to rehabilitation
   a. If patient is complaining of a headache, first check blood pressure to see whether it is elevated; it is important to know the patient's baseline blood pressure. A reading of 20–40 mmHg above baseline in adults and 15–20 mmHg in adolescents and children may confirm AD. The blood pressure with continue to rise until the cause of the irritating stimulus is removed, so check blood pressure frequently, about every 5 minutes until resolved (Maddox, 2013).
   b. Sit the patient up in bed or in wheelchair at 90 degrees to allow gravity to lower the blood pressure. Lower legs if possible. Remove tight clothing.
   c. Do not leave the patient alone.
   d. Search for and remove the irritating stimulus. Most common causes are a distended bladder or bowel. Check urinary catheter for kinks, catheterize bladder using lidocaine jelly, check rectal vault for stool, inspect body for skin irritation or pinching.
   e. Provide medications if the stimulus cannot be located or removed. Antihypertensive medications with a rapid onset and a short half-life, such as nitropaste, nifedipine, and nitrates, are commonly prescribed (Milligen et al., 2012).
   f. Monitor blood pressure for 2–48 hours after an episode of AD.
   g. Provide patient and family education about the signs, symptoms, and treatment of AD.
   h. Ensure that patients and families have the necessary equipment at home to treat an episode of AD (blood pressure cuff, lidocaine jelly, medications).
5. Outcomes and long-term considerations:
   a. Untreated, AD can lead to seizures, stroke, and potentially death (Milligen et al., 2012).
   b. Many health professionals are not familiar with this condition, so patients and families must know the patient's baseline blood pressure readings and be able to verbalize the treatment options to caregivers.
   c. Educate patients and families as to their specific triggers and premedicate if necessary (e.g., sexual activity, menstruation) to prevent occurrences.
   d. Educate patients and families about the importance of establishing appropriate bladder, bowel, and skin care practices to prevent episodes of AD.

III. Infections

A. Suture Line or Surgical Site Infection (SSI)

1. Definition: Bacteria introduced into the surgical site either during or shortly after surgery causes an infection in the part of the body where surgery occurred. The high bacteria count in the incision prevents the formation of healthy granulation tissue. Microbial growth invades into the host tissue and leads to cellular injury and immunological reactions that interrupt healing. The edges of the incision do not adhere and begin to break down, causing the incision line to open, called dehiscence. Dehiscence can occur in the first 5–8 days postoperatively or when an infection is present (Vuola, 2006). SSIs are an unintended and preventable consequence of surgery and considered the second most common healthcare-associated infection (HAI). In a 2011 study, superficial

wound infections occurred in 5.3% of patients and in 9.3% of cases that required a patient's return to surgery (Belmont et al., 2011).

2. Common rehab populations at risk
   a. Lower extremity amputations
   b. Below-the-knee amputation (BKA)
   c. Above-the-knee amputation (AKA)
   d. Postoperative craniotomies after brain tumor resections and TBI
   e. Multitrauma patients with surgical intervention or external fixator
   f. Postoperative orthopedic procedures such as total hip arthroplasty (THA) and total knee arthroplasty (TKA)
   g. SCIs with surgical intervention or stabilization hardware
3. Assessment
   a. Check temperature to assess for fever.
   b. Monitor laboratory values for elevated white blood cell count (WBC).
   c. Assess for erythema around incision site.
   d. Monitor closely for elevated local skin temperature around incision site.
   e. Assess for increased drainage, particularly malodorous drainage.
   f. Watch for presence of purulent drainage, discolored exudate.
   g. Assess for pain or tenderness at site.
   h. Determine presence of delayed healing.
   i. Monitor and measure degree of swelling or edema at site.
   j. Assess wound for tissue breakdown or enlargement of involved area.
   k. Be alert for a sudden onset of confusion (i.e., delirium), especially in older adults, which may signal infection without other signs being observable.
4. Nursing interventions specific to rehabilitation
   a. Recognize signs and symptoms of infection early.
   b. Use adequate hand hygiene before patient contact.
   c. Cleanse the wound using aseptic technique to remove bacteria and surface contaminants, with saline-soaked gauze for minimal trauma to the site, pat dry.
   d. Gently irrigate wound with normal saline.
   e. Apply appropriate dressings to absorb excess exudates.
   f. Administer oral or intravenous antibiotics as prescribed.
   g. Provide adequate nutritional support to promote healing.
   h. Appropriate pin site care, usually twice daily using cotton swabs and sterile water or a mixture of half normal saline and half hydrogen peroxide (Lethaby, Temple, & Santy-Tomlinson, 2013).
   i. Provide patient and family education on signs, symptoms, and treatment of infections.
5. Outcomes and long-term considerations
   a. Surgical site infections are a cause of increased healthcare costs, increased readmission rates, increased hospital lengths of stay, and increased mortality. These infections can also slow or prolong rehabilitation.
   b. In amputees, an infection may necessitate revision of the residual limb, which influences potential functional status.
   c. Patients with malnutrition are more at risk for infection (Vuola, 2006).

B. Central Line–Associated Bloodstream Infections (CLABSI)

1. Definition: A *CLABSI* is a bacterial infection in the bloodstream. It is a laboratory-confirmed bloodstream infection that is not secondary to an infection at another site (Centers for Disease Control and Prevention [CDC], 2014). Any patient with a central venous catheter is at risk for a bloodstream infection because his or her own skin flora can contaminate the catheter, causing a central line infection (Medina, Serratt, Pelter, & Brancamp, 2014).
2. Common rehabilitation populations at risk: Any hospitalized rehabilitation patient with a central venous catheter or other invasive device that breaches the skin barrier
3. Assessment
   a. Fever higher than 38°C
   b. Chills
   c. Hypotension
   d. Pain and tenderness at catheter insertion site
   e. Redness around catheter insertion site
   f. Drainage at catheter insertion site
   g. Delirium
   h. Elevated WBC
4. Nursing interventions specific to rehabilitation
   a. Treat fever by administering acetaminophen as prescribed. Remove all excess blankets. Cool body using a cooling blanket or ice packs if necessary for a high fever.
   b. Increase fluid intake.
   c. Administer antibiotics as prescribed.
   d. Prevention is best strategy; follow facility protocols for central line care and use.

e. Remove central line as soon as it is no longer needed.
f. Minimize manipulation of central line by patient or during therapy.
g. Educate patient and family on the signs, symptoms, and treatment of the bloodstream infection.

5. Outcomes and long-term considerations
   a. Central line use is a major risk factor for CLABSI. All central lines should be closely monitored and removed as soon as possible. Central lines should not be kept in for convenience or lab draws (Medina et al., 2014).
   b. The CDC has identified evidence-based strategies to prevent CLABSI, including proper hand hygiene, the use of insertion checklists, aseptic barrier precautions, skin cleansing, and proper line maintenance (Medina et al., 2014).
   c. Daily bathing in 2% chlorhexidine gluconate (CHG) is recommended by the CDC as an evidence-based strategy for preventing bloodstream infections by decreasing the amount of bacteria on the skin (Medina et al., 2014).
   d. CLABSI is a major source of morbidity and mortality and leads to increased length of stay. Annually more than 250,000 cases of hospital-acquired bloodstream infections are linked to central line use (Medina et al., 2014).

C. Sepsis

1. Definition: *Sepsis* is the body's systemic inflammatory response to an infection, usually bacterial, in any part of the body. Sepsis can rapidly progress to severe sepsis and septic shock unless the condition is recognized early and treatment started quickly. Sepsis is often diagnosed too late and is underreported because it is not always recognized by clinicians (Nelson, LeMaster, Plost, & Zahner, 2009). This overwhelming response of the immune system to the infection causes vasodilatation, leading to increased vascular permeability from the damaged blood vessels. This increase of blood rushing to the site of the infection and capillary leakage allows body fluids and white blood cells to leak out and accumulate in the tissues and organs, causing decreased tissue perfusion and increased clot formation. Decreased tissue perfusion contributes to tissue ischemia and hypoxia in organs. This condition progresses through four worsening phases—systemic inflammatory response syndrome (SIRS), sepsis, severe sepsis, and septic shock—unless recognized and treated. The progression may be rapid, subtle, and easily missed. Early recognition and emergency treatment within the "golden hour" after the onset of the condition are essential to successful treatment of sepsis (Privette Nelson, LeMaster, Plost, & Zahner, 2009; Rivera, 2009). Progression through the sepsis cascade can lead to organ dysfunction, organ failure, and death without treatment (Powers & Burchell, 2010). Sepsis is often mistaken for other conditions such as influenza, gastrointestinal virus, and UTIs because the symptoms can present in a subtle way, and the vital signs of many patients fit the SIRS criteria (Powers & Burchell, 2010).
2. Common rehabilitation populations at risk: Infections that involve the lungs, intraabdominal cavity, central nervous system, genitourinary system, skin or wound infections, and intravascular catheters are most commonly associated with sepsis (Rivera, 2009). In many cases, the actual cause of the infection is never known (Nelson et al., 2009).
3. Assessment: To promote early recognition of sepsis, rehabilitation patients should be assessed routinely for
   a. Fever or hypothermia
   b. Tachycardia
   c. Hypotension
   d. Tachypnea and shortness of breath
   e. Hypoxia: oxygen saturation <92%
   f. Decreasing urine output
   g. Change in mental status
   h. Warm extremities and bounding pulses
   i. Abnormal lab values: platelet count, bilirubin, serum lactate levels, creatinine, alkaline phosphate, aspartate aminotransferase level, alanine aminotransferase level
   j. Elevated, normal, or subnormal WBCs
4. SIRS
   a. Definition: This phase is the body's inflammatory reaction to a noninfective process, such as trauma, MI, or burns. Tissue damage or ischemia triggers inflammation. SIRS alters capillary endothelium, increasing nitric oxide production and impairing vasodilation. The interplay between inflammatory cells and mediators leads to a cascade of endothelial injury, global tissue hypoxia, microthrombus formation, and abnormal oxygen use (Powers & Burchell, 2010). Symptoms include at least two of the following conditions:
      1) Core body temperature higher than 38 °C or less than 36 °C
      2) Heart rate greater than 90 beats per minute
      3) Respiratory rate greater than 20 breaths per minute

4) WBC greater than 12,000

5. Sepsis: The second phase includes at least two of the SIRS criteria along with a known or suspected infection. Treating the infection with antibiotics should not be delayed until the culture is completed. The patient should start antibiotic therapy and be monitored closely for signs and symptoms of organ failure (**Table 28-1**), which indicates that the patient has moved into severe sepsis (Privette Nelson et al., 2009). Additional early signs and symptoms of sepsis are
   a. Narrow pulse pressure
   b. Tachycardia
   c. Altered tissue perfusion (hypotension, decreased urine output, decreased skin perfusion)
   d. Indication of impaired coagulation (decreased platelets, petechiae)
   e. It is crucial to monitor patients closely once sepsis is suspected because it can rapidly progress to severe sepsis. The progression to severe sepsis and septic shock can sometimes be halted by early recognition and treatment of sepsis (Kleinpell, 2004; Powers & Burchell, 2010).
6. Severe Sepsis
   a. Definition: The systemic inflammatory response profoundly affects the delivery of oxygen to the tissues. The condition now progresses to cellular dysfunction, evidence of hypoperfusion, and organ damage from tissue hypoxia. Patients need aggressive critical care medical treatment and still have a mortality rate of 30%–50% (Powers & Burchell, 2010; Privette Nelson et al., 2009).
   b. Assess for symptoms including:
      1) Body temperature > 38.3°C
      2) Heart rate > 90 beats per minute
      3) Tachypnea 20 breaths per minute
      4) Altered mental status
      5) Significant edema or positive fluid balance of 20 mL/kg over 24-hour period
      6) Hyperglycemia.
7. Septic Shock
   a. Definition: The final phase has limited chances for recovery, with a mortality rate of 50%–60% (Kleinpell, Aitken, & Schorr, 2013). In this situation, the person has persistent hypotension (systolic blood pressure below 90 mmHg), contributing to hypoperfusion that does not respond to fluid resuscitation (Privette Nelson et al., 2009). Common complications of septic shock include MI, acute renal failure (ARF), chronic renal dysfunction, disseminated intravascular coagulation (DIC), and liver failure (Powers & Burchell, 2010).
   b. Common rehabilitation populations at risk
      1) Extremes of age: very young and very old
      2) Presence of invasive devices that breach the skin barrier
      3) Use of immunosuppressants (cancer treatment, organ transplants, rheumatic disorders)
      4) Presence of comorbid conditions such as diabetes, obstructive lung disease
      5) Recent limb amputation: Sepsis is blamed for 9.3% of cases that return to the operating room and 31.7% of deaths (Belmont et al., 2011).
      6) Postsurgical patients: multitrauma
      7) Patients with existing infections (UTIs, pneumonia, suture line infection, or pressure ulcer)
   c. Assessment:
      1) Monitor vital signs and oxygenation closely.

Table 28-1. Signs and Symptoms of Organ Failure

Cardiovascular	Systolic blood pressure < 90 mmHg Mean arterial pressure < 65 mmHg A drop from baseline pressure > 40 mmHg
Hematologic	Platelets < 100,000 Platelets decreased by 50% over 3 days Acutely abnormal prothrombin time or partial thromboplastin time (PTT) without anticoagulation therapy (international normalized ratio >1.5, PTT > 60 seconds)
Hepatic	Bilirubin level > 2 mg/dL Alkaline phosphatase level > 250 units per liter Aspartate aminotransferase level > 100 units per liter Alanine amino transferase level > 100 units per liter
Metabolic	Serum lactate levels > 2 mmol/L (most sources including Surviving Sepsis Campaign guidelines agree on a serum lactate level > 4 mmol/L, but hospital data indicate an increased risk of death with serum lactate levels > 2 mmol/L)
Neurologic	Mental state acutely altered from baseline A Glasgow Coma Scale score of < 15
Pulmonary	A respiratory rate > 24 breaths per minute Oxygen saturation level < 92% with patient on oxygen at 6 L/minute using face mask
Renal	Urine output < 0.5 mL/kg per hour despite volume resuscitation Increase in creatinine level of 0.5 mg/dL

Dellinger, R. P., Carlet, J., Masur, H., Gerlach, H., Calandra, T., Cohen, J., ... Levy, M. M. (2004). Signs and Symptoms of Organ Failure. *Critical Care Medicine, 32*(3), 858–873.

2) Monitor response to intravenous fluid resuscitation.
3) Monitor urine output. Place an indwelling catheter to accurately monitor output.
4) Obtain blood cultures from two sites before initiating intravenous antibiotics.
5) Start antibiotic treatment within 45 minutes of sepsis identification (Kleinpell et al., 2013).
6) Educate patient and family about the signs, symptoms, and treatment of sepsis.
7) Prepare patient and family for probable transfer to acute hospital.

d. Nursing interventions specific to rehabilitation: Early identification of sepsis and the source of infection in the rehabilitation setting are critical to containing the infection and initiating appropriate interventions. In approximately 20%–30% of sepsis cases the source of infection cannot be easily identified (Kleinpell, 2004).

3. Outcomes and long-term considerations
1) The nurse's role in prevention of infection and sepsis is important. Use the best infection control practices of hand hygiene, central line catheter care, indwelling urinary catheter care, and wound or surgical site care to prevent infections (Kleinpell et al., 2013).
2) Early identification of symptoms and early treatment result in the best outcomes.
3) Monitor patient for seeded infection to implants such as artificial joints, defibrillators, pacemakers, heart valves, shunts, and any implanted hardware.

D. Hospital-Acquired Pneumonia

1. Definition: Hospital-acquired pneumonia is caused by an increase in thick secretions, leading to a secondary infection in the lungs. Atelectasis, the reversible closure or collapse of alveoli, occurs when a person has difficulty mobilizing thick secretions and clearing the airway because of an ineffective or weak cough (Ferreyra, Long, & Ranieri, 2009). As a result of aspiration, these secretions become infected with bacteria that normally inhabit the upper airway and stomach (nasal, oropharyngeal, or gastric flora) or their own saliva. These pneumonias are often attributed to the use of ventilators (ventilator-associated pneumonia [VAP]), weak respiratory muscles, or dysphagia. Pneumonia can inhibit the respiratory system's ability to effectively perform gas exchange, resulting in acute respiratory failure.

2. Common rehabilitation populations at risk

a. Stroke
1) Pneumonia causes the highest mortality rate of all medical complications after stroke (Armstrong & Mosher, 2011).
2) Most poststroke pneumonias are a result of aspiration because of impaired swallowing caused by the neurologic insult (Armstrong & Mosher, 2011).
3) Incidence of stroke-associated pneumonia during rehabilitation is 3.2%–11% (Hannawi, Hannawi, Rao, Suarez, & Bershad, 2013).
4) Approximately 50% of people with stroke have a dysfunctional swallow or dysphagia, and of those who aspirate, approximately one-third will develop aspiration pneumonia (Armstrong & Mosher, 2011).

b. Traumatic or acquired brain injuries: A dysfunctional swallow results in aspiration from the neurological insult.

c. SCI
1) Leading cause of death for each age group and level of injury, up to 72.3% of deaths, particularly high for patients with tetraplegia (Chiodo et al., 2007).
2) Newly injured patients with tetraplegia are often on ventilators, at least initially increasing the risk of developing hospital-acquired pneumonia. These people are also at a higher risk for developing aspiration pneumonia because of impaired or weak swallowing muscles (Laffont et al., 2008).
3) Decreased respiratory muscle strength leads to a weak and ineffective cough and difficulty clearing secretions and airways (Berry, Johnson, & Vander Ploerg, 2002). The accessory muscle strength may improve over time, although patients are still at higher risk of developing pneumonia throughout their lifetime.
4) People with tetraplegia are unable to fully expand their lungs, decreasing their vital capacity and contributing to microatelectasis (Laffont et al., 2008).

d. Neurologic conditions (e.g., MS, ALS, Guillain–Barré, Parkinson's disease, postpolio syndrome)
1) Decreased respiratory muscle strength contributes to decreased airflow and a decreased vital capacity, which leads to a rapid, shallow breathing pattern and a weak and ineffective cough (Berry et al., 2002).

2) Many neurological conditions affect a person's ability to swallow, increasing the risk for aspiration pneumonia (Mangera, Panesar, & Makker, 2012).
3) The patient's ability to protect his or her airway becomes compromised, leading to chest infections (Mangera et al., 2012).
4) Pneumonia is the cause of 20% of deaths in patients with Parkinson's disease because of weakness in facial, oropharyngeal, and laryngeal muscles, leading to compromised swallow and secretion clearance (Mangera et al., 2012).

e. Burns: Pneumonia results from extended mechanical ventilation, loss of chest wall elasticity, and thermal burns (Boots, Dulhunty, Paratz, & Lipman, 2009).

f. Postsurgical patients (amputation, multitrauma)
   1) Atelectasis is a common respiratory complication after surgery and general anesthesia (Ferreyra et al., 2009).

g. Any patient who had been previously mechanically ventilated is at risk for a hospital-acquired pneumonia because of immobility and sedation. Meticulous oral care and adherence to VAP bundles is essential for prevention (Kumar et al., 2010).

3. Assessment
   a. Pneumonia is suspected when the patient has:
      1) Shortness of breath
      2) Difficulty maintaining oxygenation
      3) Fever
      4) Increased chest congestion
      5) Increased sputum production: Could be thick and discolored, with a foul odor
      6) Abnormal breath sounds (wheezes, coarse) on auscultation
      7) Presence of cough (may be very weak)
      8) Fatigue
      9) Chest radiograph demonstrating presence of new or progressive infiltrates
      10) A WBC higher than 12,000

4. Nursing interventions specific to rehabilitation
   a. Prevention
      1) Patients at high risk for aspiration, including anyone on a ventilator or receiving enteral feedings, must be out of bed or have the head of the bed elevated greater than 45 degrees, and preferably 90 degrees if tolerated, during feeding and 1 hour after feeding. At all other times head of bed should be at least 30 degrees for all patients (even those who are NPO) (Kumar et al., 2010).
      2) Ensure that the patient receives frequent good oral care and dental hygiene, including tooth brushing and oral suctioning to decrease amount of bacteria in the mouth (Kumar et al., 2010).
      3) If a tracheostomy is in place, the site should be cleansed per hospital policy. If suctioning is necessary, sterile technique should be maintained.
      4) Consider broad-spectrum antibiotic therapy as a prophylactic measure for high-risk patients (Kumar et al., 2010).
      5) Ensure proper hand washing by patient and caregiver.
      6) Caregivers and visitors with upper respiratory infection should wear masks at all times.
      7) Encourage deep breathing exercises, use of incentive spirometry, and other respiratory treatments to expand the lungs and mobilize secretions.
      8) Promote influenza and pneumonia shots as prescribed.
   b. The focus of treatment for pneumonia is to clear the lungs of secretions, open airways, and treat the infection with antibiotics.
   c. Methods of clearing secretions and opening airways include
      1) Mucolytics to thin and loosen secretions or inhalers to open airways
      2) Increasing fluid intake (hydration) to thin and loosen secretions
      3) Ensuring that the patient receives frequent good oral care and dental hygiene, including tooth brushing to decrease amount of bacteria in the mouth (Kumar et al., 2010). Basic oral care protocols have been proven to decrease nonventilator hospital-acquired pneumonia (NV-HAP) by 37% during a 12-month intervention period (Quinn et al., 2014). Avoidance of NV-HAP cases resulted in an estimated eight lives saved, $1.72 million in costs avoided, and 500 extra hospital days averted.
      4) Assisted cough techniques to create and strengthen a cough through increased abdominal pressure
      5) Using full 12 positions of postural drainage, getting patient out of bed, and turning every 2–4 hours while in bed to mobilize secretions

6) Percussion or vibration to loosen congestion in the lungs
7) Mechanical devices to expand the lungs, loosen secretions, and trigger a cough response, such as intermittent positive pressure breathing, insufflator/exsufflator, or intrapulmonary percussive ventilation (McKinley, Gittler, Kirshblum, Stiens, & Groah, 2002; Roth et al., 2010).
8) Administering oral or intravenous antibiotic therapy such as macrolides, tetracyclines, fluoroquinolones, cephalosporins, penicillins, or vancomycin as prescribed
9) Supplementing oxygen as needed. May need short-term ventilatory support.
10) Tracheostomy decannulation should be initiated as soon as the patient is no longer ventilator dependent for at least 24 hours, unless there is an irreversible condition. Progression begins with cuff deflation after assessment of hemodynamic stability, swallowing, cough strength, and aspiration risk, management of secretions, and toleration of cuff deflation and measuring cough strength (Morris, McIntosh, & Whitmer, 2014).
11) Educating all patients on need for annual flu shots and pneumonia vaccine per schedule

5. Outcomes and long-term considerations
   a. Patients and families should be educated to aggressively treat all colds and respiratory infections by promoting lung expansion and clearing secretions to prevent lung congestion (Maddox, 2013).
   b. Promote the use of exercises to strengthen inspiratory muscles to improve the cough response, thereby decreasing risk of pneumonia (McKinley et al., 2002). Abdominal binders can stabilize the abdomen and generate pressure through the thorax to increase inspiratory and expiratory muscle activation and improve lung volumes (Wadsworth, Haines, Cornwell, Rodwell, & Paratz, 2012).
   c. Ensure that a formal swallow evaluation is completed on all patients at high risk for aspiration or dysphagia and modify food and fluid consistently as appropriate. Keep the patient NPO until the risk has been adequately assessed (Kumar et al., 2010). If enteral feeding is advised, assess patient's and caregiver's acceptance of short-term nasogastric tube versus longer duration through gastrostomy tube.
   d. Advancing paralysis with Guillain–Barré syndrome can occur after the initial onset of neurological deterioration. Monitoring of neurological level of involvement is important to recognize decline early so that additional doses of intravenous immunoglobulin or steroids can be administered.
   e. Aging postpolio patients can experience neurological decline long after the initial disease occurred. Continued monitoring of neurological level is important to detect changes in order to provide additional measures to prevent functional decline or include modifications to preserve quality of life.
   f. Patients with high-level SCI, advancing paralysis with Guillain–Barré, or aging with postpolio syndrome can experience decreased oxygenation long after the initial injury or onset of disease. Oxygen needs may change as the person ages, especially when intercostal muscle tone decreases. Monitoring of pulmonary function is important over time to determine needs. Some patients need respiratory support at night through the use of bilevel positive airway pressure or continuous positive airway pressure. Sleep apnea studies may be necessary to determine respiratory function, particularly when respiratory status is compromised.
   g. People aging with a disability, such as those who have had polio or cerebral palsy, and those who are sedentary in a wheelchair are at an increased risk for pneumonia as they age.

IV. Neurological Complications

A. Spasticity

1. Definition: A motor disorder characterized by increase in muscle tone, exaggerated tendon reflexes, and clonus. Spasticity can occur as a result of an upper motor neuron lesion in the spinal cord or brain rather than in peripheral nerves. Spasticity is characterized by a velocity-dependent increase in tonic stretch reflexes, known as muscle tone, with exaggerated tendon jerks, resulting from hyperexcitability of the stretch reflex as one component of the upper motor neuronal syndrome (Lance, 1980).
2. Muscle spasticity can interfere with motor function and may lead to soft tissue shortening (fixed contractures) or can cause distressing symptoms such as painful muscle spasms (Bakheit, 2012). Conversely, spasticity can benefit patients as the extensor muscle braces the lower limb in a rigid position. Other benefits include maintaining muscle bulk and bone mineral density and possibly

reducing risk of lower limb deep vein thrombosis. Several factors aggravate spasticity, such as pressure ulcers, fecal impaction, UTIs, and stones in the urinary bladder. Spasticity may contribute to activity limitations, caregiver burden, pain, and reduced quality of life (Demetrios, Khan, Turner-Stokes, Brand, & McSweeney, 2013).

3. Common rehabilitation populations at risk
   a. Stroke
   b. SCI
   c. TBI and nontraumatic brain injury
   d. Parkinsonism
   e. MS
4. Assessment
   a. Spasticity management and control of pain associated with spasticity management have changed significantly in the past two decades through new therapies such as botulinum toxin and surgical techniques (Bensmail, 2013).
      1) Evaluate return of reflex function after spinal shock: Rectal response to digital stimulation or bowel program.
      2) Penile erection with catheterization
      3) Observe for evidence of lower extremity spasticity.
   b. Limited data are available about clinical muscle changes that occur after stroke or about measurement tools found to be useful to address denervations, disuse, inflammation, remodeling, and spasticity (Scherbakov, von Haehling., Anker, Dirnagl, & Doehner, 2013).
   c. Evaluate impact spasticity has on functional activities, positive or negative.
      1) Does spasticity limit ability to use upper extremity to perform ADLs?
      2) Does lower extremity spasticity improve or limit patient's ability to perform transfers?
      3) Does spasticity pose a potential safety risk? Is patient able to maintain safe and functional position when sitting in wheelchair? Do spasms increase risk for injury in wheelchair or bed?
   d. Consider therapists' ratings on the Ashworth Scale as a quantitative measure of spasticity.
   e. Evaluate effectiveness of antispasmodic medications, patient compliance with medication regimen, and safety.
5. Nursing interventions specific to rehabilitation
   a. Physical activity and pharmacological measures should be promoted by rehabilitation nurses to achieve optimal function, prevent complications, and minimize distress to patients, families, and caregivers (Stevenson & Playford, 2012).
   b. Move extremities slowly to inhibit spasticity and reduce tone. Rapid stretching will increase spasticity.
   c. Note when spinal shock subsides and reflex activity is observable. Modify bowel and bladder programs because sensory stimulation provokes a predictable reflex response as spinal shock subsides, typically 8–12 weeks after damage to the central nervous system.
   d. Complementary or alternative interventions, oral medications, chemodenervation (peripheral nerve or neuromuscular junction blockade), and implantation of intrathecal baclofen pumps should be supported as viable options for patients with disabling symptom.
      1) Use of botulinum toxin A is associated with improvements in activity capacity and has been known to improve performance (Foley et al., 2013).
      2) Long-term outcomes of intrathecal baclofen therapy (ITB) for treatment of spasticity have been examined using surveys (McCormick, Chu, Mathur, & Marciniak, 2013). The efficacy and favorable side effect profile of ITB therapy was sustained in a 10-year period of using this modality. Pharmacological treatment initiated 6 months after stroke reduced lower limb spasticity (McIntyre et al., 2012).
   e. Rehabilitation nurses assist patients in making informed treatment choices hinging on the extent of symptoms, individual preference, and availability of services (Hughes & Howard, 2013).
   f. Rehabilitation nurses support and assist patients in participation and carryover of exercises such as serial casting, splinting, or positioning initiated by therapists.
   g. Enhanced communication between patient and provider improves the effect of treatment regimens for patients with poststroke spasticity (PSS) rehabilitation (Sunnerhagen & Francisco, 2013).
   h. Combinations of modalities such as repetitive transcranial magnetic stimulation and physical therapy to reduce upper limb spasticity after stroke have been documented in the literature (Barros Galvao et al., 2014).
   i. Multidisciplinary rehabilitation approaches after botulinum toxin and other focal intramuscular treatments such as phenol have been

studied to determine the effect of a team approach on activity levels, outcomes, and quality of life (Demetrios, Khan, Turner-Stokes, Brand, & McSweeney, 2013).

j. Nonpharmacological interventions for treating spasticity in adults with MS include whole body vibration, physical therapy, structured exercise programs, transcranial magnetic stimulation, repetitive transcranial magnetic stimulation, and electrical magnetic therapy (Amatya, Khan, LaMantia, Demetrious, & Wade, 2013).

k. Baclofen, tizanidine, benzodiazepine, and dantrolene sodium are first-line or adjunctive agents. Modalities such as intrathecal drug therapy contribute to accomplishment of treatment goals such as passive and active function, pain, decreased impairment, and increased mobility (Turner-Stokes, Fheodoroff, & Jacinto, 2013).

l. Conservative methods include self-management using stretching, heat, ice, vibration, electrical stimulation, extracorporeal shockwave therapy, and complementary or alternative methods such as acupuncture, cannabis and cannabinoids, nutritional supplements, massage, use of splints and orthoses, chiropractic, and exercises such as yoga.

m. The effect of controlled passive stretching and active movement training using a portable rehabilitation robot on stroke survivors with ankle and mobility impairments was evaluated in comparison to an instructed exercise program at home (Waldman et al., 2013). The robot-assisted passive stretching and active movement training are considered effective in improving motor function and mobility after stroke.

n. Visual feedback and training was studied to obtain a reliable measure for the mechanical properties of the affected upper limb during robotic therapy. The study investigated the effects of robot-assisted training and visual feedback on arm stiffness and viscosity and determined that the degree of stiffness and its relationship with training or visual feedback depended on arm position, speed, and level of resistance (Piovesan, Morasso, Giannoni, & Casadio, 2013).

o. Spasticity can be overcome actively through attempts to use the affected arm and hand. Use of the affected arm can be facilitated by adopting positions to reduce the effect of gravity on the arm or enable gravity to assist in the movement. Specific skills can be attained by repeatedly attempting specific component movements of tasks in the context of performing a variety of different activities. Frustration impedes task performance, but a mental state of detached focus can improve motivation to use the affected arm (Sabini, Dijkers, & Raghavan, 2013).

6. Outcomes and long-term considerations
   a. Spasticity is minimized through mobilization and medications.
   b. Complications can be prevented by coordination of an interdisciplinary team approach.
   c. Instruct patients to report changes in spasticity to their healthcare provider because a change in spasticity may be early sign of a complication below the level of injury.
   d. Remove noxious stimuli.
   e. Instruct patients with SCI above T6 of signs and symptoms of autonomic reflex activity, which may be caused by severe spasticity.

B. Cerebrospinal Fluid Leak

1. Definition: Meningeal tears or tears of the ventricle can result in leakage of cerebrospinal fluid (CSF) into the cortical tissue. When the CSF leaks from the nasal passages it may appear as rhinorrhea and may be unilateral. CSF may leak from other orifices as well, including the ears (otorrhea) and the postnasal sinuses. Patients with a CSF leak are at risk of developing infections, which can lead to meningitis, abscess formation in close proximity to the brain or the spinal cord, and signs or symptoms of osteomyelitis.
2. Common rehabilitation populations at risk
   a. Basal skull fractures often result in damage to the ventricles, and because of the proximity of the ventricles to the nasal passages, leakage of CSF through the nares can occur.
   b. Brain injuries with dural tears may also lead to CSF leaks. Prolonged leakage of CSF poses a significant risk for infection because organisms in the nares, ears, and paranasal sinuses may enter through the dural tear. Infections such as meningitis, brain abscess, and osteomyelitis can occur as a result of CSF leaks. Patients who have incurred penetrating head injuries from knife or gunshot wounds may be at risk as well.
3. Assessment
   a. Observe for signs of CSF drainage most commonly from the nose and the ears. CSF drainage may appear clear to light yellow in color. Bloody drainage encircled by a yellowish stain

is called the halo sign. The halo sign is commonly seen with a CSF leak.
   b. Headache
   c. Fever
   d. Intracranial pain with movement, dizziness
4. Nursing interventions specific to rehabilitation
   a. Assess patients at risk and notify the physician if there is evidence of CSF fluid in any drainage.
   b. Do not insert any objects into an orifice or irrigate the orifice because this may introduce bacteria into the leak.
   c. Caution patients with CSF leaks to avoid blowing their nose because the increase in pressure can lead to an infection.
   d. Obtain specimen for laboratory analysis.
5. Outcomes and long-term considerations
   a. Most tears associated with a basal skull fracture will heal on their own.
   b. In cases of complicated fractures that include CSF leaks, surgery may be necessary to close the leak.
   c. Antibiotic therapy may be initiated to reduce the occurrence of infection.
   d. Failure to address initial changes in motor and sensory function can result in permanent damage to the spinal cord and corresponding loss of function.

C. Syringomyelia
1. Definition: Posttraumatic syringomyelia is a disorder characterized by the formation of a fluid-filled cyst in the spinal cord. The cyst or syrinx expands and enlarges over time. Typically the syrinx occurs at or within a few segments of the traumatic lesion in the cord. If it enlarges upward, the person will complain of severe pain and progressive impairment and loss of motor function or sensation above the level of the spinal cord lesion. Other symptoms associated with syrinx formation include headaches, inability to distinguish temperature, and loss of bladder or bowel function (National Institute of Neurological Disorders and Stroke [NINDS], 2014a). If the syrinx enlarges downward, the person with an incomplete SCI may experience pain, whereas people with a complete SCI may not be aware of the presence of a syrinx until reflex activity is impaired. The most common site for a syrinx to occur is in the cervical region of the spinal cord. If there is motor or sensory loss, generally surgery is recommended to drain the syrinx. A shunt may be necessary to drain the excess CSF and reduce pressure on the surrounding tissue in the spinal cord to preserve function. If the syrinx has developed as a result of a tumor, radiation may be used to halt the growth of the tumor and reduce the pressure in the syrinx. If the syrinx is found during radiological studies and the person is asymptomatic, no treatment may be needed.
2. Common rehabilitation populations at risk
   a. People who have sustained trauma to the cerebellum or the spinal cord
   b. TBI
   c. SCI
   d. Myelomeningocele
3. Assessment
   a. Monitor and assess for changes in motor, sensory, or reflex activity after SCI. Suspect syringomyelia when there is a slow, progressive loss of function above the injury or deterioration of reflex activity below the level of the lesion. A syrinx can develop at any time after injury. Therefore, this should be considered as a potential lifetime complication.
4. Nursing interventions specific to rehabilitation
   a. Ongoing assessments of motor and sensory function after SCI are important.
   b. Assessment of patient's pain is critical. Monitoring and assessing reflex activity is part of the rehabilitation nurse's role, especially related to bladder and bowel function.
   c. If symptoms of syringomyelia are suspected, refer patient to a physician for evaluation.
5. Outcomes and long-term considerations
   a. Failure to address initial changes in motor and sensory function can result in permanent damage to the spinal cord and corresponding loss of function. A syrinx can develop at any time after injury. In a review by Perrouin-Verhe et al. (1998) involving 75 patients with SCI, a syrinx occurred in approximately 28% of the population, with the onset of the syrinx found at 1 month to 29 years.

D. Seizures
1. Definition
   a. A *seizure* is a clinical presentation of the central nervous system characterized by abnormal cerebral electrical discharges. There are many different types of seizures, and the clinical presentation of each type is associated with the location of the abnormal discharges (American Association of Neuroscience Nurses [AANN], 2007, p. 5). Status epilepticus, a medical emergency, occurs when the person experiences recurrent seizures without complete recovery of consciousness between attacks, resulting in

continuous seizure activity for more than 30 minutes (Epilepsy Foundation of America's Working Group on Status Epilepticus, 1993).

b. Physiological changes, increased central venous pressure, hyperglycemia, cardiac dysrhythmias, and respiratory collapse that occur with status epilepticus can have serious consequences.

2. Classification
   a. The International Leagues Against Epilepsy (ILAE) developed the classification system used to describe different seizure types in 1981 and revised it in 2005 (Berg et al., 2010). A second classification system, the International Classification of Epilepsy Syndromes, includes not only seizure type but also age and cause of the seizure.
   b. The ILAE table (**Table 28-2**) lists the type of seizures, common characteristics, and typical duration.
3. Common rehabilitation populations at risk
   a. TBI, especially if loss of consciousness greater than 30 minutes occurred at time of injury (Annegers, Rocca, & Hauser, 1996)
   b. Nontraumatic brain injuries
   c. Space-occupying lesions: Brain tumors, arteriovenous malformation (AVM), subdural hematoma, neurofibromatosis
   d. Cerebral infections, bacterial or viral meningitis, encephalitis, brain abscess
   e. Anoxia
   f. Cerebral vascular disorders including stroke
   g. Febrile states
   h. Hypoxic acidosis
4. Assessment
   a. The incidence of posttraumatic seizures has been reported to be anywhere from 4% to 53% (Frey, 2003). There is a higher incidence of posttraumatic seizure in patients with hemorrhages or penetrating injuries (Whyte et al., 2013).
   b. Note provoking stimuli, report of any aura and senses involved, document initial symptoms and motor activity pattern during the seizure and postictal responses.
   c. Observe for signs and symptoms of respiratory distress, which may be a precursor to status epilepticus.
5. Nursing interventions specific to rehabilitation
   a. Provide for a safe environment in bed and wheelchair and during ambulation.
      1) In bed, turn patient on side and remove any harmful objects in the vicinity, raise side rails, and stay with the patient.
      2) In wheelchair, ensure safety belt is in place, and do not attempt to transfer the patient. If possible, tilt chair backwards on rear wheels and place a pillow under the patient's head to protect the head from injury. Elevating lower extremities higher than the head will increase cerebral blood flow. Stay with the patient.
      3) If ambulating, gently lower to the floor and use a pillow or towels to protect the head. Stay with the patient.
   b. Do not restrain the person's extremities.
   c. Loosen clothing and remove eyeglasses. Do not attempt to insert anything into the person's mouth.
   d. If patient has had a craniotomy and a portion of the cranium has been removed, a protective helmet is recommended when out of bed or per surgeon's orders.
   e. Monitor for signs of respiratory compromise and status epilepticus (SE).
   f. Document time of onset, progression of symptoms, length of seizure, preceding events or symptoms, and postseizure responses.
   g. During the seizure, turn patient onto one side, open the airway, suction after, if necessary, and check vital signs.
   h. Check oxygen saturation and if low, initiate oxygen therapy as ordered.
   i. Obtain a blood glucose reading to assess whether patient is hypoglycemic.
   j. Obtain blood sample to check for medication levels if ordered.
   k. Administer medications as ordered. Common medications used to treat postinjury seizures include:
      1) Phenytoin (Dilantin)
      2) Carbamazepine (Tegretol)
      3) Valproic acid (VPA)
      4) Gabapentin (Neurontin)
      5) Levetiracetam (Keppra)
   l. Educate patient and family on measures to prevent seizures (medications to maintain therapeutic levels), safety measures (medical ID bracelet), and prohibited activities such as driving, use of power tools, swimming, and bathing safety. Check with the state Department of Motor Vehicles on reporting requirements and guidelines for issuing a driving license to people with a seizure history.

Consider a referral to vocational rehabilitation services for job counseling and training.

m. Educate patient and family on medicines prescribed to reduce the incidence of seizures and instruct how to take medications and ensure a consistent dose is given. (For liquid phenytoin, make certain to thoroughly shake bottle at time of administration.)

n. Educate patient and family on importance of routine blood work to monitor medication levels.

o. Educate family members on signs and symptoms of seizure activity and actions to take to maintain safety. Family members should be aware of signs and symptoms of status epilepticus and actions to take.

p. Instruct on safety measures and prohibited activities such as driving, use of power tools, swimming, and tub baths.

6. Outcomes and long-term considerations: Seizure activity may subside over time. Ambulatory electroencephalograms may be used to identify patients who may be weaned off antiseizure medications.

E. Hydrocephalus

1. Definition: *Hydrocephalus* is a clinical syndrome characterized by dilatation of the ventricles as a result of excess accumulation of CSF. The excess CSF may result from overproduction of CSF or impaired reabsorption (Hickey, 2003, pp. 315–316).

2. Classifications

a. Onset

1) Congenital hydrocephalus is present at birth as a result of impairment in fetal development or genetic abnormalities (NINDS, 2013, p. 2).

2) Acquired hydrocephalus occurs at birth or over the course of a person's lifetime as a result of disease or trauma.

b. Mechanism

1) Communicating hydrocephalus is a condition that occurs as a result of inadequate reabsorption of CSF within the ventricles. This may occur secondary to subarachnoid hemorrhage, aneurysm rupture, or TBI.

2) A common type of communicating hydrocephalus is normal-pressure hydrocephalus. Normal-pressure hydrocephalus is characterized by ventricular enlargement and compression on cortical tissue without changes in ventricular pressure.

3) Noncommunicating hydrocephalus occurs when an obstruction or mass impairs circulation of CSF within the ventricles. This may be seen with brain tumors, cortical infections, or structural abnormalities.

3. Common rehabilitation populations at risk

a. TBI

b. Nontraumatic brain injuries such as tumors

c. Subarachnoid hemorrhage

d. Adults older than age 70 years

e. Infants with congenital abnormalities of the spinal cord

f. Children with birth injuries such as cerebral palsy

4. Assessment

a. Symptoms may progress slowly, or it may take weeks to months to become apparent. Most common symptoms are changes in mental status often characterized by "slow, fuzzy thinking" and delayed responses. Patients may display signs of confusion or disorientation, lethargy, irritability, urinary incontinence, increased reflex activity in lower extremities, and gait disturbances.

b. In infants, a common symptom is head enlargement and delayed closure of the cranium. Treatment involves relief of the obstruction or placement of a ventricular shunt to drain CSF from the ventricles. Typically, the shunt terminates in the abdomen or other part of the body where the fluid can be absorbed into the circulatory system.

5. Nursing interventions specific to rehabilitation

a. Monitor patients for common triad of symptoms including slow thinking, recent onset of disorientation, and urinary incontinence.

b. Educate patient and caregivers about signs and symptoms and actions to take.

c. Prepare patient and family for surgical placement of ventricular shunt, if necessary.

d. Educate patient and family, if necessary, on postoperative shunt care and the need for ongoing monitoring and return of symptoms as a result of shunt malfunction.

6. Outcomes and long-term considerations

a. Patients and families should be educated to recognize signs and symptoms of shunt failure.

b. Failure may occur as a result of tissues or other anatomical structures pressing on the shunt or occlusion within the shunt. In either case, the flow of ventricular fluid through the shunt is impaired. Symptoms may appear when fluid

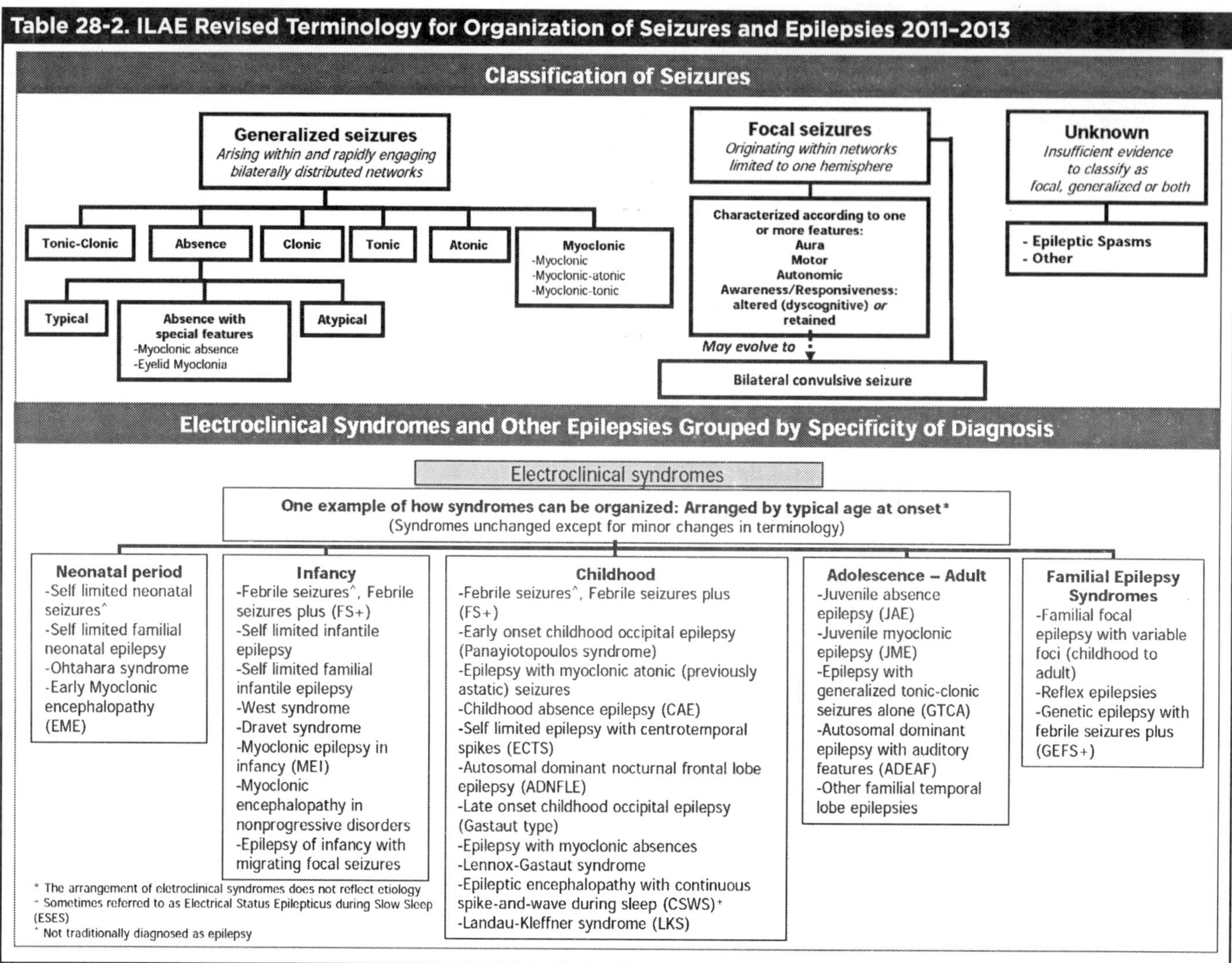

backs up in the ventricles and presses on surrounding cortical tissue.

F. Malfunctioning or Infected CSF Shunts or Ventriculoperitoneal (VP) Shunts

1. Definition: CSF shunts are the primary treatment for hydrocephalus. The CSF pathways become blocked or obstructed in the ventricular system, necessitating a shunt to drain the excess CSF off the brain to minimize damage. These CSF shunts, which may be ventriculoperitoneal (VP), lumbar-peritoneal (LP), ventriculoatrial (VA), or ventriculopleural shunts, occasionally malfunction because of obstruction, equipment error, or infection. On occasion, they may necessitate surgical revision. There is an increased risk and exposure to shunt infection with each placement or revision (Simon et al., 2009).
2. Common rehabilitation populations at risk
   a. Those with an existing shunt who are at risk for hydrocephalus
   b. TBI
   c. Brain tumors
   d. Subarachnoid hemorrhage
   e. Adults older than age 70 years
   f. Infants with congenital abnormalities of the spinal cord
   g. Children with birth injuries such as cerebral palsy
3. Assessment
   a. Most common symptoms are
      1) Drainage or odor from incision site
      2) Tenderness or bogginess at incision site
      3) Fever
      4) Headaches
      5) Nausea or vomiting
      6) Abdominal pain
      7) Personality changes
      8) Sleepiness or drowsiness
      9) Delayed verbal responses or motor reflexes
      10) Signs of confusion or disorientation, lethargy, or irritability
      11) CSF culture positive for bacteria, most often person's own skin flora, *Staphylococcus epidermis* (Langley et al., 2009).

Table 28-2. ILAE Revised Terminology for Organization of Seizures and Epilepsies 2011–2013 (continued)

Major changes in terminology and concepts		
New Term and Concept	**Examples**	**Old Term and Concept**
Etiology (an individual may fit into more than one group)		
Genetic: *genetic defect directly contributes to the epilepsy and seizures are the core symptom of the disorder*	*Channelopathies, GLUT1 deficiency, etc*	**Idiopathic:** *presumed genetic*
Structural: *caused by a structural disorder of the brain*	*Tuberous sclerosis, cortical malformations, mesial temporal lobe epilepsy with hippocampal sclerosis (MTLE with HS), gelastic seizures with hypothalmic hamartoma*	**Symptomatic:** *secondary to a known or presumed disorder of the brain*
Metabolic: *caused by a metabolic disorder of the brain*	*Pyroxidine deficiency, GLUT1 deficiency , etc*	**Symptomatic**
Immune: *epilepsy with evidence of autoimmune mediated CNS inflammation*	*NMDA receptor antibody encephalitis, voltage gated potassium channel antibody encephalitis*	**Symptomatic**
Infectious*: an infectious etiology refers to a patient with epilepsy, rather than seizures occurring in the setting of acute infection such as meningitis or encephalitis. These infections sometimes have a structural correlate.*	*Tuberculosis, HIV, cerebral malaria, neurocysticerosis, subacute sclerosing panencephalitis, cerebral toxoplasmosis*	
Unknown*: the cause of epilepsy is unknown*		**Cryptogenic:** *presumed symptomatic*

Terminology	Terms no longer recommended
Self-limited: *tendency to resolve spontaneously over time*	**Benign**
Pharmacoresponsive: *highly likely to be controlled with medication*	**Catastrophic**
Focal seizures: *seizure semiology described according to specific subjective (auras), motor, autonomic, and dyscognitive features*	**Complex Partial**
	Simple Partial
Evolving to a bilateral convulsive seizure	**Secondary generalized**

We would welcome your thoughts on this proposal. Please visit the "Request for Comments" page on the ILAE website to read the full document and register your comments.

http://www.ilae.org/Visitors/Centre/Organization.cfm

References: 1.Berg AT et al. Revised terminology and concepts for organization of seizures and epilepsies: report of the ILAE Commission on Classification and Terminology, 2005-2009. *Epilepsia* 2010;51:676-685. 2.Blume WT et al. Glossary of descriptive terminology for ictal semiology: Report of the ILAE task force on classification and terminology. *Epilepsia* 2001:42;1212-1218. 3. Scheffer IE et al. The Organisation of the Epilepsies: Report of the ILAE Commission on Classification and Terminology (ILAE website as above)

4. Nursing interventions specific to rehabilitation
   a. Maintain aseptic technique when performing incision line care.
   b. Monitor patients for symptoms of shunt malfunction or infection: slow thinking, recent onset of disorientation, and urinary incontinence.
   c. Educate patient and caregivers about signs and symptoms of infection or malfunction and appropriate actions to take.
   d. Prepare patient and family for surgical placement of ventricular shunt. Review preoperative routine of site preparation, aseptic technique, and use of prophylactic antibiotics as prescribed.
   e. Prepare patient and family for shunt tap procedure by neurosurgeon to obtain a CSF specimen to send for a culture.
   f. Educate patient and family on postoperative shunt care such as meticulous hand washing, use of strict aseptic technique with dressing changes, and universal precautions. Reinforce the need for ongoing monitoring for the return of symptoms as a result of shunt malfunction. Timely treatment of infections is extremely important. If symptoms occur, the patient should immediately contact his or her neurosurgeon (Simpkins, 2005).
   g. Prepare patient and family to transfer from the rehabilitation setting to the operating room for shunt removal.
   h. Administer antibiotics as prescribed.
   i. Educate patients and families how to maintain optimal health and nutrition, including nutritional support and ongoing rehabilitation therapies.
5. Outcomes and long-term considerations
   a. Patients and families should be educated to recognize signs and symptoms of shunt failure and how to proceed.
   b. Shunt infections are more common with children and occur sooner after surgery (Langley et al., 2009).

c. Failure may occur as a result of tissues or other anatomical structures pressing on the shunt or an occlusion within the shunt. In either case the flow of ventricular fluid through the shunt is impaired and necessitates revision. Brain damage may occur when fluid backs up into the ventricles and presses on surrounding brain tissue.
d. Shunt infections may result in shunt malfunction, short- or long-term cognitive impairments, or surgical replacement of the device (Langley et al., 2009).

G. Dysautonomia and Dystonia

1. Definition: Dysautonomia, commonly known as sympathetic storming, is characterized by severe, paroxysmal increases in heart rate, temperature, and blood pressure with decerebrate or decortical posturing (NINDS, 2014b). "Storming" is a commonly used term to describe this syndrome. It is associated with severe diffuse axonal injury and tends to occur more frequently in children and young adults. The exaggerated sympathetic response is triggered by some type of noxious stimuli. Unlike AD, which is limited to segments of the spinal cord, dysautonomia stems from damage at the cortical level.
2. Common rehabilitation populations at risk
   a. Patients with severe diffuse axonal injury, typically seen after rotational brain injury
   b. Patients with brainstem injury or history of hypoxia at time of injury
3. Assessment: Once the elevation in vital signs with concomitant posturing is identified, the next step is to identify possible noxious stimulus triggering this reaction. Assess for presence of pressure ulcer, tissue pressure associated with casting, infection, heterotopic ossification or undiagnosed fractures, and distended bladder or bowel.
4. Nursing interventions specific to rehabilitation
   a. Recognize common symptoms of storming.
   b. Look for possible noxious stimuli.
   c. Elevate head of bed or position upright, with lower extremities in dependent position, to assist with reducing blood pressure.
   d. Loosen constrictive clothing.
   e. Administer medications to lower blood pressure, such as propranolol, bromocriptine, or oral antispasticity agents.
   f. For long-term problems associated with increased tone, consider use of baclofen, either orally or intrathecally (Demetrios et al., 2013).
5. Outcomes and long-term considerations: Generally occurs during the early and acute phase after injury then subsides over time

V. Dehydration and Electrolyte Imbalance Complications

A. Definitions

1. *Dehydration* is defined as deficient fluid volume related to etiology in a specific situation, which may be evidenced by dry mucous membranes, poor skin turgor, decreased pulse volume and pressure, and thirst. Deficient fluid volume is a result of diarrhea or vomiting, endocrine dysfunction, renal dysfunction, medications (e.g., diuretics), or inadequate fluid intake.
2. *Electrolyte imbalance* occurs when minerals become concentrated in the body or are depleted from the body as a result of reduction of fluid intake, the use of diuretic medications, diarrhea, vomiting, endocrine or renal dysfunction, or excessive sweating. Dehydration is often a complication of stroke, caused by dysphagia (swallowing disorder), combined with use of diuretics. Dehydration on admission is an independent predictor of poor discharge outcomes and higher admission rates after stroke (Liu et al., 2014).
3. Dehydration after stroke has been associated with increased blood viscosity, which can lead to venous thromboembolism and stroke mortality at 3 months (Rowat, Smith, Graham, Horsburgh, & Dennis, 2011). Hyponatremia can occur after brain injury, which may lead to the syndrome of inappropriate antidiuretic hormone (SIADH) and cerebral salt wasting (CSW) (Kirkman, Albert, Ibrahim, & Doberenz, 2013).

B. Common Rehabilitation Populations at Risk

1. Stroke
2. SCI
3. Parkinsonism
4. MS
5. TBI and nontraumatic brain injury
6. Parkinsonism
7. Guillain–Barré
8. ALS
9. Burns
10. *C. difficile* infection

C. Assessment

1. Assess for dehydration: mucous membranes, fatigue, thirst, decreased urine output, decreased tear production, dry skin, headache, constipation, dizziness, decreased blood pressure, rapid pulse, rapid breathing, fever, "sunken" eyes, delirium, and loss of consciousness.
2. Assess for electrolyte imbalance: lethargy, confusion, weakness, swelling, seizures, coma, irregular

heartbeat, kidney stones, muscle spasms, hallucinations, nausea, and vomiting. Noninvasive methods such as urine specific gravity and urine color charts for detection of water loss after acute stroke have not been found to be useful (Kafri et al., 2013).

3. Assess: urinalysis, blood electrolytes, and electrocardiogram.
4. Dysphagia, nutrition, and hydration status in ischemic stroke patients were studied using laboratory testing of prealbumin and blood urea nitrogen (BUN) and creatinine. Elevated BUN and creatinine are associated with poor outcome in people with ischemic stroke (Crary et al., 2013).
5. Assess cognitive function because dehydration can cause cognitive deficits due to impaired cerebral oxygen delivery, which can contribute to worsened clinical outcomes in people with acute ischemic stroke (AIS), detectable even in the emergency room (Schrock, Glasenapp, & Drogell, 2012).
6. Hyponatremia and polyuria are important to detect because they are potentially harmful, and diagnosis is often challenging. SIADH, CSW, and diabetes insipidus must be appropriately diagnosed to correct the hydroelectrical imbalance (Corradetti et al., 2013).

D. Nursing Interventions Specific to Rehabilitation

1. Adequate fluid intake either orally, through feeding tube, or intravenously to meet hydration needs is critical to prevention and recovery.
2. Concerns for adequate oral fluid intake are especially focused on people with dysphagia who are restricted to thickened liquids. In addition, patients who have expressive aphasia are at risk because they cannot make their need for hydration known to caregivers. Patients with impaired arm movement or grasp need assistance with obtaining and drinking oral fluids.
3. Promotion of treatment for hyponatremia includes mineralocorticoids and vasopressin 2 receptor antagonists. Adequate sodium and volume balance can prevent worsening complications after the initial injury.
4. The nurse promotes hydration by assessing beverage preference, scheduling frequency of beverages, offering beverages between therapy sessions, and accurately preparing thickened beverages. These measures can increase fluid intake (McGrail & Kelchner, 2012).
5. By identifying malnutrition and dehydration in patients, nurses intervene to prevent complications and improve patient outcomes (Rowat, 2011).
6. Address diarrhea or constipation; administer electrolyte replacement as prescribed, ensure access to oral fluids, continue to monitor symptoms, and assess pattern of steroid use.

E. Outcomes and Long-Term Considerations

1. Fluids and electrolytes must be balanced to promote wellness for people with disabilities.
2. The rehabilitation nurse is in a position to educate and encourage patients who have experienced a stroke with dysphagia to ensure adequate fluid intake, even through the use of thickened liquid or tube feeding with free water.
3. People with SCI may need fluid restriction to control urinary output, but they need sufficient fluids to prevent UTIs.
4. People with cognitive impairment or aphasia must be monitored, reminded, and assisted in maintaining adequate fluid intake.

VI. Alterations in Body Composition Such as Obesity

A. Definition

1. *Body composition* is the percentage of bony minerals, cell mass, lean body mass, body fat, and body water in an organism and their distribution through the body. Obesity is defined as body mass index (BMI) of > 30 kg/m^2. An imbalance between food eaten and energy expended leads to an unhealthy accumulation of body fat. Obesity contributes to an increased risk for diabetes mellitus, hypertension, heart disease, stroke, and other illnesses. Stroke can occur at significantly younger age in patients with higher BMI. Studies have been conducted to evaluate the association of BMI with mortality and nonfatal outcome in patients with acute stroke and TIA (Lackland et al., 2014).
2. Mortality risk was shown to be lower in overweight patients and lowest in obese and very obese patients (Kim, Ryu, Kim, & Lee, 2013; Skolarus et al., 2014). Lower rates of institutional care and death were also shown to occur. Conversely, another study showed no obesity paradox (Dehlendorff, Andersen, & Olsen, 2014). BMI and changes in motor impairment and functional mobility after gait rehabilitation intervention have been studied in subjects with chronic stroke (Sheffler, Knutson, Gunzler, & Chae, 2012). Those with higher BMI demonstrated less improvement in motor impairment and functional mobility performance in response to ambulation training.
3. People with acute traumatic SCI were four times more likely to have obesity, 2.7 times more likely to have heart disease, two times more likely to

have hypertension, and 1.7 times more likely to have diabetes at the onset of TSCI than a comparable population with lower extremity fractures (Selassie, Snipe, Focht, & Welldaregay, 2013). Complications such as obesity after SCI can lead to malnutrition, which can affect mortality (Dionyssiotis, 2012). Weight management in the SCI population is important for the rehabilitation nurse to promote for quality of life, routine exercise, and prevention of complications.

B. Common Rehabilitation Populations at Risk
   1. SCI
   2. Stroke
   3. MS

C. Assessment
   1. Ensure that appropriate scales are available to safely weigh patient. Ensure that staff knows how to use scales safely. Monitor weight periodically over time.
   2. Monitor thyroid function.
   3. Follow blood glucose and HgbA1c.
   4. Collaborate with dietitian to calculate weight adjustments to BMI and caloric needs if an amputation is present.
   5. Consult with dietitian to determine current caloric intake versus needs, taking into account variables such as wounds, activity level, and muscle atrophy due to disuse or disease.
   6. Measure neck and waist circumference as a guide to determine degree of obesity.

D. Nursing Interventions Specific to Rehabilitation
   1. Promotion of normal weight should be the aim for obese patients with stroke, SCI, and MS (Dehlendorff et al., 2014). Education about the role of nutrition in health status after SCI can have an impact on overall health, which can help to prevent obesity, cardiovascular disease, diabetes, and metabolic syndrome (Khalil et al., 2013).
   2. Rehabilitation nurses are in ideal settings to provide opportunities to address complex, serious underlying etiologies of obesity (Brewer-Smyth, 2014).
   3. Monitoring body mass, food intake, and daily physical activity during and after inpatient rehabilitation is important to prevent obesity and related cardiovascular risk factors (de Groot et al., 2014). BMI should be incorporated into the formulation of rehabilitation goals by the interdisciplinary team.
   4. Early mobilization reduces risk of multiple comorbid factors (Epstein, 2014).
   5. Waist circumference (WC) can be used as an alternative to measuring BMI in people with SCI (Ravensbergen, Lear, & Claydon, 2014). A WC greater than 94 centimeters is considered the optimal cutoff for identifying adverse cardiovascular disease risk.
   6. Enlarged neck circumference may indicate risk of sleep apnea.

E. Outcomes and Long-Term Complications: Obesity can be addressed and possibly prevented through mobilization of people with disability. The rehabilitation nurse helps patients maintain healthy diet and exercise in order to prevent complications of obesity and reach determined parameters for healthy weight.

VII. Genitourinary Complications

A. UTI, Renal Calculus, Hydronephrosis, and Chronic Kidney Disease
   1. Definitions
      a. *UTI*: Bladder dysfunction can occur as a result of diminished bladder capacity and urethral compliance, increase in uninhibited detrusor contractions, residual bladder volumes, and decline in kidney function. These processes are exaggerated in people with stroke, SCI, and MS beyond the normal human aging process and can lead to UTIs characterized by elevated bacterial count in the urine.
         1) Sensory motor impairment and anatomical obstruction can lead to retention. Lumbosacral SCI and chronic indwelling urethral and suprapubic catheterization have been found to be predictors of UTI after SCI (Zhang, & Liao, 2014). The main causes of death in patients with SCI are infection or septicemia and UTIs (Lalwani et al., 2014).
         2) Infections such as urinary tract and kidney infections that occur in the pediatric population with severe TBI are known to increase medical costs and worsen patient outcomes (Alharfi, Charyk Stewart, Al Helali, Daoud, & Fraser, 2014). Recurrent symptomatic UTIs remain a major complication of long-term chronic indwelling catheter use. An International Spinal Cord Injury Urinary Tract Infection Basic Data Set has been developed to standardize the format for collecting and reporting information on UTIs. The instrument includes date of data collection, length of time of signs and symptoms, results of urine dipstick test for nitrite and leukocyte esterase, urine culture results, and resistance patterns (Brackett, Lynne, Ibrahim, Ohl, & Sonksen, 2010). People needing neurologic intensive care unit (ICU) admission tend to

have concomitant immune suppression that makes them more prone to nosocomial infections (Dayts, 2014). Urinary bladders of people with an SCI fail to create a characteristic inflammatory response to E. coli infection and cannot suppress inflammation after infection is eliminated. This may cause increased susceptibility to UTI and persistent chronic inflammation (Chaudhry et al., 2014).

b. *Renal calculus* is defined as a pebble or stone, usually composed of mineral salts, that occurs in the kidneys, ureters, bladder, or urethra. Incidence, management, and outcome of surgically treated kidney stones after SCI were described in a recent study (Welk et al., 2013). Ureteroscopy with lithotripsy was the preferred treatment. Minimally invasive surgeries prevent complications, especially in people who have had SCIs. Recurrent stones, staghorn calculi, and bilateral stone disease occur often in spinal cord injured patients. The risk of developing a renal stone after SCI is between 7% and 20% over an 8- to 10-year period (Ramsey & McIlhenny, 2011). Stone formation may be related to early demineralization of bone or chronic infection. Risk factors are related to lesion level, bladder management strategy, specific metabolic changes, and frequency of UTIs (Welk, Fullerr, Razv, & Denstedt, 2012).
   1) Patients with musculoskeletal anomalies such as MS are prone to renal calculi caused by immobility and have an increased incidence of UTIs (Gnessin, Mandeville, Handa, & Lingeman, 2011).
   2) Renal calculi that block urine flow in the upper or lower tract can lead to distension of the kidneys, bladder, urethra, or ureters, leading to increased risk of hydronephrosis and even acute renal failure.

c. *Hydronephrosis* is stretching of the renal pelvis as a result of obstruction to urinary outflow. Hydronephrosis and renal failure result from inadequate management of neurogenic bladder or from renal stones blocking urine outflow. Use of a penile sheath drainage system in a person with SCI should not be ordered when urinary retention is present.

d. *Chronic kidney disease* includes any illness in which kidney function is diminished for at least 3 months, without returning to normal.
   1) Common causes of chronic kidney disease are diabetes, hypertension, and age.
   2) Cumulatively, changes in loss of volitional control over micturition and lack of coordination of detrusor and sphincter reflexes can cause dyssynergia and elevated lower urinary tract pressure, which can then lead to hypertrophy of detrusor muscles and decreased bladder compliance, hydronephrosis, and upper urinary tract deterioration.

2. Common rehabilitation populations at risk
   a. SCI
   b. Stroke
   c. Brain injury
   d. MS
   e. Diabetes mellitus
3. Assessment
   a. Obtain urologic history to determine bladder and kidney function.
   b. Bladder function assessment is subjectively obtained.
   c. Urodynamic tests include uroflowmetry, post-void residual measurement, cystometric tests, leak point pressure measurement, pressure flow study, electromyography, and video urodynamic tests.
   d. Ultrasound should be performed by a radiologist to determine the presence of stones, grit, or crystals in urine.
4. Nursing interventions specific to rehabilitation
   a. Education programs must be provided to patients and family members about proper methods of bladder management, catheterization technique, fluid volume restrictions if appropriate, and maintenance of adequate hydration and perineal cleanliness in an effort to reduce the incidence of UTIs after SCI (Mays, McIntyre, Mehta, Hill, Wolfe, & Teasell, 2013).
   b. Intermittent catheterization is known to cause fewer complications than indwelling catheters.
   c. Many patients with SCI are placed on prophylactic oral antimicrobials or methenamine/ascorbic acid (Edokpolo, Stavris, & Foster, 2012).
   d. Early mobilization protocols are known to reduce the rate of complications and morbidity from UTIs, sepsis, or infection, which reduces the average length of stay (Epstein, 2014).
   e. Interventions used to promote bladder emptying and maintain low-pressure voiding have variable risks for UTI (Nicolle, 2014). Because bacteriuria is common in the spinal cord injured population, many experts indicate that asymptomatic bacteriuria should not be treated.

f. Rehabilitation nurses must promote evidence-based practice such as removal of indwelling catheters as soon as there is no justification for continued use, replaced by intermittent catheterization to prevent complications. Promoting intermittent catheterizations according to the urinary output and oral intake throughout a 24-hour period prevents bladder infections. A pattern of monitoring urine quality and characteristics allows patients to take ownership of their own bladder management in order to minimize complications.
g. Limiting use of indwelling catheters reduces rates of renal calculi, UTIs, and bladder cancer, and promotion of the use of anticholinergic medications may improve outcomes for these patients (Charlifue et al., 2010).
h. Patients with SCI who have high intravesical pressure should not have penile sheath drainage because they are at risk for developing hydronephrosis and renal failure. Intermittent catheterization along with antimuscarinic drugs should be the preferred option for managing neuropathic bladder (Vaidyanathan et al., 2012).
i. Bladder management methods and medical complications such as renal calculi or decubitus ulcers, number of hospital days, and psychosocial factors must be considered in rehabilitation nursing practice (Cameron et al., 2011). Rehabilitation nurses should educate physicians on evidence in the literature that correlates indwelling catheter use with the lowest levels of participation and more urological complications such as stones, urinary infection, urethral strictures, and bladder cancer (Cameron et al., 2010).
j. For people who are in the community receiving home care, bladder management with clean intermittent catheterization should be promoted when urinary retention is present in this population. Clean versus sterile intermittent catheterization technique is controversial in that although most insurance now pays for adequate supplies necessary for sterile technique to be performed, catheters that are cleaned and air dried can be reused several times if the person does not have a history of chronic bladder infections.
k. The use of ultrasound bladder scanner devices is a noninvasive method of determining bladder volume and postvoid residual volume and can be used in facilities to aid in determining whether catheterization is indicated. The use of bladder scans in institutions and in home care has resulted in a significant reduction in both indwelling and intermittent catheterizations, which has reduced the number of catheter-associated UTIs. It should be noted that ongoing competency of those performing bladder scanning should be assessed to avoid the likelihood of operator error.
l. Increasing fluid intake flushes the bladder, which is known to decrease UTIs. Acidifying urine through the use of natural products such as cranberry juice can reduce UTIs.
m. Proper technique of performing perineal hygiene by cleansing away from the meatus prevents bacteria from contaminating the bladder.
n. Antibiotic-impregnated catheters are encouraged in order to reduce bacterial count in the urethra and bladder. The nurse must select the appropriate type of catheter with size appropriate for patient's body and adequate diameter to remove sediment. Catheter care according to institutional policy includes perineal hygiene, anchoring the tubing, and changing an indwelling catheter monthly and as needed.
o. Teaching the patient to perform self-catheterization using proper technique reduces the risk of complications such as UTI and blocked catheters when patient may need to flush tubing periodically to maintain patency. Teaching the patient and caregiver signs and symptoms of UTI, renal stones, and retention is an important step in preventing complications.

5. Outcomes and long-term considerations
   a. Bladder management at the onset of injury prevents complications for people with disability.
   b. Rehabilitation nurses promote appropriate methods of urinary drainage patterns that establish healthy patterns for a lifetime.
   c. If chronic renal disease is present, the patient may be advised to avoid antiinflammatory medicines unless prescribed, and other medication dosages may be altered based on kidney function.

B. Infertility and Sexual Dysfunction
1. Definitions
   a. *Infertility* is defined as the inability to achieve pregnancy during a year or more of unprotected intercourse. Causes in men are usually failure to manufacture adequate amounts of sperm, inability to mobilize sperm to fertilize

the egg, or infection. Infertility in women can be primary, such as ovulatory failure, anatomical anomalies of the uterus, Turner's syndrome, or eating disorders. Secondary infertility can be caused by tubal scarring, as after sexually transmitted infection.

b. *Sexual dysfunction* is defined as difficulty in performing sexual activity to the satisfaction of the people involved.

3. Common rehabilitation populations at risk
   a. SCI
   b. MS
   c. Diabetes
4. Assessment
   a. Most men with SCI are infertile (Brackett et al., 2010). Erectile dysfunction, ejaculatory dysfunction, and semen abnormalities contribute to this problem. Women with SCI do not typically experience infertility.
   b. Although interventions differ, reproductive outcomes for men with SCI and infertility are similar to those of the general male population who experience infertility (Brackett, 2012). Women with SCI and infertility are similar to the general female population who experience infertility. Assessment involves use of sensitive professional interviewing techniques to subjectively collect information about pre-injury or pre-illness sexual function and activity, determine expectations of person and partner, and perform diagnostic tests to determine quality of sperm, ability to sustain erection either naturally or with adaptive devices or interventions, and the effect these interventions could have on the patient's perceived quality of life.
5. Nursing interventions specific to rehabilitation
   a. The rehabilitation team must provide information about treatment for erectile dysfunction, which includes phosphodiesterase type 5 inhibitors, intracavernous injections of alprostadil, penile prostheses, and vacuum constriction devices. Semen retrieval may be necessary in patients who are anejaculatory. Penile vibratory stimulation is the first choice intervention to collect a sperm If this fails, electroejaculation is recommended. If this approach is not possible, prostate massage is an alternative. Surgical sperm retrieval is considered a last resort. Sperm from men with SCI can induce pregnancy. Artificial intravaginal or intrauterine insemination, freezing sperm, and in vitro fertilization and intracytoplasmic sperm injection are options in cases of low total motile sperm count.
   b. The approach of the rehabilitation team to the management of sexual dysfunction in women with SCI is similar to that for men but obviously does not require treatment for erectile or ejaculatory problems (Welk et al., 2013).
6. Outcomes and long-term considerations
   a. People with disabilities who are informed of infertility options and supported to pursue assistance in conceiving during the childbearing ages will have opportunities to have a family.
   b. Quality of life can be improved by overcoming obstacles of infertility, providing resources for enhancing sexual satisfaction such as finding alternatives for positioning during sexual activity, and exploring alternative methods of enhancing psychological satisfaction during sexual activity for the individual and his or her partner.

VIII. Gastrointestinal Complications: Constipation

A. Definition

1. *Constipation* is a change in bowel pattern, inability or difficulty in passing of stool, or decreased volume or frequency of stool passage. Insufficient physical activity, insufficient fluid intake, or abdominal muscle weakness can contribute to constipation. Chronic constipation may lead to megacolon, which is expansion of large intestine. An extreme acute complication of constipation is partial or complete small bowel obstruction, which is a blockage of stool in the intestine.

B. Common Rehabilitation Populations at Risk

1. Stroke
2. MS
3. SCI
4. Parkinson's

C. Assessment

1. Assess degree of bowel dysfunction among people with MS and SCI. This was studied in an effort to objectively assess lower bowel function in clinical practice. It was found that bowel symptoms in these populations correlated with specific alterations of anorectal physiology, such as areflexic bowel pattern and incontinence. This information provided objective assessment of bowel symptoms. Obtaining detailed information led to the development of treatment plans for individual patients (Thiruppathy, Roy, Preziosi, Pannicker, & Emmanuel, 2012).
2. Explore implications of aging with SCI, which has been investigated regarding alteration in colorectal function (Charlifue et al., 2010). People who

were 20 years post-SCI in United Kingdom had increased difficulties with constipation, fecal incontinence, and gastrointestinal pain.

D. Nursing Interventions Specific to Rehabilitation

1. Positioning upright on a toilet is desirable to improve outcome of evacuation of stool if the proper equipment and skill of the caregiver permits this activity to be accomplished. Monitoring sitting balance, endurance, and safety is critical for successfully performing bowel evacuation on a toilet.
2. Monitor anxiety and quality of life issues related to bowel problems (Coggrave, Norton, & Cody, 2014).
3. Comparative studies regarding effectiveness of daily digital stimulation versus every other day have found daily practice leads to higher bowel regularity (Lim & Childs, 2013).
4. Suggest exploration of the feasibility of implanting microchips on the anterior sacral roots in patients with spinal trauma (Chia, Lee, Kour, Tung, & Tan, 1996) and electrical stimulation of the dorsal genital nerve (Worsoe, Fynne, Laurberg, Krogh, & Rijkhoff, 2012). These techniques have been studied to determine whether either of these methods actually improved bowel function. Larger studies are needed to further evaluate these techniques.
5. Determine and individualize the best method of bowel management, which may include bulk-forming laxatives, anticholinergic drug combinations, transanal irrigation (enema), oral carbonated water, and abdominal massage with lifestyle advice. These methods have been examined by researchers and clinicians for efficacy. Timing of the bowel program can be adapted to the person's lifestyle (Ng et al., 2005).
6. Encourage assessment of surgical interventions for people with SCI, such as colostomy or ileostomy, to improve bowel management. Studies have been performed to determine perceptions of patients and caregivers in Department of Veterans Affairs facilities about surgical interventions (West et al., 2013). Patient and caregiver perceptions varied, although improvement in management and control of bowel evacuation were consistent with improved quality of life in many cases.

E. Outcomes and Long-Term Considerations

1. Structured nurse-led interventions have been effective in controlling symptoms and improving the effectiveness of bowel training. Awareness of the incidence of constipation in people with neurological impairment guides rehabilitation nurses to establish standard guidelines for screening and management of bowel function to prevent complications (Lin et al., 2013).
2. Prevention of complications includes the use of medications such as stool softeners, fiber and bulk laxatives, bowel training programs, and natural products such as prune and other fiber from raw fruits and vegetables. Individualized bowel care regimens should be instituted at all levels in the continuum of care for people receiving rehabilitation services (Otegbayo et al., 2013).
3. Family and patient teaching on the importance of establishing and maintaining a regular regimen of bowel evacuation helps prevent complications.
4. Adaptive equipment such as an elevated toilet seat, appropriately sized bedside commode and shower chair for the person in his or her environment, suppository insertion devices, and other adaptive devices for toilet hygiene such as toilet paper holders increases the person's level of independence and autonomy.
5. Bowel management regimens are promoted by rehabilitation nurses to prevent the complications of constipation and bowel obstruction. Education is a key factor in promoting healthy living.

IX. Psychosocial Complications

A. Depression

1. Definition: *Depression* is a mood disorder marked by loss of interest or pleasure in living. Medical conditions that can trigger or exacerbate depression include neurologic disorders and chronic pain.
2. Common rehabilitation populations at risk
   a. Stroke
   b. Brain injury (traumatic and nontraumatic)
   c. SCI
   d. Neurological conditions such as MS, Guillain–Barré, Parkinsonism, and CP
   e. All ages and cultural groups are affected.
3. Assessment
   a. Significantly lower morale scores on the Philadelphia Geriatric Center Morale Scale (PGCMS) of people age 85 years and older after stroke have been found in a population in Sweden and Finland (Niklassom, Lovheim, & Gustafson, 2013).
   b. Assess degree of pain and nutritional status.
   c. Note that the risk of suicide is increased greatly among patients with SCI, stroke, and any debilitative condition that has the potential to negatively affect quality of life.
   d. Determine the presence of substance abuse, which is correlated with medical complications such as pressure ulcers and UTIs (Eisenberg,

1995). Substance abuse screening and history should be done with every patient.

4. Nursing interventions specific to rehabilitation
   a. Emphasis on successful interdisciplinary rehabilitation with psychological support is intended to recognize and treat depression and signs of suicide.
   b. Rehabilitation nurses, along with psychiatry staff, must help patients and families develop healthy coping strategies and social supports that encourage self-care and encourage activities such as medication compliance, diversional and recreational activities, adaptive sports, and peer support.
   c. The healthcare team across the continuum needs to be aware of the potential for depression, substance abuse, and suicide risk, especially after SCI.
   d. Depression can impair learning and decrease functional performance.
5. Outcomes and long-term considerations
   a. Depression can be prevented with early detection and treatment, which requires close monitoring throughout the continuum of care.
   b. The interdisciplinary team needs to communicate and act promptly when signs and symptoms of depression become apparent.

B. Delirium

1. Definition: *Delirium*, as defined by the American Psychiatric Association (2000), is a disturbance of consciousness characterized by impaired attention and disorganized thinking or perceptual disturbance that develops acutely and has a fluctuating course, with evidence of an underlying physiological or medical condition that may be the cause of the disorder. Unlike dementia (which is a chronic confusion), delirium is acute confusional state brought on by a medical condition or treatment. It is estimated that 50% of patients with an ICU stay greater than 2 days develop some degree of delirium (van den Boogaard, M. , 2011) In medical inpatients outside the ICU, the incidence is reported to be 3%–29% (Siddiqi, House, & Holmes, 2006).
2. Common rehabilitation populations at risk
   a. Age (older than 70 years). McAvay and colleagues (2006) found that of approximately 433 patients admitted to a general medicine service in an academic medical center, 5% of patients older than the age of 70 years met criteria for delirium at discharge, and more than 60% of the patients with delirium at discharge were admitted to nursing homes after discharge.
   b. Severity of illness and presence of a cognitive impairment
   c. Depression
   d. Sensory impairment (vision changes, hearing loss, impaired tactile sensation)
   e. Fluid and electrolyte disturbances
   f. Polypharmacy
   g. Neurological disorder
   h. Recent infection, especially UTI or pneumonia
3. Assessment
   a. Gather information on premorbid cognitive impairment.
   b. Assess cognitive status, using a standardized tool such as the Confusion Assessment Method (CAM) tool (Waszynski, 2007).
   c. Review medications with physician and pharmacist to discontinue unnecessary drugs that may cause complications.
   d. Assess pain status and effectiveness of current pain management regimen.
   e. Monitor metabolic and perfusion states.
   f. Look for the presence of infection (CBC with differential, WBCs, and cultures).
   g. Assess mobility and sensation.
   h. Perform an environmental assessment to promote safety, such as identifying environmental clutter.
   i. In collaboration with neuropsychiatrist or psychiatrist performing a Mini–Mental Examination (MMSE), nurses assess cognitive status on every shift.
      1) Alertness
      2) Attention
      3) Orientation
      4) Memory
      5) Thinking
      6) Perception
      7) Psychomotor activity
4. Nursing interventions specific to rehabilitation
   a. Eliminate or minimize risk factors
      1) Administer medications only as needed and review list for opportunities to reduce potential complications.
      2) Treat any existing infections and take necessary steps to prevent infection.
      3) Make certain patients are adequately hydrated and are eating adequate amounts of calories and nutrients.
      4) Manage pain using drugs that do not impair cognition.
      5) Provide oxygen therapy and check saturation during activities and sleep.

6) Ensure that patient is using eyeglasses and hearing aids appropriately.
7) Mobilize or ambulate the patient.

b. Provide a therapeutic environment.
1) Put clocks and calendars in room for orientation.
2) Adjust lighting at night.
3) Organize care routines to minimize waking patients at night. Consider use of back rubs, warm blankets, noise reduction, and relaxation strategies to promote sleep.
4) Minimize use of medications to induce sleep because they often have side effects that can cause confusion.
5) Provide frequent orientation and activity.

5. Outcomes and long-term considerations: Ideally, the patient will regain premorbid cognitive and functional status.

Summary

The rehabilitation nurse plays a key role in early identification of complications for patients with a new or existing disability or chronic illness. Identifying complications early will lead to early intervention and a more positive outcome for the patient. It is important to remember that the patient in a rehabilitation setting has a high potential to exhibit a medical-surgical or psychiatric complication, and it is crucial that rehabilitation nurses remain knowledgeable and up-to-date on these topics.

References

Alharfi, I., Charyk Stewart, T., Al Helali, I., Daoud, H., & Fraser, D. (2014). Infection rates, fevers, and associated factors in pediatric severe traumatic brain injury. *Journal of Neurotrauma, 31*(5), 452–458. doi:10.1089/neu.2013.2904

American Psychiatric Association. (2013). *Diagnostic and Statistical Manual* (5th ed.). Washington, DC: APA Press.

Amatya, B., Khan, F., LaMantia, L., Demetrious, M., & Wade, D. (2013). *Nonpharmacological interventions for spasticity in multiple sclerosis*. Multiple Sclerosis and Rare Diseases of the Central Nervous System Group. doi:0.1002/14651858.CD0099974pub2

Amin, A., Lin, J., Thompson, S., & Weiderkehr, D. (2013). Rate of deep-vein thrombosis and pulmonary embolism during the care continuum in patients with acute ischemic stroke in the United States. *BMC (BioMedical Center) Neurology, 13*(17). doi:10.1186/11-2377-13-17

Annegers, J. F., Rocca, W. A., & Hauser, W. A. (1996). Causes of epilepsy: Contributions of the Rochester epidemiology project. *Mayo Clinical Proceedings, 71*, 570–575.

Arbogast, S. D., Alshekhlee, A., Hussain, Z., McNeeley, K., & Chelminsky, T. C. (2009). Hypotension unawareness in profound orthostatic hypotension. *The American Journal of Medicine, 122*(6), 574–580.

Armstrong, J. R., & Mosher, B. D. (2011). Aspiration pneumonia after stroke: Intervention prevention. *The Neurohospitalist, 1*(2), 85–93.

Association of Rehabilitation Nurses (ARN). (2014). ARN competency model for professional rehabilitation nursing. Retrieved from http://www.rehabnurse.org/uploads/files/education/ARN_Rehabilitation_Nursing_Competency _Model_FINAL_-_May_2014.pdf

Bakheit, A. (2012). The pharmacological management of post-stroke muscle spasticity. *Drugs and Aging, 29*(12), 941–947. doi:10.1007/s40266-012-0032-z

Barros Galvao, S., Costa dos Santos, R., Borba dos Santos,R., Cabral, M., & Monte-Silva, K. (2014). Efficacy of coupling repetitive transcranial magnetic stimulation and physical therapy to reduce upper-limb spasticity in patients with stroke: A randomized controlled trial. *Archives of Physical Medicine and Rehabilitation, 95*(2), 222–229.

Belmont, P. J. Jr., Davey, S., Orr, J. D., Ochoa, L. M., Bader, J. O., & Schoenfeld, A. J. (2011). Risk factors for 30-day postoperative complications and mortality below-knee amputation: A study of 2,911 patients from the National Surgical Quality Improvement Program original research article. *Journal of the American College of Surgeons, 213*(3), 370–378.

Bembenek, J., & Czlonkowska, A. (2013). Venous thromboembolism prophylactic methods in acute stroke patients—current state of knowledge. *Polish Journal of Neurology and Neurosurgery, 47*(6) 564–571.

Bensmail, D. (2013). National and European consensus in spasticity management. *Annals of Physical and Rehabilitation Medicine, 56*(1), e178.

Berg, A. T., Berkovic, S. F., Brodie, M. J,. Buchalter, J., Cross, J. H., van Emde Boas, W., Engel,…Scheffer, I. E. (2010). Revised terminology and concepts for organization of seizures and epilepsieas: Report of the ILAE Commission on classification and terminology, 2005-2009. *Eplipesia, 51*(4), 676–685.

Berry, J. K., Johnson, J. H., & Vander Ploerg, K. (2002). Respiration and pulmonary rehabilitation. In S. Hoeman, *Rehabilitation nursing: Process, applications & outcomes* (3rd ed.). St. Louis: Mosby.

Biggin, A., Briody, J., Ramjan, K., Middleton, A., Waugh, M., & Munns, C. (2013). Evaluation of bone mineral density and morphology using pQCT in children after spinal cord injury. *Developmental Neurorehabilitation, 16*(6), 391–397.

Boots, R. J., Dulhunty, J. M., Paratz, J., & Lipman, J. (2009). Respiratory complications in burns: An evolving spectrum of injury. *Clinical Pulmonary Medicine, 16*(3), 132–138.

Borschmann, K., Pang, M., Iuiano, S., Churiloy, L., Brodtmann, A., Ekinci, E., & Bernhardt, J. (2013). Changes to volumetric bone mineral density and bone strength after stroke: A prospective study. *International Journal of Stroke*. doi:10.1111/ijs.12228

Bouvette, C., McPhee, B., & Opfer-Gehrking, T. (1994). Role of physical countermaneuvers in the management of orthostatic hypotension: Efficacy and biofeedback augmentation. *Mayo Clinic Proceedings, 71*, 847–853.

Brackett, N. (2012). Infertility in men with spinal cord injury: Research and treatment. *Scientifica (Cairo)*. doi:10.6064/2012/578257

Brackett, N., Lynne, C., Ibrahim, E., Ohl, D., & Sonksen, J. (2010). Treatment of infertility in men with spinal cord injury. *National Review of Urology, 7*(3), 162–172. doi:10.1038/nrurol.2010.7

Brewer-Smyth, K. (2014). Obesity, traumatic brain injury, childhood abuse, and suicide attempts in females at risk. *Rehabilitation Nursing*. doi:10.1002/rnj.150

Cameron, A., Wallner, L., Forchheimer, M., Clemens, J., Dunn, R., Rodriguez, G., . . . Tate, D. (2011). *Archives of Physical Medicine & Rehabilitation, 92*(3), 449–456. doi:10.1016/j.apmr.2010.06.028

Cameron, A., Wallner, L., Tate, D., Sarma, A., Rodriguez, G., & Clemens, J. (2010). Bladder management after spinal cord injury in United States 1972–2005. *Journal of Urology, 184*(1), 213–217.

Cardenas, D., Hoffman, J., Kirshblum, S., & McKinley, W. (2004). Etiology and incidence of rehospitalization after traumatic spinal cord injury: A multicenter analysis. *Archives of Physical Medicine Rehabilitation, 85*, 1757–1763.

Centers for Disease Control and Prevention. (2014). *Central line-associated bloodstream infection (CLABSI) event*. Retrieved from www.cdc.gov/nhsn/PDFs/pscManual/4PSC_CLABScurrent.pdf

Chang, K., Liou, T., Sung, J., Wang, C., Genamt, J., & Chan, W. (2014). Femoral neck bone mineral density change is associated with shift in standing weight in hemiparetic stroke patients. *American Journal of Physical Medicine & Rehabilitation, 93*(6), 477–485.

Chappell, F., Crawford, F., Amdras, A., Goodacre, S., McCaslin, J., Welch, K., & Oates, C. (2014). Duplex ultrasound for the diagnosis of symptomatic deep vein thrombosis in the lower limb. *Cochrane Database of Systematic Reviews, 1* (CD010930). doi:10.1002/14651858.CD010930

Charlifue, S., Jha, A., & Lammertse, D. (2010). Aging with spinal cord injury. *Physical Medicine & Rehabilitation Clinics of North America, 21*(2), 383–402.

Chaudhry, R., Madden-Fuentes, R., Ortiz, T., Balsara, Z., Tang, Y., Nseyo, U., Seed, P. (2014). Inflammatory response to Escherichia coli urinary tract infection in the neurogenic bladder of the spinal cord injured host. *Journal of Urology, 191*(5), 1454–1461. doi:10.1016/juro.2013.12.013

Chen, C. F., Lai, C. L., Lin, H. F., Liou, L. M., & Lin., R. T. (2011). Reappraisal of heart rate variability in acute ischemic stroke. *Kaohsiung Journal of Medical Sciences, 27*(6), 215–221.

Chia, Y., Lee, T., Kour, N., Tung, K., & Tan, E. (1996). Microchip implants on the anterior sacral roots in patients with spinal trauma: Does it improve bowel function? *Diseases of the Colon & Rectum, 39*(6), 690–694.

Chiodo, A. E., Scelza, W. M., Kirshblum, S. C., Wuermser, L. A., Ho, C. H., & Priebe, M. M. (2007). Spinal cord injury medicine. 5. Long-term medical issues and health maintenance. *Archives of Physical Medicine and Rehabilitation, 88*(3), 76–83.

Chung, S., Lee, S., Kim, E., & Echo, W. (2011). Incidence of deep vein thrombosis after spinal cord injury: A prospective study in 37 consecutive patients with traumatic or nontraumatic spinal cord injury treated by mechanical prophylaxis. *Journal of Trauma, 71*(4), 867–870.

Chung, W., Lin, C., Chang, S., Chung, H., Sung, F., & Kao, C. (2014). Increased risk of deep vein thrombosis and pulmonary thromboembolism in patients with spinal cord injury: A nationwide cohort prospective study. *Thrombosis Research, 133*(4), 579–584.

Coggrave, M., Norton, C., & Cody, J. (2014). Management of faecal incontinence and constipation in adults with central neurological diseases. *Cochrane Database of Systematic Reviews, 1* (CD010930). doi:10.1002/14651858.CD002115

Corradetti, V., Esposito, P., Rampino, T., Gregorini, M., Lebetta, C., Bosio, F.,Dal Canton, A. (2013). Multiple electrolyte disorders in a neurosurgical patient: Solving the rebus. *BMC Nephrology, 10*(14), 140. doi:10.1186/1471-2369-14-140

Crary, M., Humphrey, J., Carnaby-Mann, G., Sambandam, R., Miller., L., & Silliman, S. (2013). Dysphagia, nutrition, and hydration in ischemic stroke patients at admission and discharge from acute care. *Dysphagia, 28*(1), 69–76.

Cunha, J. P. (2014). *Edema facts.* Retrieved from www.medicinenet.com/edema

Davenport, R., Dennis, M., Wellwood, B., & Warlow, C. (1996). Complications after acute stroke. *Stroke, 27,* 415–420.

Dayts, O. (2014). Evidence-based protocol: Diagnosis and treatment of catheter-associated urinary tract infection within adult neurocritical care patient population. *Nursing Clinic of North America, 49*(1), 29–43.

de Groot, S., Post, M., Hoekstra, T., Valent, L., Faber, W., & van der Woude, L. (2014). Trajectories in the course of body mass index after spinal cord injury. *Archives of Physical Medicine Rehabilitation, 95*(6), 1083–1092. doi:10.1016/j.apmr.2014.01.024

Dehlendorff, C., Andersen, K., & Olsen, T. (2014). Bone mass index and death by stroke: No obesity paradox. *JAMA Neurology.* doi:10.1001/jamaneurol.2014.1017

de Jong, L., Dijkstra, P., Gerritsen, J., Geurts, A., & Postema, K. (2013). Combined arm stretch positioning and neuromuscular electrical stimulation during rehabilitation does not improve range of motion, shoulder pain or functioning patients after stroke: A randomized trial. *Journal of Physiotherapy, 50*(4), 245–254.

Dellinger, R. P., Carlet, J., Masur, H., Gerlach, H., Calandra, T., Cohen, J., … Levy, M. M. Signs and Symptoms of Organ Failure. *Critical Care Medicine, 32*(3), 858–873.

Demetrios, M., Khan, F., Turner-Stokes, L., Brand, C., & McSweeney, S. (2013). Multidisciplinary rehabilitation following botulinum toxin and other focal intramuscular treatment for post-stroke spasticity. *Cochrane Database Systems Review, 5*(6). doi:10.1002/14651858.CD009689.pub2

Dionyssiotis, Y. (2012). Malnutrition in spinal cord injury: More than nutritional deficiency. *Journal of Clinical Medicine Research, 4*(4), 227–236. doi:10.4021/jocmr924w

Doehner, W., Schenkel, J., Anker, S., Springer, J., & Audebert, H. (2013). Overweight and obesity are associated with improved survival, functional outcome, and stroke recurrence after acute stroke or transient ischaemic attack: Observations from the TEMPiS trial. *European Heart Journal, 34*(4), 268–277.

Dohle, C., Rykman, A., Chang, J., & Volpe, B. (2013). Pilot study of a robotic protocol to treat shoulder subluxation in patient with chronic stroke. *Journal of NeuroEngineering and Rehabilitation, 10,* 88.

Dolbow, J., Dolbow, D., Gorgey, A., Adler, R., & Gater, D. (2013). The effects of aging and electrical stimulation exercise on bone after spinal cord injury. *Aging and Disease, 4*(3), 141–153.

Douds, G., Helkamp, A., Olson, D., Fonarow, G., Smith, E., Schwamm, L., & Cockroft, K. (2014). Venous thromboembolism in the Get With the Guidelines–Stroke acute ischemic stroke population: Incidence and patterns of prophylaxis. *Journal of Stroke and Cerebrovascular Diseases, 23*(1), 123–129. doi:10.1016/j.jstrokecerebrovasdis.2012.10.018

Edokpolo, L., Stavris, K., & Foster, H. (2012). Intermittent catheterization and recurrent urinary tract infection in spinal cord injury. *Topics in Spinal Cord Injury Rehabilitation, 18*(2), 187–192. doi:10.1310/sci1802-187

Edwards, W., Schnitzer, R., & Troy, K. (2013). Bone mineral loss at the proximal femur in acute spinal cord injury. *Osteoporosis International, 24*(9), 2461–2469.

Edwards, W., Schnitzer, T., & Troy, K. (2014). The mechanical consequence of actual bone loss and simulated bone recovery in acute spinal cord injury. *Bone, 60,* 141–147.

Eisenberg, M. (1995). *Substance abuse and medical complications following spinal cord injury.* Retrieved from http://psycnet.apa.org/journals/rep/40/2/125.html

Epilepsy Foundation of America's Working Group on Status Epilepticus, (1993). Treatment of convulsive status epilepticus. Recommendations of the Epilepsy Foundation of America's Working Group on Status Epilepticus. *JAMA, 270*(7), 854–859.

Epstein, N. (2014). A review article on the benefits of early mobilization following spinal surgery and other medical-surgical procedures. *Surgical Neurology International, 16*(5 Suppl. 3), S66–S73. doi:10.4103/2152-7806.130674

Fehing, M., & Singh, A. (2009). The timing of surgery in patients with central spinal cord injury. *Journal of Neurosurgery: Spine, 10,* 1–2.

Ferreyra, G., Long, Y., & Ranieri, V. M. (2009). Respiratory complications after major surgery. *Current Opinion in Critical Care, 15*(4), 342–348.

Figueroa, J., Basford, J., & Low, P. (2010). Preventing and treating orthostatic hypotension: As easy as A, B, C. *Cleveland Clinic Journal of Medicine, 77*(5), 298–306.

Foley, N., Pereira, S., Salter, K., Fernandez, M., Speechley, M., Sequeira, K., . . . Teasell, R. (2013). Treatment with botulinum toxin improves upper-extremity function post stroke: A systematic review and meta-analysis. *Archives of Physical Medicine and Rehabilitation, 94*(5), 977–989.

Frey, L. C. (2003). Epidemiology of posttraumatic epilepsy: A critical review. *Epilepsia, 44*(10), 11–17.

Gisiason, M., Coupaud, S., Sasagawa, K., Tanabe, Y., Purcell, M., Allan, D., & Tanner, K. (2014). Prediction of risk of fracture in the tibia due to altered bone mineral density distribution resulting from disuse: A finite element study. *Proceedings of the Institution of Mechanical Engineers (Part H), Journal of Engineering in Medicine, 228*(2), 165–174.

Gnessin, E., Mandeville, J., Handa, S., & Lingeman, J. (2011). Changing composition of renal calculi in patients with musculoskeletal anomalies. *Journal of Endourology, 25*(9), 1519–1523. doi:10.1089/end.2010.0698

Gupta, V., & Lipsitz, L. A. (2007). Orthostatic hypotension in the elderly: Diagnosis and treatment. *The American Journal of Medicine, 120*(10), 841–847.

Halim, T., Chhabra, H., Arora, M., & Kumar, S. (2014). Pharmacological prophylaxis for deep vein thrombosis in acute spinal cord injury: An Indian perspective. *Spinal Cord.* doi:10.1038/sc.2014.71

Hammond, F., Horn, S., Smout, R., Chen, D., DeJong, G., Scelza, W., Bloomgarden, J. (2013). Acute rehospitalizations during inpatient rehabilitation for spinal cord injury. *Archives of Physical Medicine and Rehabilitation, 94*(4), S98–S105.

Hannawi, Y., Hannawi, B., Rao, C. P., Suarez, J., & Bershad, E. M. (2013). Stroke-associated pneumonia: Major advances and obstacles. *Cerebrovascular Diseases, 35*(5), 430–443.

Hayner, K. (2013). Effectiveness of the California tri-pull taping methods for shoulder subluxation post-stroke: A single subject ABA design. *American Journal of Occupational Therapy, 66*(6), 727–736.

Hickey, J. (Ed.). (2003). *The clinical practice of neurological and neurosurgical nursing* (5th ed.). Philadelphia: Lippincott Williams & Wilkins.

Hughes, C., & Howard, I. (2013). Spasticity management in multiple sclerosis. *Physical Medicine & Rehabilitation Clinics of North America, 24*(4), 593–604.

Kafri, M., Myint, P., Doherty, D., Wilson, A., Potter, J., & Hooper, L. (2013). The diagnostic accuracy of multi-frequency bioelectrical impedance analysis in diagnosing dehydration after stroke. *Medical Science Monitor, 10*(19), 548–570.

Kazakia, G., Tjong, W., Nirody, J., Burghardt, A., Carballido-Gami, J., Patsch, J., Ma, C. (2014). The influence of disuse on bone microstructure and mechanics assessed by HR-pACT. *Bone, 63,* 132–140.

Khalil, R., Gorgey, A., Janisko, M., Dolbow, D., Moore, J., & Gater, D. (2013). The role of nutrition in health status after spinal cord injury. *Aging and Disease, 4*(1), 14–22.

Kim, C., Ryu, W., Kim, B., & Lee, S. (2013). Paradoxical effect of obesity on hemorrhagic transformation after acute ischemic stroke. *BMC Neurology, 13,* 123. doi:10.1186/1471-2377-13-123

Kim, Y., Jung, S., Yang, E., & Paik, N. (2014). Clinical and sonographic risk factors for hemiplegic shoulder pain: A longitudinal observational study. *Journal of Rehabilitation Medicine, 46*(1), 81–87. doi:10.2340/16501977-1238

Kirkman, M., Albert, A., Albert, A., Ibrahim, A., & Doberenz, D. (2013). Hyponatremia and brain injury: Historical and contemporary perspectives. *Neurocritical Care, 18*(3), 406–416.

Kleinpell, R. M. (2004). Working out the complexities of severe sepsis. *Nursing Management, 35*(5), 48A–48E.

Kleinpell, R., Aitken, L., & Schorr, C. A. (2013). Implications of the new international sepsis guidelines for nursing care. *American Journal of Critical Care Nursing, 22*(3), 212–222.

Krassioukov, A., Eng, J. J., Warburton, D. E., & Teasell, R. (2009). A systematic review of the management of orthostatic hypotension after spinal cord injury. *Archives of Physical Medicine and Rehabilitation, 90,* 876–885.

Kumar, S., Selim, M. H., & Caplan, L. R. (2010). Medical complications after stroke. *The Lancet Neurology, 9*(1), 105–118.

Kuptniratsaikul, V., Kovindha, A., Suethanapornkul, S., Manimmanakorn, N., & Archongka, Y. (2013). Long-term morbidities in stroke survivors: A prospective multicenter study of Thai stroke rehabilitation registry. *BMC (BioMedical Central) Geriatric, 13*(1), 33.

Lackland, D., Roccella, E., Deutsch, A., Fornage, M., George, M., Howard, G., Towfinghi, A. (2014). Factors influencing the decline in stroke mortality: a statement from the American Heart Association/American Stroke Association. *Stroke, 45*(1), 315–353.

Laffont, I., Bensmail, D., Lortat-Jacob, S., Falaize, L., Hutin, C., LeBomin, E., Lofaso, F. (2008). Intermittent positive-pressure breathing effects in patients with high spinal cord injury. *Archives of Physical Medicine and Rehabilitation, 89,* 1575–1579.

Lalwani, S., Punia, P., Mathur, P., Trikha, V., Satyarthee, G., & Misra, M. (2014). Hospital acquired infections: Preventable cause of mortality in spinal cord injury patients. *Journal of Laboratory Physicians, 6*(1), 36–39. doi:10.4103/0974-2727.129089

Lance, J. (1980). *Spasticity: Disordered motor control.* Chicago: Year Book Medical Publishers.

Langley, J. M., Gravel, D., Moore, D., Matlow, A., Embree, J., MacKinnon-Cameron, D., & Conly, J. (2009). Study of cerebrospinal fluid shunt–associated infections in the first year following placement, by the Canadian nosocomial infections surveillance program. *Infection Control and Hospital Epidemiology, 30*(3), 285–288.

Lethaby, A., Temple, J., & Santy-Tomlinson, J. (2013). *Pin site care for preventing infections associated with external bone fixators and pins.* Retrieved from www.nlm.nih.gov/medlineplus/fractures.htm

Li, K., Murai, N., & Chi, S. (2011). Clinical reasoning in the use of slings for patients with shoulder subluxation after stroke: A glimpse of the practice phenomenon in California. *Occupational Therapy Journal of Research, 33*(4), 228–235.

Lim, S., & Childs, C. (2013). A systematic review of the effectiveness of bowel management strategies for constipation in adults with stroke. *International Journal of Nursing Studies, 50*(7), 1004–1010.

Lin, C., Cho, C., Tseng, C., Chen, H., Lin, F., & Li, C. (2013). Post-stroke constipation in the rehabilitation ward: Incidence, clinical course and associated factors. *Singapore Medical Journal, 54*(11), 624–629.

Liu, C., Lin, S., Lin, J., Yang, J., Chang, Y., Chang, C., Lee, T. (2014). Acute ischemic stroke. *European Journal of Neurology.* doi:10.1111/ene.12452

Maddox, S. (2013). *Paralysis resource guide* (3rd Ed.). Short Hills, NJ: Christopher and Dana Reeve Foundation.

Mangera, Z., Panesar, G., & Makker, H. (2012). Practical approach to management of respiratory complications in neurological disorders. *International Journal of General Medicine, 5,* 255–263.

Marshal, C., & Stansby, G. (2010). Amputation and rehabilitation. *Surgery, 28*(6), 284–287.

Mays, R., McIntyre, A., Mehta, S., Hill, D., Wolfe, D., & Teasell, R. (2013). A review of educational programs to reduce UTIs among individuals with SCI. *Rehabilitation Nursing.* doi:10.1002/rnj.130

Mazya, M., Ahmed, N., Ford, F., Hobohm, C., Mikulik, R., Nunes, A., & Wahlgren, N. (2014). Remote or extraischemic intracerebral hemorrhage—an uncommon complication of stroke thrombolysis: Results from the safe implementation of treatments in stroke. International Stroke Thrombolysis Registry. *Stroke*. doi:10.1038/sc.2014.71

McAvay, G. J., Van Ness, P. H., Bogardus, S. T., Zhang, Y., Lesie, D. L., Leo-Summers, L. S., & Inouye, S. K. (2006). Older adults discharged from the hospital with delirium 1-year outcomes. *Journal of the American Geriatrics Society, 54,* 1245–1250.

McCormick, Z., Chu, S., Mathur, S., & Marciniak, C. (2013). Long-term outcomes of intrathecal baclofen for spasticity. *Physical Medicine & Rehabilitation, 5*(9), S139.

McGrail, A., & Kelchner, L. (2012). Adequate oral fluid intake in hospitalized stroke patients: Does viscosity matter? *Rehabilitation Nursing, 37*(5), 252–257. doi:10.1002/rnj.23

McIntyre, A., Lee, T., Janzen, S., Mays, R., Mehta, S., & Teasell, R. (2012). Systematic review of the effectiveness of pharmacological interventions in the treatment of spasticity of the hemiparetic lower extremity more than six months post stroke. *Topics in Stroke Rehabilitation, 19*(6), 479–490.

McKinley, W. O., Gittler, M. S., Kirshblum, S. C., Stiens, S. A., & Groah, S. L. (2002). Spinal cord injury medicine. 2. Medical complications after spinal cord injury: Identification and management. *Archives of Physical Medicine and Rehabilitation, 83*(1), 58–64.

McKinley, W., Jackson, A., Cardenas, D., & Devivo, M. (1999). Long-term medical complications after traumatic spinal cord injury: A regional model systems analysis. *Archives of Physical Medicine Rehabilitation, 80*(11), 1402–1410.

Medina, A., Serratt, T., Pelter, M., & Brancamp, T. (2014). Decreasing central line–associated bloodstream infections in the non-ICU population. *Journal of Nursing Care Quality, 29*(2), 133–140.

Meikle, B., Devlin, M., & Garfinkel, S. (2000). Interruptions to amputee rehabilitation. *Archives of Physical Rehabilitation and Medicine, 83*(9), 1222–1228.

Milligen, J., Lee, J., McMillan, C., & Klassen, H. (2012). Recognizing a common serious condition in patients with spinal cord injury. *Canadian Family Physician, 58,* 831–835.

Morris, L. L., McIntosh, E., & Whitmer, A. (2014). The importance of tracheostomy progression in the intensive care unit. *Critical Care Nurse, 34*(1), 40–48.

Naccarato, M., Grandi, F., Dennis, M., & Sandercock, P. (2010). Physical methods for preventing deep vein thrombosis in stroke. *Cochrane Database of Systematic Reviews, 12.* doi:10.1002/14651858CD001922.pub3

Naschitz, J., & Lenger, R. (2008). Why traumatic leg amputees are at increased risk for cardiovascular diseases. *Quality Journal of Medicine, 101*(4), 251–259.

National Institute of Neurological Disorders and Stroke (NINDS). (2013). *Hydrocephalus.* Baltimore: Author.

National Institute of Neurological Disorders and Stroke (NINDS). (2014a). *Syringomyelia fact sheet.* Baltimore: Author. Retrieved from http://www.ninds.nih.gov

National Institute of Neurological Disorders and Stroke (NINDS). (2014). *Dystonias.* Baltimore: Author. Retrieved from http://www.ninda.sih.gov

Ng, C., Prott, G., Rutkowski, S., Li, Y., Hansen, R., Kellow, J., & Malcolm, A. (2005). Gastrointestinal symptoms in spinal cord injury: Relationships with level of injury and psychologic factors. *Diseases of the Colon and Rectum, 48*(8), 1562–1568.

Nickele, C., Kamps, T., & Medow, J. (2013). Safety of a DVT chemoprophylaxis protocol following traumatic brain injury: A single center quality improvement initiative. *Neurocritical Care, 18*(2), 184–192. doi:10.1007/s12028-012-9786-x

Nicolle, L. (2014). Urinary tract infections in patients with spinal injuries. *Current Infectious Disease Reports, 16*(1), 390. doi:10.1007/s11908-013-0390-9

Niklassom, J., Lovheim, H., & Gustafson, Y. (2013). Morale in very old people who have had a stroke. *Archives of Gerontology and Geriatrics, 58*(3), 408–414.

Ostwald, S. K., Godwin, K. M., & Fang, Y. (2013). Serious adverse events experienced by survivors of stroke in the first year following discharge from inpatient rehabilitation. *Rehabilitation Nursing, 38*(5), 254–263.

Otegbayo, J., Talabi, O., Akere, A., Owolabi, M., Owolabi, L., & Oguntoye, O. (2013). Gastrointestinal complications in stroke survivors. *Tropical Gastroenterology, 27*(3), 127–130.

Pang, M., Yang, R., & Jones, A. (2013). Vascular elasticity and grip strength are associated with bone health of the hemiparetic radius in people with chronic stroke: Implications for rehabilitation. *PTJ (Physical Therapy Journal), 93*(6), 774–785.

Perrouin-Verbe, B., Lenne-Aurier, K., Robert, R., Auffray-Calvier, E., Richard, I., Mauduyt de la Greve, I., & Mathe, J. F. (1998). Post-traumatic syringomyelia and post-traumatic spinal canal stenosis: A direct relationship: Review of 75 patients with spinal cord injury. *Spinal Cord, 36,* 137–143.

Picado, C., & Luengo, M. (1996a). Corticosteroid-induced bone loss. Prevention and management. *Drug Safety, 15*(5), 347–359.

Picado, C., & Luengo, M. (1996b). Pulmonary embolism without deep venous thrombosis: De novo or missed deep vein thrombosis? *Journal of Trauma & Acute Care Surgery, 7*(5), 1270–1274.

Piovesan, D., Morasso, P., Giannoni, P., & Casadio, M. (2013). Arm stiffness during assisted movement after stroke: The influence of visual feedback. IEEE Transactions on Neural Systems and *Rehabilitation Engineering, 21*(3), 454–465.

Pongmoragot, J., Rabinstein, A., Nilanont, Y., Swarz, R., Zhou, L., & Saposnik, G. (2013). Pulmonary embolism in ischemic stroke: Clinical presentation, risk factors, and outcome. *Journal of the American Heart Association, 25*(6), e000372. doi.10.1161/JAHA.113.000372

Powers, K. A., & Burchell, P. L. (2010). *Sepsis alert: Avoiding the shock. Nursing, 40*(4), 34–39.

Praeger, A., Westbrook, A., Nichol, A., Wijemunige, R., Davies, A., Lyon, S., . . . Cooper, D. (2012). Deep vein thrombosis and pulmonary embolus in patients with traumatic brain injury: A prospective observational study. *Critical Care and Resuscitation, 14*(1), 10–13.

Privette Nelson, D., LeMaster, T. H., Plost, G. N., & Zahner, M. L. (2009). Recognizing sepsis in the adult patient. *American Journal of Nursing, 109*(3), 40–45.

Quinn, B., Baker, D., Cohen, S., Stewart., J., Lima, C., & Parise, C. (2014) Basic nursing care to prevent nonventilator hospital-acquired pneumonia. *Journal of Nursing Scholarship, 46*(1), 11-19.

Ramsey, S., & McIlhenny, C. (2011). Evidence-based management of upper tract urolithiasis in the spinal cord-injured patient. Sp*inal Cord, 49*(9), 948–1054.

Ravensbergen, H., Lear, S., & Claydon, V. (2014). Waist circumference is the best index for obesity-related cardiovascular disease risk in individuals with spinal cord injury. *Journal of Neurotrauma, 31*(3), 292–300. doi:10.1089/neu.2013.3042

Rivera, C. (2009). Every minute counts: Maintain the urgency of sepsis recognition and treatment. *Nursing Management, 40*(5), 38–44.

Robertson, L., & Roche, A. (2013). Primary prophylaxis for venous thromboembolism in people undergoing major amputation of the lower extremity. *Cochrane Database of Systematic Reviews, 12.* doi:10.1002/14651858CD010525.pub2

Roth, E. J., Stenson, K. W., Powley, S., Oken, J., Primack, S., Nussbaum, S. B., & Berkowitz, M. (2010). Expiratory muscle training in spinal cord injury: A randomized controlled trial. *Archives of Physical Medicine and Rehabilitation, 91*(6), 857–861.

Rowat, A. (2011). Malnutrition and dehydration after stroke. *Nursing Standard, 26*(14), 42–46.

Rowat, A., Smith, L., Graham, C., Horsburgh, D., & Dennis, M. (2011). A pilot study to assess if urine gravity and urine colour charts are useful indicators of dehydration in acute stroke patients. *Journal of Advanced Nursing, 67*(9), 1976–1983. doi:10.1111/.1365-2648.2011.05645.x

Sabini, R., Dijkers, M., & Raghavan, P. (2013). Stroke survivors talk while doing: Development of a therapeutic framework for continued rehabilitation of hand function post stroke. *Journal of Hand Therapy, 26*(2), 124–130.

Sabour, H., Norouzi, A., Javidan, A., Latifi, S., Larijani, B., Shidfar, E.,...Emami Razavi, H. (2013). Bone biomarkers in patients with chronic traumatic spinal cord injury. *The Spine Journal, S1529-9430*(13), 01397-1

Scherbakov, N., von Haehling., S., Anker, S., Dirnagl, U., & Doehner, W. (2013). Stroke induced sarcopenia: Muscle wasting and disability after stroke. *International Journal of Cardiology, 170*(2), 89–94. doi:10.1016/j.ijcard.2013.10.031

Schrock, J., Glasenapp, M., & Drogell, K. (2012). Elevated blood urea nitrogen/creatinine ratio is associated with poor outcome in patients with ischemic stroke. *Clinical Neurology and Neurosurgery, 114*(7), 881–884. doi:10.1016/j.clineuro.2012.01.031

Selassie, A., Snipe, L., Focht, K., & Welldaregay, W. (2013). Baseline Prevalence of Heart Diseases, Hypertension, Diabetes and Obesity in Persons with Acute Traumatic Spinal Cord Injury: Potential Threats in the Recovery Trajectory. *Topics in Spinal Cord Injury Rehabilitation, 19*(3), 172–182. doi:10.1310/sci1903-172

Sheffler, L., Knutson, J., Gunzler, D., & Chae, J. (2012). Relationship between body mass index and rehabilitation outcomes in chronic stroke. *American Journal of Physical Medicine & Rehabilitation, 91*(11), 951–956. doi:10.1097/PHM.0b013e31826458c6

Siddiqi, N., House, A. O., & Holmes, J. D. (2006). Occurrence and outcome of delirium in medical in-patients: A systematic literature review. *Age and Ageing, 35,* 350–364.

Simon, T. D., Hall, M., Riva-Cambrin, J., Albert, J. E., Jeffries, H. E., LaFleur, B., Kestle, J. R. (2009). Infection rates following initial cerebrospinal fluid shunt placement across pediatric hospitals in the United States. *Journal of Neurosurgical Pediatrics, 4,* 156–165.

Simpkins, C. J. (2005). Ventriculoperitoneal shunt infections in patients with hydrocephalus. *Pediatric Nursing, 31*(6), 457–462.

Singh, R., Rohilla, R., Saini, G., & Kaur, K. (2014). Longitudinal study of body composition in spinal cord injury patients. *Indian Journal of Orthopaedics, 48*(2), 168–177.

Skolarus, L., Sanchez, B., Levine, D., Baek, J., Kerber, K., Morgenstern, L.. Kusabeth, L. (2014). Association of body mass index and mortality after acute ischemic stroke. *Cardiovascular Quality and Outcomes, 7*(1), 64–69.

Smith, M. (2012). Management of hemiplegic shoulder pain following stroke. *Nursing Standard, 26*(44), 35–44.

Smith, T. O., Hazelden, S., Parker, L., Jha, B., Youatt, M., & Haywood, R. (2012). The use of Cobantm compression bandage following below-knee free-flap surgery. *International Journal of Nursing Practice, 18,* 604–609.

Stevenson, V., & Playford, D. (2012). Neurological rehabilitation and the management of spasticity: Practice points. *Medicine Journal, 40*(9) 513–517.

Stineman, M. G., Ross, R., Maislin, G., Fiedler, R. C., & Granger, C. V. (2003). Risks of acute hospital transfer and mortality during stroke rehabilitation. *Archives of Physical Medicine and Rehabilitation, 84*(5), 712–718.

Sunnerhagen, K., & Francisco, G. (2013). Enhancing patient–provider communication for long-term post-stroke spasticity management. *Acta Neurologica Scandinavia, 128*(5), 305–310.

Tabers Medical Dictionary Online. 22nd Edition. Retrieved from www.tabers.com

Thiruppathy, K., Roy, A., Preziosi, G., Pannicker, J., & Emmanuel, A. (2012). Morphological abnormalities of the recto-anal inhibitory reflex reflects symptom pattern in neurogenic bowel. *Digestive Diseases and Sciences, 57*(70), 1908–1914.

Turner-Stokes, L., Fheodoroff, K., & Jacinto, J. (2013). Upper limb international spasticity study: Results of a large, international, prospective cohort study investigation practice and goal attainment following treatment with botulinum toxin A in real-life clinical management. *Physical Medicine and Rehabilitation, 5*(9), S238–S239.

Vaidyanathan, S., Selmi, F., Abraham, K., Hughes, P., Singh, G., & Soni, B. (2012). Hydronephrosis and renal failure following inadequate management of neuropathic bladder in a patient with spinal cord injury: Case report of a preventable complication. *Patient Safety in Surgery, 6*(1), 22. doi:10.1186/1754-9493-6-22

Van den Boogaard, M. Schoonhoven, L. van der Hoeven, J.G., van Achterberg, T., & Pickkers, P. (2011) Incidence and short term consequences of delirium in critically ill patients: A prospective observational cohort study. *International Journal of Nursing Studies, 49,* 773-783.

Van Gent, J., Zander, A. L., Olson, E. J., Shackford, S. R., Dunne, C. E., Sise, C. B., …Sise, M. J.. (2014). Pulmonary embolism without deep venous thrombosis: De nova or missed deep venous thrombosis? *Journal of Trauma & Acute Care Surgery, 76*(5), 1270–1274.

Vuola, J. C. (2006). Assessment and management of surgical wounds in clinical practice. *Nursing Standard, 20*(52), 46–56.

Wadsworth, B. M., Haines, T. S., Cornwell, P. L., Rodwell, L. T., & Paratz, J. D. (2012). Abdominal binder improves lung volumes and voice in people with tetraplegic spinal cord injury. *Archives of Physical and Medical Rehabilitation, 93*(2), 189–197.

Waldman, G., Yang, C., Ren, Y., Liu, L., Guo, X., Harvey, R., Zhang, L. (2013). Effects of robot-guided passive stretching and active movement training of ankle and mobility impairments in stroke. *NeuroRehabilitation, 32*(3), 625–634.

Waszynski, C. M. (2007). Detecting delirium. *American Journal of Nursing, 107*(12), 50–59.

Welk, B., Fuller, A., Razv, H., & Denstedt, J. (2012). Renal stone disease in spinal-cord-injured patients. *Journal of Endourology, 26*(8), 954–959. doi:10.1089/end.2012.0063

Welk, B., Shariff, S., Ordon, M., Catharine Craven, B., Herschorn, S., & Garg, A. (2013). The surgical management of upper tract stone disease among spinal cord–injured patients. *Spinal Cord, 51*(6), 457–460. doi:10.1038/sc.2013.15

West, J., Mohiuddin, S., Hand, W., Grossmann, E., Vergo, K., & Johnson, F. (2013). Surgery for constipation in patients with prior spinal cord injury: The Department of Veterans Affairs experience. *Journal of Spinal Cord Medicine, 3*(3), 207–212.

Worsoe, J., Fynne, L., Laurberg, S., Krogh, K., & Rijkhoff, N. (2012). Acute effect of electrical stimulation of the dorsal genital nerve on rectal capacity in patients with spinal cord injury. *Spinal Cord, 50*(6), 462–466.

Yongquiang, L., Reinhardt, J., Gosney, J., Zhang, X., Xiaoong, H., Chen, S., Li, J. (2012). Evaluation of functional outcomes of physical rehabilitation and medical complications in spinal cord injury victims of the Sichuan earthquake. *Journal of Rehabilitation Medicine, 44,* 534–540.

Young, T., Tang, H., & Hughes, R. (2010). Vena caval filters for the prevention of pulmonary embolism. *Cochrane Database of Systematic Reviews, 12.* doi:10.1002/14651858CD0106212.pub4

Zhang, Z., & Liao, L. (2014). Risk factors predicting upper urinary tract deterioration in patients with spinal cord injury: A prospective study. *Spinal Cord.* doi:10.1038/sc.2014.63

Index

A

B

C

D

E

F

G

H

I

J

K

L

M

N

O

P

Q

R

S

T

U

V

W

Y

Z